Clinical Atlas of Procedures in Ophthalmic and Oculofacial Surgery

Oxford Atlases in Ophthalmology

SERIES EDITORS

Daniel M. Albert, MD, MS, FACS, RRF Emmett A. Humble Distinguished Director of the
University of Wisconsin Eye Research Institute, F.A. Davis Professor, Department of
Ophthalmology and Visual Sciences and Professor, Department of Pathology,
University of Wisconsin School of Medicine and Public Health, Madison, WI

Peter A. Netland, MD, PhD, DuPont Guerry III Professor and Chairman, Department of Ophthalmology,
University of Virginia School of Medicine, Charlottesville, VA

Clinical Eye Atlas, 2nd ed. Edited by Daniel H. Gold and Richard Alan Lewis
Clinical Atlas of Procedures in Ophthalmic and Oculofacial Surgery, 2nd ed.
Edited by Daniel M. Albert and Mark J. Lucarelli

Clinical Atlas of Procedures in Ophthalmic and Oculofacial Surgery

SECOND EDITION

EDITED BY

Daniel M. Albert, MD, MS, FACS

Mark J. Lucarelli, MD, FACS

MANAGING EDITOR

Sarah L. Atzen, BA, MLIS

UNIVERSITY PRESS

OXFORD
UNIVERSITY PRESS

Oxford University Press, Inc., publishes works that further
Oxford University's objective of excellence
in research, scholarship, and education

Oxford   New York
Auckland   Cape Town   Dar es Salaam   Hong Kong   Karachi
Kuala Lumpur   Madrid   Melbourne   Mexico City   Nairobi
New Delhi   Shanghai   Taipei   Toronto

With offices in
Argentina   Austria   Brazil   Chile   Czech Republic   France   Greece
Guatemala   Hungary   Italy   Japan   Poland   Portugal   Singapore
South Korea   Switzerland   Thailand   Turkey   Ukraine   Vietnam

Published by Oxford University Press, Inc.
198 Madison Avenue, New York, New York 10016

www.oup.com

Oxford is a registered trademark of Oxford University Press

Library of Congress Cataloging-in-Publication Data
Clinical atlas of procedures in ophthalmic and oculofacial surgery / edited by Daniel M. Albert & Mark J. Lucarelli. — 2nd ed.
      p. ; cm. — (Oxford atlases in ophthalmology)
   Includes bibliographical references and index.
   ISBN 978-0-19-538861-9 (alk. paper)
   1. Eye—Surgery—Atlases.   I. Albert, Daniel M.   II. Lucarelli, Mark J.   III. Series: Oxford atlases in ophthalmology.
   [DNLM: 1. Ophthalmologic Surgical Procedures—methods—Atlases.   WW 17]
   RE80.C556 2012
   617.7'1—dc22   2011011769

9 8 7 6 5 4 3 2 1
Printed in the United States of America
on acid-free paper

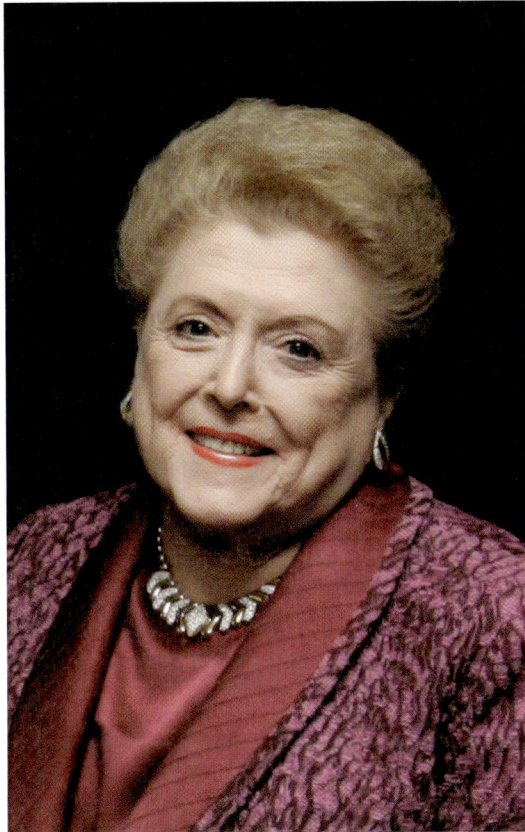

This book is dedicated to **Alice R. McPherson, M.D.**, in recognition of her many contributions to ophthalmology and for her friendship and support.

FOREWORD

I have known Dr. Daniel Albert and Dr. Mark Lucarelli as colleagues, scholars, and clinicians for many years and am well versed in their breadth of experience and high level of expertise as educators. Their publications in the past have been both prodigious and erudite, covering many different aspects of ophthalmology. Now they are publishing their 2nd Edition of *Clinical Atlas of Procedures in Ophthalmic and Oculofacial Surgery*, a hardback, single volume that is presented in seven Sections. These Sections include Cataract and Intraocular Lens Surgery, Refractive Surgery, Cornea and Ocular Surface Surgery, Glaucoma Surgery, Retina Surgery, Pediatric Ophthalmology and Strabismus Surgery, and Oculofacial Plastic, Orbital, and Lacrimal Surgery. For this book, they have carefully selected section editors, who provide editorial cohesion, and chapter authors who are experts and national leaders in their field and are able to transmit their knowledge effectively to others.

Since the 1st Edition of *Clinical Atlas of Procedures in Ophthalmic Surgery* in 2004, there have been many advances, hence the need for this volume. This 2nd Edition is broad in scope and brings the surgeon up-to-date in the major fields of ophthalmic and oculofacial surgery. It should be relevant and appealing to a wide audience from the first year resident to the experienced surgeon. All of the chapters are new. The *Atlas* includes approximately 2,500 images/illustrations with generous use of superb color intraoperative photographs that clearly indicate the important steps in each operation. New features include a uniform layout with selected references and comprehensive tables in each chapter listing indications and complications associated with various surgical procedures.

This *Atlas* has much to offer to all of those performing ophthalmic and oculofacial surgery. The uniform format with outstanding color images/illustrations and clear, concise text should make retrieval of information efficient for the reader, whether it is to note specific points or to learn a new operation. The ultimate beneficiaries of the transmission of the knowledge and skills in this excellent volume will be our patients.

Richard K. Dortzbach, MD, FACS
Professor Emeritus
Former Peter A. Duehr Chair
Department of Ophthalmology and Visual Sciences
University of Wisconsin School of Medicine and Public Health
Madison, Wisconsin

It is an acknowledged truth that surgical skills are the most challenging and difficult aspect of ophthalmology both to learn and to maintain. Ophthalmologists know that advances in ophthalmic science and technology lead to improvements and innovations in our surgical procedures. As a result, ophthalmologists require ever-higher levels of knowledge and skill to provide patients with the best treatment possible.

The staggering breadth and continual evolution of surgical techniques in comprehensive ophthalmology and the surgical subspecialties are both laudable and beneficial, but can also be overwhelming for those in the medical profession. Indeed, mastery of this full surgical repertoire has long been impossible for any individual surgeon. Accordingly, this book intends to assist the trainee, the comprehensive ophthalmologist, and the subspecialist in acquiring and maintaining command of the procedures relevant to their practice.

Specifically, the purpose of the *Clinical Atlas of Procedures in Ophthalmic and Oculofacial Surgery* is to provide an overview of a broad range of contemporary ophthalmic and oculofacial surgical procedures. The illustrations should familiarize the reader with key intraoperative and postoperative points. The *Atlas* is not intended to be a step-by-step manual or a standalone reference source to allow performance of the illustrated surgical procedures. Rather, the *Atlas* intends to illustrate surgical fundamentals clearly, with an emphasis on well-established and accepted procedures.

The first edition of the *Atlas* originated from the text, *Ophthalmic Surgery: Principles and Techniques*, which appeared in 1999. Material from that text was reorganized, updated, and expanded by a corps of capable section editors into the *Clinical Atlas of Procedures in Ophthalmic Surgery* published in 2004. The *Atlas* was well received and has proved useful to ophthalmologists for the past seven years.

Drawing on the many recommendations, comments, and criticisms that were kindly offered, the new edition of the *Atlas* has been in preparation for two years. We were gratified to be able to recruit section editors who are recognized leaders in comprehensive ophthalmology and in each of the subspecialty fields. In turn, these surgeons wrote individual chapters and attracted an outstanding group of experts to contribute the remainder. Thus, the new edition has been entirely updated and revised. The format of the chapters has been streamlined and made more uniform. The total number of illustrations has been increased to more than 2,500. Tables of indications and complications, as well as selected references, have been added to each chapter. Because of the individual preferences of the authors and their desire to utilize personal teaching material, the figures represent a variety of photographic and artistic formats.

In preparing this *Atlas*, we have been impressed by the great strides made in numerous surgical areas in the past decade. The new edition gives eloquent testimony to the cleverness, expertise, and industry of ophthalmic and oculofacial surgeons. It demonstrates the effectiveness with which the efforts of visual scientists and bioengineers support the needs of surgeons and their patients. In addition, it provides striking examples of how the ability to directly visualize diseased ocular tissue before and during intraocular surgery provides distinct advantages to ophthalmic surgeons— advantages less readily available in other fields. The *Atlas* also conveys the esthetic beauty of the eye and its adnexa, along with the refinement and intricacy that surgery in this area entails.

We sincerely hope that the new edition of the *Clinical Atlas of Procedures in Ophthalmic and Oculofacial Surgery* will continue to prove useful to the trainee, the surgeon, and the teacher.

As we review the techniques and strategies and learn the complicated maneuvers for dealing surgically with ophthalmic and oculofacial disorders, we must always let our decisions and judgments be guided by the knowledge that we operate on patients—not on diseases. Serving these patients well is our ultimate reward.

DMA
MJL

ACKNOWLEDGMENTS

The *Atlas* is very much the product of a team effort. First and foremost, the volume editors are indebted to the section editors and *Atlas* contributors, and to Sarah Atzen, our managing editor, all of whom patiently and generously gave us their time, energy, and expertise. To them belongs the principal credit for bringing this book into existence. The cataract and intraocular lens (IOL) surgery section proved a special case, with Dr. Alan Crandall helping us initially to identify and recruit contributors, and Dr. Patricia Sabb supervising completion of the section. Also, Dr. Cat Burkat and Dr. Bobby Korn stepped in as subsection editors to assist Dr. Don Kikkawa with the lengthy oculofacial plastic, orbital, and lacrimal surgery section.

The publication of the *Atlas* is a testament to the depth and resources of Oxford University Press (OUP). Catharine Carlin was the editor in the early phases of the project. Following a restructuring of the Medical Division at OUP, Catherine Barnes, vice president and publisher for OUP's Medicine Division, saw it through to completion. We are extremely grateful to Catherine for her keen judgment and organizational skills. The publisher and editors were ably assisted by a hard-working staff including Anne Dellinger, Joseph Guarino, Mallory Jensen, Rachel Mayer, Tracy K. O'Hara, Rajashri Ravindranathan, Kurt Roediger, Angelique Rondeau, and George Fuller. Barry Bowlus (AMA Press) generously provided copies of the first edition to section editors when needed.

DMA
MJL

CONTENTS

[†]Deceased

CONTRIBUTORS

Gary W. Abrams, MD
The David Barsky, MD Endowed Professor and Chair
Department of Ophthalmology
Wayne State University
Director, Kresge Eye Institute
Detroit, MI

Iqbal Ike K. Ahmed, MD, FRCSC
Assistant Professor
Department of Ophthalmology
    and Vision Sciences
University of Toronto
Toronto, Canada

Takayuki Akahoshi, MD
Director of Ophthalmology
Department of Ophthalmology
Mitsui Memorial Hospital
Tokyo, Japan

Chrisfouad R. Alabiad, MD
Assistant Professor
Ophthalmology
Bascom Palmer Eye Institute,
University of Miami
Miami, FL

Lama A. Al-Aswad, MD
Assistant Professor of Clinical Ophthalmology
Department of Ophthalmology
Edward S. Harkness Eye Institute
Columbia University College of Physicians and
    Surgeons
New York, NY

Daniel M. Albert, MD, MS, FACS
RRF Emmett A. Humble Distinguished
    Director of the University of Wisconsin Eye
    Research Institute
F.A. Davis Professor, Department of Ophthalmology
    and Visual Sciences and Professor,
    Department of Pathology
University of Wisconsin School of Medicine and
    Public Health
Madison, WI

Jeanine A. Baqai, MD
Resident
Department of Ophthalmology
Rush University Medical Center
Chicago, IL

Kleyton Barella, MD
Fellow, Glaucoma Service
Department of Ophthalmology
University of Campinas
Campinas, Brazil

Graham W. Belovay, BCmp, MD
Ophthalmology Resident
Department of Ophthalmology and Visual Sciences
University of Toronto
Toronto, Canada

Brenda L. Bohnsack, MD, PhD
Clinical Instructor
Department of Ophthalmology and Visual Sciences
Kellogg Eye Center, University of Michigan
Ann Arbor, MI

Jamin S. Brown, MD
Clinical Assistant Professor
Department of Ophthalmology
SUNY Upstate Medical University
Syracuse, NY

Adam G. Buchanan, MD
Assistant Professor of Surgery
Uniformed Services University of the Health
    Sciences
F. Edward Hebert School of Medicine
Assistant Chief
Department of Ophthalmology
Madigan Army Medical Center
Tacoma, WA

Edward G. Buckley, MD
Banks Anderson, Sr. Professor of Ophthalmology
    and Pediatrics
Vice Dean for Medical Education
Department of Ophthalmology
Duke University Medical School
Durham, NC

Cat Nguyen Burkat, MD, FACS
Oculoplastics Service, Department of Ophthalmology and
    Visual Sciences
University of Wisconsin-Madison
Madison, WI

Antonio Capone, Jr., MD, FACS
Clinical Professor
Oakland University/William Beaumont Hospital School of
    Medicine
Auburn Hills, MI
Professor
European School for Advanced Studies
    in Ophthalmology
Lugano, Switzerland
Partner
Associated Retinal Consultants
Royal Oak, MI
Director
Vision Research Foundation
Novi, MI

Daniel S. Casper, MD, PhD
Associate Clinical Professor of Ophthalmology
Columbia University
College of Physicians & Surgeons
Director of Ophthalmology
Naomi Berrie Diabetes Center
New York, NY

JoAnn C. Chang, MD
Department of Ophthalmology
University of Utah
Salt Lake City, UT

Stanley Chang, MD
Department of Ophthalmology
Edward S. Harkness Eye Institute
Columbia University
New York, NY

Leon D. Charkoudian, MD
Fellow in Vitreoretinal Disease and Surgery
Department of Ophthalmology
Emory Eye Center
Atlanta, GA

Weerawan Chokthaweesak, MD
Department of Ophthalmology
Ophthalmic Plastic and Reconstructive Surgery Service
Faculty of Medicine
Ramathibodi Hospital
Mahidol University
Bangkok, Thailand

Steven R. Cohen, MD, FACS
Clinical Professor, Plastic Surgery
University of California, San Diego
Director, Craniofacial Surgery
Rady Children's Hospital
Private Practice, FACES+ Plastic Surgery,
    Skin and Laser Center
La Jolla, CA

Kathryn A. Colby, MD, PhD
Surgeon in Ophthalmology
Massachusetts Eye and Ear Infirmary
Assistant Professor, Department of Ophthalmology,
    Harvard Medical School
Boston, MA

Joseph Colin, MD
Professor and Chairman
Department of Ophthalmology
University of Bordeaux
Bordeaux, France

Vital Paulino Costa, MD
Professor of Ophthalmology
Department of Ophthalmology, Glaucoma Service
University of Campinas
Campinas, S ão Paulo, Brazil

Stephen S. Couvillion, MD
California Retinal Consultants
Santa Barbara, CA

Philip L. Custer, MD
Professor
Department of Ophthalmology and Visual Sciences
Washington University School of Medicine
St. Louis, MO

Craig N. Czyz, DO, FACOS
Chair, Division of Ophthalmology
Section Head, Oculofacial Plastic and Reconstructive
    Surgery
OhioHealth Doctors Hospital
Clinical Faculty, Ohio University College of Osteopathic
    Medicine, Doctors Hospital Ophthalmology Residency
    Program
Eye Center of Columbus
Columbus, OH

Roger A. Dailey, MD, FACS
Lester T. Jones Endowed Chair and Director Division of
    Oculofacial Plastic Surgery
Casey Aesthetic Facial Surgery Center
Oregon Health & Sciences University
Portland, OR

Pouya N. Dayani, MD
Clinical Associate
Vitreoretinal Surgery and Ocular Inflammation
Retina-Vitreous Associates Medical Group
Beverly Hills, CA

Martin H. Devoto, MD
Director
Oculoplastic and Orbital Surgery
Consultores Oftalmológicos
Buenos Aires, Argentina

Mohit A. Dewan, MD
Clinical Instructor of Ophthalmology, Division of
    Ophthalmic Plastic Surgery
Lions Eye Institute, Department of Ophthalmology
Albany Medical Center
Albany, NY

Ali R. Djalilian, MD
Assistant Professor
Department of Ophthalmology
    and Visual Sciences
University of Illinois at Chicago
Chicago, IL

Peter J. Dolman, MD, FRCSC
Clinical Professor, Division Head
Department of Ophthalmology,
Division of Oculoplastics and Orbit,
University of British Columbia
Vancouver, Canada

Steven C. Dresner, MD
Associate Clinical Professor
The University of Southern California
Keck School of Medicine
Director ASOPRS Fellowship
Eyesthetica
Los Angeles, CA

Jay S. Duker, MD
Professor and Chair
Department of Ophthalmology
Tufts Medical Center and Tufts University School of
    Medicine
Boston, MA

Daniel S. Durrie, MD
Clinical Professor
Department of Ophthalmology
University of Kansas Medical Center
Kansas City, KS

Saad El-Naggar, MD
Ophthalmologist
TLC Eye Care of Michigan
Jackson, MI

Bita Esmaeli, MD, FACS
Professor of Ophthalmology
Section of Ophthalmology
Department of Head and Neck Surgery
The University of Texas M.D. Anderson Cancer Center
Houston, TX

Fatema Esmail, MD
Associate in Ophthalmology
Department of Ophthalmology
Emory University
Atlanta, GA
Marietta Eye Clinic
Marietta, GA

Marjan Farid, MD
Assistant Professor of Ophthalmology
Gavin Herbert Eye Institute
University of California, Irvine City
Irvine, CA

Nabeel Farooqui, MD
Instructor
Department of Medicine
The University of Tennessee Health Science Center
Memphis, TN

Mike Feilmeier, MD
Medical Director, International Division of Ophthalmology
Department of Ophthalmology and Visual Sciences
University of Nebraska Medical Center
Omaha, NE

Carlton R. Fenzl, MD
Resident
Department of Ophthalmology
New York Medical College (Brooklyn-Queens)
New York, NY

William J. Fishkind, MD, FACS
Fishkind, Bakewell, & Maltzman
Eye Care and Surgical Center
Tucson, AZ

Harry W. Flynn, Jr., MD
Professor of Ophthalmology
Department of Ophthalmology at the Miller School of
    Medicine
University of Miami
Miami, FL

Jill A. Foster, MD, FACS
Associate Clinical Professor
Ohio State University Department of Ophthalmology
Division of Oculofacial Plastic and Reconstructive Surgery
Medical Director, Plastic Surgery Ohio
Eye Center of Columbus
Columbus, OH

Ryan C. Frank, MD, FRCSC
Pediatric, Craniofacial, Aesthetic and Reconstructive Plastic
    Surgeon
Division of Plastic Surgery, Department of Surgery
Alberta Children's Hospital
University of Calgary,
Calgary, Canada

Sharon F. Freedman, MD
Professor of Ophthalmology and Pediatrics
Chief, Division of Pediatric Ophthalmology
Department of Ophthalmology
Duke Eye Center
Durham, NC

Matthew F. Gardiner, MD
Director, Emergency Ophthalmology Services
Department of Ophthalmology
Massachusetts Eye and Ear Infirmary,
    Harvard Medical School
Boston, MA

Sumit (Sam) Garg, MD
Assistant Professor – Cataract, External Disease/Corneal
    Surgery, & Refractive Surgery
The Gavin Herbert Eye Institute
University of California, Irvine City
Irvine, CA

Roberta E. Gausas, MD
Associate Professor
Department of Ophthalmology
University of Pennsylvania School of Medicine
Philadelphia, PA

Gregg S. Gayre, MD
Chief of Ophthalmology, Assistant Physician-in-Chief
    Kaiser San Rafael
Department of Ophthalmology
Kaiser Permanente
San Rafael, CA

Neelofar Ghaznawi, MD
Assistant Clinical Professor of Ophthalmology
Department of Ophthalmology
New York University
New York, NY

Shubhra Goel, MD
Associate Consultant
Ex- Fellow Ophthalmic Facial Plastic Surgery
    and Aesthetics
University of Wisconsin–Madison
Madison, WI
Department of Orbit, Trauma and Oculofacial Aesthetics
Medical Research Institute, Sankara Nethralaya
Chennai, India

Kenneth M. Goins, MD
Professor, Clinical Ophthalmology
Department of Ophthalmology and Visual Sciences
University of Iowa
Iowa City, IA

Gregory J. Griepentrog, MD
Instructor of Ophthalmology
Department of Ophthalmology and Visual Sciences
University of Wisconsin–Madison
Madison, WI

Anita Gupta, MD
Assistant Professor of Clinical Ophthalmology
Bascom Palmer Eye Institute
University of Miami Miller School of Medicine
Miami, FL

Preeya K. Gupta, MD
Assistant Professor of Ophthalmology
    Cornea and Refractive Surgery Services
Duke University School of Medicine
Duke University Eye Center
Durham, NC

David L. Guyton, MD
Director, The Krieger Children's Eye Center at The Wilmer
    Institute
Zanvyl Krieger Professor of Pediatric Ophthalmology
The Wilmer Ophthalmological Institute
The Johns Hopkins University School of Medicine
Baltimore, MD

Kristin M. Hammersmith, MD
Director, Cornea Fellowship Program
Attending Surgeon, Wills Eye Institute
Philadelphia, PA

Dennis P. Han, MD
Jack A. and Elaine D. Klieger Professor
Department of Ophthalmology
Medical College of Wisconsin
Milwaukee, WI

Sadeer B. Hannush, MD
Attending Surgeon, Cornea Service,
    Wills Eye Institute
Department of Ophthalmology, Jefferson Medical College,
    Thomas Jefferson University
Medical Director, Lions Eye Bank of Delaware Valley
Scientific Program Chair, The Cornea Society
Philadelphia, PA

Andrew R. Harrison, MD
Director of Oculoplastic and Orbital Surgery
University of Minnesota
Minneapolis, MN

Morris E. Hartstein, MD, FACS
Clinical Associate Professor
Department of Ophthalmology and Division of Plastic
    Surgery
Saint Louis University
St. Louis, MO
Chief, Ophthalmic Plastic Surgery
Assaf Harofeh Medical Center
Zerifin, Israel

Lawrence W. Hirst, MD, MPH
CEO, The Australian Pterygium Centre
Faculty, Queensland Eye Institute
Professor, University of Queensland
Brisbane, Australia

David E.E. Holck, MD
Department of Ophthalmology/MCST
Wilford Hall Medical Center
San Antonio, TX

John B. Holds, MD, FACS
Clinical Professor
Departments of Ophthalmology and Otolaryngology/
    Head and Neck Surgery
Saint Louis University
St. Louis, MO

Joel Hunter, MD
Refractive Surgeon
Hunter Vision
Orlando, FL

Srinivas S. Iyengar, MD
ASOPRS Fellow
Eyesthetica
Santa Monica, CA

Glenn J. Jaffe, MD
Professor of Ophthalmology
Chief, Vitreoretinal Service
Director, Duke Reading Center
Duke Eye Center
Durham, NC

Bennie H. Jeng, MD
Associate Professor of Ophthalmology UCSF Department of
    Ophthalmology and F. I. Proctor Foundation Co-Director,
    UCSF Cornea Service Chief
Department of Ophthalmology
San Francisco General Hospital
San Francisco, CA

Thomas E. Johnson, MD
Professor of Clinical Ophthalmology
Bascom Palmer Eye Institute
University of Miami Miller School of Medicine City
Miami, FL

Daniel P. Joseph, MD, PhD
Associate Clinical Professor
Barnes Retina Institute/Washington University
Department of Ophthalmology and Visual Sciences
Saint Louis, MO

Alon Kahana, MD, PhD
Helmut F. Stern Career Development Professor of
    Ophthalmology and Visual Sciences
Eye Plastic, Orbital and Facial Cosmetic Surgery
Kellogg Eye Center, University of Michigan
Ann Arbor, MI

Carol L. Karp, MD
Professor of Clinical Ophthalmology
Bascom Palmer Eye Institute
University of Miami Miller School of Medicine
Miami, FL

William R. Katowitz, MD
Assistant Professor of Clinical Ophthalmology
Division of Ophthalmology
The Children's Hospital of Philadelphia
The University of Pennsylvania
Philadelphia, PA

Sang In Khwarg, MD
Professor
Department of Ophthalmology
Seoul National University Hospital
Seoul, Republic of Korea

Don O. Kikkawa, MD
Chief, Division of Ophthalmic Plastic and Reconstructive
    Surgery
Shiley Eye Center
La Jolla, CA

Nancy Kim, MD, PhD
Ophthalmologist
Massachusetts Eye and Ear Infirmary
Boston, MA

Terry Kim, MD
Professor of Ophthalmology
Duke University School of Medicine
Director of Fellowship Programs
    Cornea and Refractive Surgery Services
Duke University Eye Center
Durham, NC

Douglas D. Koch, MD
Professor and Allen, Mosbacher, and Law Chair
Department of Ophthalmology
Cullen Eye Institute, Baylor College of Medicine
Houston, TX

Bobby S. Korn, MD, PhD
Associate Professor of Ophthalmology
Division of Oculofacial Plastic
    and Reconstructive Surgery
UCSD Shiley Eye Center
La Jolla, CA

Amol D. Kulkarni, MD
Clinical Instructor
Department of Ophthalmology and Visual Sciences
University of Wisconsin–Madison
Madison, WI

Scott R. Lambert, MD
R. Howard Dobbs Professor of Ophthalmology and
    Pediatrics
Department of Ophthalmology
Emory University Chief of Pediatric Ophthalmology
Children's Healthcare of Atlanta at Egleston Emory
    University Atlanta
Atlanta, GA

Stephen S. Lane, MD
Medical Director, Associated Eye Care
Stillwater, MI
Adjunct Clinical Professor, University of Minnesota
Minneapolis, MI

Scott D. Lawrence, MD
Assistant Professor
Department of Ophthalmology
University of North Carolina, Chapel Hill
Chapel Hill, NC

Min Joung Lee, MD
Clinical Instructor
Department of Ophthalmology
Hallym University Sacred Heart Hospital
Anyang, Republic of Korea

Bradley N. Lemke, MD
Lemke Facial Plastic and Cosmetic Surgery
Madison, WI

Jeffrey M. Liebmann, MD
Clinical Professor of Ophthalmology
Director, Glaucoma Services
Manhattan Eye, Ear and Throat Hospital
New York University Medical Center
New York, NY

Richard L. Lindstrom, MD
Founder and Attending Surgeon
Minnesota Eye Consultants
Adjunct Professor Emeritus
Department of Ophthalmology
University of Minnesota
Associate Director
Minnesota Lions Eye Bank, Minneapolis, MI

Manuel A. Lopez, MD, FACS
Lopez Plastic Surgery
San Antonio, TX

Mark J. Lucarelli, MD, FACS
Professor; Chief, Oculoplastics Service
Oculoplastic, Facial Cosmetic & Orbital Surgery
Department of Ophthalmology and Visual Sciences
University of Wisconsin–Madison
Madison, WI

David B. Lyon, MD
Associate Professor
Department of Ophthalmology
Eye Foundation of Kansas City and Vision Research Center
    Kansas City, MO
University of Missouri–Kansas City School of Medicine
Kansas City, MO

Vanessa Vera Machado, MD
Advanced Anterior Segment Surgery and Glaucoma
    Specialist
Department of Ophthalmology and Glaucoma
Unidad Oftalmologica de Caracas
Caracas, Venezuela

Tamer H. Mahmoud, MD, PhD
Associate Professor
Vitreoretinal Division
Program Director, Vitreoretinal Fellowship
Kresge Eye Institute
Wayne State University
Detroit, MI

Boris Malyugin, MD, PhD
Professor of Ophthalmology
Deputy Director General
Chairman, Cataract & Implant Surgery Department
S. Fyodorov Eye Microsurgery Complex State Institution
Moscow, Russian Federation

Anil K. Mandal, MD
Director, Jasti V. Ramanamma Children's Eye Care Center
Consultant, Pediatric and Adult Glaucoma Services
L.V. Prasad Eye Institute
Hyderabad, India

Geva E. Mannor, MD, MPH
Head of Oculoplastic Surgery
Division of Ophthalmology
Scripps Clinic and Research Foundation
Assistant Clinical Professor of Ophthalmology
University of California San Francisco
La Jolla, CA

Ron Margolis, MD
Retina Consultants, PC
Hartford, CT

Douglas P. Marx, MD
Department of Ophthalmology, Oculofacial Plastic and
    Reconstructive Surgery Division
Oculofacial Plastic Surgery
Oregon Health & Science University
Portland, OR

Timothy J. McCulley, MD
Associate Professor
The Wilmer Eye Institute
Johns Hopkins School of Medicine
Director of Oculoplastic Surgery
King Khaled Eye Specialist Hospital
Riyadh, Saudi Arabia

Peter M. McGannon, MD
Associate Staff
Department of Ophthalmology, Lorain Institute
Cleveland Clinic Foundation/Lakeland Eye Surgeons
Lorain, OH

Stephen D. McLeod, MD
Theresa M. and Wayne M. Caygill, M.D. Endowed Chair
    Professor and Chairman
Department of Ophthalmology
    University of California San Francisco
San Francisco, CA

Dale R. Meyer, MD, FACS
Director, Ophthalmic Plastic Surgery; Professor of
    Ophthalmology
Lions Eye Institute, Department of Ophthalmology
Albany Medical Center
Albany, NY

Monte D. Mills, MD
Director of Ophthalmology
The Children's Hospital of Philadelphia
Associate Professor
Department of Ophthalmology
University of Pennsylvania School of Medicine
Philadelphia, PA

Yair Morad, MD
Departments of Pediatrics, Ophthalmology,
    and Pediatric Neurology
Assaf Harofeh Medical Center
Tel Aviv, Israel

Majid Moshirfar, MD, FACS
Professor of Ophthalmology
Director of Cornea and Refractive Surgery Services,
    Corneal Transplantation, Cataract Surgery,
    Implants and LASIK
Department of Ophthalmology and Visual Sciences
John A. Moran Eye Center
University of Utah Health Sciences Center
Salt Lake City, UT

Timothy G. Murray, MD, MBA, FACS
Professor of Ophthalmology
Department of Ophthalmology
Bascom Palmer Eye Institute
University of Miami School of Medicine
Miami, FL

Frank L. Myers, MD
Department of Ophthalmology and Visual Sciences
University of Wisconsin–Madison
Madison, WI

Jonathan S. Myers, MD
Associate Attending Surgeon
Wills Eye Institute
Philadelphia, PA

Nariman Nassiri, MD
Research Fellow
Department of Ophthalmology and Visual Sciences
University of Illinois at Chicago
Chicago, IL

Christine C. Nelson, MD, FACS
Professor of Ophthalmology
Professor of Surgery
Eye Plastic, Orbital and Facial Cosmetic Surgery
Kellogg Eye Center, University of Michigan
Ann Arbor, MI

Peter A. Netland, MD, PhD
Professor and Chair
Department of Ophthalmology
University of Virginia School of Medicine
Charlottesville, VA

Cynthia P. Nix, MD
Cornea, Cataract, and Refractive Surgery Specialist
Ophthalmology
West Georgia Eye Care Center
Columbus, GA

Sang-Rog Oh, MD
Department of Ophthalmology
Mount Sinai School of Medicine
New York, NY

Timothy W. Olsen, MD
F. Phinizy Calhoun Sr. Professor
Chairman of Ophthalmology
Director Emory Eye Center
Department of Ophthalmology
Emory University
Atlanta, GA

Paul F. Palmberg, MD, PhD
Professor
Bascom Palmer Eye Institute
University of Miami Health System
Miami, FL

D.J. John Park, MD
Resident Physician
Aesthetic and Plastic Surgery Institute
University of California, Irvine City
Orange, CA

Dante J. Pieramici, MD
Director, California Retina Research Foundation
Assistant Clinical Professor
Doheny Eye Institute
University of Southern California
Santa Barbara, CA

David A. Plager, MD
Professor of Ophthalmology
Director of Pediatric Ophthalmology and Adult Strabismus
Department of Ophthalmology
Indiana University Medical Center
Indianapolis, IN

Karim G. Punja, MD
Clinical Associate Professor
Department of Surgery, Division of Ophthalmology
University of Calgary
Calgary, Alberta, Canada

Shetal M. Raj, MS
Consultant Ophthalmologist
Iladevi Cataract & IOL Research Centre
Raghudeep Eye Clinic
Ahmedabad, India

Tushar M. Ranchod, MD
Vitreoretinal Surgeon
Bay Area Retina Associates
Walnut Creek, CA

Matthew P. Rauen, MD
Associate
Virdi Eye Clinic
Rock Island, IL

James C. Robinson, MD
Associate Professor of Ophthalmology
   The Eye Institute
Milwaukee, WI

**Geoffrey E. Rose, DSc, MS, MBBS, BSc,
FRCOphth, FRCS, FRCP**
Consultant Surgeon,
Oculoplastic, Orbital and Lacrimal Service,
Moorfields Eye Hospital,
London, United Kingdom

John G. Rose, Jr., MD
Oculoplastic, Orbital & Facial Cosmetic Surgery
   Departments of Ophthalmology and Plastic Surgery
Dean Health Systems Board of Directors, Finance Chair and
   Treasurer
Madison, WI

Arthur L. Rosenbaum, MD†
Brindell and Milton Gottlieb Chair in Pediatric
   Ophthalmology and Strabismus
Professor of Ophthalmology
Vice-Chairman, Department of Ophthalmology
David Geffen School of Medicine at UCLA
Jules Stein Eye Institute, UCLA
Los Angeles, CA

E. Victor Ross, MD
Director of Laser and Cosmetic Dermatology Center
Scripps Clinic
San Diego, CA

Jonathan B. Rubenstein, MD
Deutsch Family Professor and Vice-Chairman
Department of Ophthalmology
Rush University Medical Center
Chicago, IL

Patricia C. Sabb, MD
Assistant Professor
Department of Ophthalmology
   and Visual Sciences
University of Wisconsin–Madison
Madison, WI

Robert M. Schertzer, MD, MEd, FRCSC
Associate Clinical Professor
Department of Ophthalmology
   and Visual Sciences
The University of British Columbia
Vancouver, Canada

Stephen G. Schwartz, MD, MBA
Associate Professor of Clinical Ophthalmology
Medical Director
Bascom Palmer Eye Institute
University of Miami Miller School of Medicine
Naples, FL

Hosam Sheha, MD, PhD
Director of Clinical Research
Ocular Surface Center
Miami, FL

M. Bruce Shields, MD
Marvin L. Sears Professor
Chairman Emeritus
Department of Ophthalmology and Visual Science
Yale University School of Medicine
New Haven, CT

Kimiya Shimizu, MD, PhD
Professor and Chairman
Department of Ophthalmology
Kitasato University School of Medicine
Sagamihara, Japan

Bryan S. Sires, MD, PhD, FACS
Clinical Associate Professor
Department of Ophthalmology
University of Washington
Allure Facial Laser Center
Kirkland, WA

William E. Smiddy, MD
Professor of Ophthalmology
Bascom Palmer Eye Institute
University of Miami Miller School of Medicine
Miami, FL

Seaver L. Soon, MD
Staff Physician
Division of Dermatology & Dermatologic Surgery
Scripps Clinic
La Jolla, CA

Janet R. Sparrow, PhD
Anthony Donn Professor of Ophthalmic Science
    Departments of Ophthalmology, Pathology & Cell
    Biology
Department of Ophthalmology
Columbia University
New York, NY

Roger F. Steinert, MD
Irving H. Leopold Professor and Chair
Director, Gavin Herbert Eye Institute
University of California, Irvine City
Irvine, CA

Geoffrey C. Tabin, MD
Associate Professor
Director of the International Division
    of Ophthalmology
Co-founder/Co-director Himalayan Cataract Project
John A. Moran Eye Center
University of Utah
Salt Lake City, UT

Tasha Y. Tanhehco, MD
Staff Ophthalmologist
Department of Ophthalmology
Krieger Eye Institute, Sinai Hospital
Baltimore, MD

Jeremiah P. Tao, MD, FACS
Director, Oculofacial Plastic & Orbital Surgery
Department of Ophthalmology
University of California, Irvine City
Irvine, CA

Christopher C. Teng, MD
Clinical Assistant Professor
Department of Ophthalmology
The New York Eye and Ear Infirmary
New York, NY

Mark A. Terry, MD
Director, Corneal Services
Devers Eye Institute
Legacy Health Systems
Professor, Clinical Ophthalmology
Oregon Health Sciences University
Portland, OR

Scheffer C.G. Tseng, MD, PhD
Director
Ocular Surface Center
Miami, FL

Abhay R. Vasavada, MS, FRCS
Director
Iladevi Cataract & IOL Research Centre
Memnagar, Ahmedabad, India

Vaishali Vasavada, MS
Consultant Ophthalmologist
Iladevi Cataract & IOL Research Centre
Ahmedabad, India

Viraj A. Vasavada, MS
Consultant OphthalmologistIladevi Cataract
    & IOL Research Centre
Ahmedabad, India

Federico G. Velez, MD
Assistant Clinical Professor of Ophthalmology
Pediatric Ophthalmology and Strabismus
Department of Ophthalmology
UCLA School of Medicine
Jules Stein Eye Institute
Los Angeles, CA

Rengaraj Venkatesh, MD
Chief Medical Officer
NIL
Aravind Eye Hospital, Pondicherry
Pondicherry, India

David H. Verity, MD, MA, FRCOphth
Consultant Eyelid, Lacrimal and Orbital Surgeon
Moorfields Eye Hospital
London, United Kingdom

Mitchell P. Weikert, MD, MS
Assistant Professor of Ophthalmology
Baylor College of Medicine
Houston, TX

Bryan J. Winn, MD
Assistant Professor of Clinical Ophthalmology
Associate Residency Program Director
Director of Medical Student Education for Ophthalmology
Department of Ophthalmology
Division of Ophthalmic Plastic and Reconstructive Surgery
Columbia University Medical Center
Edward S. Harkness Eye Institute
New York, NY

Schonmei Wu, MD
Intern
Internal Medicine
New York Hospital Queens
Flushing, NY

Charles C. Wykoff, MD, PhD
Chief Resident & Co-Director of Ocular Trauma
Department of Ophthalmology
Bascom Palmer Eye Institute, University of Miami
Miami, FL

Tammy L. Yanovitch, MD, MHSc
Assistant Professor of Ophthalmology
Department of Ophthalmology
Duke Eye Center
Durham, NC

Michael T. Yen, MD
Associate Professor
Department of Ophthalmology
Cullen Eye Institute,
   Baylor College of Medicine
Houston, TX

Elizabeth Yeu, MD
Assistant Professor
Department of Ophthalmology
Cullen Eye Institute, Baylor College of Medicine
Houston, TX

Sonia H. Yoo, MD
Professor of Ophthalmology
Bascom Palmer Eye Institute
University of Miami Miller School of Medicine
Miami, FL

Steven J. Yoon, MD
Clinical Instructor, Oculofacial Plastic & Orbital Surgery
Department of Ophthalmology
University of California, Irvine City
Gavin Herbert Eye Institute
Irvine, CA

Daniel E. Zelac, MD
Department of Mohs and Dermatologic Surgery
Laser and Cosmetic Center
Scripps Clinic
La Jolla, CA

SECTION EDITORS

Edward G. Buckley, MD
Banks Anderson, Sr. Professor of
    Ophthalmology and Pediatrics
Vice Dean for Medical Education
Department of Ophthalmology
Duke University Medical School
Durham, NC

Jay S. Duker, MD
Professor and Chair
Department of Ophthalmology
Tufts Medical Center and Tufts University
    School of Medicine
Boston, MA

Bennie H. Jeng, MD
Associate Professor of Ophthalmology
    UCSF Department of Ophthalmology
    and F. I. Proctor Foundation Co-Director,
    UCSF Cornea Service Chief
Department of Ophthalmology
San Francisco General Hospital
San Francisco, CA

Don O. Kikkawa, MD
Chief, Division of Ophthalmic Plastic and
    Reconstructive Surgery
Shiley Eye Center
La Jolla, CA

Douglas D. Koch, MD
Professor and Allen, Mosbacher,
    and Law Chair
Department of Ophthalmology
Cullen Eye Institute, Baylor College of Medicine
Houston, TX

Stephen D. McLeod, MD
Theresa M. and Wayne M. Caygill, M.D.
    Endowed Chair Professor and Chairman
    Department of Ophthalmology
University of California San Francisco
San Francisco, CA

Peter A. Netland, MD, PhD
Professor and Chair
Department of Ophthalmology
University of Virginia School of Medicine
Charlottesville, VA

Patricia C. Sabb, MD
Assistant Professor
Department of Ophthalmology and Visual
    Sciences
University of Wisconsin–Madison
Madison, WI

Mitchell P. Weikert, MD, MS
Assistant Professor of Ophthalmology
Baylor College of Medicine
Houston, TX

MANAGING EDITOR

Sarah L. Atzen, BA, MLIS
Editor
Department of Ophthalmology and Visual Sciences
University of Wisconsin–Madison
Madison, WI

VOLUME EDITORS

Daniel M. Albert, MD, MS, FACS
RRF Emmett A. Humble Distinguished Director of the University of Wisconsin Eye Research Institute
F.A. Davis Professor, Department of Ophthalmology and Visual Sciences and Professor, Department
   of Pathology
University of Wisconsin School of Medicine and Public Health
Madison, WI

Mark J. Lucarelli, MD, FACS
Professor; Chief, Oculoplastics Service
Oculoplastic, Facial Cosmetic & Orbital Surgery
Department of Ophthalmology and Visual Sciences
University of Wisconsin–Madison
Madison, WI

Cataract and Intraocular Lens (IOL) Surgery

Edited by **Patricia C. Sabb**

1 Anesthesia for Cataract Surgery

Patricia C. Sabb, MD

TABLE 1.1 *Agents for Topical Anesthesia*

Anesthetic	Dose
Proparacaine	1 or 2 drops to operative eye prior to antiseptic prep
Tetracaine	1 or 2 drops to operative eye prior to antiseptic prep
Lidocaine gel	Small amount to operative eye prior to antiseptic prep
Preservative-free intracameral 1% lidocaine	Inject 0.1–0.5 mL through the paracentesis after administration of topical anesthetic

TABLE 1.2 *Indications for Topical Anesthesia*

Indications	Relative and Absolute Contraindications
Short procedures	Long procedures
Clear cornea incisions	Deaf patients
Cooperative patient	Nystagmus
Monocular patient	Tremors
High Myopia (decrease risk of globe injury)	Anxious patient
Need for rapid recovery of vision	Dementia
	Language barrier
	Uncooperative patient
	Allergy to topical drops/preservatives

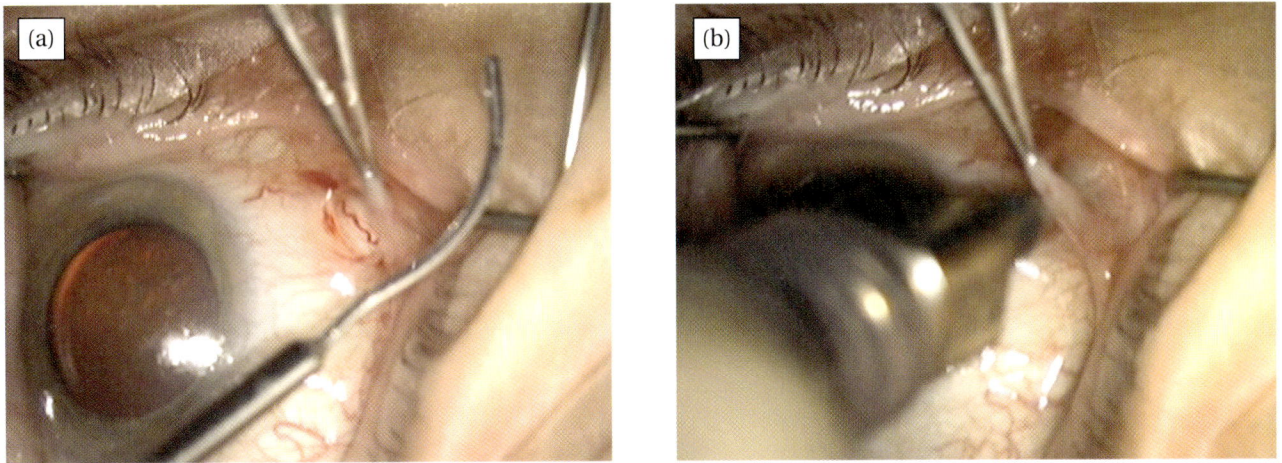

FIGURE 1.1 (a) Topical anesthetic drops are placed on the eye, and the patient is asked to look away from the chosen quadrant. The lateral quadrant is most commonly used. A small opening in the conjunctiva and Tenon's capsule is created using 0.12 forceps for conjunctival retraction, and Westcott scissors to bluntly dissect down to sclera. (Credit: EyeRounds.org, University of Iowa.) (b) The specially designed curved cannula for sub-Tenon injection is placed through the opening along the globe, extending posterior to the equator. Approximately 2 mL of a 50:50 mixture of 4% lidocaine and 0.75% bupivacaine or 1% lidocaine/0.375% bupivacaine is injected using a 3cc syringe. Sub-Tenon's injection is contraindicated if the patient has conjunctival or Tenon's scar tissue from previous surgeries, or trauma due to poor spread of anesthetic through the adhesions. Patching is required post surgery. (Credit: EyeRounds.org, University of Iowa.)

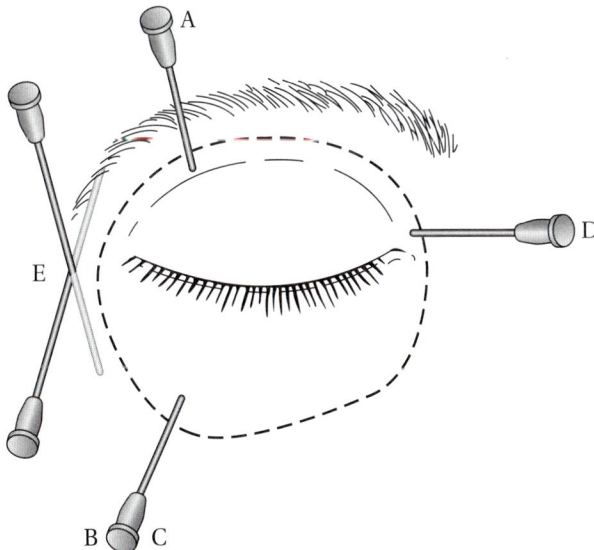

FIGURE 1.2 Schematic of the possible injection sites for a supertemporal peribulbar injection (A), for an inferotemporal peribulbar (B) or a retrobulbar injection (C), for an extremely medial peribulbar injection (D), and for a Van Lindt facial block (E).

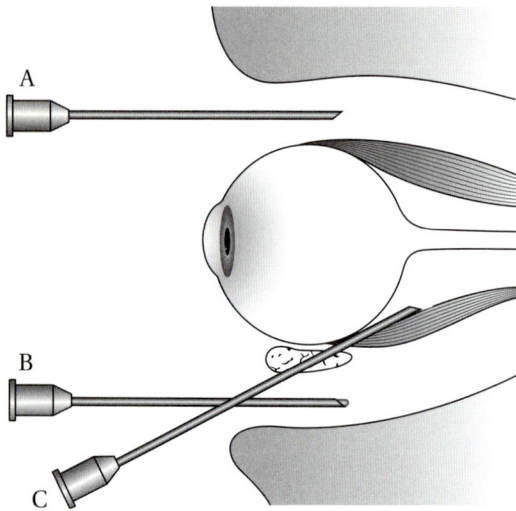

FIGURE 1.3 Schematic in a sagittal view of the needle position in a supertemporal peribulbar block (A), an inferotemporal peribulbar block (B), and a retrobulbar block (C). The bevel of the needle is directed toward the globe. The angle in a retrobulbar injection is shallow, and the needle may easily deliver anesthetic into the inferior rectus muscle.

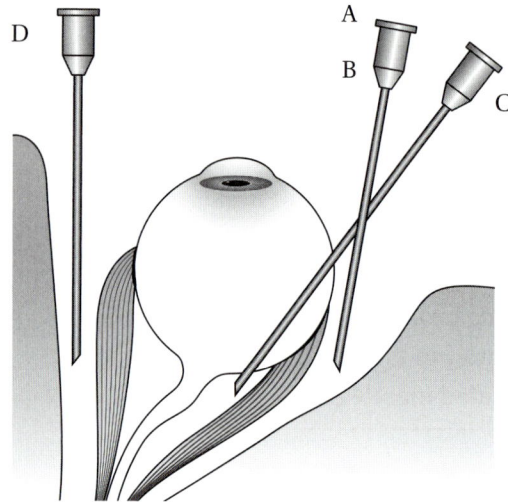

FIGURE 1.4 Schematic in a horizontal view of the needle position in a supertemporal or an inferotemporal peribulbar block (A, B), a retrobulbar block (C), and an extremely medial peribulbar block (D). The optic nerve moves away from the needle in an outward and downward gaze, but approaches the needle in an upward and inward gaze.

TABLE 1.3 *Peribulbar and Retrobulbar Anesthesia*

Method	Technique
Peribulbar injection	Most commonly, a needle is placed parallel to the orbital axis, inferotemporally, and aspiration is performed to ensure the needle is not in a blood vessel. Approximately 4–5 mL of a mixture of 1% lidocaine and 0.375% bupivacaine and ± hyaluronidase without epinephrine is injected. A pressure patch must be applied postoperatively.
Retrobulbar injection	A *blunt* retrobulbar needle, such as a 23 gauge Atkinson needle, should be used. A mixture of 1% lidocaine and 0.375% bupivacaine and ± hyaluronidase without epinephrine is introduced either through the lower lid or the inferior fornix in the inferotemporal quadrant at the junction of the middle and lateral thirds of the inferior orbital rim. The eye should be in primary position and the needle is directed to the superior orbital fissure, not the orbital apex. The needle will pass through the septum, there will be a "pop," and then into muscle cone, for the second "pop." Advance the needle approximately 1–1½ inches.
	Aspiration is performed to insure the needle is not in a blood vessel, and approximately 3–4 mL of anesthetic is injected. Gentle massage is performed to spread the anesthetic. A pressure patch must be applied postoperatively.

TABLE 1.4 *Indications for General Anesthesia*

Open globe—must use general endotracheal tube rather than laryngeal mask airway
Claustrophobia
Severe anxiety
Significant head tremor
Children
Nystagmus
Long procedure anticipated
Allergy to topical or injectable anesthesia
Altered mental status

TABLE 1.5 *Anesthesia Complications*

Method	Mild Complications with No Long-Term Effect on Visual Acuity	Complications with Potential Vision Loss	Systemic Complications
Topical	Epithelial toxicity Burning and stinging Discomfort during surgery Allergy to medicine	None	None
Topical plus Intracameral	Transient vision loss Epithelial toxicity	Corneal decompensation if preserved formulation used	None
Sub-Tenon's	Subconjunctival hemorrhage Chemosis	Diplopia secondary to extraocular muscle trauma	None
Peribulbar	Chemosis Ecchymosis Ptosis	Diplopia Globe perforation—rare	Oculocardiac reflex stimulation
Retrobulbar	Chemosis Ecchymosis Ptosis	Diplopia Globe perforation CRAO Optic nerve injury Retrobulbar hemorrhage	Oculocardiac reflex stimulation/bradycardia Seizures due to intra-arterial injection Brain stem anesthesia due to intradural injection

SELECTED REFERENCES

Chuang LH, Yeung L, Ku WC, et al. Safety and efficacy of topical anesthesia compounded with a lower concentration of intracameral lidocaine in phacoemulsification: a paired human eye study. *J Cat Ref Surg.* 2007;33:293–296.

Gills JP, Cherchio M, Raanan MG. Unpreserved lidocaine concentrations to control discomfort during cataract surgery using topical anesthesia. *J Cat Ref Surg.* 1997;23:545–550.

Khoo BK, Lim TH, Yung V. Sub-Tenon's vs. retrobulbar anesthesia for cataract surgery. *Ophthalmol Surg Lasers.* 1996;27: 773–777.

Patel BC, Burns TA, Crandall A, et al. A comparison of topical and retrobulbar anesthesia for cataract surgery. *Ophthalmology.* 1996;103:1196–1203.

Roman S, Auchlin F, Ullern M. Topical vs. peribulbar anesthesia in cataract surgery. *J Cat Ref Surg.* 1996;22:1121–1124.

Saude G, Jonas JB. Topical vs. peribulbar anesthesia for cataract surgery. *Acta Ophthalmol Surg Lasers.* 2003;81:596–599.

2 Incisions for Cataract Surgery

Patricia C. Sabb, MD

TABLE 2.1   *Indications for Incision Type*

Clear Cornea Incision	Scleral Tunnel Incision	Limbal Incision
Common technique for phacoemulsification with topical anesthesia Preserves conjunctiva for future bleb if needed	Phacoemulsification	Large incision extracapsular cataract extraction

Figures

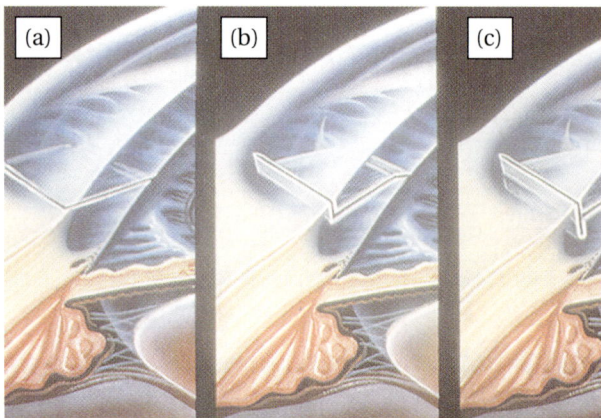

FIGURE 2.1   Clear cornea incisions are useful for phacoemulsification with topical anesthesia. These are commonly placed temporally and are self-sealing. Either a diamond blade or a single-use metal keratome are used to create either a single plane incision (a) or a shallow partial-thickness groove (b and c). (Image from Fine, IH. J. Cat Ref Surg. 2007 and Fine, IH, Clear Corneal Lens Surgery, Slack, Inc., 1999).

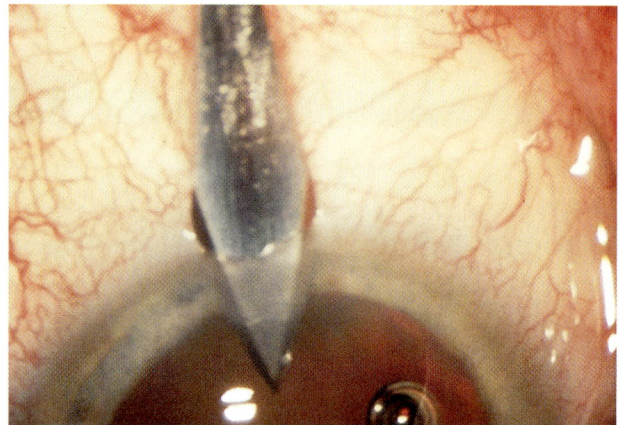

FIGURE 2.2   A single plane incision is fashioned in temporal clear cornea, after insertion of viscosurgical material, with a steel keratome blade. The globe is stabilized with either a toothed-forceps or scleral fixation ring. This method avoids bleeding and preserves the conjunctiva for future trabeculectomy, if needed. Care is taken to avoid placing the wound too anterior, which may result in corneal striae, inhibiting the surgical view. A posterior wound may cause conjunctival chemosis and bleeding. A tight wound may result in a wound burn.

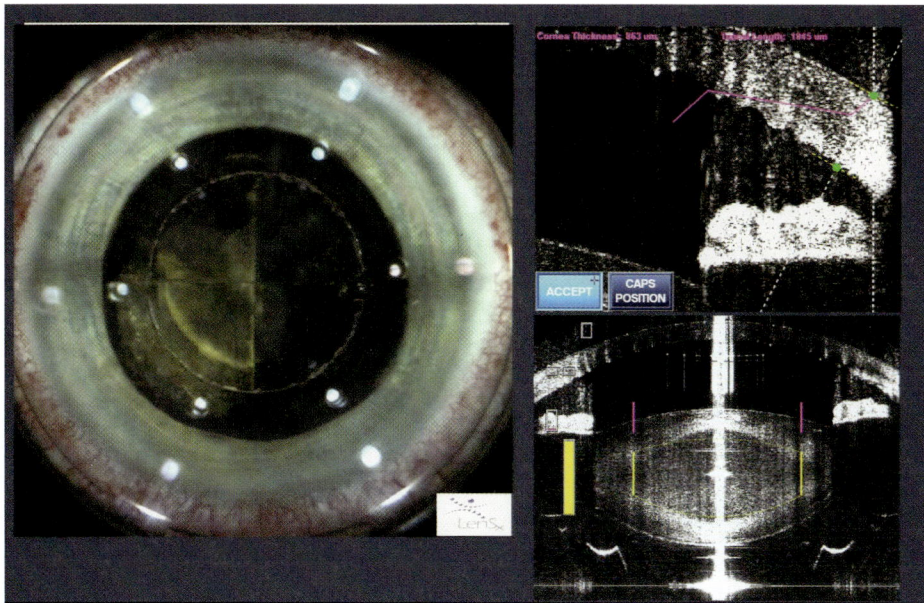

FIGURE 2.3 A graphic user interface of femtosecond laser. The left side of the picture shows the positioning of the primary clear cornea incision and the paracentesis. The OCT image in the upper right shows the customization of the size, shape, and design of the corneal incisions. (Credit: Alcon LenSx)

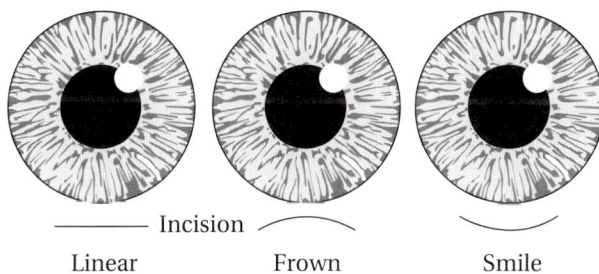

FIGURE 2.4 Optional configurations for scleral tunnel incisions. These incisions are useful for phacoemulsification but usually require more than topical anesthesia because a conjunctival peritomy and cautery are performed. These are most commonly placed superiorly, but can be placed temporally and are typically self-sealing or require only 1 suture.

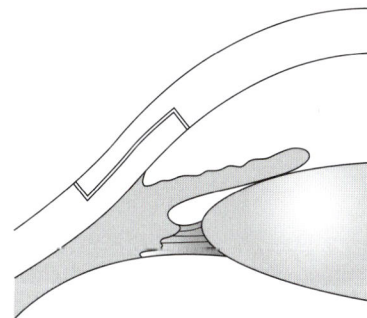

FIGURE 2.5 Cross section demonstrating the configuration of the self-sealing triplanar square wound.

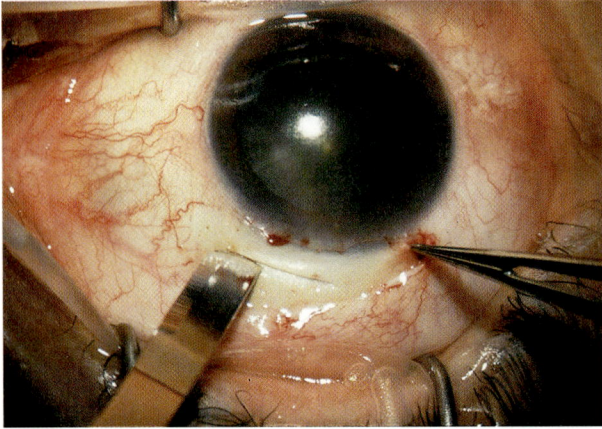

FIGURE 2.6 After the conjunctival peritomy and cautery, an initial vertical groove 1–2 mm posterior to the limbus is created with a steel crescent blade or diamond blade.

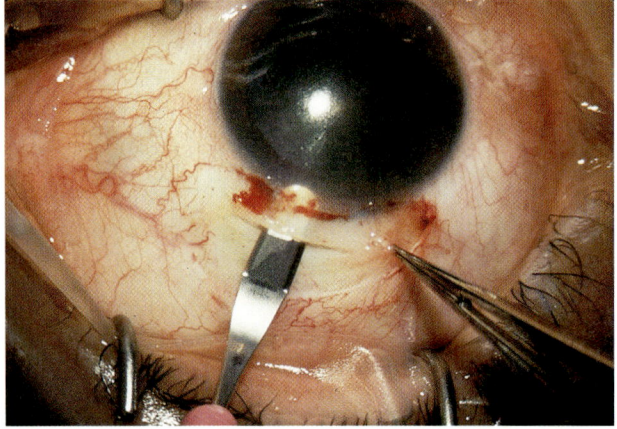

FIGURE 2.7 A crescent blade is used to dissect a lamellar flap through the sclera, toward the limbus, into peripheral cornea.

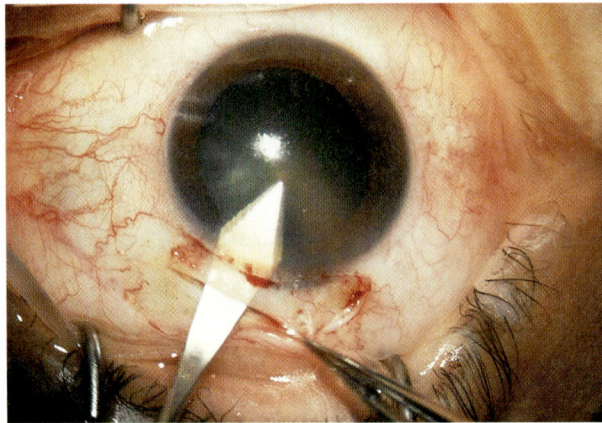

FIGURE 2.8 Advancement of the keratome blade is performed by pressing down through Descemet's and entering into the anterior chamber. This creates a self-sealing square incision. Care is taken to avoid an incision that is too anterior, which causes striae, or too posterior, which may result in iris prolapse.

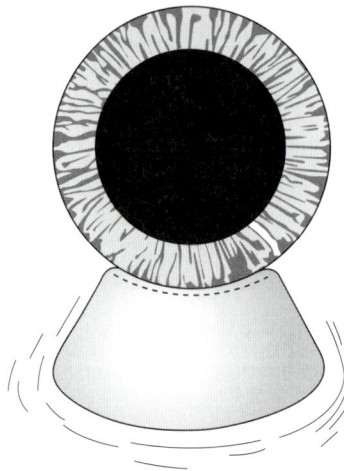

FIGURE 2.9 After conjunctival peritomy and cautery at the superior or 12 o' clock position, an incision is made at the gray-white junction, or surgical limbus, for large incision extracapsular cataract extraction. The initial groove is made with a crescent or keratome blade, and can be enlarged in either direction with corneoscleral scissors or a blade. This incision is not self-sealing and requires multiple interrupted sutures or running sutures.

TABLE 2.2 *Complications of Clear Corneal and Scleral Tunnel Incisions*

Method	Incision Too Anterior	Incision Too Posterior	Incision Too Tight	Incision Too Thin	Incision Too Wide
Clear cornea	Corneal striae obstructing surgical view	Conjunctival ballooning inhibiting surgical view Bleeding	Striae Wound burn Descemet's tear Difficult to maneuver phaco tip/instruments through incision	Tear roof of incision	Chamber instability
Scleral tunnel	Corneal striae obstructing surgical view	Iris prolapse Poor seal/wound leak Bleeding	Striae Wound burn Difficult to maneuver Phaco tip/instruments through incision Descemet's tear	Tear roof of incision	Chamber instability

TABLE 2.3 *Complications of Limbal Incisions*

Wound gape

Wound leak

Astigmatism—especially against the rule drift

Exposed sutures
Loose sutures } Leading to infection/giant papillary conjunctivitis/irritation

Increased risk of suprachoroidal hemorrhage

Caution with scleral thinning disorders

Iris prolapse

SELECTED REFERENCES

Fine IH, ed. *Clear Corneal Lens Surgery.* Thorofare, NJ: Slack, Inc; 1999

Fine IH, Hoffman RS, Packer M. Profile of clear corneal cataract incisions demonstrated by ocular coherence tomography. *J Cat Refract Surg.* 2007;(1):94–97.

Kershner RM. Clear corneal cataract surgery & the correction of myopia, hyperopia and astigmatism. *Ophthalmology.* 1997;104:381–389.

Olsen T, Dam-Johansen M, Bek T, Hjortdal J. Corneal vs. scleral tunnel incision in cataract surgery: a randomized study. *J Cat Ref Surg.* 1997;(3):337–41.

3 Anterior Capsulotomy Techniques

Patricia C. Sabb, MD

TABLE 3.1 *Indications for Anterior Capsulotomy Techniques*

Continuous Curvilinear Capsulorhexis	Can-Opener Capsulotomy
Phacoemulsification	Planned extracapsular cataract extraction
Utilize capsular staining techniques with mature, white cataracts	Useful for mature, white cataracts if capsular stain not available

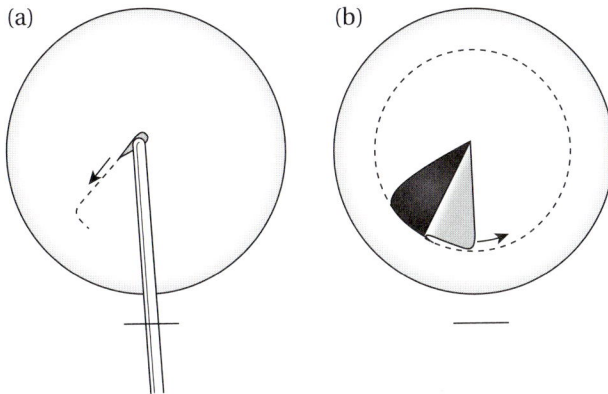

FIGURE 3.1 Formation of continuous curvilinear capsulorhexis. (a) Initiation of capsular tear with a cystotome. (b) Folding over edge of capsular flap.

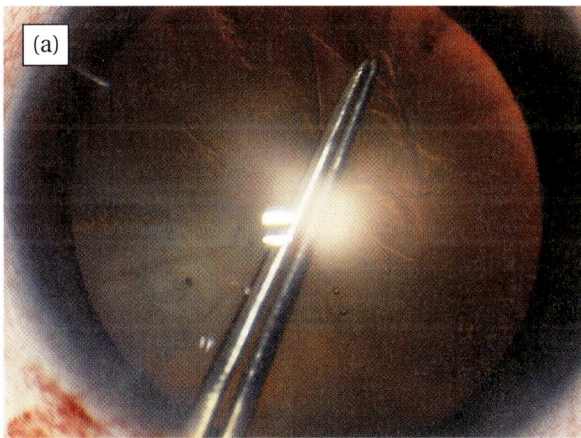

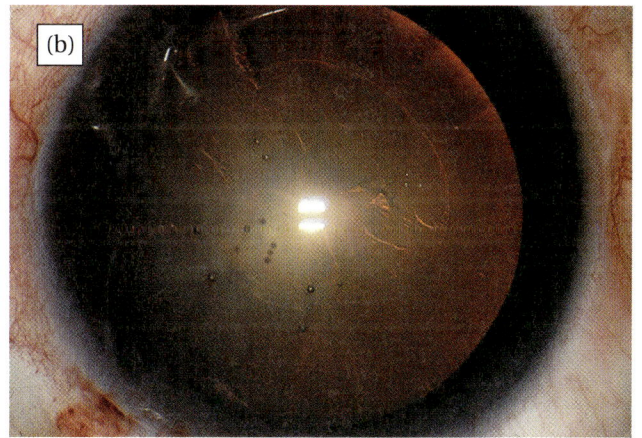

FIGURE 3.2 Completion of continuous curvilinear capsulorhexis. (a) Advancement of capsular tear with forceps. (b) Completed continuous curvilinear capsulorhexis. A continuous curvilinear capsulorhexis (CCC) increases the resistance of the bag to tearing. The CCC should overlap the optic edges to decrease the incidence of posterior capsular opacification (PCO) and anterior capsular opacification, optimize centration, and reduce dysphotopsias. The anterior capsule is incised and torn with either a bent 26 gauge needle, cystotome, or capsulorhexis forceps.

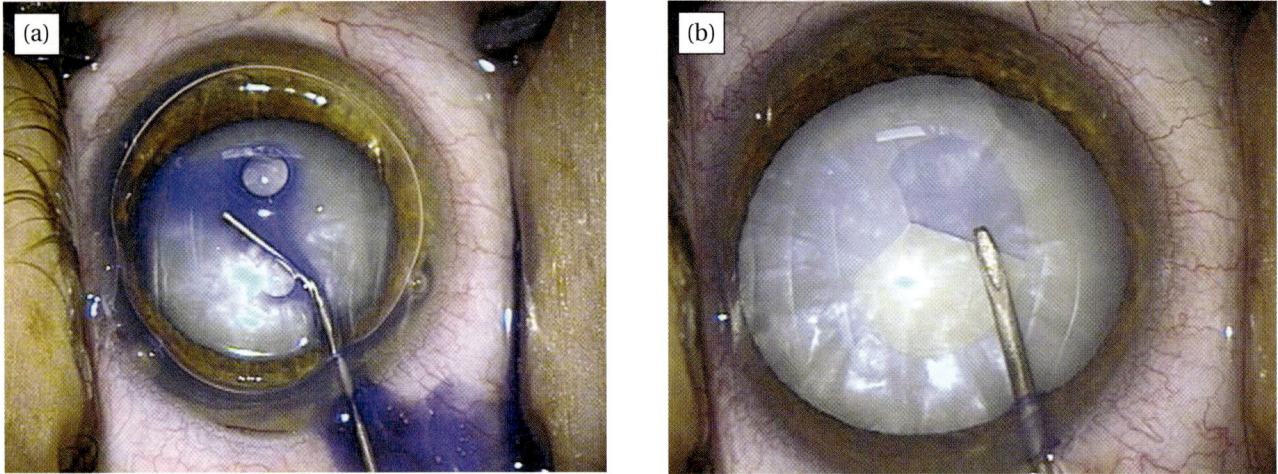

FIGURE 3.3 Trypan blue can be used to stain the anterior lens capsule when the red reflex is compromised, such as in this mature white cataract. (a) A filtered air bubble is injected into the anterior chamber. Filtered, premixed trypan blue is inserted, using a 30 gauge cannula, under the air bubble to stain the anterior lens capsule. (b) Trypan blue provides intense staining of the anterior capsule, improving visualization for the capsulorhexis. (Photographs courtesy of Dr. David F. Chang.)

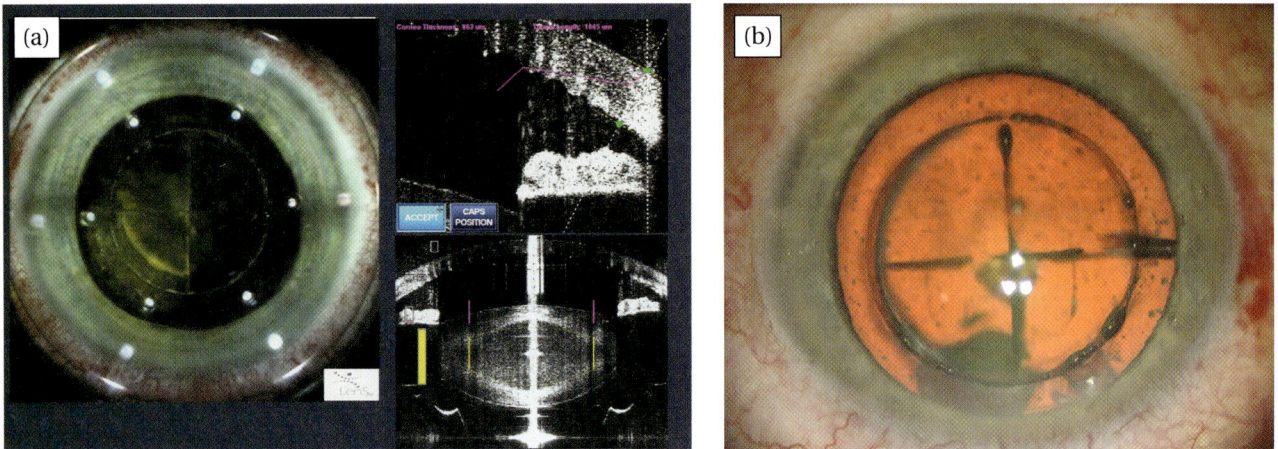

FIGURE 3.4 (a) Femtosecond laser graphic user interface showing X–Y axis shape and positioning of the capsulorhexis on the left, and the OCT images used to position and design the capsulorhexis on the right. (b) Capsulorhexis created by a femtosecond laser. Femtosecond laser capsulotomy may improve the centration, safety, and consistency of the anterior capsulorhexis. The size and shape of the capsulorhexis may be precisely adjusted with this technique. (Images courtesy of Alcon LenSx.)

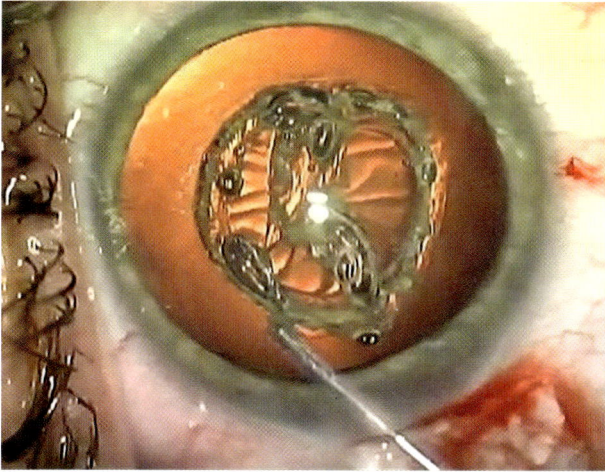

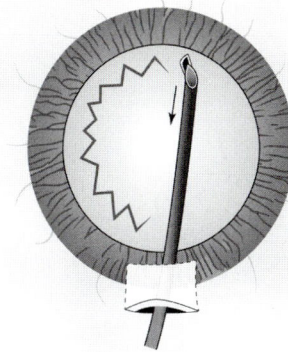

FIGURE 3.5 A plasma ablation capsulotomy (PAC) is performed in several seconds employing the plasma cloud that surrounds the blunt, hair-thin cutting filament at the end of the Fugo plasma blade hand piece. This capsulotomy can be quickly modified by merely tracing over unwanted capsule along the capsulotomy rim, such as removing inadvertent tears in the capsule rim. (Credit: Medisurg R&M Corp., Norristown, PA.)

FIGURE 3.6 A can-opener capsulotomy is performed with a bent needle or cystotome when a large-diameter capsulotomy is required for manual extracapsular cataract extraction, or when no red reflex is visible.

TABLE 3.2 *Complications of Continuous Curvilinear Capsulorhexis (CCC)*

Radial tear to periphery

Anterior capsule tear by phacoemulsification tip or other instrument

Small CCC inhibits cortical clean up and implant insertion, increases risk of anterior capsule fibrosis

Large CCC will not overlap the IOL edge and increases risk of PCO and dysphotopsias

Decentration of CCC prohibits centration of IOL, especially critical with multifocal IOLs

SELECTED REFERENCES

Assia EI, Apple DJ, Barden A, et al. An experimental study comparing various anterior capsulotomy techniques. *Arch Ophthalmol.* 1991;109:642–647.

Horiguchi M, Miyake K, Ohta I, Ito Y. Staining of the lens capsule for circular continuous capsulorhexis in eyes with white cataract. *Arch Ophthalmol.* 1998; 116:535–537.

Nagy Z. Intraocular femtosecond laser applications in cataract surgery: Precise laser incisions may enable surgeons to deliver more reproducible outcomes. *CRSToday.* Sept 2009:29–30.

Wilson ME. Anterior lens capsule management in pediatric cataract surgery. *Trans Am Opththalmol Soc.* 2004 Dec;102:391–422.

4

The New Iris Management Technique in Small Pupil Cataract Surgery

Boris Malyugin, MD, PhD

TABLE 4.1 *Indications: Main Reasons for Poor Pupil Dilation in Cataract Patient*

Glaucoma

Pseudoexfoliative syndrome

Ocular trauma

Uveitis

Previous ocular surgery

Diabetes

Senile iris atrophy

Pharmacotherapy (alpha-1a receptor blockers, cholinergic receptor stimulators, etc.)

The Malyugin Ring

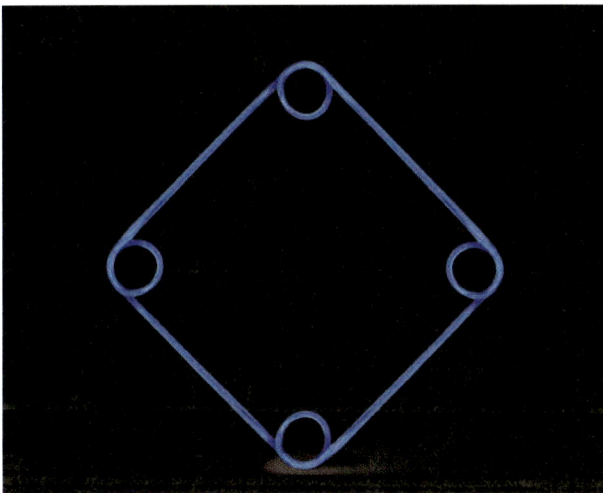

FIGURE 4.1 General view of the Malyugin Ring. The Malyugin Ring is made of 5-0 polypropylene, has one-piece design with square shape and four equidistantly located circular loops. The device comes with two sizes: 6.25 and 7.0 mm. The advantage of the smaller ring is that it is easier to insert and to retract. 6.25 mm ring cause less stress to the iris margin. The advantage of the 7.0 mm ring is that one can use it if the pupil starts of bigger, and also in IFIS cases. The 7.0 mm ring provides larger exposition of the lens nucleus and is preferable for the surgeons using phaco flip nucleus removal technique, and also for the 6.5 mm optic IOL users. Evacuation of the cortical material with 7.0 mm Malyugin Ring is also easier.

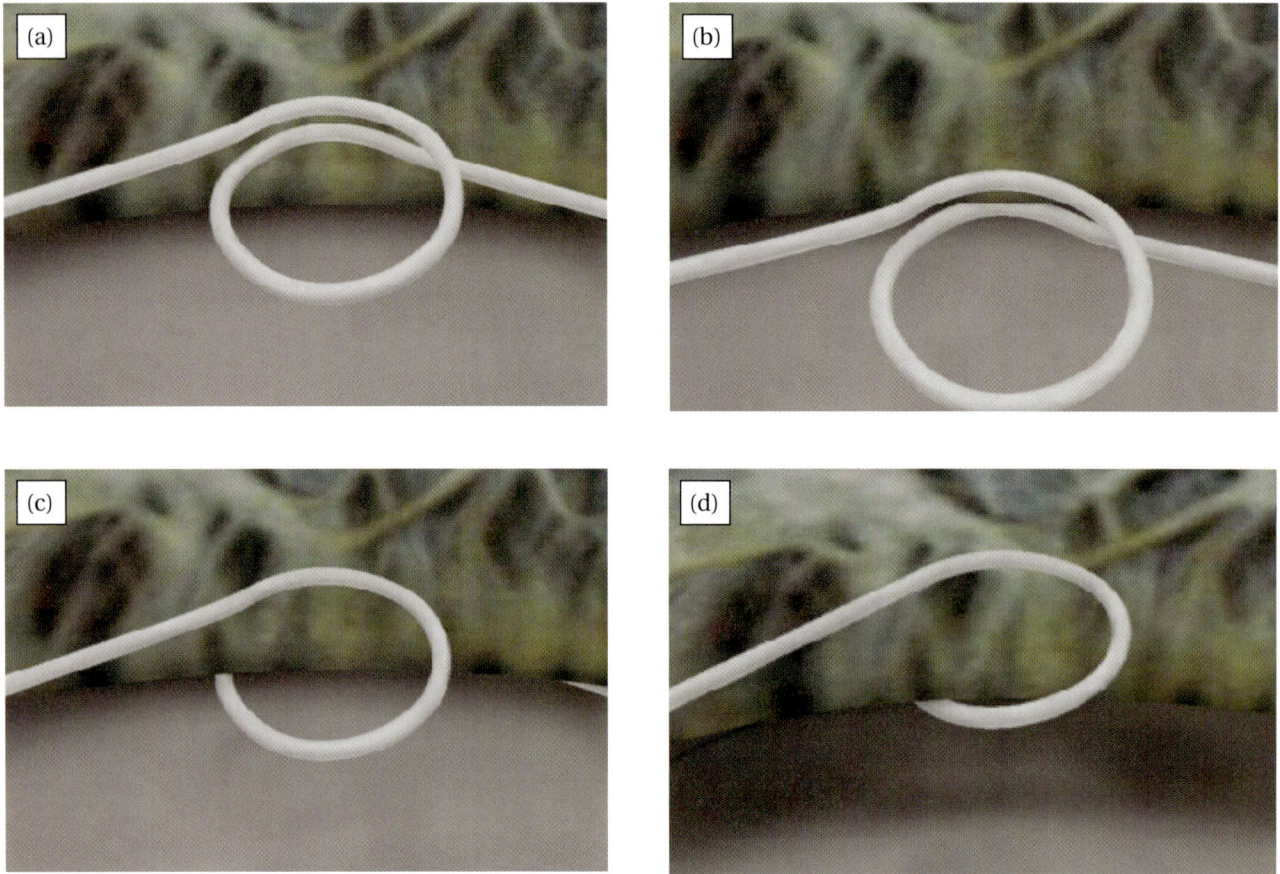

FIGURE 4.2 The basic concept of the Malyugin Ring iris fixation mechanism is based on the loops located at each angle of the device, each loop having a gap used to accommodate the iris tissue and to hold and retract the pupillary margin (a–d).

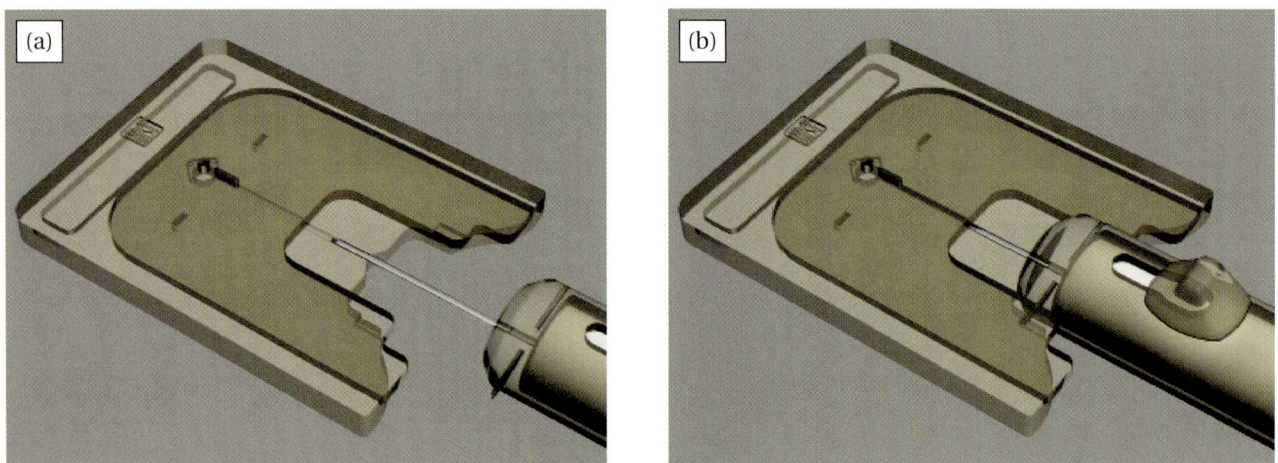

FIGURE 4.3 The Malyugin Ring produced by MST (Microsurgical Technology Inc., USA) consists of a presterilized single-use holder containing the ring and injector.

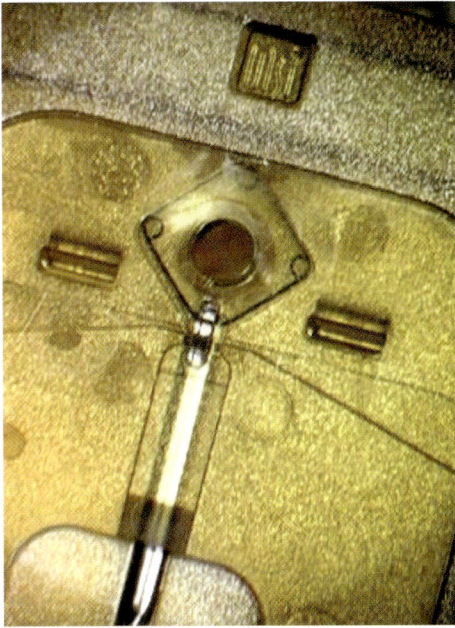

FIGURE 4.4 View of the Malyugin Ring holder with the ring inside. The dark blue ring is located inside the holder and can be visualized through its upper portion.

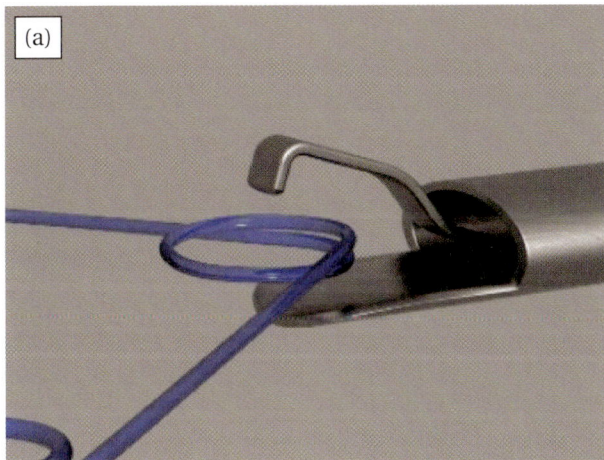

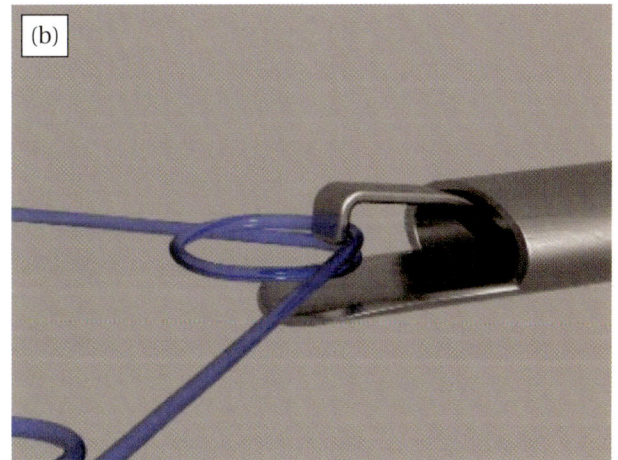

FIGURE 4.5 The hook of the injection device catches the proximal loop of the Malyugin Ring and is used to retract it inside the tube.

Insertion of the Malyugin Ring

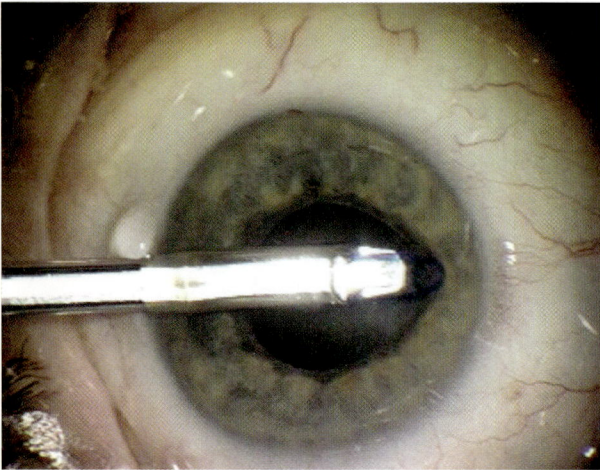

FIGURE 4.6 Engagement of the iris with the distal scroll of the Malyugin Ring. Surgical steps of Malyugin Ring implantation are demonstrated in the patient with the cataract complicated by pseudoexfoliation syndrome and small pupil. After topical anesthesia is applied, clear corneal incision is performed and ophthalmic viscosurgical device (OVD) is injected in the anterior chamber to stabilize it and protect the corneal endothelium. The Malyugin Ring is loaded into the injector. Then it is inserted through a 2.0 mm or wider clear corneal incision. The tip of the injector is positioned at the center of the anterior chamber. While pushing on the thumb button, the ring is released from the tip approximately 2.0 mm forward, and the distal scroll is engaged with the distal iris.

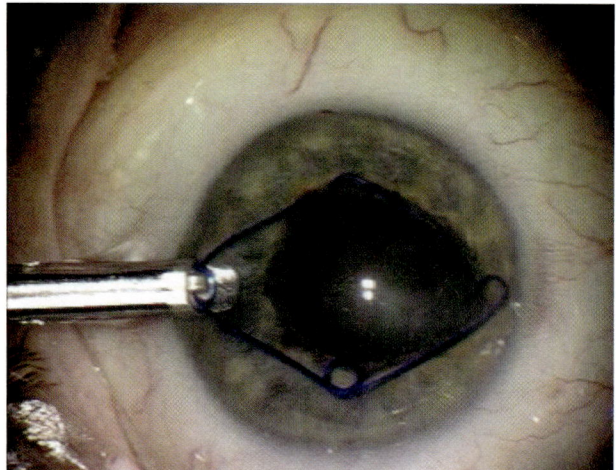

FIGURE 4.7 Engagement of the pupillary margin with the two lateral scrolls. The Ring is injected while simultaneously retracting the injector. Lateral scrolls emerge from the tube of the injector and one (or both) of them simultaneously catch(es) the iris margins. The proximal scroll is expelled from the cannula/injector, and the injector is moved until the injector hook is no longer holding the ring. In some cases it is useful to disengage the proximal scroll from the injector with the help of the instrument introduced through the paracentesis. The surgeon may push the ring slightly to the side to allow the injector exiting out of the eye.

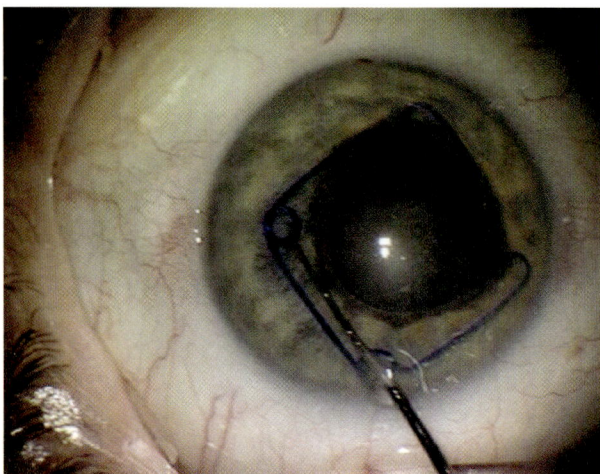

FIGURE 4.8 The proximal and lateral scrolls are now lying on top of the iris. Osher/Malyugin ring manipulator (Kuglen or Lester hook) is used to engage iris margin with the proximal scroll.

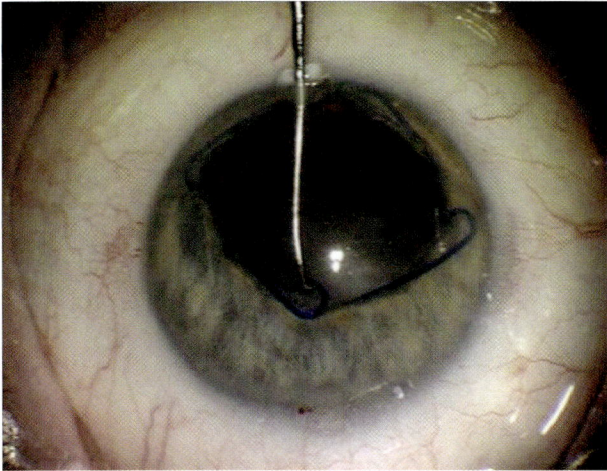

FIGURE 4.9 The Osher/Malyugin ring manipulator introduced through the sideport is used to engage iris margin with Malyugin Ring lateral scroll.

Surgical Steps of Phacoemulsification Cataract Surgery with the Malyugin Ring

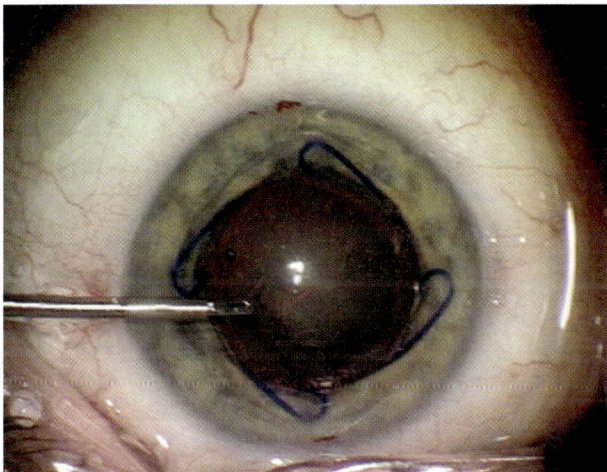

FIGURE 4.10 Anterior capsule is punctured with microforceps and capsular flap is created. The flap is pulled in the clockwise direction to complete the circular capsulorhexis opening.

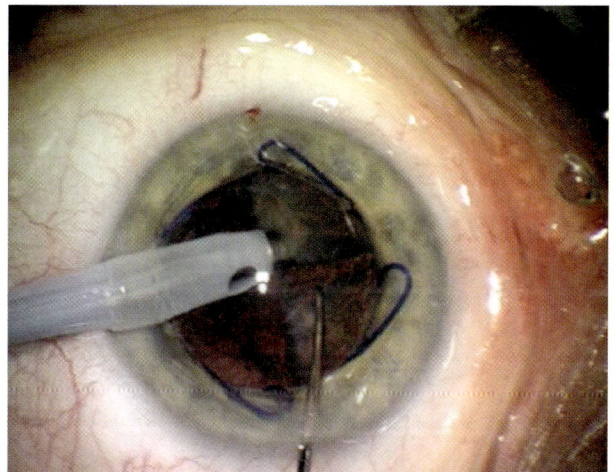

FIGURE 4.11 After hydrodissection and hydrodelineation with BSS, phacoemulsification is performed utilizing a chop technique.

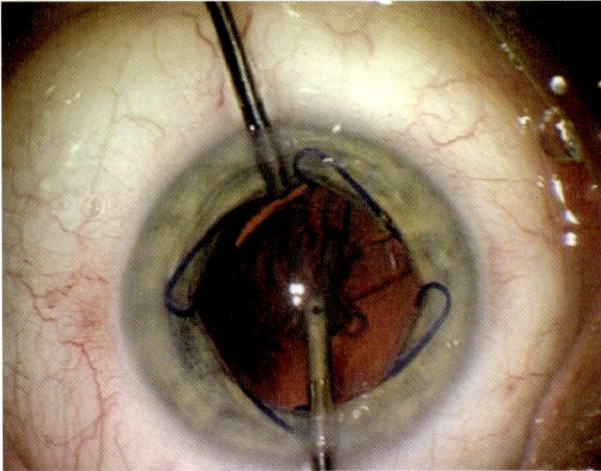

FIGURE 4.12 Bimanual irrigation/aspiration is used to clean capsular bag from the residual cortical fibers.

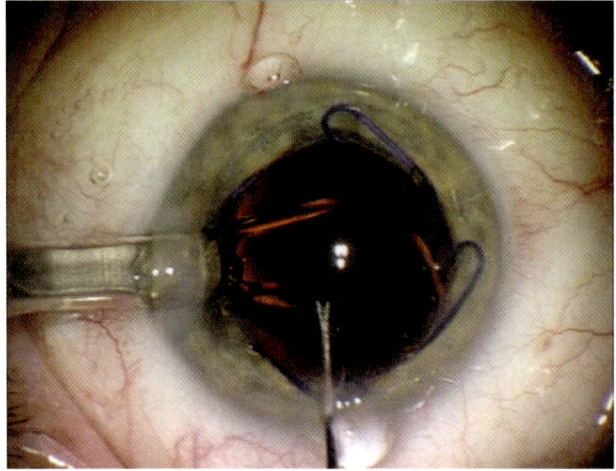

FIGURE 4.13 Capsular bag is filled with the cohesive OVD and the foldable intraocular lens (IOL) is inserted using the injector.

Removal of the Malyugin Ring

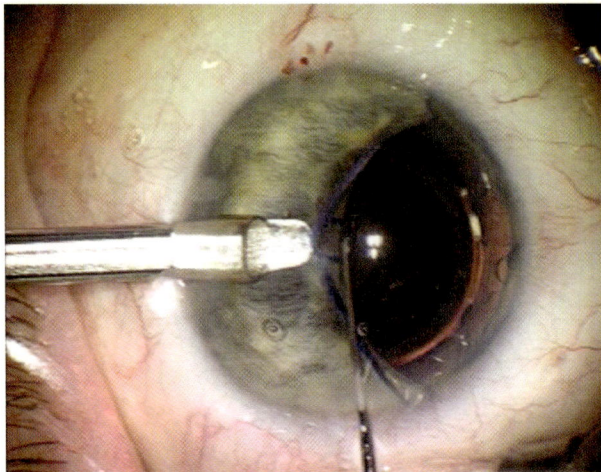

FIGURE 4.14 The Malyugin Ring is removed from the eye in the reverse order. The injector is inserted through the corneal incision. Proximal scroll is disengaged from the iris and lifted with the second instrument slightly above the iris plane. In some cases it is useful to disengage both distal and proximal scrolls before retracting the ring inside the injector.

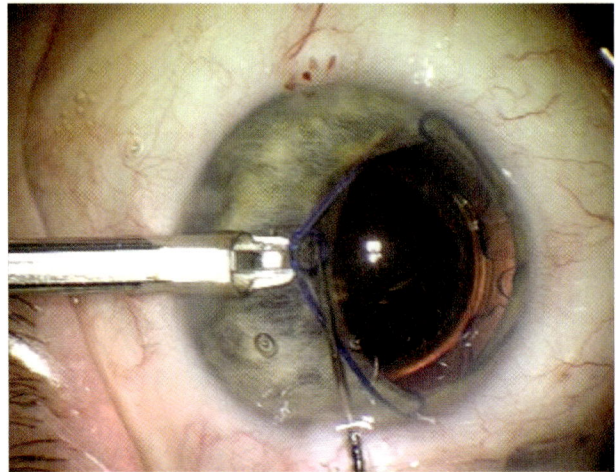

FIGURE 4.15 The injector's platform is positioned under the proximal scroll of the Malyugin Ring. The injector button is moved forward and the proximal scroll is catched with the hook of the injector. In this photo, the sideport instrument is helping to engage the proximal scroll with the injector hook.

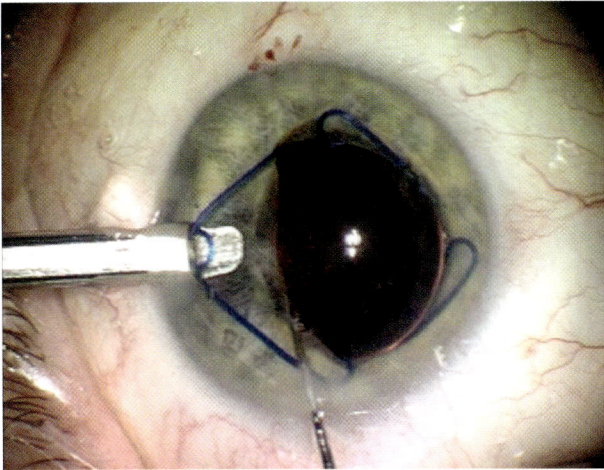

FIGURE 4.16 After engaging the proximal scroll with the hook, the injector button is pushed backward and the ring starts retracting into the injector.

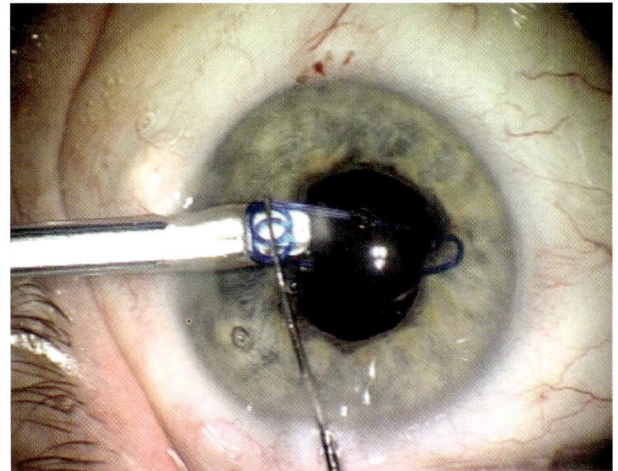

FIGURE 4.17 In order to retract the Ring completely inside the injector, it is necessary to press with the side port instrument on the lateral scrolls when they merge together, as shown here. With this maneuver the surgeon can avoid catching the rim of the injector with the lateral scroll, which is located above, and subsequent twisting of the ring. If the corneal incision size is over than 2.2 mm, the surgeon can alternatively, decide not to retract the ring completely in the injector and stop retracting when the left scroll rides above the cannula and then remove the entire assembly.

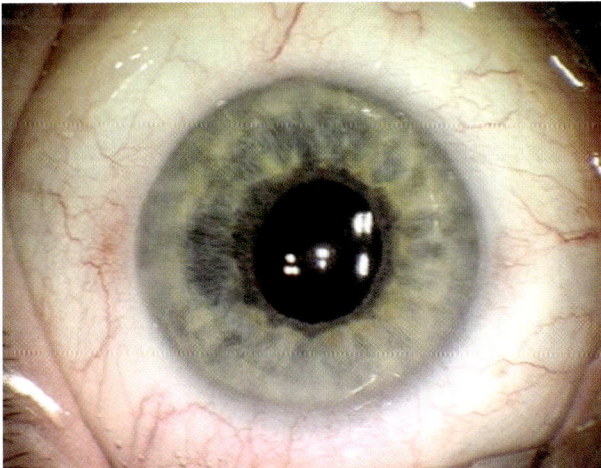

FIGURE 4.18 After ring removal the pupil constricts spontaneously.

The Malyugin Ring System (MST) is a very useful tool in phacoemulsification surgery. The easy to insert and remove device expands the pupil, protects the iris sphincter during surgery, and allows the pupil to return to its normal shape, size, and function postoperatively.

TABLE 4.2 *Potential Complications of the Malyugin Ring*

Scroll dislocation leading to ring decentration

Iris sphincter microtears

Bleeding from the pupillary margin

SELECTED REFERENCES

Chang D. Use of Malyugin pupil expansion device for intraoperative floppy-iris syndrome: Results in 30 consecutive cases. *J Cat Refract Surg.* 2008;34(5):835–841.

Malyugin B. Review of surgical management of small pupils in cataract surgery: use of the Malyugin Ring. *Techni Ophthalmol.* 2010;8(3):104–118.

Malyugin B. Russian solution to small pupil phaco Tamasulosin-induced floppy-iris syndrome. Video presented at the ASCRS 2006 Congress, S.Francisco, USA

Malyugin B. Small pupil phaco surgery: a new technique. *Ann Ophthalmol.* 2007; (3):185–193.

5

The Phaco Prechop Method for Dividing the Nucleus before Phacoemulsification

Takayuki Akahoshi, MD

TABLE 5.1 *Indications for Phaco Prechop*

Indication of Phaco Prechop
- Any cataract

Indication of Karate Prechop
- Soft cataract with rotatablte nucleus

Indication of Sector Prechop
- Soft cataract with non-rotatable nucleus

Indication of Counter Prechop
- Dense cataract too hard to insert Combo Prechopper blades
- Weakened ciliary zonules
- Incomplete CCC

Karate Prechop (Phaco Prechop for Rotatable Soft Nucleus)

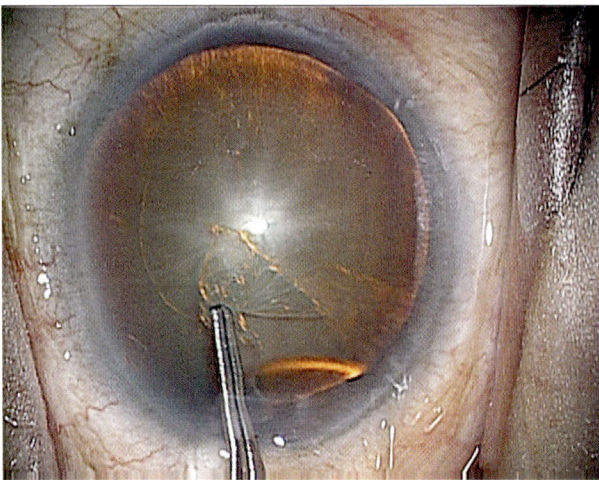

FIGURE 5.1 Make a complete curvilinear capsulorhexis (CCC) slightly smaller than the IOL optic size. For the better visibility of the nuclear surface, CCC should be made with the minimal touching of the lens cortex by forceps. If the CCC is not completed, *Karate Prechop* is not the method of choice. In such a case, alternative *Counter Prechop* should be carefully performed.

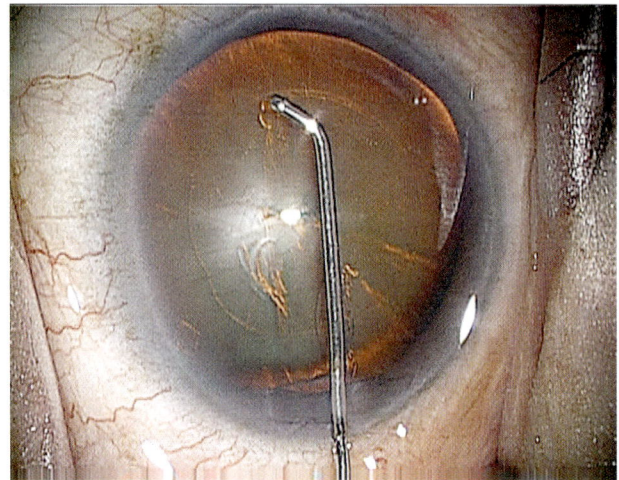

FIGURE 5.2 Perform cortical cleaving hydrodissection and ascertain that the nucleus can be rotated freely in the capsular bag. If the nucleus could not be rotated at this point, the bisected nucleus with larger volume will never be rotated. For very soft cataract where hydrodissection and/or nuclear rotation could not be performed, *Sector Prechop* is the method of choice.

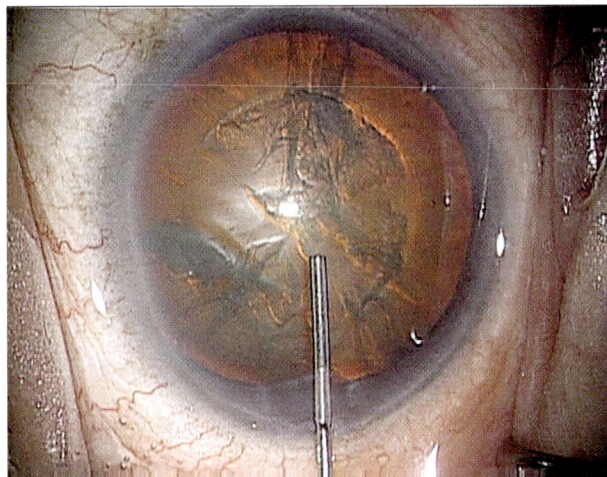

FIGURE 5.3 Fill up the anterior chamber with dispersive OVD to maintain the space and clear the nuclear surface for better visibility.

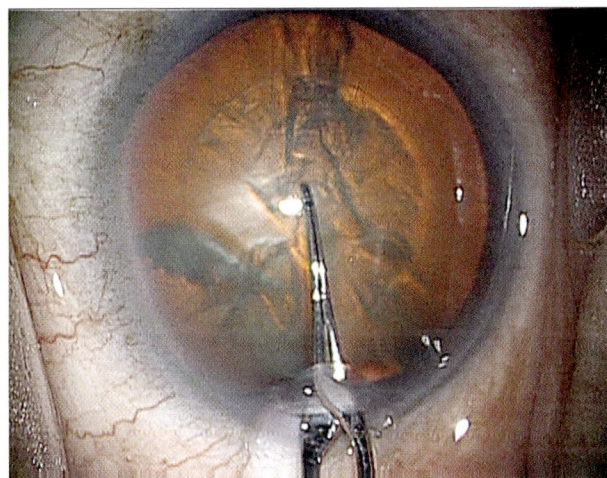

FIGURE 5.4 Place the angular side of the Combo prechopper (ASICO AE-4190) at the center of the nucleus. By placing the blades at this position, the stress on the ciliary zonules is equalized and minimized. Insert the whole blade vertically into the core of the nucleus. The blades should be inserted precisely perpendicular to the nucleus, keeping the right angle to the incision. If the nucleus is too hard to insert the blades, or if there are any signs of weakened ciliary zonules, Karate Prechop should not be performed. Those cases include severe pseudoexfoliation syndrome, nuclear cataract after vitrectomy and traumatic cataract, etc. If you force insertion of the Combo prechopper into a too-dense nucleus, it will stress the zonules to cause the serious complication of zonules rupture. In such cases, the prechopper should not be inserted without nuclear support. Hard nucleus, cases with weakened ciliary zonules, or incomplete CCC should be prechopped with the support of a Nucleus Sustainer (ASICO AE-2530) using the *Counter Prechop* technique.

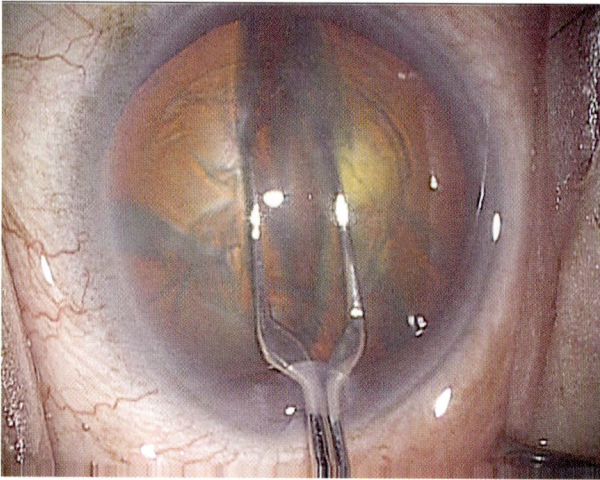

FIGURE 5.5 When the whole blades are inserted into the nucleus, they can be opened. While pushing the nucleus downward, open the blades slowly. If you open the blades too quickly, the nucleus will not be divided. It is important to apply the pressure along the lens fiber structure of the nucleus. Repeat the opening action to attain the complete nuclear crack which reaches to its bottom.

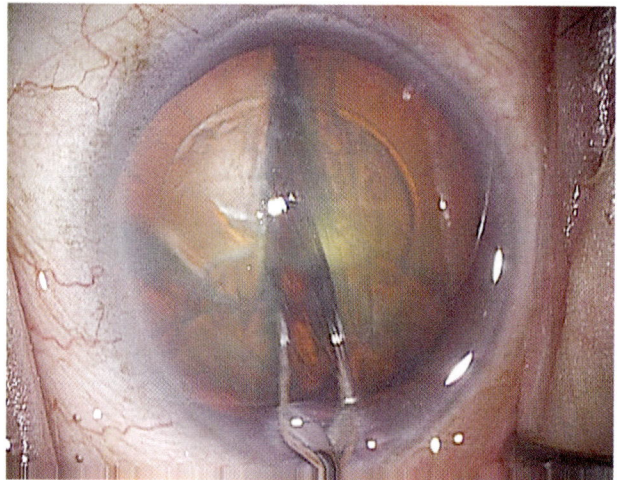

FIGURE 5.6 Place the blades at the proximal part of the nucleus to separate its equator completely.

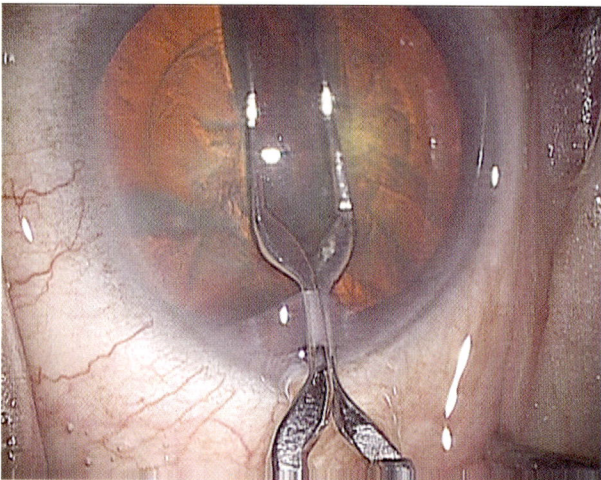

FIGURE 5.7 Place the blades at the distal part of the nucleus to attain the complete division.

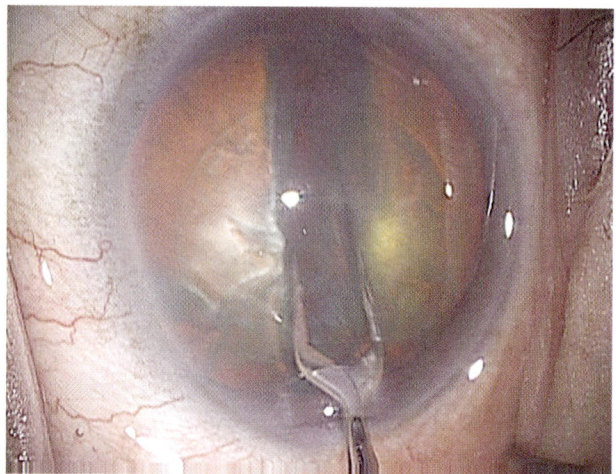

FIGURE 5.8 Using the rounded, blunt side of the Combo prechopper blades, attain the complete division from the surface to the bottom.

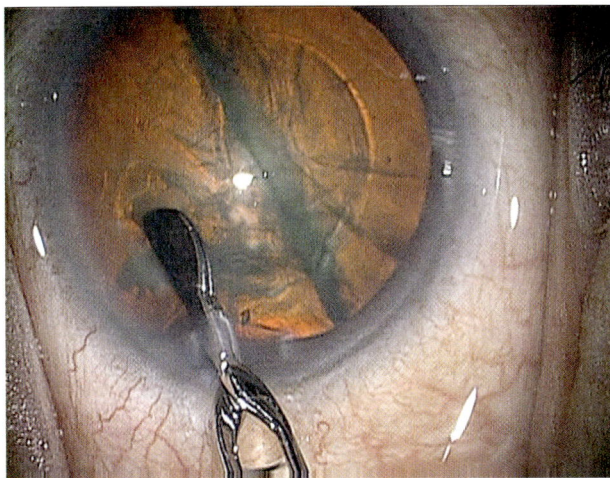

FIGURE 5.9 After restoring the bisected nuclear fragments to their original position, rotate the nucleus by 60 degrees for prechopping into six pieces, or by 90 degrees for prechopping into four pieces.

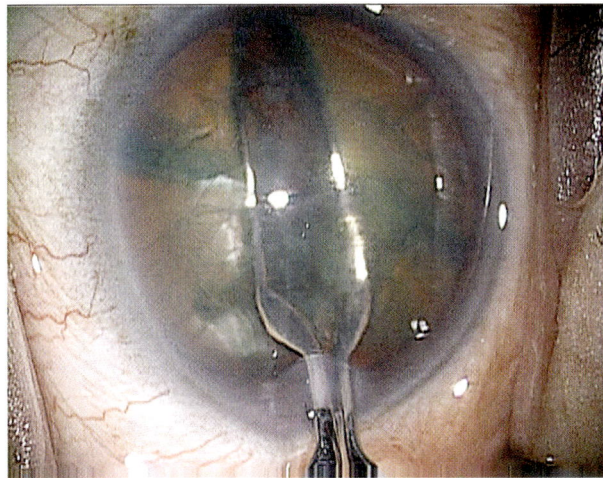

FIGURE 5.10 Prechop the nucleus into four pieces in the same way. If the cortical material hindered the visibility of the nuclear surface, additional OVD can improve the visibility. Pre-aspiration of the anterior cortex followed by the OVD injection will also improve the visibility of the nuclear division.

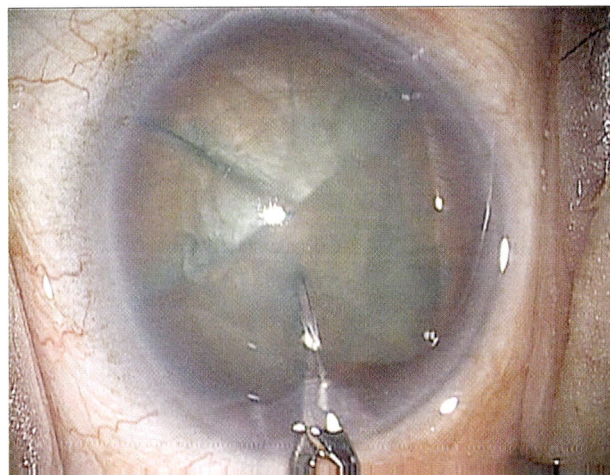

FIGURE 5.11 Rotate the nucleus by 60 degrees again and prechop into six pieces. The nucleus may be prechopped into four pieces if it is soft and easy to phacoemulsify.

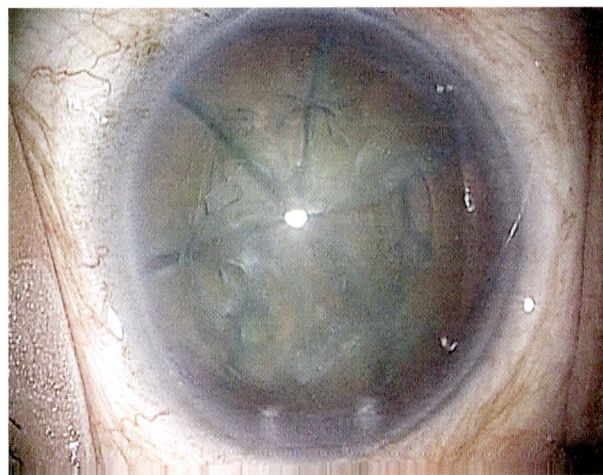

FIGURE 5.12 The nucleus is completely divided into six pieces and now ready for the phacoemulsification. *Visco Dissection*, a procedure to inject small amount of cohesive OVD, can attain perfect separation of the prechopped nuclear fragments, which will facilitate the following phacoemulsification.

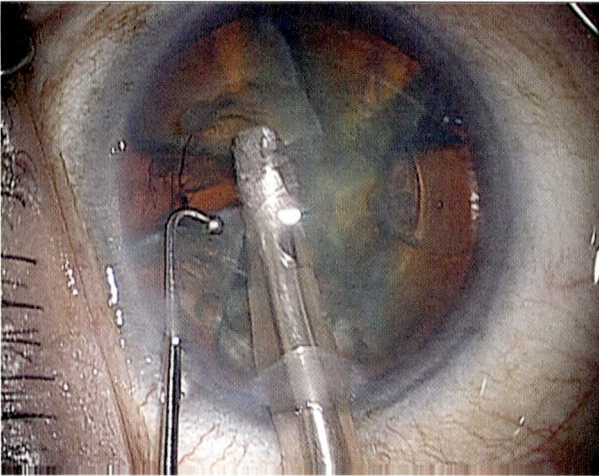

FIGURE 5.13 Each prechopped nuclear fragment is aspirated and phacoemulsified, one by one. The phaco tip is used with its bevel facing downward to the nucleus. The Nucleus Sustainer (ASICO AE-2530) is used to control the nuclear fragments in the anterior chamber. As the disassembled nuclear fragments can easily move into the anterior chamber and damage the corneal endothelium, controlling the nuclear fragments with a second instrument is mandatory.

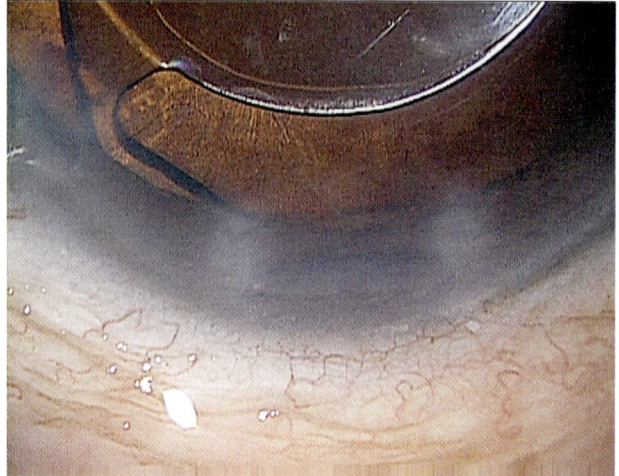

FIGURE 5.14 By prechopping the nucleus, the ultrasound energy required for the phacoemulsification can be markedly reduced. Accordingly, there is no thermal damage even in a sub-2 mm small incision. Consequently, it can be sealed easily without performing a stromal hydration.

Sector Prechop (Phaco Prechop for Non-Rotatable Soft Nucleus)

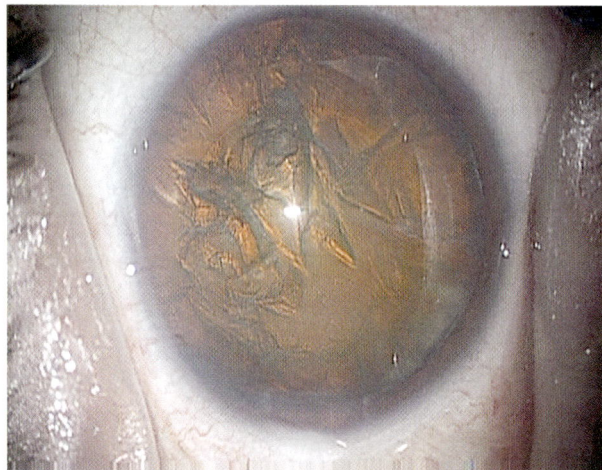

FIGURE 5.15 Make a complete curvilinear capsulorhexis (CCC) slightly smaller than the IOL optic size. If the CCC is not completed or the case has weakened ciliary zonules, the nucleus should be prechopped with the support of a Nucleus Sustainer. Try to perform cortical cleaving hydrodissection. If it was successful, prechop the nucleus using *Karate Prechop* technique, which requires nuclear rotation. If it was not successfully rotated, *Sector Prechop* is the method of choice.

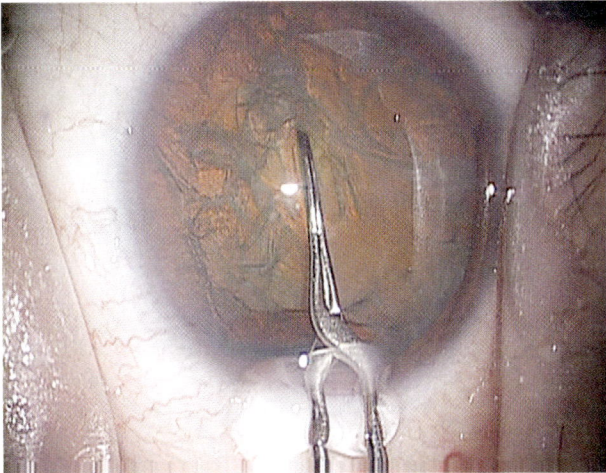

FIGURE 5.16 Fill up the anterior chamber with dispersive OVD. Place the angular side of the Combo Prechopper at the center of the nucleus. Insert the whole blade vertically into the nucleus. If the nucleus is very soft, the rounded side of the blade can be safely used.

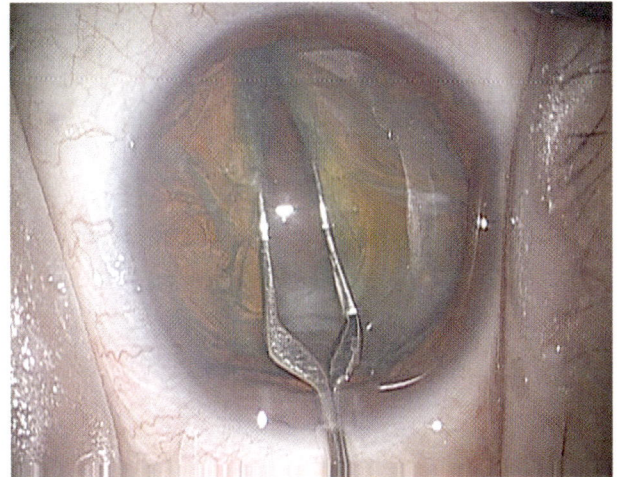

FIGURE 5.17 While pushing the nucleus downward, open the blades slowly to attain the complete division from the surface to the bottom. When the perfect division has been attained, the inner surface of the posterior capsule can be observed.

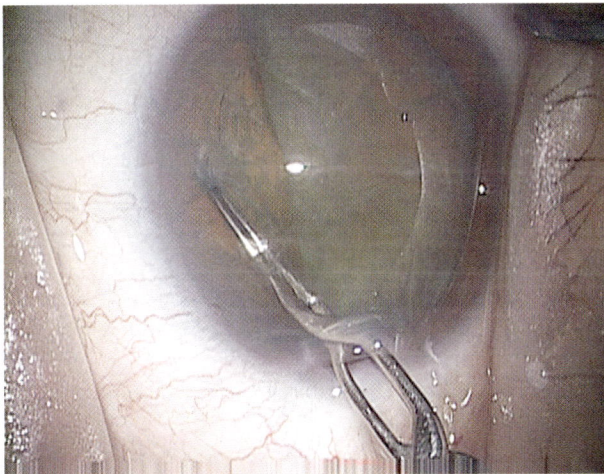

FIGURE 5.18 Insert the blades at 45 degrees to the initial crack. If the nucleus is not so hard, insertion of the blades against the lens fiber structure will be possible.

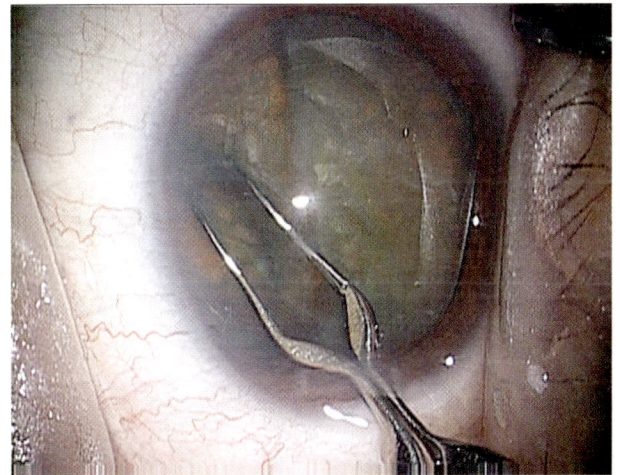

FIGURE 5.19 While pushing the nucleus downward, open the blades slowly to bisect the nucleus into fan shapes.

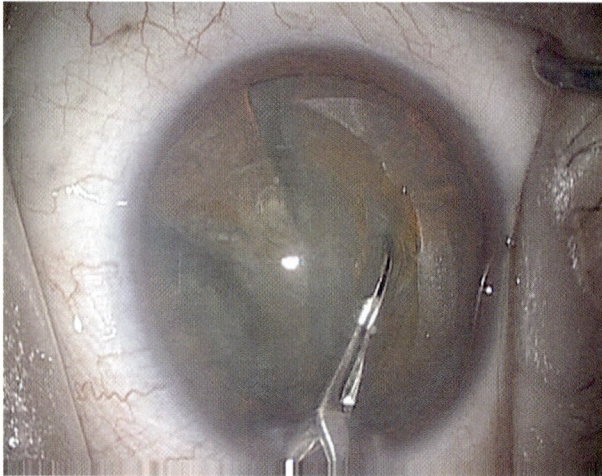

FIGURE 5.20 Insert the blades into the other half of the nucleus at 45 degrees to the initial crack. There is no need of the nuclear rotation before next prechop procedure.

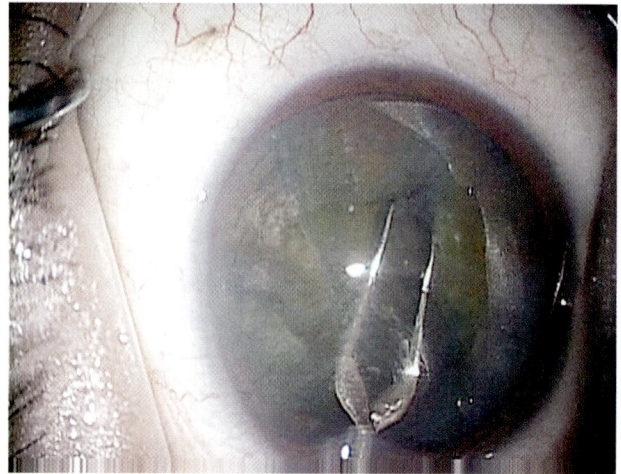

FIGURE 5.21 By opening the blades several times, attain the complete division from the surface to the bottom, as well as from the proximal to the distal end of the nucleus. The rounded side of the blade can be used safely to ascertain the complete division.

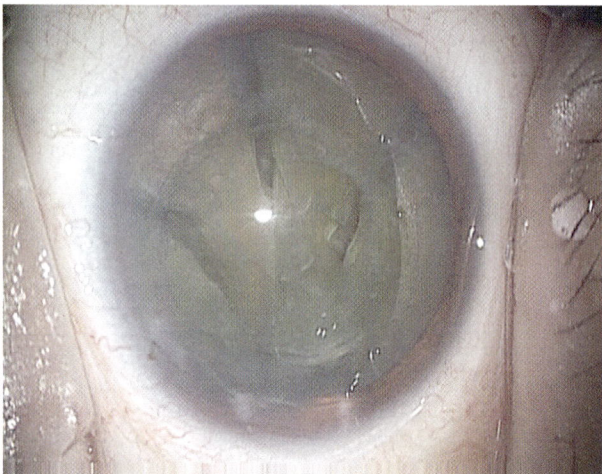

FIGURE 5.22 Without performing hydrodissection or rotation, the nucleus can be prechopped into four pieces in fan shapes.

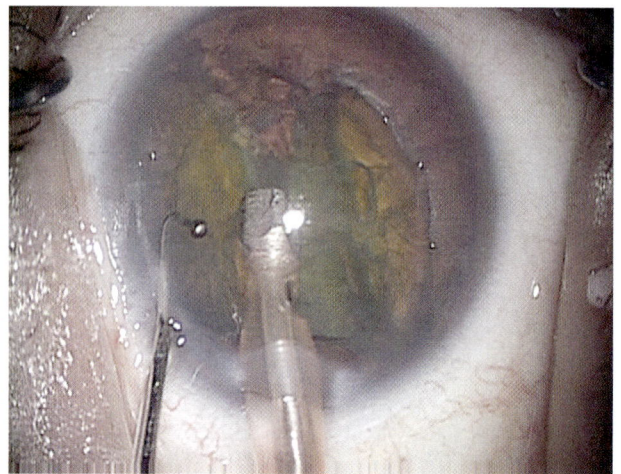

FIGURE 5.23 Using the phaco tip with its bevel down, the central two sectors of the nucleus can be easily removed. Then the lateral two sectors can be slid into the center of the capsular bag to phacoemulsify safely.

Counter Prechop (Phaco Prechop for Dense Nucleus)

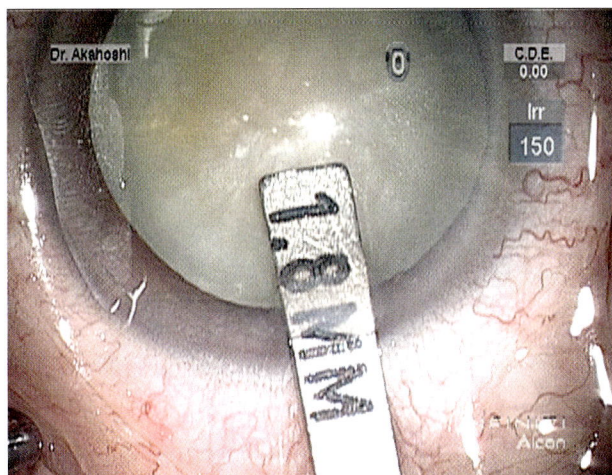

FIGURE 5.24 For the micro incision cataract surgery (MICS), either with a sleeve or without, it is critical to remove the cataract with the minimum ultrasound energy to protect the incision from the thermal damage. For this purpose, phaco prechop is mandatory in the MICS of the dense cataract.

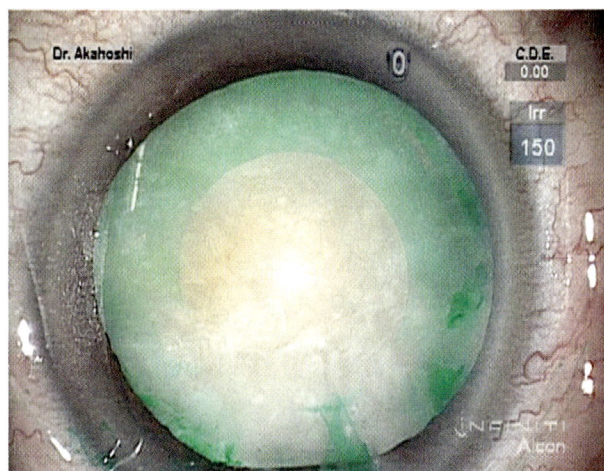

FIGURE 5.25 To identify the capsulorhexis edge, staining of the capsule with an appropriate dye is helpful during insertion of a Nucleus Sustainer in cases with a white or very dense cataract. Especially, the distal half of the capsulorhexis edge should be clearly identified. Fill up the anterior chamber with dispersive OVD and clear the nuclear surface. Making a complete CCC without tears or notches is the first important prerequisite. However, once you are accustomed to the prechop procedures, you may perform Counter Prechop very carefully even in the case of incomplete CCC. Pre-aspiration of the anterior cortex followed by the OVD injection will expose the nuclear surface clearly, which will facilitate the visibility of the nuclear division.

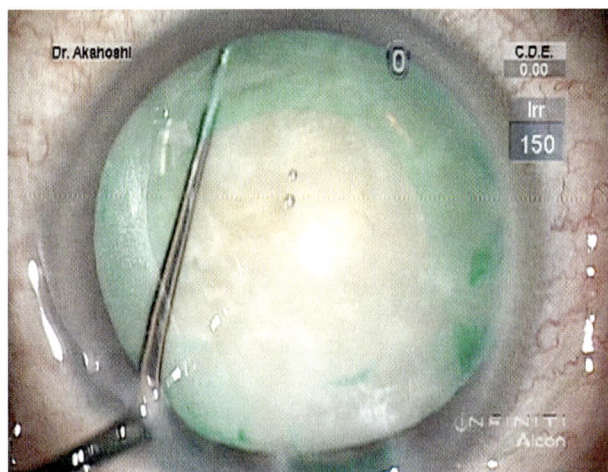

FIGURE 5.26 Insert a Nucleus Sustainer carefully into the equator to provide counterforce against the prechopper. If you support the nucleus over the capsule, focal zonules rupture or a tear in the anterior capsule will occur. For the appropriate insertion of a Nucleus Sustainer, capsular staining is helpful. It is important to support the nucleus at its deep equatorial portion. For myopic eyes with larger lens volume, AE-2530L, which has a longer tip, can support the nucleus better than the conventional one.

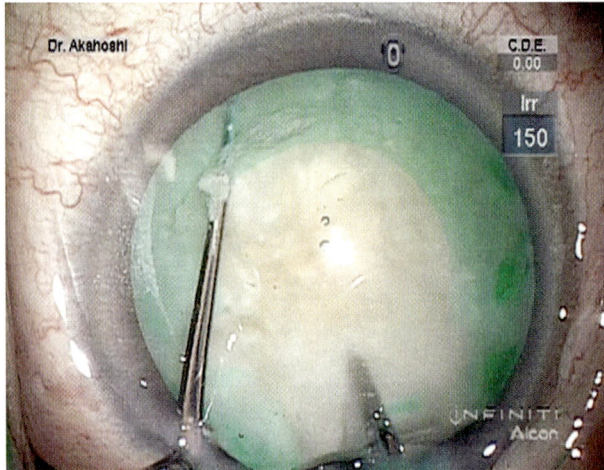

FIGURE 5.27 Insert the Universal Prechopper (AE-4192) from the periphery of the nucleus close to the proximal capsulorhexis edge. The direction of the insertion is toward the tip of the Nucleus Sustainer. The tip of the prechopper blade, the hardest core of the nucleus, and the tip of the sustainer should be aligned on the same axis. Accordingly, the sustainer should be inserted into the deep equatorial portion of the nucleus. If you support the nucleus too superficially and the prechopper is inserted to the center of the nucleus, there will be a stress on the proximal ciliary zonules. The alignment of the three points is a key for success of this technique.

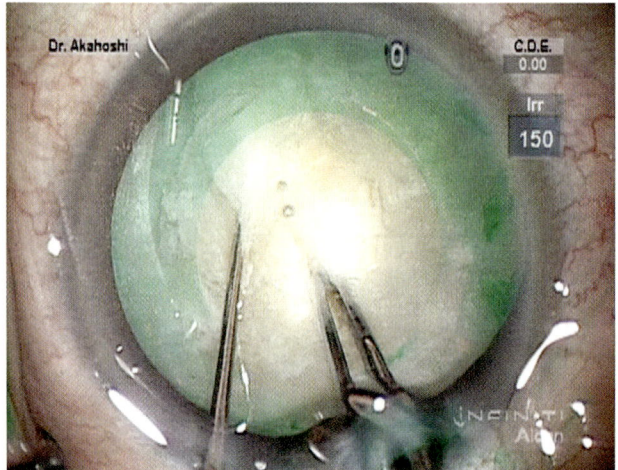

FIGURE 5.28 By bringing the Nucleus Sustainer toward the prechopper blade, it can chop the nucleus. In this situation, the prechopper is used like a phaco tip to fix the nucleus, and the sustainer as a phaco chopper to chop.

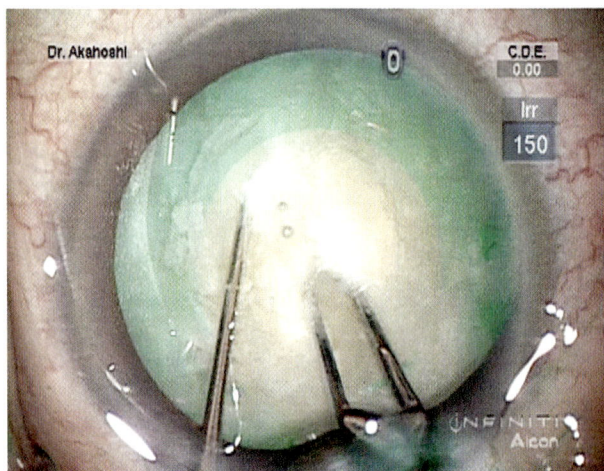

FIGURE 5.29 While supporting the nucleus with a Nucleus Sustainer, the nucleus can be prechopped by opening the prechopper blades. By opening the blades repeatedly, prechop the nucleus until you reach the bottom.

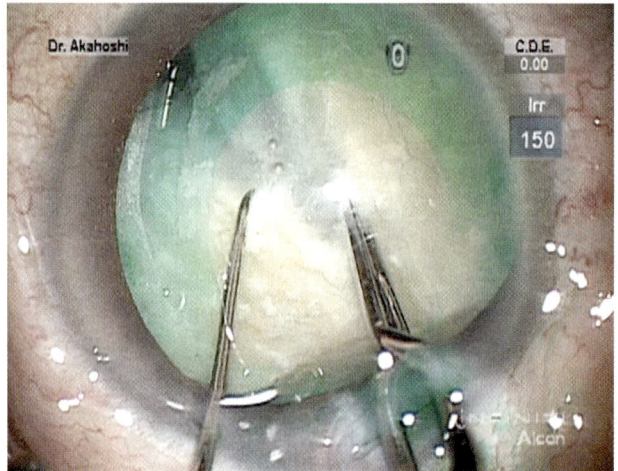

FIGURE 5.30 The most important point of the prechop is to break the posterior plate of the nucleus completely. Using the sustainer and closed prechopper blades, bisect the nucleus completely.

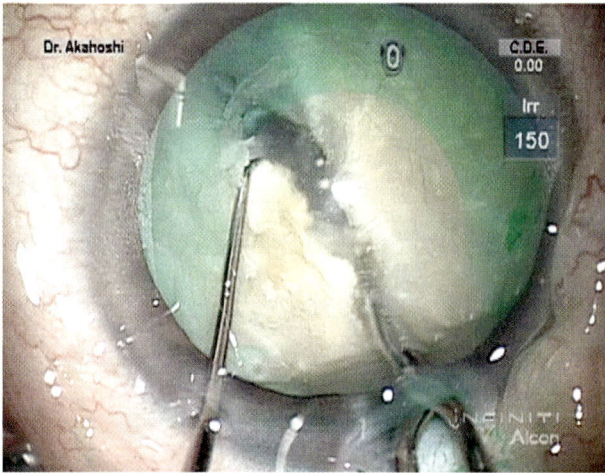

FIGURE 5.31 When the complete nuclear division has been attained, the inner surface of the posterior capsule can be observed between two prechopped nuclear fragments. Open the prechopper blades repeatedly after inserting into deeper position, and attain complete division. To prevent the posterior capsule rupture, the prechopper blades should be carefully manipulated close to the capsule.

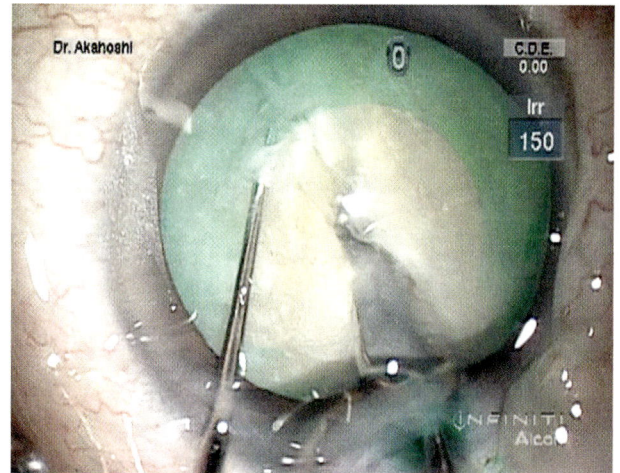

FIGURE 5.32 Merely making a crack into the nucleus is not sufficient, Complete nuclear division from the surface to the bottom, as well as from the periphery to the distal end of the equator, is mandatory.

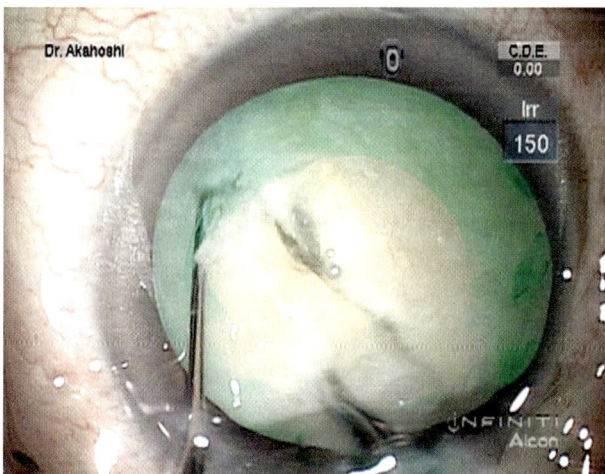

FIGURE 5.33 Using two instruments, rotate the nucleus. There may be some difficulties in rotation if the anterior chamber is collapsed. By filling up the chamber with sufficient OVD, rotation can be performed smoothly.

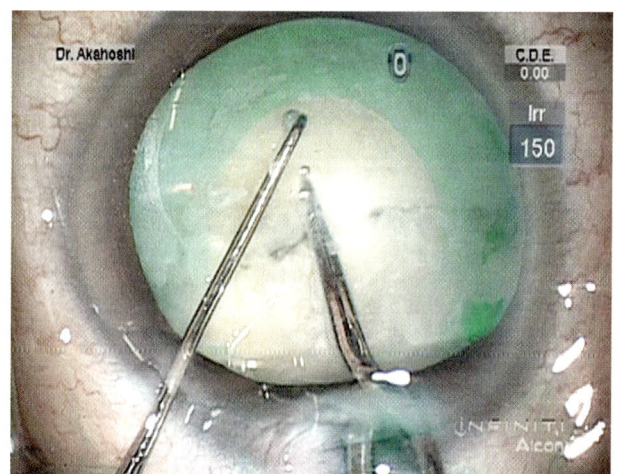

FIGURE 5.34 After rotating the nucleus by 90 degrees, insert the sustainer carefully under the capsulorhexis edge. The nuclear fragments may be stabilized by the closed prechopper blades.

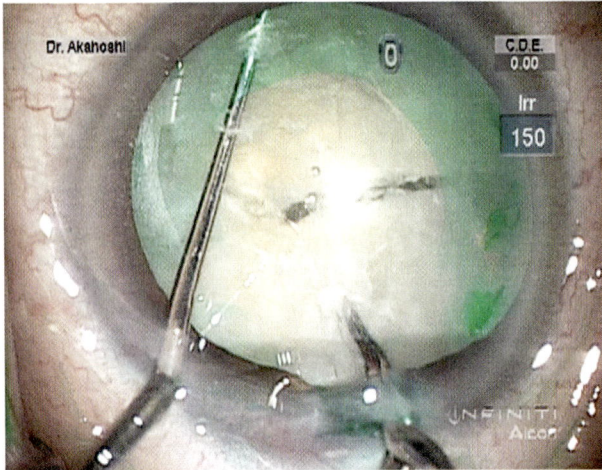

FIGURE 5.35 By supporting the nucleus at its equator, insert the prechopper blade from the periphery of the nucleus. The tip of the prechopper, the core of the nucleus, and the tip of the sustainer should be aligned on the same axis. If this alignment is not correct, the nucleus will rotate and the sustainer cannot provide proper counterforce against the prechopper blade.

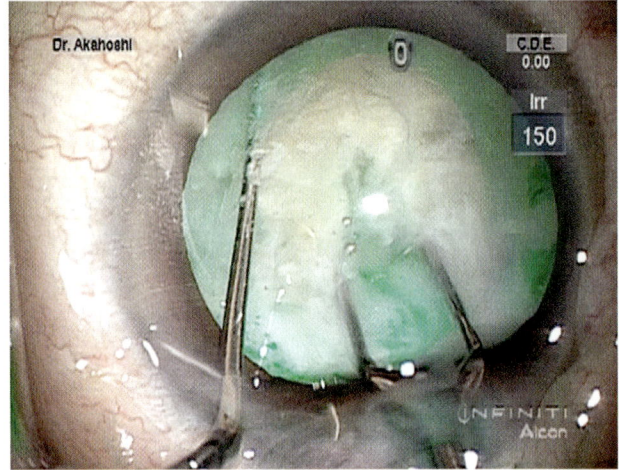

FIGURE 5.36 By opening the blades, the proximal nuclear fragment is prechopped into two pieces. In this situation, the distal half of the nucleus is used to support the proximal fragment, and thus the stress on the ciliary zonules is reduced.

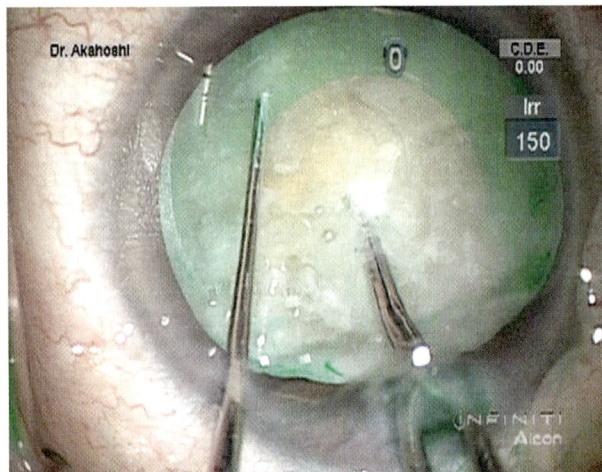

FIGURE 5.37 Then the distal half of the nucleus is prechopped. In this situation, the tip of the prechopper blade is placed at the center of the nucleus. By pushing the periphery of the distal nuclear fragment towards the prechopper , the blade is inserted into the nucleus. The tip of the sustainer, the hardest part of the nucleus, and the blade tip should be aligned on the same axis.

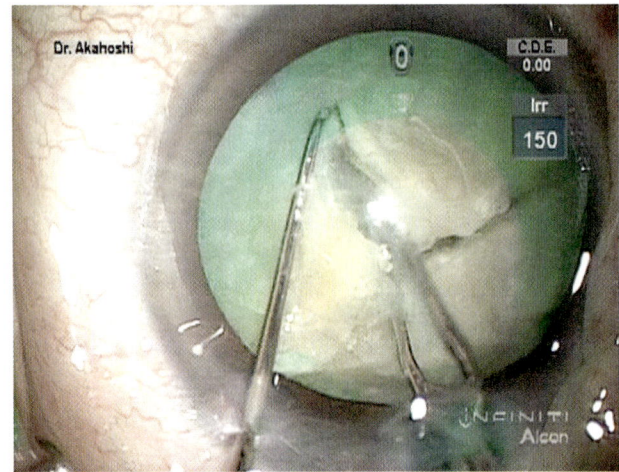

FIGURE 5.38 Attain the complete division of the distal half of the nucleus. Additional OVD may be injected to improve the nuclear visibility and maintain the anterior chamber if necessary.

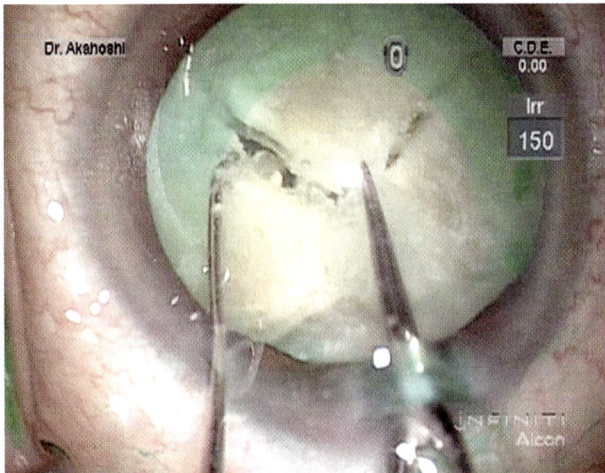

FIGURE 5.39 In advanced dense cataract, prechopping the nucleus into smaller pieces will facilitate the subsequent phacoemulsification. In cases that require shorter aspiration time, such as glaucoma, floppy iris syndrome, or decreased corneal endothelium, etc., additional prechopping into smaller fragments will be advantageous. Rotate the nucleus by 45 degrees.

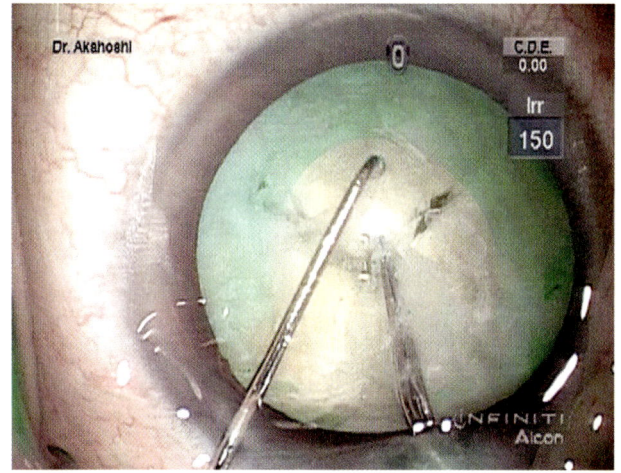

FIGURE 5.40 Each quadrant is further prechopped into two pieces. The Nucleus Sustainer should be always inserted under the capsulorhexis edge to support the nucleus at its equator.

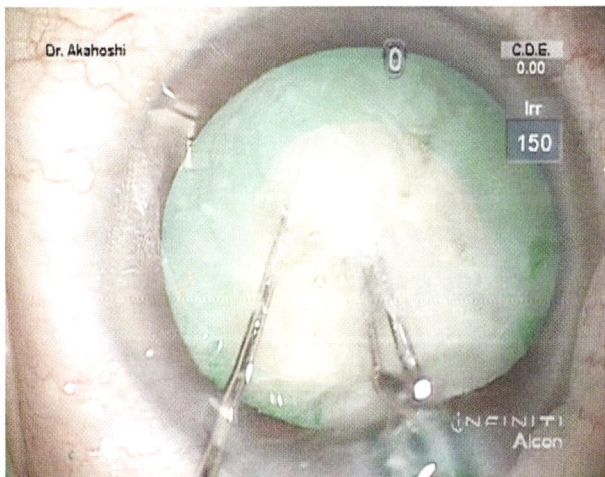

FIGURE 5.41 By holding the core of the nuclear fragment with the tips of the two instruments, even a dense nucleus can be safely divided into smaller pieces.

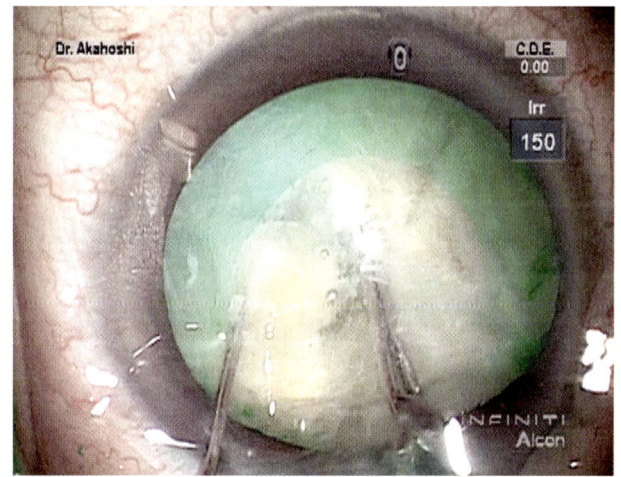

FIGURE 5.42 As all these prechopping procedures are performed under the OVD, the surgeon can take enough time, until the nucleus is completely divided.

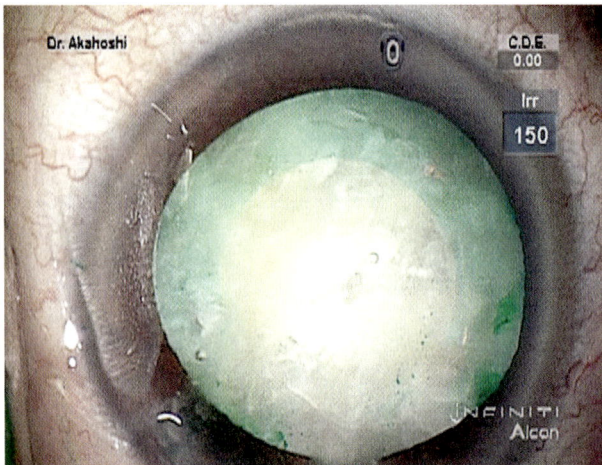

FIGURE 5.43 Without using any ultrasound energy, the nucleus is prechopped into eight pieces completely. By this simple procedure, total ultrasound energy required for the phacoemulsification will be markedly reduced.

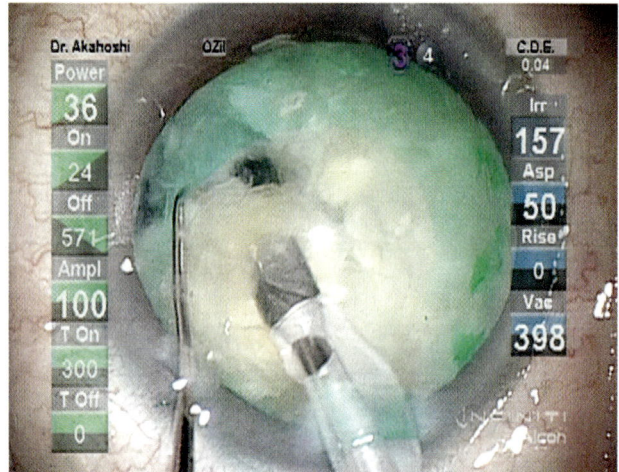

FIGURE 5.44 Each prechopped nuclear fragment is sucked out, aspirated, and phacoemulsified, one by one. Using an Akahoshi style phaco tip, which has a tip head bent toward its bevel (reverse to the Kelman tip), complete occlusion of the tip to the nucleus can be easily attained. Consequently, all the ultrasound energy is effectively used to emulsify the nucleus. High vacuum and high flow settings of the phaco machine will facilitate the safe and efficient phacoemulsification after the prechop.

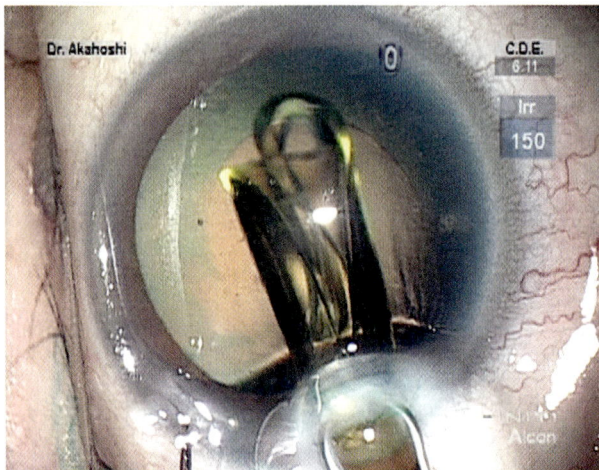

FIGURE 5.45 6.0 mm optic hydrophobic acrylic IOL can be implanted through the 1.8 mm incision with a D-cartridge using the counter traction implant technique.

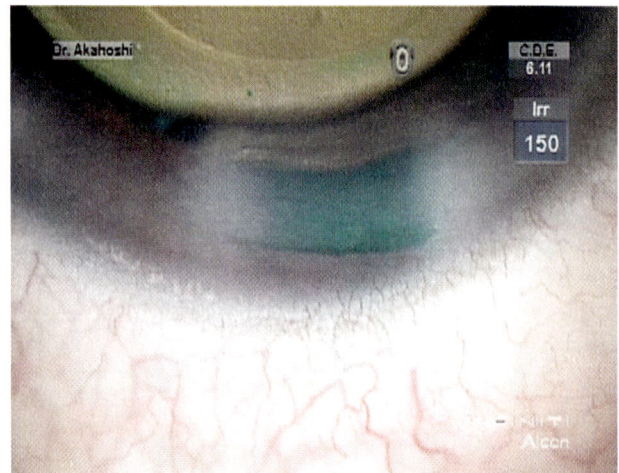

FIGURE 5.46 By prechopping the nucleus, thermal damage of the incision can be eliminated. Just by increasing the intraocular pressure, the incision can be easily self-sealed without stromal hydration.

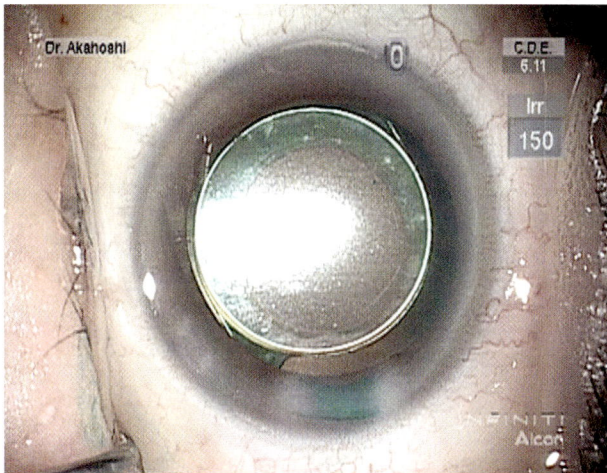

FIGURE 5.47 End of the surgery. The phaco prechop can realize the safest and most efficient micro incision cataract surgery.

Instruments for Phaco Prechop

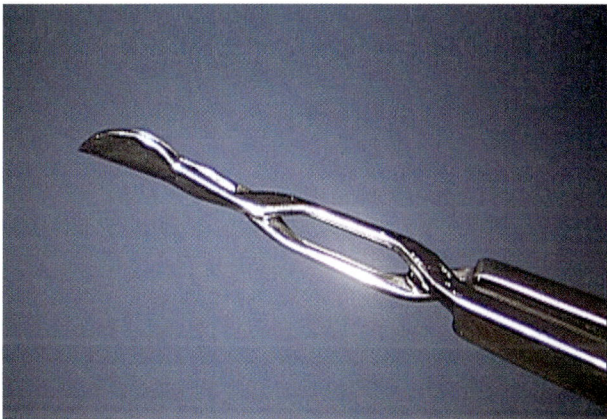

FIGURE 5.48 Combo Prechopper (ASICO AE-4190). The rounded side of the blade is blunt and suitable for ascertaining the complete division. The angular side of the blade is sharp and suitable for inserting into the nucleus.

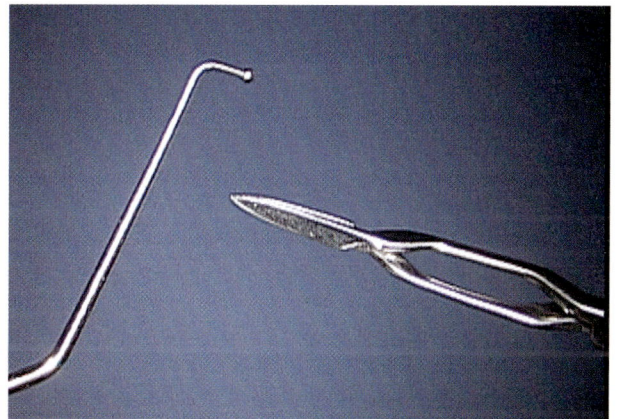

FIGURE 5.49 Universal Prechopper (ASICO AE-4192) has sharp blades that are suitable for dense nuclei. There is a micro ball attached at the tip of the Nucleus Sustainer (ASICO AE-2530). Any kind of nucleus can be prechopped using these three instruments.

TABLE 5.2 *Complications of Phaco Prechop*

Zonule rupture (only if the indication and/or procedure was wrong)

Posterior capsule rupture (only if the procedure was wrong)

SELECTED REFERENCES

Akahoshi T. Phaco Prechop: Manual nucleofracture prior to phacoemulsification. *Op Tech Cat Ref Surg.* 1998;1:69–91.

Akahoshi T. Phaco Prechop: mechanical nucleofracture prior to phacoemulsification. In: Yuan Jia-Qin, Arthur Lim Siew Ming, eds. *The Frontier of Ophthalmology in the 21st Century.* Tianjin Science and Technology Press, China 2001:288–322.

Akahoshi T. Farewell to Bimanual. Developing a sub-2 mm coaxial phaco and IOL insertion technique. *Cat Ref Surg Today*, June 2005 (Suppl):1–4.

Akahoshi T. The countertraction technique. Implanting a 6 mm AcrySof lens through a sub-2 mm incision. *Cat Ref Surg Today*, April 2006 (Suppl):1–3.

Lucio Buratto, Liliana Werner, Maurizio Zanini, David Apple. *Phacoemulsification principles and techniques.* 2nd ed. SLACK Incorporated; 2002:333–346.

6

Innovative Enhancement of Phaco Energy Production: Non-Longitudinal Phaco

William J. Fishkind, MD, FACS

SELECTED REFERENCES

Non-Longitudinal Phaco

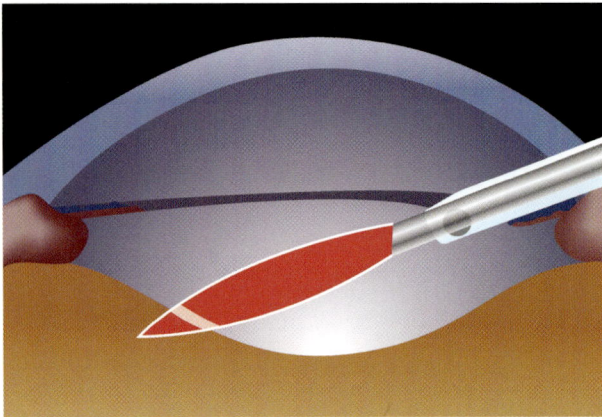

FIGURE 6.1 A major revision of phaco energy delivery is the development of non-longitudinal phaco. Since the innovation of phaco by Dr. Charles Kelman, phaco energy has been delivered in a longitudinal fashion. This means that the phaco needle moves forward and backward at the manufacturer defined frequency. Longitudinal movement of the needle creates a thrusting vector, which pushes material away from the phaco tip. Therefore the influence of fluid flow and vacuum are required to overpower this tendency, allowing nuclear material to be held at the phaco tip for emulsification. Longitudinal phaco creates cores of emulsified material.

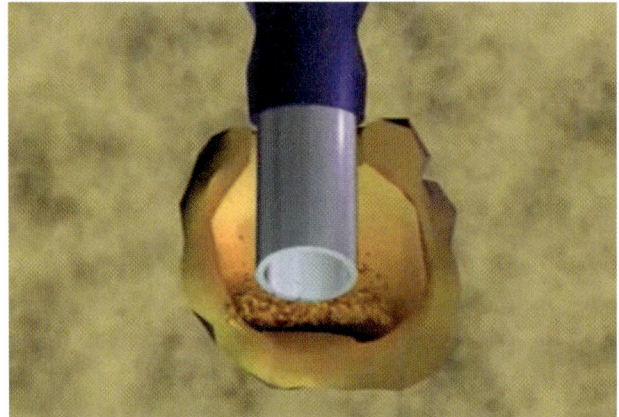

FIGURE 6.2 In the past few years, both Abbott Medical Optics and Alcon Laboratories have developed non-longitudinal phaco. In this design of phaco energy delivery, the movement of the needle is either pendular or elliptical. This mode of energy delivery does not drive nuclear material away from the phaco tip. On the contrary, it holds material in close proximity to the phaco tip, thus enhancing follow-ability. Non-longitudinal energy shaves nuclear material.

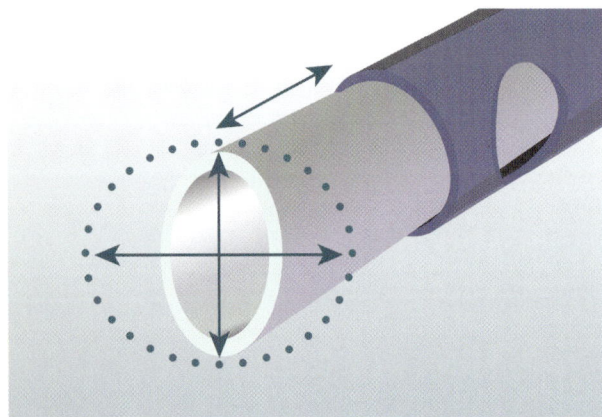

FIGURE 6.3 Abbott Medical Optics has developed elliptical energy, entitled *Signature Fx*. Any phaco tip can be utilized. The tip moves alternatively both elliptically and longitudinally at 38 KHz. (Image courtesy of Abbott Medical Optics, Inc.)

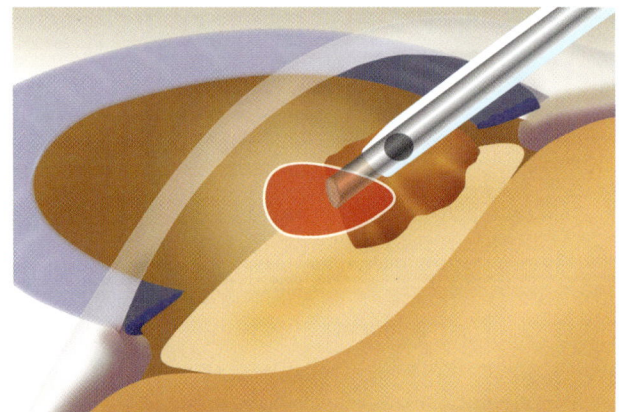

FIGURE 6.4 This creates an elliptical energy pulse.

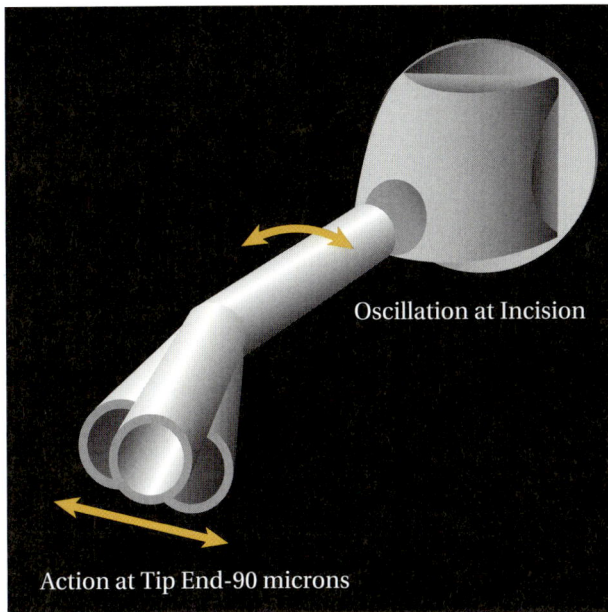

FIGURE 6.5 Alcon Laboratories has developed *"Torsional with the Ozil Handpiece."* This is a pendular needle movement, at 32 KHz, generated by an angled Kelman tip. In the IP addition of software, the pendular movement is augmented by longitudinal movement at 44 KHz. (Image courtesy of Alcon Surgical, Inc.)

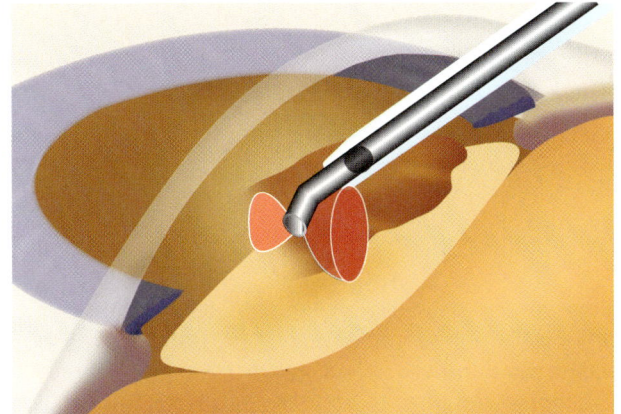

FIGURE 6.6 This creates a lateral bow tie pattern of ultrasonic energy distribution.

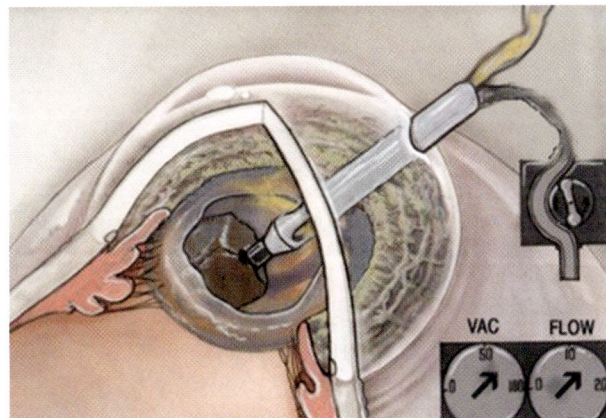

FIGURE 6.7 In both machines, some longitudinal movement is necessary to create cavitation within the lumen of the needle, to clear particulate material and prevent clogging. Both variations are extremely effective at increasing follow-ability of fragments and maintaining a deep and stable anterior chamber. When combined with micro-pulse phaco, the quantity of energy delivered to the anterior chamber is strikingly reduced when compared to typical phaco. Interestingly, these modes of phaco power delivery are not only a power modulation but also a noteworthy fluidic modulation. By retaining the fragment in close proximity to the phaco tip, but not allowing occlusion, this is a potent source of partial occlusion phaco. In partial occlusion phaco, the nuclear material is near, but not occluding, the phaco tip, thus avoiding occlusion, and subsequent post occlusion surge. It is this modification of fluid flow that is responsible for both increased follow-ability and a deep and stable anterior chamber.

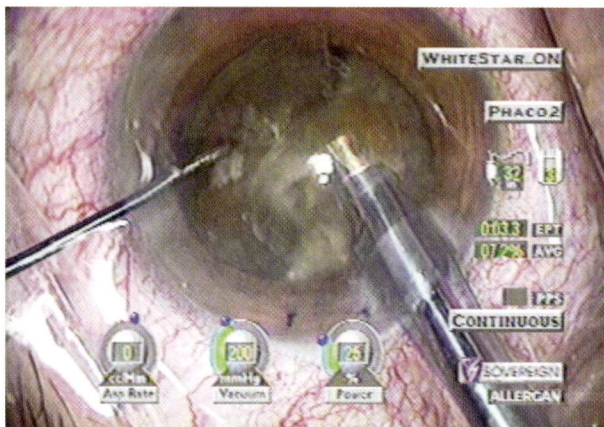

FIGURE 6.8 Therefore, in this surgical photo demonstrating longitudinal energy, occlusion phaco is occurring. The aspiration rate (Asp Rate) gauge is at 0, and the vacuum gauge at 200, the maximum. The nuclear fragment is covering the phaco tip, causing occlusion. Phaco has been energized, as seen in the power gauge, at 25%. When the fragment clears the phaco tip, potential energy stored during this instant of phaco will be transformed to kinetic energy. The inflow through the tip will become unequal in relation to the outflow through the handpiece, and a surge must occur.

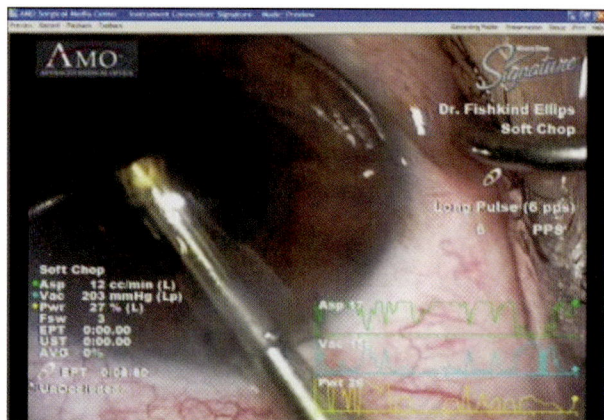

FIGURE 6.9 In this surgical photo, elliptical phaco is energized. The nuclear fragment is immediately adjacent to the phaco tip. Only in this example, on analysis, we see the Asp (Aspiration Rate–Green Dot) is 12 cc/min, and the Vacuum (Blue Dot) 203 mmHg. Occlusion has not come about, as there is both fluid flow and vacuum. Neither value is not at the maximum preset value. Therefore, when power is energized, as shown here at 27%, the lack of occlusion will not give rise to surge. The chamber remains stable and the effectiveness of phaco is significantly improved.

TABLE 6.1 *Complications*

Problem	Solution
Poor follow-ability	Increase flow by 2 cc/min increments
	Increase the off time of the cycle in micro-pulse phaco
Poor holding	Increase vacuum by 25 mm increments
	Increase the off time of the cycle in micro-pulse phaco
	Turn down power in elliptical or Torsional phaco (linear foot-pedal less foot-pedal excursion)
Events occur too quickly at some point in phaco	Decrease flow in 2 cc/min increments
	Decrease rise time (Venturi pump)
	Decrease pump speed (peristaltic pump)
Chamber shallowing during phaco	Increase bottle height in 2 in or 4 cm increments
	Check for wound leak
	Decrease flow by 2 cc/min increments
	Increase off time of the cycle of micro-pulse phaco
	Decrease rise time (Venturi Pump)
	Decrease pump speed (peristaltic pump)

(*continued*)

TABLE 6.1 *(continued)*

Problem	Solution
Disproportionate surge	Use micro-pulse, torsional, or elliptical phaco
	Raise bottle height in 2 in or 4 cm increments
	Depending on machine, use anti-surge technology
	Decrease rise time (Venturi pump)
	Decrease pump speed (peristaltic pump)
Clogging	Use IP on Alcon Infinity
	Use increased power and longer power on cycle in micro-pulse
	Irrigate handpiece
	Irrigate aspiration tubing
Difficulty attracting fragment to phaco tip	Increase flow by 2 cc/min increments
	Increase pump speed (peristaltic)
	Increase vacuum (Venturi)

SELECTED REFERENCES

Fishkind, William J. The phaco machine: physical fundamentals governing its interaction with the eye. In Garg A et al., eds. *Mastering the phacodynamics* (Chapter 3). New Delhi: Jaypee Brothers; 2007.

Fishkind WJ, Neuann TF, SteinertRF. The phaco machine: the physical principles guiding its operation. In Steinert R, ed. *Cataract surgery,* 3rd ed. (Chapter 7). China: Saunders Elsevier; 2010.

Seibel BS. *Phacodynamics: Mastering the tools and techniques of phacoemulsification surgery,* 4th ed. Thorofare, NJ: Slack Inc.; 2005.

7 Manual Small Incision Cataract Surgery

Rengaraj Venkatesh, MD, Geoffery Tabin, MD,
and Mike Feilmeier, MD

TABLE 7.1 *List of Instruments Necessary for Manual Small Incision Cataract Surgery*

Dish for gauze pads	Toothed forceps (0.12 or 0.3)	Cautery (low-temp or wet-field)
Gauze pads	Bevel-up crescent blade	25–27 gauge needle
5% povidone-iodine	Microkeratome blade	Vannas scissors
Eyelid speculum	Viscoelastics	3 mL syringe
4-0 Silk	Cystotome needle	Sinskey hook
Needle driver	27 gauge cannula	PCIOL
Superior rectus forceps	Simcoe I/A cannula	Sideport blade
Wescott scissors	Tying forceps	

Steps of Manual Small Incision Cataract Surgery

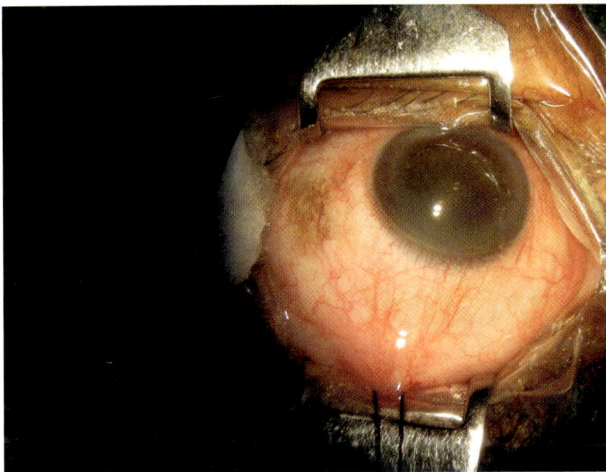

FIGURE 7.1 **Bridle Suture.** Manual Small Incision Cataract Surgery (MSICS) can be performed through either a superior scleral tunnel or a temporal scleral tunnel. When using a superior tunnel, a bridle suture may be placed beneath the tendon of the superior rectus muscle to facilitate surgical exposure. Many surgeons elect not to place a bridal suture. If the surgeon elects to utilize this step, they will find that a bridle suture is useful in the following ways: (1) To maneuver the globe and to fix it during the steps of surgery like tunneling. (2) To provide counter traction force during procedures such as nucleus removal and epinucleus delivery, thereby making these procedures easier and less traumatic.

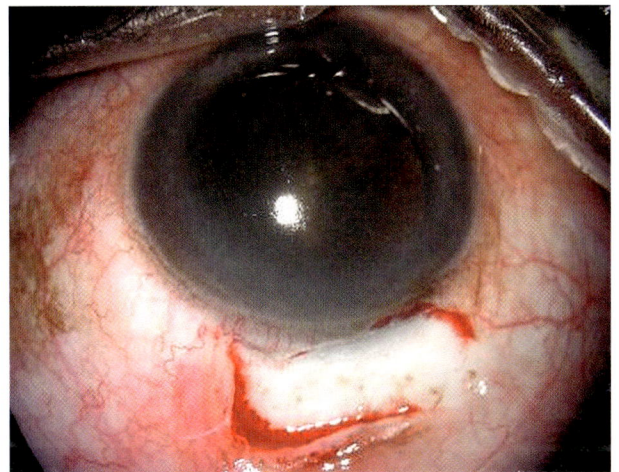

FIGURE 7.2 **Conjunctival Relaxing Incision**. A fornix based conjunctival flap of around 7 mm is made. After Tenon's capsule is dissected out, light cautery is applied to maintain hemostasis.

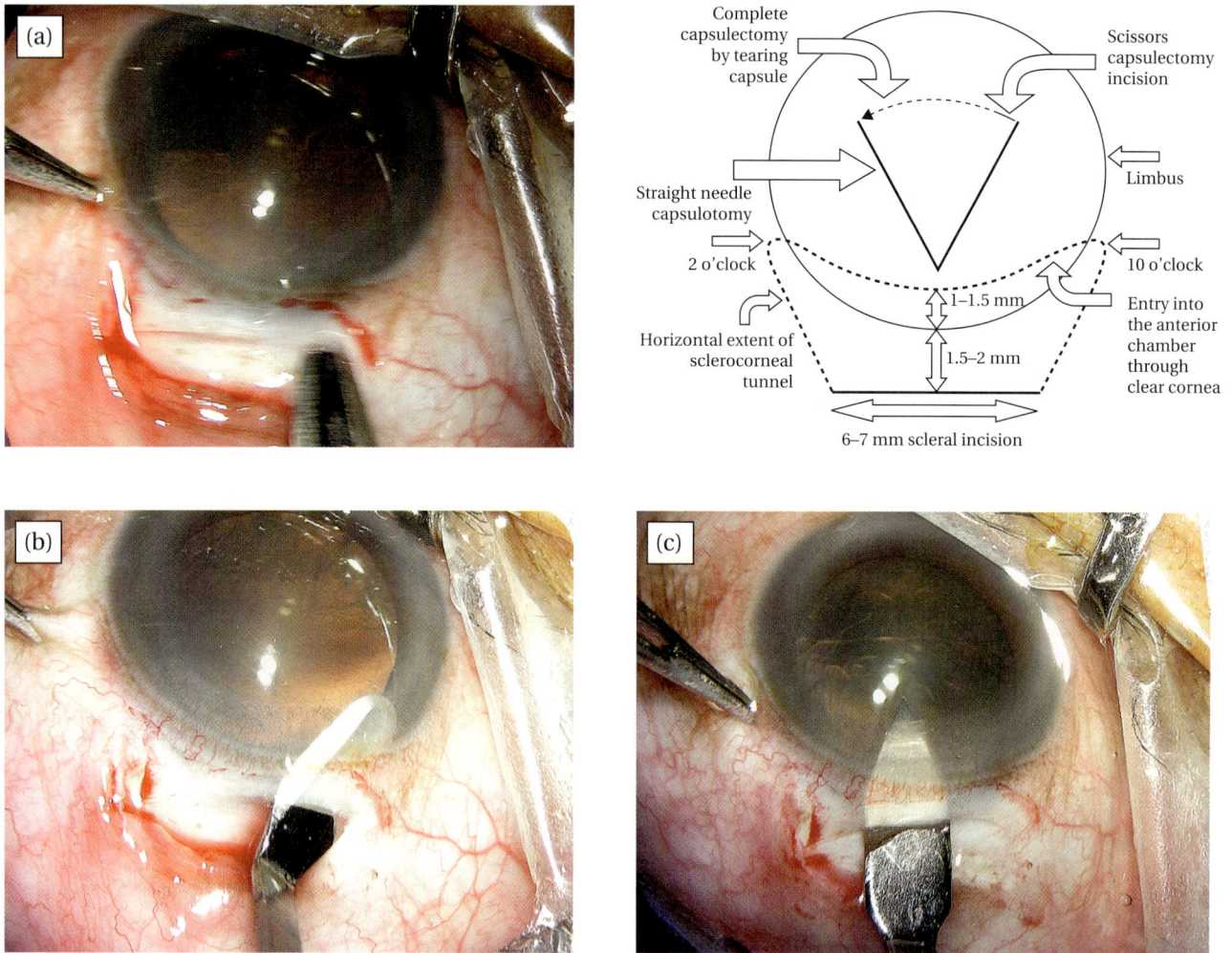

FIGURE 7.3 **Scleral Tunnel Construction.** (a) External Scleral Incision: A 30%–50% depth scleral incision is created using a sharp blade. This incision should be approximately 6–7 mm in length and approximately 2 mm posterior to the limbus. The incision should be tangential to the limbus or frown shaped to limit postoperative astigmatism and improve wound stability. (b) Sclerocorneal Tunneling: A sclerocorneal tunnel is created using an angled bevel-up crescent blade. The blade is gently advanced from the starting point of the scleral incision in a fashion parallel to the ocular surface. The tunnel is ideally located at a 30–50% scleral depth, and care is taken to create a single plane tunnel of uniform thickness. The tunnel should be advanced anteriorly approximately 1.5 mm into the clear cornea. The wound should be trapezoidal in appearance, with the internal portion of the tunnel extending from limbus to limbus. (c) Internal Corneal Entry: Viscoelastic is injected through a sideport incision into the anterior chamber for stabilization, and a sharp-angled keratome blade is used to enter the anterior chamber. The heel of the keratome is raised until the blade becomes parallel to the iris plane, resulting in a dimple on the corneal surface. The keratome is then advanced anteriorly in the iris plane until the anterior chamber is entered and the internal wound is visualized as a straight line. During extension of the incision, care should be taken to keep the internal incision in the same plane.

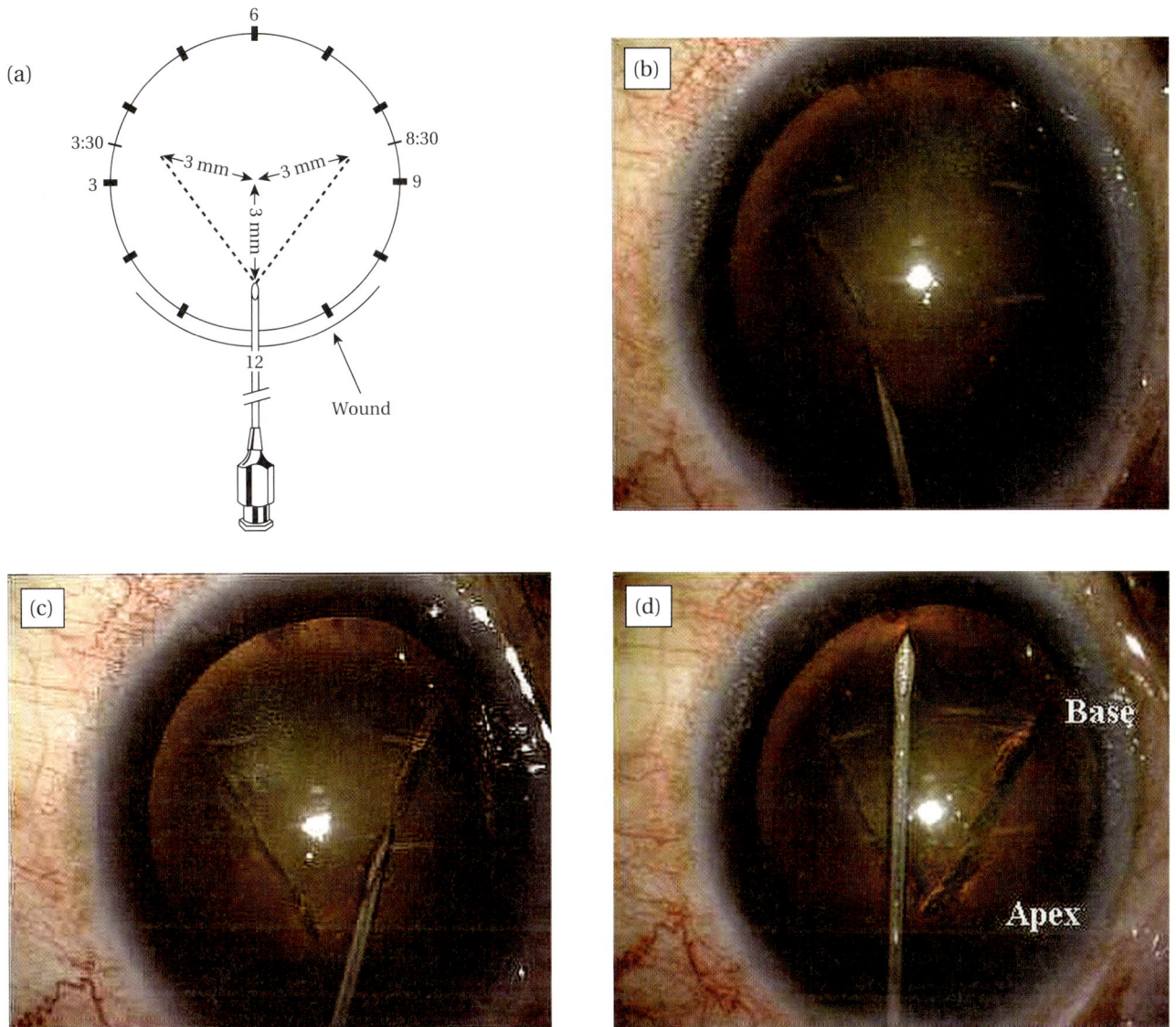

FIGURE 7.4 **Triangular Capsulotomy**. MSICS can also be safely performed using a can opener or triangular (or V-shaped) capsulotomy. In cases of mature and hypermature cataracts, a can opener or V-shaped capsulotomy is a good option, because it facilitates prolapse of the nucleus into the anterior chamber. The triangular capsulotomy and can-opener capsulotomy can be particularly useful in these suboptimal surgical settings, especially when capsular staining techniques are not available. If the surgeon uses a triangular capsulotomy, (a) this step should be performed prior to creation of the internal corneal incision and entry into the AC. A straight 25–27 gauge needle attached to a 1 mL syringe filled with balanced saline solution (BSS) is advanced in the scleral tunnel just anterior to the limbus, angled parallel to the iris plane, and advanced into the anterior chamber. Using the bevel tip of the needle, a linear cut is made from 4 o'clock to 12 o'clock (b) and then from 8 o'clock to 12 o'clock (c) so the two incisions meet at 12 o'clock (d). Thus, a triangular or V-shaped flap of anterior lens capsule is created with its base still attached. The apex of the V should be oriented toward the surgeon, and the base of the capsulotomy away from the surgeon. Each point of the triangle should be approximately 3 mm from the center of the pupil. Next, the apex is lifted with the tip of the needle and peeled away from the surgeon. This confirms the capsulotomy incisions are complete (d).

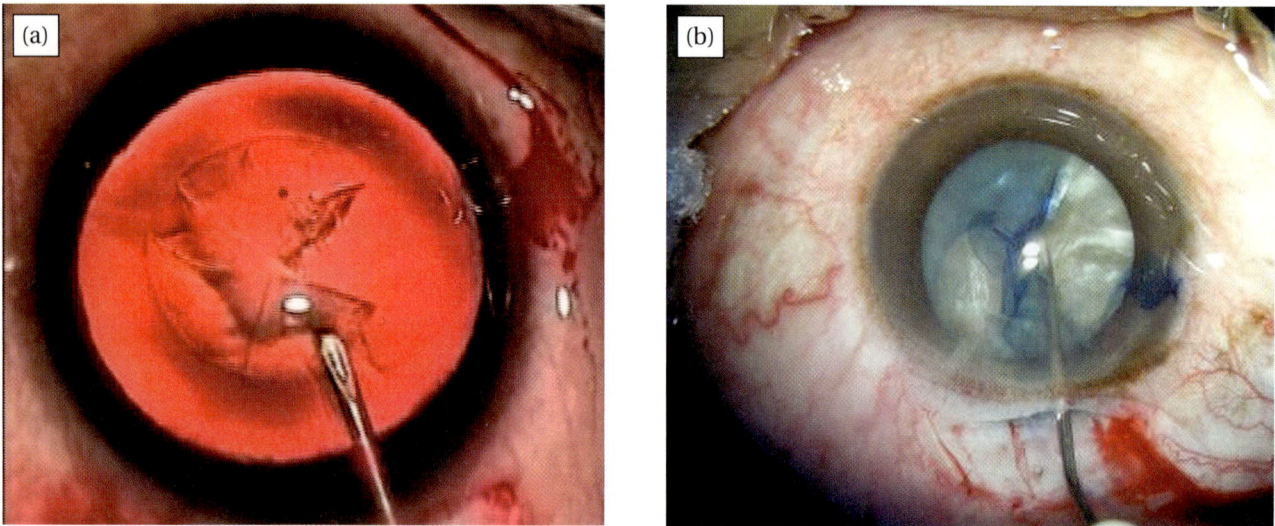

FIGURE 7.5 Continuous Curvilinear Capsulorhexis. Continuous curvilinear capsulorhexis (CCC) may provide optimal IOL positioning, but can be difficult in the setting of large mature, hypermature, or morgagnian cataracts and in the setting of poor surgical visibility due to corneal scars, pterygium, and suboptimal operating microscopes, all of which are common circumstances in the developing world. The size of the CCC is based upon the size and density of the cataract. It should have a minimum diameter of 5–6 mm and may need to be as large as 7–8 mm in diameter for more mature cataracts (a). If the CCC is too small for prolapse of the lens into the anterior chamber, the surgeon should make 8 or more radial relaxing incisions or convert to can-opener capsulotomy. Capsular staining will be helpful in cases with white cataracts and dense brown cataracts (b).

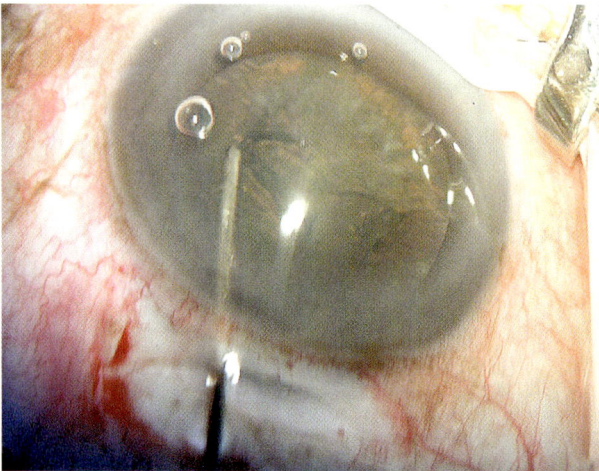

FIGURE 7.6 Hydroprocedures. Hydrodissection is performed using a 27 gauge bent tip cannula attached to a syringe filled with BSS. In the presence of a capsulorhexis, this procedure is completed in one smooth step by injecting the fluid beneath the anterior capsular rim. In the presence of a can opener or V-shaped capsulotomy, small amounts of fluid can be injected in multiple areas so as to "unshackle" the nucleus from the confines of the cortical hug. At the end of a successful hydrodissection, the nucleus should be freely mobile within the capsular bag.

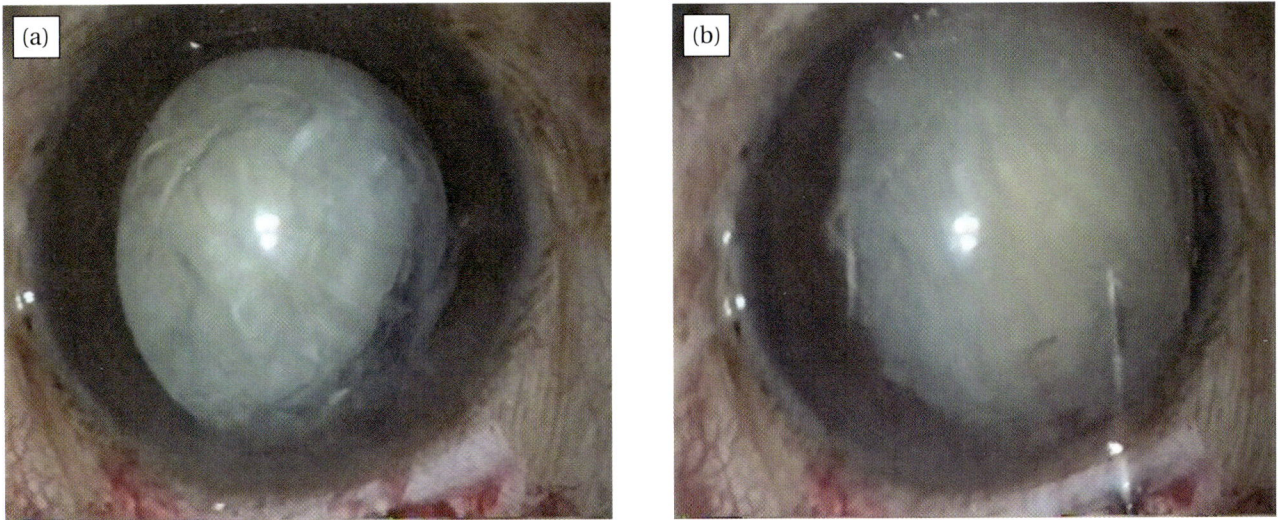

FIGURE 7.7 **Nuclear Prolapse into the Anterior Chamber**. Commonly, when the hydrodissection is performed, one pole of the nucleus will prolapse into the anterior chamber along with the fluid wave. At the sight of this prolapse, hydrodissection can be stopped and under the cover of an adequate amount of viscoelastics, the remainder of the nucleus can be delivered by rotating the prolapsed pole with a Sinskey hook.

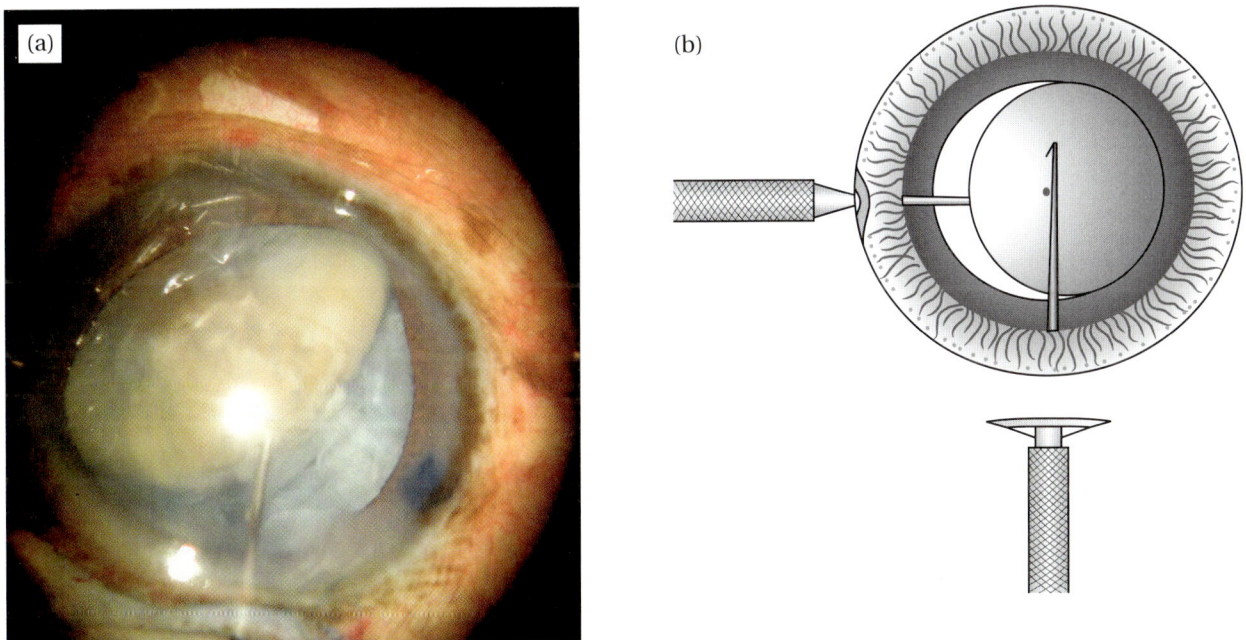

FIGURE 7.8 **Nuclear Prolapse into the Anterior Chamber in Special Situations**. (a) White and Brown Cataract: In these cases, the safest technique is to perform a can-opener or V-shaped capsulotomy and prolapse the nucleus. If the surgeon is keen to perform a capsulorhexis, it is necessary to stain the anterior capsule and perform a larger capsulorhexis (6.0–7.5 mm) followed by a less forceful hydrodissection. As the capsule is stained, it will be easy to retract the capsule and lever out a part of the nucleus with a Sinskey hook. The nucleus is then gently wheeled out, watching the movement of the capsular bag throughout the procedure. (b) Subluxated Cataracts: In cases with zonular compromise, a bimanual prolapse technique is employed: in this technique, a cyclodialysis spatula and Sinskey hook is used for the prolapse. The nucleus is retracted to one side (temporal in right eye or nasal in left eye) with a Sinskey hook from the scleral tunnel. Following this, a spatula is introduced through the sideport incision and placed under the nucleus. Using this as a fulcrum, the nucleus is rotated with the Sinskey hook out of the capsular bag. By this technique, the cyclodialysis spatula absorbs the rotational forces, minimizing stress on the zonules.

(a)

Irrigating vectis

Internal hydrostatic pressure

Depression of posterior lip

Scleral stretching by the nucleus

Mechanical direction by the vectis

(b)

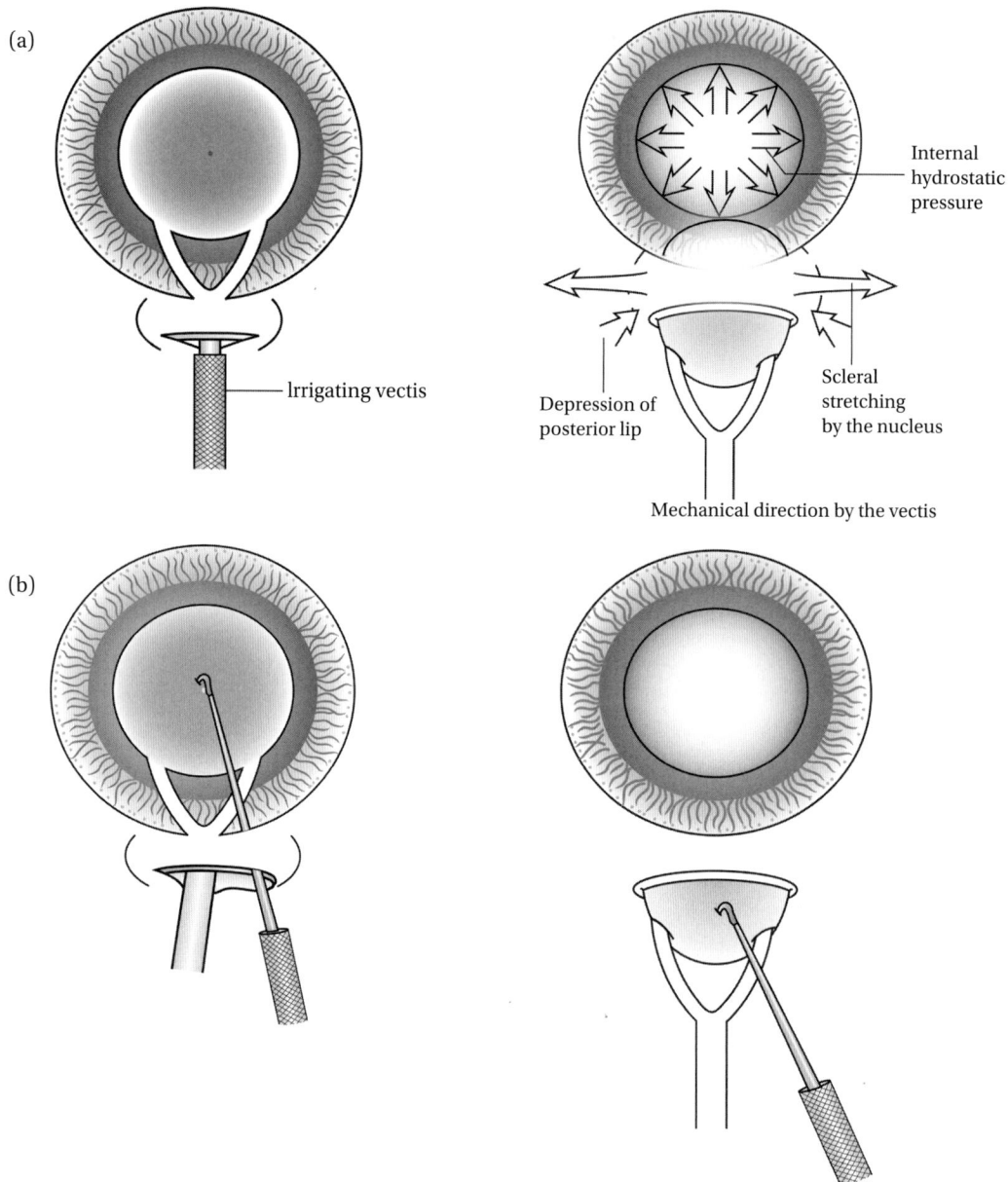

FIGURE 7.9 Nuclear Delivery using Different Techniques. Several techniques can be employed with success in delivery of the nucleus. These techniques include (a) Irrigating Vectis Technique: After the nucleus is prolapsed into the anterior chamber, viscoelastics are liberally injected, first above and then below the nucleus. The upper layer shields the endothelium, while the lower layer pushes the posterior capsule and iris diaphragm posteriorly. This maneuver creates adequate space in the anterior chamber for atraumatic nuclear delivery. As the superior rectus bridle suture is pulled tight, the irrigating vectis is slowly withdrawn without irrigating, until the superior pole of the nucleus is engaged in the tunnel. Gentle irrigation is then started and the vectis is slowly withdrawn, while pressing down gently on the posterior lip of the scleral incision. (b) Sandwich Technique: In this technique, a Sinskey hook is used in addition to the vectis. The key requisite is that the anterior chamber is adequately filled with viscoelastics. Once the vectis is placed beneath the nucleus, the Sinskey hook is carefully introduced and placed on top of the nucleus, sandwiching it between the vectis and the Sinskey hook. The tip of the Sinskey hook is placed beyond the central portion of the lens to get a better grip using a two-handed technique. With the Sinskey hook in the dominant hand and vectis in the other, the nucleus is sandwiched and extracted. This technique is particularly helpful with delivery of a large nucleus.

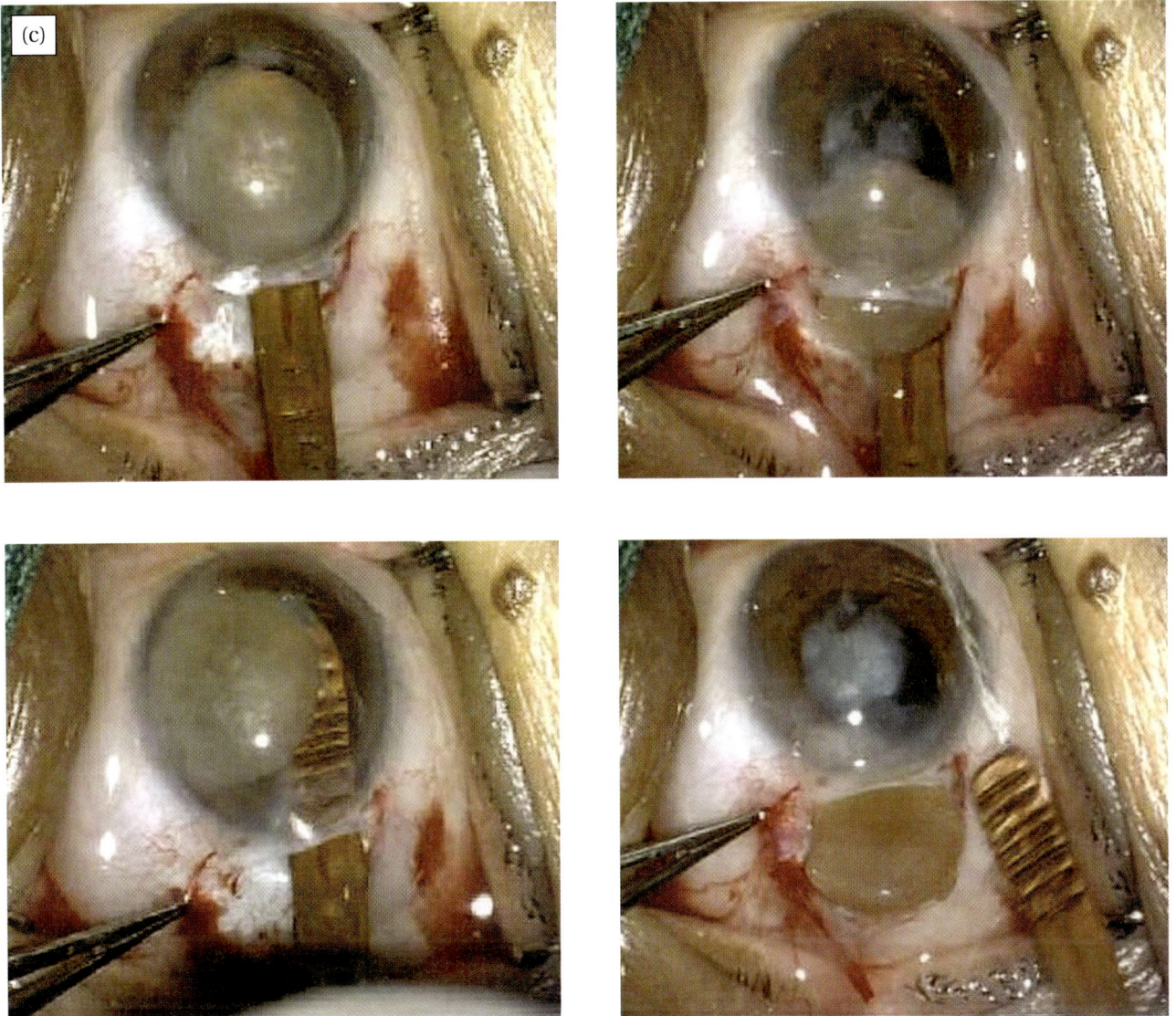

FIGURE 7.9 (*continued*) (c) *Simcoe Technique*: After delivery of the lens into the AC and injection of viscoelastics anterior and posterior to the lens, the sclera or tenons is grasped with a 0.12 forceps and the globe is rotated away from the surgeon. The Simcoe is introduced and centered posterior to the lens and anterior to the iris, and the irrigation is turned on. The tip of the cannula should be visualized distal to the nucleus. The hydrostatic forces will bring the nucleus to the internal incision. Once the nucleus engages in the tunnel, slight downward pressure is applied to the external lip of the wound using the cannula, while slowly withdrawing the cannula. Upon nuclear delivery, the Simcoe is used for cortical cleanup.

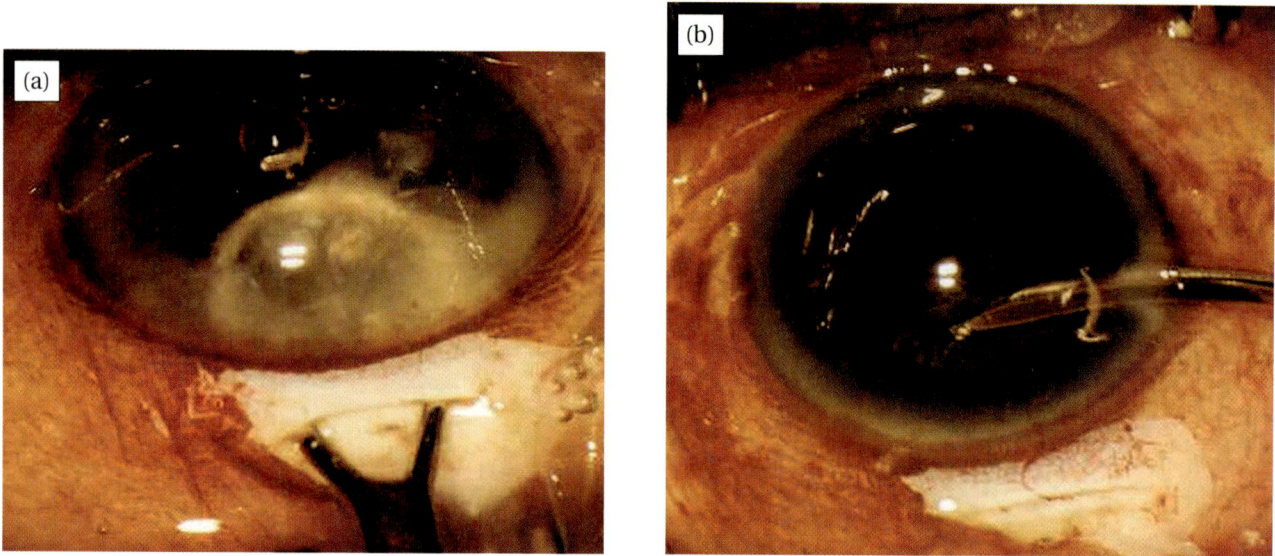

FIGURE 7.10 Epinucleus and Cortex Removal. The epinucleus can be flipped out of the bag by placing the Simcoe cannula under the anterior capsular rim and lifting out the epinucleus into the anterior chamber. The prolapsed epinucleus can then be extracted using again an irrigating vectis, or by depressing the inferior scleral lip with the Simcoe cannula and pulling the superior rectus bridle suture at the same time. The remaining cortex, including the subincisional cortex, can be safely removed through either the sideport incision or main wound, using the Simcoe cannula.

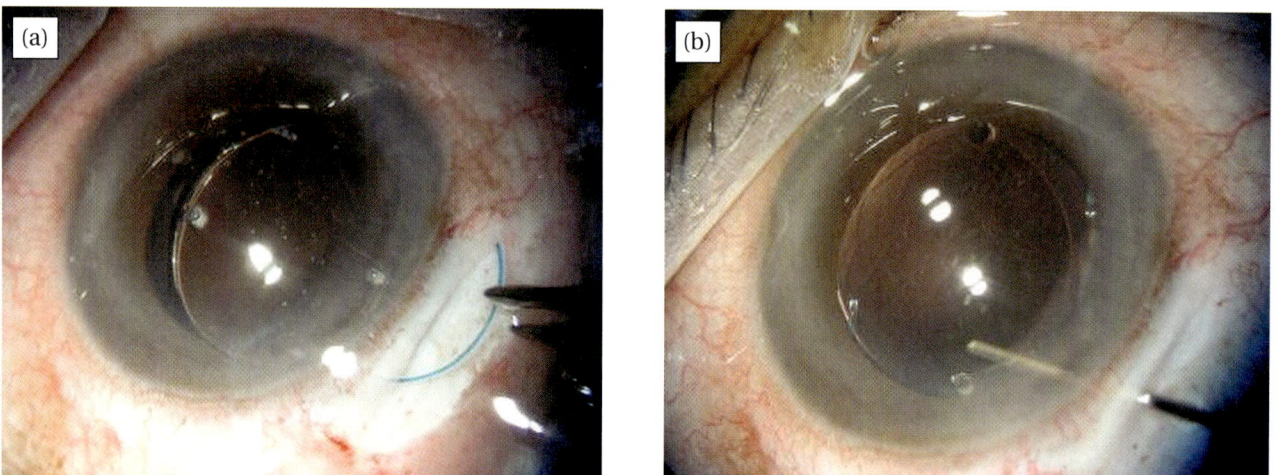

FIGURE 7.11 Intraocular Lens Insertion. As the size of the wound becomes greater than 6 mm, it is preferable to place a 6 mm optic rigid PMMA IOL, especially with a can-opener capsulotomy. If a CCC has been performed, a foldable lens can be implanted in the bag.

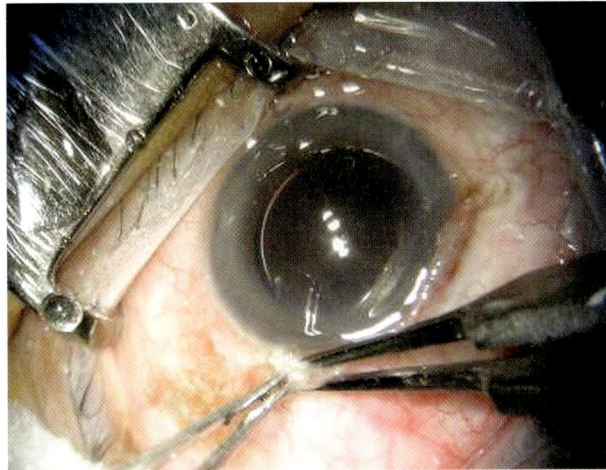

FIGURE 7.12 **Conjunctival Closure**. BSS is injected through the sideport incision to form the anterior chamber. If the wound is constructed properly, a watertight closure is observed, and no sutures are necessary. Otherwise, interrupted 10-0 nylon sutures may be placed to secure the wound. After watertight closure is ensured, the conjunctiva should be replaced to cover the external scleral incision. This can be performed on superior and temporal incisions using cautery. In cases of superior incisions, injection of subconjunctival antibiotics can be utilized to balloon the conjunctiva over the superior scleral incision. Alternatively, a suture can be placed to secure the conjunctiva.

TABLE 7.2 *Potential Complications of Nucleus Extraction with an Irrigating Vectis and their Causes*

Potential Complications	Cause
Corneal endothelial damage	• Misjudged nuclear size leading to disproportion between nucleus and wound size • Inadequate use of viscoelastics • Improper technique in handling the vectis • Surgeon's ego leading to repeated attempts at extraction
Trapped nucleus	• Improper bridle suture • Misjudged nuclear size • Improperly designed vectis; i.e., not having a concavity • Poor technique
Iris trauma/Iris stretching or dialysis	• Premature entry causing iris to be washed out through the weak site • Premature injection of fluid • Vectis insinuated under the 6 o'clock iris • Vectis not pressed down on the posterior scleral lip
Posterior capsular rent with vitreous loss	• Sharp edges of the vectis • Forceful extrusion of the nucleus • Enlargement of a preexisting zonular dialysis caused while prolapsing the nucleus

SELECTED REFERENCES

Ruit S, Tabin GC, Nissman SA, Paudyal G, Gurung R. Low-cost high-volume extracapsular cataract extraction with posterior chamber intraocular lens implantation in Nepal. *Ophthalmology.* 1999;106:1887–1892.

Venkatesh R, Das MR, Prashanth S, Muralikrishnan R. Manual small incision cataract surgery in eyes with white cataracts. *Ind J Ophthalmol.* 2005;53:173–176.

Venkatesh R, Tan CSH, Singh GP, Veena K, Krishnan KT, Ravindran RD. Safety and efficacy of manual small incision cataract surgery for brunescent and black cataracts. *Eye* 2009;23(5):1155–1157.

8 Managing Dense Cataract Emulsification

Abhay R. Vasavada MS, FRCS, Vaishali Vasavada, MS,

Shetal M. Raj, MS, and Viraj A. Vasavada, MS

Surgical Technique: Microcoaxial Phacoemulsification

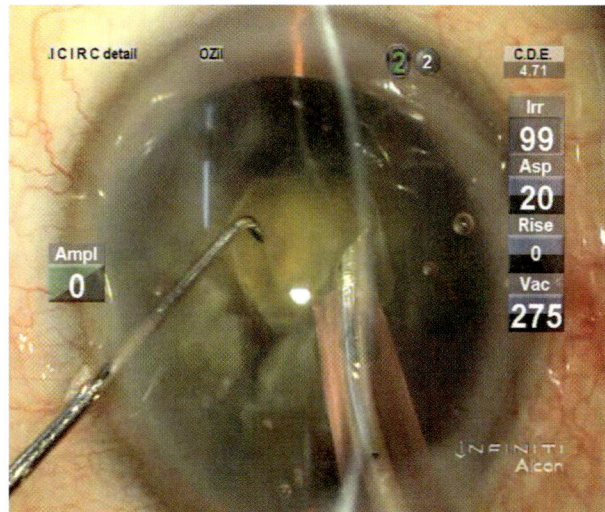

FIGURE 8.1 As cataract surgical techniques and technology have evolved, surgeons are now switching to smaller and smaller incisions for phacoemulsification. Small incisions have several benefits, including faster patient rehabilitation, improved prognosis for visual acuity, and reduced surgically induced astigmatism. Currently, there are two popular small incision phacoemulsification techniques: bimanual phacoemulsification and microcoaxial phacoemulsification. Microcoaxial phacoemulsification is a modification of the existing conventional coaxial phacoemulsification technique. Here, a sleeved tip is passed through a valvular incision that ranges from 2.0 to 2.4 mm in width, to allow coaxial irrigation and aspiration. A silicone sleeve on the phaco tip acts to cool the tip, and it also seals and protects the incision from thermal injury when performing phacoemulsification. In this chapter, we describe microcoaxial phacoemulsification for emulsification of dense cataracts.

Clear Corneal Incision

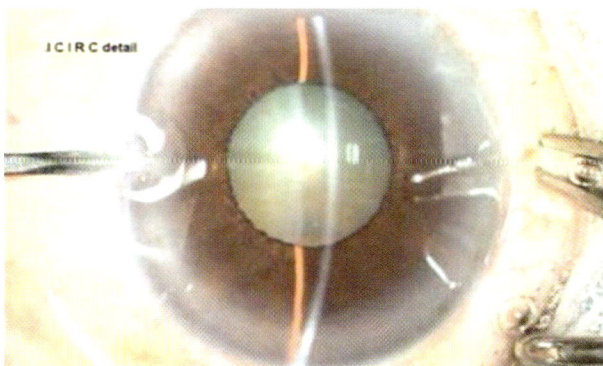

FIGURE 8.2 A 1.0mm clear corneal paracentesis incision is created using a dual bevel knife. Before making the main incision, a sideport incision is created through which ophthalmic viscosurgical device (OVD) is injected to form the anterior chamber.

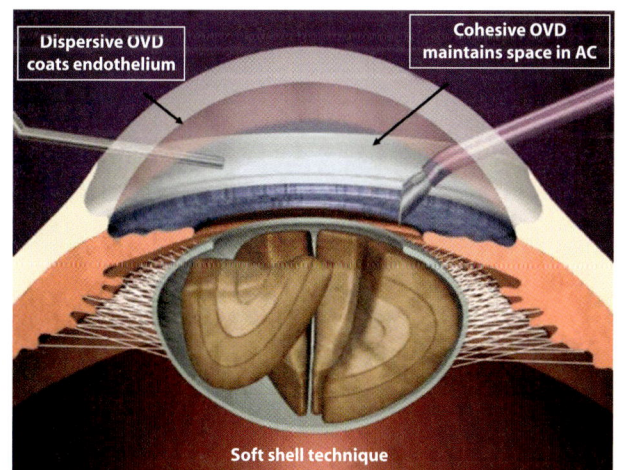

FIGURE 8.3 Following initial paracentesis, a dispersive OVD is injected, and then a cohesive OVD is injected below it, as per the soft shell technique. The dispersive OVD coats the endothelium, and the cohesive OVD maintains space in the anterior chamber.

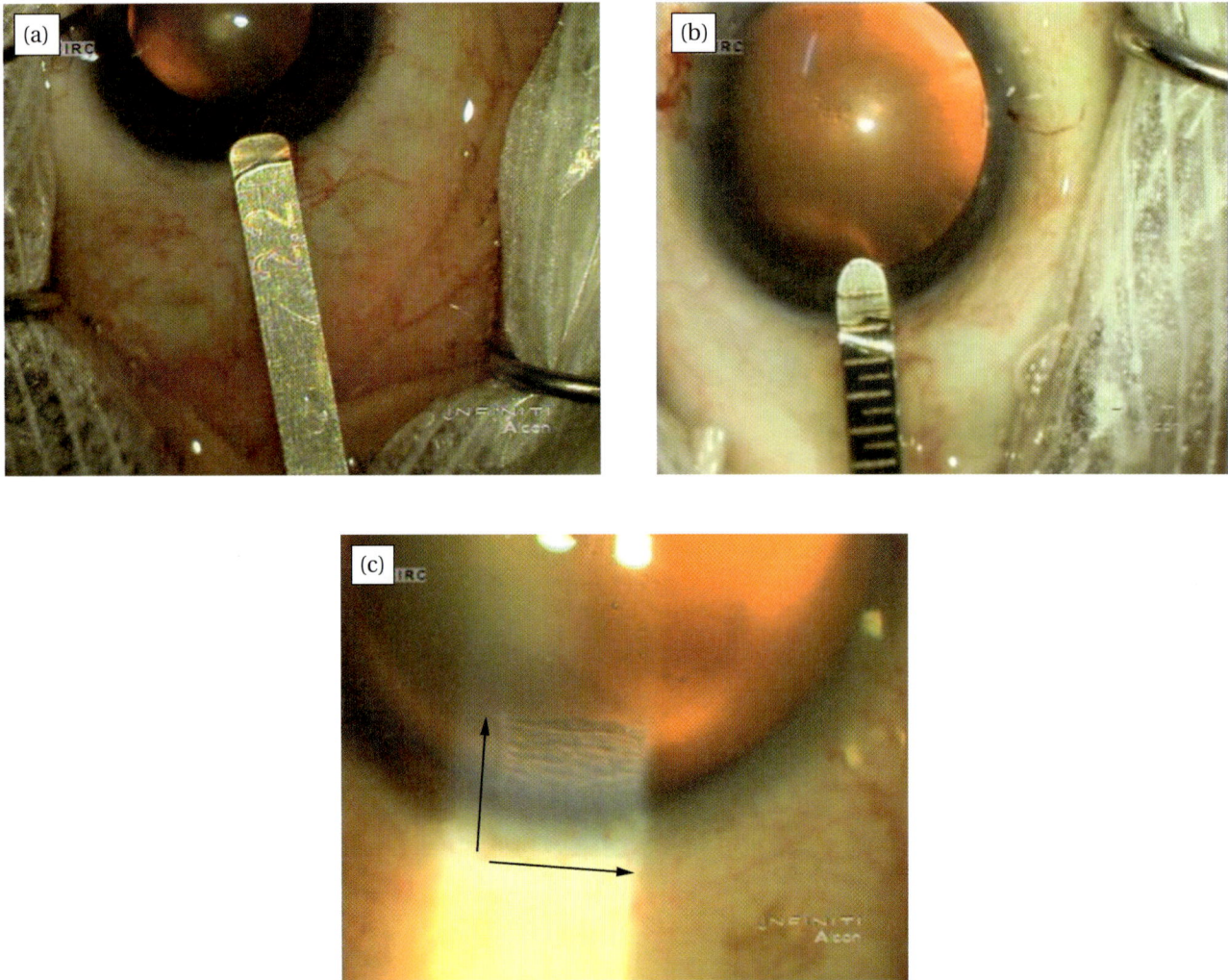

FIGURE 8.4 The single-plane, clear corneal phaco incision should have a square, or near-square architecture. (a) A clear corneal incision of 2.0 to 2.2 mm is created using a sharp trapezoidal keratome placed parallel to the dome of the cornea, making the internal entry in a single motion. (b) The internal length of the incision is crucial in determining the square configuration. For an incision of 2.2 mm width, an internal entry of at least 1.5 mm is mandatory to ensure good self-sealing of the wound. It has been suggested that poorly constructed and distorted wounds may increase the risk of postoperative endophthalmitis. Therefore, paying attention to wound geometry is crucial even with these small incisions. (c) Having an incision width of 2.2 mm with an internal entry length of 1.5 mm or more ensures a square or near square configuration of the incision.

Capsulorhexis

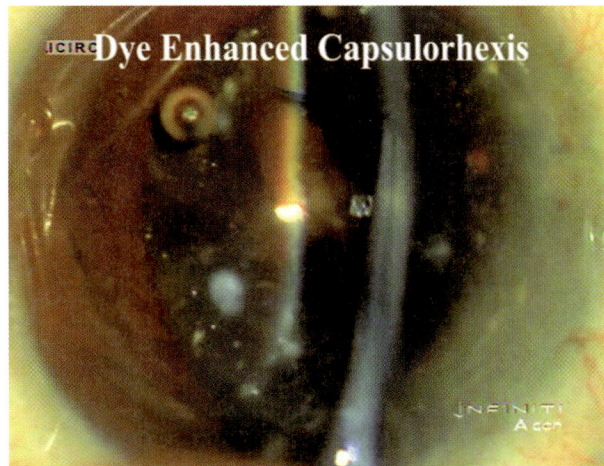

FIGURE 8.5 Often, in dense, brunescent cataracts, there is absence of fundal glow that may make capsulorhexis difficult. In these cases, staining of the anterior capsule with trypan blue aids in visualization of capsule. Balanced salt solution is injected beneath the OVD, and thereafter, small quantities of 0.0125% trypan blue are injected in the plane created by the fluid. This restricts the dye into that specific plane, and allows localized "painting" of the capsule.

Cortical-Cleaving Hydrodissection

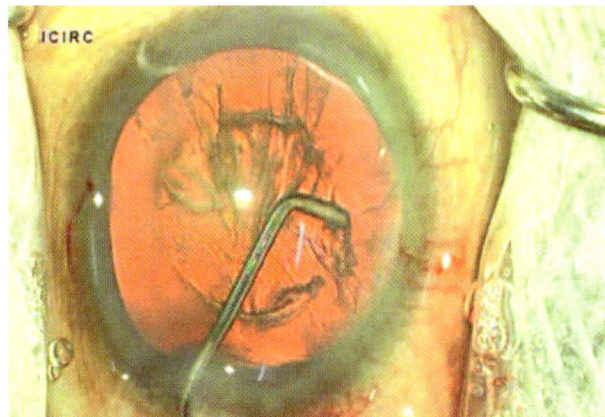

FIGURE 8.6 In these dense cataracts, there is the possibility of a sudden blow-out of the posterior capsule during cortical cleaving hydrodissection, because a bulky nucleus does not allow egress of the injected fluid, especially in eyes where the capsulorhexis is small. In these eyes, immediate decompression of the nucleus upon its forward bulge can prevent an intraoperative capsular block. Also, careful and gentle cortical-cleaving hydrodissection should be performed in these eyes. Dense cataracts often resist rotation after single quadrant cortical cleaving hydrodissection because of corticocapsular adhesions. Multi-quadrant hydrodissection helps to cleave the corticocapsular adhesions, making rotation easier.

Nucleus Emulsification: Phases of Phacoemulsification

TABLE 8.1 *Phacoemulsification Parameters during Each Stage of the Surgery*

Surgical Parameters			
	Parameters		
Stage of Surgery	Torsional Amplitude – Burst mode %	Aspiration Flow Rate cc/minute	Vacuum mm Hg
Sculpting	80 (100) preset amplitude with linear control, 300 milliseconds on time	25	120
↓		↓	↓
Approach posterior	↓	20	60
Chopping	60 amplitude 70 preset amplitude with linear control, 300 milliseconds on time	20	650+ (maximum machine vacuum)
1ˢᵗ Fragment Removal	80–100 preset amplitude with linear control, 300 milliseconds on time	25	450
		↓	↓
↓		20	300
	↓	↓	↓
Last Fragment Removal	60	18	150
	↓		
	50		

* According to the principles of the step-down technique, the vacuum, AFR, and ultrasound energy are progressively reduced as more and more nuclear fragments are removed and posterior capsule is exposed. This allows emulsification safely in the capsular bag without danger of aspiration of the posterior capsule or uveal tissue.

Stage 1: Creation of a Central Space (Sculpting)

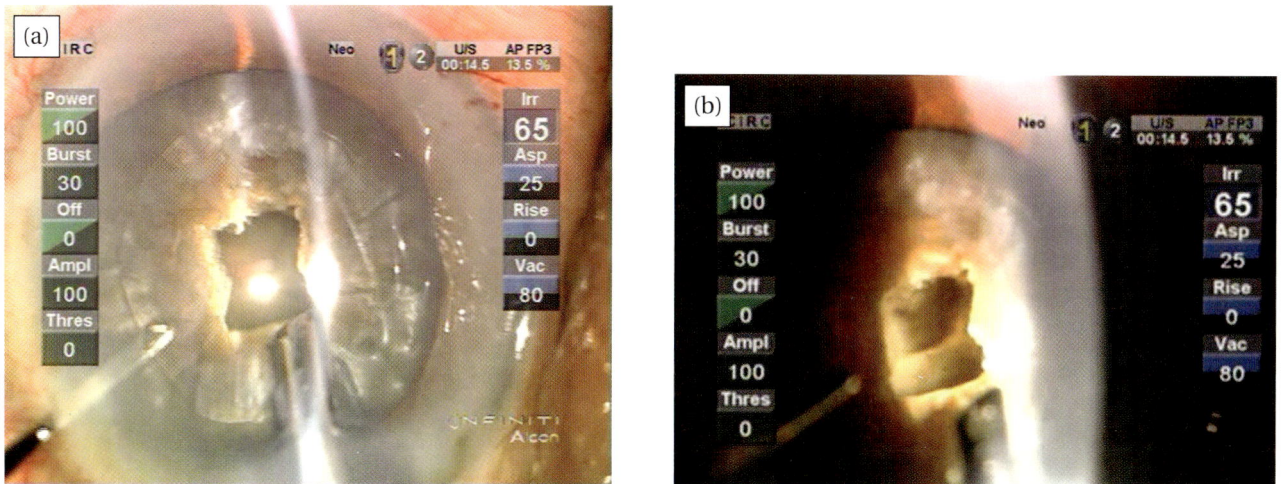

FIGURE 8.7 (a, b) It is important to create a central, deep area of sculpting within the confines of the rhexis margin. This central space will provide space to emulsify the nuclear fragments within the capsular bag, away from the corneal endothelium. Also, creating a thin trench will help in complete division of the nuclear fragments, so that they do not remain attached in the center.

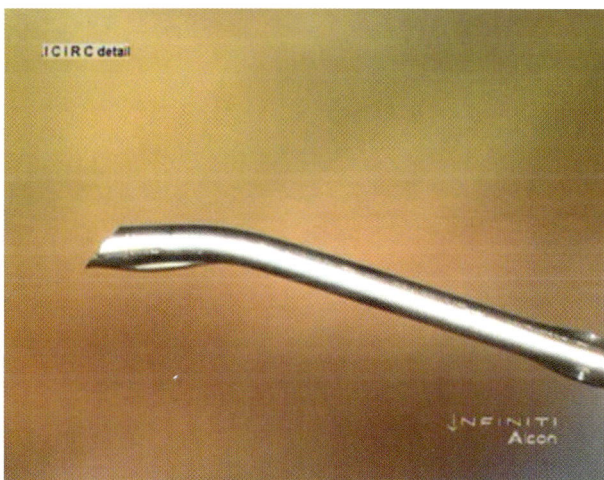

FIGURE 8.8 A bent Kelman tip allows sculpting in the depth of the trench without any incisional stress or undue zonular stress. If a straight tip is used, often there is compression of the sleeve when sculpting the subincisional area, which can cause wound site thermal injury (WSTI).

Stage 2: Creation of Multiple Nuclear Fragments (Chopping)

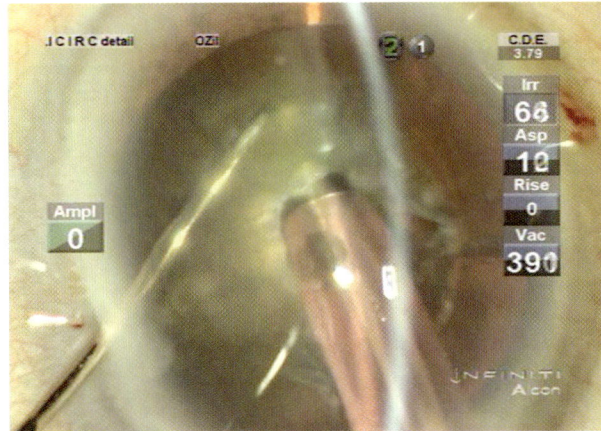

FIGURE 8.9 Whatever the chopping technique, multiple small, nuclear fragments must be created. This allows easy emulsification at a desired posterior plane. To initiate the chopping, the foot pedal is depressed to the third position and the phaco probe is advanced toward the wall of the trench. If the wall of the trench is arbitrarily divided into 3 equal parts, the tip is buried at the junction of the anterior 1/3 and posterior 2/3 of the trench. The foot pedal immediately switches from the third position to the second position and remains there till an occlusion (indicated by the machine as a ringing bell) is achieved. This produces a vacuum seal, resulting in an effective hold on the nucleus with the phaco probe.

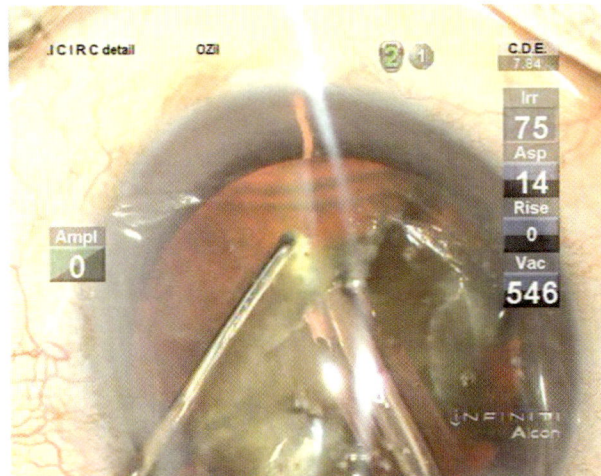

FIGURE 8.10 As a next step, the vertical element of the chopper is depressed. This initiates a partial thickness crack. No attempt is made at this time to extend the crack completely until the bottom of the nucleus. This avoids undue stress to the capsulo-zonular complex.

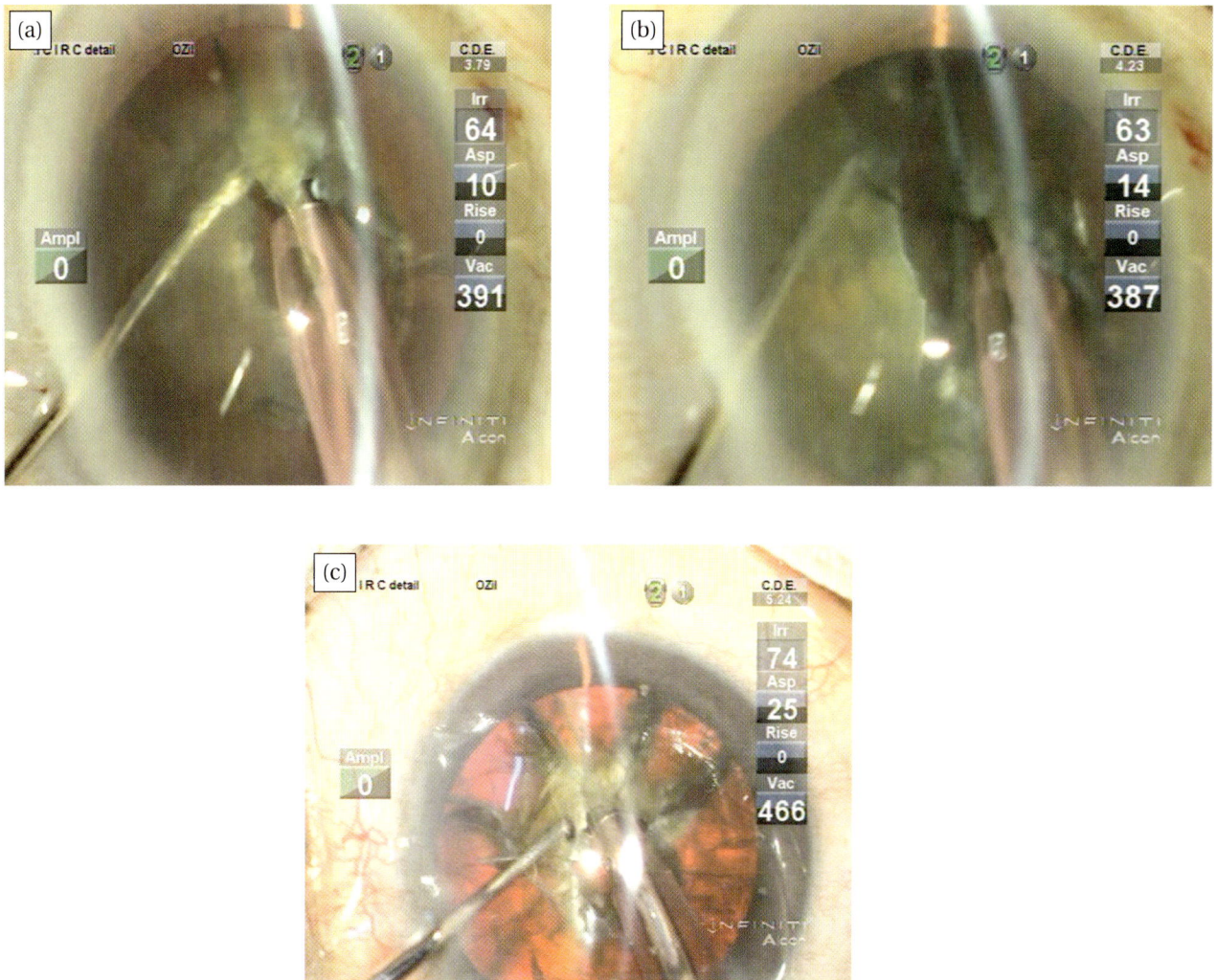

FIGURE 8.11   (a) Once a partial thickness crack has been initiated, the chopper is repositioned in the depth of the crack and gentle lateral separating movements are performed to achieve lateral separation of the fragments. (b) Thereafter, the chopper is moved from center to periphery and from superficial to deep. Similar movements are performed by repeatedly placing the chopper in the depths of the crack to achieve complete separation of nuclear fragments. (c) The aim should be to create multiple nuclear fragments which can be easily emulsified away from the corneal endothelium.

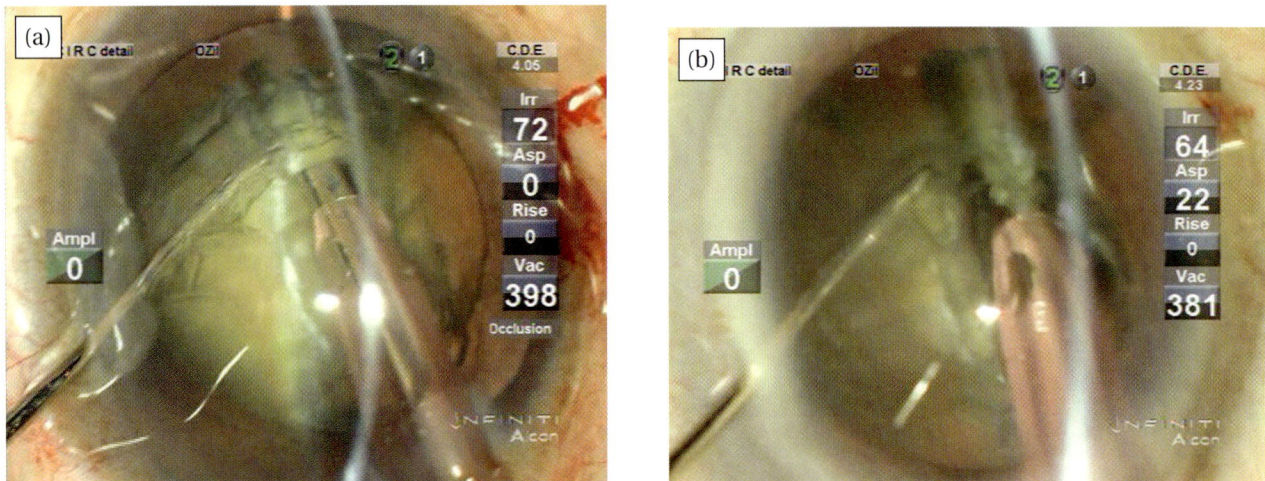

FIGURE 8.12 (a, b) In spite of all efforts, often the very dense cataracts will resist complete division of nuclear fragments. We use the technique called *multilevel chop* in these brunescent, leathery cataracts. After deep sculpting, an initial vacuum seal is achieved and a chop is initiated adjacent to the phaco tip, achieving a partial crack, as described above. This is followed by minimal lateral separating movements within the crack. Subsequently, the phaco tip is occluded at multiple levels, from anterior to posterior. Fibers adjacent to the tip are chopped, followed by minimal lateral separating movements in every plane. Alternating between in-situ vacuum seal and lateral separation maneuvers allows division to be extended posteriorly, facilitating complete division of posterior plate . Multiple fragments can be created by repeating this technique every 1–2 clock hours. This technique minimizes the separation-induced stress to the capsular bag and zonules. It allows complete antero-posterior division of all nuclear fragments. It also eliminates the possibility of partially divided nuclear fragments remaining attached to a central posterior plate.

Stage 3: Nuclear Fragment Removal

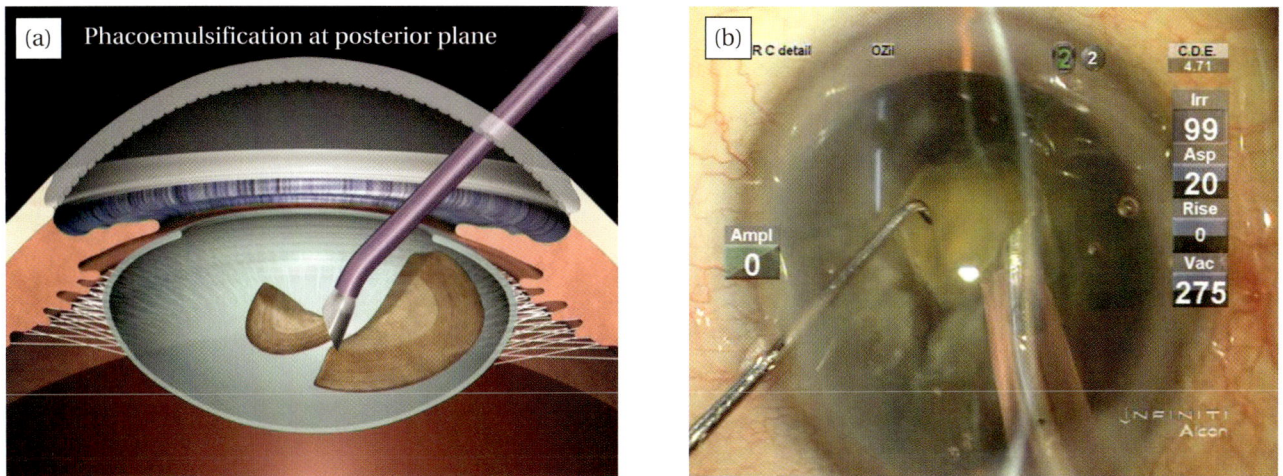

FIGURE 8.13 (a, b) It is vital to emulsify fragments in the posterior plane, to avoid the undesirable consequences of anterior plane emulsification that may be caused by energy dissipation close to the endothelium, and mechanical damage to the endothelium by the hard fragments. The surgeon must always be conscious of the plane at which he/she is performing emulsification. On the other hand, emulsification in the posterior plane increases the risk of inadvertent posterior capsule rupture if very high fluidic parameters are used. Therefore, in order to achieve posterior plane emulsification safely, without risking posterior capsule rupture, we use the step-down technique. In this technique, we reduce all the parameters in a step by step manner, after removal of every two fragments. (Table 8.1) This technique is a judicious combination of using appropriate parameters for an appropriate stage of surgery, and slow motion phacoemulsification. This provides for additional safety during fragment removal. The preset low energy allows judicious consumption of ultrasound energy and prevents WSTI. Further, the use of low energy and vacuum prevent sudden post-occlusion chamber instability, and the low AFR reduces the turbulence in the anterior chamber. We find that the use of torsional ultrasound makes low parameters dramatically effective. Normally, there is a conflict between aspiration forces on the one hand, which attract the nuclear material, and ultrasound energy on the other, which tends to repel the fragments. However, with the torsional ultrasound, there is a perfect harmony between these two opposing forces, and, therefore, even modest aspiration flow rates and bottle heights become very effective. We now no longer have to use high flow rates and bottle heights, even with these dense cataracts.

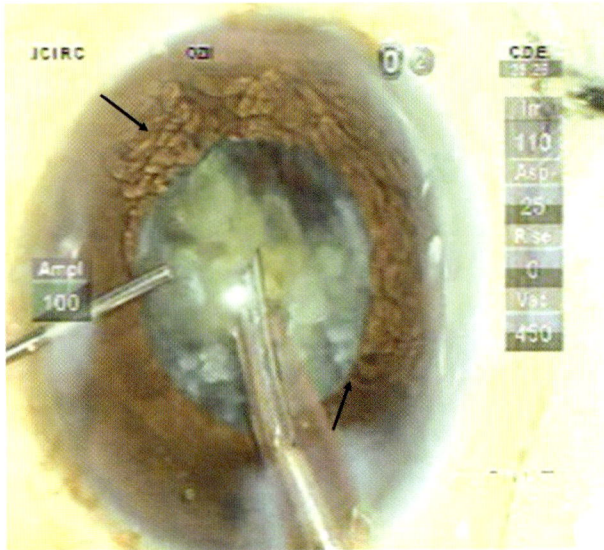

FIGURE 8.14   It is very important to repeat injection of dispersive OVD (Viscoat ®) during fragment removal to protect the corneal endothelium. After every 2–3 fragments, repeat injection of dispersive OVD should be performed in order to coat and protect the corneal endothelium.

Intraocular Lens (IOL) Implantation

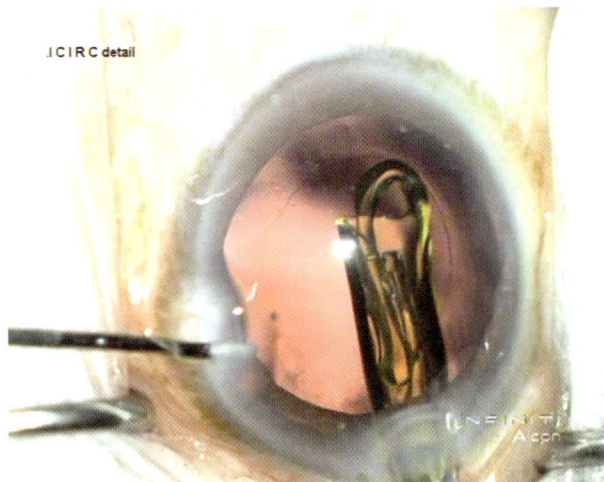

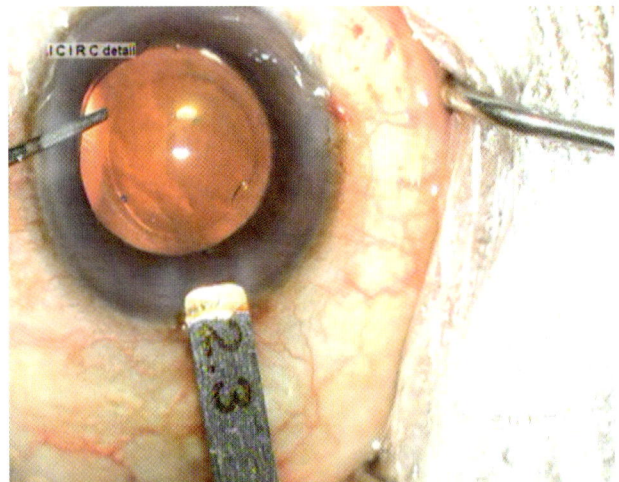

FIGURE 8.15   IOL implantation can be performed using a plunger type injection system and the appropriate cartridge, with the wound-assisted injection technique. Even though the cartridge does not pass through the internal entry of the 2.2 mm incision, it suffices to place the cartridge at the outer edge of the incision and use the plunger to implant the lens into the eye. The key point is to provide counterforce to the cartridge. Keeping a rigid ocular tension during implantation is another important point.

FIGURE 8.16   Typically, there is an enlargement by about 1 mm following implantation of the IOL. However, newer cartridges that allow IOL implantation through these incisions are now available, which cause minimal wound distortion.

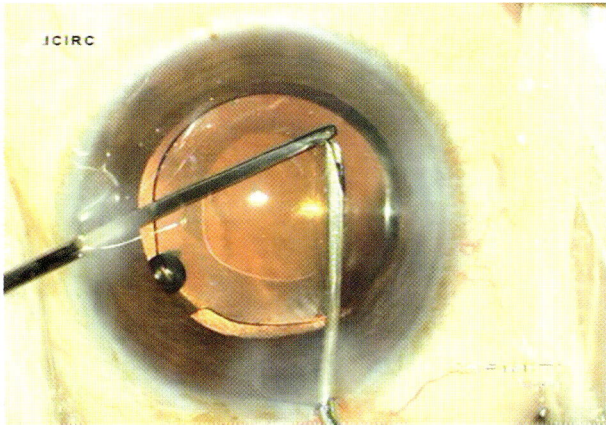

FIGURE 8.17 After cortex aspiration and IOL implantation, an initial small rhexis may be enlarged to a definitive large size. A high-viscosity cohesive OVD is injected over the anterior capsule, to push it posteriorly. An iris spatula is introduced through the sideport and placed under the anterior capsule to support it. The cystotome needle is introduced through the main incision to cause a break in the continuous margins of the capsulorhexis.

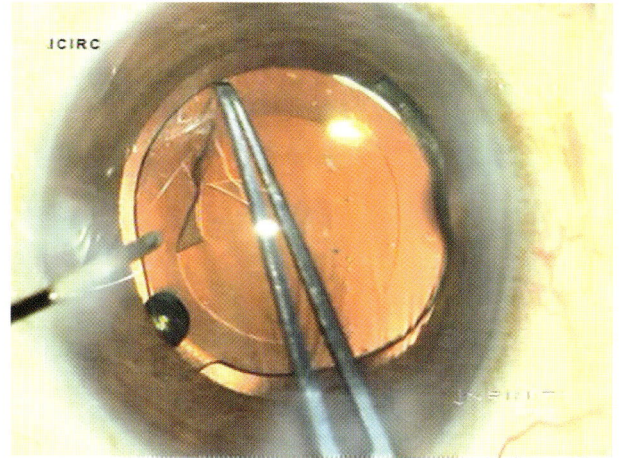

FIGURE 8.18 Following the initial nick, the rhexis is enlarged using Uttrata's capsulorhexis forceps.

Ophthalmic Viscosurgical Device (OVD) Removal

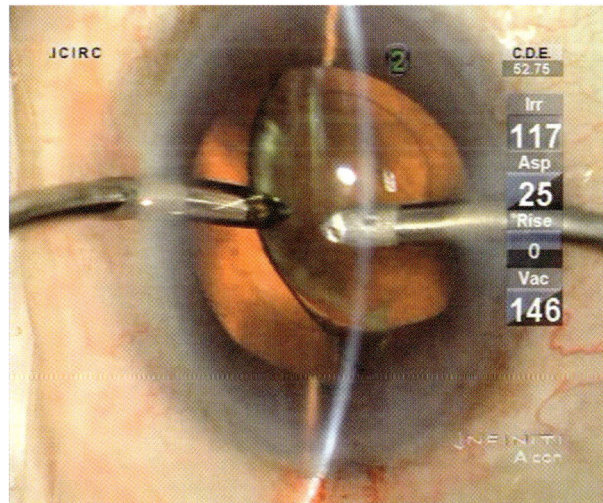

FIGURE 8.19 The residual OVD is aspirated by performing bimanual irrigation/aspiration. It is very important to perform a thorough removal of the OVD, even going behind the IOL to ensure that there is no residual OVD or nuclear fragment trapped behind the iris or in the anterior chamber angles. Finally, all incisions are hydrated with a balanced salt solution before completing the surgery. It is of utmost importance to closely inspect the incision at the end of surgery to look out for incision distortion/wound site thermal injury. In case of doubt, the incision should be sutured.

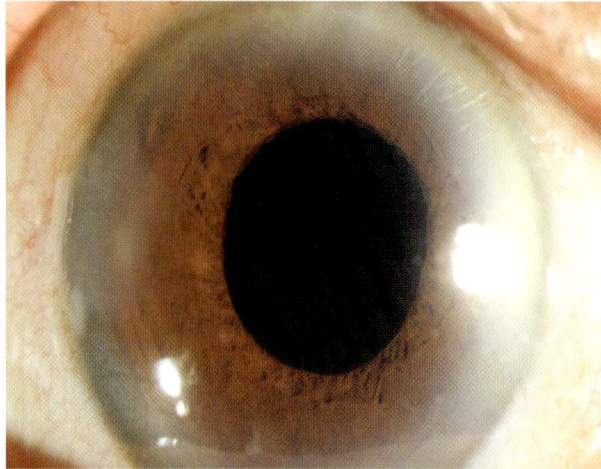

FIGURE 8.20 Clear cornea on postoperative day 1 following emulsification of a brunescent cataract. Adhering to the following strategies can help achieve clear corneas consistently after dense cataract emulsification. The technology must complement the surgeon's technique when emulsifying a dense cataract. Posterior plane emulsification during dense cataract emulsification can be safely and consistently achieved by: (a) use of newer ultrasound energy delivery modalities such as the torsional ultrasound and interrupted energy delivery modes with longitudinal ultrasound; (b) dividing the nucleus into multiple small fragments: step-by-step chop in situ, and lateral separation; (c) multilevel occlusion for complete division of fragments; (d) breaking the occlusion gradually; and (e) applying the step-down technique.

TABLE 8.2 *Complications*

Intraoperative Complications

Nucleus drop

Posterior capsule rupture

Incomplete division of fragments

Postoperative Complications

Corneal edema

Retained nuclear fragment

Anterior chamber inflammation

Postoperative IOP spike

SELECTED REFERENCES

Arshinoff SA. Dispersive-cohesive viscoelastic soft shell technique. *J Cataract Refract Surg.* 1999; 25:167–173.

Fine IH, Packer M, Hoffman RS. New phacoemulsification technologies. *J Cataract Refract Surg.* 2002; 28:1054–1060.

Fine IH. Cortical cleaving hydrodissection. *J Cataract Refract Surg.* 1992; 18:508–512.

Liu Y, Zeng M, Liu X, et al. Torsional mode versus conventional ultrasound mode phacoemulsification: Randomized comparative clinical study. *J Cataract Refract Surg.* 2007;33:287–292.

Osher RH. Slow motion phacoemulsification approach. *J Cataract Refract Surg* 1993;19:667

Singh R, Vasavada AR. Phacoemulsification of brunescent and black cataracts. *J Cataract Refract Surg.* 2001;27:1762–1769.

Singh R, Vasavada AR. Step-by-step chop in situ and separation of very dense cataracts. *J Cataract Refract Surg.* 1998;24:156–159.

Vasavada AR, Goyal D, Shastri L, Singh R. Cortico capsular adhesions and their effect during cataract surgery. *J Cataract Refract Surg.* 2003;29:1–6.

Vasavada AR, Raj S. Step down technique. *J Cataract Refract Surg.* 2003;29:1077–1079.

Vasavada AR, Raj SM, Patel U, et al. Comparison of torsional (ozil) versus microburst longitudinal (traditional) phacoemulsification—A prospective, randomized, masked clinical trial. *Ophthalmic Surg Lasers Imaging.* 2010;41:109–114.

Vasavada AR, Raj SM, Praveen MR, et al. Associations of corticocapsular adhesions in an Indian population. *Indian J Ophthalmol.* 2008;56:103–108.

Vasavada AR, Shastri L. Initial and definitive capsulorhexes: An extended application. *J Cataract Refract Surg.* 2000;26:634.

Vasavada V, Vasavada V, Raj SM, Vasavada AR. Intraoperative performance and postoperative outcomes of microcoaxial phacoemulsification: Observational study. *J Cataract Refract Surg.* 2007;33:1019–1024.

Yeoh R. The 'pupil snap' sign of posterior capsule rupture with hydrodissection in phacoemulsification (letter). *Br J Ophthalmol.* 1996;80:486.

Refractive Surgery

Edited by **Douglas D. Koch** and **Mitchell P. Weikert**

9

Laser-Assisted In Situ Keratomileusis (LASIK)

Cynthia P. Nix, MD and Sonia H. Yoo, MD

TABLE 9.1 *Indications/Contraindications*

Indications

Dependence on optical correction for refractive error and desire to reduce or eliminate dependence on spectacles or contact lenses

Must be 18 years of age or older

Demonstrate stable refractive errors

Refractive errors treated:

(Ranges differ between laser platforms.[1] Extremes beyond those listed in parenthesis below may lead to unpredictability of outcomes.)

    Myopia (<−14.0 D)

    Myopia with astigmatism (≤5.0 D)

    Hyperopia (<+5.0 D)

    Hyperopia with astigmatism (≤3.0 D)

    Mixed astigmatism (<6.0 D)

Contraindications

Unstable refractive errors

Patients under 18 years of age

Women who are pregnant or nursing

Ocular

Untreated dry eye syndromes

Uveitis

Scarring

Active infection

Keratoconus

Systemic

Collagen vascular diseases

Immunodeficiency syndromes

Autoimmune diseases

Severe atopy

Use of amiodarone or isotretinoin

Relative Contraindications

Diabetes mellitus

History of ocular herpes simplex or zoster

Deep-set eyes or narrow interpalpebral fissure

Screening

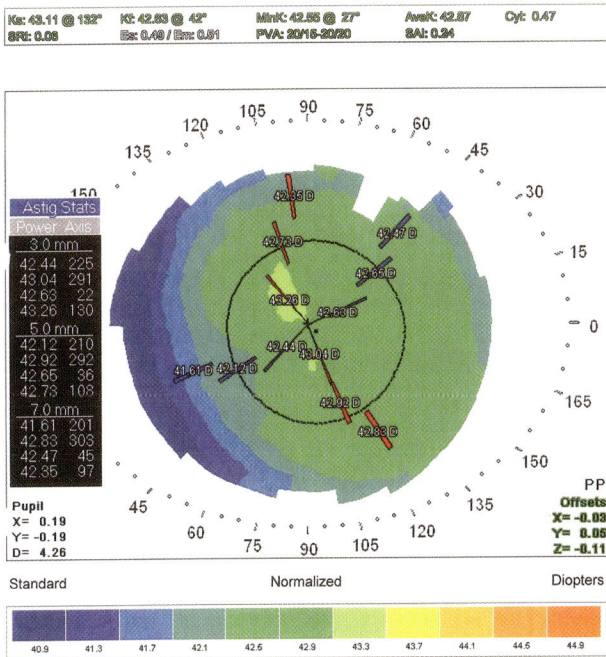

Ks: 43.11 @ 132°	Kf: 42.63 @ 42°	MinK: 42.56 @ 27°	AveK: 42.87	Cyl: 0.47
SRI: 0.06	Es: 0.49 / Em: 0.51	PVA: 20/16-20/20	SAI: 0.24	

FIGURE 9.1 **Topography**. Normal corneal topography with minimal astigmatism.

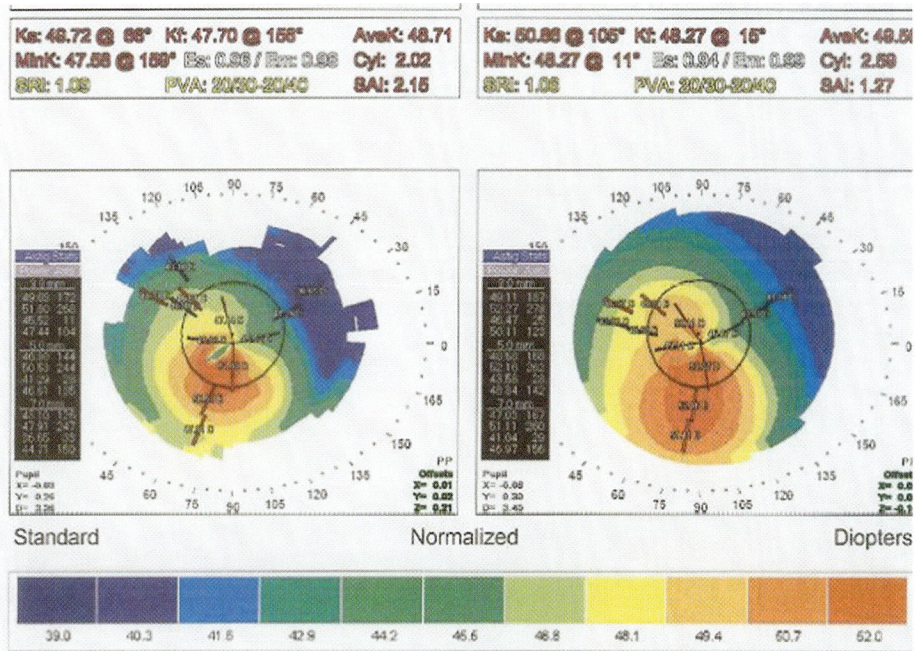

Ks: 48.72 @ 66°	Kf: 47.70 @ 156°	AveK: 48.71	
MinK: 47.56 @ 156°	Es: 0.96 / Em: 0.96	Cyl: 2.02	
SRI: 1.06	PVA: 20/30-20/40	SAI: 2.15	

Ks: 50.86 @ 105°	Kf: 48.27 @ 15°	AveK: 49.56	
MinK: 48.27 @ 11°	Es: 0.94 / Em: 0.92	Cyl: 2.59	
SRI: 1.06	PVA: 20/30-20/40	SAI: 1.27	

FIGURE 9.2 **Topography—Forme Fruste Keratoconus**. Certain types of asymmetric astigmatism are potential signs of forme fruste keratoconus. Forme fruste keratoconus may also be demonstrated by thin corneas and corneas with pachymetry that is significantly thinner inferiorly than superiorly. The topography map can be useful to visualize these changes. A helpful screening tool is the degree of inferior steepening, or the inferior/superior ratio. A value of 1.40 D or more is suspicious. Steep corneas (above 47 D) are also suggestive of early keratoconus. A skewing of the steep semi-meridians or abnormal posterior elevation may also be suggestive.

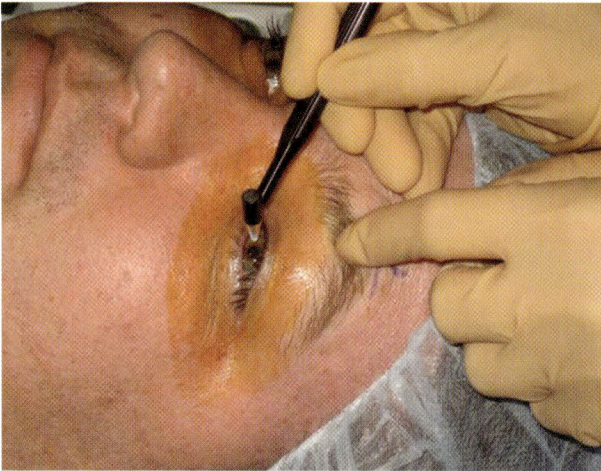

FIGURE 9.3 **Pachymetry**. Central corneal thickness – thickness of flap – depth of ablation = residual bed thickness. It is recommended to have >250 μm of residual bed thickness in order to decrease the risk of post-LASIK ectasia.

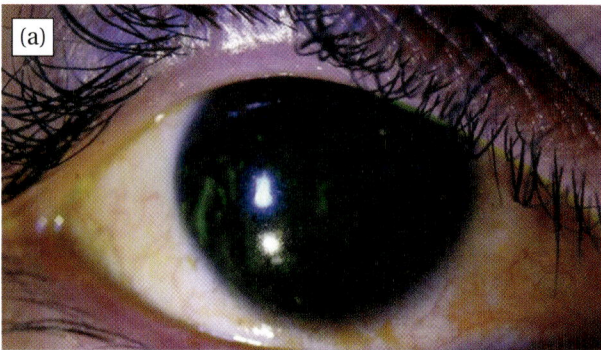

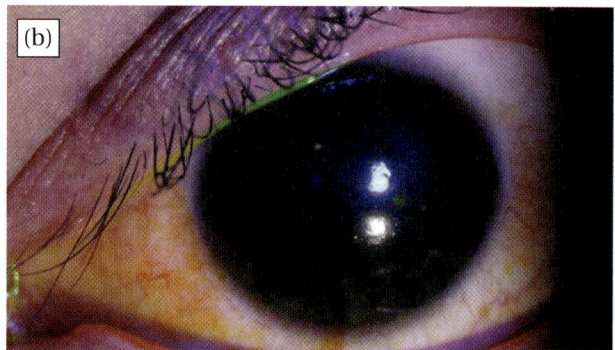

FIGURE 9.4 **Dry Eye**. Dry eye syndrome can be a significant problem post-LASIK. It is important to look for signs of this when evaluating patients preoperatively. Two examples of dry eye are shown (a, b). In addition to a thorough history, one may also evaluate the tear meniscus, tear breakup time, rose bengal staining and Schirmer testing. Evidence of blepharitis, meibomian gland dysfunction, and ocular rosacea should be noted and treated prior to LASIK surgery. Patients should be counseled on the risk of worsening symptoms after LASIK, and the procedure should be avoided in patients with severe dry eye symptoms refractory to treatment.

Treatment Options

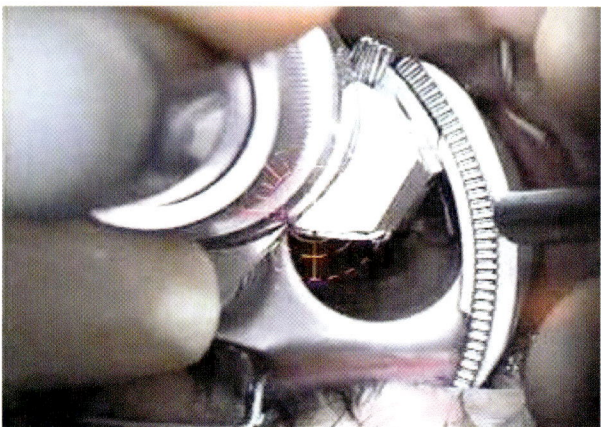

FIGURE 9.5 **Treatment Option 1: Microkeratome Flap Creation**. Whether the flap is created using a microkeratome blade or the femtosecond laser, patients receive a mild sedative 30 minutes prior to the procedure. At the time of the procedure, topical anesthetic is applied; then the skin prepped with providone-iodine, draped, and an eyelid speculum placed. A corneal suction ring is applied, which holds the eye in place and causes a transient dimming of vision in the treated eye due to the suction pressure. Next, the flap is cut.

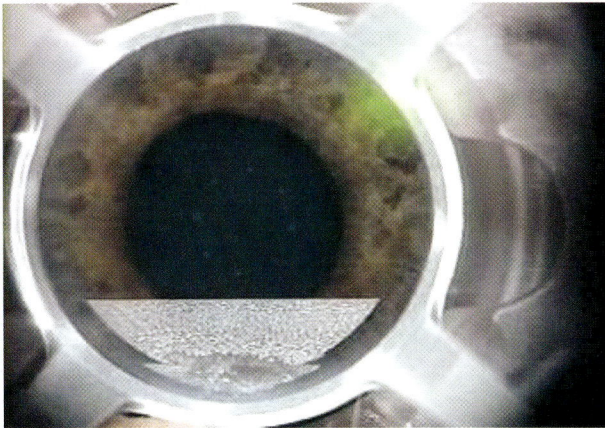

FIGURE 9.6 **Treatment Option 2: Femtosecond Laser Flap Creation**. The suction ring of the femtosecond laser (Intralase 30 kHz shown here) is in place and the laser flap creation is in progress. In this case, the hinge is being placed superiorly.

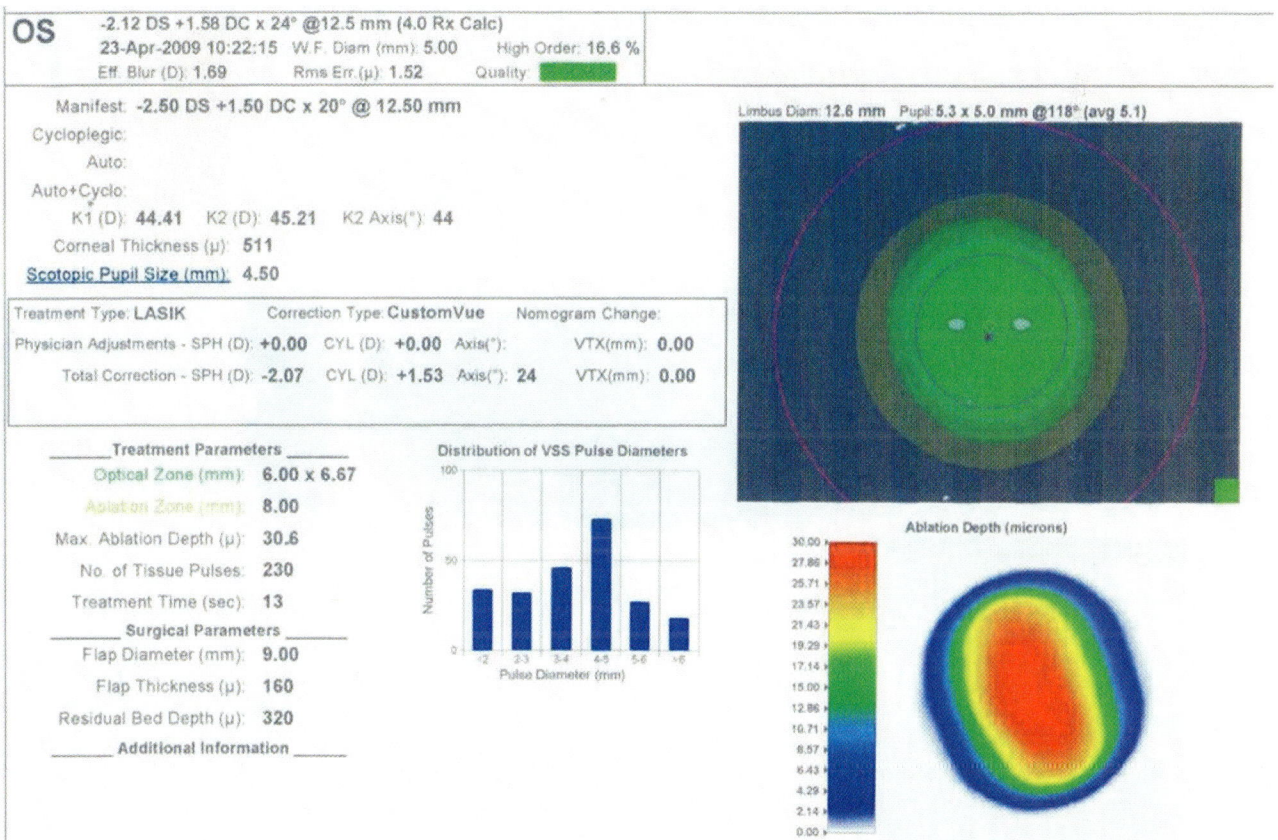

FIGURE 9.7 **Treatment Option 3: Wavefront-guided Ablation**. Wavefront-guided LASIK is a type of LASIK surgery that applies a spatially varying correction to the cornea stroma. This is done using the excimer laser with measurements from a wavefront sensor. The goal is to achieve a more optically perfect eye and decrease symptoms of higher order aberrations such as glare and haloes. This figure shows the computer generated measurements for degree and location of higher order aberrations on the patient's cornea.

Technique

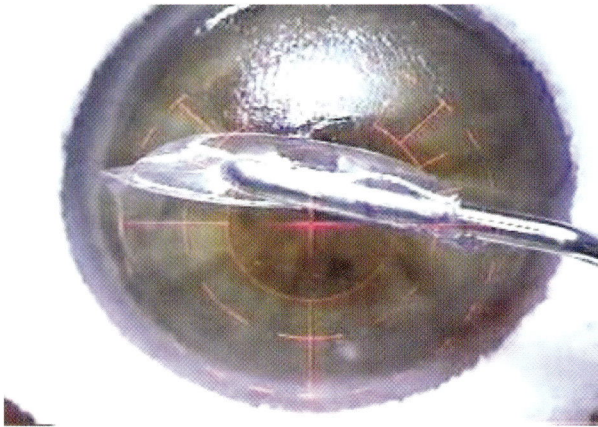

FIGURE 9.8 **Flap Lift**. A cornea marker is often used to mark the edges of the flap prior to lifting. This step helps to realign the flap edges during replacement of the flap. The flap is carefully dissected and folded back at the hinge to reveal the stroma. Next, the excimer laser is used to remodel the corneal stroma. The laser photoablates tissue in a finely controlled manner without damaging the adjacent stroma.

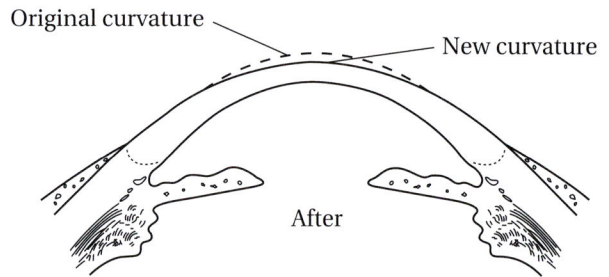

FIGURE 9.9 **Myopic Ablation**. Schematic drawing of correction of myopia by flattening of the central cornea with the excimer laser.

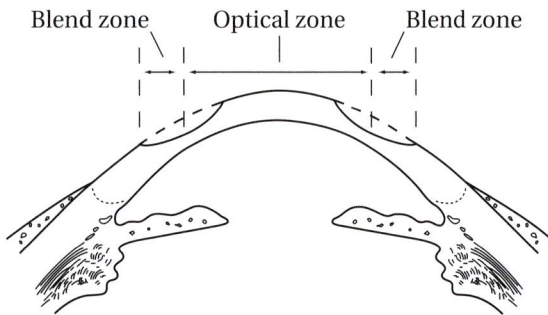

FIGURE 9.10 **Hyperopic Ablation**. Schematic drawing of correction of hyperopia by steepening of the central cornea with blending of the periphery.

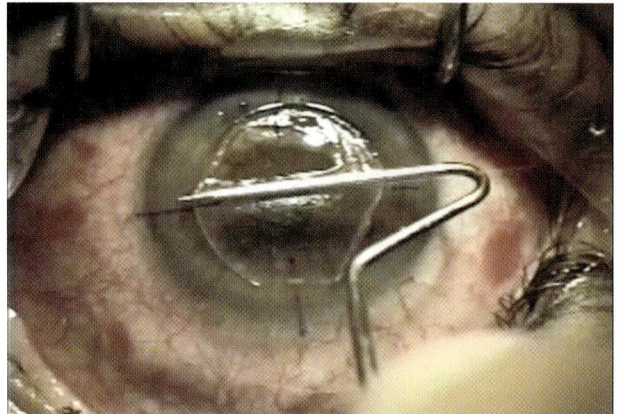

FIGURE 9.11 **Replacement of Flap**. The flap is carefully replaced over the corneal stroma ensuring that the markings realign and the flap is flat, in good position, and without interface debris. This helps to prevent complications such as epithelial ingrowth, striae, or dehiscence from the hinge. Once the flap is determined to be in correct position, an antibiotic drop, corticosteroid drop, and occasionally a bandage contact lens is placed. The flap is rechecked at the slit lamp one hour after the procedure. The patient is instructed to wear protective shield/goggles when sleeping. A postoperative regimen of topical antibiotic and corticosteroid is given for 5–7 days post-op. Patients return on post-op day 1 to recheck the flap.

Complications

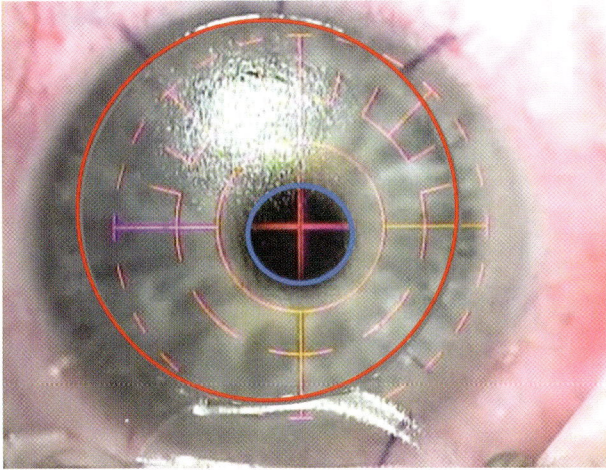

FIGURE 9.12 **Decentered Flap**. Decentration of the LASIK flap from the center of the pupil. The flap edge is indicated by the solid red circle.

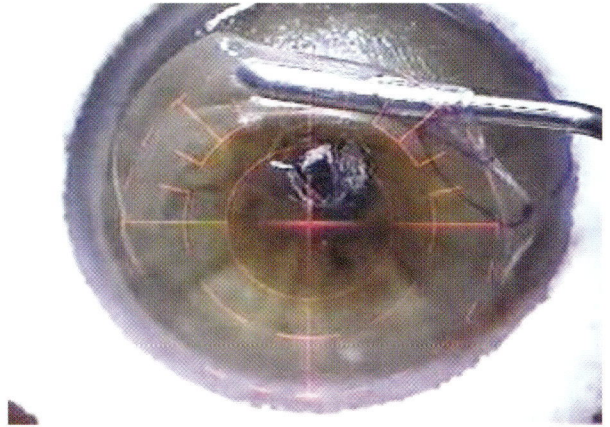

FIGURE 9.13 **Buttonhole of Flap**. Creation of a buttonhole in the LASIK flap using a microkeratome blade. A steep corneal curvature is a risk factor for this complication. A buttonholed flap should be replaced and allowed to heal without performing the ablation.

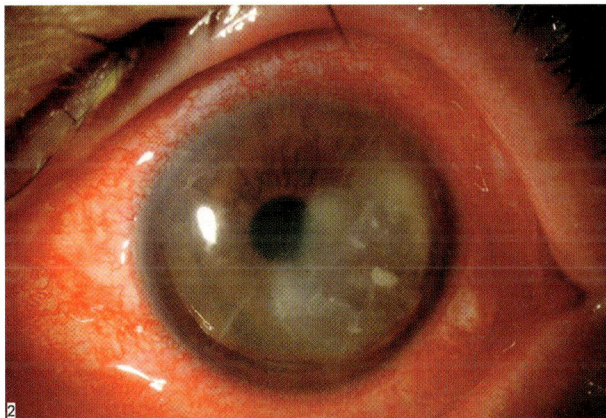

FIGURE 9.14 **Infectious Keratitis**. Infectious keratitis in the LASIK flap caused by methicillin-resistant *Staphylococcus aureus*. Such infections should be treated aggressively with flap lift, culture, and appropriate topical antibiotic therapy.

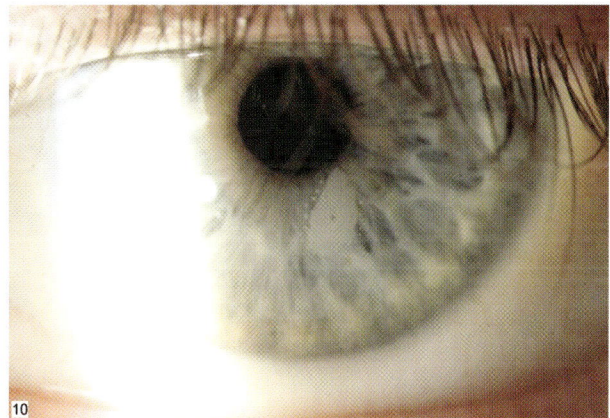

FIGURE 9.15 **Epithelial Ingrowth**. Epithelial ingrowth demonstrating central nests of epithelial cells in the interface under the LASIK flap. If the visual axis is involved, or if corneal melt or irregular astigmatism results, the flap may be lifted and scraped to remove the epithelial cells.

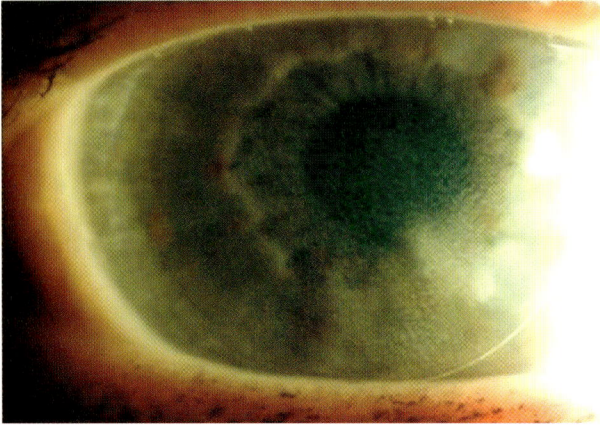

FIGURE 9.16 Diffuse Lamellar Keratitis. Diffuse lamellar keratitis with dense accumulation of inflammatory cells. Mild or moderate disease may improve with corticosteroid treatment. Severe cases require flap lift and irrigation.

TABLE 9.2 *Complications of LASIK*

Central islands

Corneal perforations

Decentration

Diffuse lamellar keratitis

Dry eye syndrome

Epithelial erosions

Epithelial ingrowth

Flap irregularities (button hole, free flap)

Infectious keratitis

Striae

Traumatic flap dislocations

SELECTED REFERENCES

Basic and Clinical Science Course, 2006–2007. Section 13: Refractive surgery. San Francisco: American Academy of Ophthalmology; 2006:87–135.

FDA. U.S. Department of Health and Human Services, Medical Devices, LASIK (2009, Nov 27). List of FDA-Approved Lasers for LASIK. Retrieved from http://www.fda.gov/MedicalDevices/ProductsandMedicalProcedures/SurgeryandLifeSupport/LASIK/ucm192109.htm.

Haft P, Yoo SH, Kymionis GD, Ide T, O'Brien TP, Culbertson WW. Complications of LASIK flaps made by the IntraLase 15- and 30-kHz femtosecond lasers. *J Refract Surg.* 2009 Nov;25(11):979–984.

Kymionis GD, Bouzoukis D, Diakonis V, Tsiklis N, Gkenos E, Pallikaris AI, Giaconi JA, Yoo SH. Long-term results of thin corneas after refractive laser surgery. *Am J Ophthalmol.* 2007 Aug;144(2):181–185.

Lee JK, Nkyekyer EW, Chuck RS. Microkeratome complications. *Curr Opin Ophthalmol.* 2009 Jul;20(4):260–263.

Panday VA, Reilly CD. Refractive surgery in the United States Air Force. *Curr Opin Ophthalmol.* 2009 Jul; 20(4):242–246.

Randleman JB, White AJ Jr, Lynn MJ, Hu MH, Stulting RD. Incidence, outcomes, and risk factors for retreatment after wavefront-optimized ablations with PRK and LASIK. *J Refract Surg.* 2009 Mar;25(3):273–276.

10 Photorefractive Keratectomy (PRK)

Peter McGannon, MD, Douglas D. Koch, MD, and Mitchell P. Weikert, MD, MS

Photorefractive keratectomy is a safe and effective photoablation technique to reduce or eliminate spectacle dependence, especially for those individuals who may not be ideal candidates for LASIK.

TABLE 10.1 *Indications and Contraindications for Photorefractive Keratectomy*

Indications

Myopia and myopic astigmatism up to 10–12 diopters

Hyperopia and hyperopic astigmatism up to 4 diopters

Thin corneas where residual bed following LASIK would be less than 300 micrometers

Predisposition to trauma (military, law enforcement, martial arts, etc.)

Mild to moderate dry eye syndrome

Epithelial basement membrane dystrophy or recurrent erosions

If using a mechanical microkeratome, flat (<40 D) corneas to reduce risk of free flap and steep (>48 D) corneas to reduce risk of buttonhole

Previous corneal refractive surgery

Inexperienced refractive surgeon

Patient preference

Contraindications

Thin corneas where residual bed following PRK would be less than 300 micrometers

Signs of keratoconus

Severe dry eye syndrome

Collagen vascular, autoimmune, or immunodeficiency diseases

Patients who are pregnant or breastfeeding

A history of ophthalmic herpes simplex or herpes zoster

Significant corneal scarring

Patients taking isotretinoin, amiodarone, sumatriptan, topical, or oral corticosteroids

Visually significant cataracts

Uveitis

Screening

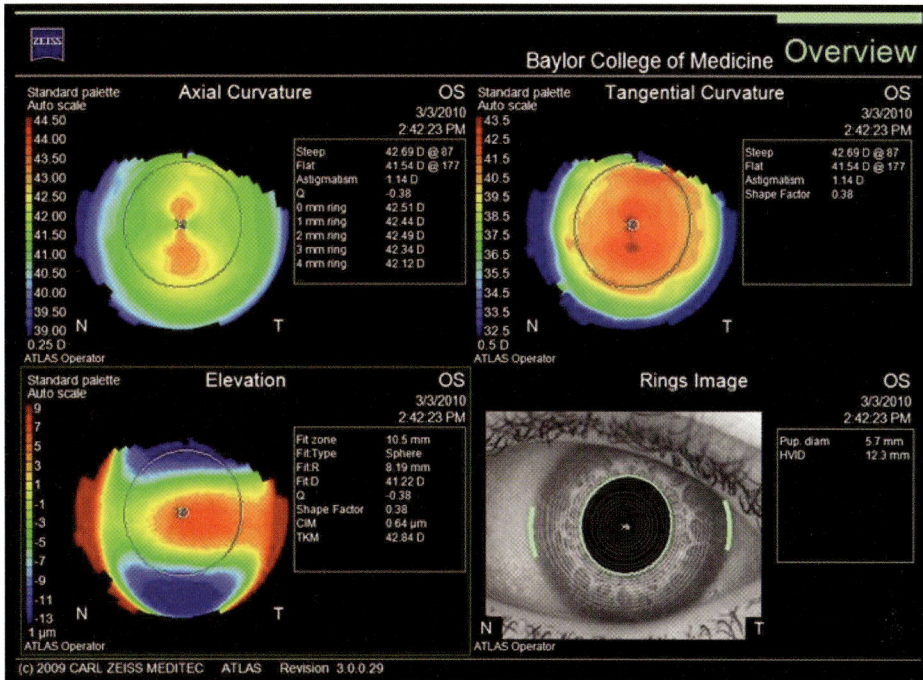

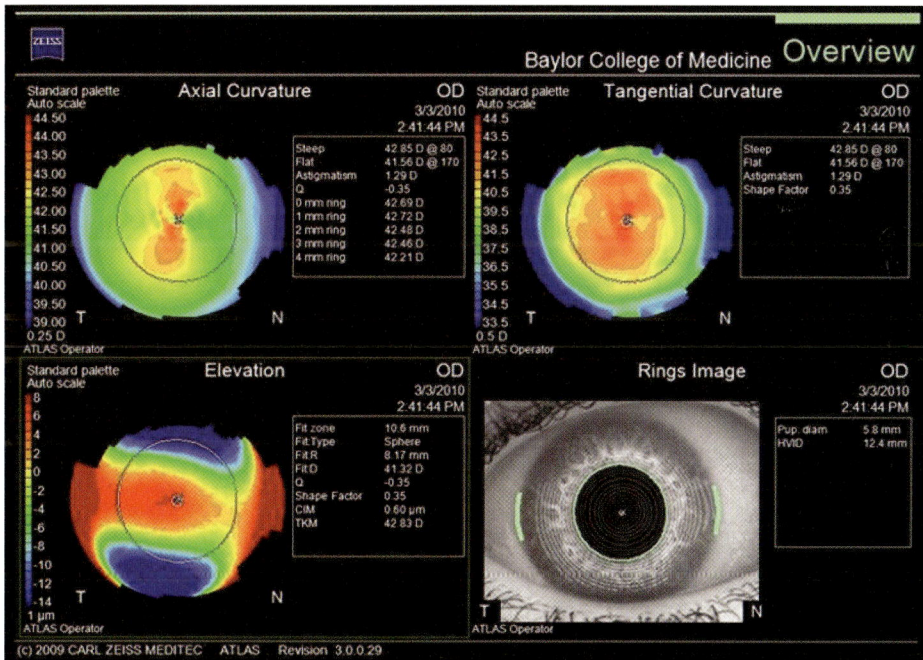

FIGURE 10.1 **Topography**. Obtaining topography is an essential component of the screening process to identify patients with forme fruste keratoconus and those at risk for post-refractive ectasia. It also serves as a data source for surgical planning. Currently popular topographers include: (a) Humphrey Atlas (placido disk imaging).

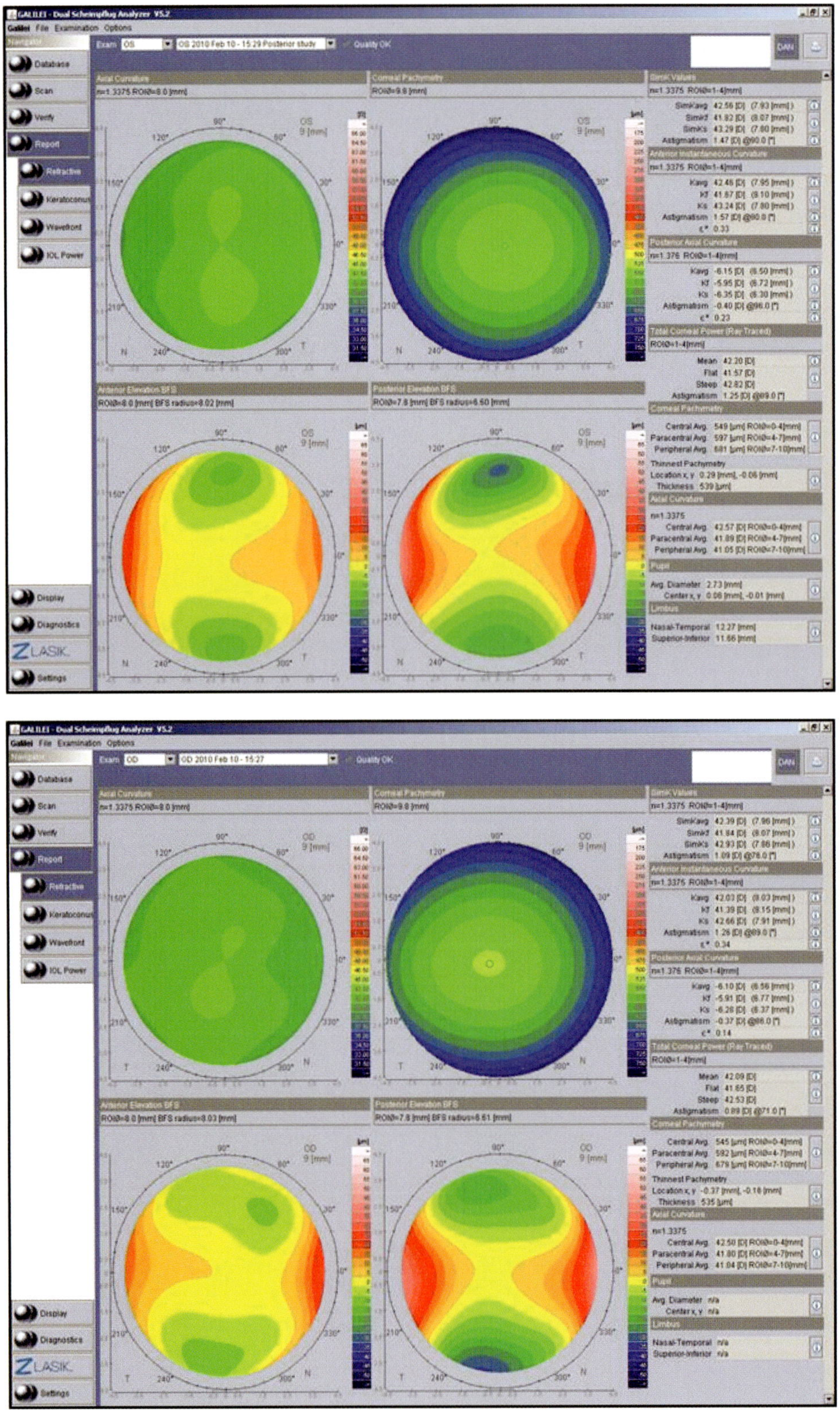

FIGURE 10.1 (*continued*) (b) Galilei Dual Scheimpflug Analyzer (Placido disk combined with dual scheimpflug imaging).

OS

Date: 2/10/2010 3:32:49 PM   Exam 2

Ks: 43.46 @ 84°	Kf: 41.72 @ 174°	MinK: 41.64 @ 4°	AveK: 42.59	Cyl: 1.74
SRI: 0.07	Es: 0.69 / Em: 0.49	PVA: 20/15-20/20	SAI: 0.24	

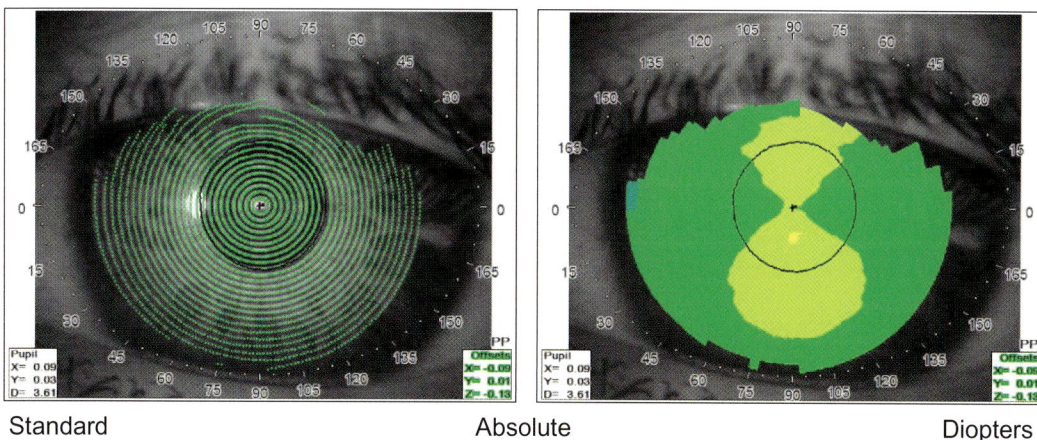

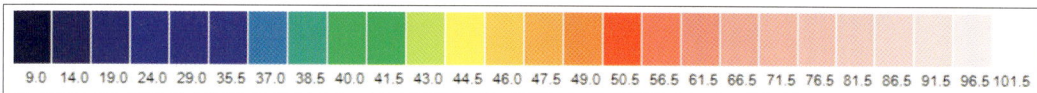

Standard   Absolute   Diopters

9.0 14.0 19.0 24.0 29.0 35.5 37.0 38.5 40.0 41.5 43.0 44.5 46.0 47.5 49.0 50.5 56.5 61.5 66.5 71.5 76.5 81.5 86.5 91.5 96.5 101.5

Klyce / Maeda
KCI
0.0% Similarity

**Keratoconus
Pattern not
Detected**

Smolek / Klyce
KSI
0.0% Severity

**Keratoconus
Pattern not
Detected**

Keratoconus
Screening
System

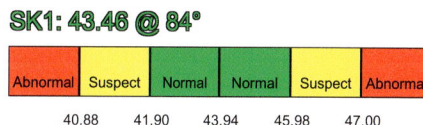

SK1: 43.46 @ 84°

Abnormal	Suspect	Normal	Normal	Suspect	Abnormal
	40.88	41.90	43.94	45.98	47.00

Related Indices:

SK1 : 43.46	SK2 : 41.72	CYL : 1.74
SAI : 0.24	DSI : 2.56	SRI : 0.07
OSI : 0.20	CSI : 0.37	SDP : 0.80
IAI : 0.33	KPI : 0.17	AA : 75.35%

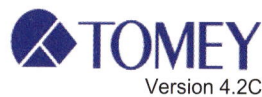

TOMEY
Version 4.2C

FIGURE 10.1 (*continued*) (c) Tomey topography (placido disk imaging).

OD

Date: 2/10/2010 3:32:43 PM   Exam 1

Ks: 43.39 @ 84°   Kf: 41.63 @ 174°   MinK: 41.63 @ 176°   AveK: 42.51   Cyl: 1.75
SRI: 0.41   Es: 0.68 / Em: 0.53 PVA: 20/20-20/25   SAI: 0.19

Standard   Absolute   Diopters

9.0 14.0 19.0 24.0 29.0 35.5 37.0 38.5 40.0 41.5 43.0 44.5 46.0 47.5 49.0 50.5 56.5 61.5 66.5 71.5 76.5 81.5 86.5 91.5 96.5 101.5

Klyce / Maeda   Smolek / Klyce   Keratoconus
KCI   KSI   Screening
0.0% Similarity   0.0% Severity   System

Keratoconus   Keratoconus   SK1: 43.39 @ 84°
Pattern not   Pattern not
Detected   Detected | Abnormal | Suspect | Normal | Normal | Suspect | Abnormal |
                                                       40.88   41.90   43.94   45.98   47.00

Related Indices:
SK1 : 43.39   SK2 : 41.63   CYL : 1.75
SAI : 0.19   DSI : 3.03   SRI : 0.41
OSI : 0.67   CSI : 0.40   SDP : 0.83
IAI : 0.33   KPI : 0.18   AA : 79.87%

TOMEY
Version 4.2C

FIGURE 10.1 *(continued)*.

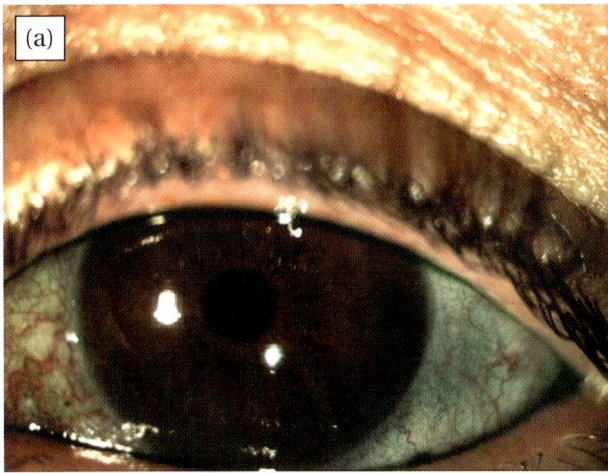

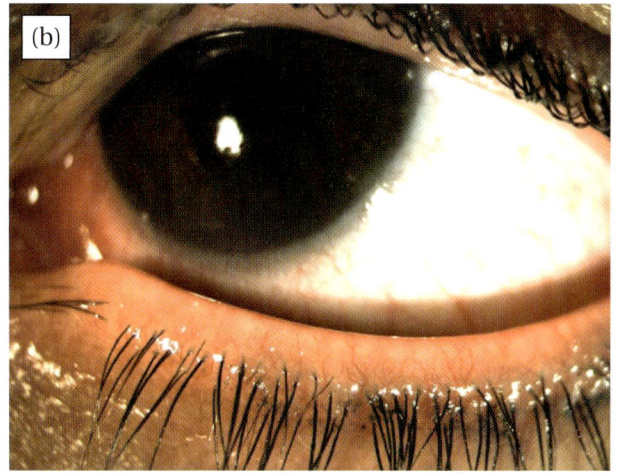

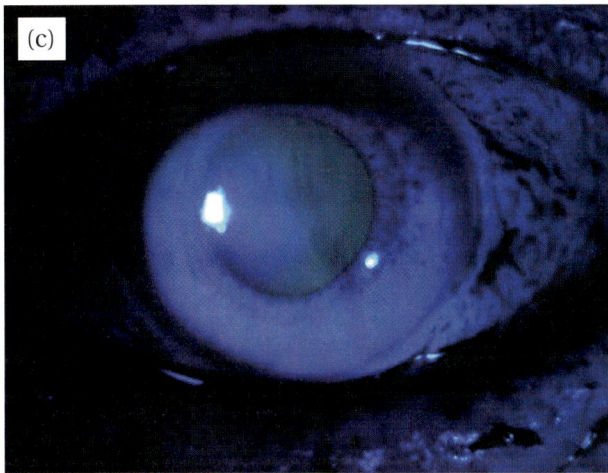

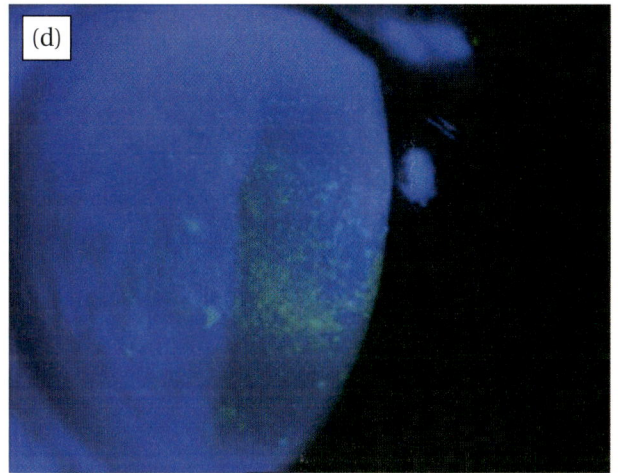

FIGURE 10.2 **Dry Eye**. Although surgically induced dry eye is extremely rare following PRK, uncontrolled dry eye could affect healing. Therefore, it is important to screen refractive surgical candidates for dry eye, and, if present, control preoperatively or eliminate those with severe forms. Important findings in potential post-refractive dry eye candidates include a reduced tear meniscus (a), meibomian gland disease with dilated lid margin vessels (brush marks) (b), reduced tear breakup time (<7 seconds) (c), and punctate epithelial erosions (d).

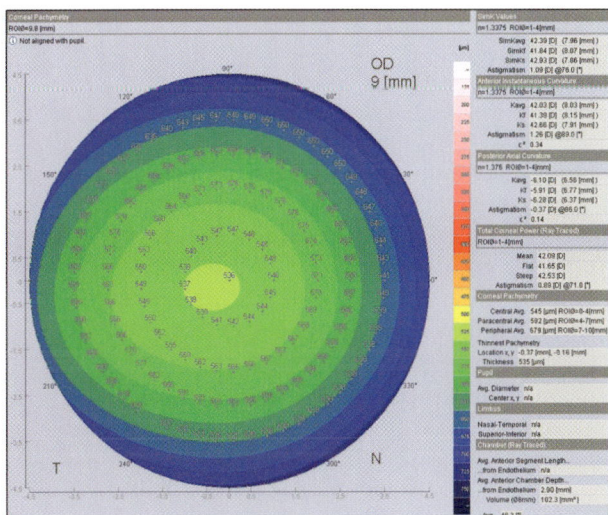

FIGURE 10.3 **Pachymetry Map**. A corneal thickness or pachymetry map will help to predict the residual bed thickness and is also helpful for keratoconus screening.

Treatment Decision

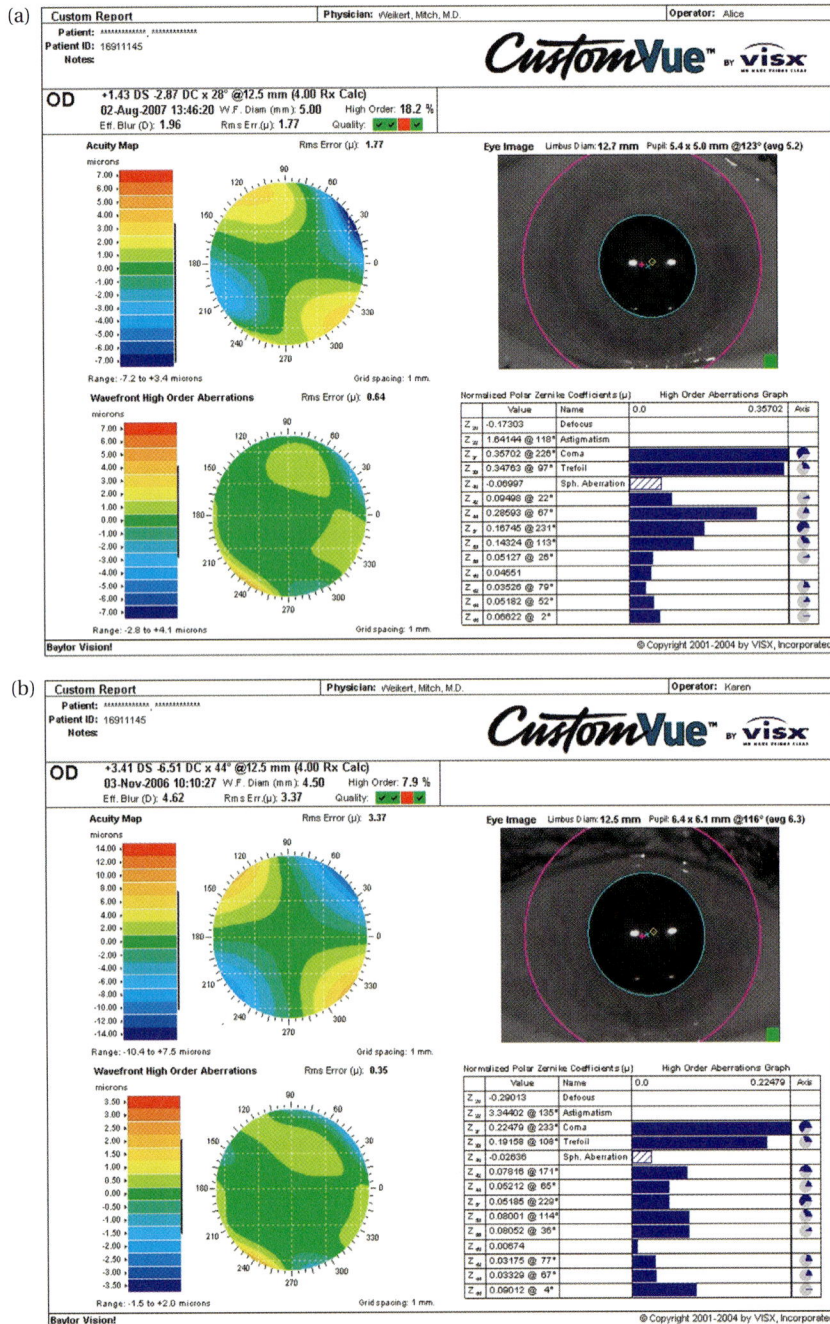

FIGURE 10.4 **Wavefront Guided vs. Conventional Ablation.** Depending on the laser platform, the desired refractive correction, FDA approval status, the ability to obtain a useful wavefront measurement, and other factors, one will use wavefront-guided (a), wavefront-optimized, or a conventional ablation pattern. Wavefront-guided ablations have the advantage of enlarged optical zones, reduced higher-order aberrations, and iris registration with torsional tracking. Most patients will qualify for a wavefront-guided ablation, except those with high levels of astigmatism (b) or hyperopia, which may require conventional ablation. Different laser platforms differ in their ability to treat high hyperopia and astigmatism. Please refer to your specific laser manual for your laser's hyperopia and astigmatism limits.

Epithelial Removal

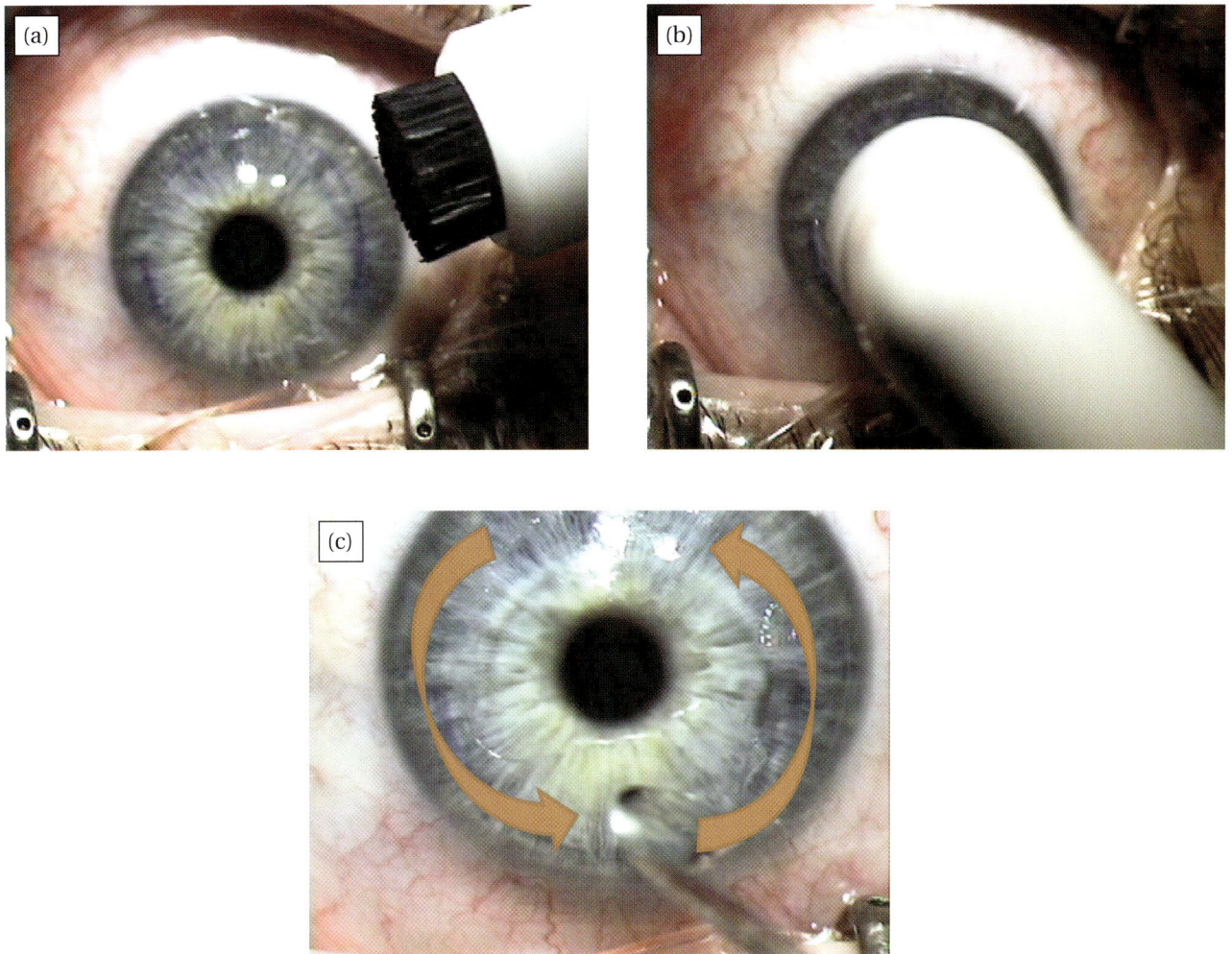

FIGURE 10.5 **Brush**. Prior to beginning any procedure, the patient's eyes should be prepped. Then, after instilling topical 0.5% proparacaine or equivalent, the eyelashes should be isolated from the surgical field and a lid speculum placed. Once the patient is properly anesthetized and correctly positioned, the ablation zone is marked. Then a motorized brush (a) can quickly and evenly remove the epithelium. Because the brush heads typically are flat, it is important to "rock" the brush in all directions to remove the peripheral epithelium up to the markings (b). After using the brush, any remaining epithelium within the ablation zone should be removed with a spatula or blade. A circumferential motion, rather than radial, typically provides the most efficient removal (c).

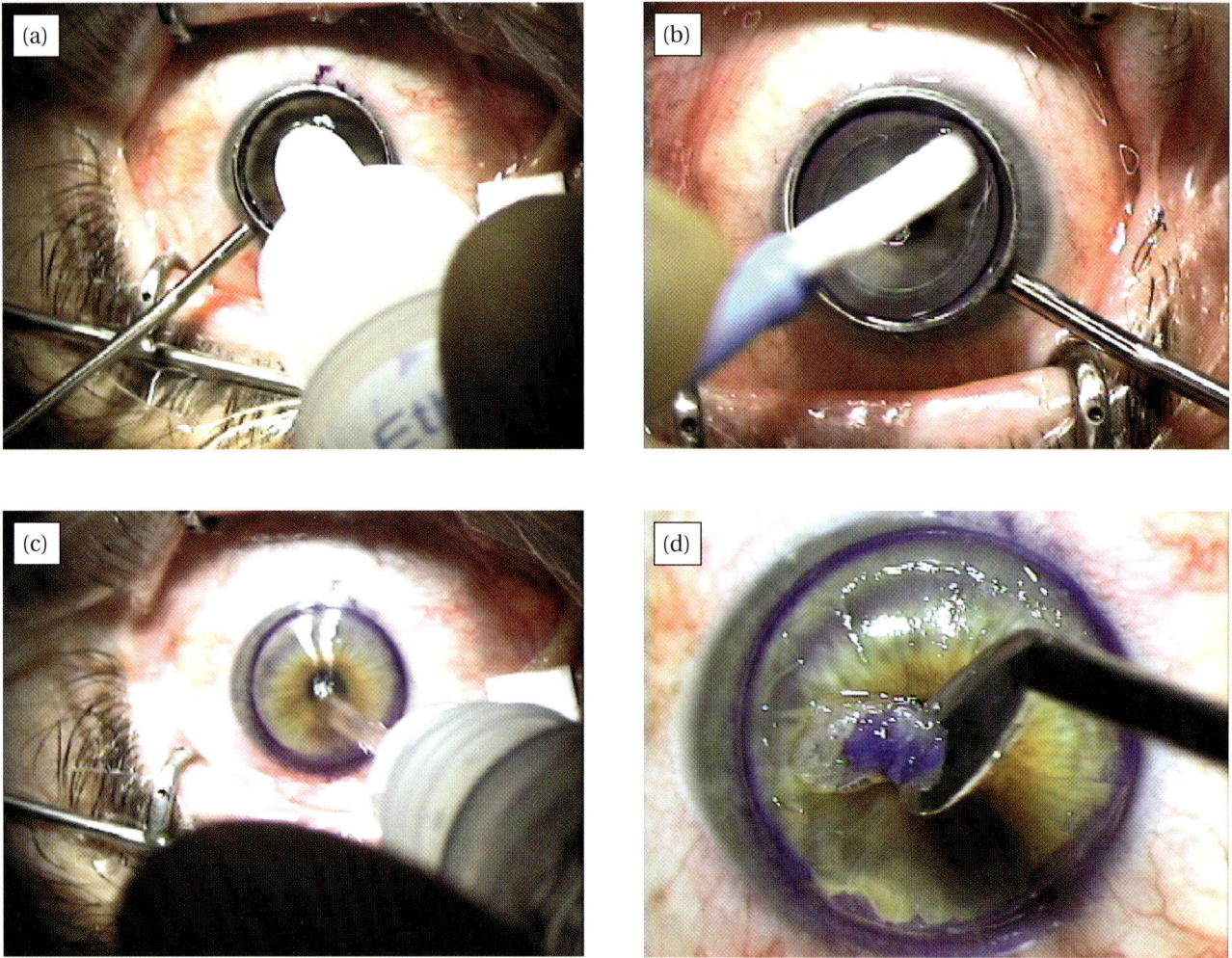

FIGURE 10.6 **Alcohol**. Initially, the ablation zone is marked. An 18–20% ethanol solution can then be applied to the epithelium using a well or corneal light shield (a), typically for 30–45 seconds (longer in cases of prior surgery, such as LASIK or radial keratotomy). The ethanol is absorbed using a sponge (b), and the cornea is copiously irrigated (c) with at least 15 cc of balanced salt solution (BSS). The epithelium can then be easily removed using a spatula or sponge (d).

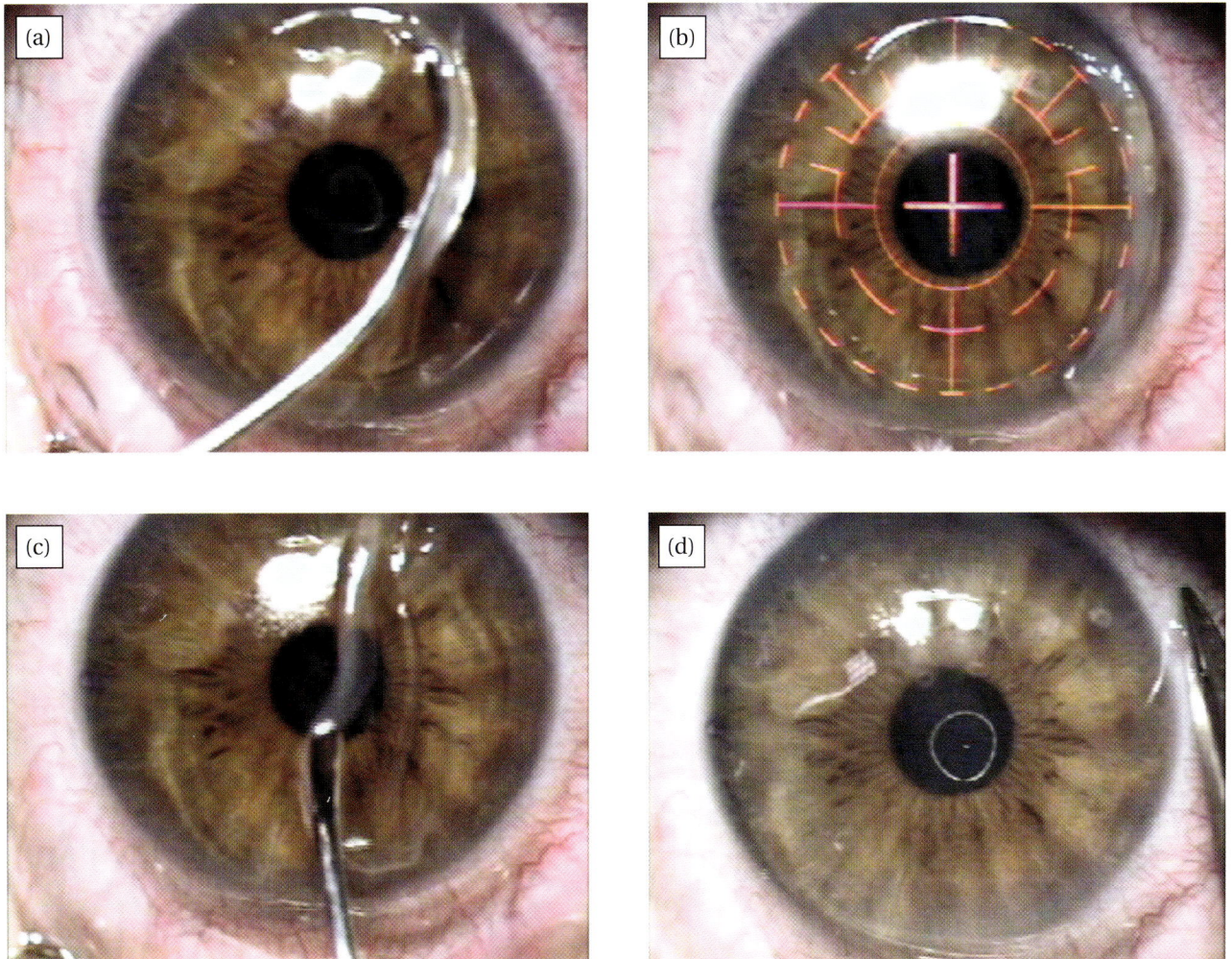

FIGURE 10.7 **LASEK**. Start by marking the epithelium as in LASIK to aid in realignment. An 18–20% ethanol solution is then applied to the epithelium for 20–40 seconds using a well or corneal light shield (see above). Then, a flap consisting only of epithelium is created by cutting the edge with a modified trephine or other device. The epithelium is carefully retracted using a spatula (a) or sponge. The ablation is performed after the bed is dried (b). Following the ablation the bed is hydrated with a drop of BSS and the epithelium is replaced using the spatula (c) or sponge. Finally, a contact lens is placed (d).

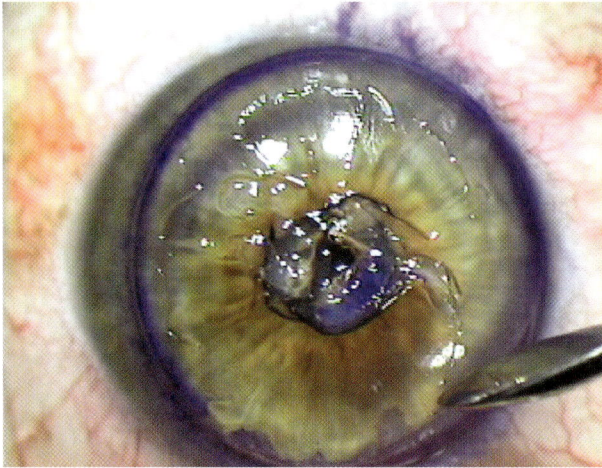

FIGURE 10.8 **Manual Scraping**. The ablation zone is marked. A spatula or blade is used to remove epithelium without the use of alcohol or epikeratome system. Although this approach requires minimal instrumentation, the untreated epithelium may be quite adherent and hence more difficult to remove.

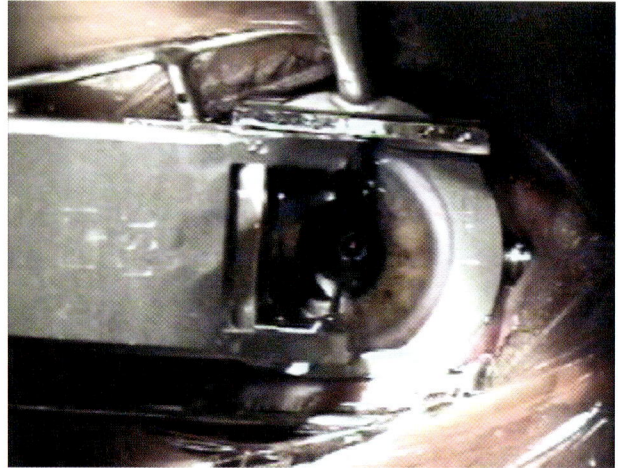

FIGURE 10.9 **Epikeratome**. An epikeratome system, similar to a microkeratome in LASIK but with a duller blade, can be used to free the epithelium. The epikeratome lifts the epithelium in one pass. As in LASEK (see above), a spatula or sponge is used to retract the epithelium. After the ablation, the stromal bed is hydrated, and the epithelium is replaced with the spatula. A contact lens should be placed after the epithelium is repositioned. Some surgeons discard rather than replace the epithelial flap.

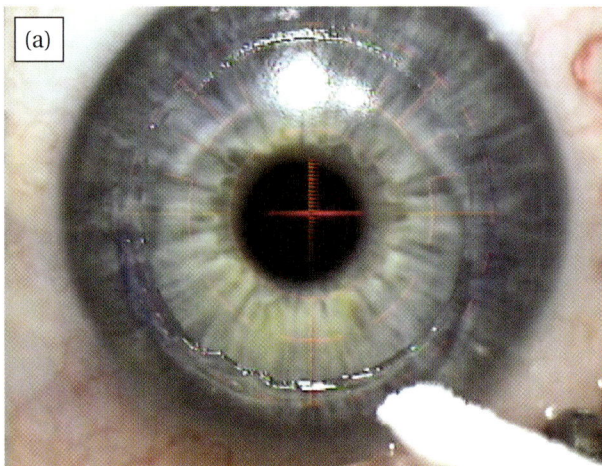

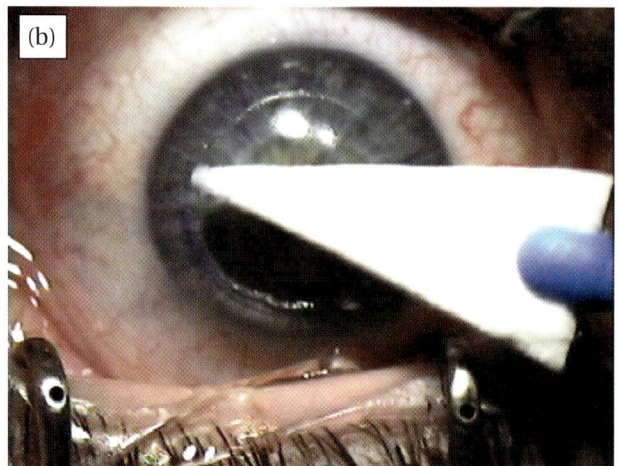

FIGURE 10.10 **Ablation Zone Preparation**. Sufficient epithelial removal can be confirmed using the reticule overlay as a guide (a). After epithelial removal, the ablation zone should be dried evenly using a sponge (b). Uneven stromal bed hydration can result in irregular ablations. Care should be taken not to leave any fragments of sponge in the ablation zone. If sponge fragments or epithelium are left behind, they will light up during the ablation and should be removed.

Ablation

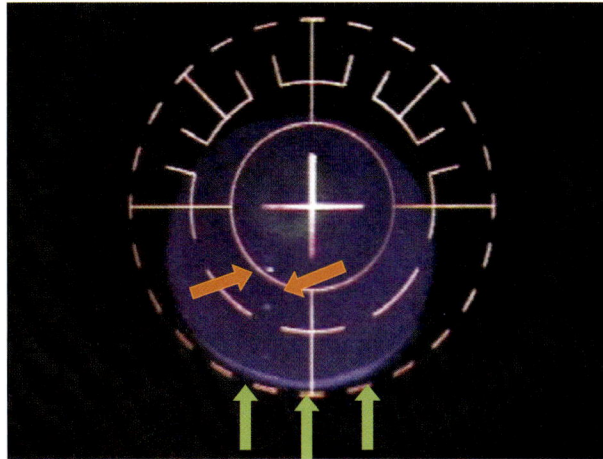

FIGURE 10.11 **Ablation**. When the stromal bed is clean and dry, activate the pupil tracking system and iris registration, if applicable. Proper head positioning, focusing on the corneal surface, and steady patient fixation can increase the likelihood of successful iris registration. Reduce the light source to a dim setting to help the patient fixate on the target light. Begin the ablation. Pay attention to the ablation zone during the laser treatment to look for debris (orange arrows) or residual epithelium (green arrows), which will fluoresce when struck by the laser, and remove if present. In addition, condensation may accumulate on the stromal bed, especially for longer ablations. Pause the laser and dry with a sponge if this occurs.

Haze Prevention

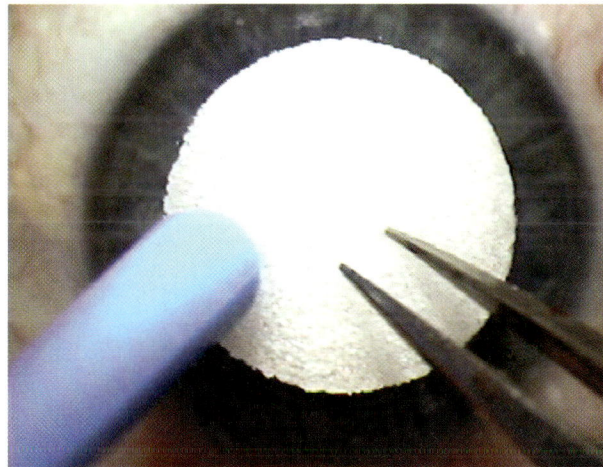

FIGURE 10.12 **Haze Prevention: Mitomycin-C**. Conditions that pose an increased risk of developing visually significant postoperative corneal haze include: (1) greater ablation depths, (2) corneas that have undergone prior surgery, including PRK, LASIK, radial keratotomy, and penetrating keratoplasty, and (3) scarred corneas. To minimize this risk, mitomycin-C 0.02% can be applied for intervals as short as 12 seconds in "virgin" corneas, ranging up to 2 minutes in corneas with dense preexisting haze. Apply with a 6-mm corneal light shield moistened with mitomycin-C until damp, and then copiously irrigate with 20–30 cc of BSS. Mitomycin-C may be considered in (1) myopic ablations greater than 6 diopters, (2) smaller corrections with larger ablation zones, when greater than 75 microns of tissue is ablated, and (3) any corneas with prior surgery (e.g., LASIK, PRK, radial keratotomy, penetrating keratoplasty). Forceps or a sponge can be used to maintain light shield contact with the corneal surface while applying the mitomycin-C.

Post-ablation Care

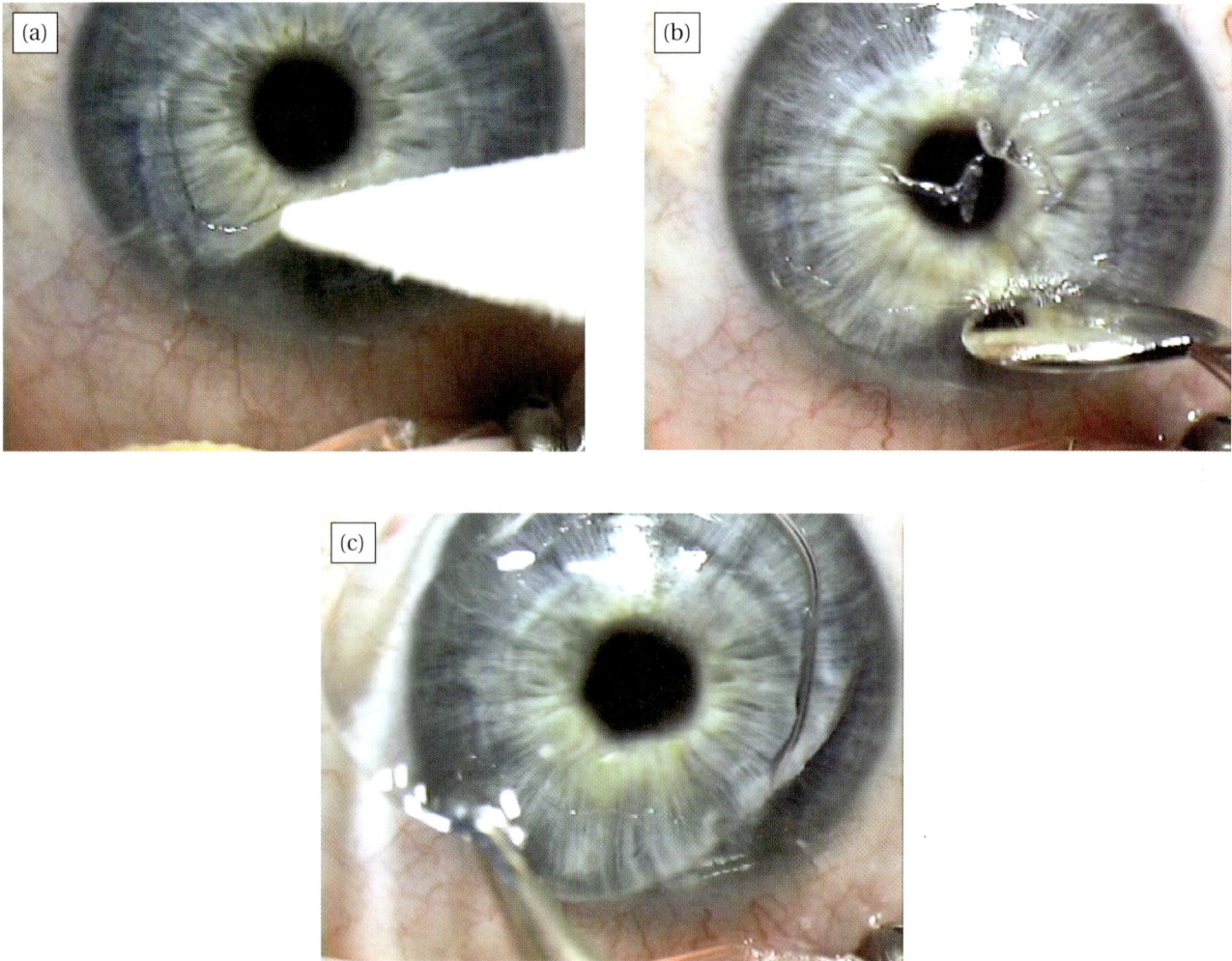

FIGURE 10.13 **Post-ablation Care**. After completing the ablation, use a sponge or spatula to replace small amounts of folded or loose epithelium at the border of the ablation zone (a) or remove it, especially if excessive (b). Finally, place a bandage contact lens over the cornea (c).

Complications

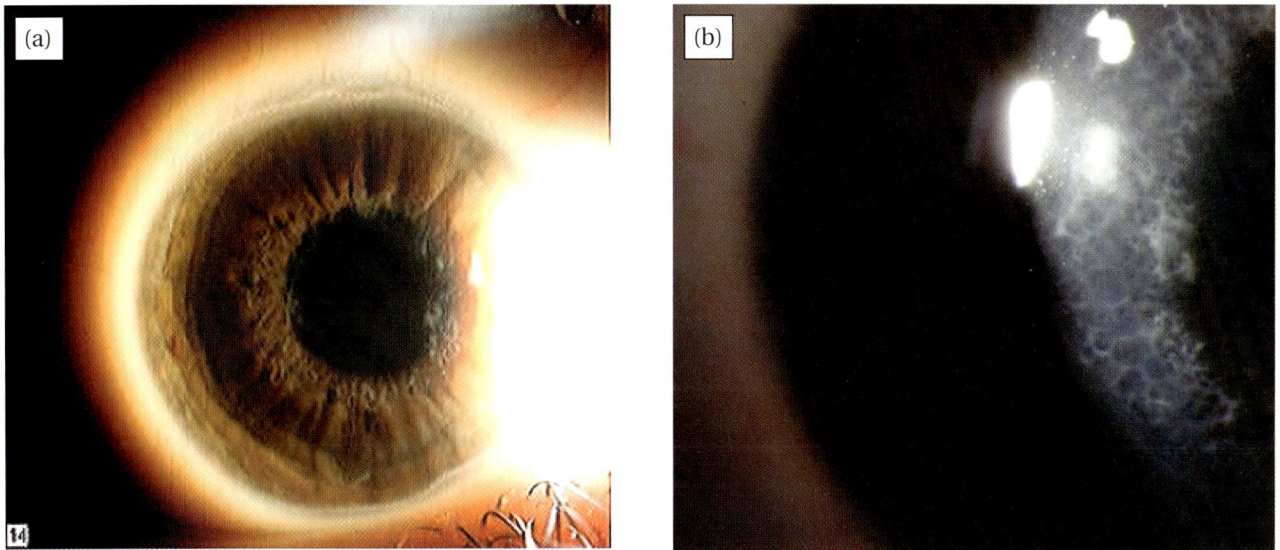

FIGURE 10.14 **Haze**. Mild anterior stromal haze may develop as a normal healing response and can be seen a few weeks after surgery (a). Visually significant haze typically is first noted 3 months postoperatively, but often develops 6–12 months after surgery. It has a reticular pattern (b) and can obscure the view of the underlying iris. Treatment options include topical corticosteroids (which may halt but rarely reverse the haze formation), PTK, and observation, as the haze may regress over several months.

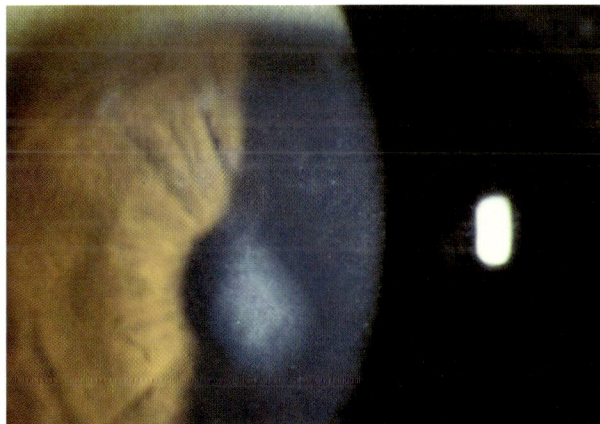

FIGURE 10.15 **Infection or Sterile Infiltrates**. Infection after PRK is a rare (0.2%) but potentially vision-threatening complication. All infiltrates, as seen in the figure above, should be treated as a possible infection and followed closely. If there is a high clinical suspicion of an infectious etiology, the bandage contact lens and infiltrate should be cultured. Sterile corneal infiltrates can also rarely occur, with a typical onset of 2–3 days following surgery. They can often be distinguished from infection by their peripheral corneal location (often outside the original zone of the epithelial defect), intact epithelium, and multiple foci.

TABLE 10.2 *Complications*

Over/undercorrection

Glare

Haloes

Monocular diplopia

Image ghosting

Haze/scarring

Regression

Recurrent erosions

Infection

Sterile infiltrates

Central islands

Eccentric ablation and decentration

Dry eye syndrome

Irregular astigmatism

Ectasia

Complications associated with topical steroid use:

- Raised intraocular pressure
- Cataract
- Stromal thinning

SELECTED REFERENCES

Munnerlyn CR, Koons SJ, Marshall J. Photorefractive keratectomy: a technique for laser refractive surgery. *J Cat Refract Surg*. Jan 1988;14(1):46–52.

Rajan MS, Jaycock P, O'Brart D. A long-term study of photorefractive keratectomy; 12-year follow-up. *Ophthalmology*. Oct 2004;111(10):1813–1824.

Slade, Stephen G., Richard N. Baker, and Dorothy Kay Brockman. *The Complete Book of Laser Eye Surgery*. Naperville, IL: Sourcebooks; 2000.

11 Phototherapeutic Keratectomy (PTK)

Jeanine A. Baqai, MD and Jonathan B. Rubenstein, MD

TABLE 11.1 *Indications for Surgery*

Corneal opacity (scars, nodules, band keratopathy, anterior dystrophies)

Irregular astigmatism (basement membrane abnormalities, Salzmann's nodular degeneration, irregular scars, band keratopathy, anterior dystrophies)

Surface breakdown/Recurrent erosions

Any pathology within the anterior 100 microns

TABLE 11.2 *Preoperative Considerations*

In the presence of HSV, consider treatment with oral anti-virals preoperatively and postoperatively

The pathology should be anterior such that the remaining corneal thickness is at least 350 microns after the procedure is performed

Treatment should be deferred in patients with active disease until the disease process has become quiescent

Avoid in severe limbal stem cell disease or neurotrophic corneas

Clinical Indications

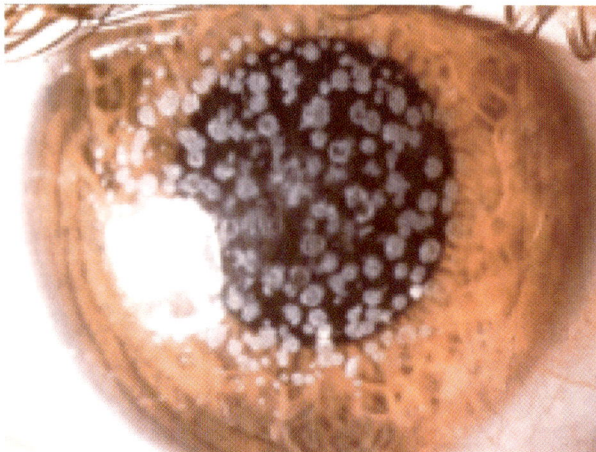

FIGURE 11.1 Granular Dystrophy.

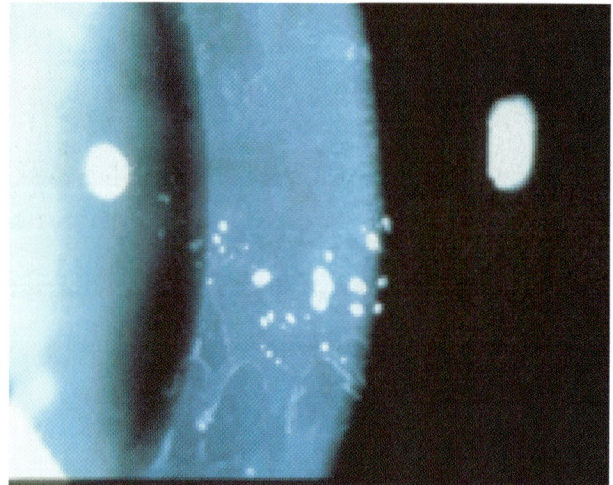

FIGURE 11.2 Epithelial Basement Dystrophy.

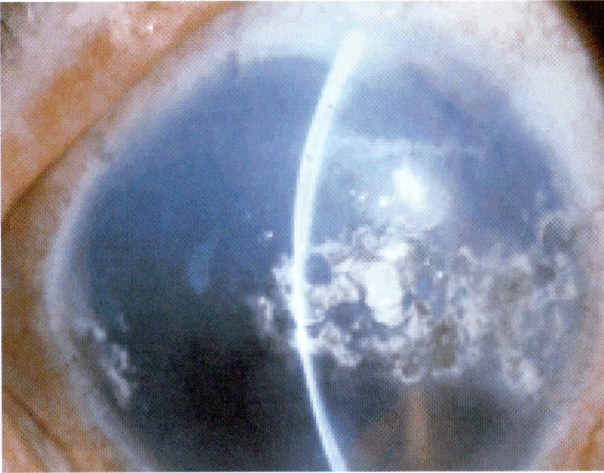

FIGURE 11.3 Band Keratopathy.

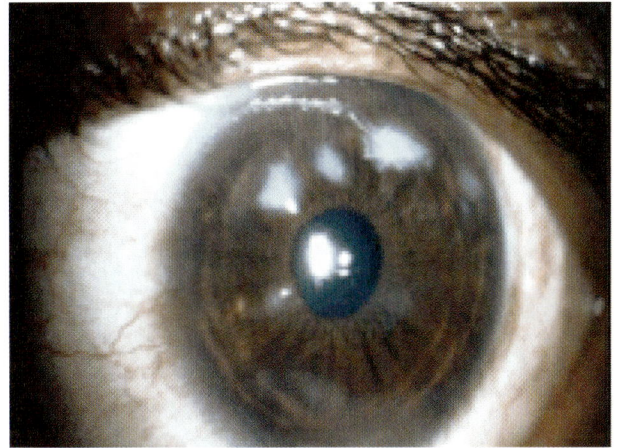

FIGURE 11.4 Salzmann's Nodular Degeneration.

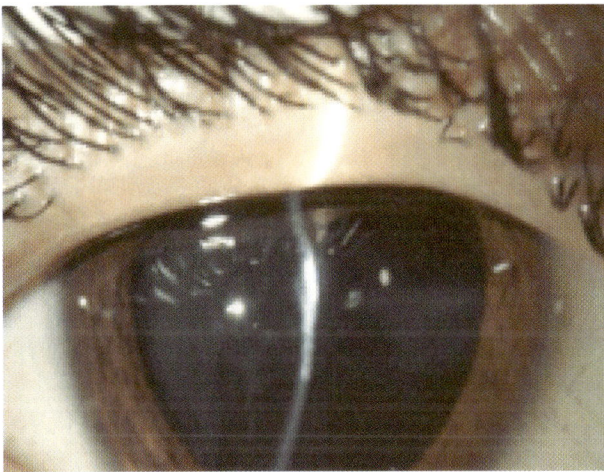

FIGURE 11.5 Scar within the Anterior 100 Microns.

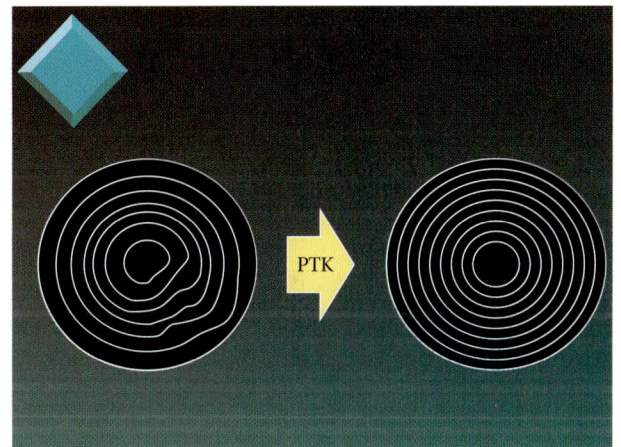

FIGURE 11.6 Topographic Smoothing Utilizing PTK.

Surgical Procedure and Application of Laser

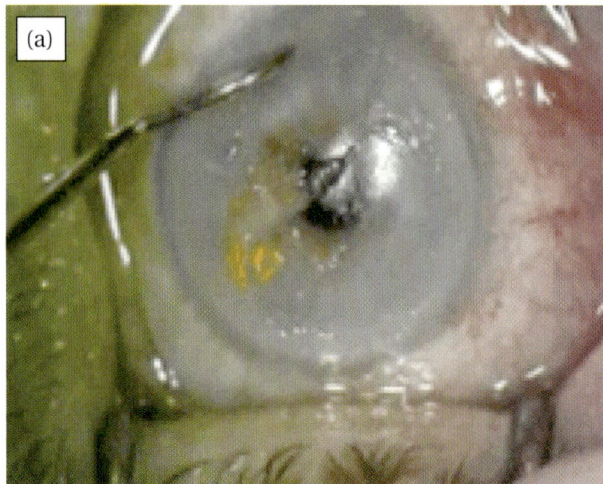

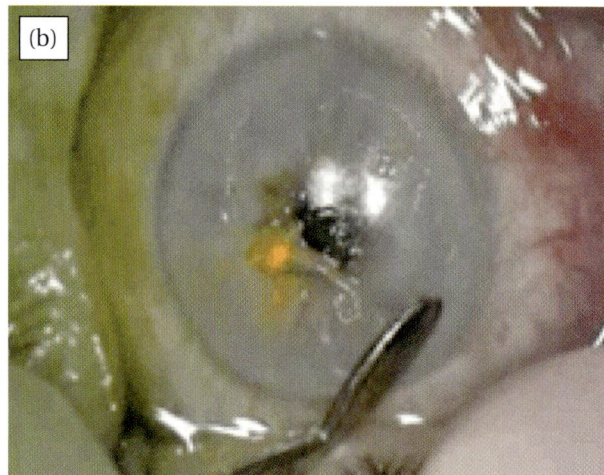

FIGURE 11.7 **Epithelial Removal**. (a, b) After application of topical anesthetic, corneal epithelium is removed using a Maloney blunt spatula.

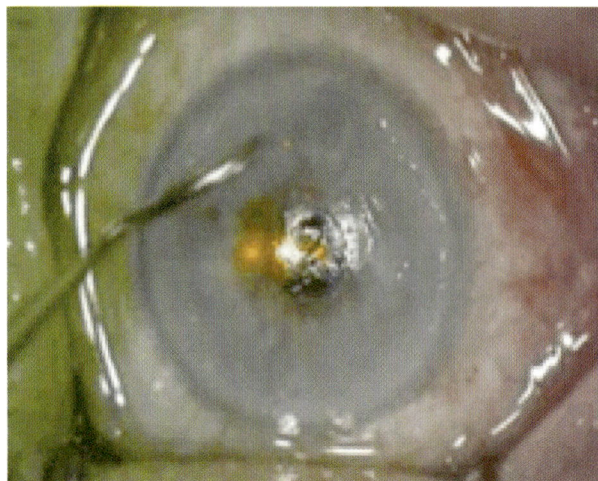

FIGURE 11.8 **Mechanical Surface Preparation**. Anterior stromal opacities are removed, and the corneal surface is mechanically polished using a Maloney blunt spatula or 64 Beaver blade. It is preferable to remove as much of the pathology as possible mechanically and only use the laser as a means for a final smoothing or polishing.

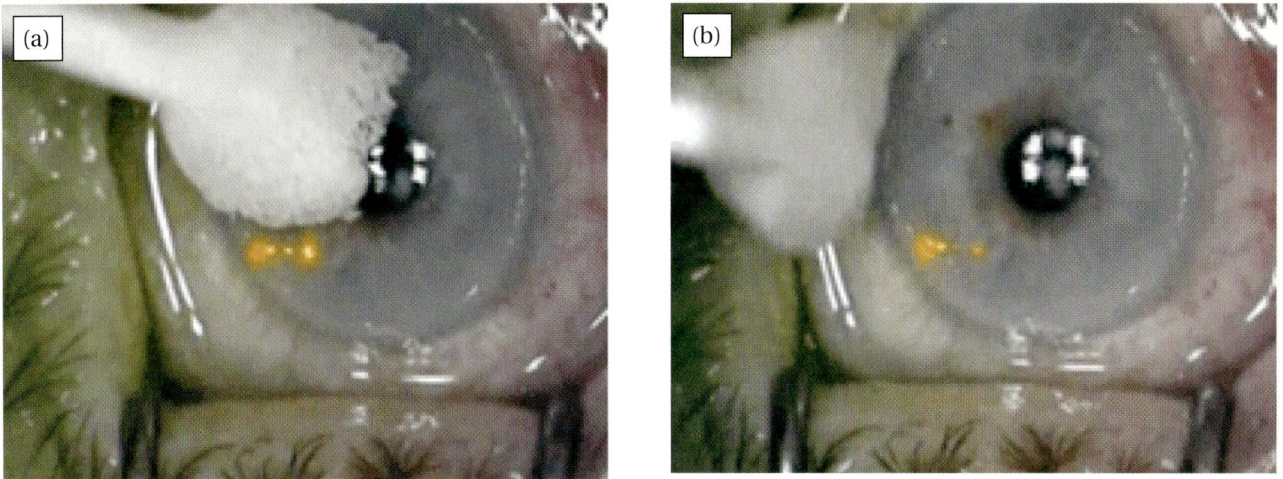

FIGURE 11.9 **Applying Masking Agents**. (a, b) A thin film of smoothing or masking agent (e.g., methylcellulose 1–2%) is applied to the cornea with a spearhead sponge to neutralize the irregular surface and achieve a smooth ablation zone. Only apply enough masking agent to barely cover any elevations or surface abnormalities. The masking agent should only be reapplied if obvious dry spots are present during treatment.

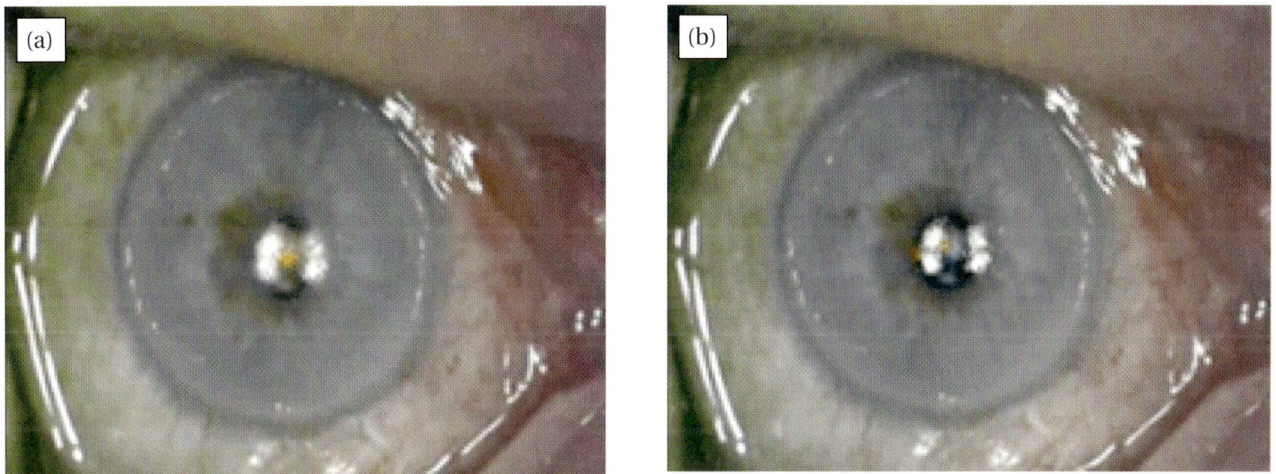

FIGURE 11.10 **Excimer Laser Ablation**. (a, b) Excimer laser emitting high-energy ultraviolet radiation of wavelength 193 nm is applied to the designated ablation zone. Use the least amount of laser energy possible to smooth the corneal surface. The depth should be just sufficient to ablate the lesion or irregularity, usually the equivalent of –0.50 diopters or 12–24 microns of laser ablation after the majority of the pathology is removed mechanically with a spatula or blade. If the masking agent is used minimally as described above, it should not alter treatment depth. A maximum beam width should be used across at least a 6.5 mm optical zone (OZ), preferably with peripheral blending to a 9.0 mm OZ to apply an even treatment and avoid refractive power change. Tracking or manual spot delivery may be used and applied with either a broad beam or flying spot laser. The use of a masking agent to smooth irregularities and the uniform delivery of the laser with a wide optical zone will decrease the chance of irregular astigmatism and refractive error change.

Postoperative Considerations

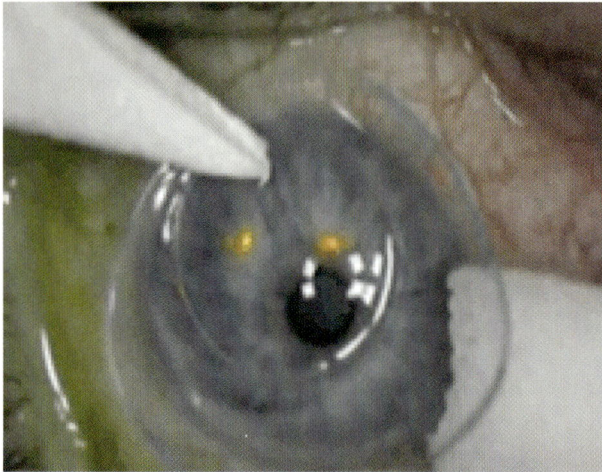

FIGURE 11.11 Procedure Completion and Postoperative Care. A Bandage contact lens is placed. Mitomycin-C is not routinely used for minimal ablations. For deep ablations (>100 microns), mitomycin-C can be applied for 10–12 seconds after the laser treatment to prevent the formation of haze. Postoperative topical antibiotics (fourth generation fluoroquinolone), nonsteroidal anti-inflammatory agents, and steroids are administered during the postoperative period.

TABLE 11.3 *Complications*

Hyperopic shift

Delayed epithelialization
Bacterial or viral keratitis
Recurrence of pathology
Irregular surface
Sub-epithelial haze

SELECTED REFERENCE

Stasi K, Chuck R. Update on phototherapeutic keratectomy. *Curr Opin Ophthalmol.* 2009;20:272–275.

12   Corneal Inlays

Daniel S. Durrie, MD, Richard Lindstrom, MD, and Joel Hunter, MD

TABLE 12.1 *Indications for the Procedure*

Indication	Example
Refractive error	Myopia
	Hyperopia
	Astigmatism
Presbyopia	
Corneal pathology	Keratoconus

TABLE 12.2 *Types of Corneal Inlays*

Mechanism	Example
Change Corneal Curvature	Intacs—Additions Technologies
	Presbylens—ReVision Optics
	Keratophakia (historical)
Change Corneal Power	Polysulfones (historical)
	Chiron Hydrogel Inlay (historical)
	BioVision
	Presbia
Change Depth of Focus	Kamra—Acufocus

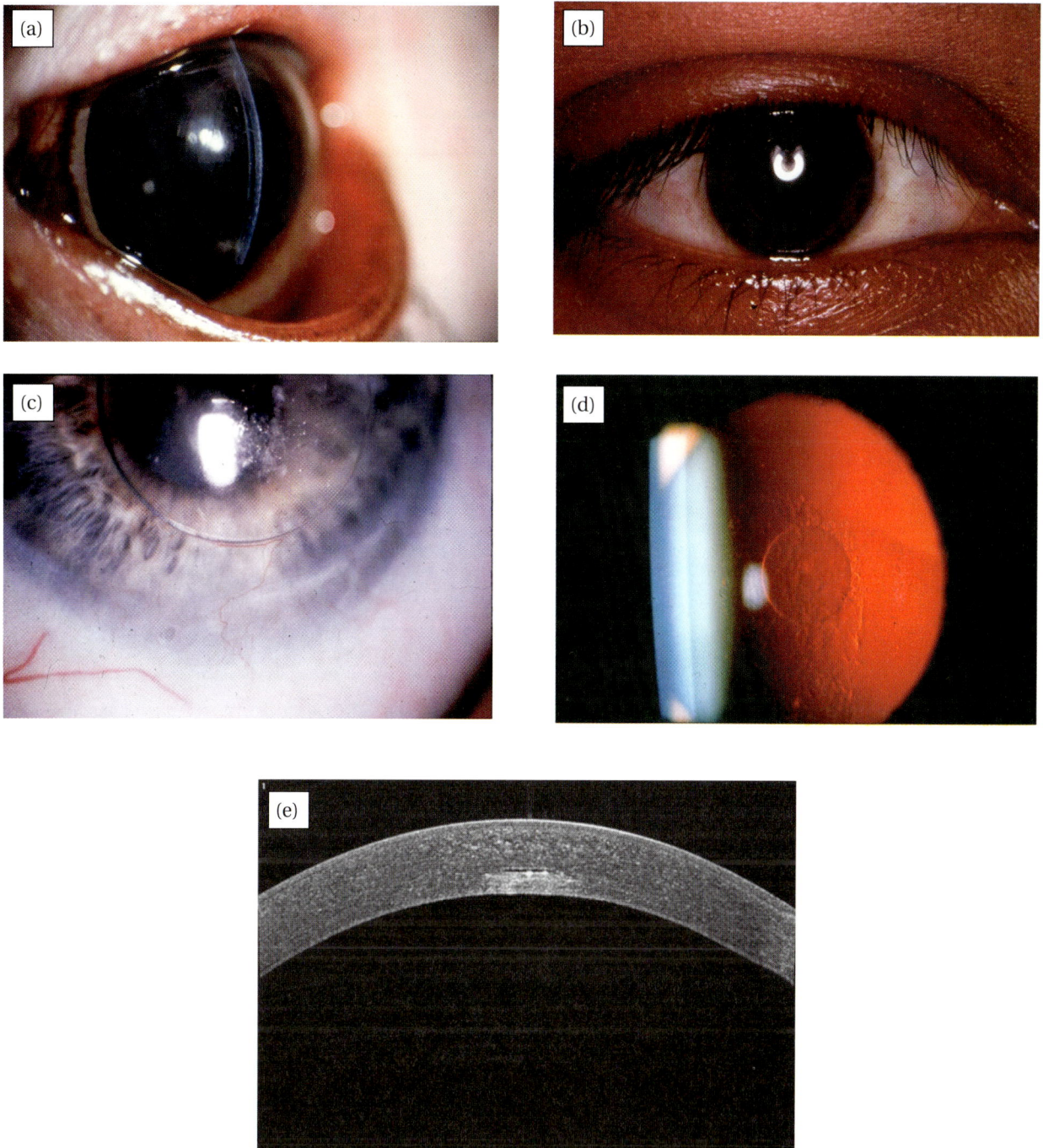

FIGURE 12.1 Previous corneal inlays had complications secondary to impaired corneal metabolism caused by blockage of gradient flow from the aqueous through the corneal stroma. Historical corneal implants including complications. (a) Well-tolerated hydrogel 4-years post-op in a monkey. (b) Well-tolerated polysulfide inlay. (c) Corneal neovascularization in response to polysulfide implant with epithelial breakdown. (d) Well-tolerated Chiron inlay 1 month post-op. (e) OCT showing Chiron inlay 16 years post-op. (Images courtesy of: [a–d] Bernie McCarey PhD and Peter Choyce MD; [e] Daniel Durrie MD.)

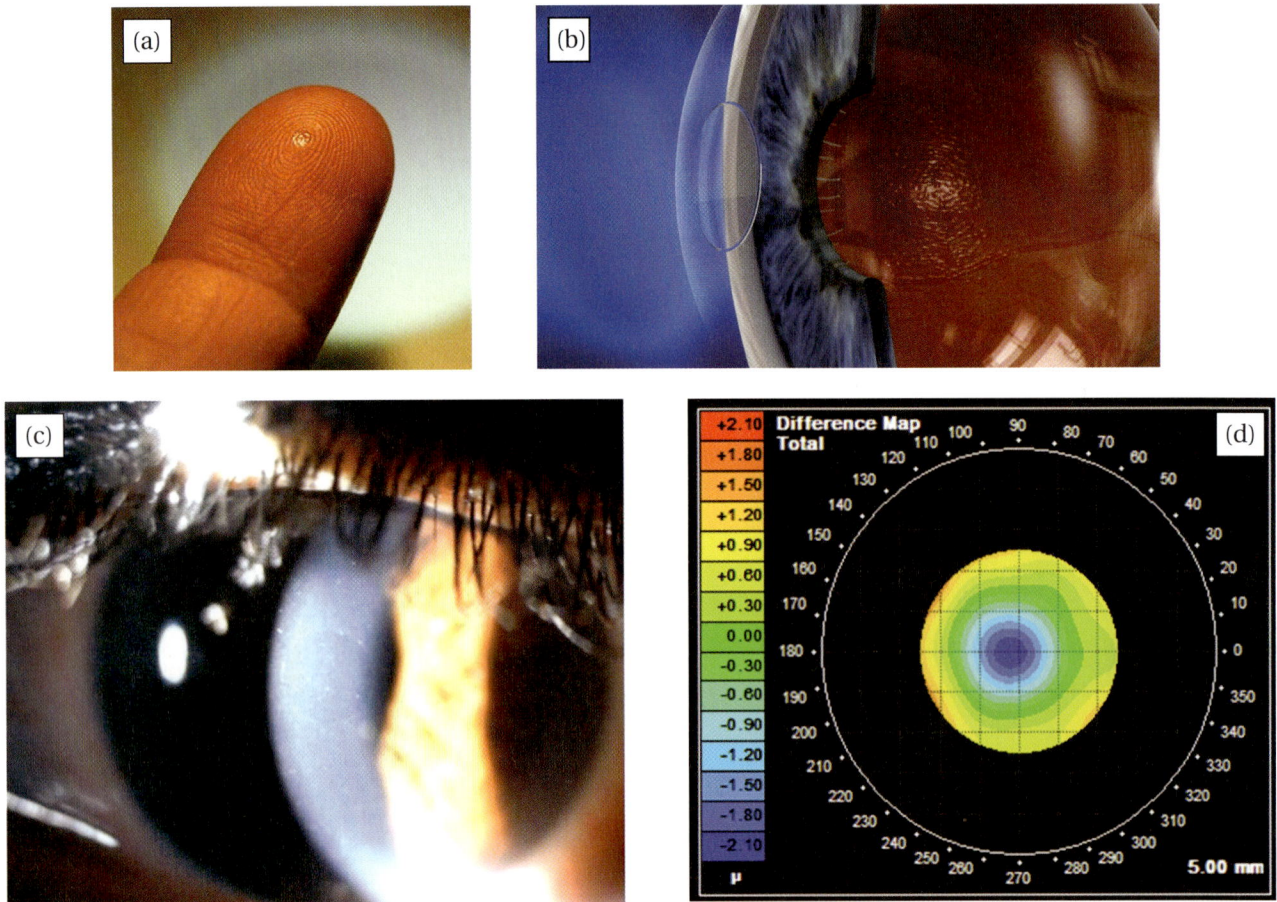

FIGURE 12.2 Corneal inlays implanted in the anterior stroma can change the corneal curvature to increase corneal power centrally and improve near vision in presbyopic patients. The Prebylens by ReVision Optics increases the anterior corneal curvature to add power to the central cornea. (a) 2 mm and 30 micron thick Presbylens on a fingertip. (b) Illustration of Presbylens implant position in cornea. (c) Slit lamp photo of Presbylens centered in anterior corneal stroma. (d) Wavefront difference map from subtraction two Tracey iTrace scans of the same cornea preoperatively and postoperatively. (Images courtesy of: [a–d] Stephen Slade M.D. and Revision Optics).

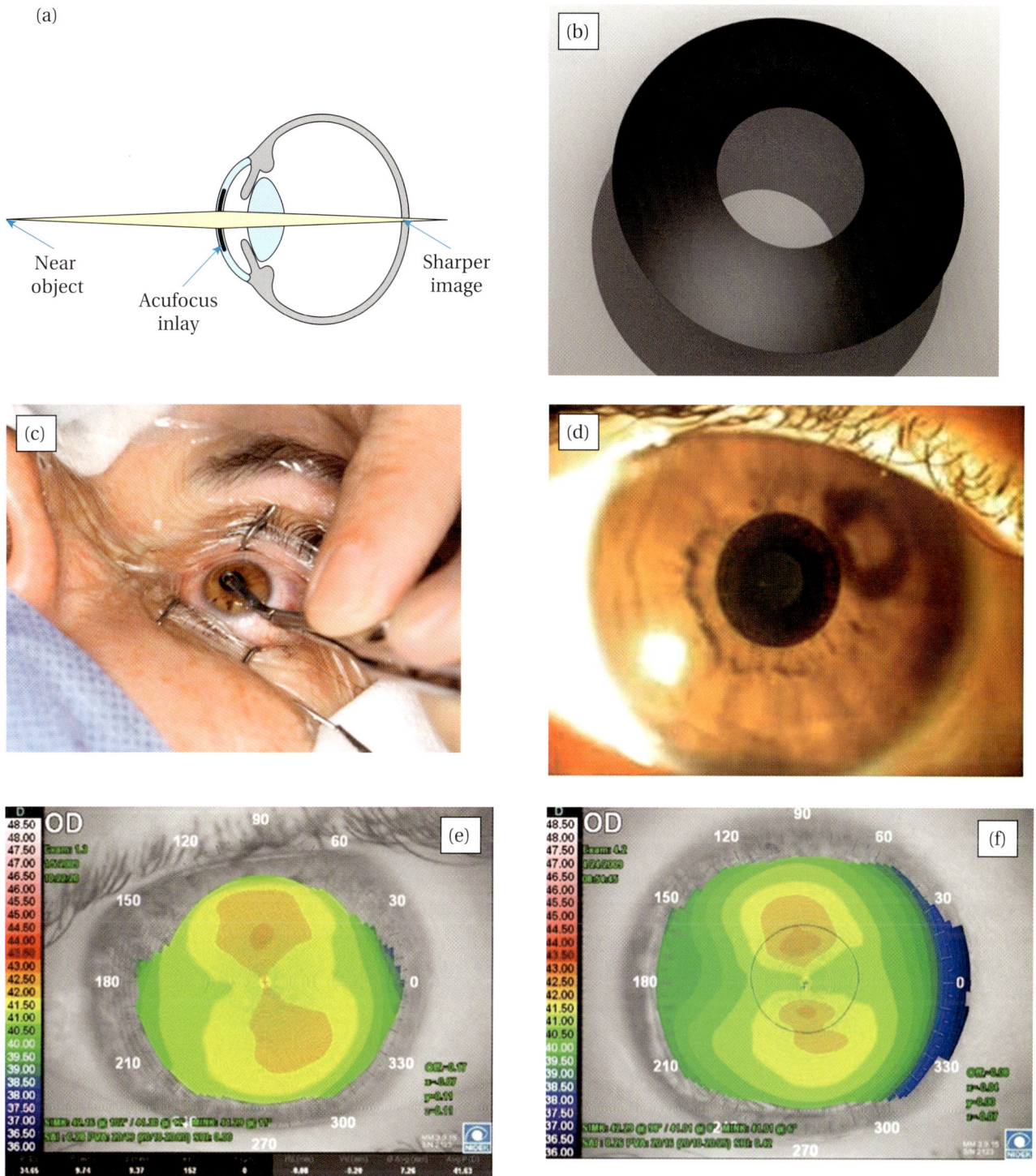

FIGURE 12.3 By creating small aperture optics, the Kamra by Acufocus increases the depth of focus in a presbyopic eye. (a) Schematic of Kamra inlay by Acufocus showing small aperture optics to increase depth of focus using a (b) 1.6 mm central aperture in 3.8 mm inlay with a 5 micron thickness. There are 8400 micro-perforations to enable gradient flow of stromal nutrients. (c) Implantation of Kamra in 200 micron deep corneal pocket with temporal wound edge. This is created by femtosecond laser technology. (d) Eye implanted with Kamra. There is little to no change in corneal topography from (e) preoperative to (f) 6 months postoperatively. Optical quality analysis system (OQAS) laser interferometry demonstrates improved depth of focus in a 49-year-old patient's.

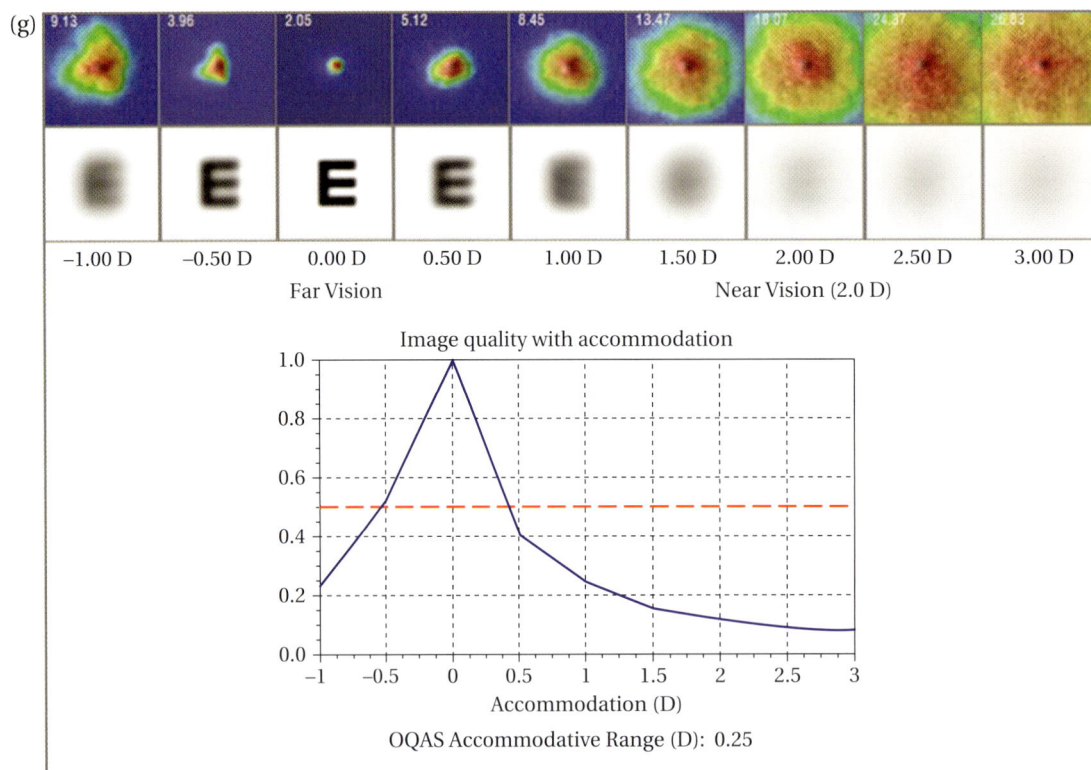

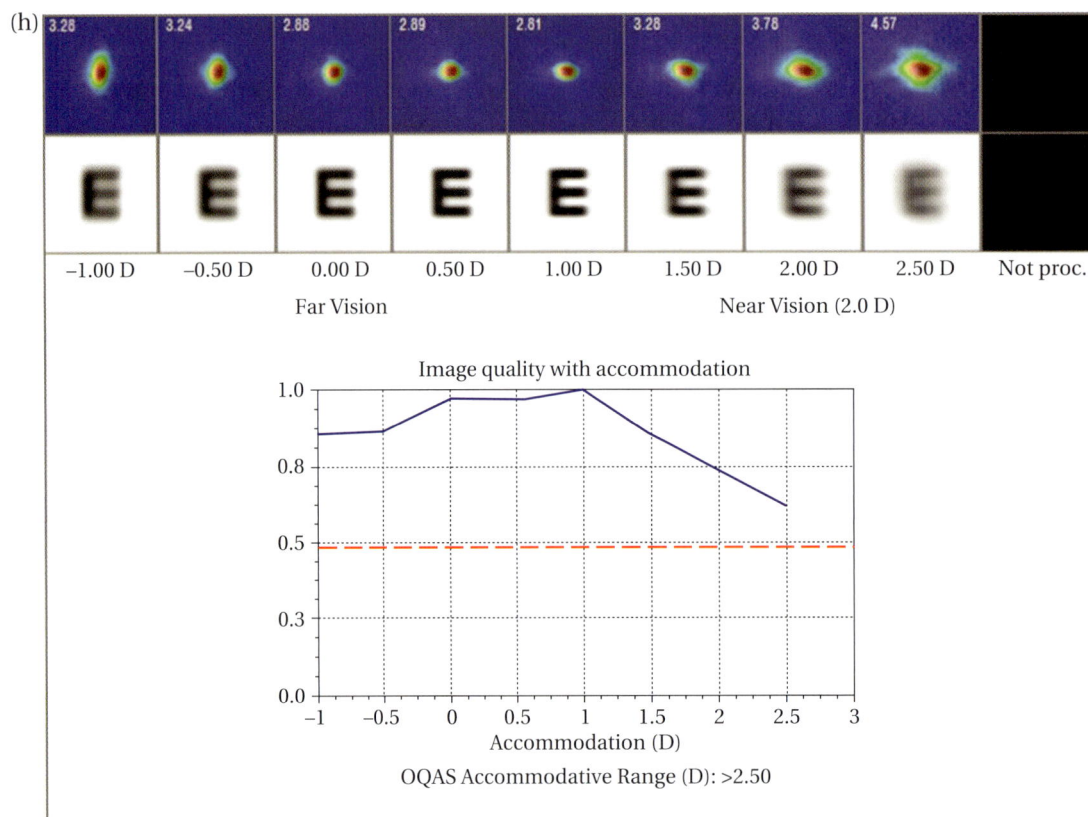

FIGURE 12.3 (*continued*) (g) non-operative left eye and (h) Kamra-implanted right eye. (Images courtesy of: [a–h] Acufocus.)

TABLE 12.3 *Complications*

Complication	Cause
Anterior stromal necrosis	Poor nutrient flow
Corneal neovascularization	Corneal ischemia
Decentration of device	Operator error
Interface opacity	Healing haze, debris

SELECTED REFERENCES

Alió JL, Mulet ME, Zapata LF, Vidal MT, De Rojas V, Javaloy J. Intracorneal inlay complicated by intrastromal epithelial opacification. *Arch Ophthalmol.* 2004 Oct;122(10):1441–1446.

Barraquer JI. Modification of refraction by means of intracorneal inclusions. *Int Ophthalmol Clin.* 1966;6:53–78.

Barraquer JI. Queratoplatica Refractiva. Estudios e informaciones. *Oftalnologicas* 1949; 2:10.

Choyce P. The present status of intracorneal implants. *J Cat Ophth.* 1968;3:295.

Dohlman CH, Refojo MF, Rose J. Synthetic polymers in corneal surgery: glyceryl methacylate. *Arch Ophthalmol.* 1967; 177:52–58.

Klyce SD, Dingeldein SA, Bonanno JA, McDonald MB, Kaufman HE. Hydrogel implants: Evaluation of first human trial. *Invest Ophthalmol Vis Sci Suppl.* 1988;29:393.

Klyce SD, Russell SR. Numerical solution of coupled transport equations applied to corneal hydration dynamics. *J Physiol.* 1979;292:107–134.

Larrea X, De Courten C, Feingold V, Burger J, Büchler P. Oxygen and glucose distribution after intracorneal lens implantation. *Optom Vis Sci.* 2007 Dec;84(12):1074–1081.

McCarey BE. Alloplastic Refractive Keratoplasty. In: Sanders DR, Hofmann RF, Salz JJ, eds. *Refractive Corneal Surgery.* SLACK Inc. 1986:531–548.

Mulet ME, Alio JL, Knorz MC. Hydrogel intracorneal inlays for the correction of hyperopia: outcomes and complications after 5 years of follow-up. *Ophthalmology.* 2009 Aug;116(8):1455–1460.

Seyeddain O, Riha W, Hohensinn M, Nix G, Dexl AK, Grabner G. Refractive surgical correction of presbyopia with the AcuFocus small aperture corneal inlay: two-year follow-up. *J Refract Surg.* 2010 Oct;26:1–9.

Werblin TP, Patel AS, Barraquer JI. Initial human experience with Permalens myopic hydrogel intracorneal lens implants. *Refract Corneal Surg.* 1992;8:23–26.

Yilmaz OF, Bayraktar S, Agca A, Yilmaz B, McDonald MB, van de Pol C. Intracorneal inlay for the surgical correction of presbyopia. *J Cataract Refract Surg.* 2008 Nov;34(11):1921–1927.

13

Corneal Relaxing Incisions

Elizabeth Yeu, MD, Mitchell P. Weikert, MD, MS and Douglas Koch, MD

Complications

SELECTED REFERENCES

TABLE 13.1 *Indications for Corneal Relaxing Incisions*

Regular corneal astigmatism

In eyes undergoing cataract surgery

In phakic eyes to treat mixed astigmatic refractive error

Regular astigmatism following corneal transplant surgery

No evidence of peripheral corneal thinning disorder

No evidence of ectasia

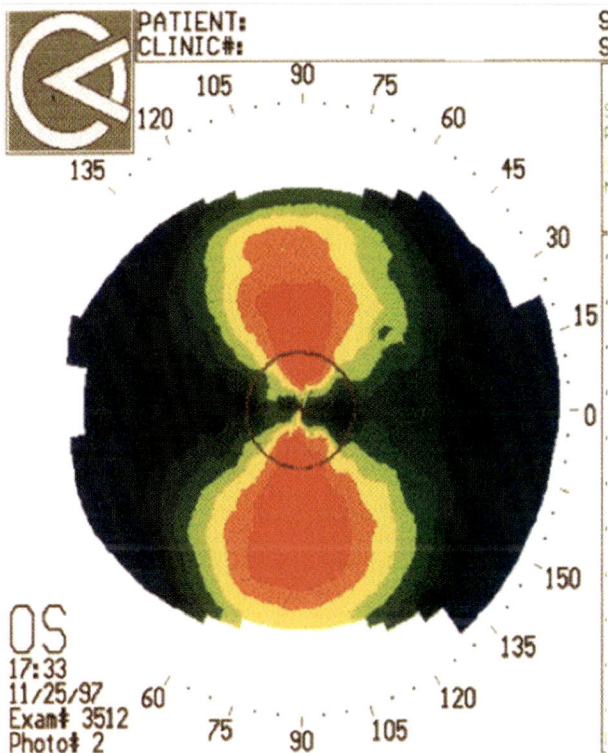

FIGURE 13.1 Astigmatism is a condition in which light passing through a lens system is not focused to a single point. Astigmatism may be regular or irregular, and in the phakic eye can be produced by the cornea and/or the lens. Regular astigmatism occurs when the curvature of the steep and flat meridia is relatively constant throughout its course and the steep and flat meridia are oriented 90 degrees apart, or "orthogonal." Corneal relaxing incisions can effectively correct regular corneal astigmatism. The figure shows a corneal topographic map demonstrating regular, with-the-rule (i.e., steep along vertical meridian) astigmatism.

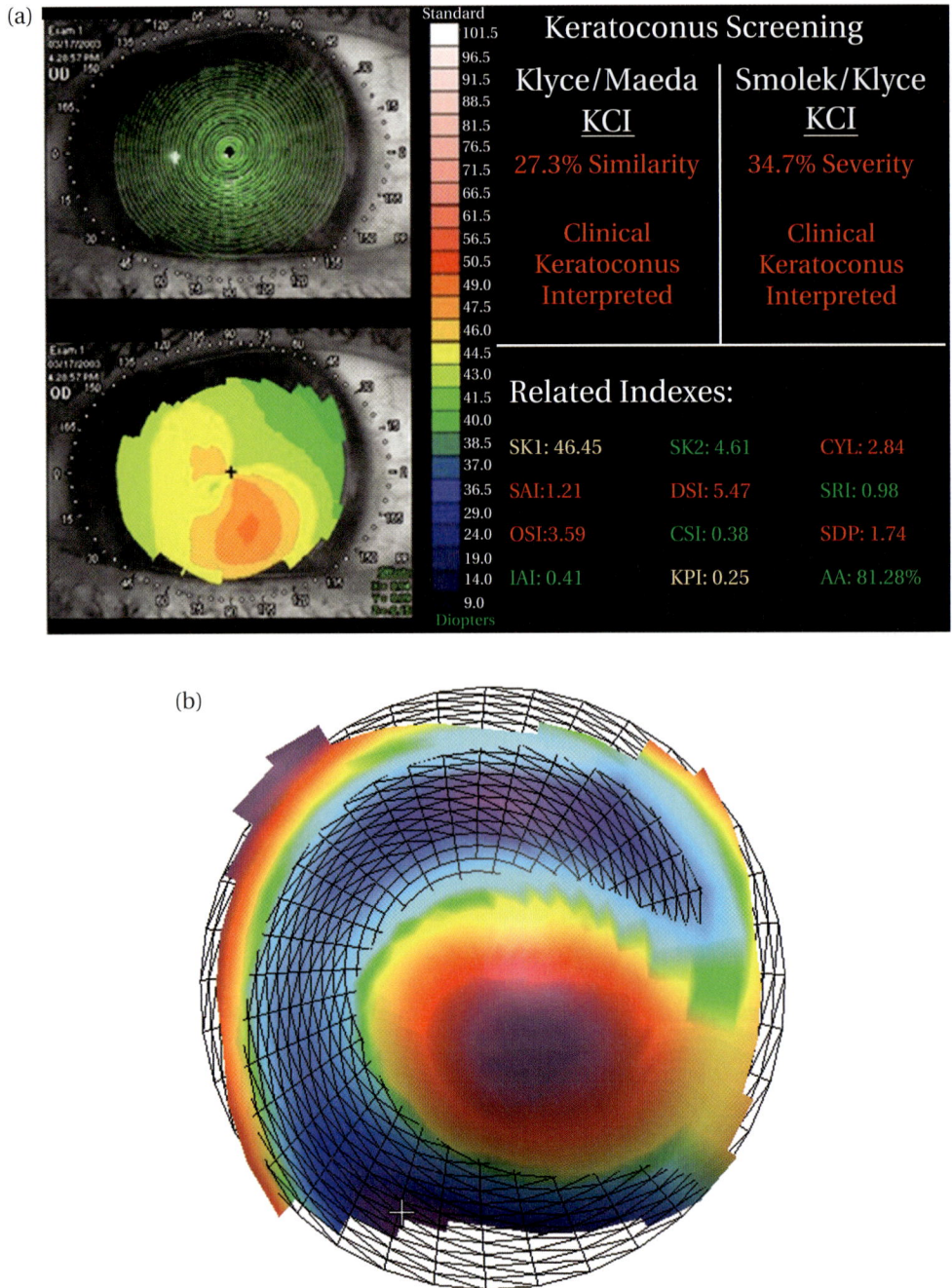

FIGURE 13.2 Astigmatism is considered *irregular* when the steep and flat meridia are unevenly distributed throughout the cornea, deviating from the classic, symmetric "bowtie" appearance. In general, relaxing incisions should not be used (or used with great caution) to correct irregular astigmatism. Doing so may increase corneal irregularity and/or further destabilize the cornea. These corneal topographic images demonstrate irregular astigmatism with (a) an asymmetric bowtie and (b) inferior steepening, specifically in the setting of keratoconus.

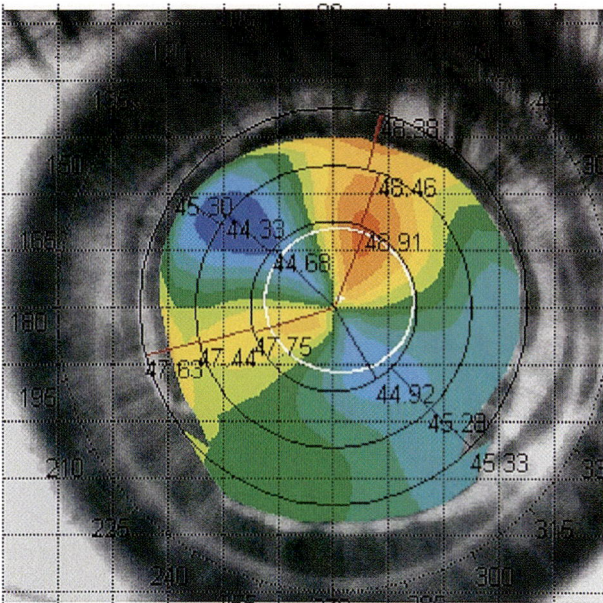

FIGURE 13.3 Irregular astigmatism also exists when the two meridia of curvature are skewed, or "non-orthogonal" (i.e., no longer 90 degrees apart).

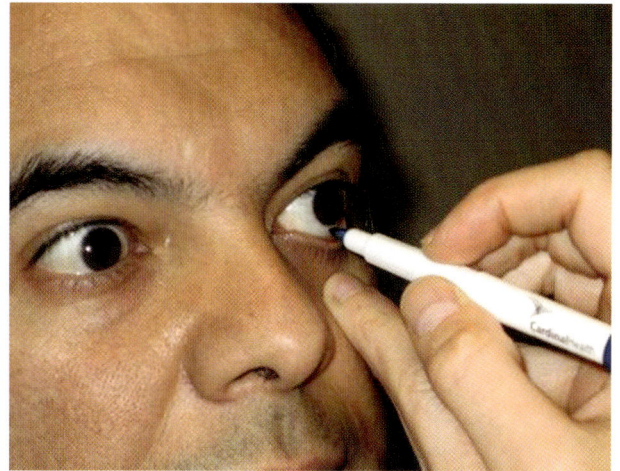

FIGURE 13.4 In preparation for performing corneal relaxing incisions , mark 2 points along either the 90 degree (12, 6 o'clock) or 180 degree (3, 9 o'clock) meridia on the patient's limbus while the patient is sitting upright and fixing straight ahead with the operative eye. Alternatively, one can identify prominent landmarks along the horizontal or vertical meridia of the conjunctiva, cornea, or iris; these landmarks will serve as a reference for identifying the steep meridian during surgery. The reference points are essential for proper alignment since cyclotorsion of the eye commonly occurs when moving from an upright to a supine position.

AE-2811S Koch LRI Marker II
• Marks in degrees of 45°, 60° and 80°
• Diameter 10.5mm

AE-2814 Kraff-Zaldivar LRI Marker
• Marks arcuate segments for chord lengths of 5.5mm & 7.5mm
• Diameter 10.5mm

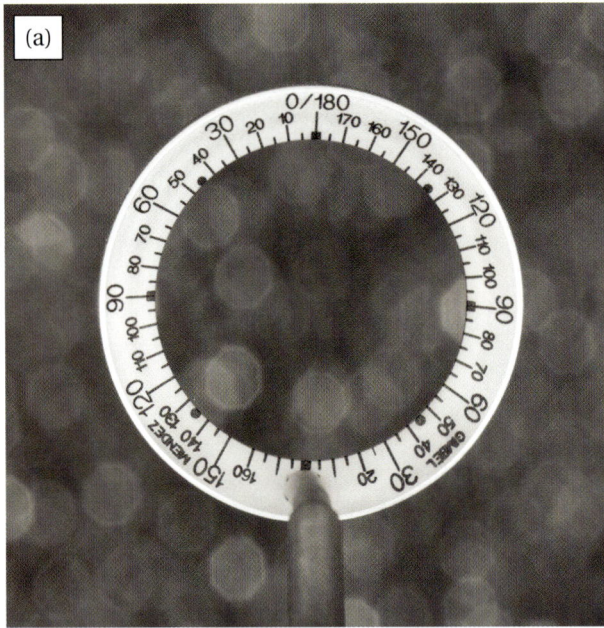

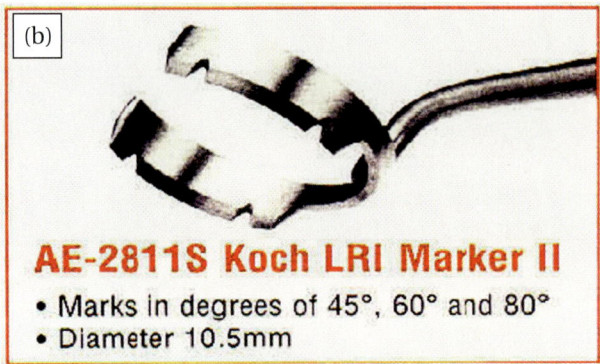

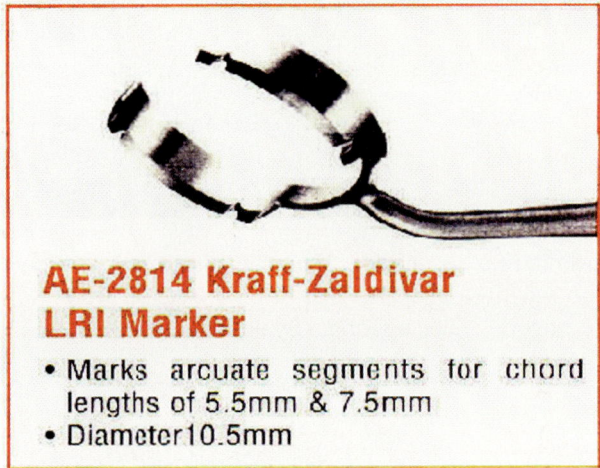

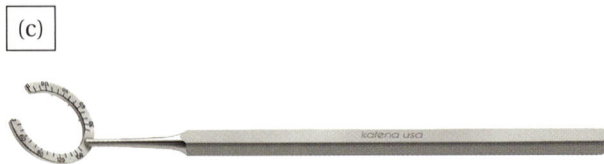

FIGURE 13.5 Many types of astigmatic markers are available, labeled in either millimeters or degrees, depending on which type of nomogram is utilized. (a) Gimbel Mendez Ring (Mastel). (b) Koch LRI Marker II (Asico) (top) and Kraff-Zaldivar LRI Marker (Asico) (bottom). (c) Lu-Mendez LRI Marker (Katena).

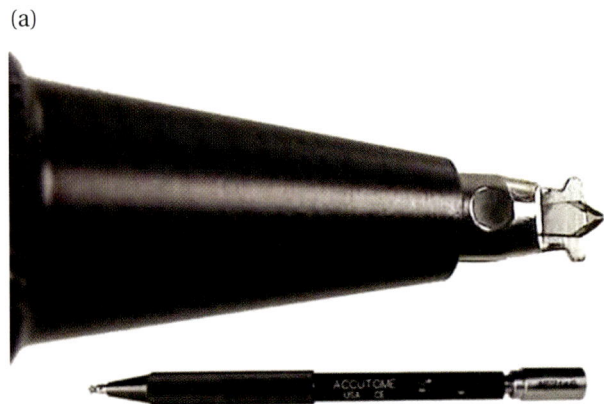

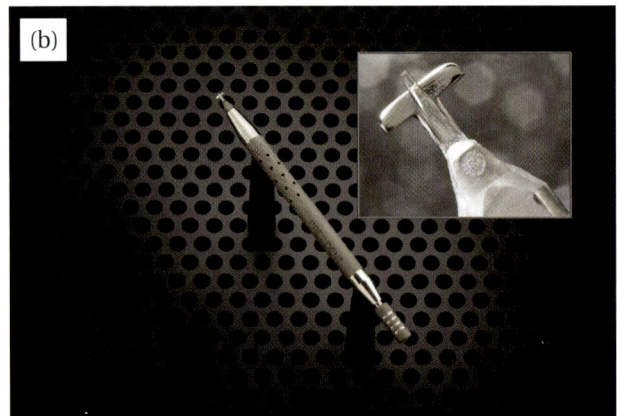

FIGURE 13.6 Various AK knives are available. Figures (a) and (b) demonstrate 600-micron preset diamond knives. (a) Rubenstein LRI Diamond Knife (Accutome). (b) Nichamin Classic 600 Scalpel (Mastel). Diamond knives with adjustable depths are also available.

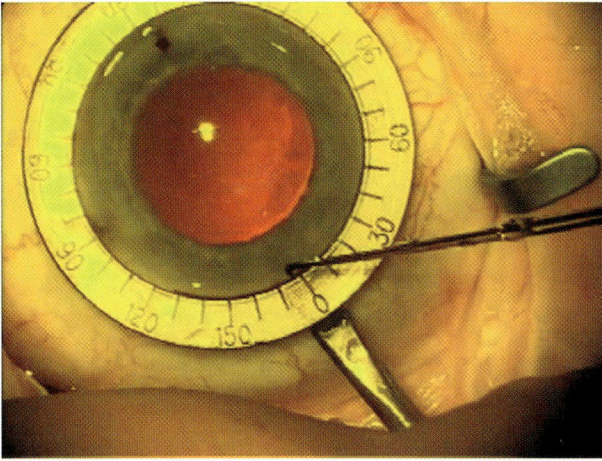

FIGURE 13.7 Intraoperatively, the premarked limbal 90 degree and 180 degree meridia serve as the reference points for the astigmatic gauge or marker. The patient's steep meridian can then be identified and marked. Here, the steep meridian is at 178 degrees.

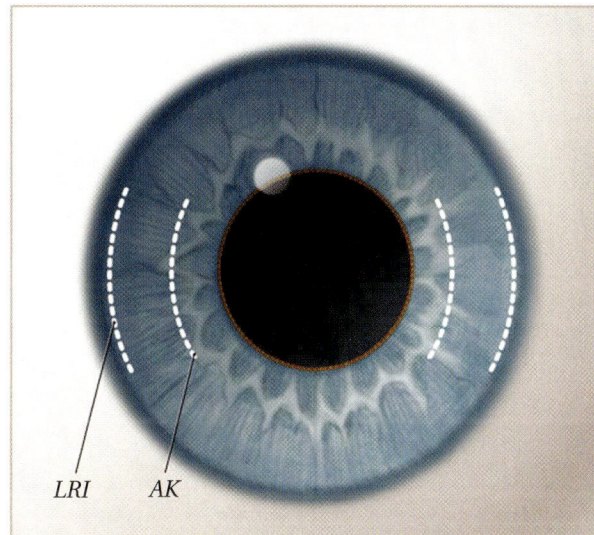

LRI   AK

FIGURE 13.8 Regarding corneal relaxing incisions, nomograms exist for both *astigmatic keratotomy* (AK) and *peripheral corneal relaxing incisions* (PCRI), which are also referred to as *limbal relaxing incisions* (LRI). In both procedures, incisions are typically made to a depth of 90%–95% in the cornea in order to flatten the steep meridian. The basic principles of astigmatic correction hold true with both types of keratotomy surgeries: a greater effect is achieved with longer incisions, smaller optical zones, and deeper incisions, and in older patients. Hence, the more central AK incisions have a greater effect and can correct upwards of 6–7 diopters of astigmatism. PCRIs have a weaker effect because of their more peripheral location, and generally can correct 2–3 diopters of astigmatism. Because the incisions are made closer to the limbus, they may heal faster; thus, the refractive effect stabilizes more quickly. Given their peripheral location, the coupling ratio (flattening in meridian of incision and steepening in the orthogonal meridian) is usually 1:1. Furthermore, patients experience less irregular astigmatism, glare, and foreign body sensation as compared to their more central counterparts. Technically, PCRIs are easier to perform, and are more forgiving as well.

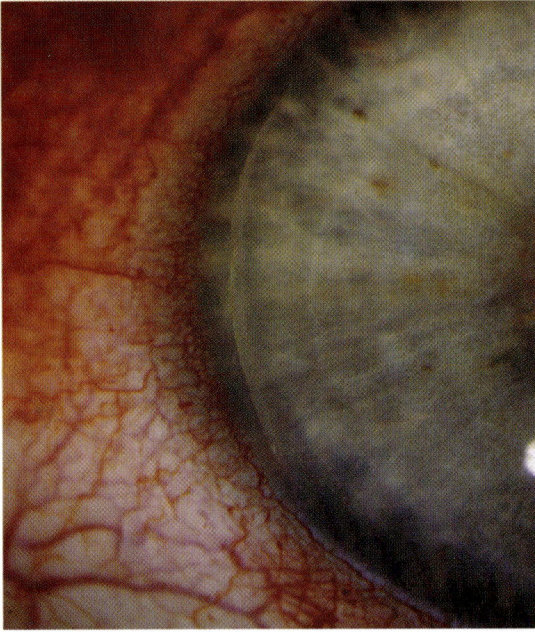

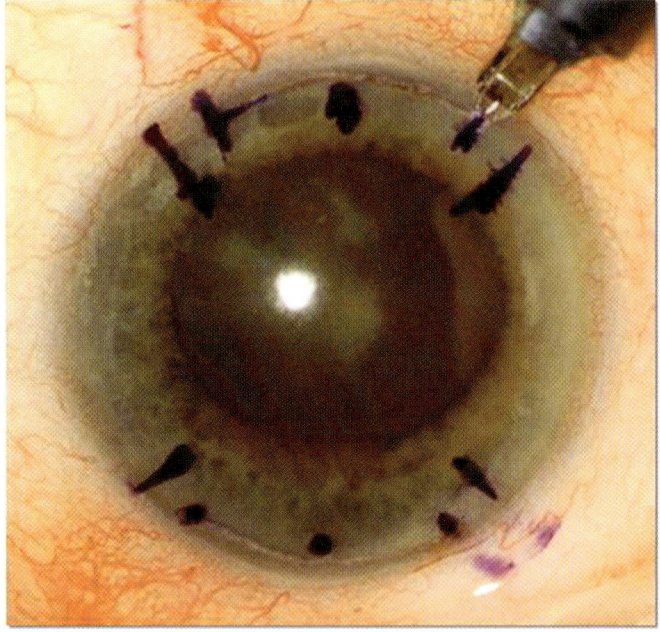

FIGURE 13.9 PCRIs should be placed within the peripheral cornea, inside of the surgical limbus. Depending on the nomogram and the amount of the patient's astigmatism, single or paired incisions may be required. In creating the incision, the knife should be held perpendicular to the corneal surface. (a) Single PCRI. (b) Paired 6-mm PCRIs.

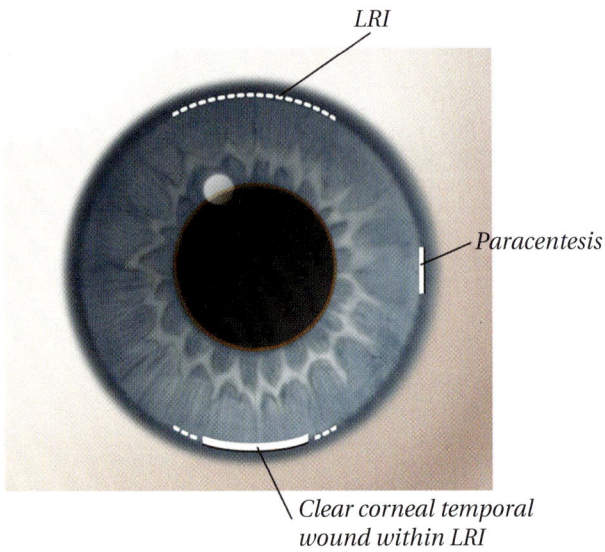

LRI

Paracentesis

Clear corneal temporal wound within LRI

FIGURE 13.10 In the correction of against-the-rule astigmatism during cataract surgery, a single PCRI can be created nasally, so as to not interfere with the temporal surgical wound. If paired PCRIs are indicated, create the clear corneal temporal wound at the beginning of the case as usual, after identifying the steep meridian and intended length of the relaxing incisions. After the cataract surgery is performed, prior to stromal hydration, extend the length of the temporal wound with the diamond knife on either side until the desired PCRI length and location are achieved.

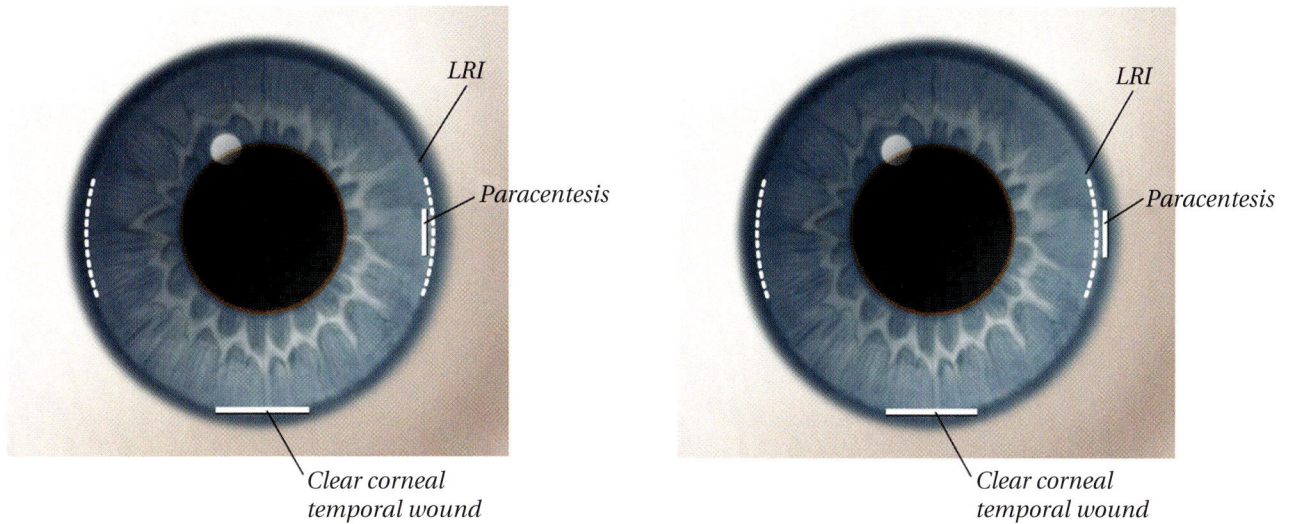

FIGURE 13.11 In the correction of with-the-rule astigmatism during cataract surgery, the PCRI will often be coincident with the location of the paracentesis. The PCRI should not intersect the paracentesis site. Rather, the relaxing incisions should be placed either more peripheral to, or central to the paracentesis site(s). This should be planned out carefully, and the paracentesis wound(s) should be strategically created during the beginning of cataract surgery with the latter PCRIs in mind.

Complications

TABLE 13.2 *Complications of Corneal Relaxing Incisions*

Foreign body sensation

Glare with more central incisions

Decreased corneal sensation

Dry eye syndrome

Infection, inflammation

Undercorrection

Overcorrection: Flipped meridian of astigmatism

Irregular astigmatism

Wound gape, perforation

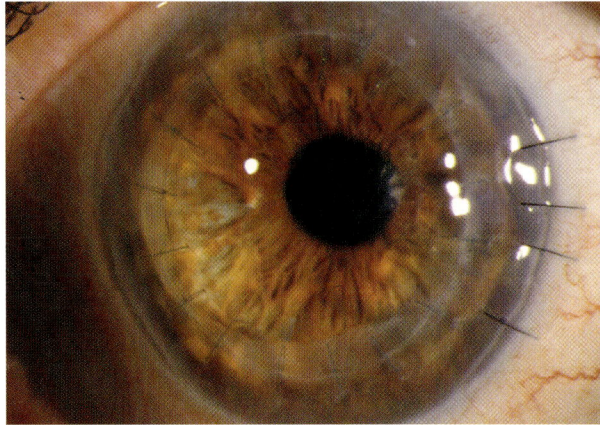

FIGURE 13.12 A preset diamond knife set at 550 or 600 microns is commonly used for PCRIs, although this technique potentially increases the risk of perforation if the cornea possesses an area of peripheral thinning. A trapezoidal blade, as compared to a triangular blade, may increase the risk of perforation. Also, the relaxing incision can leak if it intersects the path of other penetrating wounds, such as a paracentesis site. The photo below demonstrates paired against-the-rule PCRIs that were created intraoperatively at the time of cataract surgery in a Fuchs' dystrophy patient. Secondary to the dense lens, the cornea developed bullous keratopathy post-operatively. At the time of the penetrating keratoplasty, one of the PCRIs gaped open excessively, necessitating suturing.

SELECTED REFERENCES

Price FW, Grene RB et al. Astigmatism reduction clinical trial: a multicenter prospective evaluation of the predictability of arcuate keratotomy. Evaluation of surgical nomogram predictability. ARC-T Study Group. *Arch Ophthalmol.* 1995 Mar;113(3):277–282.

Rowsey JJ. Ten caveats in corneal astigmatism following cataract surgery. *Ophthalmology.* 1983;90:148–155.

Wang L, Misra M, Koch DD. Peripheral corneal relaxing incisions combined with cataract surgery. *J Cat Refract Surg.* 2003 Apr;29(4):712–722.

Yeu E, Rubenstein JB. Management of astigmatism in lens-based surgery. *Focal points: Clinical modules for ophthalmologists.* American Academy of Ophthalmology. 2008:2.

<table>
<tr><td>14</td></tr>
</table>

Phakic IOLs: Angle-supported—AcrySof® Cachet™

Stephen S. Lane, MD

ACKNOWLEDGMENTS

SELECTED REFERENCES

The AcrySof® Cachet™ Phakic Lens (Alcon Laboratories, Inc., Fort Worth, TX) is intended to be positioned in the angle of the anterior chamber of a phakic eye in order to provide refractive correction to patients with moderate to high myopia.

TABLE 14.1 *Recommended Preoperative Indications and Limitations for use of the AcrySof® Cachet™ Phakic Lens.**

Patient Indication/Limitation	Requirement
Age	21 years or older
Anterior chamber depth	≥3.2 mm, including corneal thickness
Mesopic pupil diameter	≤7 mm
Central endothelial cell density	Minimum cell density, cells/mm^2
Age 21–25 years	2800
Age 26–35 years	2600
Age 36–45 years	2200
Age >46 years	2000
Preoperative or expected postoperative astigmatism	≤2.0 D
Manifest refraction history	Stable ± 0.5 D for 1 year prior to surgery
Crystalline lens health	No cataract formation
Corneal health	No dystrophy, transplant, irregularity
Ocular health history	No chronic or recurrent anterior or posterior segment inflammation
	No preexisting ocular conditions which may compromise outcomes

* Based on CE mark labeling, dated 2008.

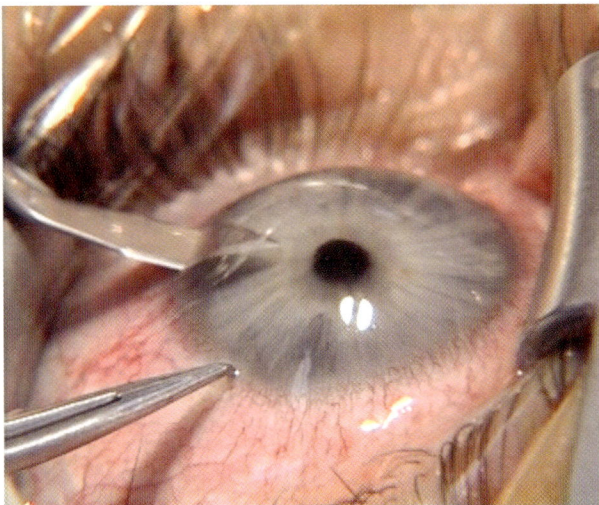

FIGURE 14.1 **Creation of a 2.6-mm Clear Corneal Self-Sealing Incision.** Pupil constriction must be verified; intraocular anesthetic–miotic combination is often injected to assure maximum miosis. A cohesive ophthalmic viscosurgical device is then instilled. Minimal bleeding may be encountered as peripheral limbal vessels are incised. If bimanual irrigation will be used, two 1-mm paracenteses are created.

(a)

"Haptics"

"Bridge"

"Side up" indicator

(b)

¼

¾

P

(c)

(d)

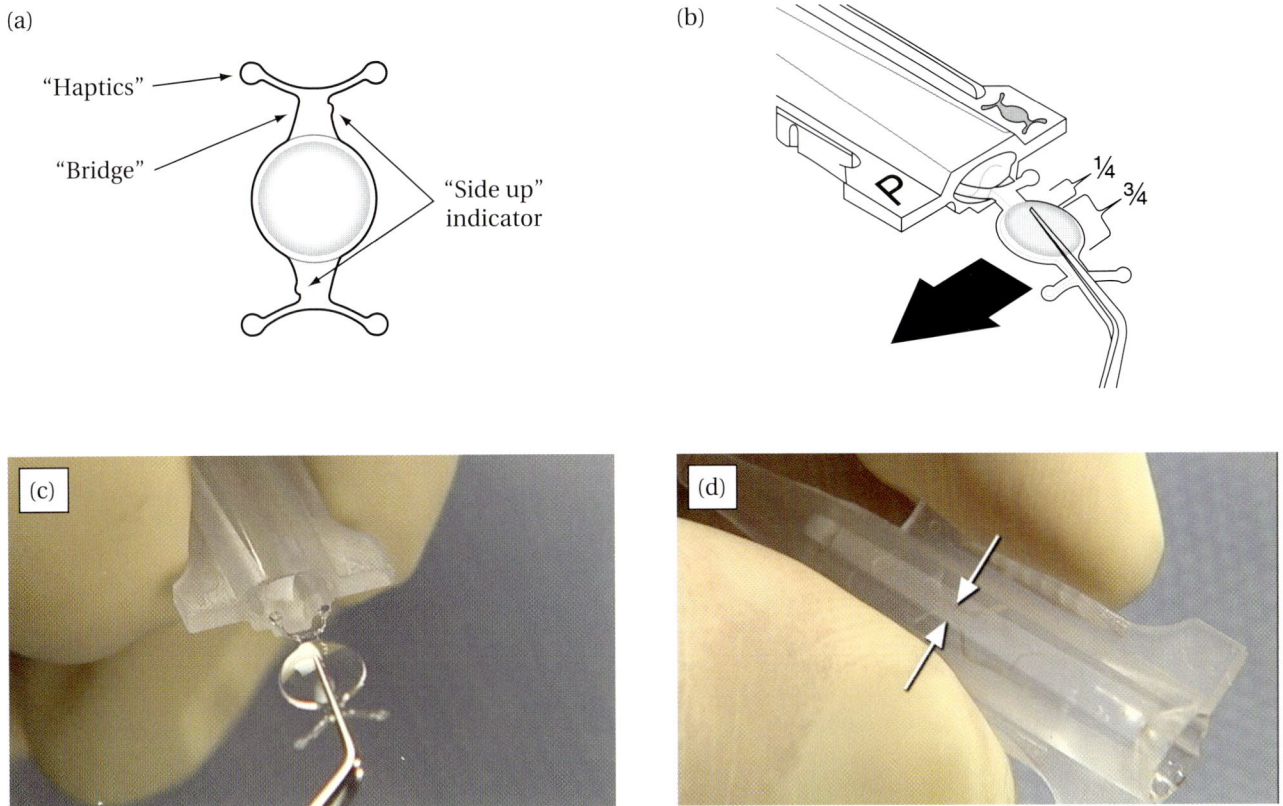

FIGURE 14.2 Loading the Intraocular Lens (IOL) into the Monarch® III P Cartridge (Alcon).
(a) Verify that the optic is right-side up by checking that the lens vaults upward and that the "side-up" indicator marks point to a clockwise direction. The "bump" should be on the right-hand side of the leading bridge. (b) Round-bladed, nonserrated forceps is used to grasp the lens, right side up, with the forceps extending across at least 3/4 of the optic. The lens is held level with a Monarch® III P cartridge that has been prefilled with a room-temperature cohesive ophthalmic viscosurgical device (OVD). One haptic is deflected forward against the inner edge of the cartridge. (c) The second leading haptic is deflected forward against the other inner edge of the cartridge. This creates a "dive" position, as shown in Figure (c). The "dive" position must be shaped before the lens can be inserted into the back of the cartridge. (d) Pushing the lens forward in the cartridge. **Step 1: Inserting the lens into the cartridge.** The lens is inserted slowly into the back of the cartridge, until the trailing haptics reach the edge of the cartridge. The optic edges are allowed to fold upwards and to conform to the shape of the cartridge. The lens then is released and the forceps is retracted. **Step 2: Biasing the lens down**. After closing the forceps, the tip of the forceps is reinserted into the back of the cartridge, on top of the optic, and the bottom surface of the closed forceps is used to induce symmetrically folded curvature in the lens. While pressing the lens downward against the floor of the cartridge with the forceps, the lens is pushed forward until it is completely inside the cartridge. The forceps is first lifted and then retracted, leaving the lens seated in place inside the cartridge. **Step 3: Advancing the lens with the tip of the forceps**. The tip of the closed forceps is reinserted into the back of the cartridge, this time engaging the trailing bridge of the lens. The forceps is glided along the floor of the cartridge while pushing the lens forward as far as the forceps will easily permit. The forceps is then removed. **Step 4: Verifying the lens position in the cartridge**. If the lens has been loaded properly, both optic edges will be visible in a semi-folded position, as shown in this image. If the lens is not in this position, the delivery should not be continued. The loading procedure should be repeated with another lens and cartridge.

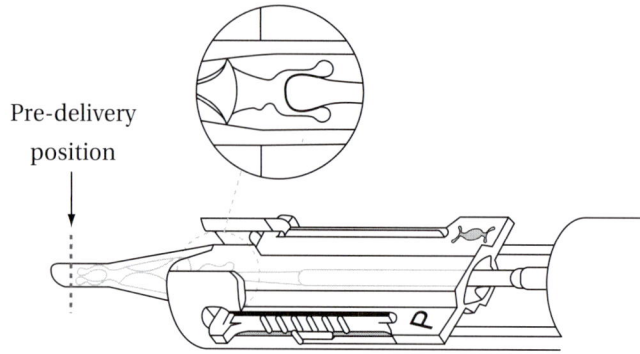

FIGURE 14.3 **Mounting the Loaded Cartridge onto the Handpiece.** The loaded cartridge is placed into the handpiece slot. In the final position, the cartridge "locks" or "clicks." The plunger is slowly advanced forward. The surgeon visually verifies that the plunger tip engages the lens at the edge of the trailing bridge between the haptics (see figure), and ensures that the lens advances slowly and freely. The handpiece knob is pushed until the threads are engaged, and then the knob is advanced clockwise half of a turn. Immediately prior to inserting the nozzle tip through the incision, the lens is advanced to the "ready," pre-delivery position, as shown by the arrow. The leading haptics should be at least 1 mm back from exiting the nozzle tip. **No part** of the lens should exit the cartridge prior to insertion of the cartridge through the incision.

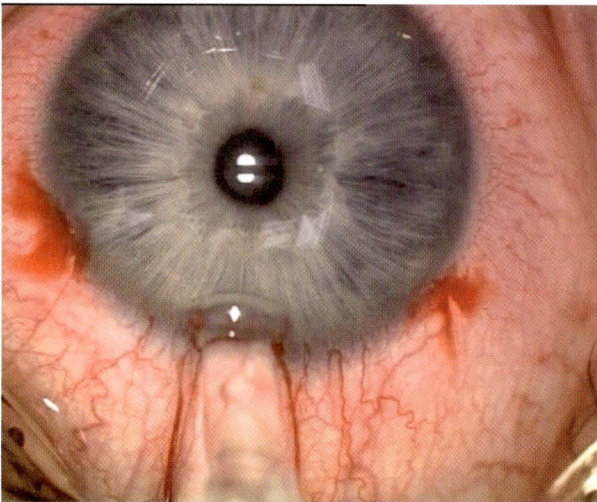

FIGURE 14.4 **The cartridge is placed through the incision completely into the anterior chamber** such that the distal end of the cartridge extends to or just beyond the distal pupil edge.

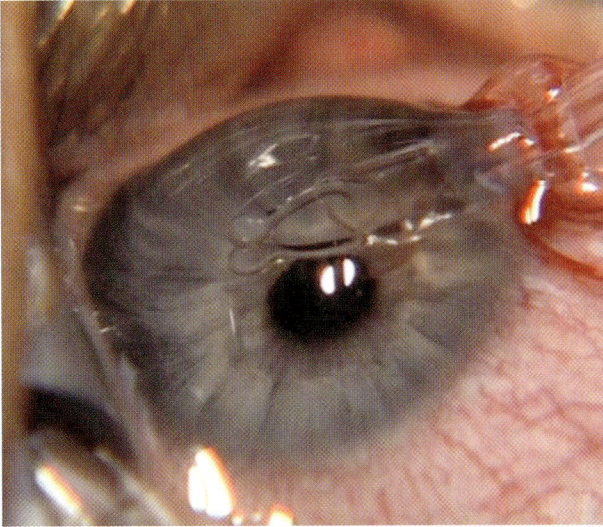

FIGURE 14.5 **The IOL is slowly injected into the eye** by turning the screw mechanism of the injector (Step 1), being sure that the haptics emerge in the dive position and that the IOL fold is facing directly up.

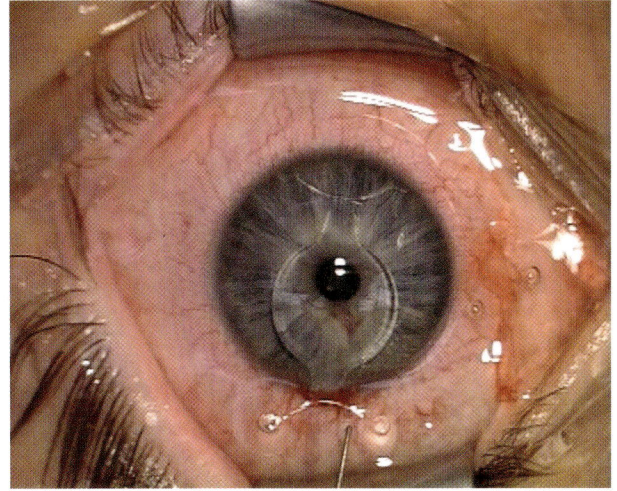

FIGURE 14.6 **Injection of the IOL is completed** when the proximal haptics are expressed out of the injector (Step 2). As the injector is removed from the eye, the proximal IOL haptics should protrude through the incision.

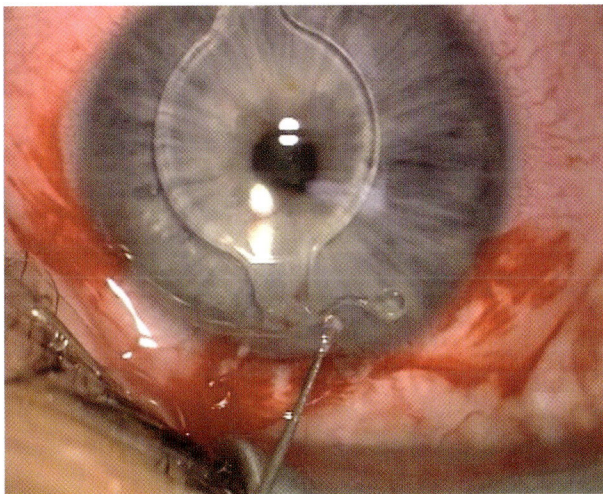

FIGURE 14.7 **A Y-hook is used to place the first haptic through the incision into the angle.**

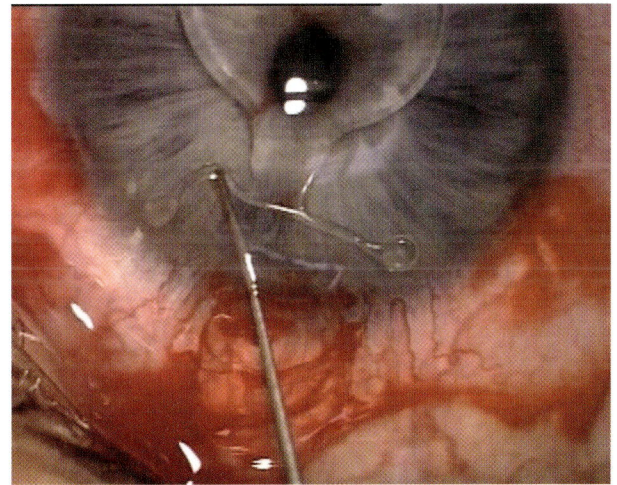

FIGURE 14.8 **Placement of the second haptic through the incision into the angle with Y-hook.**

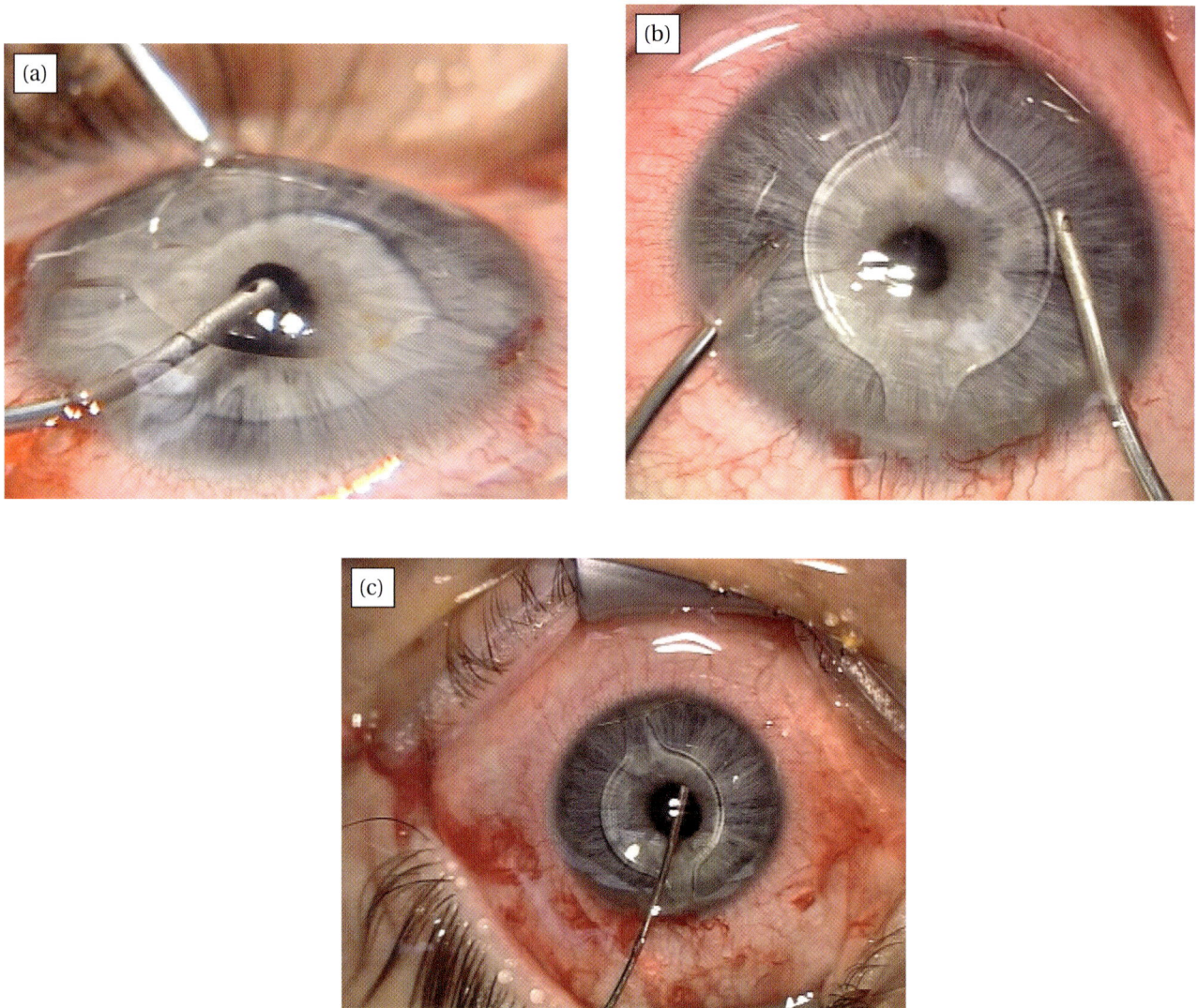

FIGURE 14.9 **Removal of OVD**. Thorough removal of OVD from around and behind the IOL is important. **Option 1**: The 2 paracenteses (as described in Figure 14.1) are used to perform bimanual OVD removal. Place the aspiration port into the eye first and gently rest it on the IOL optic as the irrigating cannula is introduced (with irrigation flowing) second. This prevents any potential movement of the IOL as irrigation is introduced into the eye. Bimanual irrigation/aspiration is used to remove OVD from behind the IOL (a) and around the IOL (b). **Option 2**: (c) Passive irrigation. Alternatively, OVD can be removed using balanced salt solution to flush the OVD out of the anterior chamber through the primary incision. The cannula is used to contact the edge of the IOL to prevent movement of the IOL and to prevent anterior lens vaulting.

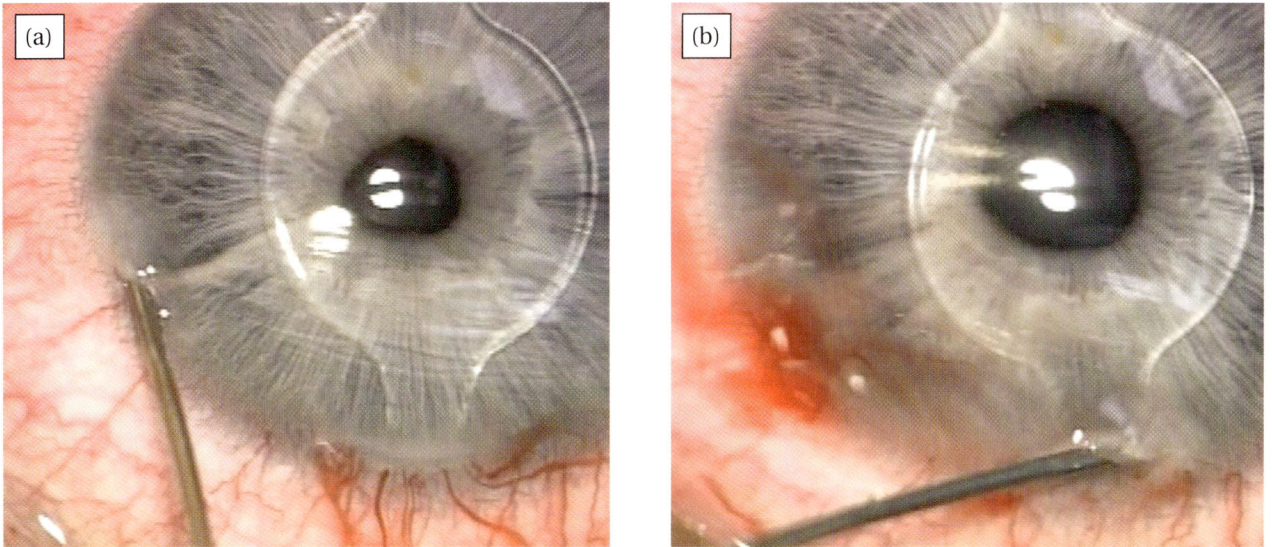

FIGURE 14.10 **Reforming the Anterior Chamber and Hydration of the Wounds.** (a) shows irrigation of the paracentesis site. (b) shows irrigation of the incision site.

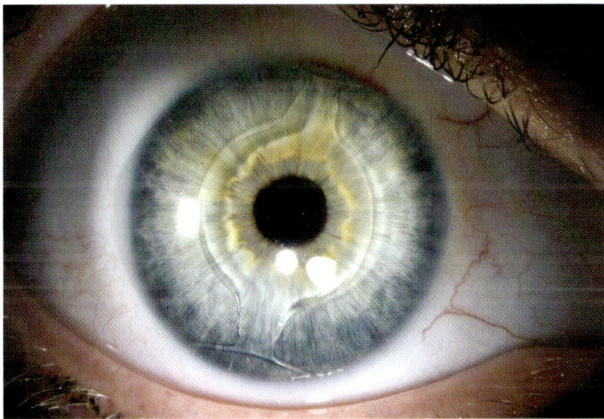

FIGURE 14.11 **The Cachet™ Lens Perfectly Centered in the Eye.** Note that a peripheral iridectomy is not required. (Image courtesy of Alcon Laboratories, Inc.)

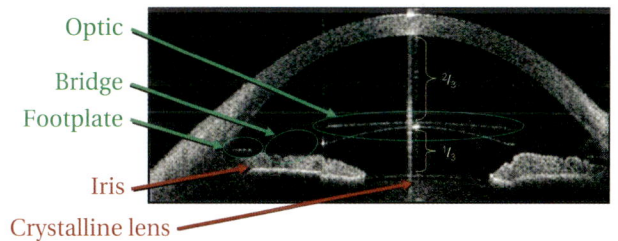

FIGURE 14.12 **Optical Coherence Tomography Image of the IOL within the Eye.** Image taken with a Visante optical coherence tomographer, Carl Zeiss Meditec Inc., Dublin, CA. (Courtesy of Alcon Laboratories, Inc.)

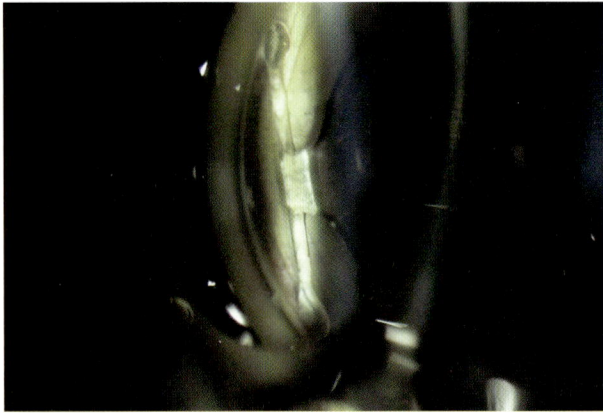

FIGURE 14.13 **Gonioscopy Image.** Demonstrating good position of the footplates at the iris insertion, lack of inflammatory reaction, and absence of iris tuck.

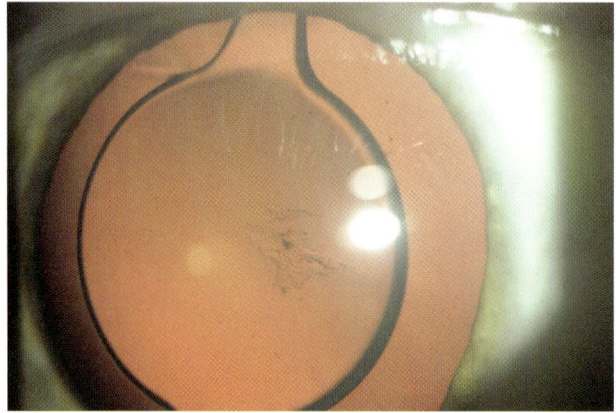

FIGURE 14.14 **Potential Complication: Anterior Subcapsular Cataract.** This can occur as a result of anterior capsular touch from the IOL, cartridge, or instruments used during the procedure.

TABLE 14.2 *Potential Complications*

Ocular Conditions and Surgical Reinterventions

- Corneal haze
- Raised intraocular pressure requiring treatment
- Cataract formation
- Synechiae
- Secondary surgical intervention, including IOL repositioning, explant, or replacement
- Loss of corrected visual acuity
- Retinal detachment/repair
- Lens dislocation
- Reduction in endothelial cell density, potentially necessitating corneal surgery
- Hyphema

ACKNOWLEDGMENTS

Surgical images were courtesy of Michael C. Knorz, MD (FreeVis LASIK Center, University Eye Clinic Mannheim, Mannheim, Germany); of Captured Light Studio, Inc. (Keene, NH); and of Alcon. Cartridge figures were adapted with permission from Alcon. Medical writing assistance was provided by Alcon.

SELECTED REFERENCES

MONARCH® III Loading Instructions: AcrySof® Cachet™ Lens and MONARCH® III P Cartridge. Alcon Laboratories, Inc. Fort Worth, Texas, USA. 2009.

Physician Labeling: AcrySof Phakic Angle-supported IOL. Alcon Laboratories, Inc. Fort Worth, Texas, USA. 2008.

15 Phakic IOLs: Iris-fixated—Verisyse™

Majid Moshirfar, MD, FACS, JoAnn C. Chang, MD,
and Carlton R. Fenzl, MD

TABLE 15.1 *Indications for Surgery*

Indications for Verisyse™ Phakic IOL

Myopia –5.00 to –20.00 D with Astigmatism ≤2.50 D

High myopia after PKP in phakic and pseudophakic eyes

High myopia associated with selected cases of keratoconus

IOL = intraocular lens; D = diopters; PKP = penetrating keratoplasty.

TABLE 15.2 *Preoperative Considerations*

Preoperative Considerations for Verisyse™ Phakic IOL

Patient age between 21–50

ACD ≥3.2 mm

ECD of at least 2000 cells/mm²

Stable manifest refraction of ≤0.50 D at two exams at least one month apart

Refractive stability for minimum 6 months (SE change < 0.50 D)

No previously diagnosed glaucoma

Clear natural crystalline lens

No significant retinal pathology limiting visual acuity (i.e., DR, ARMD, etc.)

No significant cornea pathology limiting visual acuity (i.e., central haze/scar, NV, etc.)

No abnormal iris morphology (i.e. peaked pupil, elevated iris margin, etc.)

IOL = intraocular lens; ACD = anterior chamber depth; ECD = endothelial cell density; D = diopters; SE = spherical equivalent; DR = diabetic retinopathy; ARMD = age-related macular degeneration; NV = neovascularization.

Surgical Approach

Superior Wound (Modify as needed for temporal wound)

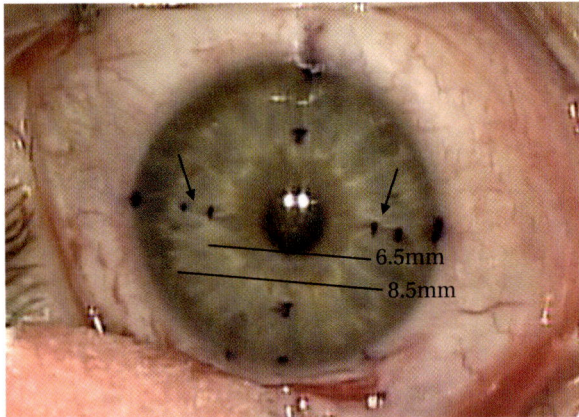

FIGURE 15.1 **Marking the Cornea for Appropriate Lens Placement.** Four perilimbal cardinal marks are made, centered on the pupil. Additional marks are made, 6.5 and 8.5 mm apart, for the eventual position of the lens (centered on the pupil). The enclavation sites will be between the latter two marks (arrows).

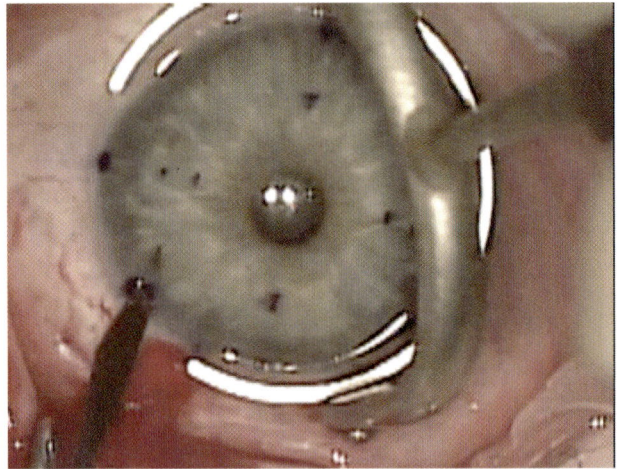

FIGURE 15.2 **Paracentesis for Enclavation Needle.** Two paracentesis ports are made at 1–2 o'clock and 10 to 11 o'clock positions. They are pointed inferiorly toward the enclavation sites. Be sure to make short stab incisions for better maneuverability of the instruments. A cohesive viscoelastic is used for ease of removal at the end of the case.

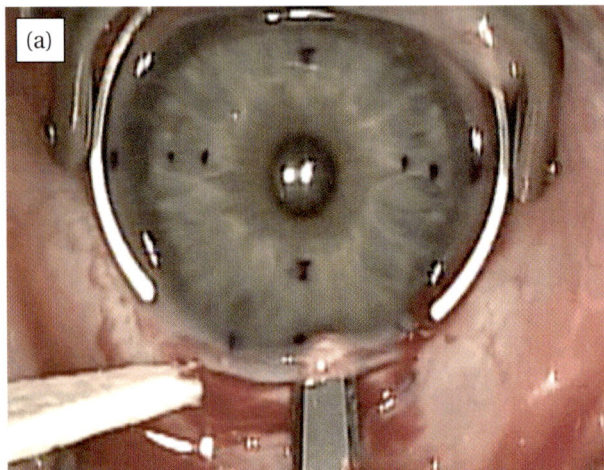

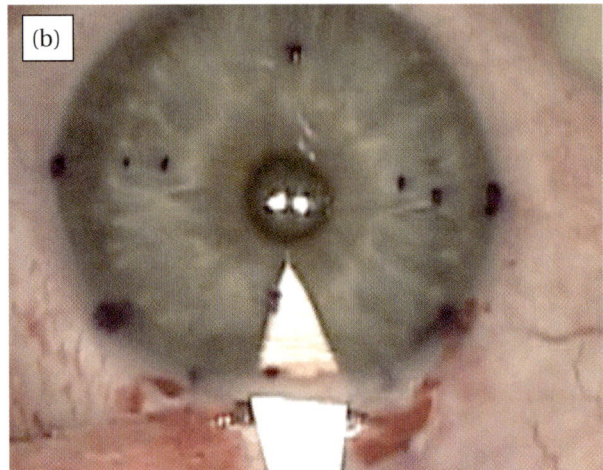

FIGURE 15.3 **Making the Primary Incision.** (a) Limbal incision. A tunnel incision can be made via the sclera, limbus, or cornea. Note that surgically induced astigmatism can be more significant for clear corneal incisions. (b) Entering the anterior chamber with a microkeratome or similar instrument. The primary incision should be slightly larger than the size of the optic (Verisyse™ comes in two sizes: 5.0 or 6.0 mm).

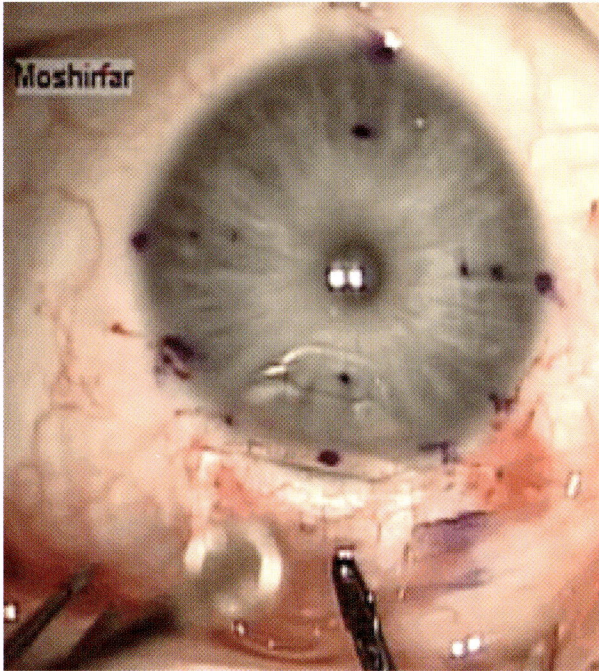

FIGURE 15.4 Placement of Verisyse™ Lens into the Anterior Chamber. Using lens forceps, slide the lens into the anterior chamber. For limbal and scleral incisions, concurrent irrigation with BSS helps wash away blood that can cause pigment deposits on the lens optic.

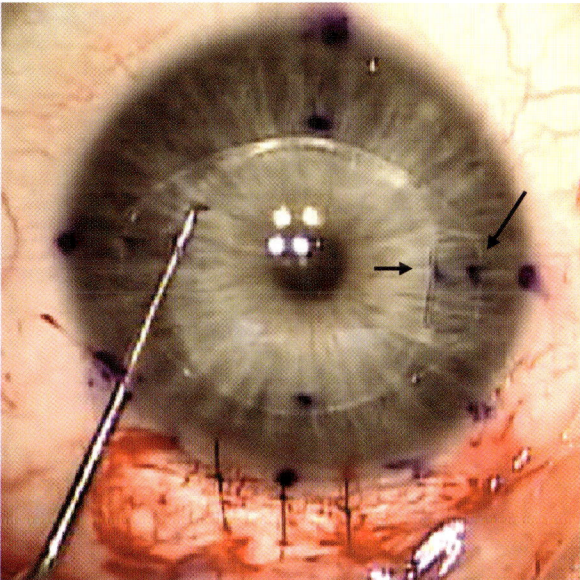

FIGURE 15.5 Repositioning of Lens in the Anterior Chamber. Using a Sinsky hook or similar instrument, move the lens so that the enclavation arms are properly aligned with the markings (arrows). Inject viscoelastic over the optic to push it more posterior to assist in enclavation.

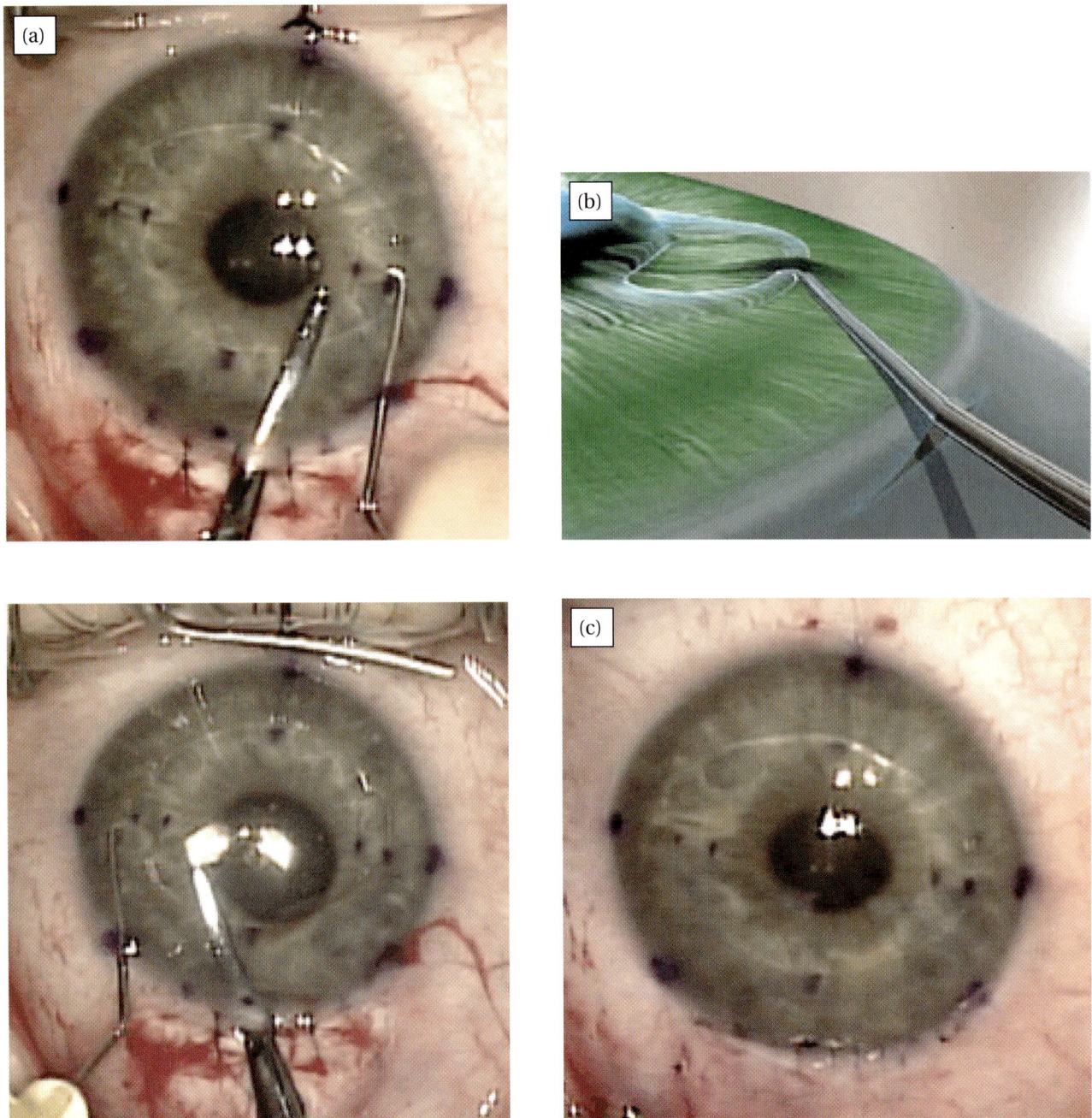

FIGURE 15.6 **Enclavation.** (a) Bimanual procedure: Right handed enclavation above, left handed enclavation below. One hand stabilizes the lens with forceps, the other holds the enclavation needle. (b) The enclavation needle is passed underneath the haptic clasp. Tug the iris with the needle and feed it through the clasp opening. It may take several attempts to get enough iris capture. Slight posterior tilt of the lens toward the iris will help in iris capture. Refill AC with viscoelastic between enclavations. (Image courtesy of AMO) (c) Minimal ovalization of the pupil (arrow) is a good indication of appropriate amount of iris capture.

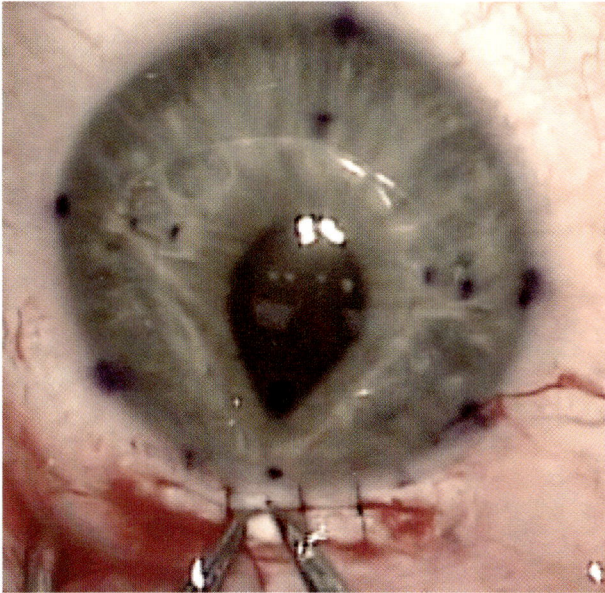

FIGURE 15.7 **Peripheral Iridectomy (PI), Intraoperative.** PI is necessary to prevent postoperative pupillary block. PI can be made preoperatively (with a yag laser) or intraoperatively. When using the yag laser, it is recommended to create two PIs.

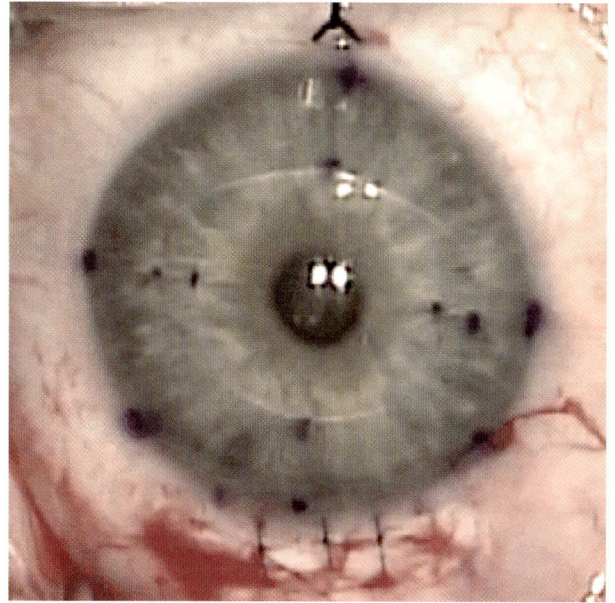

FIGURE 15.8 **Primary Wound Closure.** Three to five interrupted 10.0 nylon sutures are used to close the primary wound. Viscoelastic can be removed via a partially closed main incision or with an irrigation/aspiration bimanual handpiece via the stab incisions. Take care not to disrupt the lens. Postoperative care is similar to post-cataract surgery.

TABLE 15.3 *General Recommendations*

Intracameral Miochol®, Carbostat®, or Myostat® to assist in pupillary constriction

Care not to get viscoelastic underneath the optic

Too much iris capture creates significant pupil ovalization; too little risks IOL dislocation

Superior primary incisions for with-the-rule astigmatism; temporal incision for against-the-rule astigmatism

Lid block or equivalent is recommended to decrease positive pressure

For the first enclavation, start with dominant hand or start temporally

Early selective suture removal (about 2 weeks postoperatively) to decrease surgically induced astigmatism

TABLE 15.4 *Complications to Verisyse™ Phakic IOL surgery*

Postoperative IOP elevation

Postoperative wound leak

Cystic macular edema

Postoperative pupillary block

Hyphema

Uveitis/iritis

Decentration

Dislocation

Posterior synechiae

Pupil ovalization/irregularity

Atonic pupil

Cataract

Endophthalmitis

Retinal tear or detachment

Cornea edema/decompensation

IOP = intraocular pressure.

SELECTED REFERENCES

Stulting RD, John ME, Maloney RK, et al. Three-year results of Artisan/Verisyse phakic intraocular lens implantation. Results of the United States Food and Drug Administration clinical trial. *Ophthalmology.* 2008;115:464–472.

U.S. FDA Center for Devices and Radiological Health page. Artisan (Model 206 and 204) Phakic Intraocular Lens (PIOL), Verisyse (VRSM5US and VRSM6US) Phakic Intraocular Lens (PIOL) – P030028. Available at: http://www.fda.gov/MedicalDevices/ProductsandMedicalProcedures/DeviceApprovalsandClearances/Recently-ApprovedDevices/ucm080863.htm.

Moshirfar M, Gregoirea, FJ, Mirzaian G, et al. Use of Verisyse iris-supported phakic intraocular lens for myopia in keratoconic patients. *J Cat Refract Surg.* 2006;32:1227–1232.

Moshirfar M, Feilmeier MR, Kang PC. Implantation of verisyse phakic intraocular lens to correct myopic refractive error after penetrating keratoplasty in pseudophakic eyes. *Cornea.* 2006;25:107–111.

Phakic IOLs Posterior Chamber—Visian ICL

Kimiya Shimizu, MD, PhD

TABLE 16.1 *Indications*

Phakic patients aged 20 years or older

Myopic, hyperopic, or astigmatic patients with a stable refraction over 3.0 diopters

Anterior chamber depth of at least 2.8 mm

Exclusion Criteria

    A history of uveitis

    Diabetic retinopathy

    Glaucoma

    Pseudoexfoliation

    Prior retinal detachment

    A history of ocular surgery considered improper for this surgery

    A history of refractive surgery considered improper for this surgery

    Crystalline lens opacity considered improper for this surgery

    Patients considered improper for this surgery because of some systemic or ocular disease

Surgery

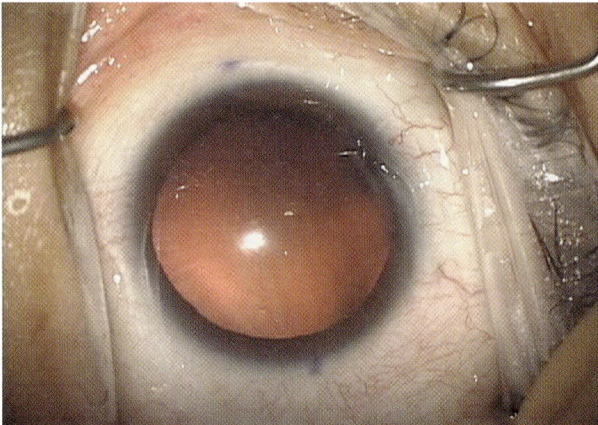

FIGURE 16.1 **Mark the 3 and 9 o'clock Positions at the Limbus.** If inserting a toric ICL or planning a corneal relaxing incision, the surgeon preoperatively marks the 3 and 9 o'clock positions at the limbus with a marking pen, with the patient in a sitting position. Marking the eye under the slit-lamp facilitates a more accurate alignment.

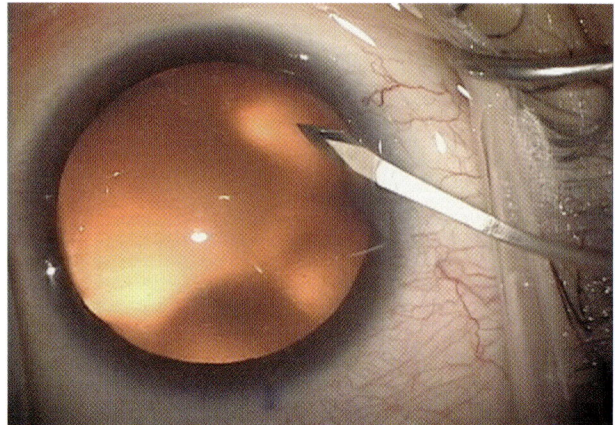

FIGURE 16.2 **Create a Sideport Incision.** Using a 1 mm slit knife, a sideport incision is made. Creating this sideport incision on the side of the surgeon's dominant hand facilitates easier manipulation of the ICL. Some surgeons make two sideport incisions, one inferonasally and the other superotemporally. These incisions can be straight, or can be angled to facilitate manipulation of the haptics. A low-molecular-weight ophthalmic viscosurgical device (OVD) is then injected.

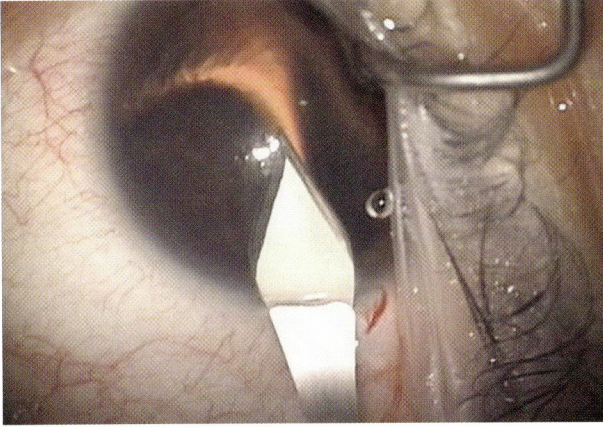

FIGURE 16.3 **Create the Main Incision**. The temporal corneal incision is made with a 3 mm slit knife. The wound must be made with extreme care to avoid contact with the crystalline lens. The outside edge is widened by approximately 0.2 mm to create a trapezoidal shape that stabilizes the injector.

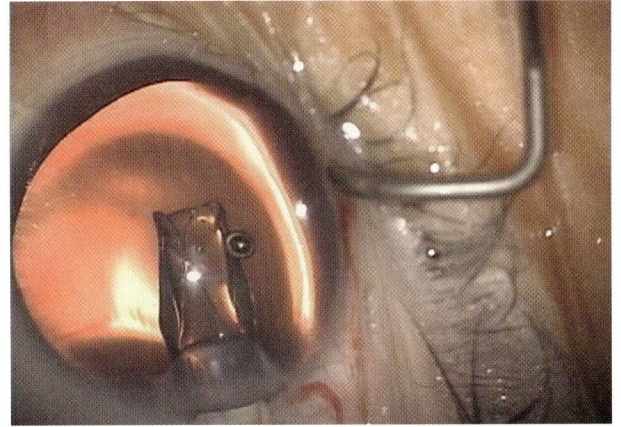

FIGURE 16.4 **Insert the ICL** With the authors' technique, the ICL is injected without inserting the injector into the anterior chamber. It is the authors' belief that this minimizes the risk of surgically induced cataract. Other surgeons find it easier to insert the injector approximately half way into the anterior chamber before injecting the ICL.

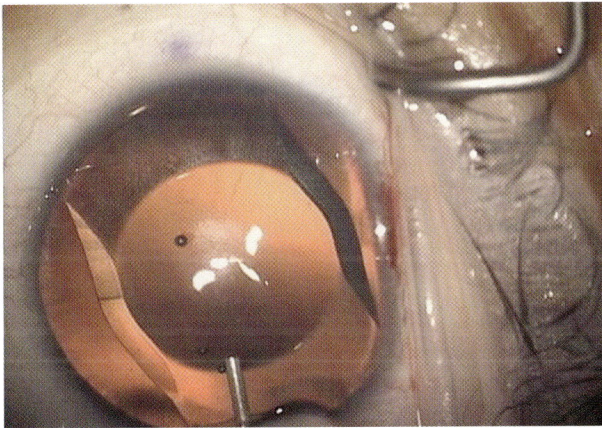

FIGURE 16.5 **Inject Additional OVD**. To maintain the anterior chamber dome, additional OVD is injected. A high-molecular-weight OVD provides even greater maintenance of anterior chamber than the low-molecular-weight OVD that was injected prior to insertion of the ICL.

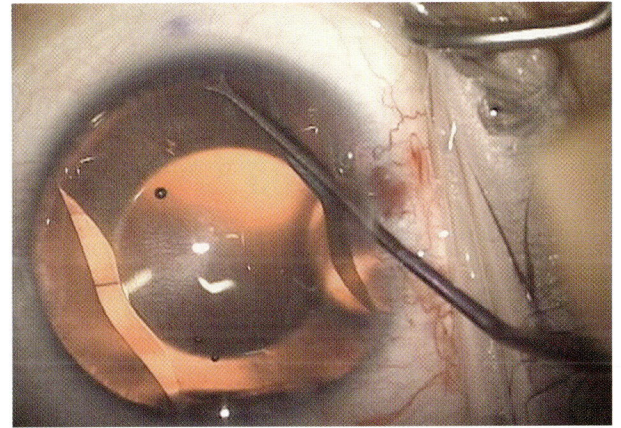

FIGURE 16.6 **Insert ICL Haptics into the Ciliary Sulcus**. Using a hook, each haptic of the ICL is gently pulled centrally (but not posteriorly) and then tucked into the ciliary sulcus. The authors use the sideport to insert the distal haptics, and the main incision for the proximal haptics.

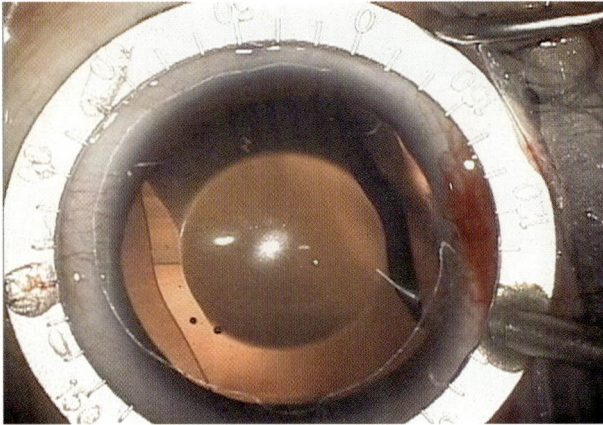

FIGURE 16.7 **Align the ICL**. Using a degree gauge, the surgeon confirms that the ICL is correctly aligned. Additional rotation of the ICL can be gently implemented as necessary to assure accurate placement or ocular alignment.

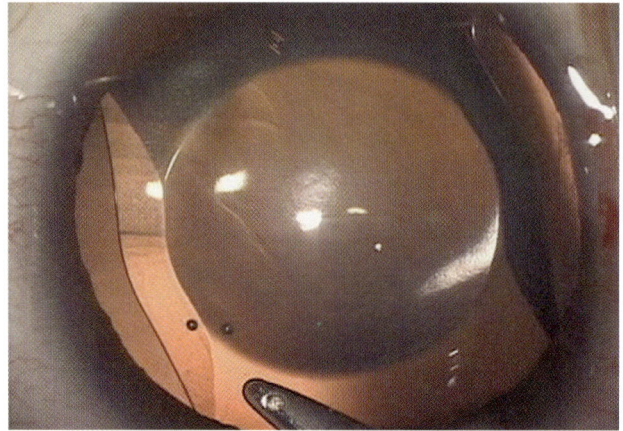

FIGURE 16.8 **Remove the OVD**. The authors remove the OVD using a Simcoe needle. This procedure should be done carefully to avoid iris prolapse. If only a low-molecular-weight OVD is used, it can be gently removed by irrigating through the sideport incision.

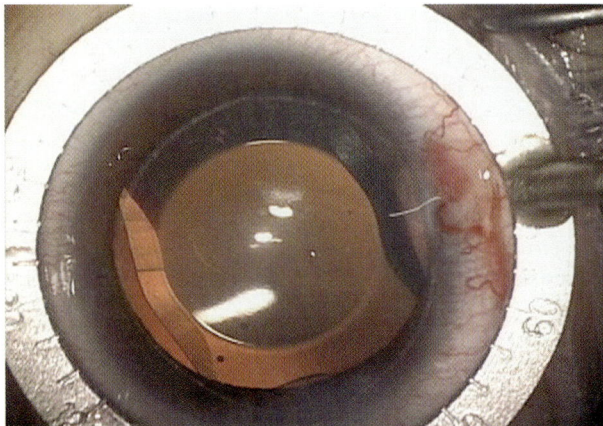

FIGURE 16.9 **Confirm ICL Alignment**. Verify correct alignment of the ICL after the OVD has been removed.

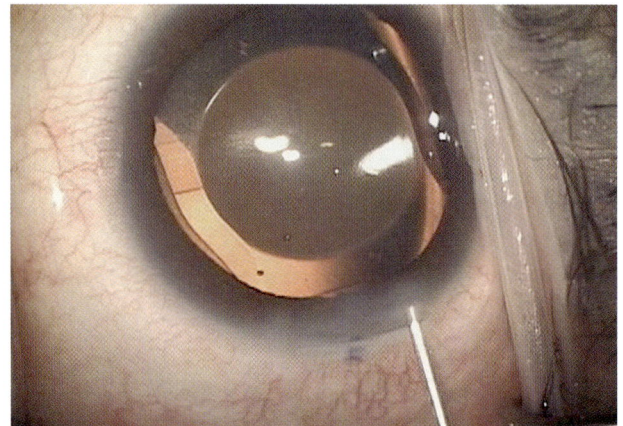

FIGURE 16.10 **Close the Wound**. The main incision and sideport incision are hydrated until watertight.

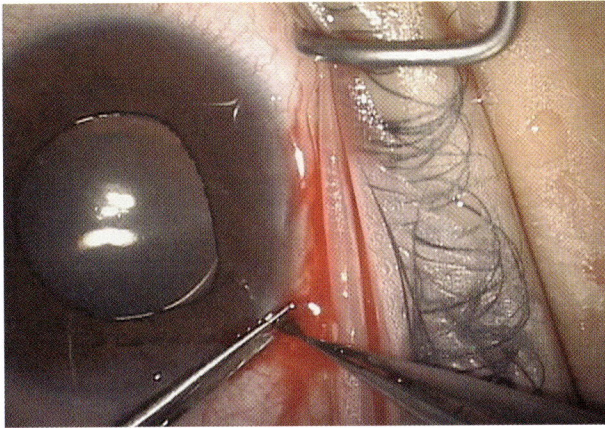

FIGURE 16.11 **Create a Peripheral Iridectomy**. A miotic is injected to constrict the pupil. Through the 1 mm sideport incision, which was made in the beginning of the surgery, the iris is gently grasped, and a peripheral iridectomy is performed. In case the existing sideport is in an improper position for peripheral iridectomy, another 1mm sideport incision is made in the limbus posterior to the clear cornea.

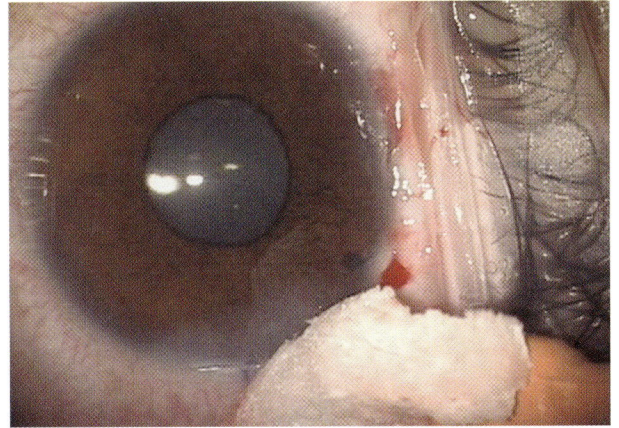

FIGURE 16.12 **Confirm Wound Closure**. The wounds are checked one final time, and the eye is left with a normal intraocular pressure. If the wound cannot be closed with hydration, a suture can be inserted.

TABLE 16.2 *Complications*

Secondary cataract

Intraocular pressure elevation

Hyphema

Iritis or cyclitis

Endophthalmitis

ICL sizing problem: too large or too small

SELECTED REFERENCES

Kamiya K, Shimizu K, Igarashi A, et al. Four-year follow-up of posterior chamber phakic intraocular lens implantation for moderate to high myopia. *Arch Ophthalmol.* 2009;127(7):845–850.

Sanders DR, Doney K, Poco M, ICL in Treatment of Myopia Study Group. United States Food and Drug Administration clinical trial of the Implantable Collamer Lens (ICL) for moderate to high myopia: three-year follow-up. *Ophthalmology.* 2004;111(9):1683–1692.

Cornea and Ocular Surface Surgery

Edited by **Stephen D. McLeod** and **Bennie H. Jeng**

17 Limbal Stem Cell Transplantation

Nariman Nassiri, MD and Ali R. Djalilian, MD

TABLE 17.1 *Indications for Limbal Stem Cell Transplantation*

Clinically significant limbal stem cell deficiency manifested by:
- Persistent/recurrent epithelial defects
- Conjunctivalization
- Neovascularization
- Corneal ulceration & scarring
- Visual loss, pain

TABLE 17.2 *Preoperative Considerations*

Consider conjunctival-limbal autograft for cases of unilateral limbal stem cell deficiency, most commonly a unilateral chemical injury.

Consider keratolimbal allograft for cases with bilateral limbal stem cell deficiency.

Consider permanent punctal occlusion in patients with aqueous tear deficiency.

Significant abnormalities such as entropion or ectropion, trichiasis or distichiasis, and palpebral conjunctival keratinization should be corrected prior to limbal transplantation.

Consider reconstruction of the fornix by autologous graft from the oral or nasal mucosa in patients with severe conjunctival deficiency and obliteration of the fornices prior to limbal transplantation.

Consider aggressive management of glaucoma in patients undergoing limbal stem cell grafting. Specifically, any patient on 2 or more drops should be referred for surgical management of glaucoma before proceeding with limbal allograft transplant.

In patients with significant inflammation (e.g., recent chemical injury, cicatricial pemphigoid, inflamed Stevens-Johnson syndrome, atopic keratoconjunctivitis), control the inflammation with systemic immunosuppression for minimum of 3–6 months.

Conjunctival-Limbal Autograft (CLAU)

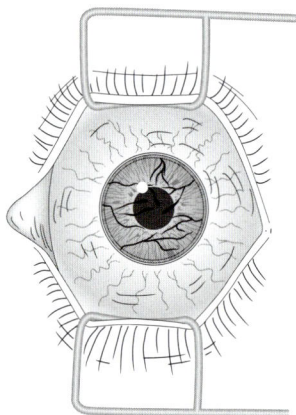

FIGURE 17.1 An eye with limbal stem cell deficiency with conjunctivalization, recurrent corneal epithelial defects, corneal neovascularization, secondary stromal scarring.

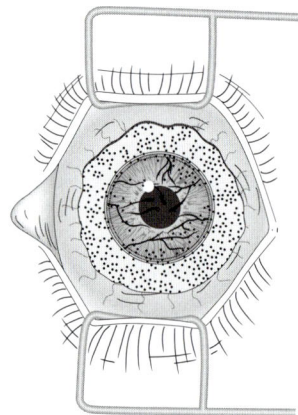

FIGURE 17.2 A peribulbar or retrobulbar block is used for the recipient (diseased) eye. A 360° limbal peritomy is performed. Topical epinephrine (1:10,000 dilution) is applied to minimize bleeding. The use of wet-field cautery is kept to a minimum.

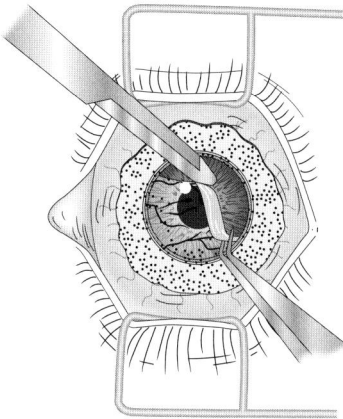

FIGURE 17.3 Removal of abnormal corneal epithelium and fibrovascular pannus by superficial keratectomy using a No. 64 Beaver blade. Care is given to avoid cutting deep into stroma because of the risk of corneal perforation and postoperative optical distortion from surface irregularity.

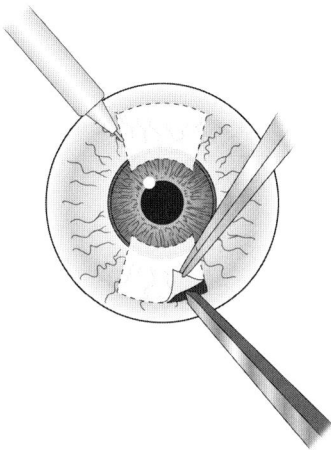

FIGURE 17.4 Topical or subconjunctival anesthesia (1%–2% lidocaine with epinephrine) is typically adequate for the donor eye. Two conjunctival limbal autografts are taken from the corresponding 12 and 6 o'clock positions of the donor eye. A gentian violet surgical marking pen is used to mark the conjunctival portions of the grafts. The limbal portion should be approximately 2 clock hours, while the conjunctival portion is extended approximately 5 mm posteriorly. The conjunctiva is elevated with a subconjunctival injection of 1% lidocaine with epinephrine. Wescott scissors are used to begin the dissection by incising along the lateral borders, with complete undermining between the lateral edges, if possible, before cutting along the posterior edge. **Notes**: This sequence helps keep the tissue on-stretch. The gentian violet markings should be included in the graft, to help delineate the epithelial surface from the undersurface. A non-toothed forceps are recommended to help avoid buttonholes and tears through the conjunctiva.

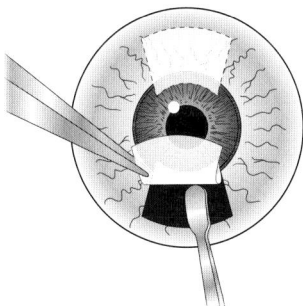

FIGURE 17.5 Once the lateral and posterior edges are released, the conjunctiva is reflected anteriorly over the cornea, and blunt dissection is continued anteriorly. When the point of conjunctival insertion at the limbus is reached, further dissection is performed mostly by blunt dissection using closed tips of a sharp Wescott scissors (occasionally, a crescent blade may be necessary). This maneuver is mostly a superficial keratectomy of peripheral limbus and cornea, and very little lamellar dissection is necessary. The dissection is carried forward into the peripheral cornea approximately 1 mm beyond the peripheral corneal vascular arcades. Finally, the anterior edge of the graft is cut free from the cornea using a Van Ness scissors. The tissue is then transferred onto a piece of sterile paper and covered with balanced salt solution. The donor sites can be left open to heal, but it may be preferred to undermine the surrounding conjunctiva, and pull the conjunctiva forward and suture to the limbus with dissolvable suture (e.g., 9-0 vicryl) to cover the defect as much as possible.

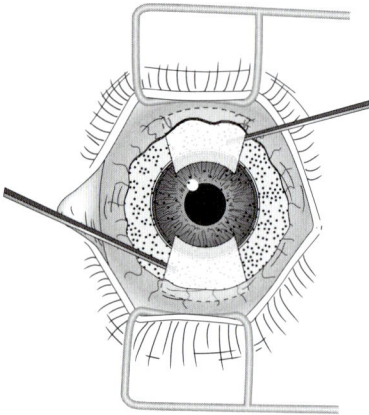

FIGURE 17.6 Each autograft is placed onto its anatomically correct position (limbus to limbus) and is attached firmly to the bed by injecting Tisseel fibrin glue (Baxter AG, Vienna, Austria) beneath the donor tissue. The excess glue is "milked" from under the graft, and the posterior edge of the graft is re-approximated with the host conjunctiva. The remaining gaps in the nasal and temporal limbus are typically left open, and the conjunctiva is allowed to stay back. At the conclusion of the operation, antibiotic and corticosteroid is injected subconjunctivally in the fornix of the recipient eye. A patch and protective shield is placed over the eye until the patient is seen the next day.

Keratolimbal Allograft (KLAL)

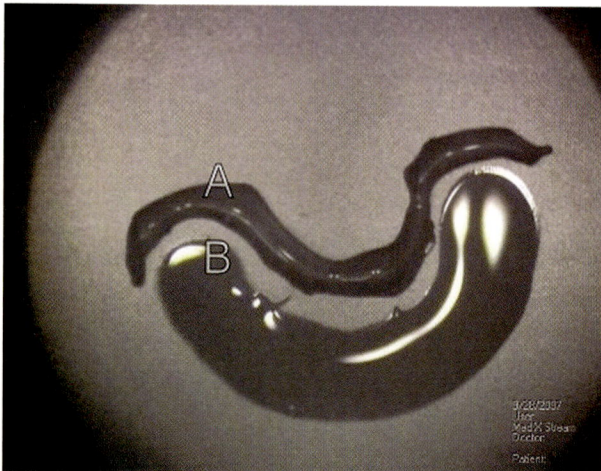

FIGURE 17.7 A thin layer of tissue N-butyl-2-cyanoacrylate adhesive (Indermil® Tissue Adhesive, Tyco Healthcare Group LP) along with a thin strip of viscoelastic (Viscoat®, Alcon Laboratories) near the anterior edge of the adhesive is spread on a sterile plastic platform. **A** refers to the viscoelastic and **B** refers to the adhesive.

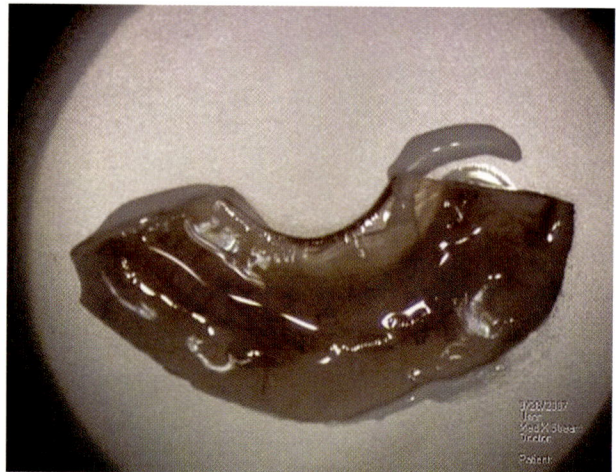

FIGURE 17.8 A 180-degree donor corneoscleral rim is placed epithelial side up on the adhesive and the viscoelastic to allow for firm attachment onto the platform. ***Note:*** The viscoelastic helps to prevent the glue from tracking up the anterior and lateral edges of the tissue.

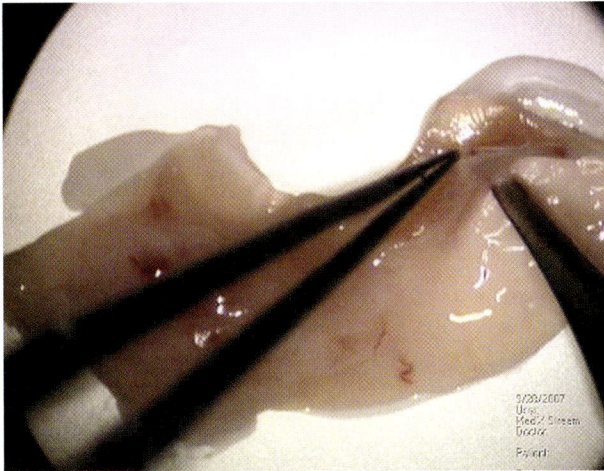

FIGURE 17.9 Starting from its free edge, the conjunctiva is lifted up and dissected off the sclera by cutting the underlying attachments using Wescott scissors leaving behind as much Tenon's capsule as possible.

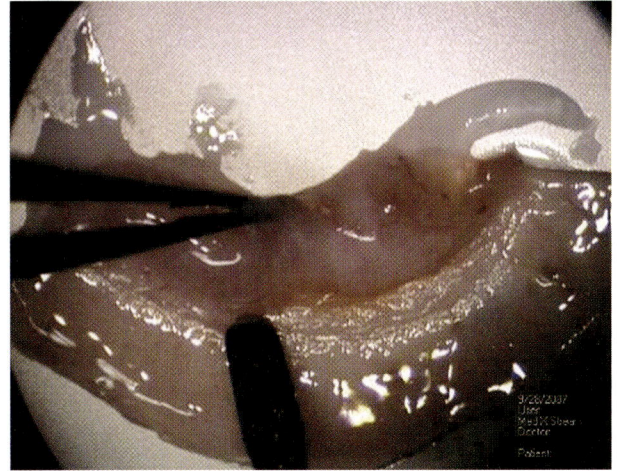

FIGURE 17.10 A superficial lamellar dissection is carried forward onto the cornea extending at least 1.5 mm anterior to the limbus using a crescent blade, keeping at a depth of approximately one-third. *Note:* The same procedure is performed on two additional donor corneoscleral crescents. The keratolimbal allograft tissue consists of a rim of conjunctiva and the peripheral corneal and limbal epithelium, with some underlying stroma.

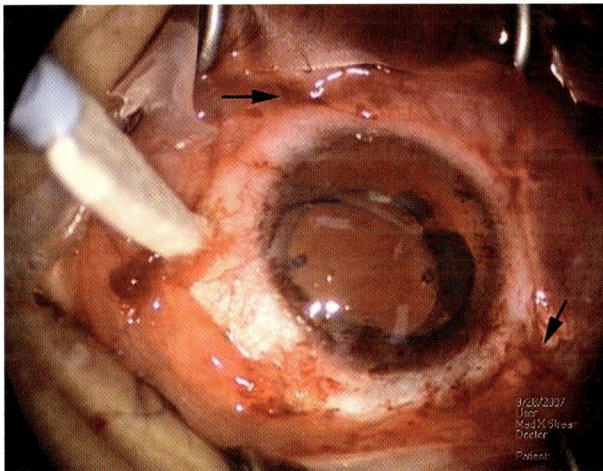

FIGURE 17.11 The recipient patient's eye is anesthetized with a peribulbar or retrobulbar injection, or occasionally general anesthesia is used if necessary. A 360-degree peritomy is performed with relaxing incisions (arrows) to allow the conjunctiva to fall back. Superficial keratectomy is also performed to remove all abnormal epithelium and superficial fibrovascular scar tissues.

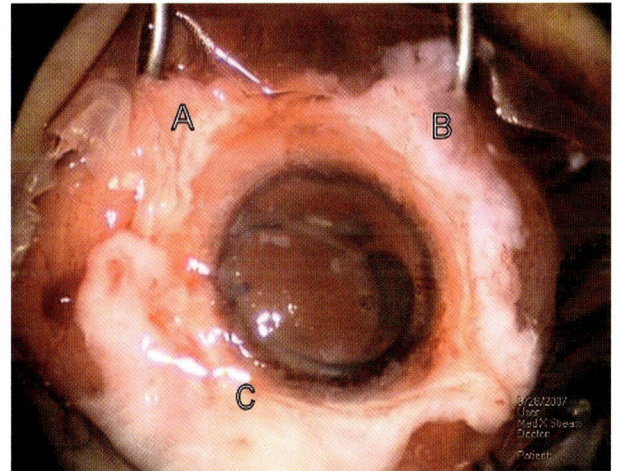

FIGURE 17.12 Three 180-degree conjunctival-limbal donor rims (A, B, C) were placed in close proximity to one another in order to cover the entire bed (piece A was slightly trimmed in order to fit).

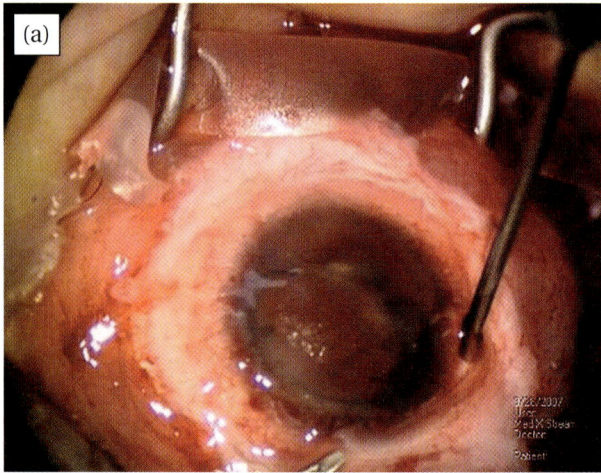

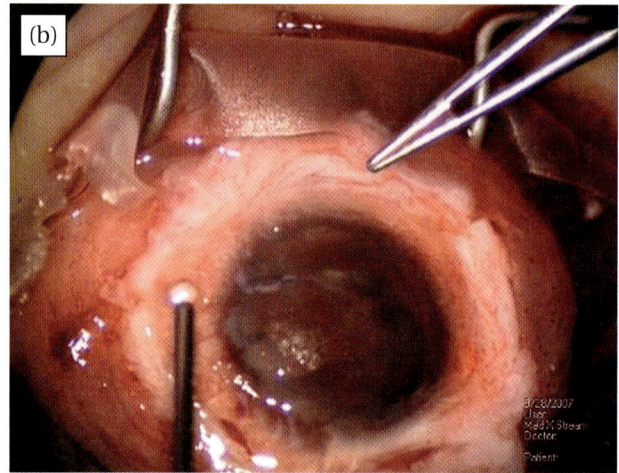

FIGURE 17.13 The Tisseel fibrin glue (Baxter AG, Vienna, Austria) is injected beneath the donor tissue in order to attach them to the bed.

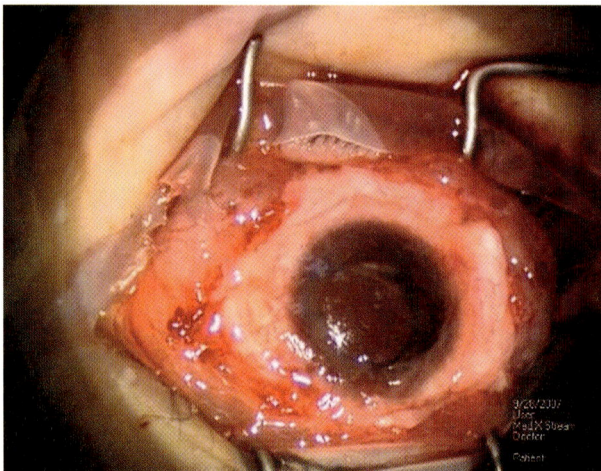

FIGURE 17.14 The excess conjunctival tissue is trimmed from the donor tissue, and the host conjunctiva is slightly pulled over on top of the donor grafts.

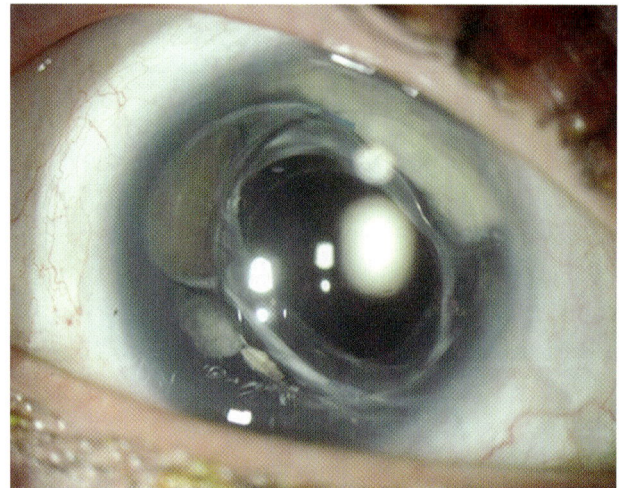

FIGURE 17.15 Slit-lamp photo of the same patient at 15 months after surgery.

TABLE 17.3 *Postoperative Considerations*

The **donor eye** (in CLAU) is treated with the antibiotic and corticosteroid drops 3–4 times daily until epithelialization is complete (usually 1–2 weeks) and inflammation has subsided.

In both KLAL and CLAU, the **recipient eye** is treated with a low-toxicity antibiotic 4 times daily as prophylaxis during re-epithelialization. Topical corticosteroids are used 4 times daily for inflammation.

In **allograft patients,** topical immunosuppression including corticosteroids (qid–qd, continued indefinitely) and cyclosporine A (CsA) (0.05% qid, indefinitely), and systemic immunosuppression consisting of oral prednisone (1 mg/kg/day, taper over 3–4 months), cyclosporine A (CsA) (3 mg/kg/day, 12–18 months) or tacrolimus (1–4 mg bid, 12–18 months), and azathioprine (100 mg/day, 12–18 months) or mycophenolate mofetil (1000 mg bid, 12–18 months) is started on the day of surgery. Immunosuppression is continued at least 12–18 months then taper is attempted. Some patients may require longer or indefinite therapy to prevent graft rejection. All patients are also followed for the side effects of the systemic immunosuppressive drugs.

All patients are instructed to use nonpreserved artificial tears every 1–2 hours. Punctal occlusion, tarsorrhaphy, and use of a bandage soft contact lens are other interventions commonly used as needed.

In rare circumstances, namely significant corneal thinning with risk of perforation, **penetrating keratoplasty** is performed concomitantly with one of the above epithelial transplantation procedures. Otherwise, it is better to wait at least 3 months for the ocular surface to appear stable before proceeding with additional surgeries, particularly penetrating keratoplasty.

TABLE 17.4 *Potential Complications for Limbal Stem Cell Transplantation*

Delayed epithelial healing

Immune mediated graft rejection

Microbial infection of the cornea

Glaucoma or worsening intraocular pressure

Adverse effects due to systemic immunosuppression

SELECTED REFERENCES

Holland EJ. Epithelial transplantation for the management of severe ocular surface disease. *Trans Am Ophthalmol Soc.* 1996;94:677–743.

Djalilian AR, Wadia HP, Balali S, Nassiri N, Holland EJ. Epithelial transplantation for the management of severe ocular surface disease. In: Brightbill FS, Mcdonnell PJ, Mcghee CJ, et al. eds. *Corneal Surgery: Theory, Technique and Tissue,* 4th ed. Missouri: Mosby, 2008:241–258.

18

Amniotic Membrane Transplantation

Hosam Sheha, MD, PhD and Scheffer C.G. Tseng, MD, PhD

TABLE 18.1 *Corneal Indications for Amniotic Membrane Transplantation*

AM as a Temporary Graft (Biological Bandage)	AM as a Permanent Graft
• Neurotrophic persistent epithelial defect without ulceration • Acute chemical/thermal burn • Acute Stevens Johnson syndrome/Toxic epidermal necrolysis • High-risk corneal graft • Post-infectious keratitis • Recurrent epithelial erosion • Following superficial keratectomy	• Neurotrophic persistent epithelial defect with ulceration • Corneal descemetocele or perforation • Bullous keratopathy • Following superficial keratectomy to remove band keratopathy, scar, or tumor • Partial limbal stem cell deficiency • In conjunction with limbal conjunctival autograft for unilateral total limbal stem cell deficiency • In conjunction with keratolimbal allograft for bilateral total limbal stem cell deficiency

Two Modes of Amniotic Membrane Transplantation

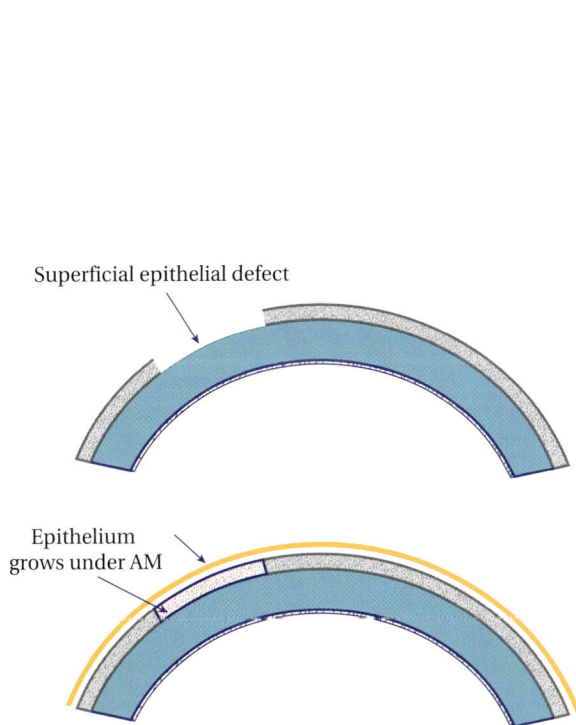

FIGURE 18.1 **Mode I: AM as a Temporary Graft (*Biological Bandage*).** When AM is used as a *temporary* graft, it is used like a *biological bandage* and is aimed to reduce either acute or chronic ocular surface inflammation, caused by various diseases and injuries, so as to promote epithelial healing with minimal or no scarring.

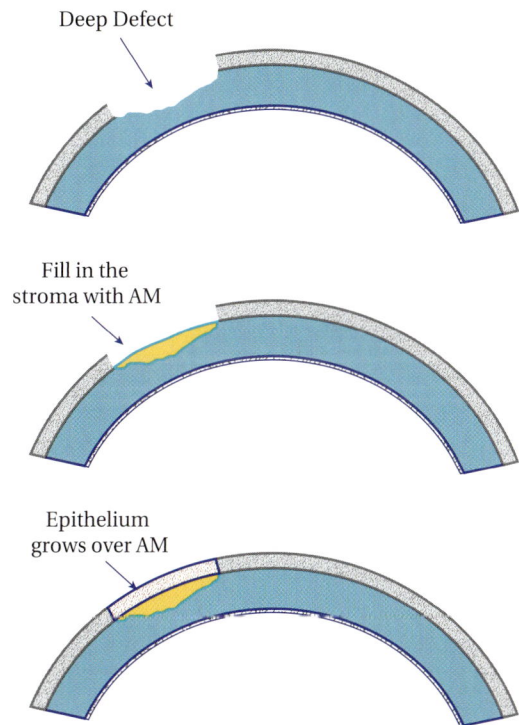

FIGURE 18.2 **Mode II: AM as a Permanent Graft.** When used as a *permanent graft*, it is aimed to fill in a stromal defect and to restore its integrity. Upon integration into the host tissue, the resultant stroma often regains clarity.

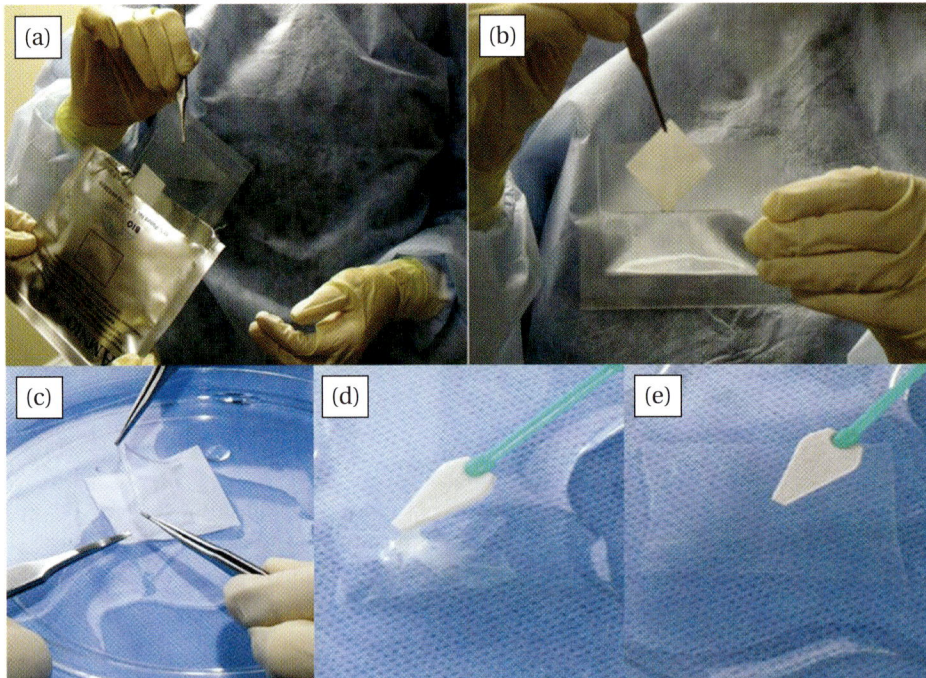

FIGURE 18.3 Handling of Cryopreserved Amniotic Membrane (Bio-Tissue, Inc., Miami, FL) After thawing at the room temperature, it can be retrieved aseptically from the inner clear plastic pouch and the membrane is attached to one side of nitrocellulose paper (a and b). Once transferred to the operating field, the membrane can be easily peeled off from the paper by two forceps grabbing the two corners while the nurse peels the paper away (c). In general, amniotic membrane graft is placed with the stromal side on the recipient bed; the side can be discerned by touching it with the tip of a dry MicroSponge™ (Alcon Surgical, Fort Worth, TX). The stromal side (d), but not epithelial side (e), sticks to MicroSponge™.

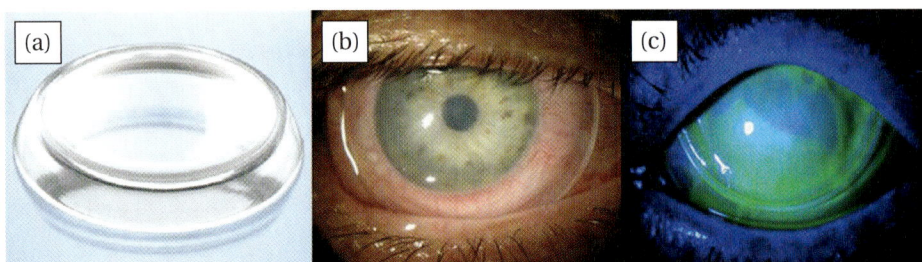

FIGURE 18.4 Handling of Sutureless Device (ProKera®, Bio-Tissue, Inc., Miami, Fl) ProKera® is a dual ring system that fastens a sheet of semitransparent cryopreserved AM (a). It enhances the ease of patient care in many difficult corneal diseases. ProKera® can be inserted in an office setting using aseptic technique to deliver the AM's biological actions on a temporary manner without sutures. For its insertion, after using topical anesthetic eye drops a lid speculum is used to open the eye. Then, it is inserted into the upper fornix first, and then tucks it under the lower lid. A slit-lamp photograph (b) depicts its appearance when inserted in the eye. During the insertion, the status of epithelialization can be monitored by fluorescein staining and the intraocular pressure can be measured by Tonopen™ without having ProKera® removed (c). After epithelial healing is completed, the membrane is dissolved and ProKera® ring can be removed.

Clinical Uses and Surgical Procedures

AM As a Temporary Graft (Biological Bandage)

Neurotrophic Persistent Epithelial Defect without Ulceration

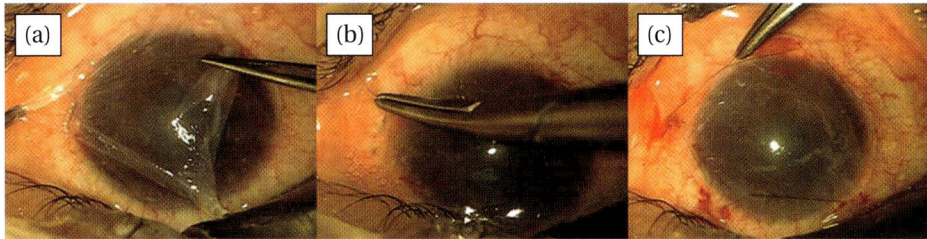

FIGURE 18.5 Cryopreserved AMT as a temporary graft to treat a corneal persistent epithelial defect caused by neurotrophic keratitis Amniotic membrane (2.5 × 2.0 cm size) is secured by a 10-0 Nylon suture at 2–3 mm from the limbus in a purse-string running fashion for a total of 6–8 episcleral bites to cover the corneal surface. As a temporary graft, AM can be sutured with the sticky stromal surface facing down or up. Corneal surface breakdown can recur if severe neurotrophic keratopathy persists. Therefore, it is advised to perform punctal occlusion before AMT and/or temporary tarsorrhaphy at the time of AMT, and add extended high DK contact lens or permanent tarsorrhaphy after healing by AMT.

Acute Stevens-Johnson Syndrome/Toxic Epidermal Necrolysis

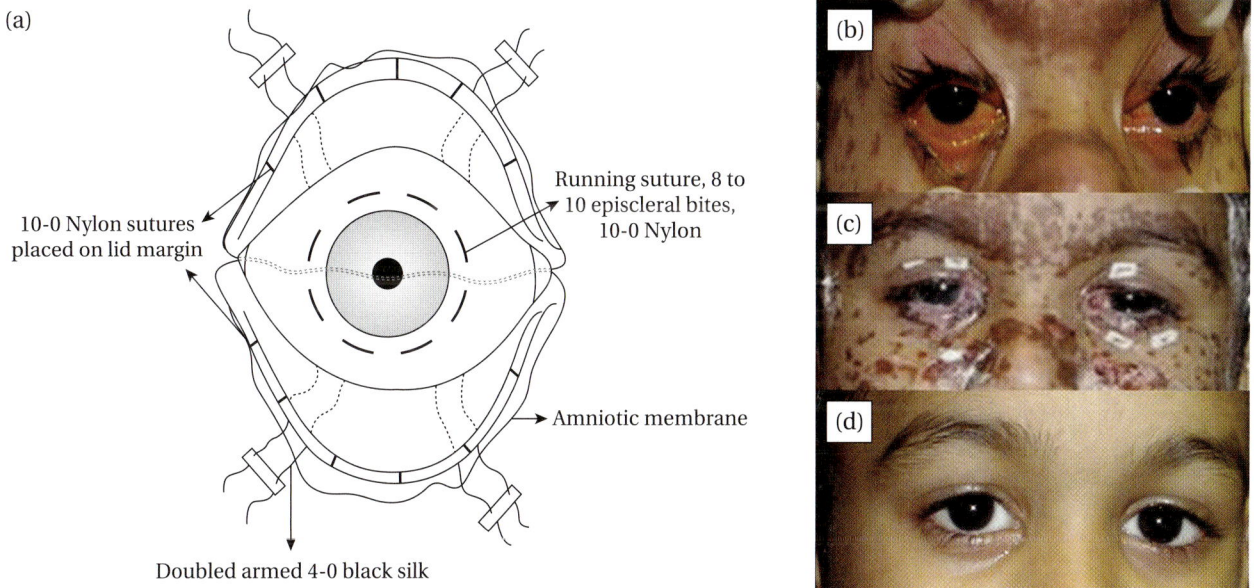

FIGURE 18.6 Early intervention by AMT (e.g., within the first week) to suppress the acute inflammatory and ulcerative stage of Stevens-Johnson syndrome/Toxic epidermal necrolysis This important modality will not only reduce inflammation and facilitate epithelial wound healing, but also prevent the late cicatricial complications that are known to cause corneal blindness. To cover both corneal and conjunctival surfaces, two large pieces of membrane (3.5 × 3.5 cm size) are needed. One of these membranes is secured to the skin surface of the upper lid margin by a 10-0 Nylon suture in an interrupted or running manner, and then tugged into the upper fornix with a muscle hook and secured there by passing a double-armed 4-0 black silk in a mattress fashion to the skin surface with a bolster. The remaining AM is spread to cover the upper bulbar conjunctiva and a part of the upper corneal surface. The other piece is secured to the lower lid and the lower fornix in the similar fashion, overlapped with the first piece on the corneal surface, and secured by a 10-0 Nylon suture placed in the same manner as described above. A temporary tarsorrhaphy is added to minimize the lid fissure if there is an exposure concern.

Recurrent Epithelial Erosion

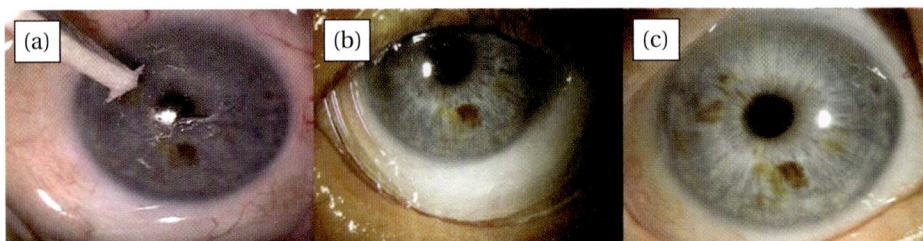

FIGURE 18.7 **AM as a Temporary Graft for Recurrent Corneal Erosion.** After removal of the loose adherent epithelium from the corneal surface (a), ProKera® was inserted to cover the cornea (b). This resulted in a stable corneal epithelium and a clear cornea with 20/20 vision two weeks after the procedure and remained stable without recurrence for a follow up of one year (c).

AM as a Permanent Graft

Neurotrophic Persistent Epithelial Defects with Superficial Ulceration

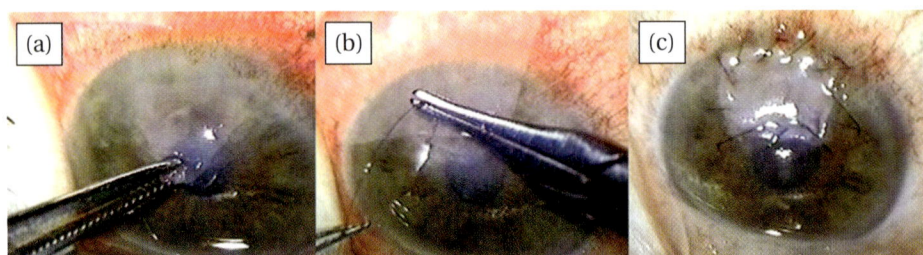

FIGURE 18.8 **Amniotic Membrane as a Permanent Graft for Superficial Corneal Ulcer.** When the corneal epithelial defect extends deeper to involve stromal ulceration (a), a temporary AM graft is not sufficient to restore the stromal integrity. If the corneal ulcer is superficial, a single layer of AM is sufficient to fill in the stromal defect, and is secured by interrupted or continuous 10-0 nylon suture (b and c).

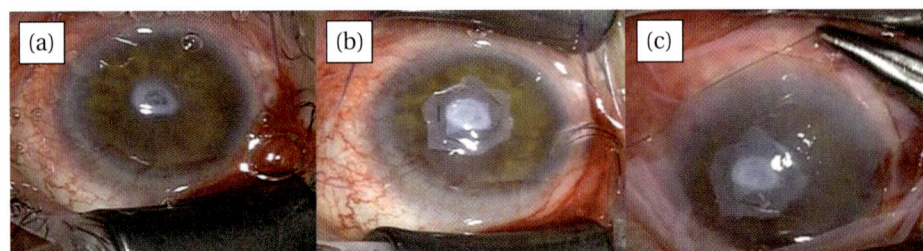

FIGURE 18.9 **AM as a Permanent Graft for Deep Corneal Ulcer**. When the corneal epithelial defect extends deeper to involve more stromal ulceration (a), a single layer of AM graft may not be enough to restore the stromal integrity. Thus, multiple layers of AM can be used as a permanent graft to restore the corneal stromal integrity, and the top layer needs to be sutured with 10-0 Nylon (b). To ensure rapid epithelialization, another AM graft is laid down as a temporary graft and secured to the perilimbal sclera (c) in the same manner as shown in Figure 18.5. The latter temporary graft can be substituted by insertion of ProKera®. A temporary tarsorrhaphy can be added to minimize the exposure problem due to the lack of blinking.

Corneal Descemetocele or Perforation

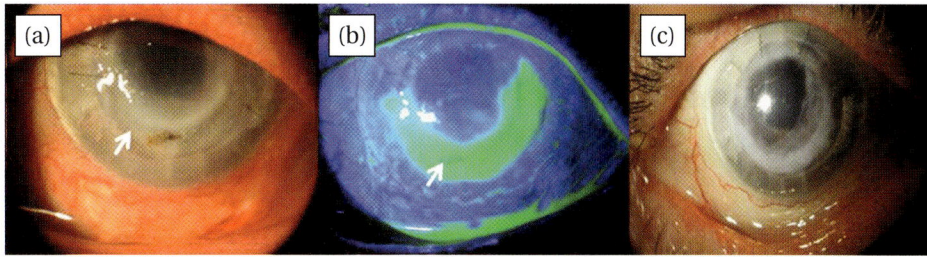

FIGURE 18.10 AM as a Permanent Graft for Deep Corneal Ulcer and Occult Perforation. In this eye that developed a circumlinear ulceration between the corneal graft and the host, there was a perforation at the 6 o'clock position (marked by arrow, a and b). Similar to what has been described in Figure 18.9, multiple layers of AM are used as a permanent graft to restore the corneal stromal integrity while the top layer is sutured with 10-0 nylon, and another AM graft is laid down as a temporary graft and secured to the perilimbal sclera. The latter temporary graft can be substituted by insertion of ProKera®. This technique results in restoration of the corneal integrity, averting the need of corneal patch graft, which will be more difficult to perform and face the risk of rejection, and avoid subsequent corneal transplantation (c).

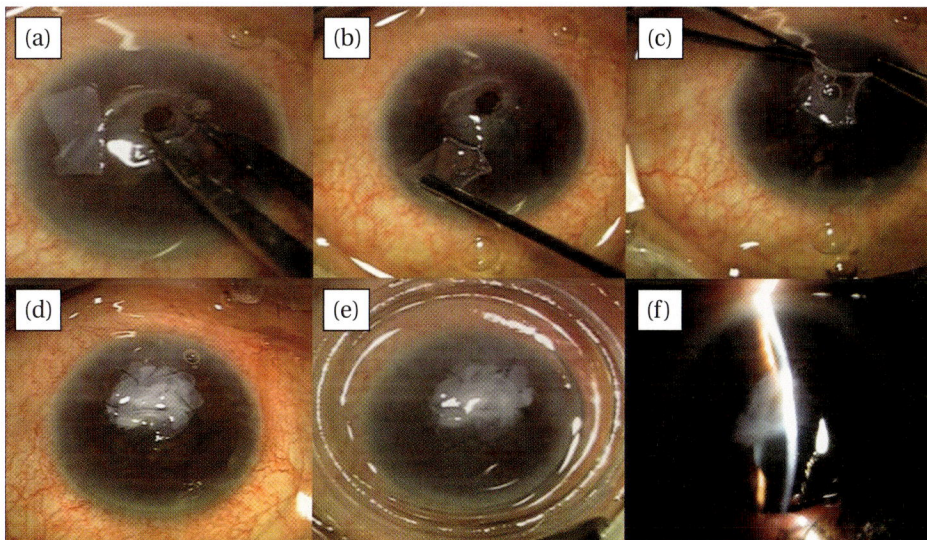

FIGURE 18.11 AM as a Permanent Graft for Deep Corneal Ulcer and Frank Perforation. When a deep corneal ulcer leads to a frank perforation up to 2 mm in diameter (a), it is still feasible to restore the corneal stromal integrity using multiple layers of AM as a permanent graft. To do so, multiple smaller pieces of AM are gelled together by fibrin glue (b, c) and sutured by 10-0 nylon (d). To ensure rapid epithelialization, another AM graft is laid down as a temporary graft and secured to the perilimbal sclera in the same manner as shown in Figure 18.5. The latter temporary graft can be substituted by insertion of ProKera® (e). A temporary tarsorrhaphy can be added to minimize the exposure problem due to the lack of blinking. This technique results in restoration of a stable corneal surface with a deep anterior chamber (f). (All pictures except (f) are displayed as a surgeon's view during surgery). AMT offers the following advantages: avoidance of potential allograft rejection and postoperative astigmatism of tectonic corneal grafts, ease and convenience of use, feasibility in the event of corneal tissue shortage, and preservation of a better aesthetic appearance.

Bullous Keratopathy with or without Band Keratopathy

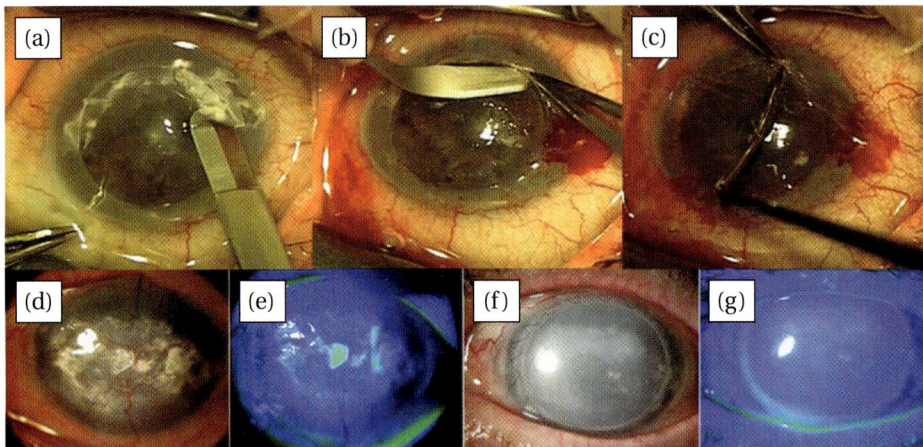

FIGURE 18.12 AM as a Permanent Graft for Bullous Keratopathy. Eyes with painful bullous keratopathy but without visual potential are not indicated for conventional corneal transplantation. If such eyes have developed recurrent pain, persistent epithelial defect, band keratopathy, or concerns of superinfection, they are indicated for AMT. The surgery starts with debridement of loose central epithelium and superficial keratectomy to remove a calcified epithelium (if associated with band keratopathy) using a #64 blade (a). A superficial trephination (a quarter-turn) of the size of 9.5–10 mm in diameter is followed by a lamellar pocket created 360 degrees toward the limbus by a crescent blade (b). AM is inserted into this pocket and can be either glued or sutured (c) to ensure that epithelialization will take place on the top, but not underneath the membrane. It is optional to insert a bandage contact lens or another layer of AM or ProKera® as a temporary graft, as shown in Figure 18.5. Such a procedure invariably results in a smooth, noninflamed, healed, and stable corneal surface without pain afterwards (before, d, e, and after, f, g).

Following Superficial Keratectomy to Remove Band Keratopathy, Scar, or Tumor

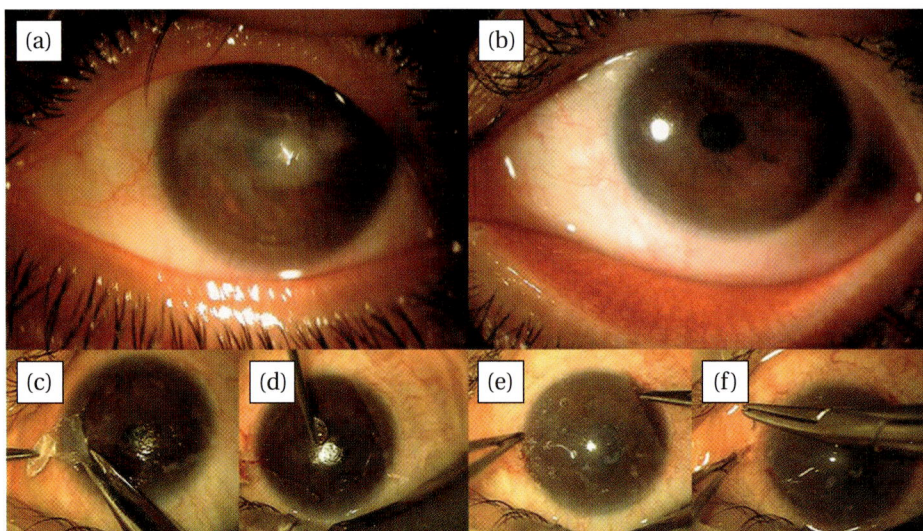

FIGURE 18.13 AMT Following Superficial Keratectomy to Remove a Scar. In an eye with superficial scar (a), the surgery starts with superficial keratectomy to remove the scar tissue (c). AM is placed as a permanent graft on the cornea and secured by fibrin glue (d, e). To ensure rapid epithelialization, another layer of AM as a temporary graft is secure with 10-0 nylon in a purse-string running fashion 2–3 mm from the limbus (similar to what has been shown in Figure 18.5) or a ProKera® is inserted. Such a procedure results in a smooth, stable, and clear corneal surface afterwards (b).

Partial Limbal Stem Cell Deficiency (LSCD)

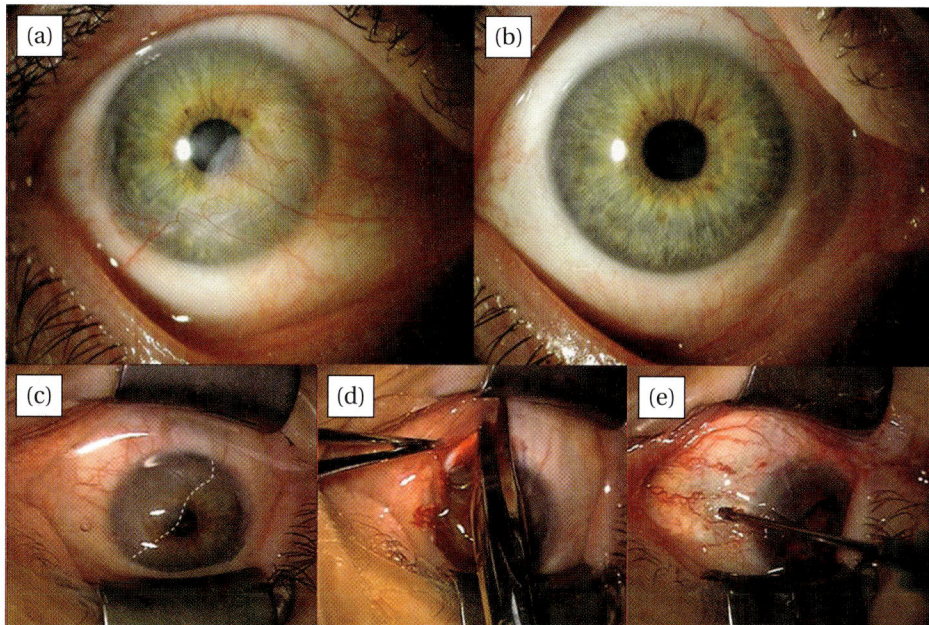

FIGURE 18.14 AMT as a Permanent Graft for Partial LSCD. The corneal epithelial stem cells are located exclusively at the limbus. Destructive loss of the limbal epithelial stem cells and/or dysfunction of the limbal stroma will lead to limbal stem cell deficiency, which is characterized by conjunctivalization of the cornea; i.e., the conjunctival epithelium migrates to cover the corneal surface, which is accompanied by vascularization, destruction of the basement membrane, chronic inflammation, and scarring of the cornea. In eyes with *partial* limbal stem cell deficiency, AMT alone can successfully reconstruct these limbal deficient corneas by expanding residual limbal stem cells from the adjacent limbus, thus avoiding transplantation of autologous or allogeneic limbal stem cells. In this eye with partial limbal stem cell deficiency involving the limbus from 3:00 to 7:00 (a), the conjunctivalized pannus is removed by superficial keratectomy (c) and the adjacent conjunctiva is recessed to the fornix (d). The entire denuded corneal and scleral surface is covered by a layer of cryopreserved AM, with the stromal surface down, using fibrin glue (e). This procedure can restore a normal, avascular smooth corneal surface without stem cell transplantation (b).

In Conjunction with Limbal Conjunctival Autograft for Unilateral Total LSCD after Superficial Keratectomy

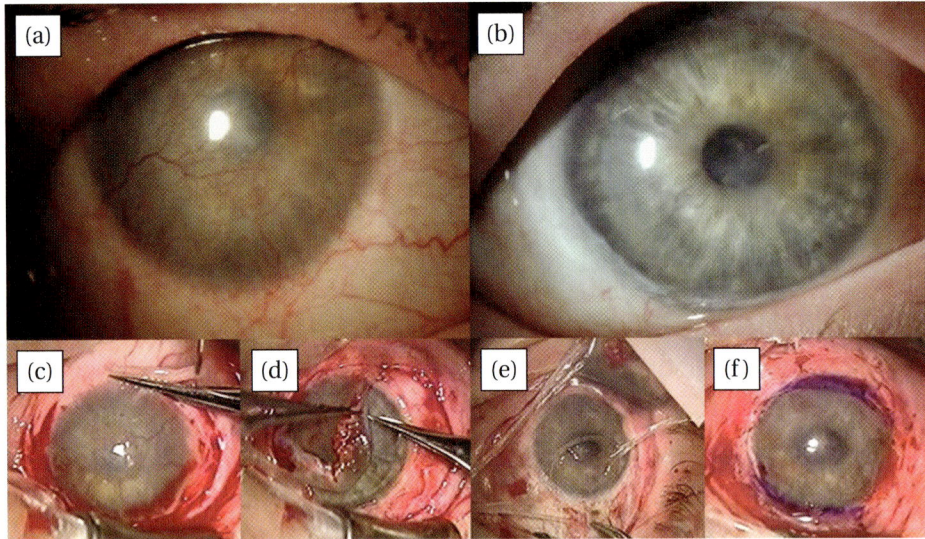

FIGURE 18.15 **AMT as a Permanent Graft for Unilateral Total LSCD**. In this eye inflicted with *unilateral total* limbal stem cell deficiency due to Stevens Johnson syndrome (a), transplantation of autologous limbal epithelial stem cells via conjunctival limbal autograft is indicated. The entire conjunctivalized pannus is removed by superficial keratectomy from the corneal surface (c, d). A large sheet of AM is placed over the cornea with the stromal surface down, and secured with fibrin glue (e) or sutures. Two strips of conjunctival limbal autograft are removed from the healthy fellow-eye (marked in blue), and transferred and secured by interrupted 10-0 nylon sutures over AM (f). To facilitate the healing process and recovery of the limbal integrity, another AM as a temporary graft is applied via insertion of ProKera® or sutured in the same manner as in Figure 18.5. This procedure results in restoration of a smooth, avascular, and stable corneal surface (b).

In Conjunction with Keratolimbal Allograft for Bilateral Total LSCD

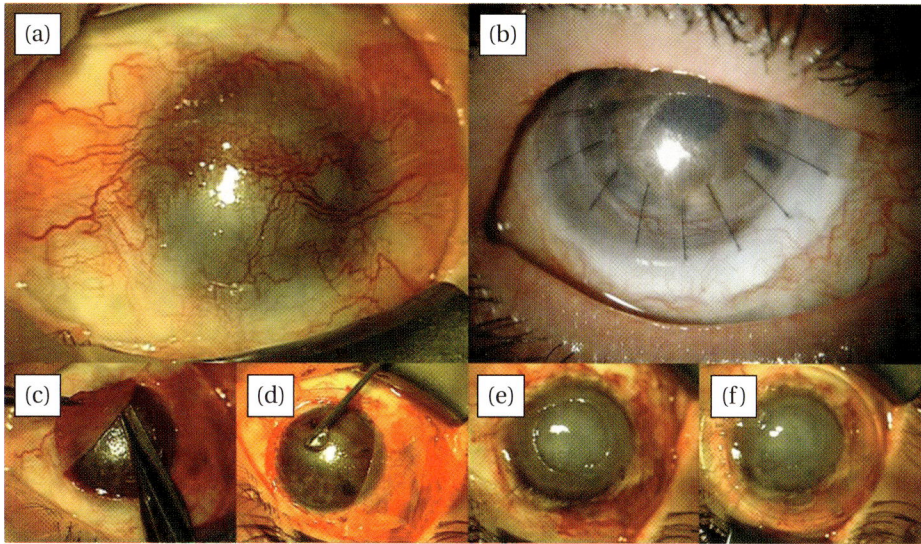

FIGURE 18.16 AMT as a Permanent Graft and Temporary grafts for Total Bilateral LSCD. In cases with *total bilateral* limbal stem cell deficiency, transplantation of allogeneic limbal epithelial stem cells is required. In this eye with total bilateral limbal stem cell deficiency caused by a chemical burn (a), the procedure starts with the removal of conjunctivalized fibrovascular tissue from the corneal surface by superficial keratectomy (c). A large sheet of AM is placed over the cornea with the stromal surface down, and secured with fibrin glue (d). A keratolimbal allograft is prepared from a donor corneoscleral rim following conventional corneal transplantation, and sutured over AM (e). A ProKera® is then inserted as a temporary graft to facilitate re-epithelialization (f). This procedure was then followed by a successful penetrating keratoplasty 4 months later (b). AMT alone cannot treat ischemia caused by radiation or MMC, or chemical burns. It can help ischemia in conjunction with tenonplasty. AMT alone cannot treat *total* limbal stem cell deficiency. It can help both the donor and recipient eyes receiving conjunctival limbal autograft (Fig. 18.15) or keratolimbal allograft (Fig. 18.16). AMT alone cannot treat exposure problems due to the lack of tear film, including dellen. It can help healing if the exposure problem is resolved by other measures, including punctal occlusion, tarsorrhaphy, etc. ProKera® should not be used in eyes with glaucoma drainage implant or scleral buckle, as its skirt might rub against the implanted tube/plate.

TABLE 18.2 *Possible Complications of Amniotic Membrane Transplantation*

General postoperative complications
Infection
Bleeding
Graft rejection
Suture related complications
Inflammation
Granuloma formation
Graft related complications
Hematoma under the graft
Graft detachment
Graft failure

SELECTED REFERENCES

Anderson DF, Ellies P, Pires, et al. Amniotic membrane transplantation for partial limbal stem cell deficiency. *Br J Ophthalmol.* 2001;85:567–575.

Dua HS, Gomes JA, King AJ, et al. The amniotic membrane in ophthalmology. *Surv Ophthalmol.* 2004;49:51–77.

Espana EM, Grueterich M, Sandoval H, et al. Amniotic membrane transplantation for bullous keratopathy in eyes with poor visual potential. *J Cat Refract Surg.* 2003;29:279–284.

Kheirkhah A, Johnson DA, Paranjpe DR, et al. Temporary sutureless amniotic membrane patch for acute alkaline burns. *Arch Ophthalmol.* 2008;126:1059–1066.

Meallet MA, Espana EM, Grueterich M, et al. Amniotic membrane transplantation with conjunctival limbal autograft for total limbal stem cell deficiency. *Ophthalmology.* 2003;110:1585–1592.

Meller D, Pires RTF, Mack RJS, et al. Amniotic membrane transplantation for acute chemical or thermal burns. *Ophthalmology.* 2000;107:980–990.

Sheha H, Liang L, Li J, Tseng SCG. Sutureless amniotic membrane transplantation for severe bacterial keratitis. *Cornea.* 2009; 28(10):1118–1123.

Solomon A, Meller D, Prabhasawat P, et al. Amniotic membrane grafts for nontraumatic corneal perforations, descemetoceles, and deep ulcers. *Ophthalmology.* 2002;109:694–703.

Tseng SCG, Espana EM, Kawakita T, et al. How does amniotic membrane work? *Ocular Surface.* 2004;2:177–187.

Tseng SCG, Prabhasawat P, Barton K, et al. Amniotic membrane transplantation with or without limbal allografts for corneal surface reconstruction in patients with limbal stem cell deficiency. *Arch Ophthalmol.* 1998;116:431–441.

19

Management of Ocular Surface Tumors

Anita Gupta, MD and Carol L. Karp, MD

Ocular Surface Tumors

There are a variety of neoplastic lesions that arise within the conjunctiva and cornea. These are classified by their tissue of origin, then subdivided as benign, preinvasive, or malignant. Distinguishing between such lesions can be challenging, and often requires multiple examinations, different imaging techniques, and biopsy for proper diagnosis.

TABLE 19.1 Neoplastic Lesions of the Conjunctiva and Cornea

	Benign	*Preinvasive*	*Malignant*
Tumors of epithelial origin	Squamous papilloma	Conjunctival and corneal intraepithelial neoplasia (CIN)	Squamous cell carcinoma (SCCA) Mucoepidermoid carcinoma
Tumors of neuroectodermal origin	Nevus Benign congenital or acquired melanosis Ocular melanocytosis	Primary acquired melanosis (PAM)	Melanoma
Tumors of vascular and mesenchymal origin	Hemangioma Pyogenic granuloma		Kaposi sarcoma
Tumors of lymphatic origin	Lymphangioma Benign reactive lymphoid hyperplasia		Lymphoma
Choristomas	Epidermoid and dermoid cyst Dermoid tumor Dermolipoma		

Nonpigmented Conjunctival Lesions

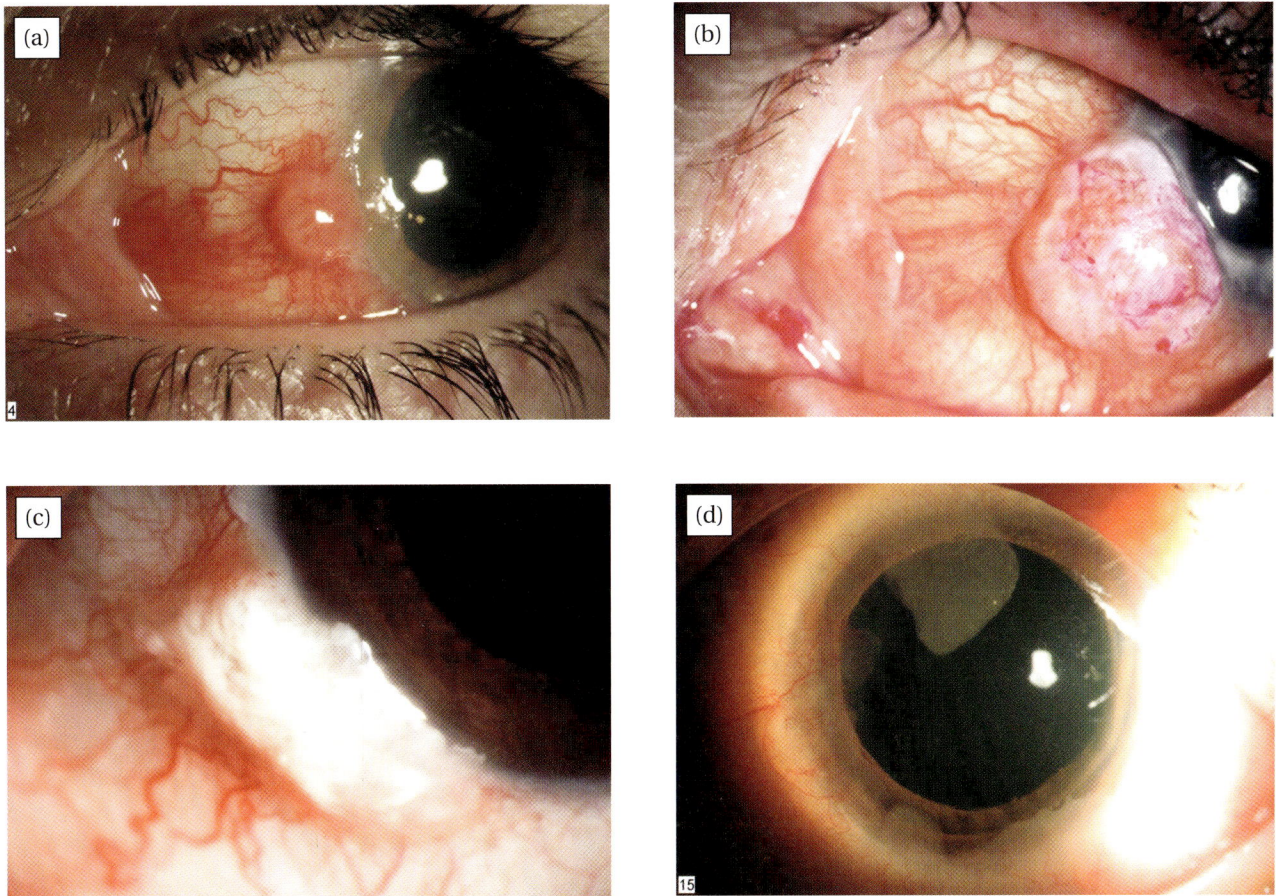

FIGURE 19.1 **Non-pigmented Conjunctival Lesions.** (a) Conjunctival and corneal intraepithelial neoplasia (CIN), papilliform; (b) CIN, leukoplakic; (c) CIN, gelatinous; (d) CIN, opalescent. Conjunctival and corneal intraepithelial neoplasia (CIN) is a preinvasive lesion that represents the most common nonpigmented tumor affecting the ocular surface. CIN is a dysplastic process limited to the epithelium. If invasion of the basement membrane occurs, it is then considered invasive squamous cell carcinoma. Factors associated with CIN include sun exposure, human papilloma virus (mainly type 16 and 18), and HIV infection. CIN presents in four main forms: papilliform (a), leukoplakic (b), gelatinous (c), and opalescent (d). Although CIN can occur anywhere on the conjunctival or corneal surface, lesions typically arise within the interpalpebral fissure, at the limbus. Staining the ocular surface with rose bengal can disclose a fine granular pattern over CIN lesions as seen in Figure (b), which can aid in diagnosis.

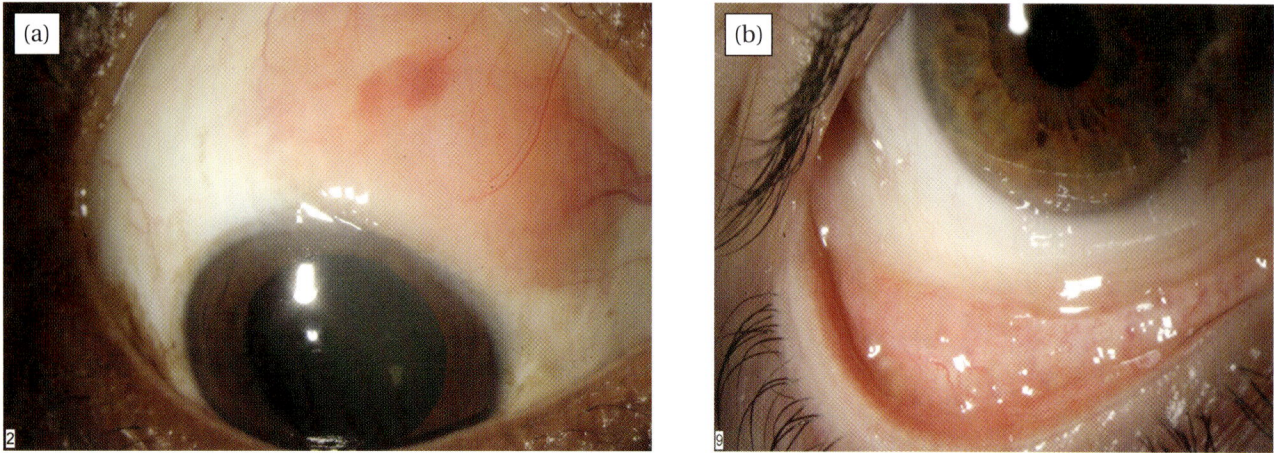

FIGURE 19.2 Conjunctival Lymphoma. (a) Epibulbar lesion; (b) Conjunctival lymphoma with follicular reaction in the inferior fornix. Conjunctival lymphoma is caused by a monoclonal proliferation of lymphocytes. The majority of conjunctival lymphomas are of the B-cell type and arise from mucosa associated lymphatic tissue (MALT). Conjunctival lymphoma often appears as a pink mobile mass on the bulbar conjunctiva (a). Lack of mobility may be suggestive of scleral extension. A follicular reaction is also typically present (b). Conjunctival lymphoma and benign reactive lymphoid hyperplasia can have the same clinical appearance; therefore biopsy with flow cytometry and gene rearrangement may be required for diagnosis. Local external beam radiotherapy is currently the gold standard treatment for localized conjunctival lymphoma. Other treatments such as monoclonal immunotherapy have also proven successful in managing this disease, when systemic.

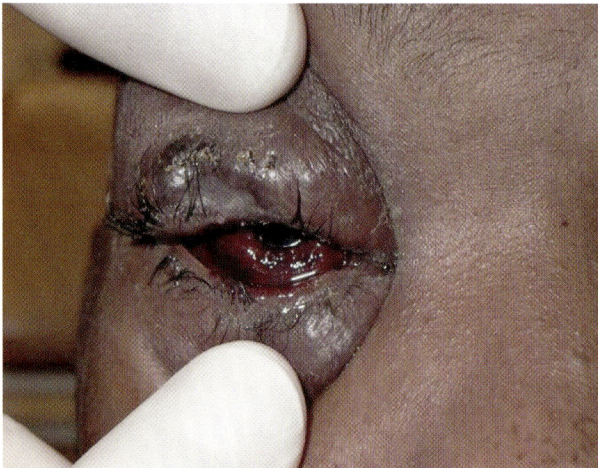

FIGURE 19.3 Kaposi Sarcoma. Kaposi sarcoma is tumor of the vascular endothelium, and is associated with herpes virus 8. The tumor can be multicentric or diffuse, affecting the eyelids, conjunctiva, and orbit. On the conjunctiva, lesions appear as bulky red lesions that are highly vascular and have a tendency to bleed, causing associated subconjunctival hemorrhages. The goal of treatment is often to control or debulk, rather than curing disease. Treatment can involve radiotherapy, cryotherapy, interferon alpha-2b, and surgical debulking, and systemic chemotherapy.

Pigmented Conjunctival Lesions

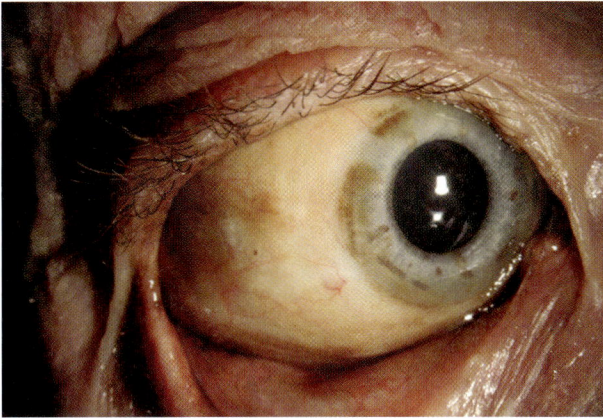

FIGURE 19.4 **Primary Acquired Melanosis (PAM).** Primary acquired melanosis (PAM) is an acquired pigmentation of the conjunctiva, where melanocytes abnormally proliferate in the basal conjunctival epithelium. Light-skinned and middle-aged individuals are most commonly affected. PAM can occur both with and without atypical cells. Diagnosis of atypia is made histologically. PAM without atypia poses minimal risk for malignant transformation, whereas PAM with atypia can increases the risk of malignant transformation up to 50%. The clinical appearance of PAM is multiple flat brown patches in the conjunctiva; however, nodularity, elevation, increase in size, and increased vascularity can represent malignant transformation.

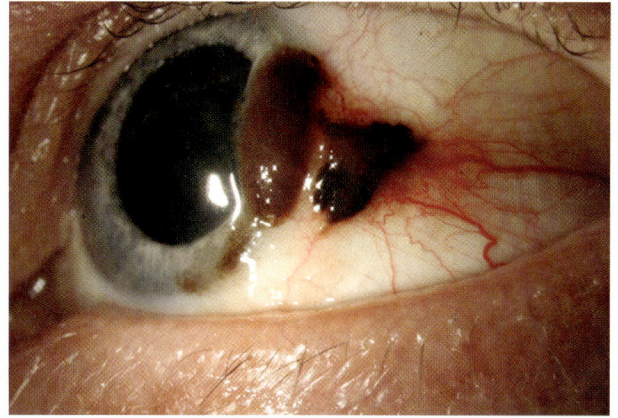

FIGURE 19.5 **Malignant Melanoma of the Conjunctiva.** Malignant melanoma can arise from PAM with atypia, acquired nevi, or de novo from normal conjunctiva. Malignant melanoma rarely arises from congenital nevi. Metastasis does occur overall, but conjunctival melanoma offers a better prognosis than that of cutaneous melanoma. Factors associated with a poorer prognosis in conjunctival melanoma include multifocality, caruncular, tarsal, or forniceal involvement, positive surgical margins, and recurrent disease.

Treatment Considerations of Ocular Surface Tumors

The goal in treating ocular surface neoplasias is eradication of all tumor cells in order to cure disease and reduce the rate of recurrence. The treatment strategies listed in the following table have been utilized successfully in management of a variety of ocular surface tumors, and include both surgical and nonsurgical techniques. Treatment choice is typically individualized case by case. Surgery can be advantageous in patients with small or well-defined tumors where excision can be performed with high likelihood of tumor-free margins. In addition, surgical interventions offer definitive treatment without risk of compliance issues that can occur with nonsurgical strategies. However, nonsurgical treatment can offer useful alternatives to surgical excision, especially in patients who cannot undergo surgery. Nonsurgical treatments also have the benefit of treating the entire ocular surface, which is particularly helpful for treating large, diffuse, or recurrent tumors where margins are not well defined and there is a risk for limbal stem cell deficiency after surgical excision.

TABLE 19.2 *Treatment Options for Ocular Surface Neoplasia*

Surgical Options
Simple surgical excision with wide margins
Surgical excision with adjuvant therapies (cryotherapy, cautery, topical chemotherapy)

Nonsurgical Options
Radiotherapy
Excimer laser
Photodynamic therapy
Topical chemotherapy (interferon alpha-2b, mitomycin C, and 5-fluorouracil)

Surgical Excision and Cryotherapy for Ocular Surface Tumors: Step-by-Step

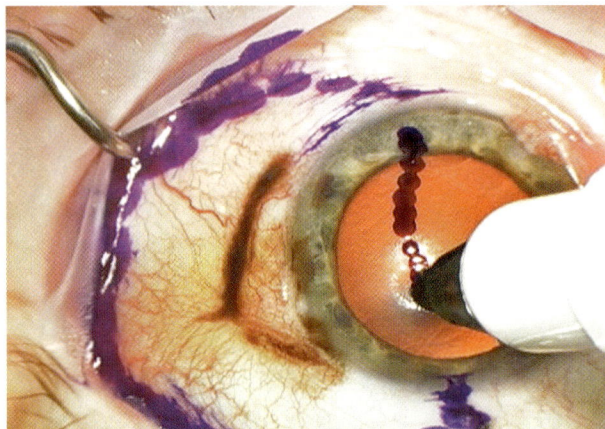

FIGURE 19.6 **Outline Lesion with 4–6 mm Margins.** Conjunctival melanoma treated with surgical excision and cryotherapy. The first step of surgery is to identify the tumor. Staining with Rose Bengal intraoperatively can help visualize subtle tumor margins. The edges of the area to be excised are marked with a marking pen, using 4–6 mm margins around the tumor.

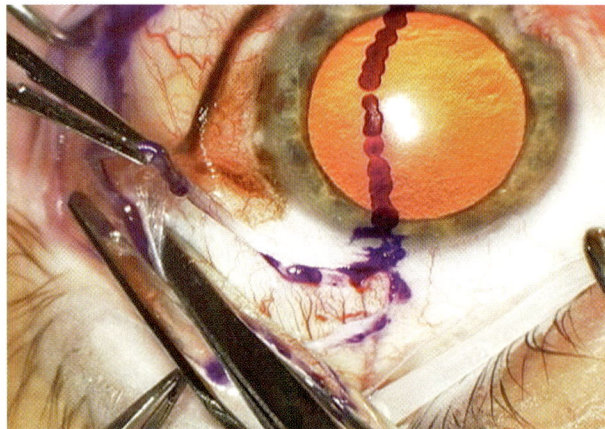

FIGURE 19.7 **Excision of Lesion Utilizing a "No Touch" Technique.** The conjunctival portion of the tumor is excised along the pre-marked margins and the limbus using Wescott scissors. During excision, spreading should be performed along the marked margins, while avoiding any spreading under the tumor. In addition, it is important to avoid manipulation of the tumor itself by using the Shield's "no touch" technique in order to avoid possible seeding of tumor cells.

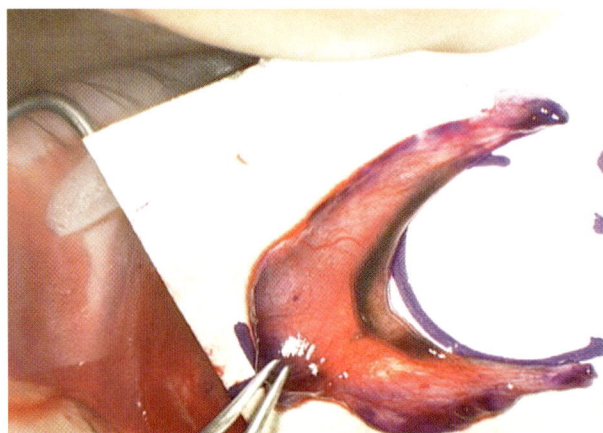

FIGURE 19.8 **Orientation of Specimen for Pathology.** The specimen is placed on a paper, with the correct orientation marked. Marking should be retraced with pencil, as ink can smear or dissolve in formalin. The specimen is allowed to dry on the paper so that it is adherent. The specimen with the paper is then placed in formalin for subsequent histopathologic analysis.

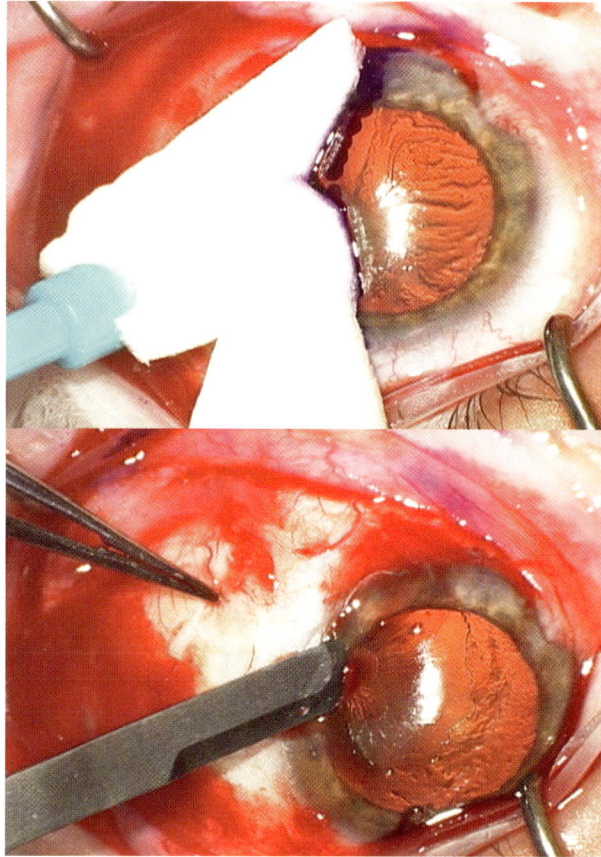

FIGURE 19.9 **Alcohol Epitheliectomy to Remove Corneal Extent of Lesion.** Excision of the corneal extent of the tumor is carried out by first loosening the corneal epithelium with absolute alcohol for 30 seconds. Alcohol is then irrigated away using copious balanced salt solution. The loosened epithelium is "scrolled" over the entire lesion, plus another 3–4 mm of epithelium to the limbus using a straight crescent blade.

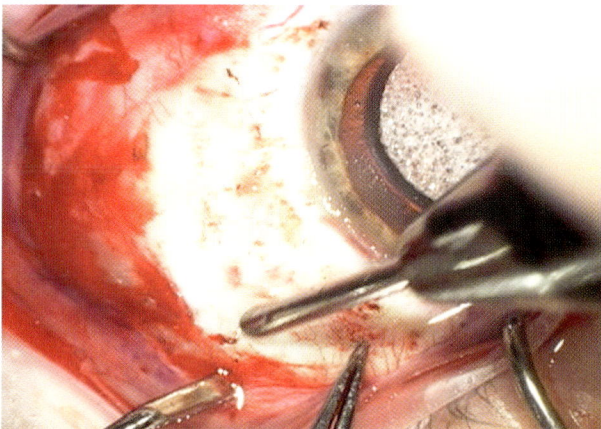

FIGURE 19.10 **Cautery to the Scleral Bed.** Once the specimen is removed, the scleral bed is scraped using a straight crescent blade. Cautery is then applied to the scleral bed in order to render any possible remaining tumor cells nonviable.

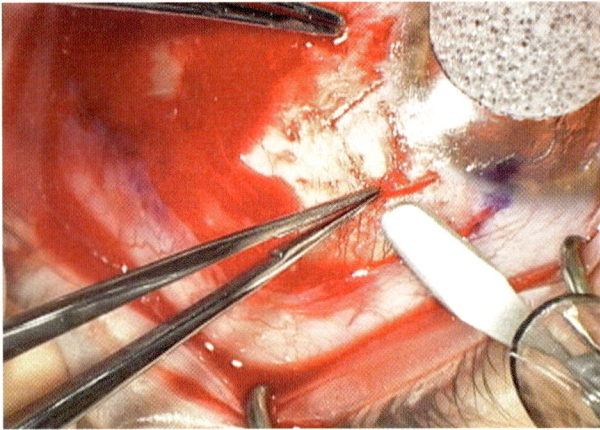

FIGURE 19.11 **Lamellar Sclerectomy when Scleral Extension is Suspected.** Scleral extension of ocular surface tumors should be suspected when tumors are not freely mobile, are adherent to underlying sclera, or have abnormal appearing sclera associated with them. If scleral extension is suspected, a 20% thickness sclerectomy should be carried out in these areas and sent for histopathological analysis.

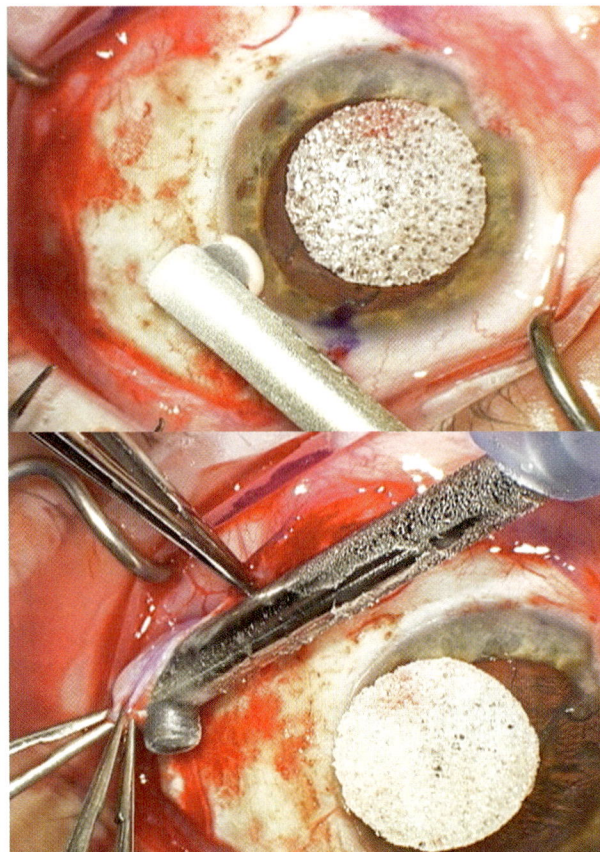

FIGURE 19.12 **Double Freeze/Slow Thaw Cryotherapy to Limbus and Conjunctival Margins.** Cryotherapy is performed in a double freeze/slow thaw cycle to the limbus and conjunctival edges. Effective cryotherapy includes rapid freezing followed by a slow thawing, which allows for maximum cell death. Once cryotherapy is complete, all instruments should be changed to avoid possible seeding of tumor cells.

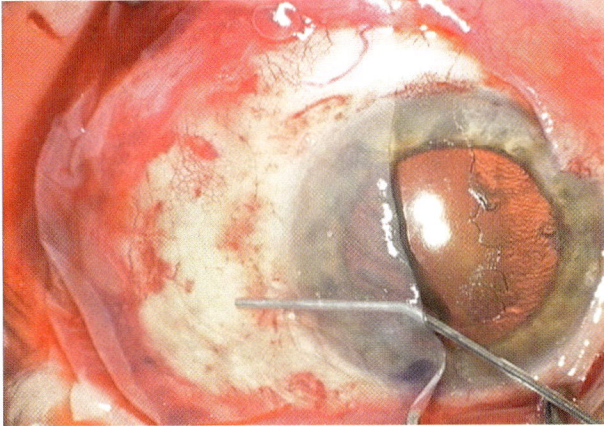

FIGURE 19.13 **Amniotic Membrane Placed over Exposed Sclera, Secured into Place with Tissue Adhesive.** Closure is typically carried out using preserved human amniotic membrane to cover the exposed sclera. This is placed with the stromal side of the membrane facing the sclera, and then secured into place using tissue adhesive. The two components of the adhesive (fibrinogen and thrombin) are placed separately between the sclera and membrane using a 30-gauge cannula. A muscle hook is used to smooth the membrane, and tuck its edges underneath the cut conjunctival edge. Excess amniotic membrane is trimmed.

Complications of Surgical Treatment

Complications of surgical excision and adjuvant cryotherapy are listed in the following table. Larger and more diffuse tumors often require more aggressive surgical intervention that can lead to a higher risk of complication.

TABLE 19.3 *Post-surgical Complications After Tumor Excision with Cryotherapy*

Limbal stem cell deficiency

Corneal thinning

Cyclodestruction/hypotony

Muscle damage

Hyphema and iritis secondary to cryotherapy

Cataract

Pyogenic granuloma

Recurrent tumor

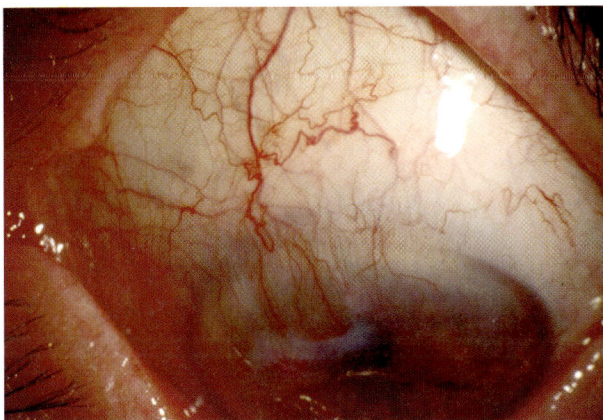

FIGURE 19.14 **Limbal Stem Cell Deficiency after Surgical Excision and Cryotherapy for CIN.** Limbal stem cell deficiency occurs when a critical amount of limbal tissue is removed or destroyed during tumor excision or cryotherapy. For this reason, large or annular tumors may be better managed with non-surgical techniques. Topical chemotherapeutic agents can be utilized as sole treatment, or initial treatment in order to decrease the tumor burden prior to surgical excision, thereby minimizing limbal stem cell loss.

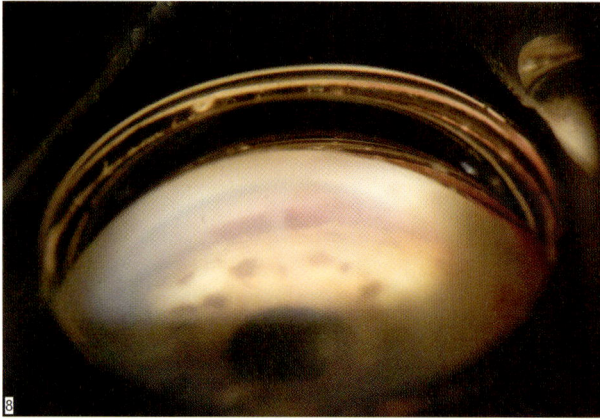

FIGURE 19.15 **Hyphema after Surgical Excision and Cryotherapy for CIN.** Aggressive cryotherapy can result in iritis and hyphema as shown above. This complication is typically self-limited, and can be treated with topical steroids.

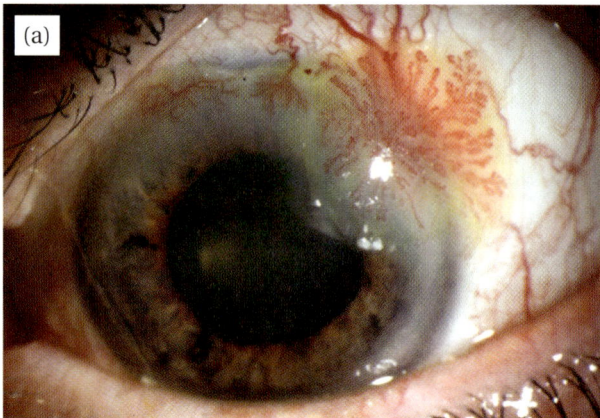

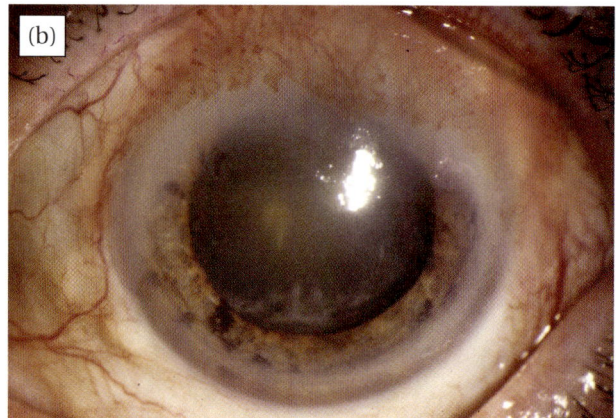

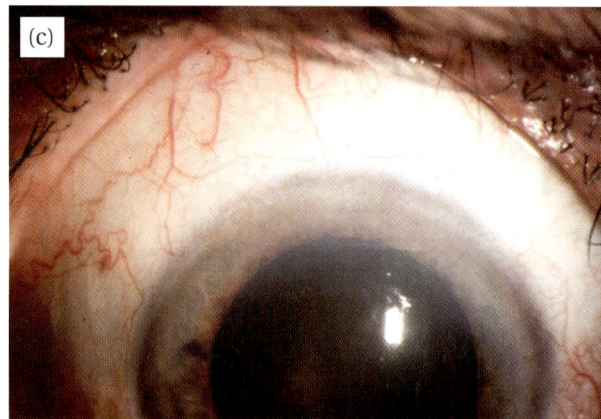

FIGURE 19.16 **Recurrence of CIN after Surgical Excision.** (a) CIN at presentation, before treatment with surgical excision and cryotherapy. (b) CIN recurrence 2 years after surgical excision and cryotherapy for CIN. (c) Resolution of recurrent CIN after treatment with subconjunctival injections of interferon alpha-2b. Recurrence of ocular surface tumors is a common complication of surgical excision. The rate of recurrence for CIN is been shown to be as high as one-third in patients who have clear surgical margins and one half in patients with positive margins. This figure shows a patient with a papilliform CIN that was treated with wide margin surgical excision and cryotherapy. Surgical margins were examined and found to be free of tumor. The patient then developed a recurrence of the tumor 2 years after surgical excision. This recurrent disease was treated successfully with 6 weekly subconjunctival injections of interferon alpha-2b, with no evidence of recurrence at 10-year follow-up.

Medical Treatment

Classically, the treatments for ocular surface tumors have been surgical excision, cryotherapy and rarely radiation. More recently, topical chemotherapeutic agents have been developed as adjuvant or primary treatment of ocular surface tumors including interferon alpha-2b, mitomycin C, and 5-fluorouracil with significant success. Medical management has advantage particularly in cases of recurrent or diffuse disease, where tumor margins are not clear, or in patients where surgery should be avoided (i.e. stem cell deficiency, compromised wound healing, or poor surgical candidate).

TABLE 19.4 *Medical Treatment Options for Ocular Surface Neoplasia*

Medication	Mechanism of Action	Route	Dose	Regimen
Mitomycin C	Alkylating agent that binds DNA, causing irreversible crosslinking and inhibiting nucleotide synthesis	Topical	0.02% or 0.04%	Qid × 1–2 weeks, then 1 week off. Continue for 2–3 cycles or until resolution
5-Fluorouracil	Antimetabolite that inhibits DNA and RNA synthesis during cell cycle S-phase	Topical	1%	Qid × 4–7 days, then 30 days off. Repeat until resolution.
Interferon alpha-2b	Indirect antiproliferative effect on tumor cells through activation of host cytotoxic effector cells	Topical or Subconjunctival	Topical: 1 MIU/mL Subconjunctival: 3 MIU/0.5 mL	Topical: qid until resolution Subconjunctival: 0.5 mL qweek until resolution

MIU = million international units.

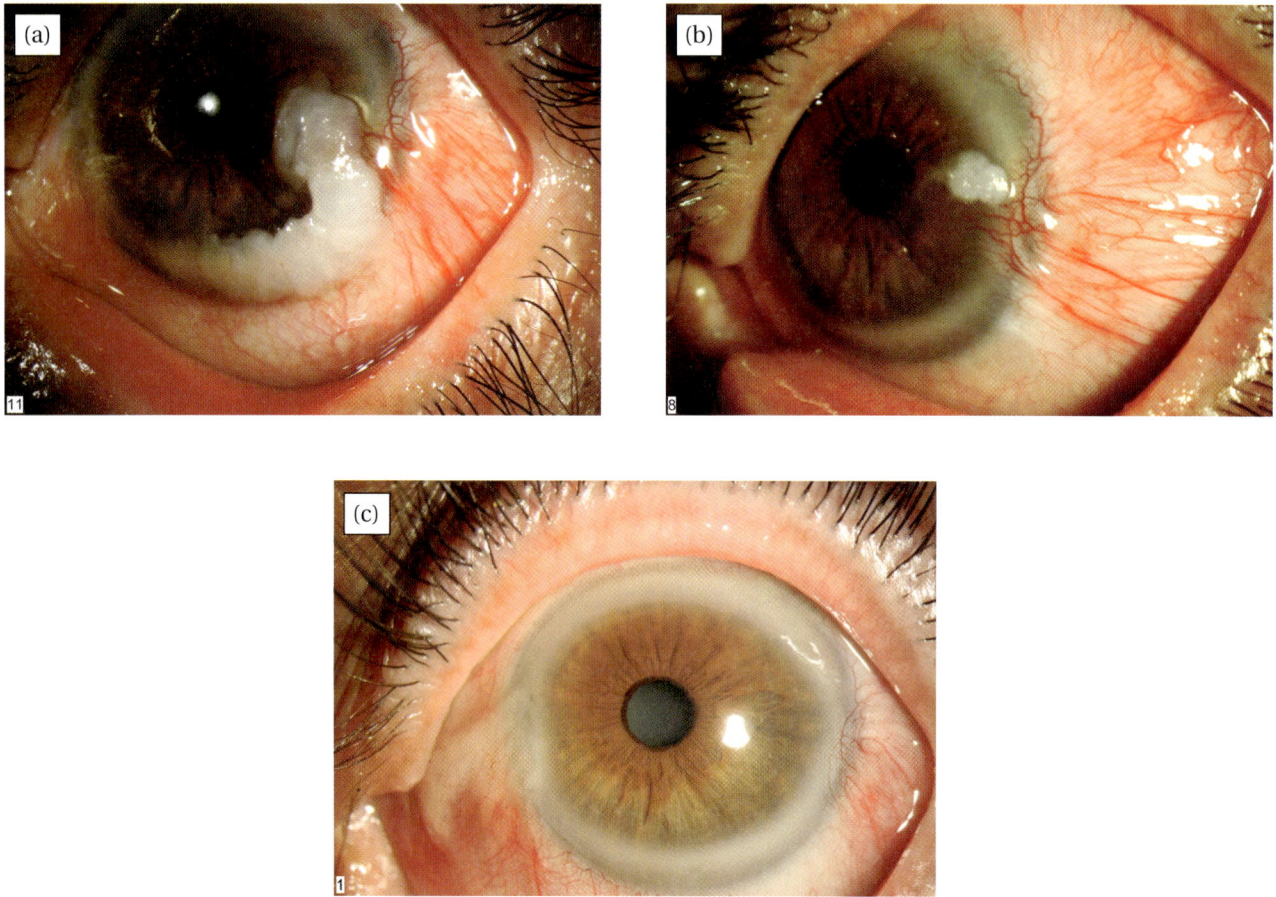

FIGURE 19.17 **CIN Before and After Treatment with Topical Mitomycin C.** (a) CIN at presentation, before treatment with topical mitomycin C (0.04%). (b) CIN after first cycle of topical mitomycin C (0.04%) therapy. (c) CIN after 3 cycles of topical mitomycin C (0.04%) therapy. Mitomycin C is an alkylating agent that inhibits DNA synthesis. It has been used successfully in treatment of several types of ocular surface tumors, both as primary treatment and as an adjunct. It can have significant toxicity, including hyperemia, blepharospasm, keratoconjunctivitis, and punctal stenosis. For this reason, it is administered in cycles of 7–14 day intervals where the treatment is stopped in order to reduce ocular surface toxicity. In addition, punctal plugging and topical steroid may also be needed to limit toxicity. The patient shown here had a large opalescent CIN that was treated with mitomycin C (0.04%). The drug was administered in cycles, qid for 7–10 days for each cycle, with 1 week of no drug between cycles. Resolution of the tumor was seen after 3 cycles.

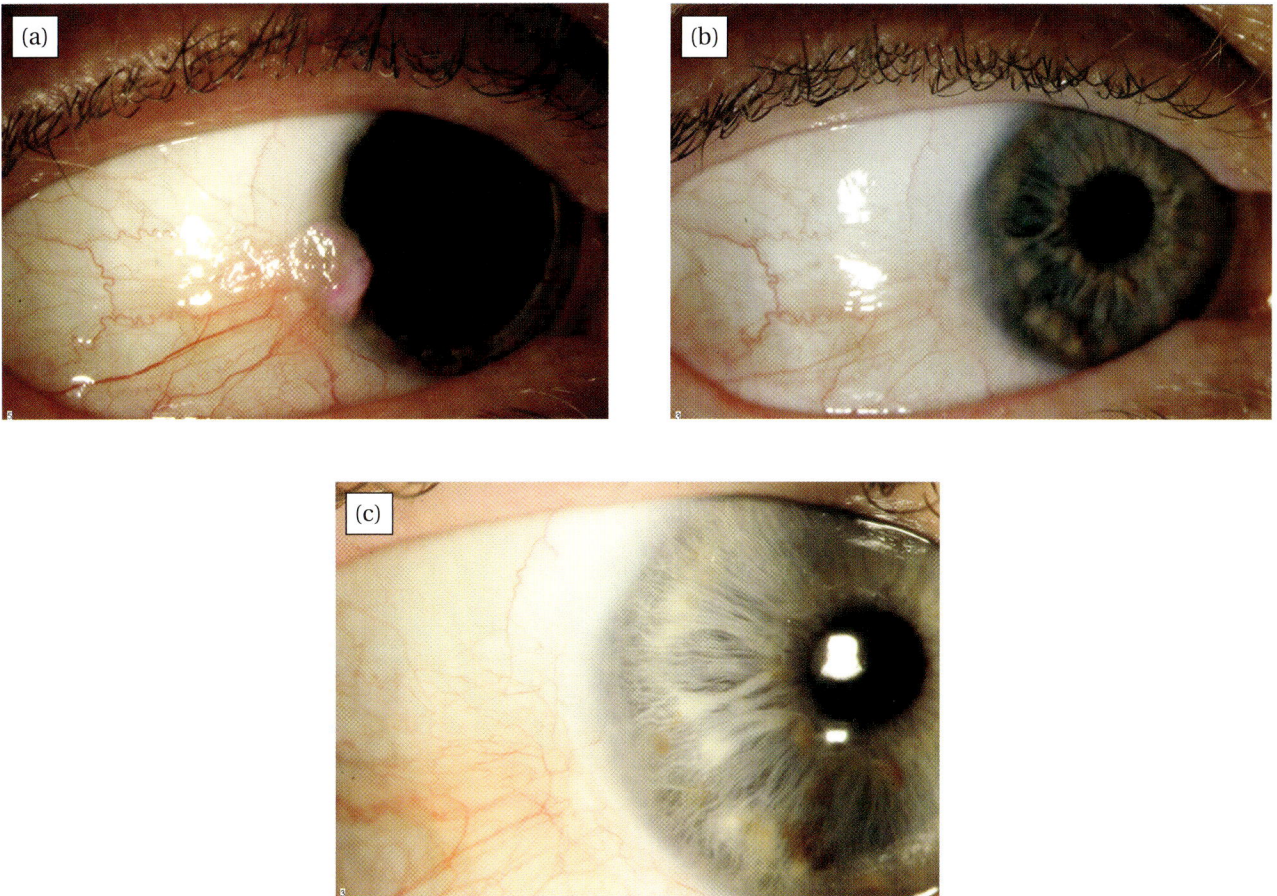

FIGURE 19.18 **CIN Before and After Treatment with Topical 5-fluorouacil.** (a) CIN at presentation, before treatment with topical 5-fluorouracil; (b) CIN after 1 cycle of treatment with topical 5-fluorouracil; (c) CIN after 3 cycles of treatment with topical 5-fluorouracil. 5-Fluorouracil is an antimetabolite that inhibits DNA synthesis in proliferating cells. It can be used topically as primary treatment or adjuvant therapy to surgical excision for many types of ocular surface tumors. It is generally better tolerated than mitomycin C, however still can cause hyperemia and pain. The above patient presented with a leukoplakic CIN which was successfully treated with topical 5-fluorouracil. The patient received 3 cycles of treatment, qid for 4 days, with 30 days off between cycles, before resolution of the tumor.

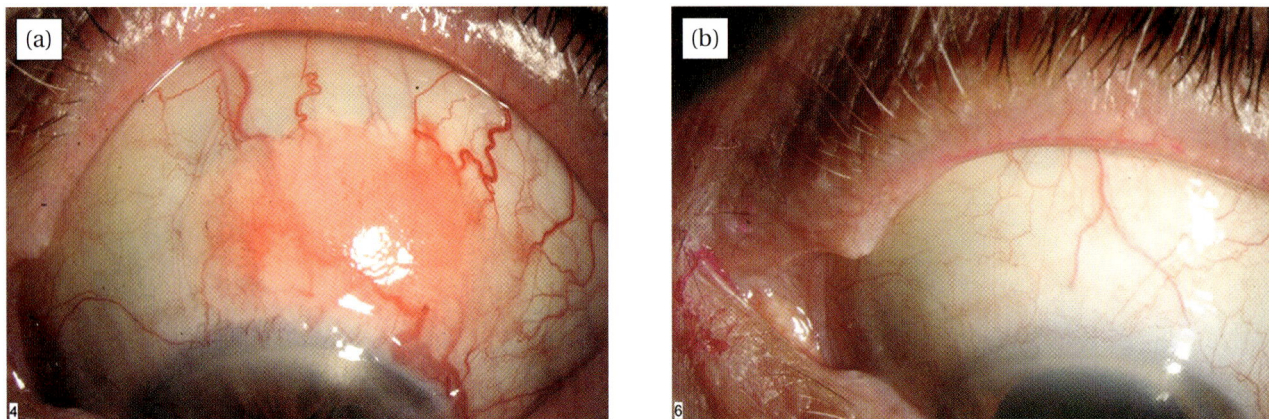

FIGURE 19.19 **CIN Before and After Treatment with Topical Interferon Alpa-2b.** (a) CIN at presentation, before treatment with topical interferon alpha-2b; (b) CIN after two months of treatment with topical interferon alpha-2b. Interferons are low molecular weight glycoproteins produced by leukocytes that have both antiviral and antineoplastic properties. They inhibit viral multiplication, directly inhibit cancer cell proliferation, and activate natural killer leukocytes. Interferons have been used to treat multiple non-ocular cancers, and more recently have been used successfully in treatment of ocular surface tumors. Interferon is generally well tolerated on the ocular surface, and therefore topical treatment involves qid dosing until the tumor resolves. The average time to resolution is 12 weeks. The above patient presented with a large CIN that was treated with topical interferon alpha-2b qid for 2 months prior to resolution of the tumor.

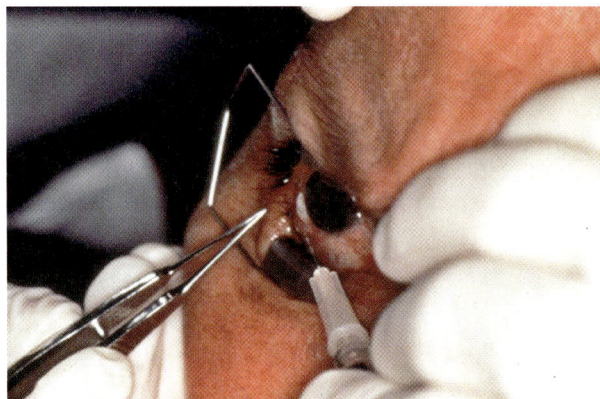

FIGURE 19.20 **Subconjunctival Injection of Interferon Alpha-2b for Treatment of Ocular Surface Neoplasia.** Subconjunctival or intralesional injection of interferon alpha-2b for the treatment of ocular neoplasia can have advantage over topical administration in that it is less expensive, ensures compliance, and shows rapid resolution of disease. It is administered as a 0.5 mL subconjunctival injection of interferon alpha-2b (3 million international units in 0.5 mL) weekly until the tumor resolves. The average time to resolution is 4–5 weeks. Side effects include fever, chills, headache, and myalgia, which are not seen with topical administration. Acetaminophen may be used after injection to ameliorate side effects.

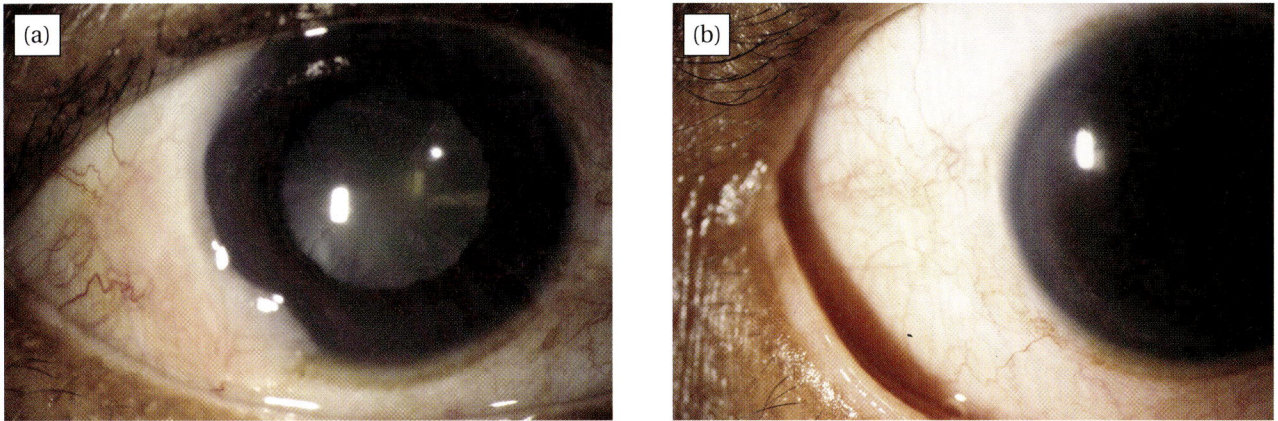

FIGURE 19.21 CIN Before and After Treatment with Subconjunctival Injection of Interferon Alpha-2b. (a) CIN at presentation, before treatment with subconjunctival injection of interferon alpha-2b; (b) CIN after treatment with eleven weekly subconjunctival injections of interferon alpha-2b. The patient pictured here presented with a large CIN with both gelatinous and papillary components. The patient underwent treatment with weekly subconjunctival injections of interferon alpha-2b. Complete resolution of the tumor was seen after 11 weeks of treatment.

SELECTED REFERENCES

Cervantes G, Rodriguez Jr AA, Leas AG. Squamous cell carcinoma of the conjunctiva: clinicohistopathological features in 287 cases. *Can J Ophthalmol.* 2002;37(1):14–20.

Dausch D, Lendesz M, Schroder E. Phototherapeutic Keratectomy in recurrent corneal intraepithelial displasia. *Arch Ophthalmol.* 1994;112:22–23.

Giaconi, JA, Karp CL. Current treatment options for conjunctival and corneal intraepithelial neoplasia. *The Ocular Surface.* 2003;1(2):66–67.

Karp CL, Scott IU, Chang TS, et al. Conjunctival intraepithelial neoplasia. A possible marker for human immunodeficiency virus infection? *Arch Ophthalmol.* 1996;114:257–261.

Pe'er J. Ocular surface squamous neoplasia. *Ophthalmol Clin N Am.* 2005;18:1–13.

Schechter BA, Koreishi AF, Karp CL, Feuer W. Long-term follow-up of conjunctival and corneal intraepithelial neoplasia treated with topical interferon alfa-2b. *Ophthalmology.* 2008;115(8):1291–1296.

Sun EC, Fears TR, Goedert JJ. Epidemiology of squamous cell conjuntival cancer. *Cancer Epidemiolo Biomarders Prev.* 1997;6(2):73–77.

Tabin G. Levin S., Snibson G, et al. Late recurrences and the necessity for long-term follow-up in corneal and conjunctival intraepithelial neoplasia. *Ophthalmology.* 1999;106:91–97.

Tabrizi SM, McCurrach FE, Drewe RH, Borg AJ, Garland SM, Taylor HR. Human papilloma virus in corneal and conjunctival carcinoma. *Aust N Z J Ophthalmol.* 1997;25(3):211–215.

20 Pterygium Surgery

Lawrence Hirst

Please note that all intraoperative images are presented as viewed by the surgeon (i.e., from a temporal approach for a nasal pterygium).

TABLE 20.1 *Indications for Surgery*

Indications For Surgery For Primary Pterygium

Ophthalmologist-Initiated Decision to Advise Surgery

Visual disturbance attributable to pterygium

- Increasing with the rule astigmatism
- Noticing flare at night

Growth

- Documented growth over one or more years of >1 mm (arbitrary limit) and > 2 mm in absolute size

Symptoms

- Irritation, redness resistant to occasional vasoconstrictors
- Regular use of vasoconstrictors of >1/day for >1 year (arbitrary limit)

Size

- Across limbus by 3 mm or greater (arbitrary limit)

Other Indications

- Unusual appearance suggestive of CIN
- Restrictive strabismus

Patient-Initiated Decision to Have Surgery

Cosmesis

Indications for Surgery for Recurrent Pterygium

As above, with possibly lower threshold for intervention

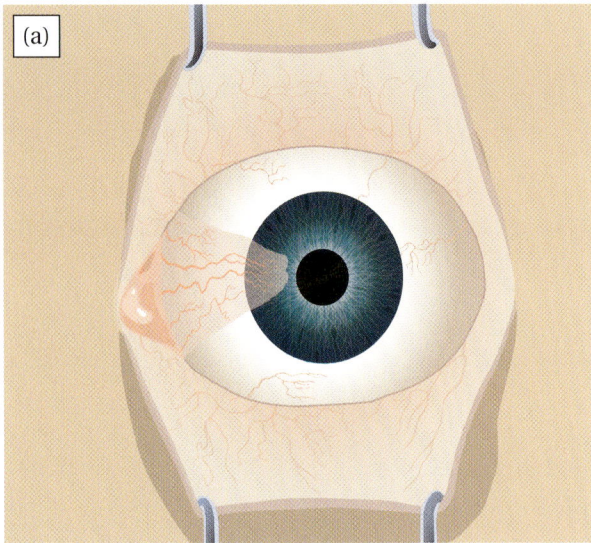

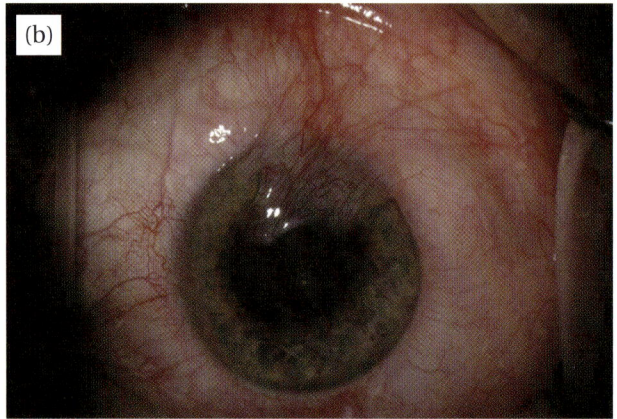

FIGURE 20.1 Left nasal pterygium. (Image (a) originally published in Hirst L. Prospective study of primary pterygium surgery using pterygium extended removal followed by extended conjunctival transplantation. *Ophthalmology* 2008;115:1663–1672. Reprinted by permission of Elsevier Ltd.)

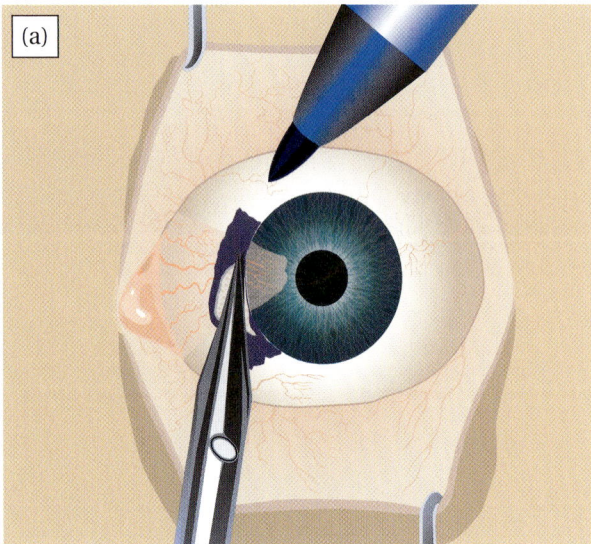

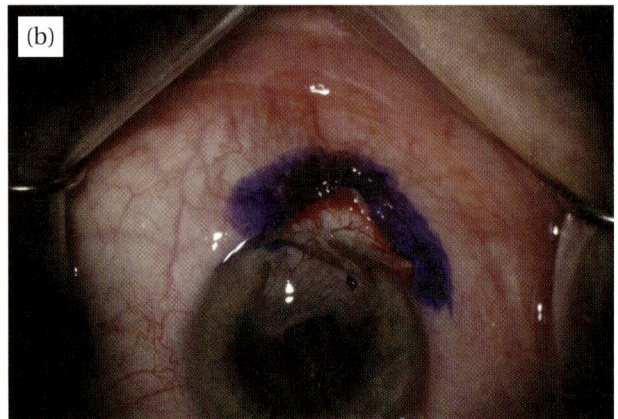

FIGURE 20.2 Marking of limbus and transection of pterygium at limbus: note early retraction of marked conjunctival edge away from limbus with release of Tenons capsule drawn up into pterygium head. (Image (a) originally published in Hirst L. Prospective study of primary pterygium surgery using pterygium extended removal followed by extended conjunctival transplantation. *Ophthalmology* 2008;115:1663–1672. Reprinted by permission of Elsevier Ltd.)

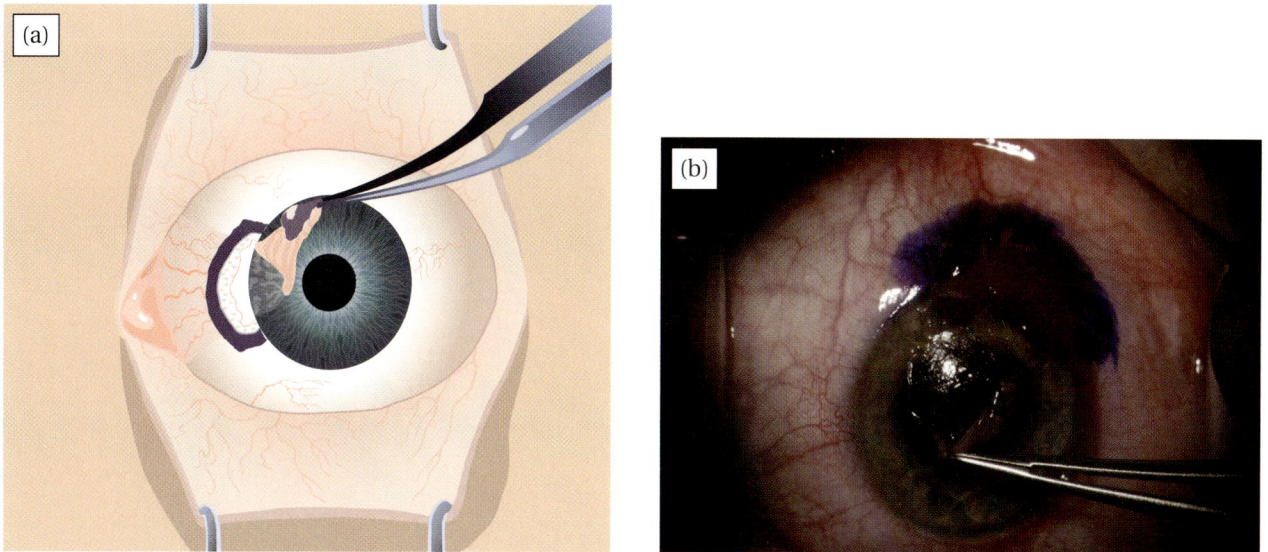

FIGURE 20.3 Stripping of pterygium head off the corneal surface with forceps: note that there has been a spontaneous retraction of the marked conjunctival edge away from the limbus without any conjunctival resection. (Image (a) originally published in Hirst L. Prospective study of primary pterygium surgery using pterygium extended removal followed by extended conjunctival transplantation. *Ophthalmology*. 2008;115:1663–1672. Reprinted by permission of Elsevier Ltd.)

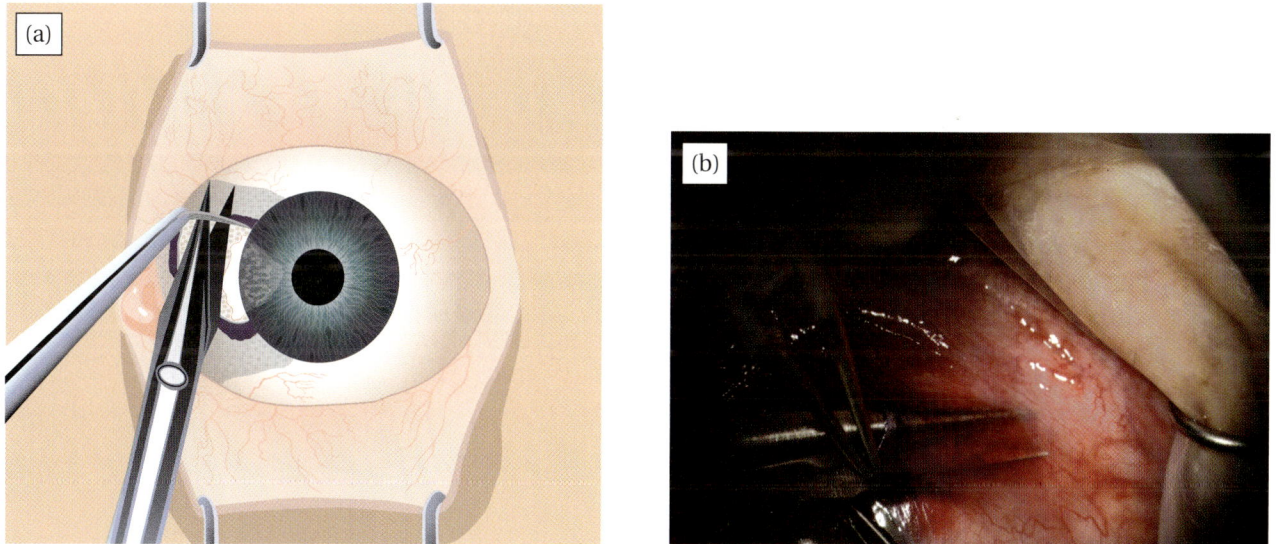

FIGURE 20.4 Extensive sharp dissection separating conjunctiva from Tenons capsule extending 5 mm near the limbus to over 10 mm towards the semilunar fold above and below the medial rectus. (Image (a) originally published in Hirst L. Prospective study of primary pterygium surgery using pterygium extended removal followed by extended conjunctival transplantation. *Ophthalmology*. 2008;115:1663–1672. Reprinted by permission of Elsevier Ltd.)

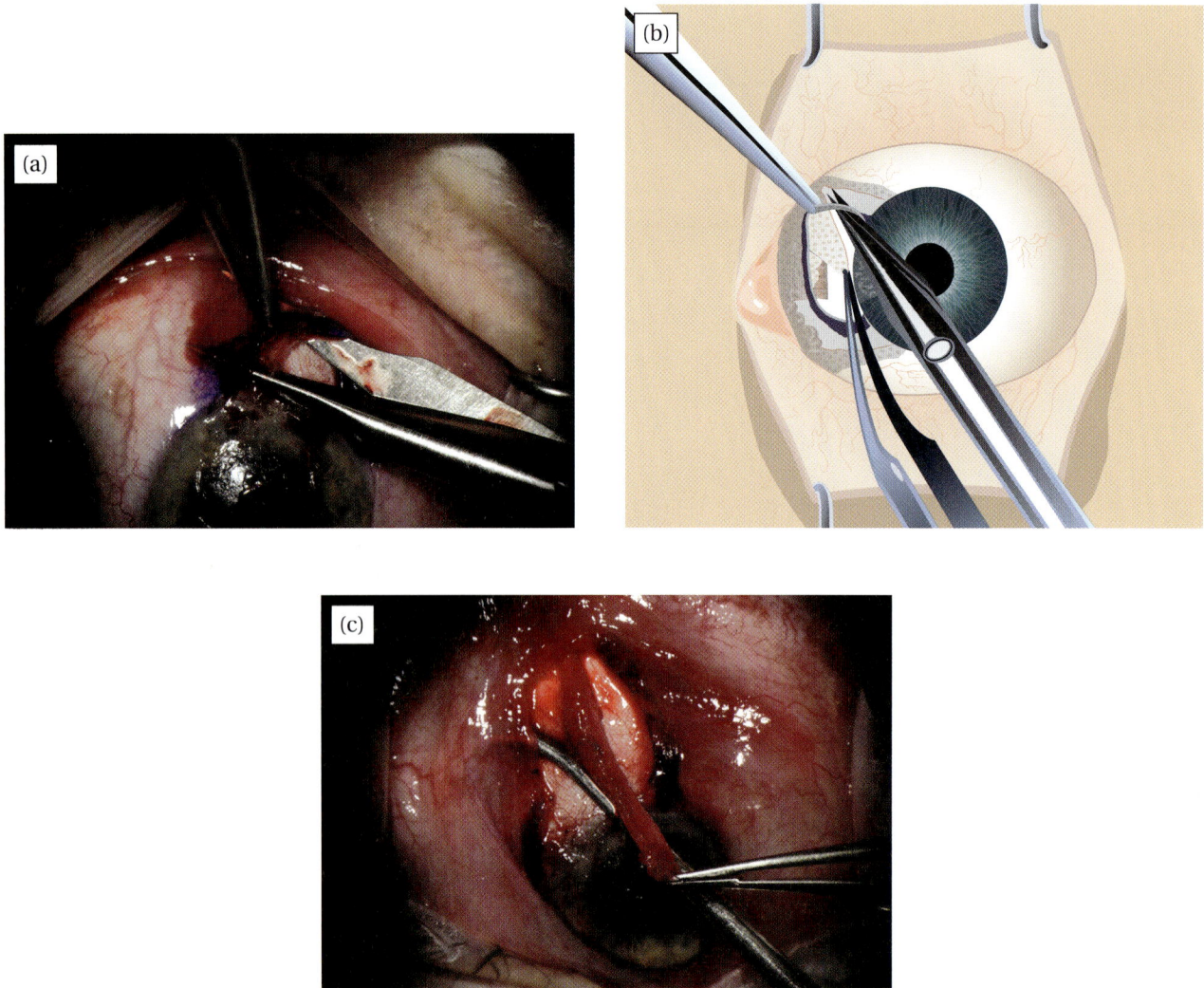

FIGURE 20.5 After separating Tenons capsule from the underlying sclera (a), the Tenons is excised without damaging or excising the overlying conjunctiva (b and c). The medial rectus may be drawn to the side with a strabismus hook to avoid any damage to its insertion (c). (Image (b) originally published in Hirst L. Prospective study of primary pterygium surgery using pterygium extended removal followed by extended conjunctival transplantation. *Ophthalmology*. 2008;115:1663–1672. Reprinted by permission of Elsevier Ltd.)

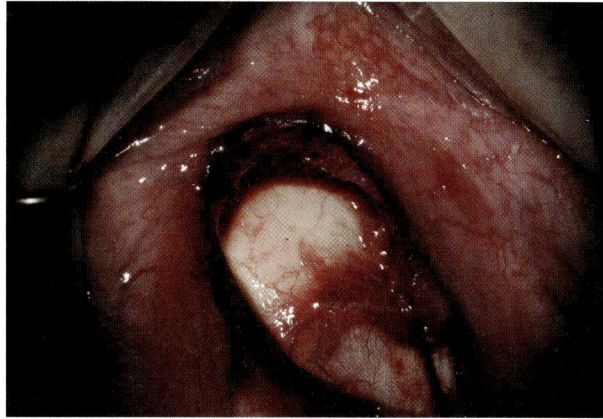

FIGURE 20.6 The sclera above and below the medial rectus is carefully examined to confirm clearance of all Tenons capsule.

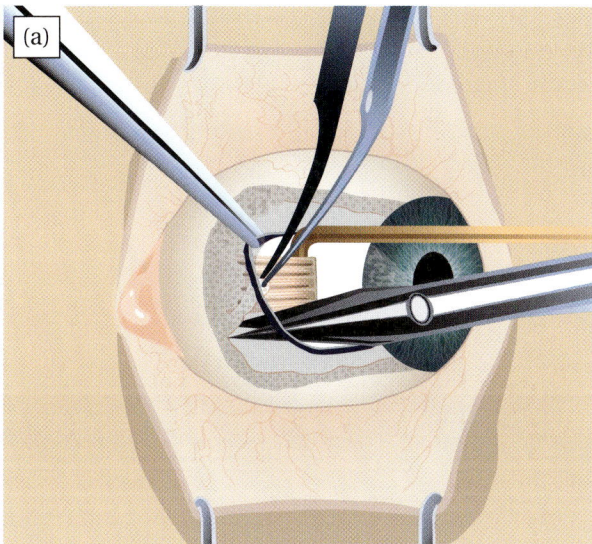

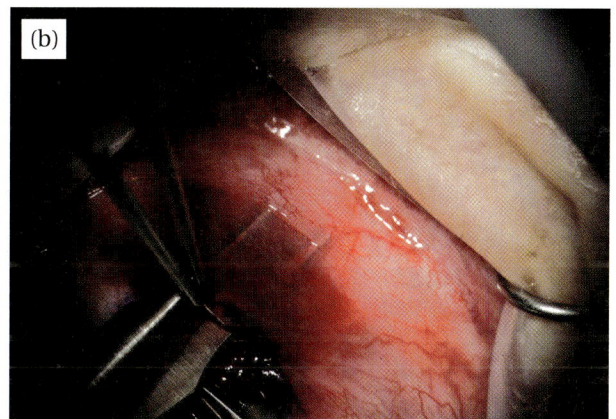

FIGURE 20.7 Tenons capsule is removed back to the caruncle. (Image (b) originally published in Hirst L. Prospective study of primary pterygium surgery using pterygium extended removal followed by extended conjunctival transplantation. *Ophthalmology.* 2008;115:1663–1672. Reprinted by permission of Elsevier Ltd.)

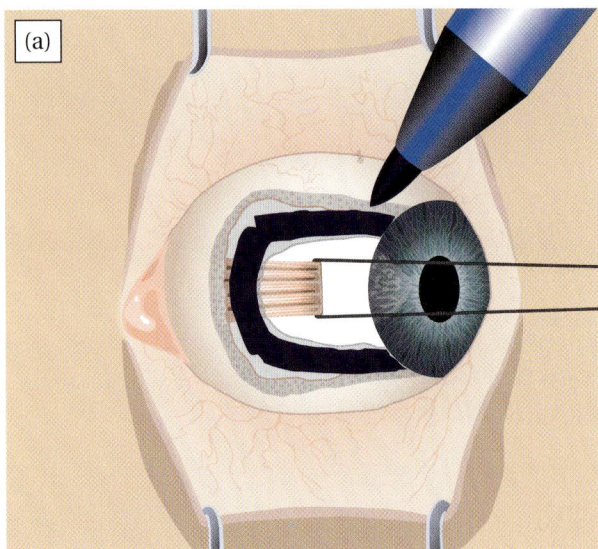

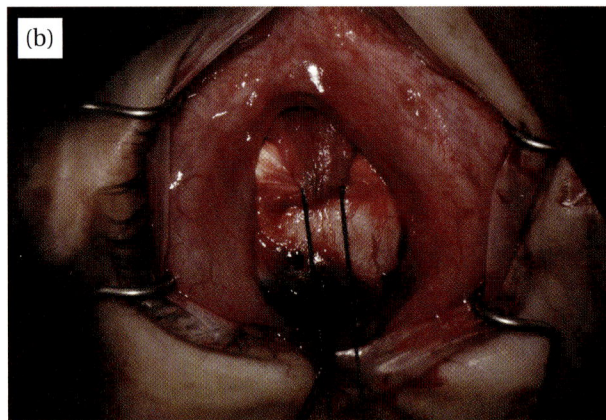

FIGURE 20.8 Heavy marking of free conjunctival edge (a). Note that at this time, no conjunctiva has been excised, apart from the pterygium head off the cornea and yet the free conjunctival edge has retracted extensively with the excision of Tenon's capsule (b). (Image (a) originally published published in Hirst L. Prospective study of primary pterygium surgery using pterygium extended removal followed by extended conjunctival transplantation. *Ophthalmology*. 2008;115:1663–1672. Reprinted by permission of Elsevier Ltd.)

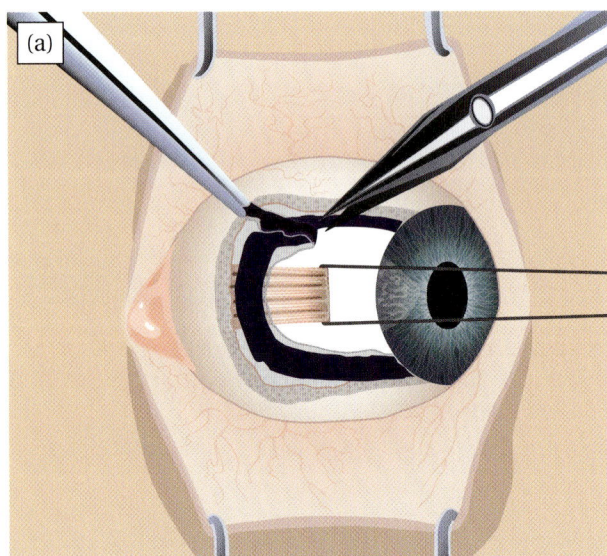

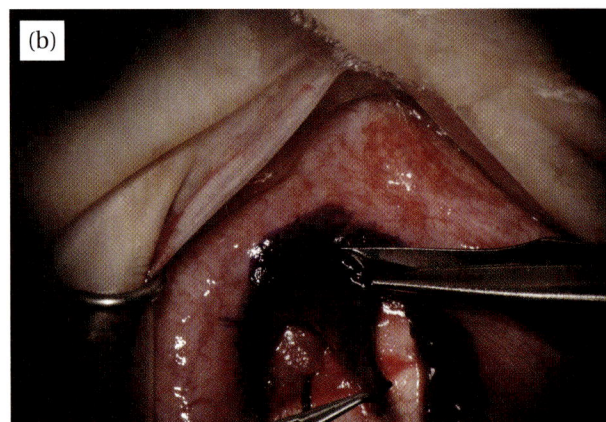

FIGURE 20.9 Excision of minimal conjunctival tissue from the superior and inferior conjunctival edges and removal of the entire semilunar fold. (Image (a) originally published in Hirst L. Prospective study of primary pterygium surgery using pterygium extended removal followed by extended conjunctival transplantation. *Ophthalmology*. 2008;115:1663–1672. Reprinted by permission of Elsevier Ltd.)

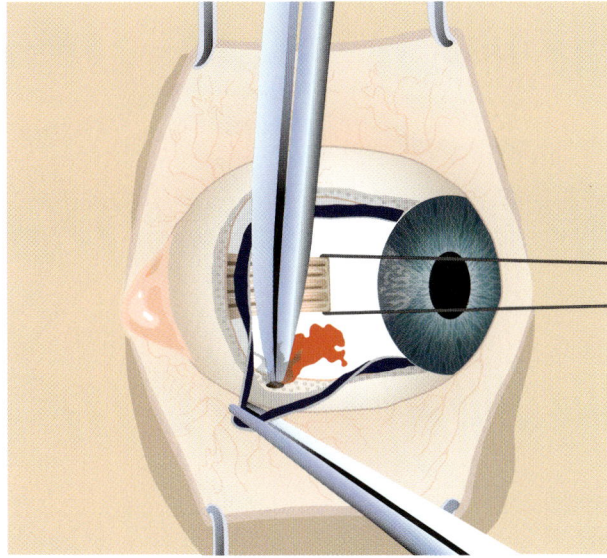

FIGURE 20.10 Wet-field cautery applied to subconjunctival bleeding vessels especially near the caruncle. (Image originally published in Hirst L. Prospective study of primary pterygium surgery using pterygium extended removal followed by extended conjunctival transplantation. *Ophthalmology.* 2008;115:1663–1672. Reprinted by permission of Elsevier Ltd.)

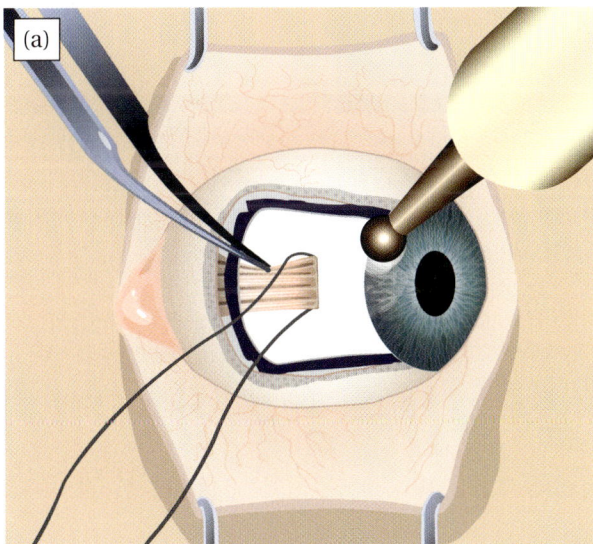

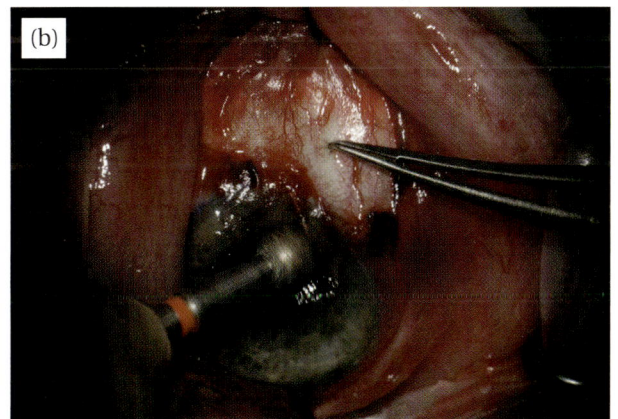

FIGURE 20.11 Diamond burr polishing of the cornea bed and limbus but care being taken not to remove any corneal or scleral tissue. (Image (a) originally published in Hirst L. Prospective study of primary pterygium surgery using pterygium extended removal followed by extended conjunctival transplantation. *Ophthalmology.* 2008;115:1663–1672. Reprinted by permission of Elsevier Ltd.)

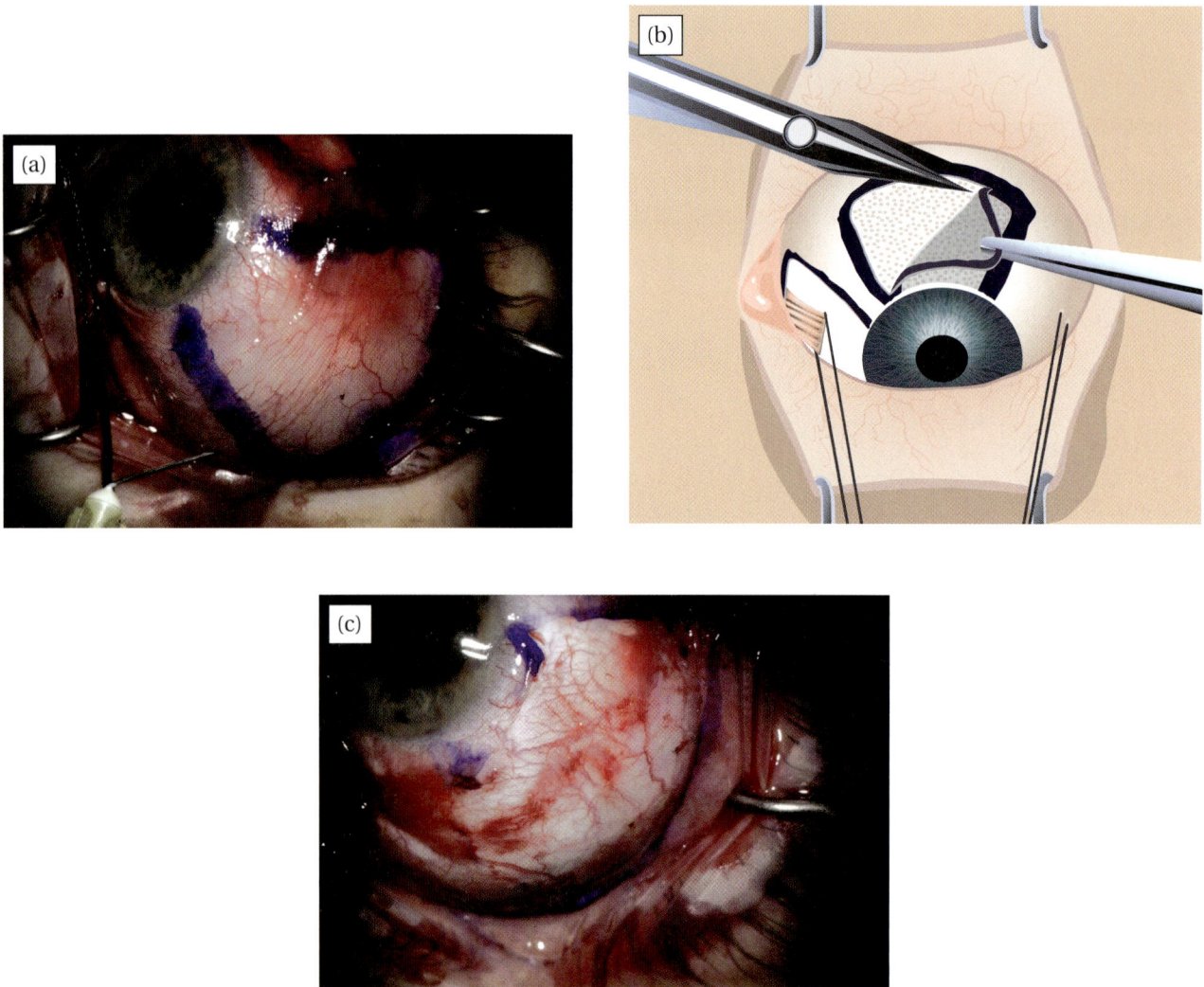

FIGURE 20.12 The size of graft required is marked heavily (a). The graft is carefully dissected from Tenon's capsule starting superiorly near the fornix and moving towards the limbus (b). Once again, emphasizing that the underlying Tenon's capsule must be left intact. 1–2 mm of limbal conjunctival fringe is left in situ (c), ensuring that the superior limbus is not made stem cell deficient: it also demonstrates that the conjunctival autograft does not require limbal stem cells to be effective. (Image (b) originally published in Hirst L. Prospective study of primary pterygium surgery using pterygium extended removal followed by extended conjunctival transplantation. *Ophthalmology*. 2008;115:1663–1672. Reprinted by permission of Elsevier Ltd.)

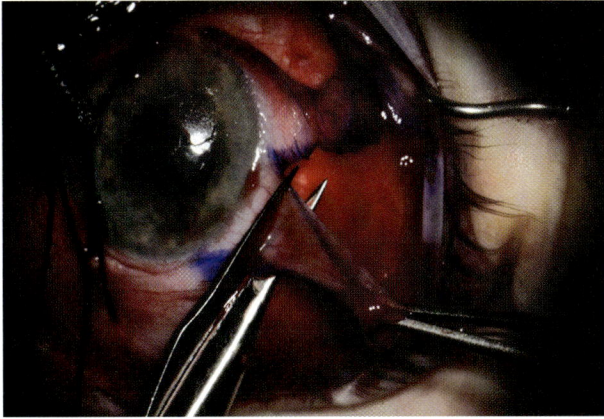

FIGURE 20.13 Removal of superior conjunctival graft with great care being taken NOT to damage underlying Tenon's capsule. This will ensure that within a year the superior conjunctiva will appear to be "untouched" and can be reharvested if a temporal pterygium on the same eye is to be removed.

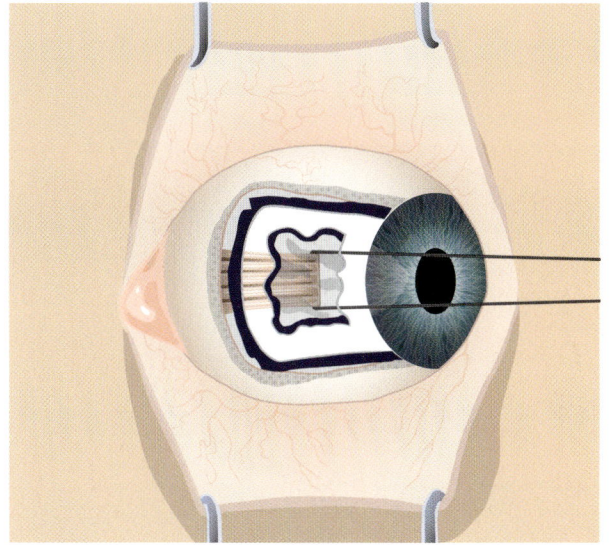

FIGURE 20.14 The graft is transferred to the pterygium bed with the marking providing orientation. (Image originally published in Hirst L. Prospective study of primary pterygium surgery using pterygium extended removal followed by extended conjunctival transplantation. *Ophthalmology*. 2008;115:1663–1672. Reprinted by permission of Elsevier Ltd.)

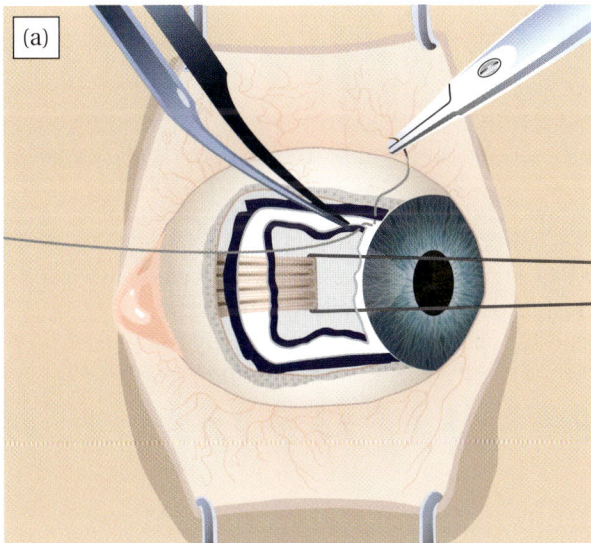

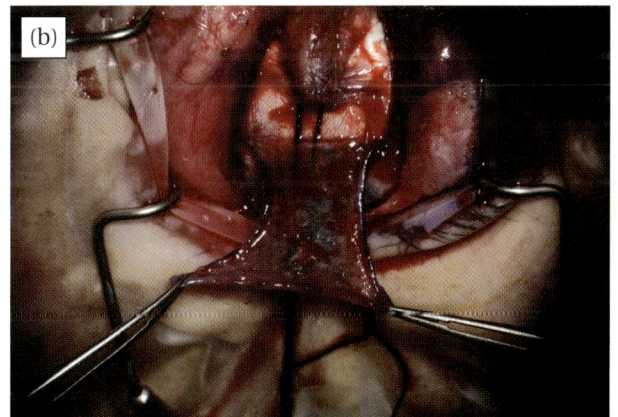

FIGURE 20.15 The corneal edge of the graft is sutured with 9/0 Vicryl to the sclera and adjacent conjunctival edge above and below under tension and 1-2 mm back from the limbus (a), and the graft flipped back to show size and orientation of graft after corneal edge sutures have been placed (b). (Image (a) originally published in Hirst L. Prospective study of primary pterygium surgery using pterygium extended removal followed by extended conjunctival transplantation. *Ophthalmology*. 2008;115:1663–1672. Reprinted by permission of Elsevier Ltd.)

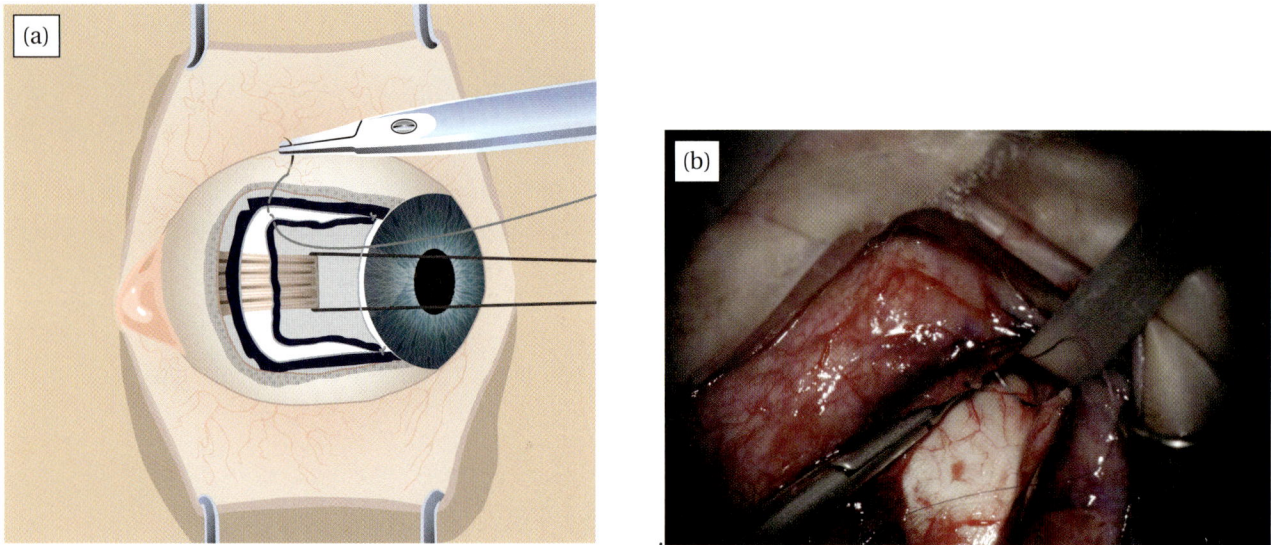

FIGURE 20.16 The superior and inferior posterior graft corners are sutured under tension to the sclera approximately 12 to 13 mm back from limbus (a). These are extremely superficial scleral bites to avoid the possibility of perforation and also to avoid the vortex veins (b). (Image (a) originally published in Hirst L. Prospective study of primary pterygium surgery using pterygium extended removal followed by extended conjunctival transplantation. *Ophthalmology*. 2008;115:1663–1672. Reprinted by permission of Elsevier Ltd.)

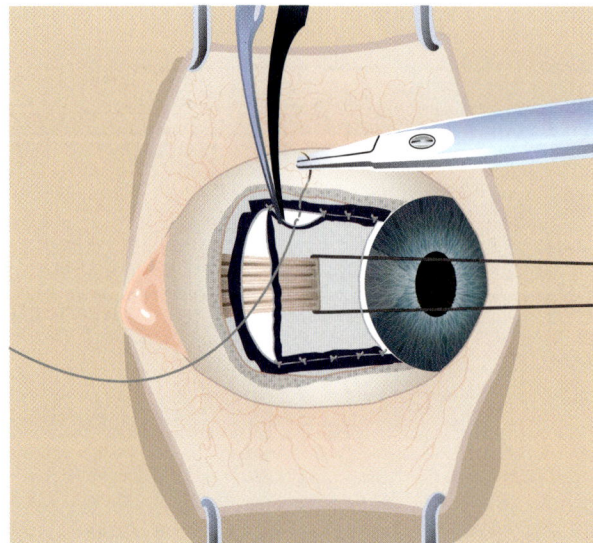

FIGURE 20.17 The suturing of the graft is completed with an additional three sutures to the sclera and adjacent free conjunctival edge along the superior and inferior margins. (Image originally published in Hirst L. Prospective study of primary pterygium surgery using pterygium extended removal followed by extended conjunctival transplantation. *Ophthalmology*. 2008;115:1663–1672. Reprinted by permission of Elsevier Ltd.)

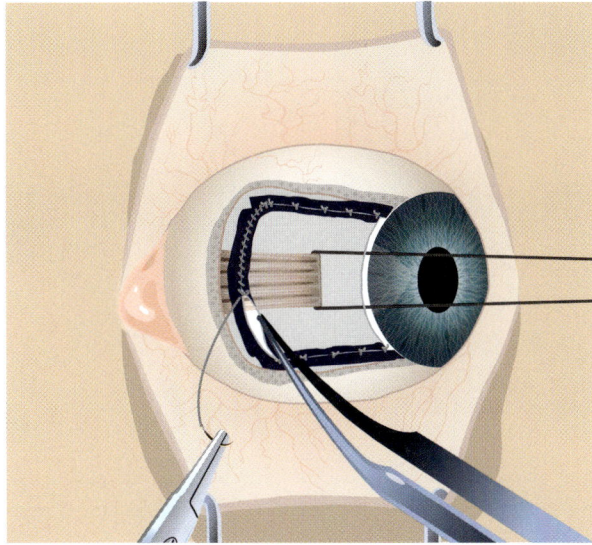

FIGURE 20.18 Then a continuous graft to caruncular conjunctival edge suture is placed to complete the reconstructed semilunar fold. (Image originally published in Hirst L. Prospective study of primary pterygium surgery using pterygium extended removal followed by extended conjunctival transplantation. *Ophthalmology*. 2008;115:1663–1672. Reprinted by permission of Elsevier Ltd.)

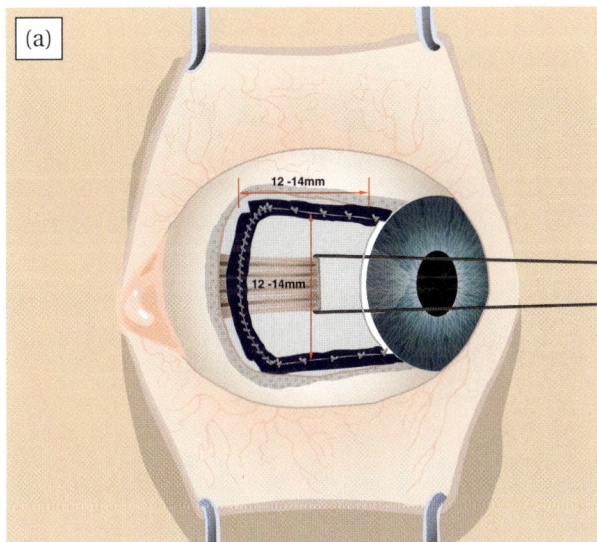

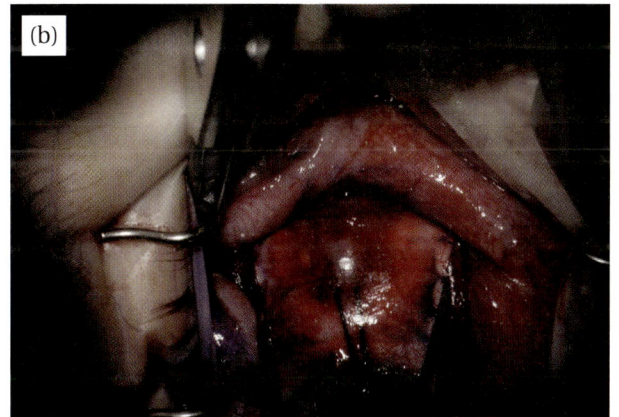

FIGURE 20.19 The average size of the graft is about 13 × 14 mm measured from the limbus to the reconstructed semilunar fold and the width of the graft at the midpoint of the graft's superior and inferior edges. (Image (a) originally published in Hirst L. Prospective study of primary pterygium surgery using pterygium extended removal followed by extended conjunctival transplantation. *Ophthalmology*. 2008;115:1663–1672. Reprinted by permission of Elsevier Ltd.)

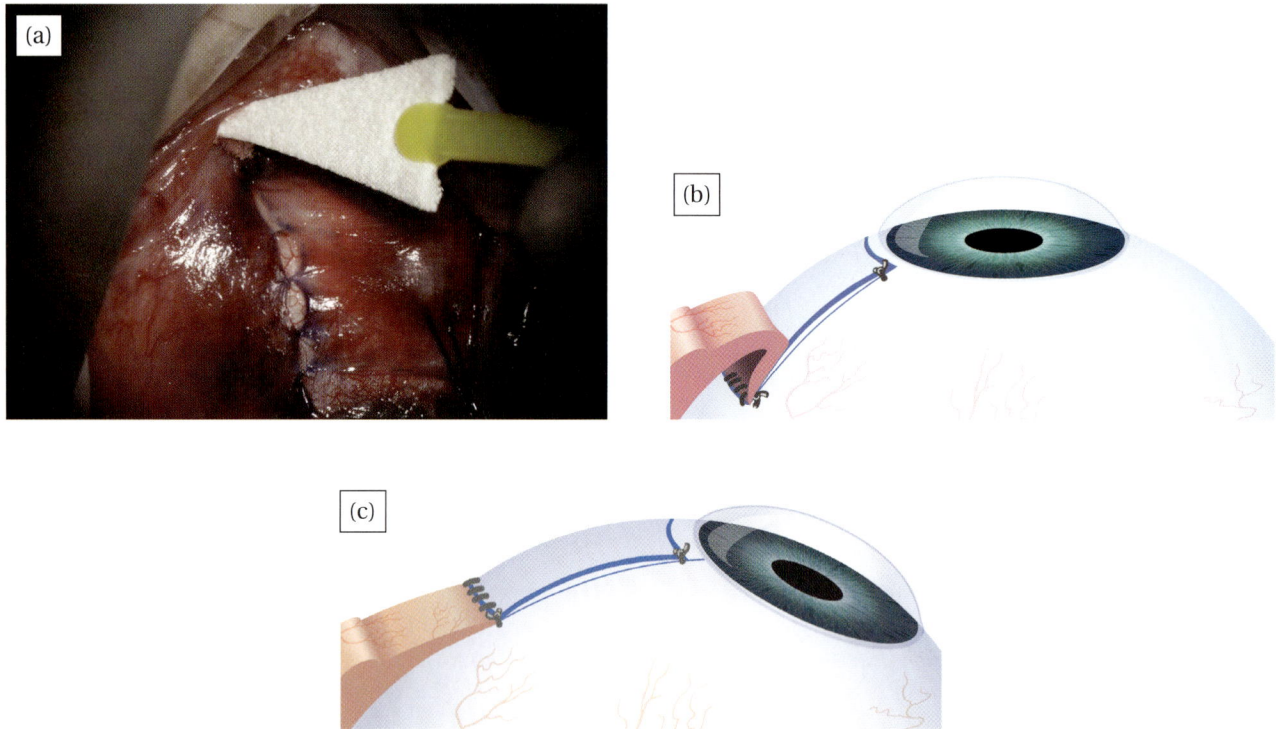

FIGURE 20.20 Figures (a), (b), and (c) explain the principle of the reconstruction of the semilunar fold created by first removing the original fold, and then suturing of the posterior graft corners to the scleral to anchor the graft to the posterior sclera. When the eye is in the primary position (b), the reconstructed semilunar is seen and hides any conjunctiva to conjunctiva scar underneath. With the eye pulled temporally the cul-de-sac created by the posterior scleral sutures is seen (c). (Images (b) and (c) originally published in Hirst L. Prospective study of primary pterygium surgery using pterygium extended removal followed by extended conjunctival transplantation. *Ophthalmology*. 2008;115:1663–1672. Reprinted by permission of Elsevier Ltd.)

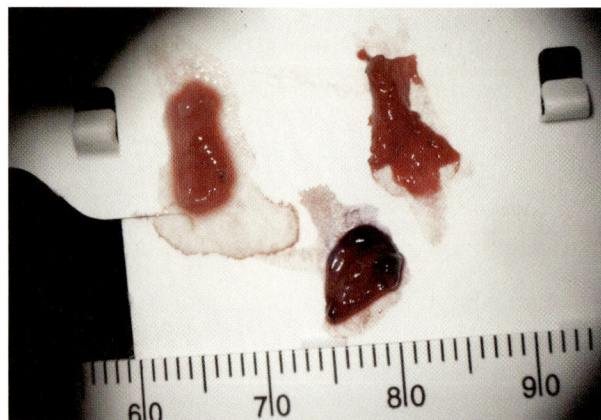

FIGURE 20.21 Excised tissue consisting of marked semilunar fold and a piece of Tenon's capsule from above and below the medial rectus.

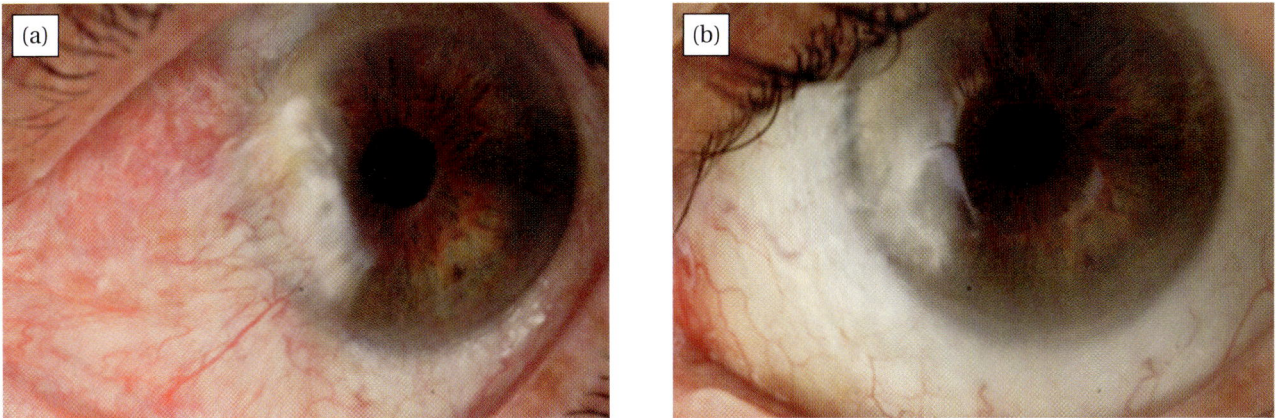

FIGURE 20.22   Before (a) and after (b) removal of a recurrent pterygium that had been removed 9 times previously. Note the corneal opacity cannot be removed.

TABLE 20.2 *Complications of Surgery*

Possible complications:
- Major
  - Recurrence
  - Medial rectus damage
  - Corneal infection
  - Scleral necrosis
  - Scleral infection
  - Endophthalmitis
  - Ocular perforation with retinal detachment
- Minor
  - Dellen
  - Autograft dislodgement
  - Autograft infection
  - Corneal thinning
  - Corneal scarring
  - Inclusion cyst
  - Pyogenic granuloma
  - Limbal deficiency at donor site

SELECTED REFERENCES

Frucht-Pery J, Siganos CS, Ilsar M. Intraoperative application of topical mitomycin C for pterygium surgery. *Ophthalmology.* 1996;103:674–677.

Hirst LW, Sebban A, Chant D. Pterygium recurrence time. *Ophthalmology.* 1994;101:755–758.

Hirst LW. The treatment of pterygium. *Surv Ophthalmol.* 2003;48:145–180.

Hirst LW. Prospective study of primary pterygium surgery using pterygium extended removal followed by extended conjunctival transplantation. *Ophthalmology.* 2008;115;1663–1672.

Hirst LW. Recurrent pterygium surgery using pterygium extended removal followed by extended conjunctival transplant recurrence rate and cosmesis. *Ophthalmology.* 2009:116;1278–1286.

Kenyon KR, Wagoner MD, Hettinger ME. Conjunctival autograft transplantation for advanced and recurrent pterygium. *Ophthalmology.* 1985;92:1461–1470.

MacKenzie FD, Hirst LW, Kynaston B, Bain C. Recurrence rate and complications after beta irradiation for pterygia. *Ophthalmology.* 1991;98:1776–1780.

Manning CA, Kloess PM, Diaz MD, Yee RW. Intraoperative mitomycin in primary pterygium excision. A prospective, randomized trial. *Ophthalmology.* 1997;104:844–848.

Oguz H, Basar E, Gurler B. Intraoperative application versus postoperative mitomycin C eye drops in pterygium surgery. *Acta Ophthalmol Scand.* 1999;77:147–150.

Prabhasawat P, Barton K, Burkett G, Tseng SC. Comparison of conjunctival autografts, amniotic membrane grafts, and primary closure for pterygium excision. *Ophthalmology.* 1997;104:974–985.

Rubinfeld RS, Pfister RR, Stein RM, et al. Serious complications of topical mitomycin-C after pterygium surgery. *Ophthalmology.* 1992;99:1647–1654.

Sanchez-Thorin JC, Rocha G, Yelin JB. Meta-analysis on the recurrence rates after bare sclera resection with and without mitomycin C use and conjunctival autograft placement in surgery for primary pterygium. *Br J Ophthalmol.* 1998;82:661–665.

Sanchez-Thorin JC. A randomized trial comparing mitomycin C and conjunctival autograft after excision of primary pterygium. *Am J Ophthalmol.* 1996;121:333–334.

Solomon A, Pires RT, Tseng SC. Amniotic membrane transplantation after extensive removal of primary and recurrent pterygia. *Ophthalmology.* 2001;108:449–460.

Tan DT, Chee SP, Dear KB, Lim AS. Effect of pterygium morphology on pterygium recurrence in a controlled trial comparing conjunctival autografting with bare sclera excision. *Arch Ophthalmol.* 1997;115:1235–1240.

21

Tissue Adhesives in Anterior Segment Surgery

Preeya K. Gupta, MD and Terry Kim, MD

TABLE 21.1 *Indications and Preoperative Considerations*

Cyanoacrylate Glue	Fibrin Glue
Indications	*Indications*
Corneal perforation/corneal thinning	Pterygium excision with amniotic membrane graft placement
Preoperative Consideration	Lamellar keratoplasty
Dry ocular surface to allow proper polymerization of glue	Flap closure in treatment of epithelial ingrowth post-LASIK
	Preoperative Considerations
Place the least amount of glue necessary to seal perforation	Prepare glue in advance of beginning the surgical procedure
	Dry ocular surface to allow greatest contact of glue to bed
Placement of bandage contact lens for post-procedure comfort	Ensure adequate mixing of fibrin and thrombin components
	Allow adequate drying time for coagulum formation

Pterygium Excision

Fibrin Glue with Amniotic Membrane Graft

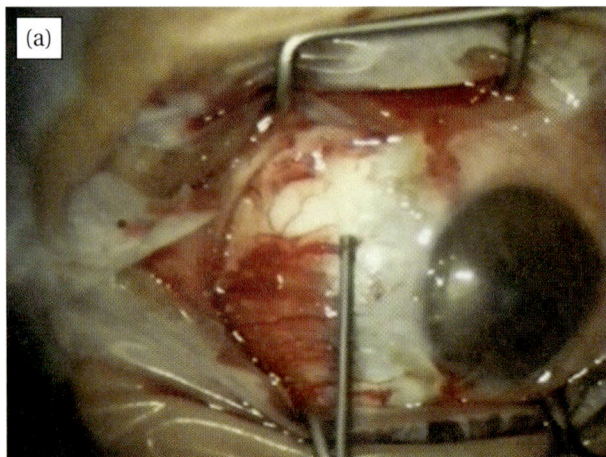

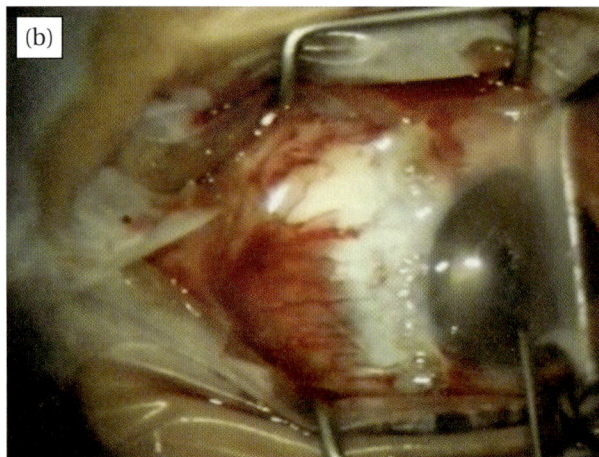

FIGURE 21.1 (a) After removal of the pterygium, the scleral bed is dried and the fibrin glue component is placed along the limbus and on the entire area of bare sclera. (b) The amniotic membrane graft is oriented on the cornea with the stromal side up and then the thrombin glue component is placed on the stromal side of the graft.

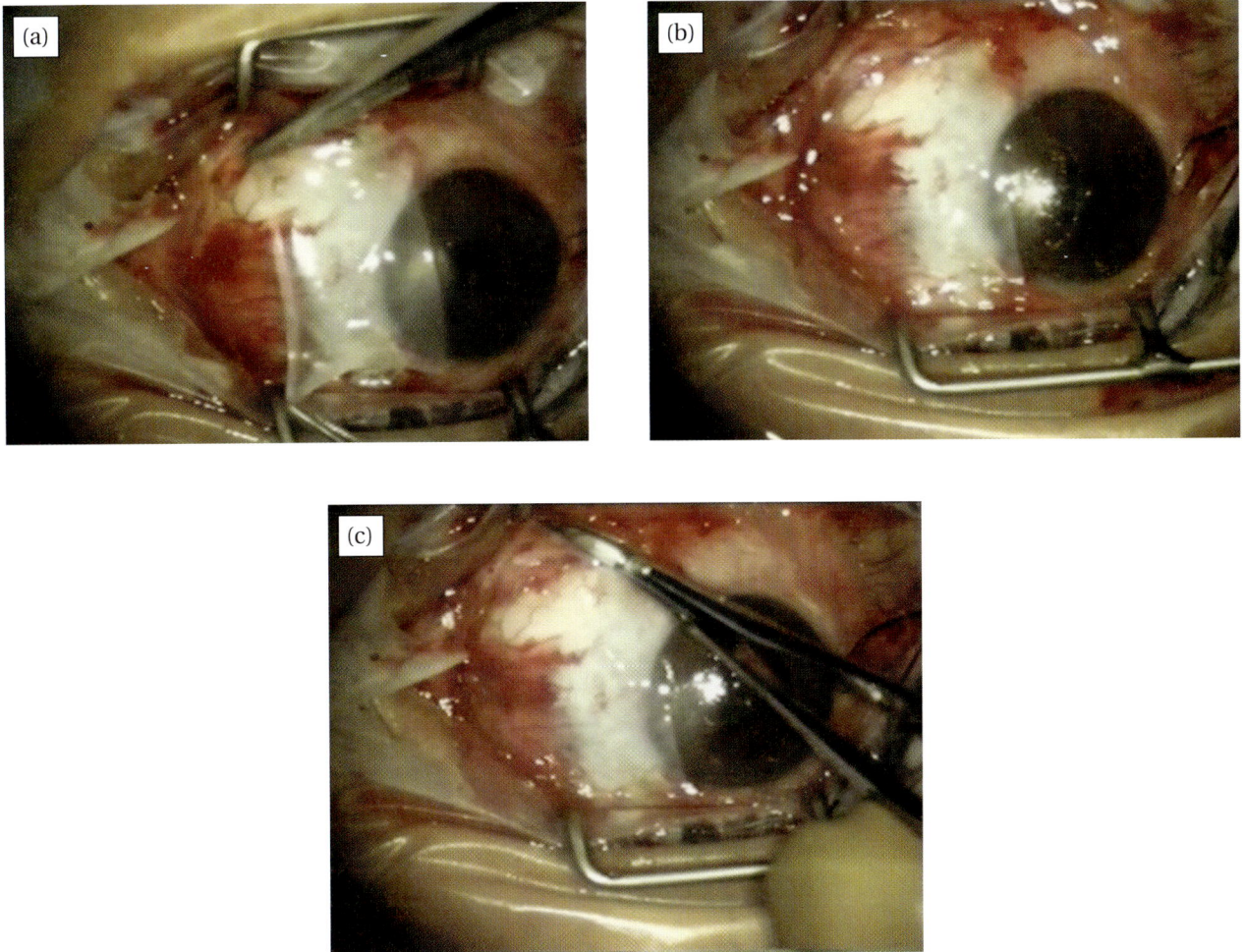

FIGURE 21.2 (a) The amniotic membrane graft is lifted with a smooth forceps and then flipped onto the area of bare sclera so that the stromal side of the graft is in contact with bare sclera, allowing the fibrin and thrombin components of the glue to combine and form a coagulum. (b) During the 5–8 minutes of drying time, the edges of the amniotic graft should be tucked under the free edges of the surrounding conjunctiva until the amniotic graft is secured into place. (c) Care should be taken when removing the lid speculum/draping to ensure no glue is attached to the speculum/draping to avoid inadvertent detachment of the graft; a Vannas scissors is used to sever any glue attachments.

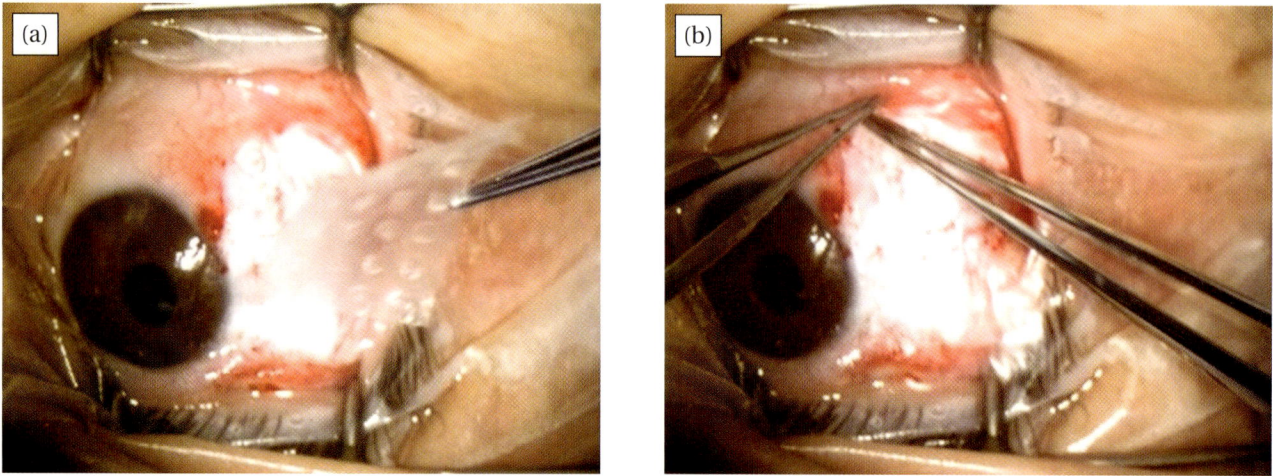

FIGURE 21.3 Pterygium excision can also be done with dehydrated amniotic membrane. (a) After removal of the pterygium and application of fibrin glue to the bare sclera, the dehydrated amniotic graft is cut to size and placed onto the bare sclera. (b) The fibrin glue component moistens and activates the amniotic graft, and the edges of the amniotic graft are tucked under the free edges of the surrounding conjunctiva.

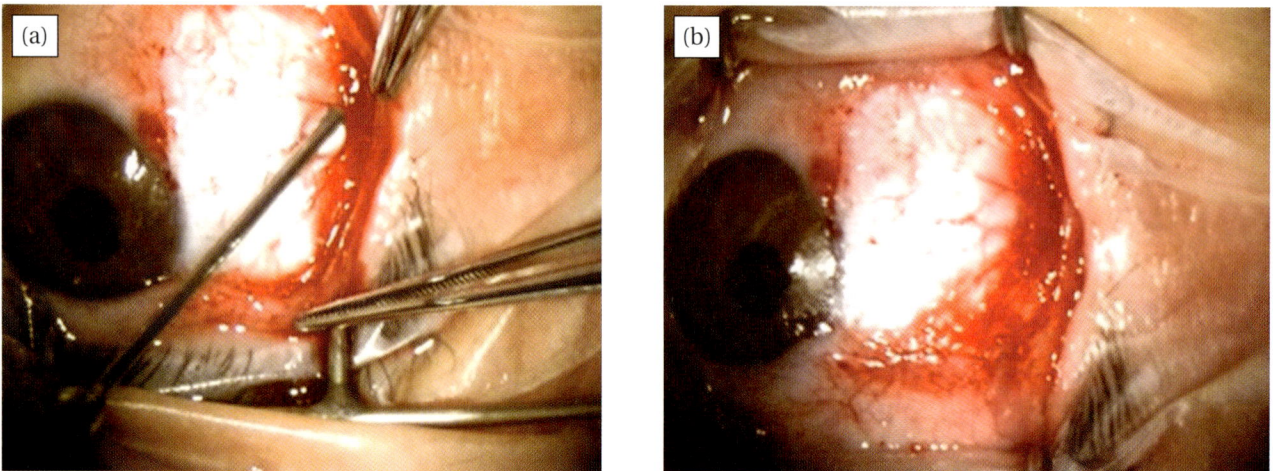

FIGURE 21.4 (a) The thrombin component is placed under and around the moistened graft, allowing it to combine with the fibrin component already present, and (b) The fibrin-thrombin coagulum is left to dry for 5–8 minutes to secure the amniotic graft onto bare sclera.

Lamellar Keratoplasty

Fibrin Glue Technique

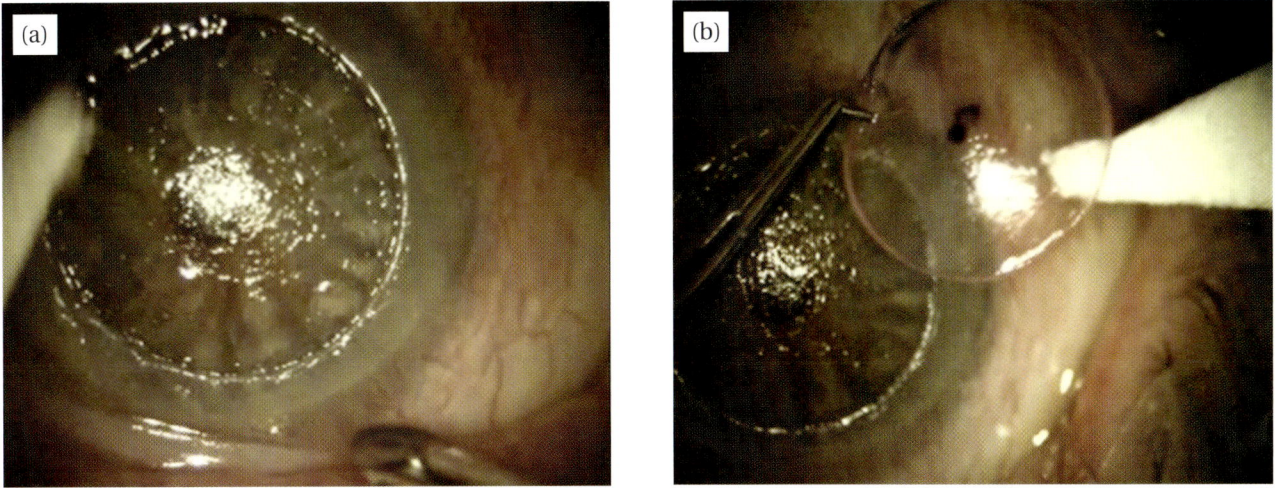

FIGURE 21.5 (a) The anterior stroma of the recipient host cornea has already been removed with a partial-thickness trephination with a Hessburg-Barron vacuum trephine. (b) The donor anterior cap has already been cut and trephined to appropriate size (typically 0.25 mm larger than the host trephine size).

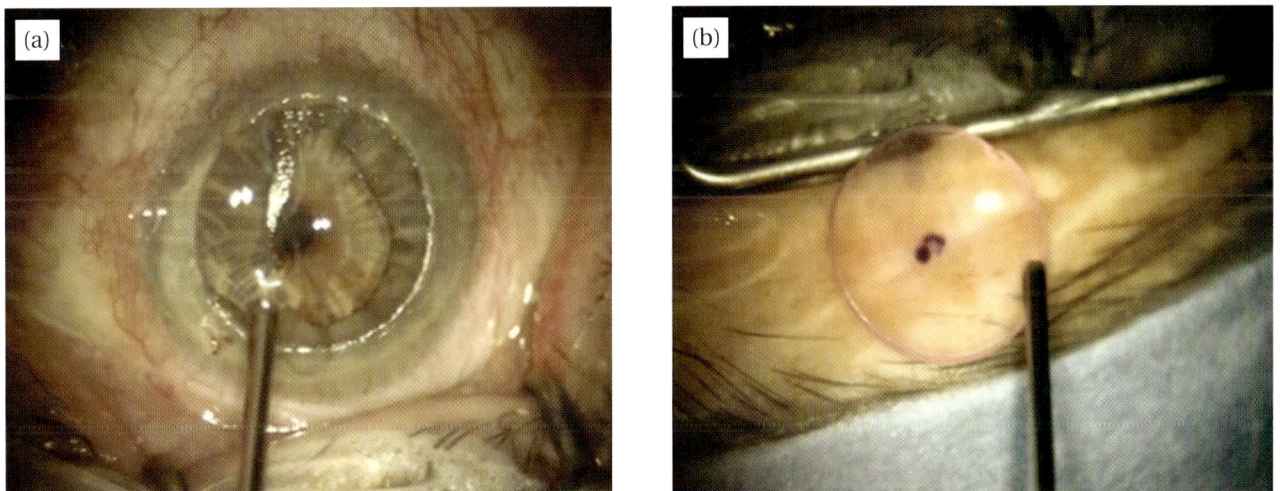

FIGURE 21.6 (a) The host bed and donor cap are dried with a weck sponge and then the fibrin component of the glue is applied to the stromal surface of the host bed. (b) The thrombin component is placed on the stromal surface of the donor cap.

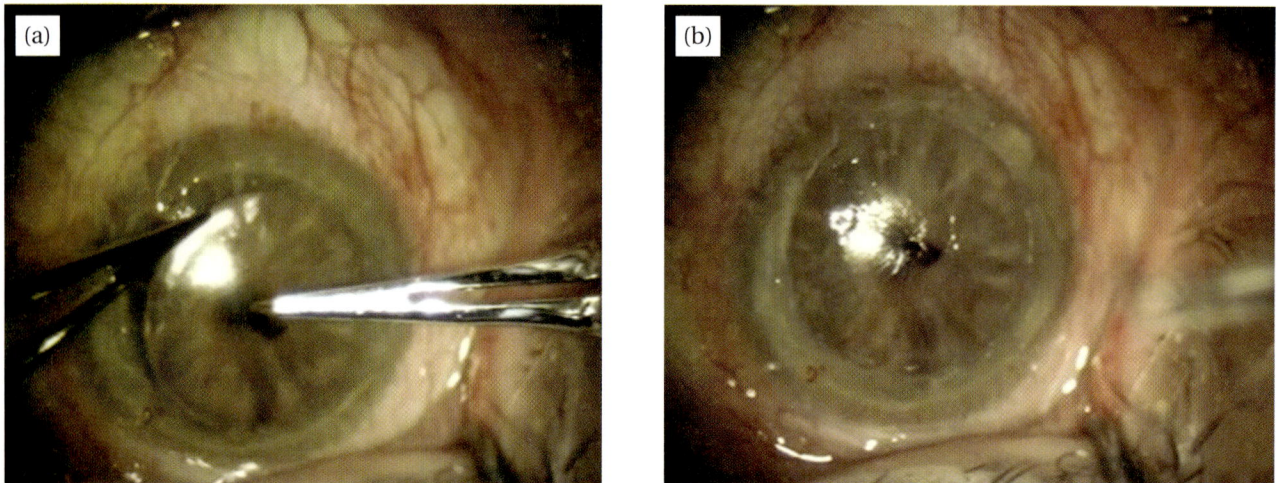

FIGURE 21.7 (a) The donor cap is then placed onto the recipient bed, allowing the fibrin and thrombin components of the adhesive to combine while a forceps can be used to "squeegee" out any excess glue. (b) The glue is allowed to dry for 5–8 minutes, after which the donor cap is securely adhered to the stromal bed.

Treatment of Epithelial In-growth after LASIK

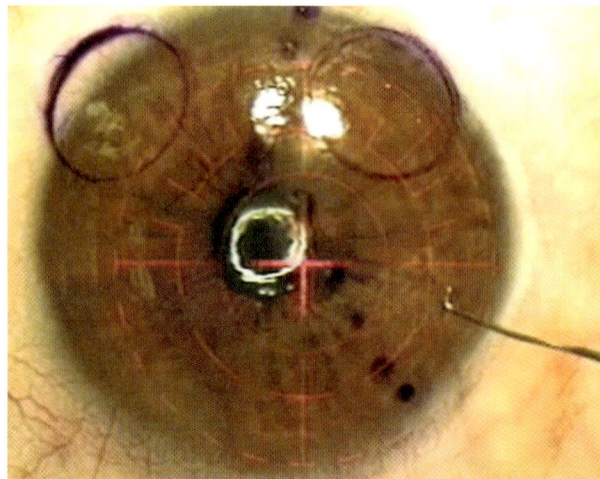

FIGURE 21.8 The areas of epithelial in-growth at the flap edge are marked with a marking pen and a Sinskey hook is used to identify and score the edge of the flap.

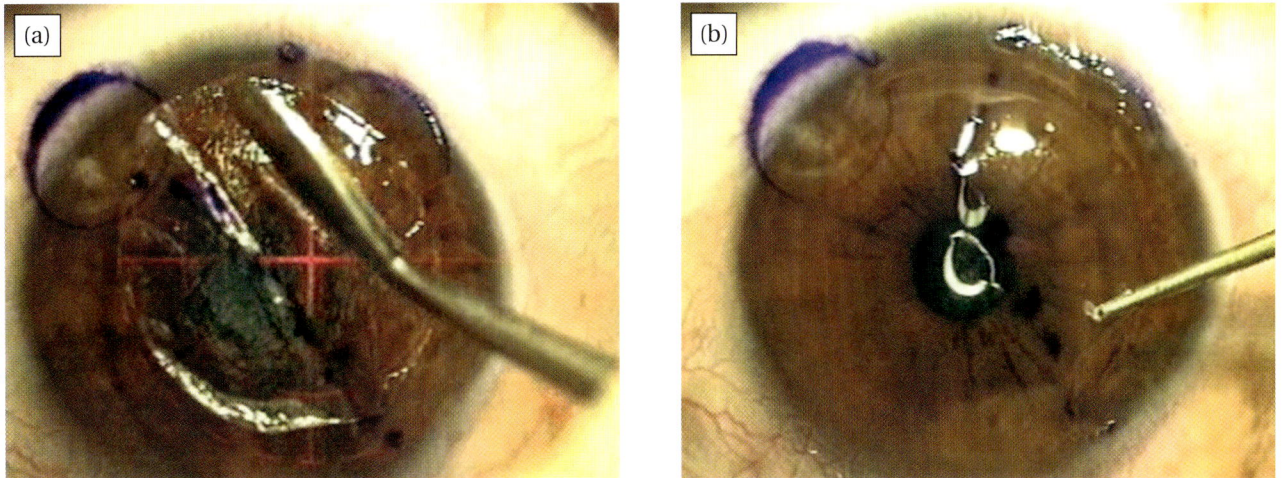

FIGURE 21.9 (a) The LASIK flap is lifted and the stromal bed and underside of the flap are scraped using a Maloney spatula to remove the epithelial ingrowth. (b) The LASIK flap is replaced to its original position using a non-toothed forceps and irrigated with balanced salt solution.

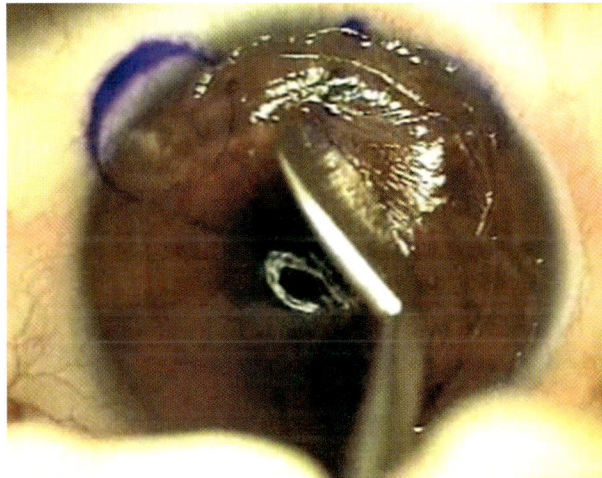

FIGURE 21.10 A Maloney spatula is used to remove the epithelium outside the flap edge as well as any loose epithelium on the surface of the flap in an effort to remove the source of potential recurrent ingrowth of surface epithelium

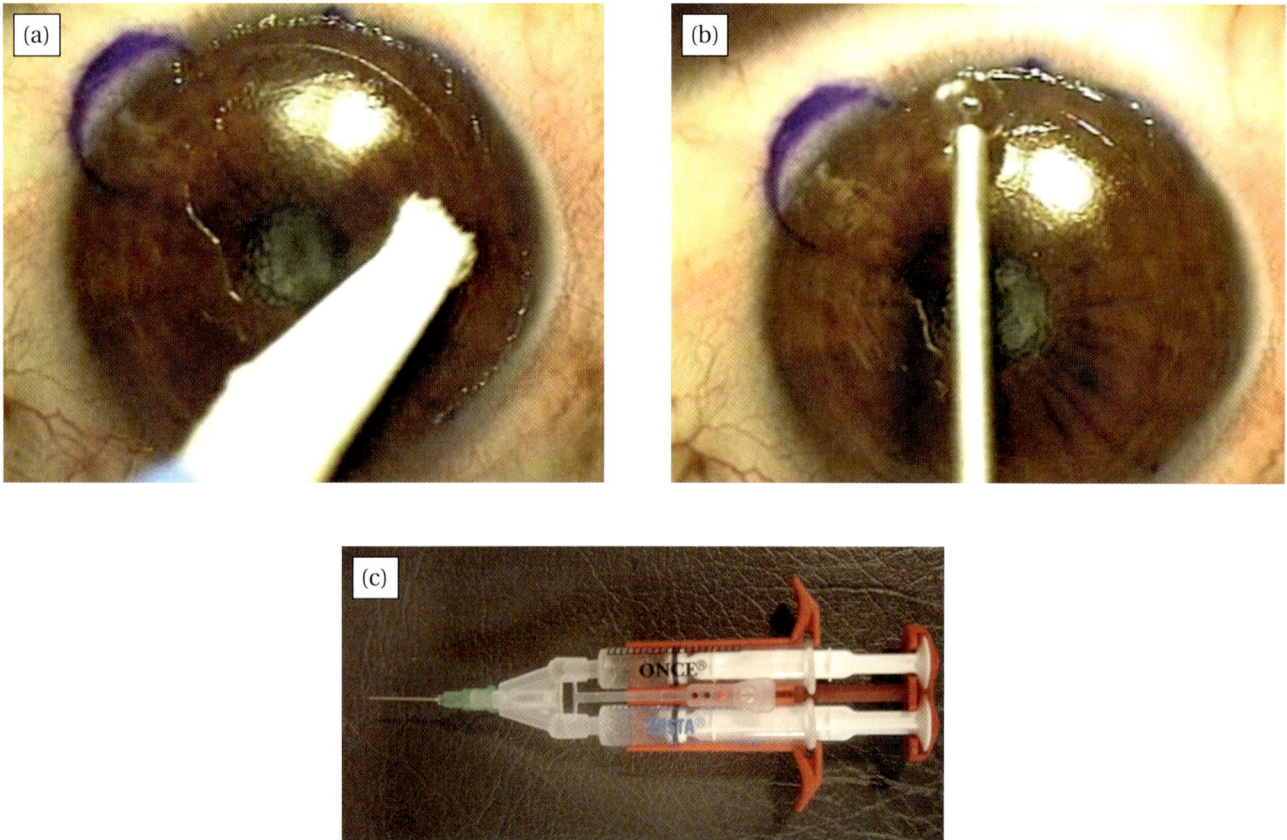

FIGURE 21.11 (a) The surface and flap edge is dried with a weck sponge. (b) The fibrin and thrombin components of the adhesive are delivered onto the dried flap edge and surface simultaneously using a dual-barreled syringe. Alternatively, these components can be applied to the flap edge/surface separately. (c) A dual-barreled syringe containing the fibrin component (labeled in light blue) in one barrel and the thrombin component (labeled in black) in the other barrel; the specially designed tip allows these two components to be mixed and delivered simultaneously.

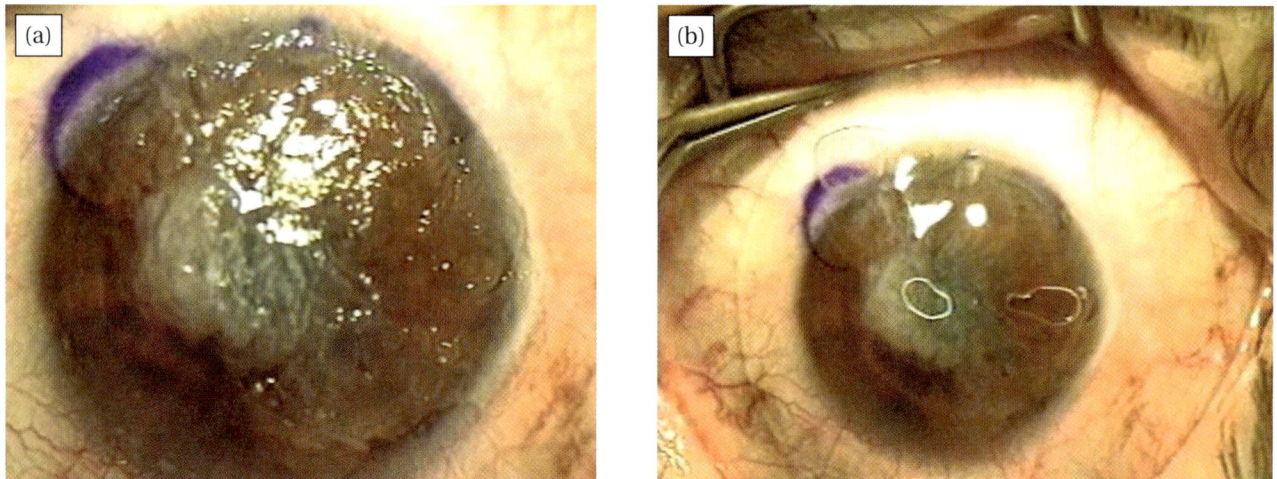

FIGURE 21.12 (a) The fibrin coagulum seals the flap edge to prevent epithelium from growing under the flap and gradually dissolutes over 1–2 weeks. (b) A bandage lens is placed over the cornea and fibrin glue.

Cyanoacrylate Glue

Corneal Perforation

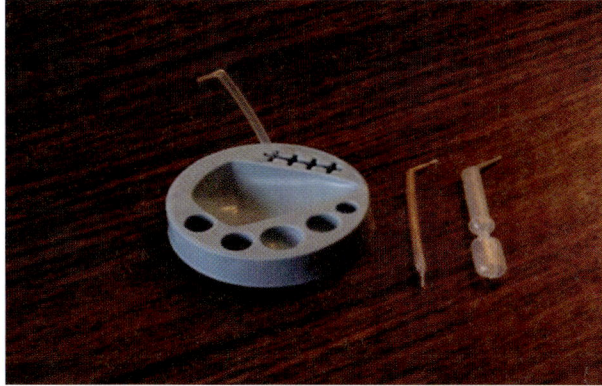

FIGURE 21.13 Cyanoacrylate glue is drawn into a plastic pipette or TB syringe. The ocular surface should be dried completely to ensure that glue polymerization occurs on the ocular surface immediately upon application.

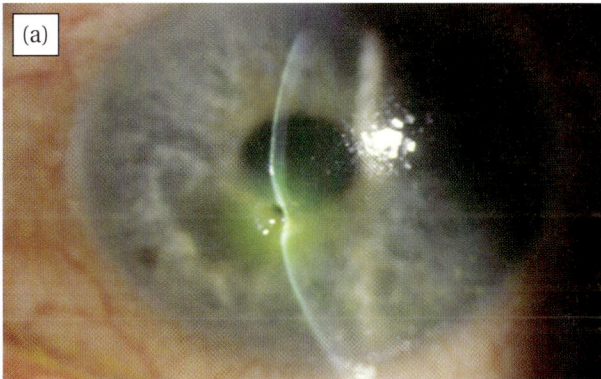

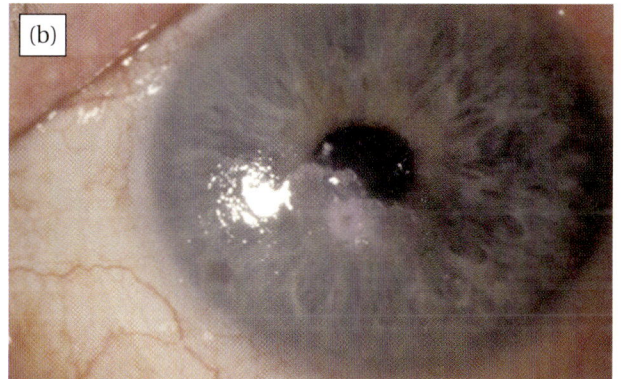

FIGURE 21.14 (a) Corneal surface is dried with a Weck sponge. (b) Cyanoacrylate glue is drawn into the pipette or syringe. After inserting the lid speculum, a small amount of glue is placed onto the cornea to seal the area of perforation. A bandage contact lens may be placed for comfort. (Images courtesy of Christopher Rapuano, MD; Wills Eye Hospital, Philadelphia, PA.)

TABLE 21.2 *Potential Complications of Tissue Adhesives*

Cyanoacrylate Glue

    Excessive accumulation of polymerized glue

    Ocular toxicity secondary to inadvertent entry of glue intraocularly

    Irregular corneal surface and surface irritation

    Run-off onto adjacent ocular structures with liberal application

Fibrin Glue

    Poor graft adhesion due to inadequate mixing of fibrin/thrombin components and/or inadequate drying time for coagulum formation

    Temporary visual obscuration secondary to coagulum formation in stromal interface

    Theoretical risk of infection (viral/prion transmission)

SELECTED REFERENCES

Anderson NJ, Hardten DR. Fibrin glue for the prevention of epithelial ingrowth after laser in situ keratomileusis. *J Cataract Refract Surg.* 2003;29(7):1425–1429.

Chan SM, Boisjoly H. Advances in the use of adhesives in ophthalmology. *Curr Opin Ophthalmol.* 2004 Aug;15(4):305–310.

Duarte MC, Kim T. Sutureless lamellar keratoplasty: a modified approach for fibrin glue application. *Cornea.* 2007; 26(9):1127–1128.

Kang PC, Carnahan MA, Wathier M, et al. Novel tissue adhesives to secure laser in situ keratomileusis flaps. *J Cataract Refract Surg.* 2005;31(6):1208–1212.

Kaufman HE, Insler MS, Ibrahim-Elzembely HA, Kaufman SC. Human fibrin tissue adhesive for sutureless lamellar keratoplasty and scleral patch adhesion a pilot study. *Ophthalmology.* 2003;110(11):2168–2172.

Koranyi G, Seregard S, Kopp ED. Cut and paste: a no suture, small incision approach to pterygium surgery. *Br J Ophthalmol.* 2004;88:911–914.

Yeh DL, Bushley DM, Kim T. Treatment of Traumatic LASIK Flap Dislocation and Epithelial Ingrowth with Fibrin Glue. *Am J Ophthalmol.* 2006;141(5):960–962.

22 Penetrating Keratoplasty

Matthew Rauen, MD and Kenneth M. Goins, MD

SELECTED REFERENCES

Indications and Contraindications for Penetrating Keratoplasty

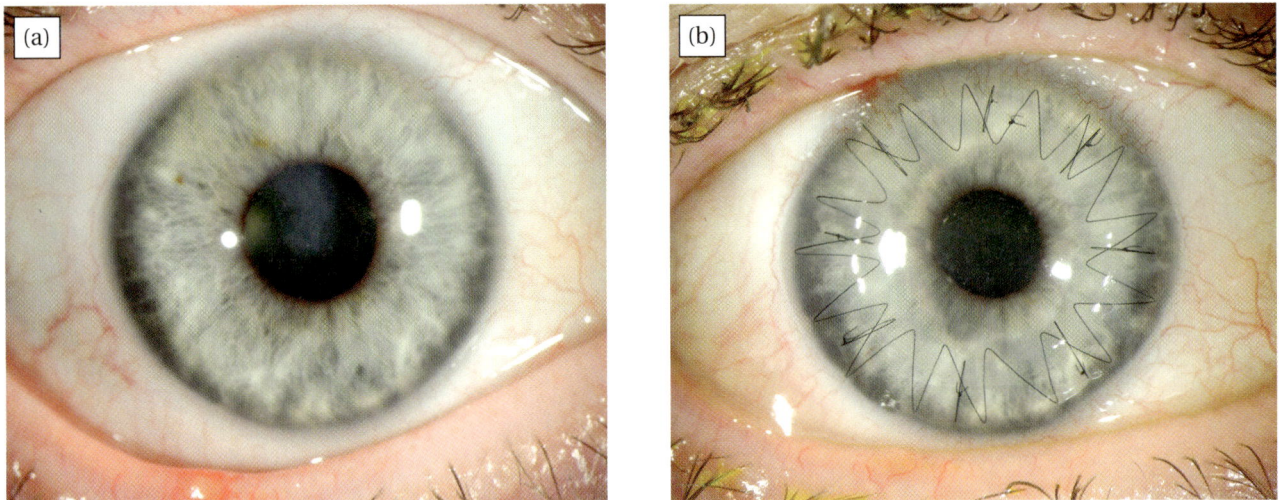

FIGURE 22.1 Optical Indication. (a) Penetrating keratoplasty will remove the scar associated with a previous HSV infection. (b) The visual axis has been cleared in this patient after surgery. The four main indications for performing penetrating keratoplasty (PKP) are optical, tectonic, therapeutic, and cosmetic.

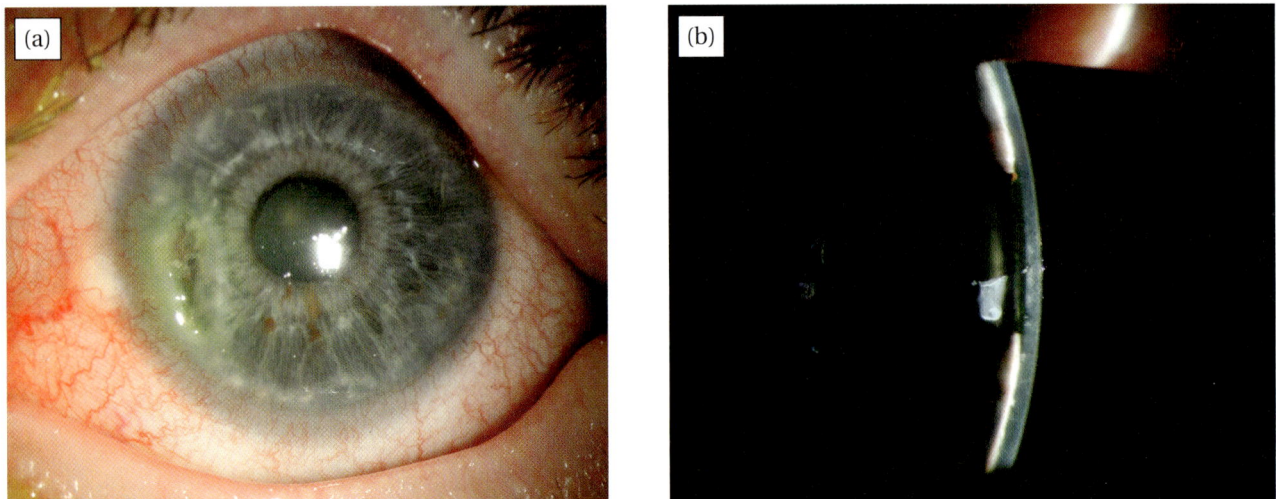

FIGURE 22.2 Tectonic Indication. (a) This eye has a full-thickness corneal melt related to an underlying autoimmune condition. (b) Anterior chamber shallowing prompted use of a PKP to restore globe integrity.

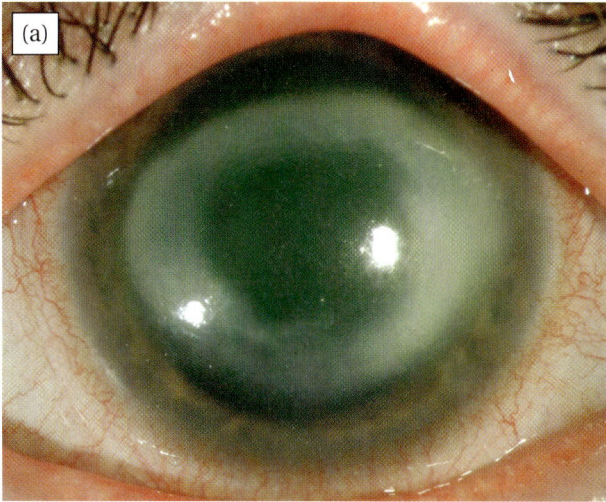

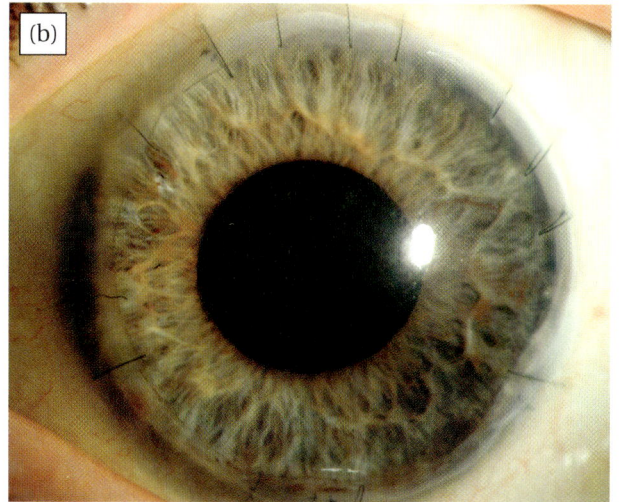

FIGURE 22.3 Therapeutic Indication. (a) A ring infiltrate in a patient with active *Acanthamoeba* keratitis. (b) After a large-diameter PKP and subsequent cataract extraction, the patient had an uncorrected visual acuity of 20/25.

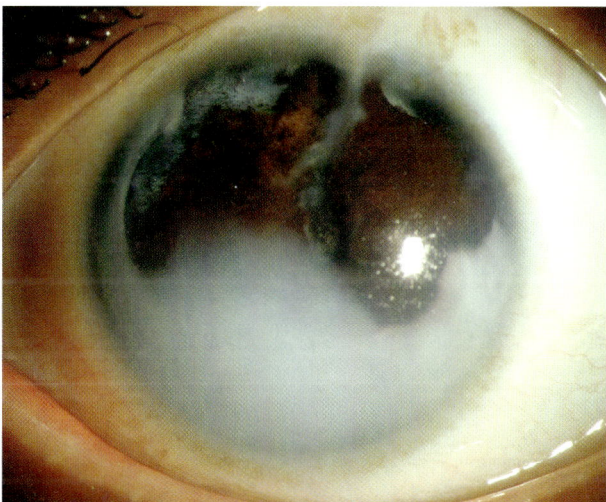

FIGURE 22.4 Optical and Cosmetic Indication. At age 3, this patient sustained an injury with a nail. No surgical intervention was performed at the time of injury. PKP with lensectomy and anterior segment reconstruction will improve the eye's appearance.

TABLE 22.1 *Indications for Penetrating Keratoplasty*

Pseudophakic corneal edema

Ectasia/Thinning

Endothelial corneal dystrophies

Regraft unrelated to allograft rejection

Aphakic corneal edema

Stromal corneal dystrophies

Noninfectious ulcerative keratitis

Corneal degenerations

Congenital opacities

Mechanical trauma

Viral/postviral keratitis

Microbial/postmicrobial keratitis

Chemical injuries

Optical (including postrefractive surgery)

Source: Eye Banking Statistics for 2004.

Preoperative Tests and Evaluations

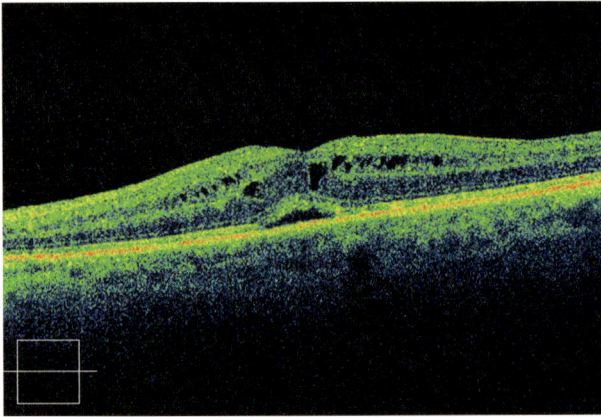

FIGURE 22.5 Macular optical coherence tomography (OCT) can be used to identify cystoid macular edema (CME) in a patient with corneal edema.

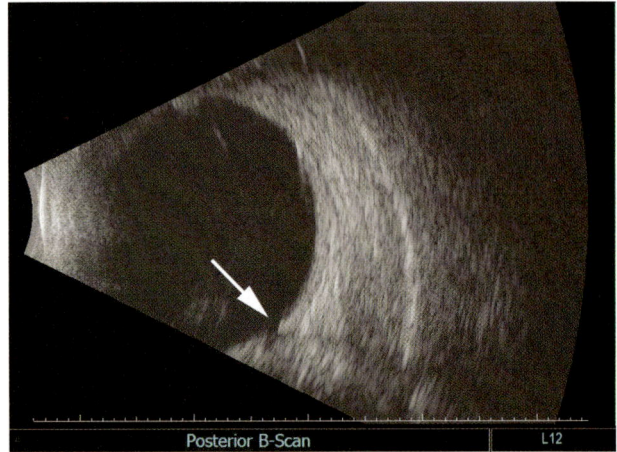

FIGURE 22.6 B-Scan ultrasonography shows glaucomatous cupping in a patient with aniridia (arrow). This same study can be used to evaluate possible retinal pathology in the setting of an opacified cornea.

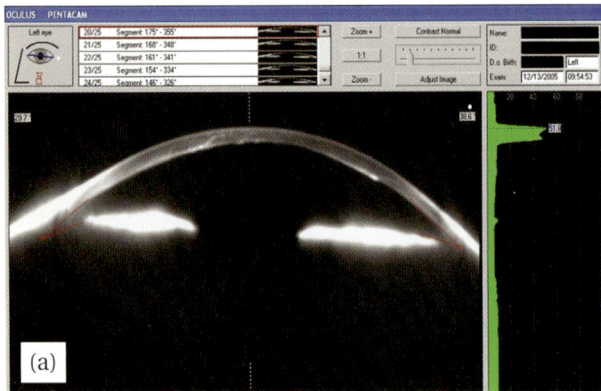

FIGURE 22.7 Anterior segment imaging can assist in planning the appropriate transplant procedure. (a) Pentacam® Scheimpflug analysis can characterize corneal opacity depth and density. (b) The Visante® anterior segment OCT can also assist in surgical planning for this patient with both pseudophakic corneal edema and anterior scaring related to limbal stem cell deficiency.

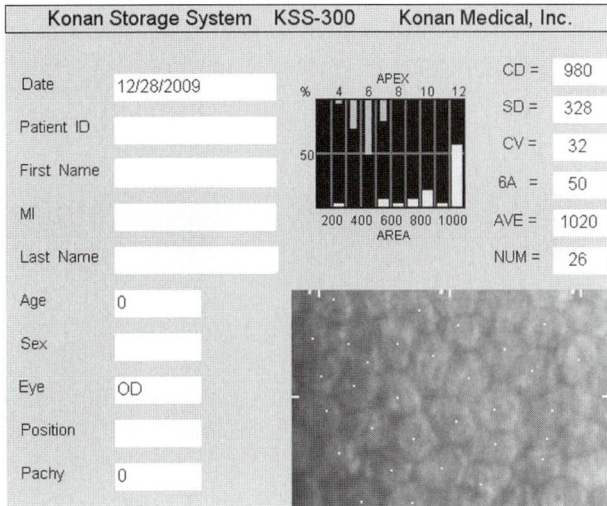

FIGURE 22.8 Specular microscopy can be performed prior to corneal transplantation. This patient had ectasia related to previous radial keratotomy (RK). Deep anterior lamellar keratoplasty (DALK) was considered, but given the low endothelial reserve a PKP was felt to be the best option.

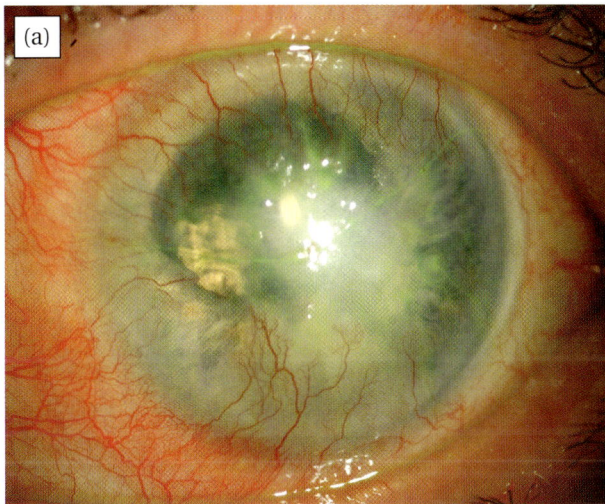

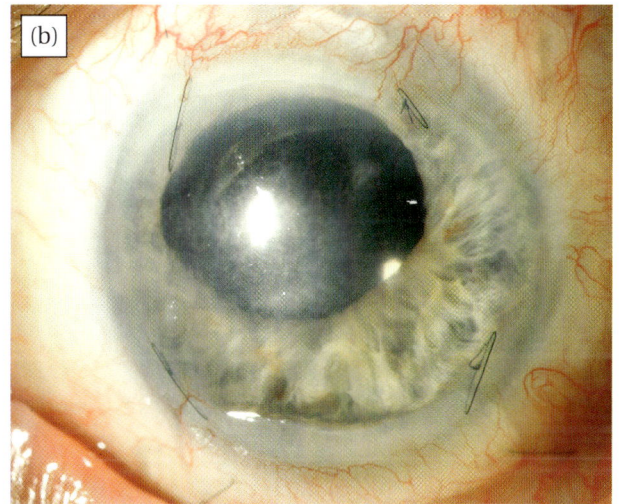

FIGURE 22.9 (a) This patient had both epithelial limbal stem cell deficiency and pseudophakic corneal edema related to combined phacoemulsification and mitomycin-C assisted trabeculectomy. (b) A limbal stem cell transplant was performed in order to prepare the patient for penetrating keratoplasty.

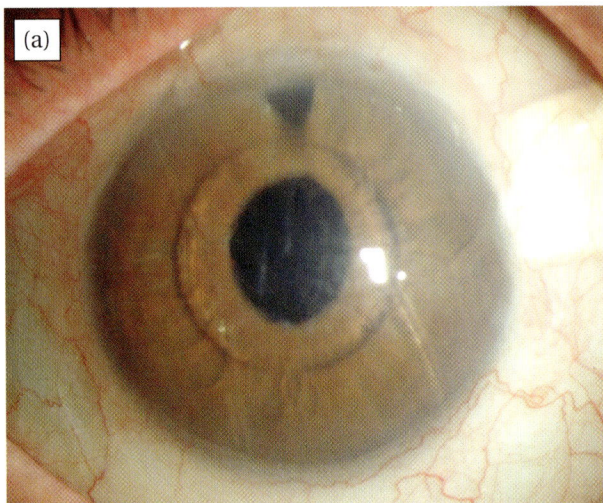
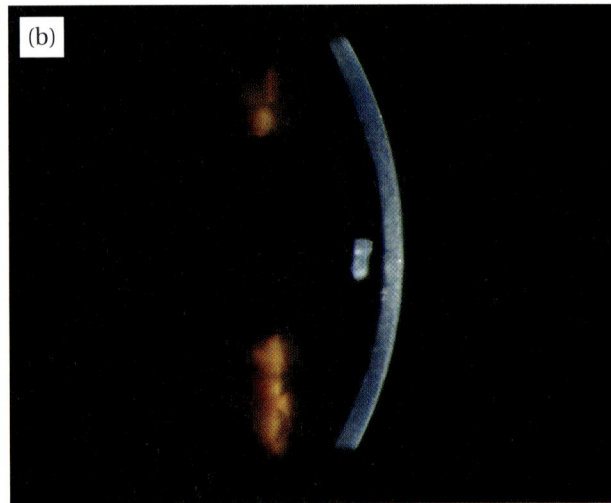

FIGURE 22.10   (a) This patient has a closed loop anterior chamber intraocular lens (IOL) and new onset pseudophakic bullous keratopathy. (b) Magnified slit-beam view of the same eye demonstrates stromal edema. Even with the advances in endothelial keratoplasty (EK), PKP could still be considered in this case, given the presence of the glaucoma drainage device and the challenges associated with lens removal in a closed system.

Phakic Corneal Transplantation

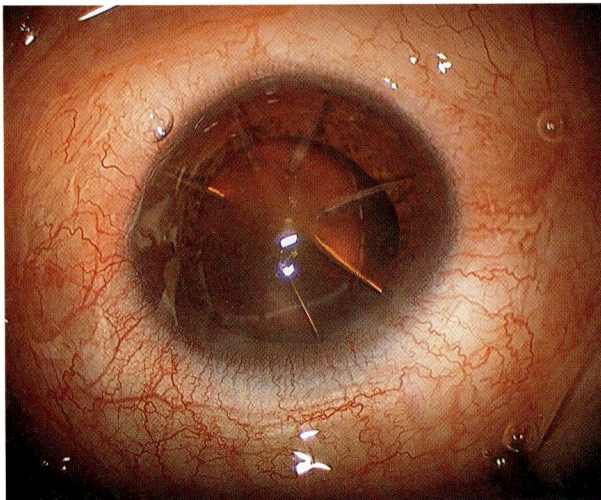

FIGURE 22.11   This patient had 8-incision RK and developed subsequent ectasia. The specular microscopy (shown in Figure 22.8) showed a low endothelial cell count, prompting the surgeon to choose phakic PKP.

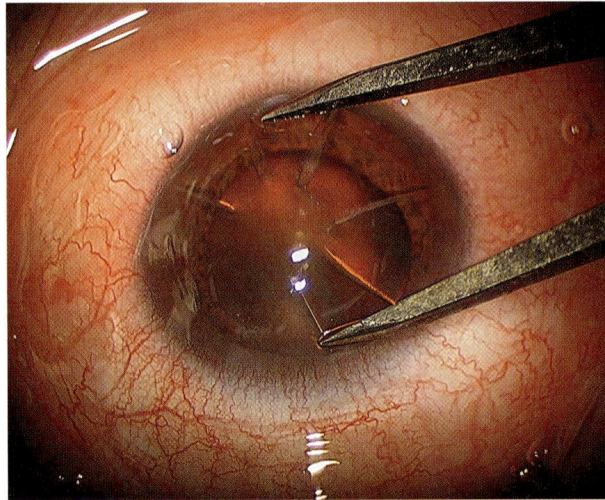

FIGURE 22.12   Calipers are used to measure the recipient cornea in order to determine a trephination size that encompasses the pathology.

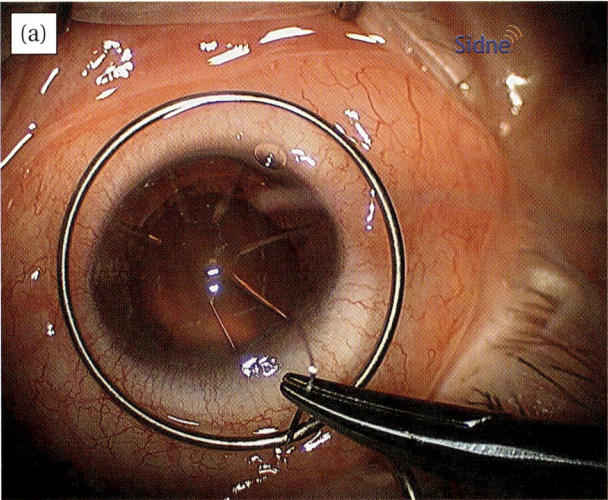

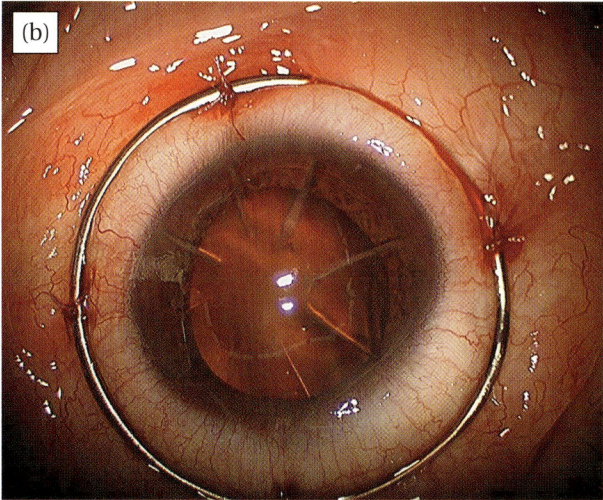

FIGURE 22.13 (a) A 6-0 vicryl suture is used to fixate the scleral support ring. (b) In this case, four interrupted sutures were used for support.

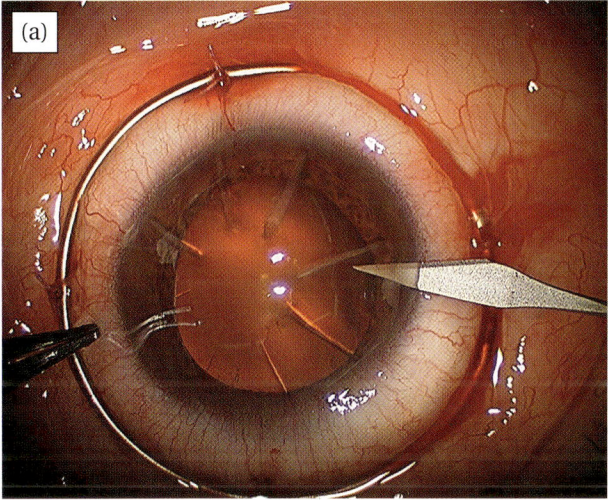

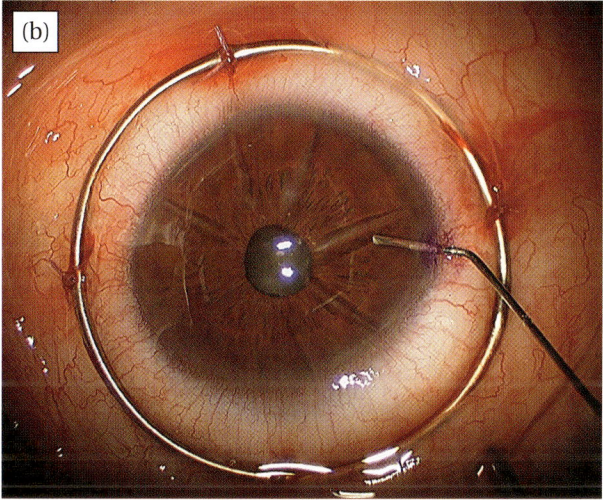

FIGURE 22.14 (a) A super-sharp blade is used to create a paracentesis. (b) In this case, miosis was obtained with intracameral acetylcholine.

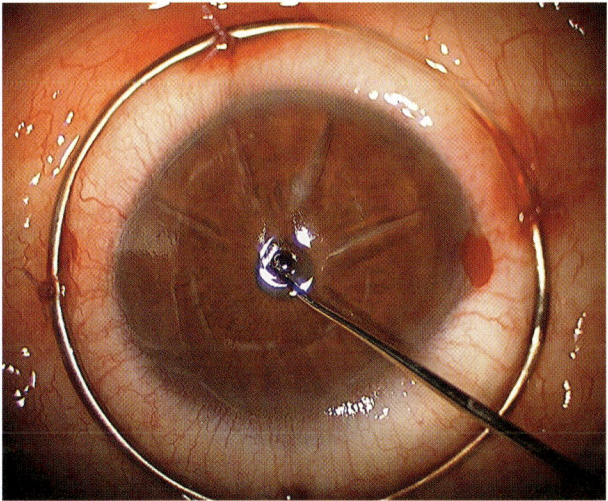

FIGURE 22.15 The visual axis is marked with an inked Sinskey hook.

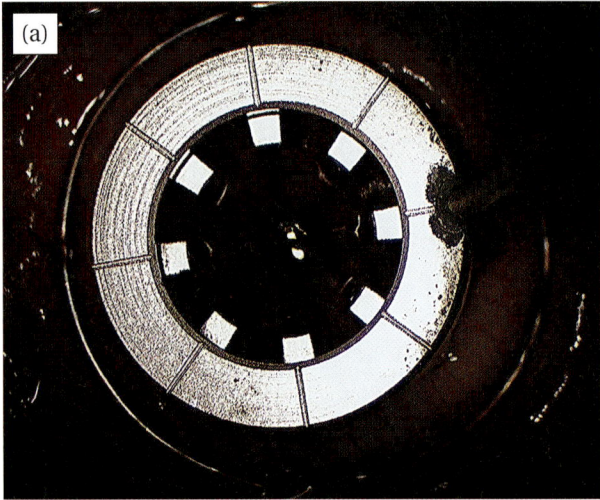

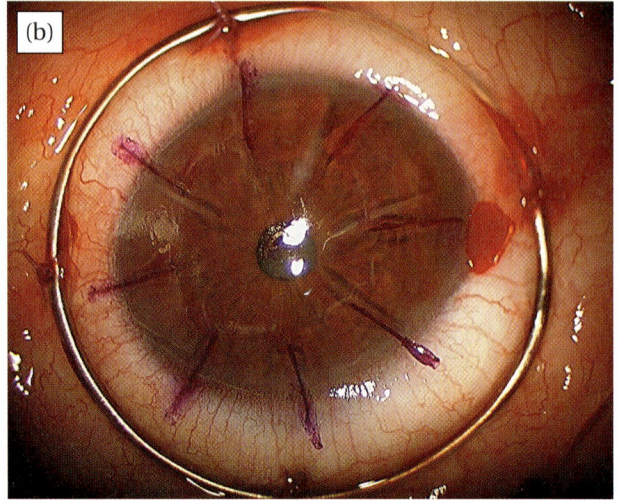

FIGURE 22.16 (a) An inked RK marker is centered on the visual axis. (b) The radial marks generated will assist in future suture placement.

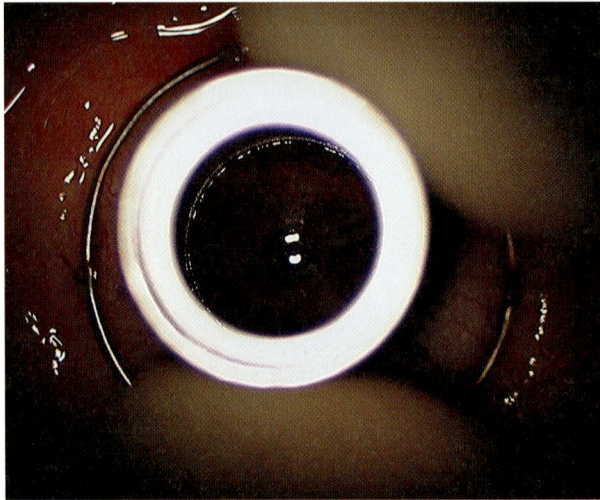

FIGURE 22.17 The host cornea is cut by hand with a manual trephine.

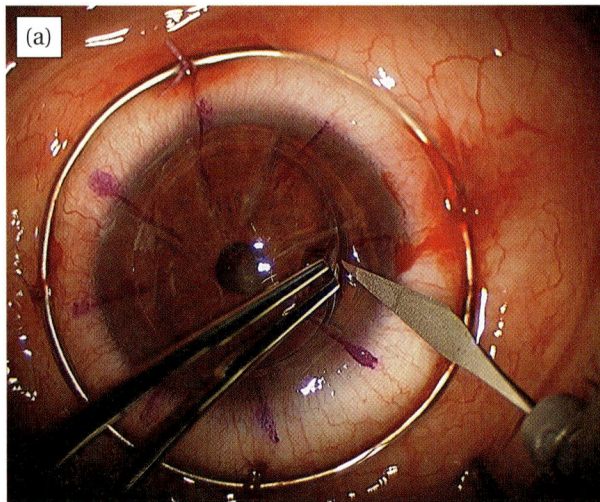

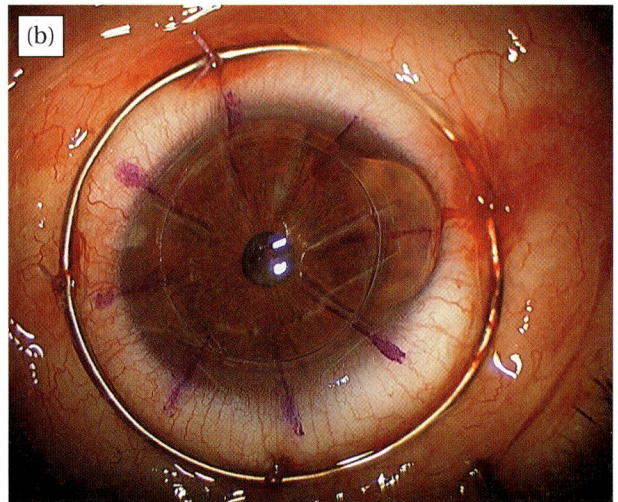

FIGURE 22.18 (a) The super-sharp blade is used to enter the anterior chamber. (b) An opening of 2.5 clock hours allows for easy insertion of the fine corneal scissors.

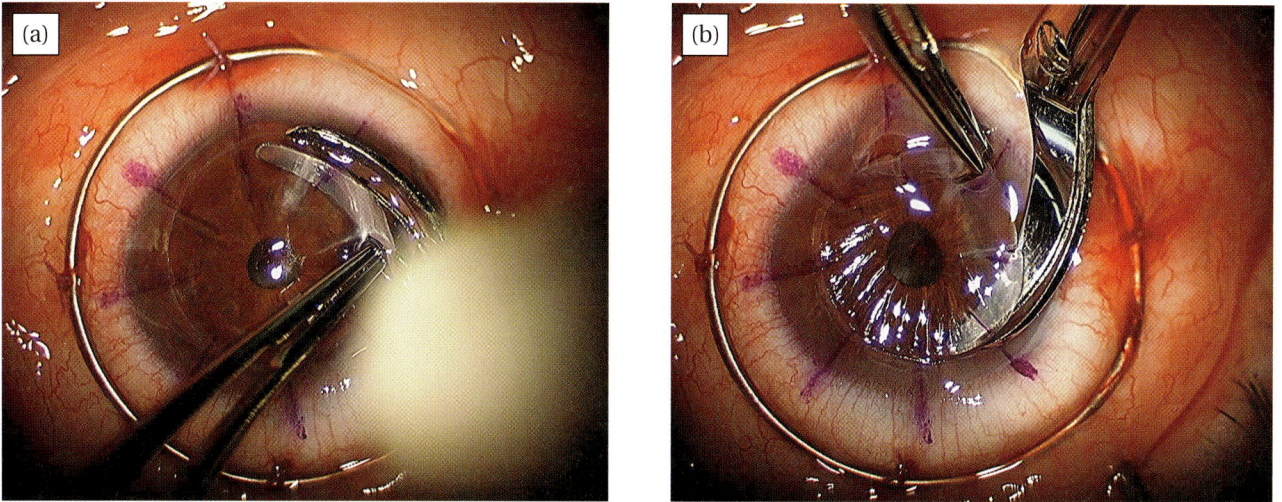

FIGURE 22.19 (a) Right-going cornea scissors are used to cut the host cornea. (b) Left-going scissors are then used to complete the removal. Care is taken to avoid damage to the iris or lens. Holding traction 90° from the scissors helps ensure a uniform cut.

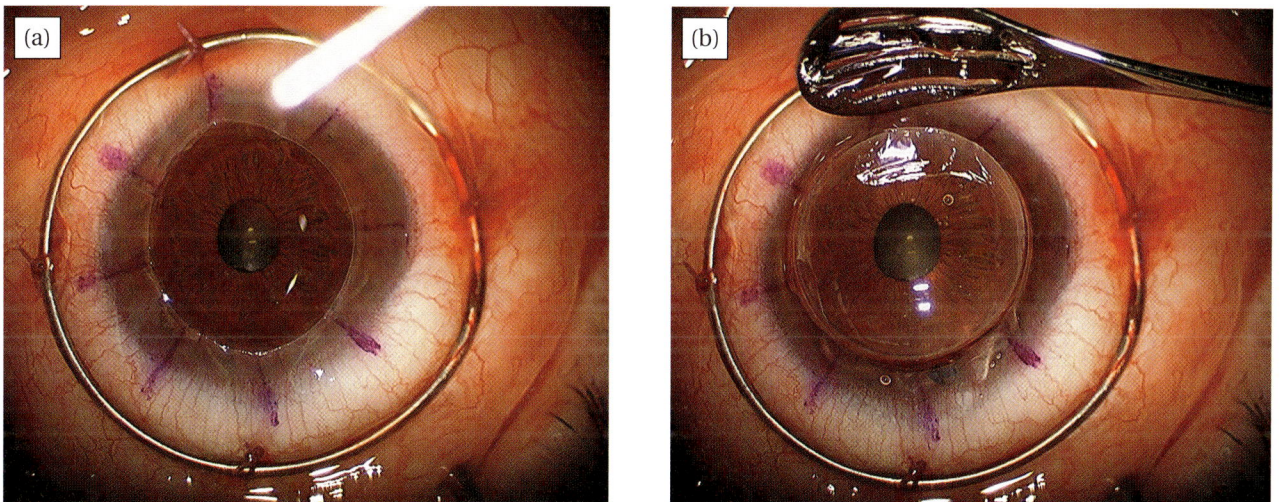

FIGURE 22.20 (a) Viscoelastic is placed on the surface of the iris and lens. (b) The donor button is then brought into position.

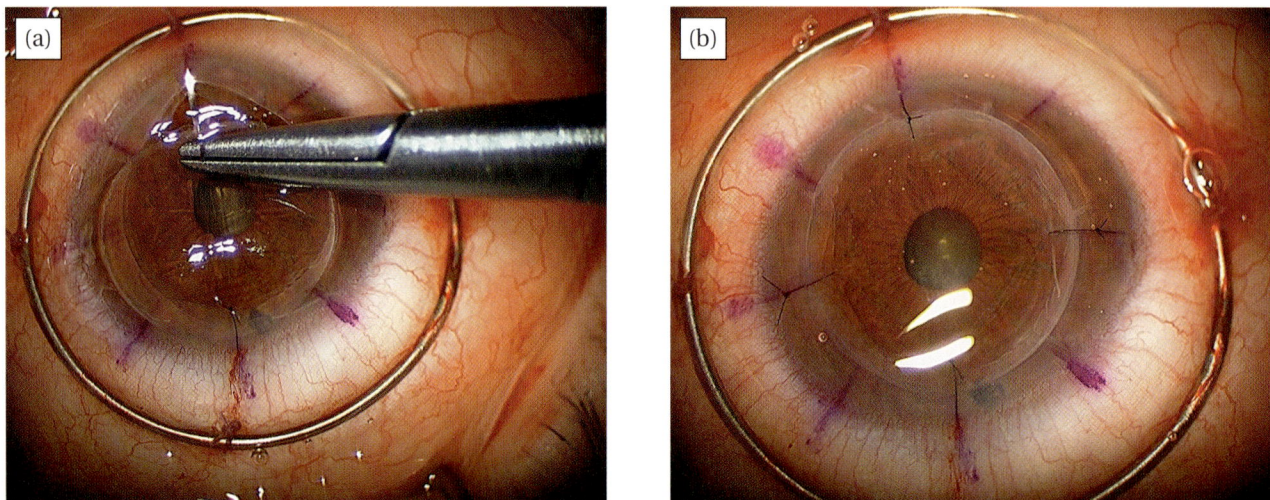

FIGURE 22.21 The donor button is secured with interrupted 10-0 nylon sutures. (a) The most important of these is arguably the 6 o'clock suture. (b) Once four cardinal sutures have been placed, a diamond crease may be apparent on the graft surface.

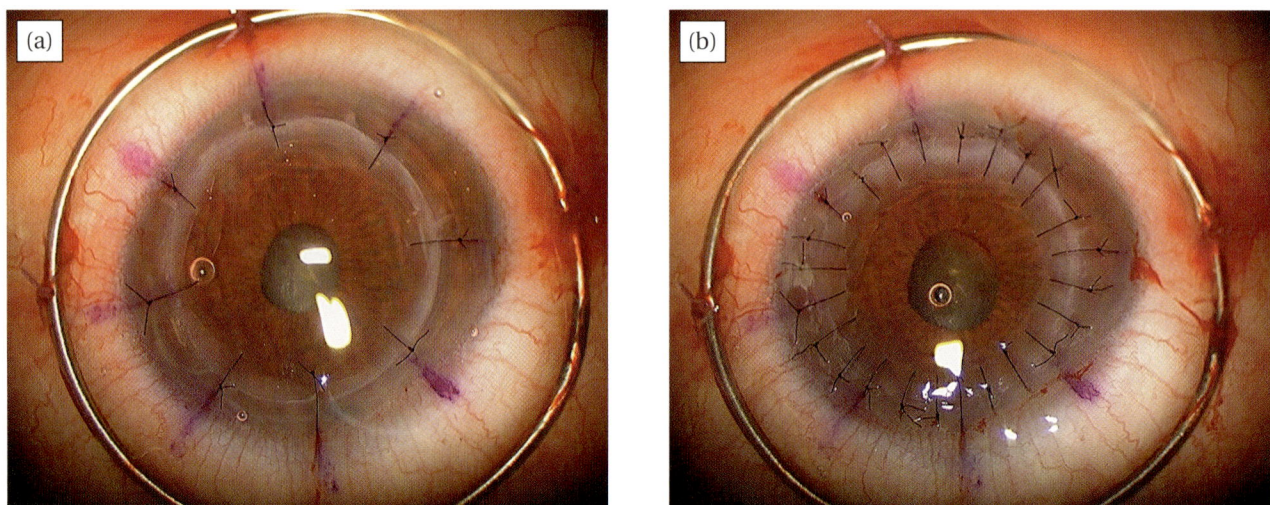

FIGURE 22.22 (a) Four additional sutures are placed. (b) In order to promote immediate and prolonged graft stability, a total of 24 interrupted sutures were placed in this case.

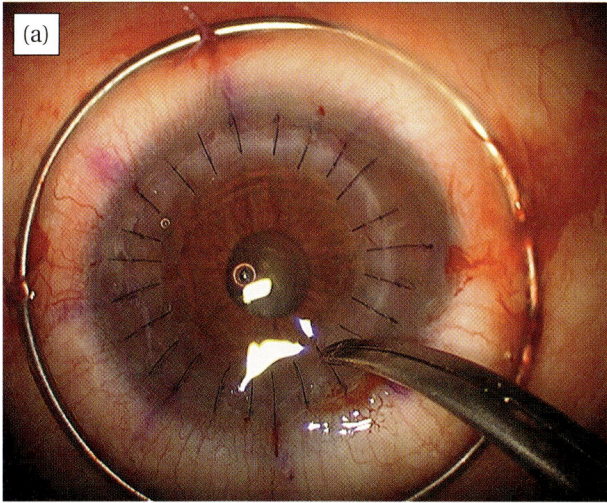

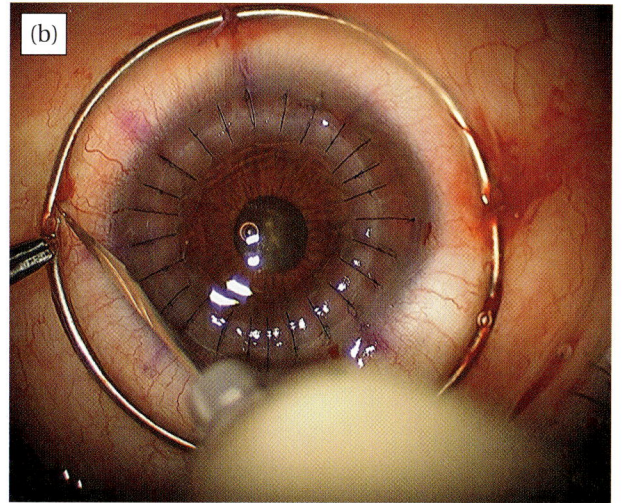

FIGURE 22.23 (a) With an angle tiers, the suture knots are buried. (b) The sutures securing the support ring are then cut with a super-sharp blade and removed.

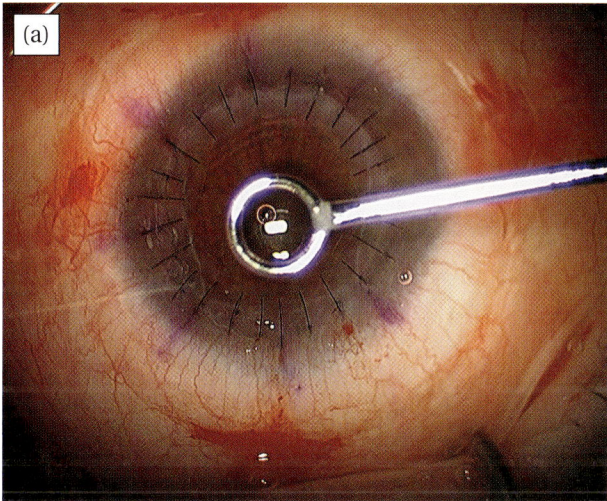

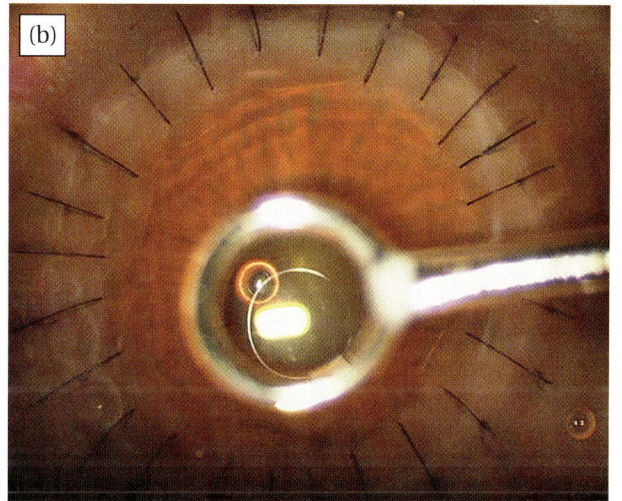

FIGURE 22.24 (a) The Mandell keratometer is brought onto the field. (b) A round keratometry reflection is reassuring at the end of surgery.

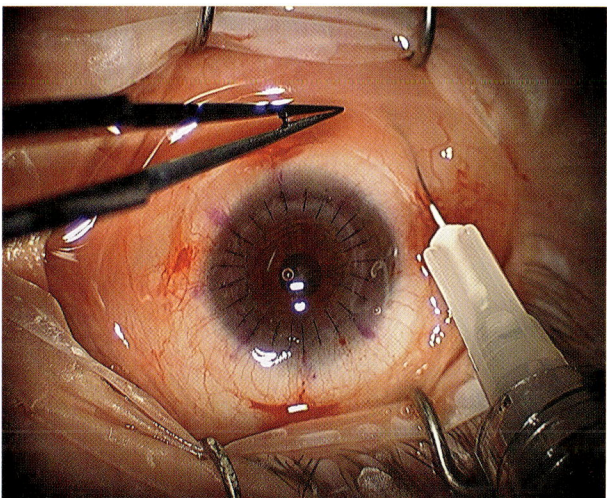

FIGURE 22.25 The case is concluded with delivery of subconjunctival antibiotic injections.

Aphakic and Pseudophakic Keratoplasty

Scleral Support

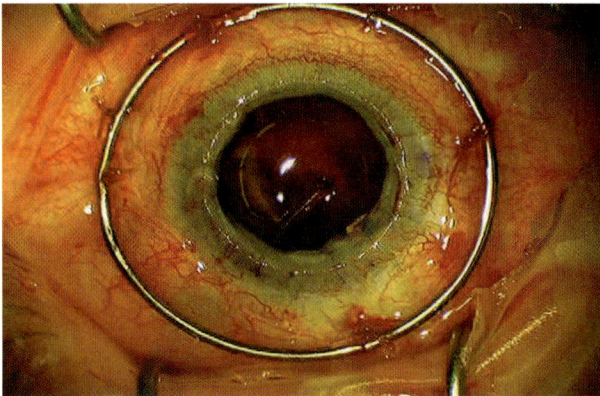

FIGURE 22.26 Because the aphakic or pseudophakic eye lacks the support of the crystalline lens and may require vitrectomy and intraocular lens (IOL) manipulation, it is important to provide intraoperative scleral support. Proper tension of the fixation ring sutures helps to make the host bed round, enabling accurate donor placement.

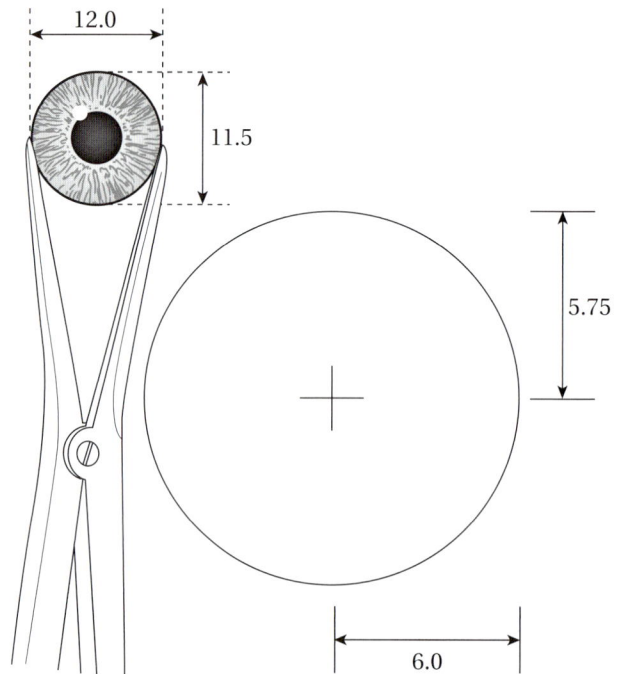

FIGURE 22.27 Centering the trephine on the host cornea requires consideration of several factors: the existing pathologic tissue to be excised, areas of corneal thinning to be avoided, and pupil position. The intersection of the horizontal and vertical diameters can be used to center the trephine.

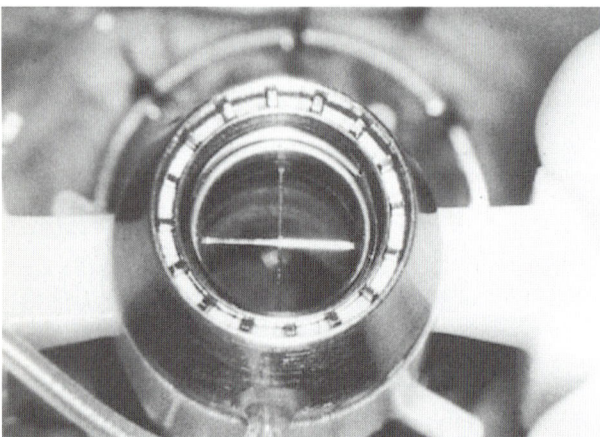

FIGURE 22.28 Use of a vacuum trephine may also assist in placement of the cardinal sutures. The teeth in the outer barrel are colored with a marking pen. The teeth leave properly aligned marks on the recipient cornea following trephination.

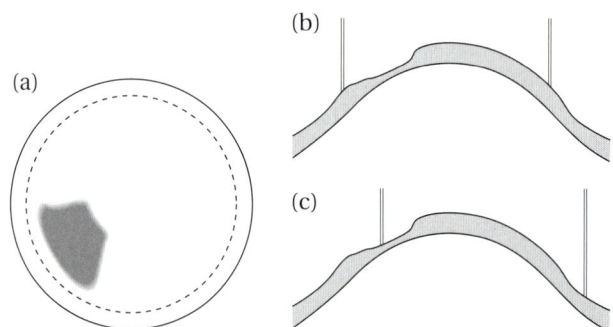

FIGURE 22.29 The size and location of the trephination site are selected to remove focal pathologic tissue and to avoid cutting through areas of corneal thinning, if possible. (a) An example of a focus of corneal thinning within the anticipated area of trephination. (b) Correct placement of the trephine to incorporate the area of thinning within the tissue to be removed. (c) Incorrect trephine placement.

(a)

Viscoelastic material
is introduced into
the AC to dissect
iris from cornea

(b)

Iris spatula is used to
sweep tissue away

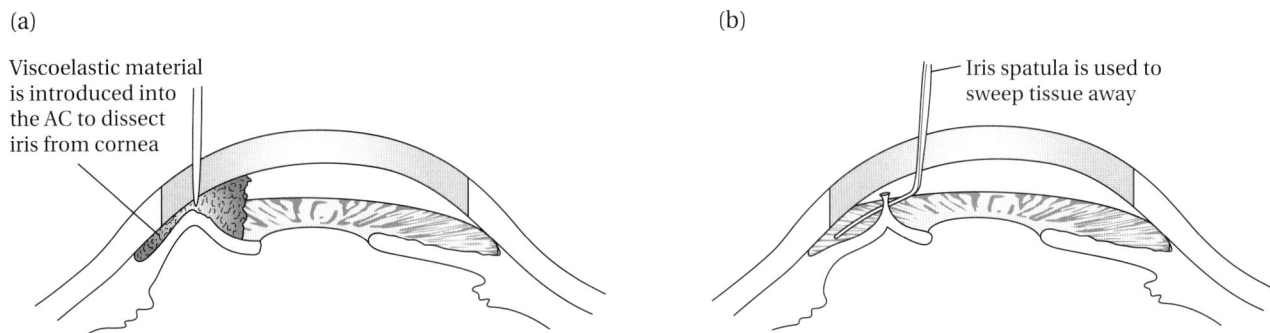

FIGURE 22.30 (a) Viscoelastic substance is injected into the anterior chamber to dissect the iris from the cornea. (b) An iris spatula may be used to help sweep tissue away.

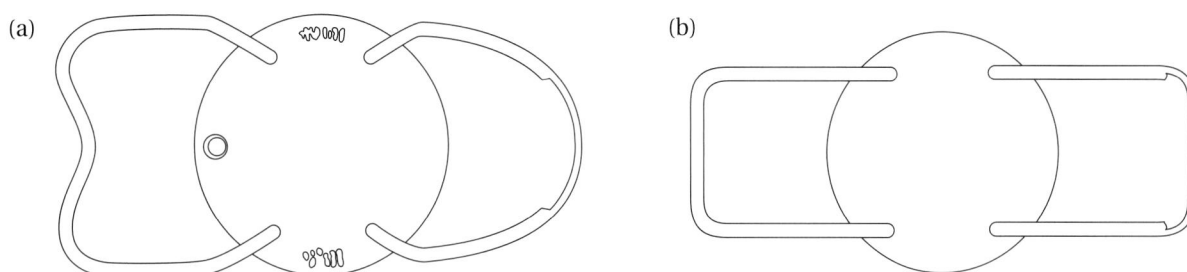

(a)

(b)

FIGURE 22.31 (a, b) Two examples of closed loop, semiflexible anterior chamber IOLs. When encountered, these should be removed and replaced.

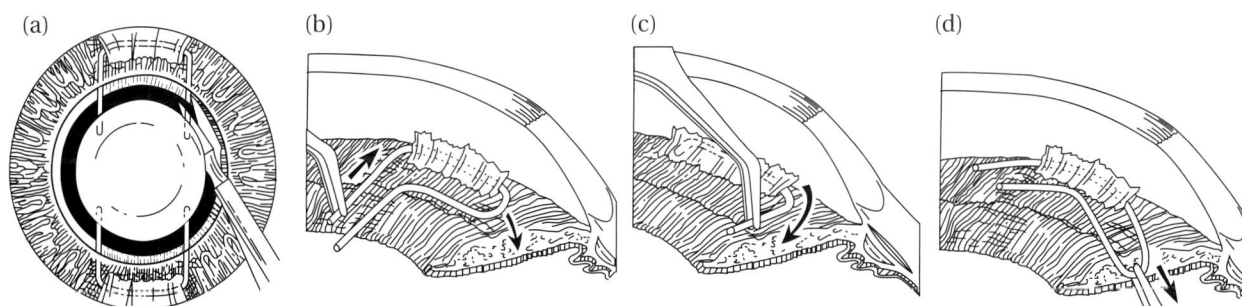

(a)   (b)   (c)   (d)

FIGURE 22.32 (a) An operating microscopic view of one method to remove a closed loop anterior chamber IOL. The portion of the haptic located in the angle is covered by multiple iris adhesions. Scissors are used to cut the haptic, as indicated. (b) Another view of a cut haptic from a stable flex IOL. Forceps are used to initiate passage of the cut haptic through the cocoon of iris adhesions. (c) Forceps are shown grasping one end of the cut haptic from the lens style in (a). A rotational movement is used to free the haptic from the cocoon-like iris adhesions. (d) Once the loop portion of the haptic is remote from the iris adhesions, it may be grasped with a forceps or Sinskey hook and slid from within the adhesions completely. (Reprinted with permission from Brightbill FS, ed. *Corneal Surgery: Theory, Technique, and Tissue*. 3rd ed. St. Louis, MO: Mosby, Inc.; 1999.)

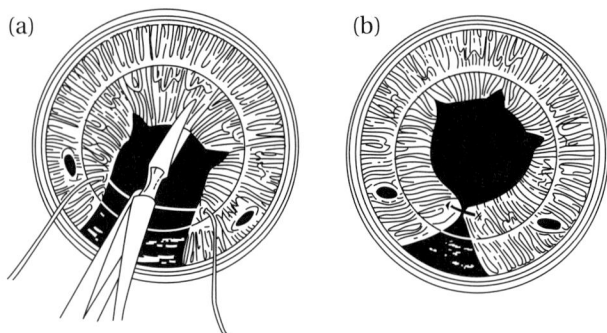

FIGURE 22.33 Reconstruction of an updrawn pupil typically seen in a patient with previous sector iridectomy. Reconstruction can be completed following placement of a posterior chamber scleral fixated IOL, or before placement of an anterior chamber IOL. (a) Small sphincterotomies are performed away from the sector iridectomy. (b) A No. 10 polypropylene (Prolene) suture is used to close the unopposed sides of the previous sector iridectomy. (Reprinted with permission from Brightbill FS, ed. *Corneal Surgery: Theory, Technique, and Tissue.* 3rd ed. St. Louis, MO: Mosby, Inc.; 1999.)

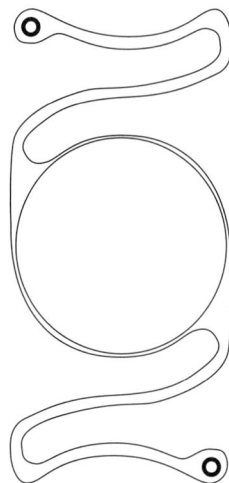

FIGURE 22.34 The flexible style anterior chamber IOL is the simplest choice for placement in the aphakic eye.

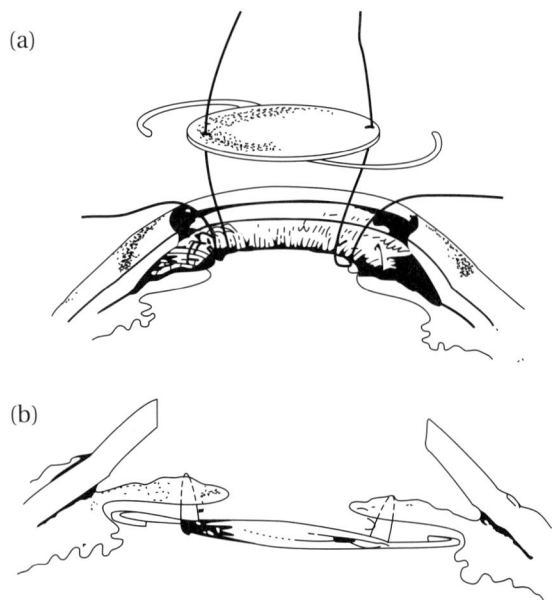

FIGURE 22.35 Fixation of a posterior chamber IOL to the iris. (a) Polypropylene (Prolene) suture is used to pass through positioning holes within the optic portion of the lens, then through the iris and is then tied. Alternatively, a McCannel-style polypropylene suture can be placed around the haptic securing it to the back of the iris. (b) Note the position of the lens with haptics in the sulcus. Sutures secure it to the iris. (Reprinted with permission from Brightbill FS, ed. *Corneal Surgery: Theory, Technique, and Tissue.* 3rd ed. St. Louis, MO: Mosby, Inc.; 1999.)

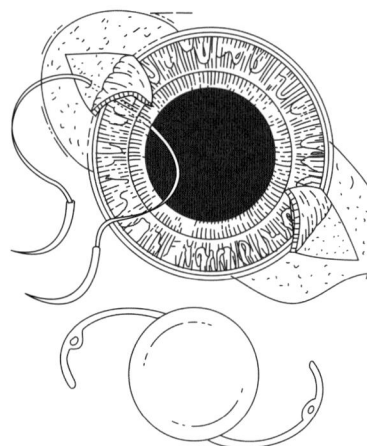

FIGURE 22.36 Previously prepared lamellar scleral flaps are shown in a triangular configuration. Through the open sky wound, a single arm of a double-armed 10-0 polypropylene (Prolene) suture is passed beneath the iris and out through the sulcus area. The second arm of this suture has been passed through the eyelet of the haptic. The end of this arm of the polypropylene suture is then passed again through the sulcus and out through the sclera, about 1 mm back from the limbus. (Reprinted with permission from Brightbill FS, ed. *Corneal Surgery: Theory, Technique, and Tissue.* 3rd ed. St. Louis, MO: Mosby, Inc.; 1999.)

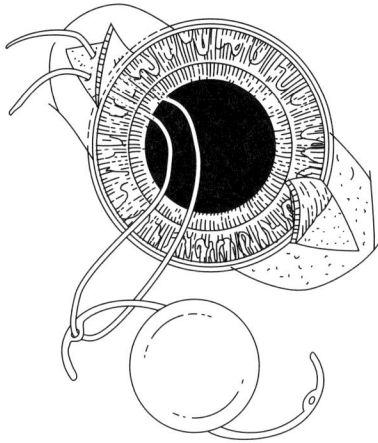

FIGURE 22.37 The other end of the double-armed suture is then passed through the positioning hole of the haptic eyelet. The second needle is passed similarly under the iris adjacent to the first pass. Passing the first suture arm and tightening the slack before traversing the lens eyelet with the second suture arm prevents entanglement in the suture. (Reprinted with permission from Brightbill FS, ed. *Corneal Surgery: Theory, Technique, and Tissue.* 3rd ed. St. Louis, MO: Mosby, Inc.; 1999.)

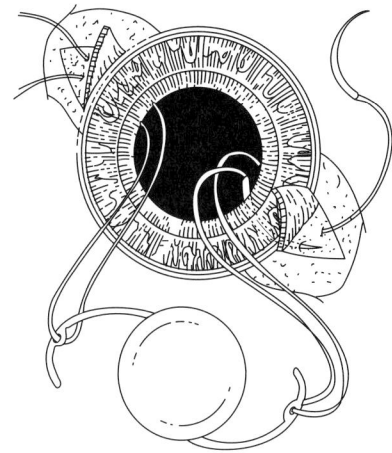

FIGURE 22.38 A 10-0 double-armed polypropylene (Prolene) suture is used to secure the second haptic in a similar fashion. The lens is guided into position and the inferior haptic is placed initially, as the suture is pulled up snug, while the haptic moves into the sulcus region. The sutures are held taut as the superior haptic is then placed in the sulcus. Those sutures also are drawn up and tied. (Reprinted with permission from Brightbill FS, ed. *Corneal Surgery: Theory, Technique, and Tissue.* 3rd ed. St. Louis, MO: Mosby, Inc.; 1999.)

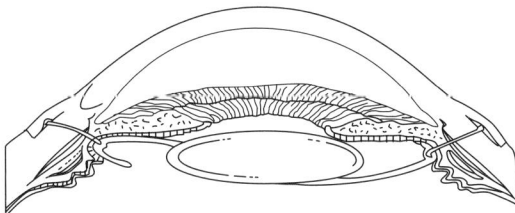

FIGURE 22.39 The haptics are observed in the sulcus. Polypropylene (Prolene) suture is transscleral and tied beneath the now reposited scleral flaps. The scleral flaps are secured with a 10-0 nylon suture, and the conjunctiva is brought back to cover the wound. (Reprinted with permission from Brightbill FS, ed. *Corneal Surgery: Theory, Technique, and Tissue.* 3rd ed. St. Louis, MO: Mosby, Inc.; 1999.)

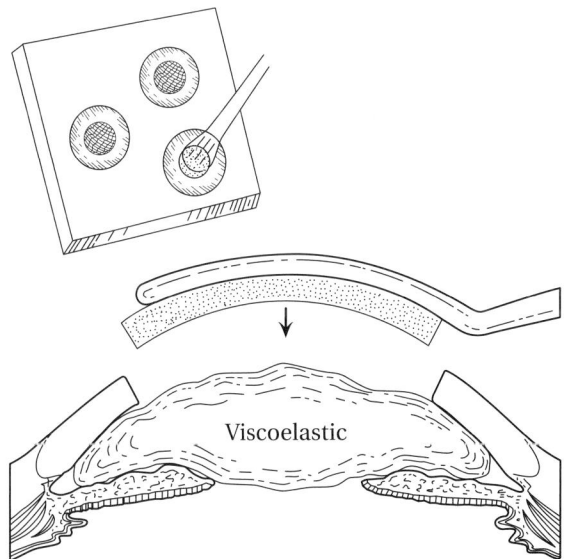

FIGURE 22.40 A Paton spatula slides beneath the epithelial surface, lifting the donor button from the cutting block. The button is then placed on a "bed" of viscoelastic material within the recipient bed. (Reprinted with permission from Brightbill FS, ed. *Corneal Surgery: Theory, Technique, and Tissue.* 3rd ed. St. Louis, MO: Mosby, Inc.; 1999.)

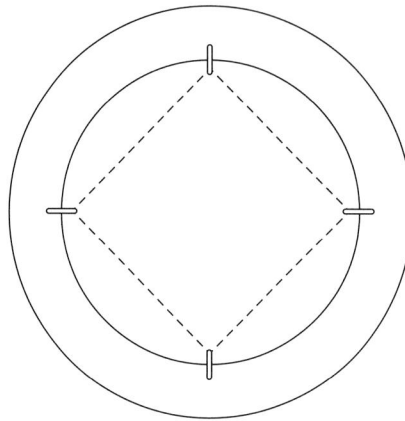

Tension lines between
four cardinal sutures form
a diamond pattern

FIGURE 22.41 The tension lines between the anterior insertion of the four cardinal sutures form a diamond pattern.

(a) Continuous running suture   (b) Continuous running suture

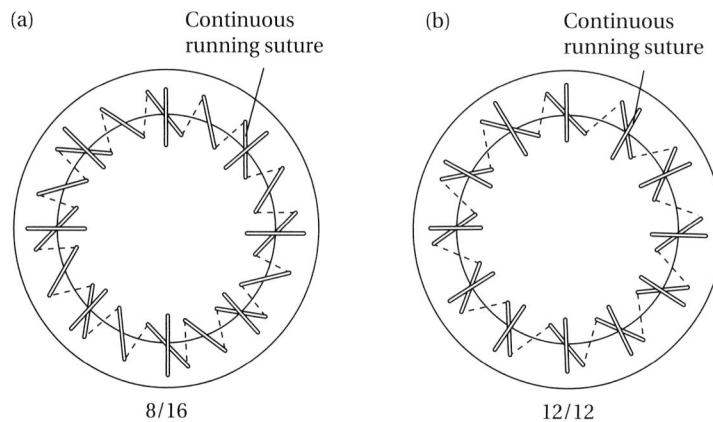

8/16   12/12

FIGURE 22.42 Patterns of combined interrupted and running sutures vary. Two popular patterns are (a) 8 interrupted sutures with a 16-bite running suture, or (b) 12 interrupted sutures with a 12-bite running closure.

Intraocular Lens Management in Penetrating Keratoplasty

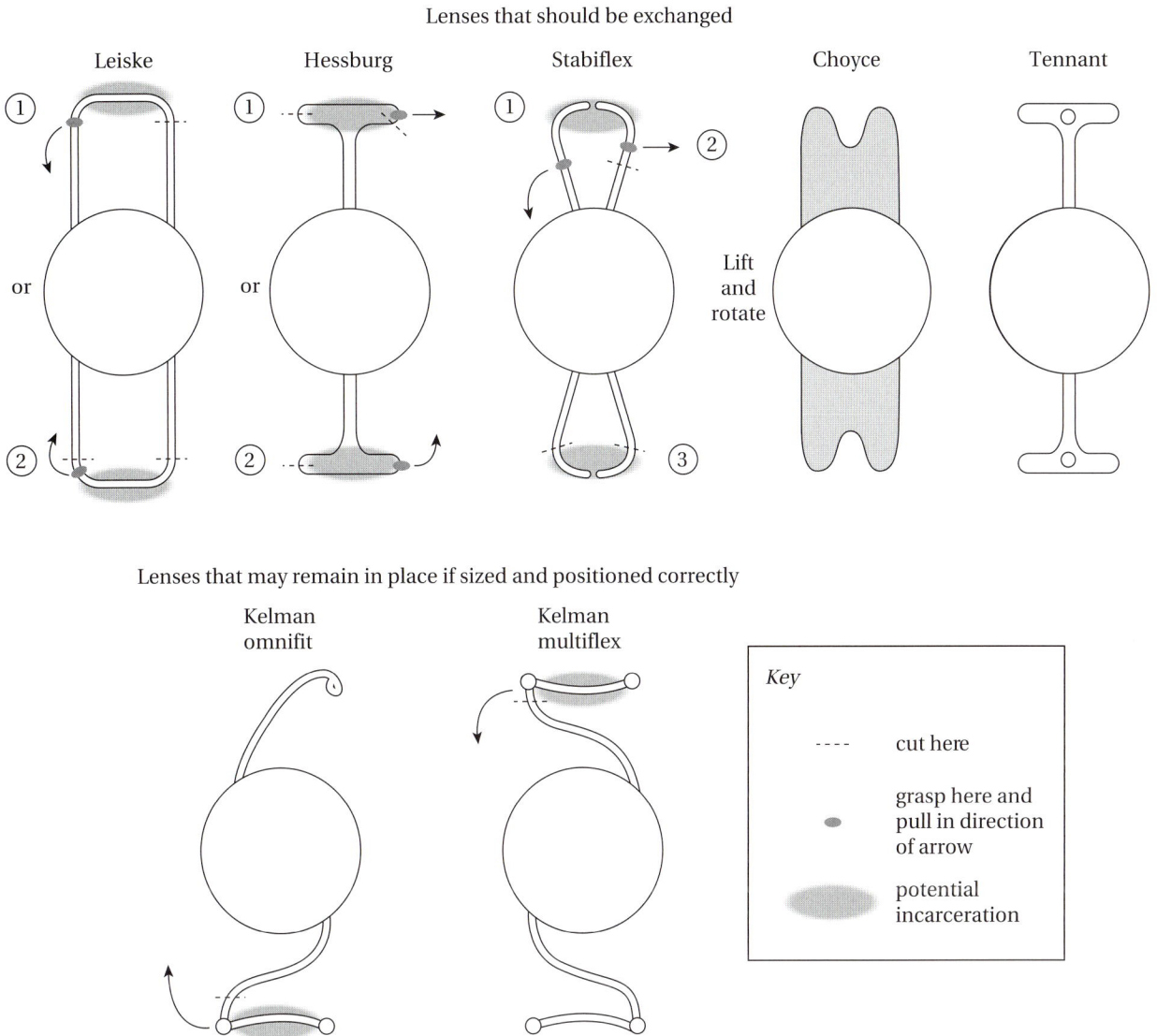

Lenses that should be exchanged

Leiske Hessburg Stabiflex Choyce Tennant

Lift
and
rotate

Lenses that may remain in place if sized and positioned correctly

Kelman
omnifit

Kelman
multiflex

Key

---- cut here

grasp here and
pull in direction
of arrow

potential
incarceration

FIGURE 22.43 The IOL styles that should be removed if found in the anterior chamber are shown in the top row. The dotted line indicates where the haptic should be cut. The broad gray area shows the locations of partial incarceration, and the small dot or gray area indicates where one should grasp to remove the cut haptic. In the bottom row of lenses, flexible-style anterior chamber IOLs are demonstrated. While it is unusual for these lenses to be removed at the time of keratoplasty, on occasion an undersized or oversized lens may need to be exchanged. If areas of incarceration exist, as shown, the proper location for cutting the haptic and direction of removal of the haptic are demonstrated. If the haptic incorporation into iris adhesions is significant, it may be necessary to leave some haptic material to avoid inadvertent bleeding.

Corneal Sutures, Trephines, and Cutting Blocks

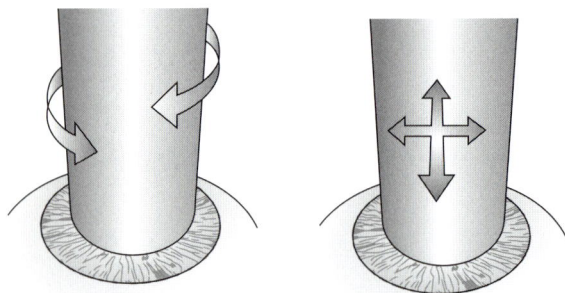

FIGURE 22.44 Direction of trephine motion. (Reprinted with permission from Bruner WE, Stark WJ, Maumenee AE, eds. *Manual of Corneal Surgery.* New York, NY: Churchill Livingstone; 1987, p. 21.)

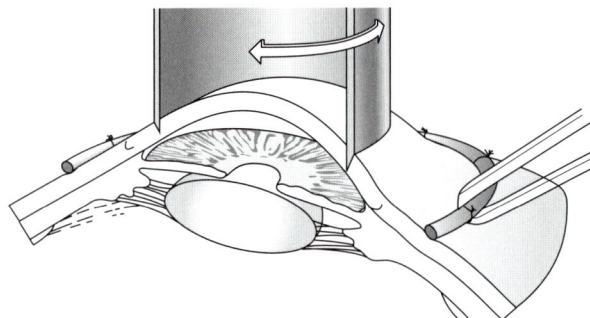

FIGURE 22.45 The trephine is used to make an incision to approximately 80% depth. (Reprinted with permission from Waltman SR. Penetrating keratoplasty. In: Waltman SR, Keates RH, Hoyt CS, et al., eds. *Surgery of the Eye.* New York, NY: Churchill Livingstone; 1988, p. 202.)

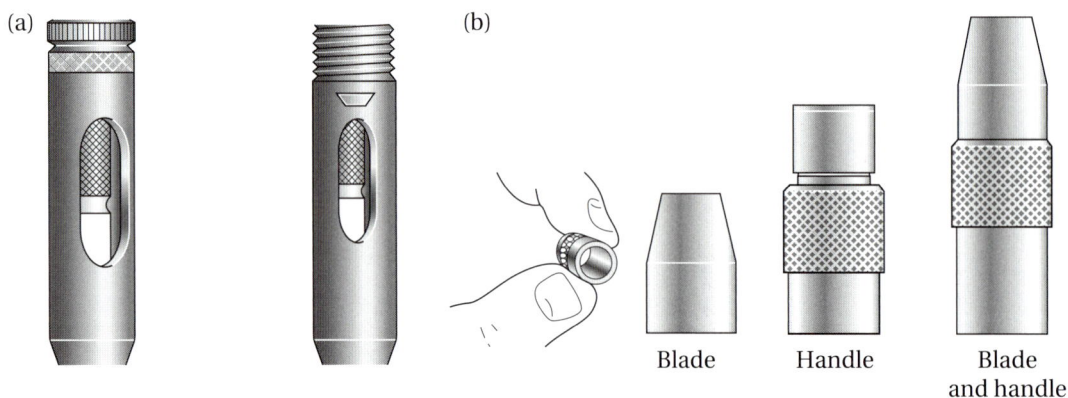

(a)   (b)

Blade   Handle   Blade and handle

FIGURE 22.46 (a) Castroviejo corneal trephine. Modified trephine also is used with the corneal graft punch, shown here with a Weck disposable blade. (b) A "see-through" handle is available for each size to allow the surgeon to fully visualize the cutting process through the center of the blade and handle. (Figure [a] reprinted with permission from Brightbill FS, Pollack FM, Slappey T. A comparison of two methods for cutting donor corneal buttons. *Am J Ophthalmol.* 1973;75:501. [b] Reprinted with permission from Katena Products, Inc.)

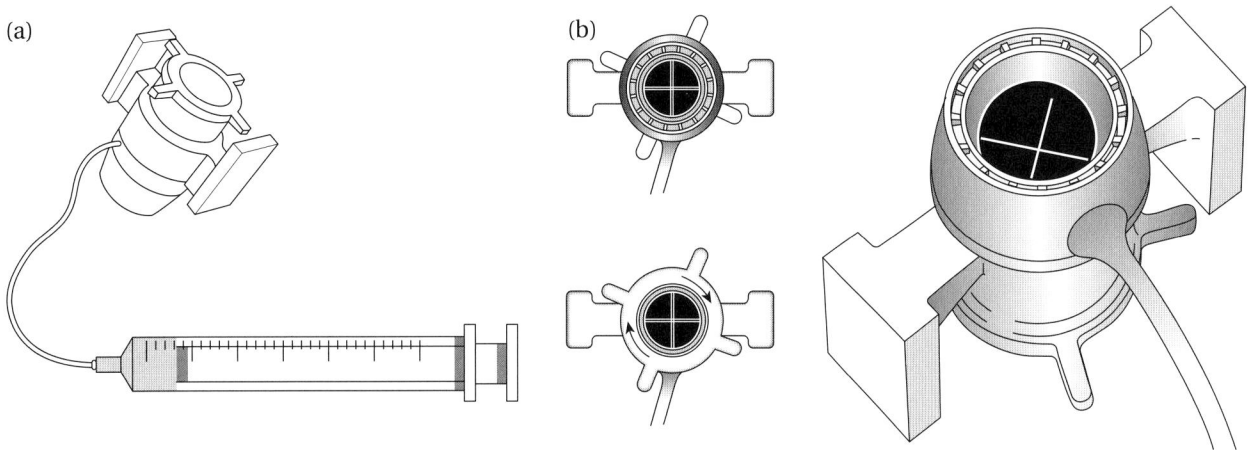

FIGURE 22.47 (a) Diagram of a Hessburg-Barron vacuum trephine. (b) Corneal distortion is reduced by this suction chamber device. Extra-fine crosshairs are centered inside the trephine blade for accurate alignment with the visual axis of the recipient. A precisely calibrated rotating mechanism allows the surgeon to advance the blade depth 0.25 mm with each 360° rotation for lamellar or penetrating keratoplasty. (Figure [a] Reprinted with permission from Bruner WE, Stark WJ, Maumenee AE, eds. *Manual of Corneal Surgery.* New York, NY: Churchill Livingstone; 1987, p. 22. [b] Reprinted with permission from Katena Products, Inc.)

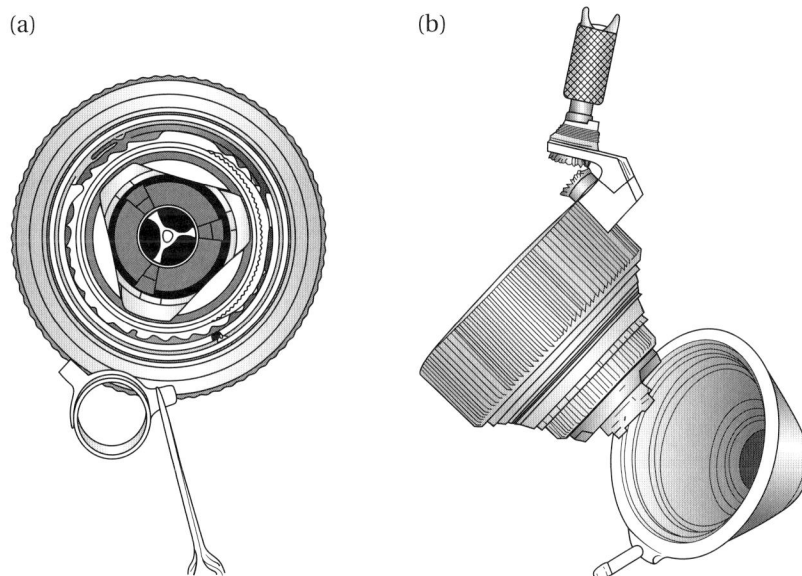

FIGURE 22.48 (a, b) The trephine features a 360° limbal suction ring that secures the trephine to the eye. Support surfaces on both sides of the trephine blade stabilize the cornea during trephination; a manually operated gear mechanism provides smooth, uniform cutting, and a calibration device governs the blade extension and also allows cutting without descent. The trephine produces a symmetric and nearly vertical incision. (Reprinted with permission from Moria catalog, on the Hanna corneal trephine system, France.)

(a)

(b)

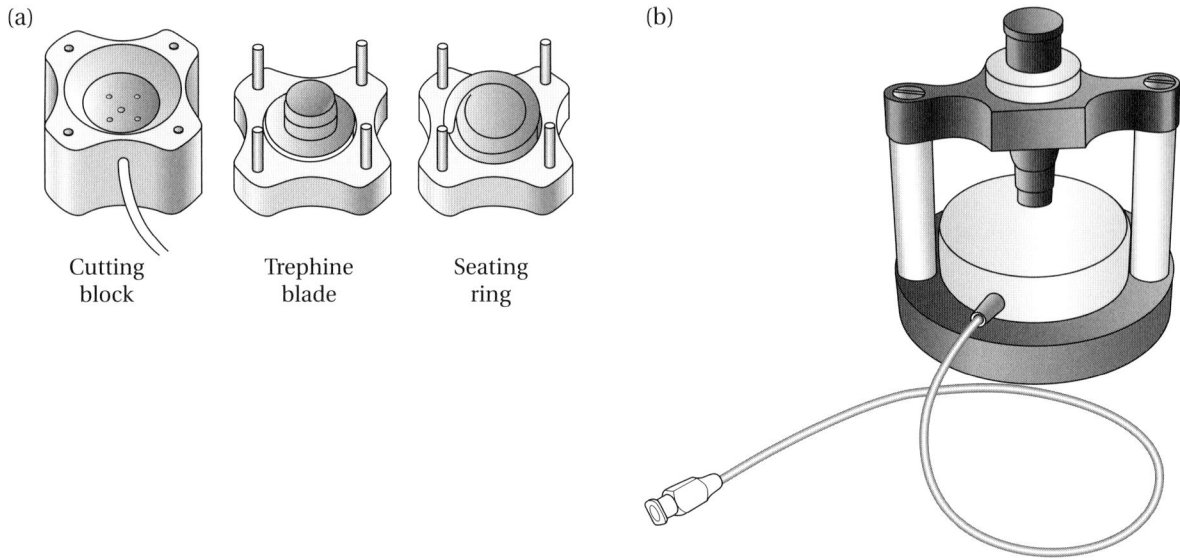

Cutting block

Trephine blade

Seating ring

FIGURE 22.49 (a) The base of the Barron vacuum punch features a circular groove for aspirating the epithelial side of the cornea and immobilizing it for cutting the button. The seating ring is used to ensure complete contact between the peripheral part of the cornea and the aspirating groove, for positive vacuum. Immobilizing the donor cornea in this manner allows the surgeon to cut a perfectly round button from the center of the cornea every time. (b) The Rothman-Gilbard corneal punch uses a specially designed suction cutting block with 8 precisely placed suction holes. These holes are inked, the cornea is placed in the well, suction is applied, and the button is punched. (Figure [a] reprinted with permission from Katena Products, Inc., 1996 catalog. [b] Reprinted with permission from Storz Ophthalmics.)

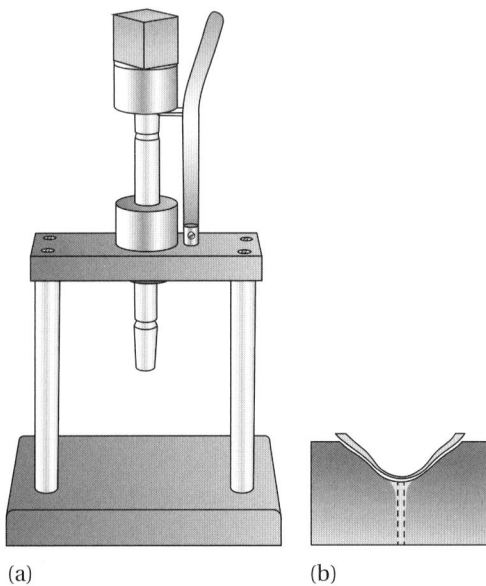

FIGURE 22.50 (a) The Lieberman gravity action corneal donor button punch is made of solid stainless steel and produces a symmetric, smooth, vertical cut. The punch accepts blade sizes 7.5 to 9.0 mm. The cutting block is made of black nylon and its concavity features multiple radii to most closely approximate the shape of the average corneoscleral surface. A black nylon cutting block was chosen for better visualization of the clear cornea. The block is vented to the outside to release air and fluid beneath the donor button. (b) Lieberman donor button cutting block features multiple radii to closely approximate the corneoscleral profile. (Reprinted with permission from Katena Products, Inc.)

(a)

(b)

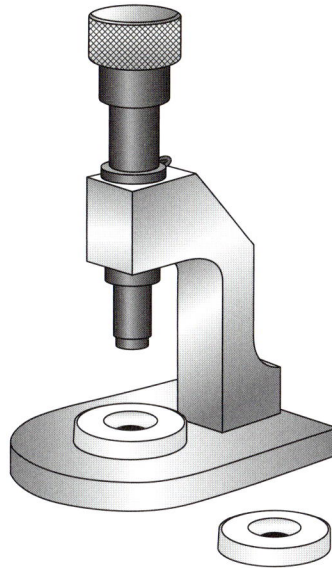

FIGURE 22.51 The Iowa PK press punch was designed for precise punching of the donor corneal button. A unique 2-color cutting block aids in centration of the donor tissue. A recessed base ensures that the block is held centrally under the trephine blade. (Reprinted with permission from Storz Ophthalmics.)

TABLE 22.2 *Corneal Transplantation: Early Postoperative Management*

There are probably as many postoperative care regimens as there are surgeons performing corneal transplantation. Each surgeon will be influenced by his or her training and experience, the nature of the condition requiring surgery, and even the availability of the patient for follow-up care. Whatever the specific approach taken, the following must be monitored in the early postoperative period:

1. Infection
2. Wound leak and suture problems
3. Persistent epithelial defect
4. Anterior synechiae
5. Iritis
6. Glaucoma
7. Vascularization
8. Primary graft failure

Early Postoperative Management

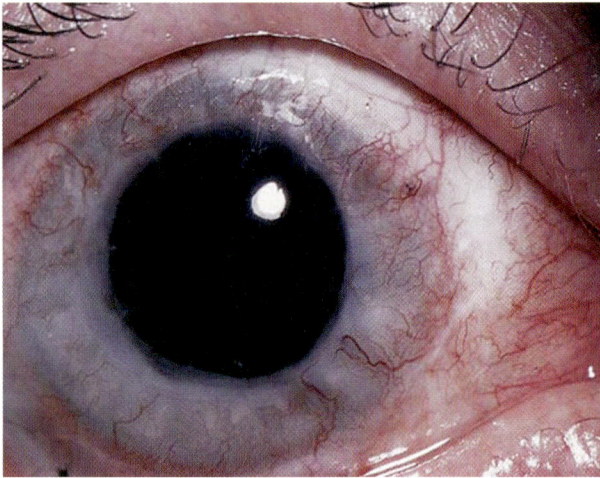

FIGURE 22.52 When a graft is placed in a vascularized bed, steroids must be continued indefinitely to prevent rejection.

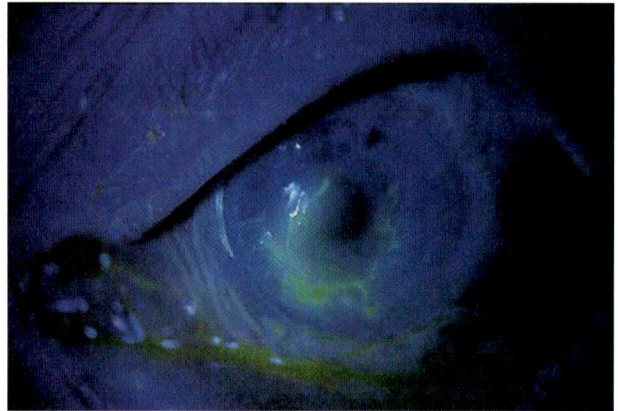

FIGURE 22.53 Although not universally accepted, the use of an antiviral agent is recommended for a patient with a history of herpes simplex keratitis. Recurrent herpes dendritic keratitis in a graft is shown. The patient was receiving steroids but no antiviral coverage.

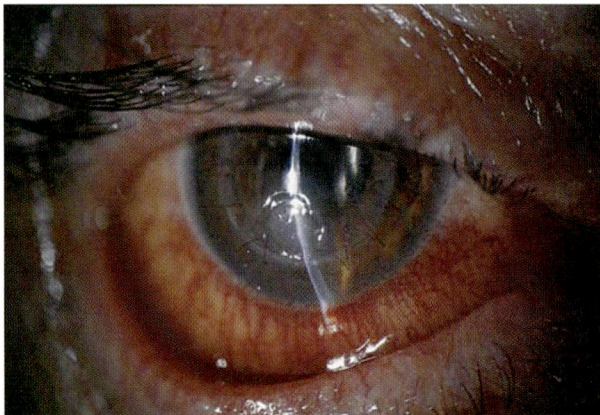

FIGURE 22.54 Complications in the period following corneal transplantation can vary from the minor postoperative issue to the true ophthalmic disaster that results in the loss of an eye. What is certain for all the potential complications is that the best chance for a successful outcome occurs with early intervention. Corneal epithelial defect shown here has become infected.

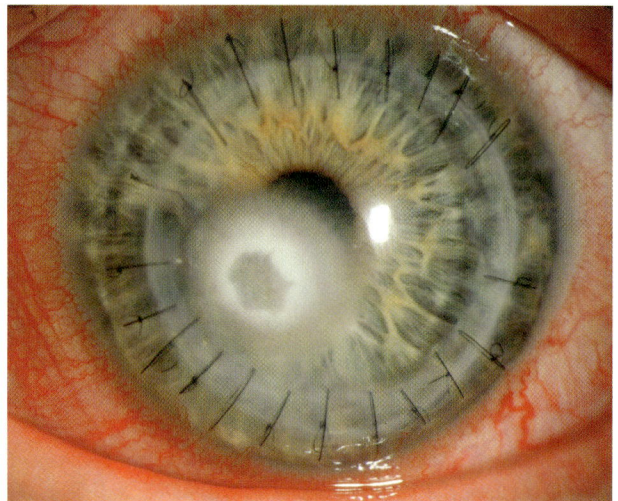

FIGURE 22.55 Fungal keratitis is found in the wound margin; a mass of hyphae extends into the anterior chamber.

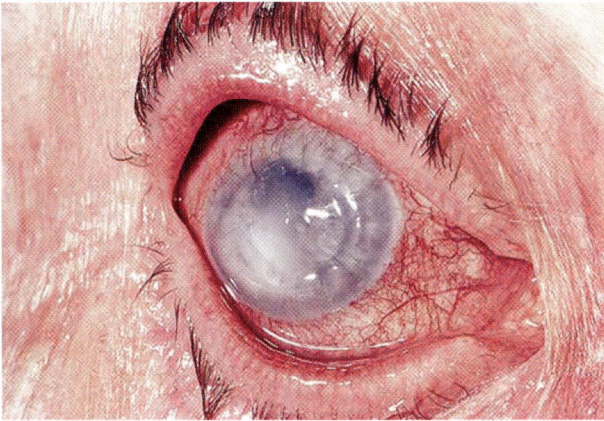

FIGURE 22.56 A neglected corneal ulcer has led to perforation. Note the relatively mild inflammatory reaction due to use of topical steroids.

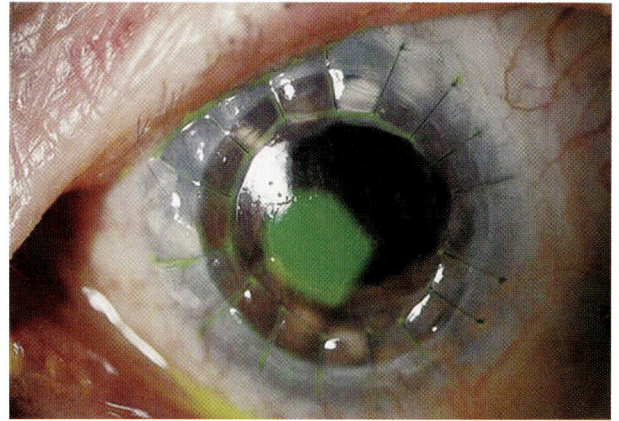

FIGURE 22.57 An epithelial defect requires prompt treatment to prevent secondary complications.

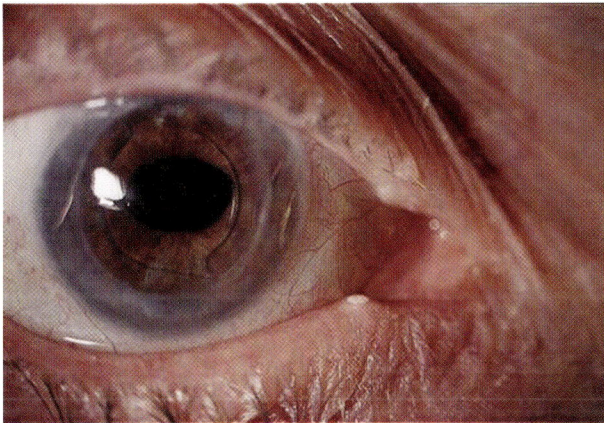

FIGURE 22.58 Punctal plug is placed to help protect the graft epithelium in a patient with dry eye.

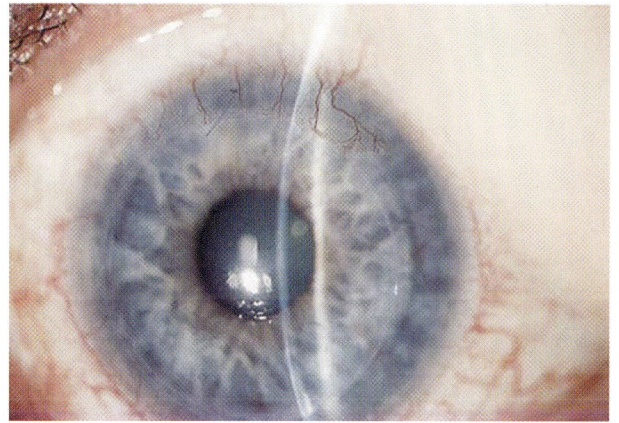

FIGURE 22.59 Superficial vascularization of the cornea follows placement of a bandage soft contact lens for chronic filamentary keratitis.

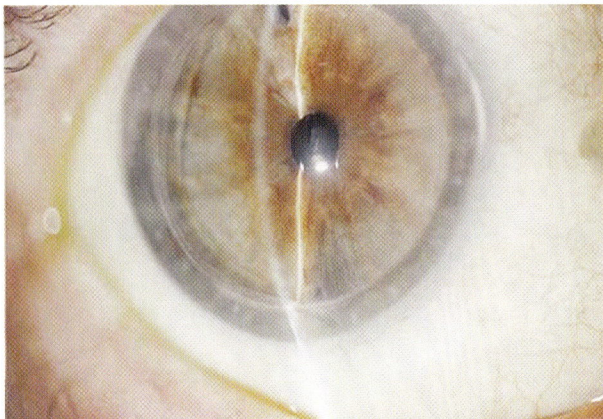

FIGURE 22.60   Limited anterior synechia to the graft wound has been present for years without adversely affecting graft survival.

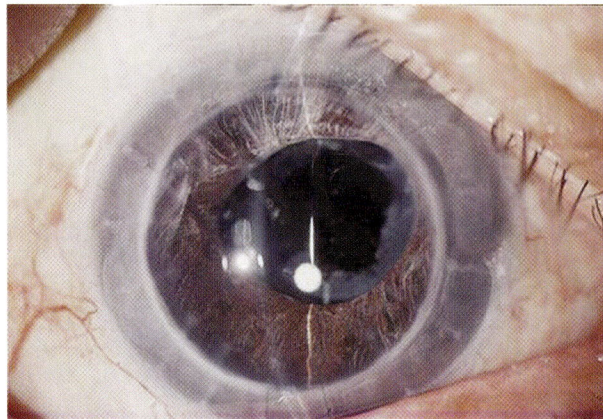

FIGURE 22.61   Total angle closure from progressive anterior synechial formation was found in this patient with marked postoperative inflammation. The graft remained clear, and the intraocular pressure was controlled with medication.

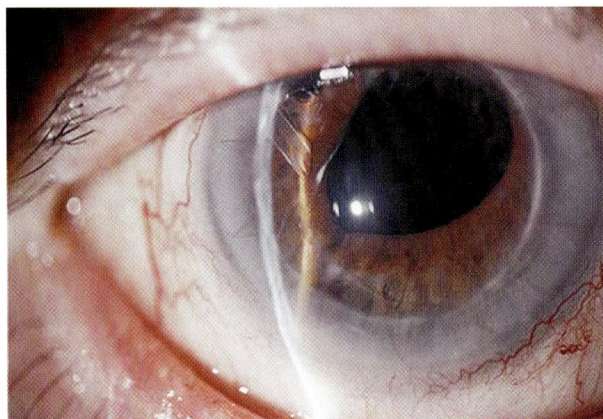

FIGURE 22.62   Note that the tube from this valve has been positioned well away from the back of the graft.

SELECTED REFERENCES

Brightbill FS, McDonnell PJ, McGhee CNJ, Farjo AA, Serdarevic O. *Cornea surgery: Theory technique and tissue.* 4th ed. St. Louis: Mosby; 2008.

Bruner WE, Stark WJ, Maumenee AE. *Manual of corneal surgery.* New York, NY: Churchill Livingstone; 1987.

Krachmer JH, Mannis MJ, Holland EJ. *Cornea: Fundamentals, diagnosis, and management.* 3rd ed. St. Louis: Mosby; 2010.

<table>
<tr><td>23</td><td># Deep Anterior Lamellar Keratoplasty</td></tr>
</table>

Deep Anterior Lamellar Keratoplasty

Sadeer B. Hannush, MD

TABLE 23.1 *Indications for Deep Anterior Lamellar Keratoplasty (DALK)*

Conditions causing corneal clouding or optical interference that do not involve Descemet's membrane and endothelium

A. Corneal ectasias

Keratoconus

Keratoglobus

Pellucid marginal degeneration

Post-corneal refractive surgery ectasias

B. Corneal stromal dystrophies

Granular

Lattice

Macular (only in the absence of Descemet/endothelial involvement)

Other stromal dystrophies

C. Corneal scars sparing Descemet's membrane

Infection

Non-penetrating trauma

TABLE 23.2 *Contraindications to Deep Anterior Lamellar Keratoplasty (DALK)*

Absolute Contraindications

Conditions associated with endothelial dysfunction (Procedure of choice: endothelial keratoplasty)

Posterior dystrophies: Fuchs' endothelial dystrophy, posterior polymorphous corneal dystrophy, congenital hereditary endothelial dystrophy

Corneal edema and bullous keratopathy secondary to endothelial cell loss/dysfunction

Iridocorneal endothelial (ICE) syndromes

Relative Contraindications

Previous rupture of Descemet's membrane (hydrops, traumatic perforation): may be amenable to DALK with increased surgeon experience

Limbal stem cell deficiency states and severe surface disease: aniridia, chemical injury, neurotrophic keratitis, keratoconjunctivitis sicca, etc. DALK may be combined with other ocular surface reconstructive procedures (e.g., limbal stem cell transplantation, amniotic membrane transplantation, tarsorrhaphy, punctal occlusion, etc.)

Surgical Technique

There is more than one technique for deep anterior lamellar keratoplasty (DALK). Manual dissection can usually be performed to near 90% depth. Viscodissection may be performed at a deeper lamellar plane, but may or may not find the pre-Descemet space. The "big bubble technique" (BBT) can usually and reliably cleave off Descemet's membrane from the posterior stroma. It is the technique we describe below.

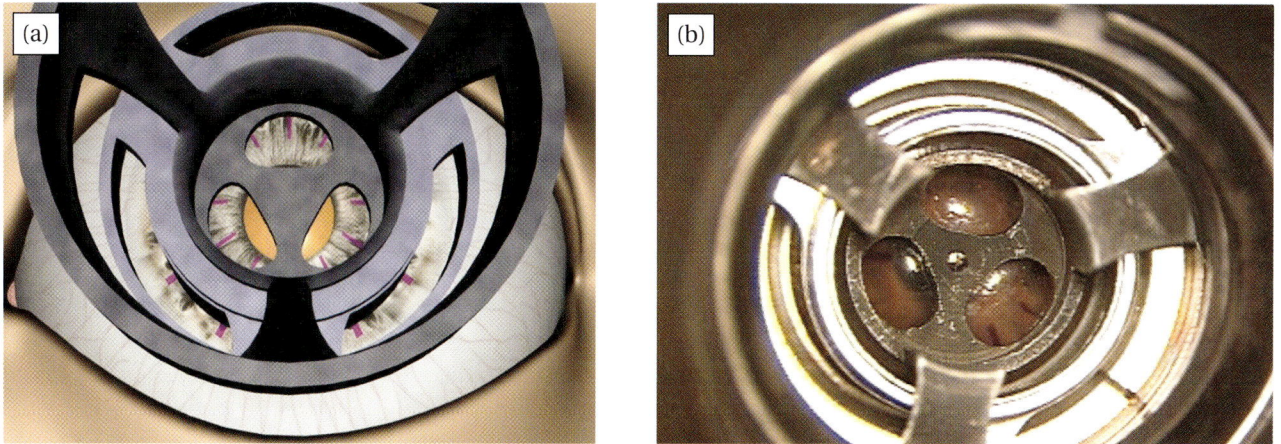

FIGURE 23.1 Partial trephination: 70%–80% of local pachymetry. (Drawing (a) by and courtesy of Eric J. Fleischer, MD.)

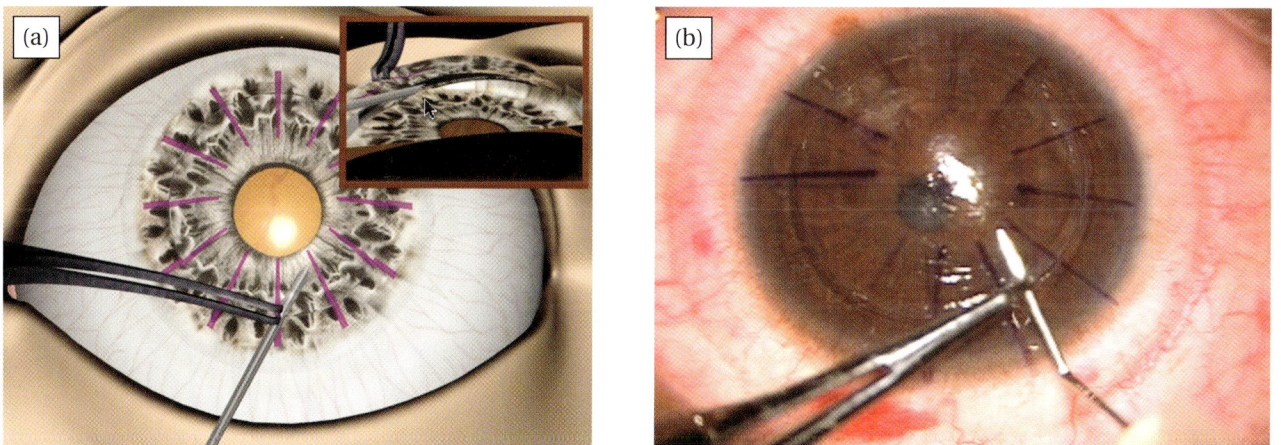

FIGURE 23.2 Placement of the hypodermic needle (27 gauge) bevel down. The needle or a probe followed by cannula with an inferior opening (Tan, Sarnicola, Fogla) is placed, at the bottom of the trephination wound, or slightly deeper, and advanced 4–5 mm into clear cornea, making every effort to stay in the same plane, directed away from both corneal center and trephination groove (45 degrees from the tangent to the trephination groove at the site of entry). The needle/cannula should be placed deep enough in the corneal stroma so that the pathway of least resistance for the injected air is posteriorly through the deep stromal lamellae into the pre-Descemet potential space and not out around the needle/cannula, but not so deep as to risk perforation. (Drawing (a) by and courtesy of Eric J. Fleischer, MD.)

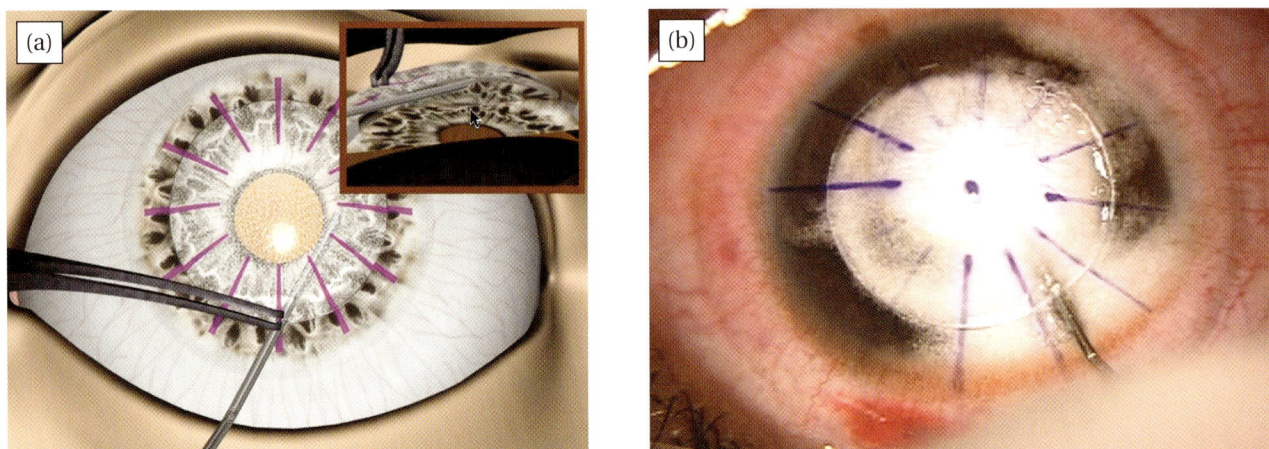

FIGURE 23.3 Creation of the big bubble with slow, but steady injection of air. The speed of air injection should be adjusted to force air posteriorly through the deep stromal lamellae, more so than laterally or around the needle/cannula, in order to expand the air bubble in the pre-Descemet space, but not too forcefully, so as to avoid rupture of Descemet's membrane. (We usually use a 5 cc syringe and inject air at the rate of 1 cc second). Horizontal/lateral air dissection through the corneal stroma is a side effect of the attempted creation of a big bubble, and not the goal or endpoint of air injection. If the big bubble development can be visualized, stop when the bubble reaches the edges of the trephination wound. Further enlargement of the big bubble in the pre-Descemet space towards the limbus may lead to disinsertion of Descemet's membrane at Schwalbe's line, or delivery of unwanted air into the anterior chamber through Schlemm's canal. Avoid decompressing the eye by placing a paracentesis prematurely. Most DALK surgeons prefer to wait until the big bubble is developed. A soft eye may lead to uncontrolled expansion of the air in the pre-Descemet's space at the time of air injection and a tear in Descemet's membrane or disinsertion at Schwalbe's line. (Drawing (a) by and courtesy of Eric J. Fleischer, MD.)

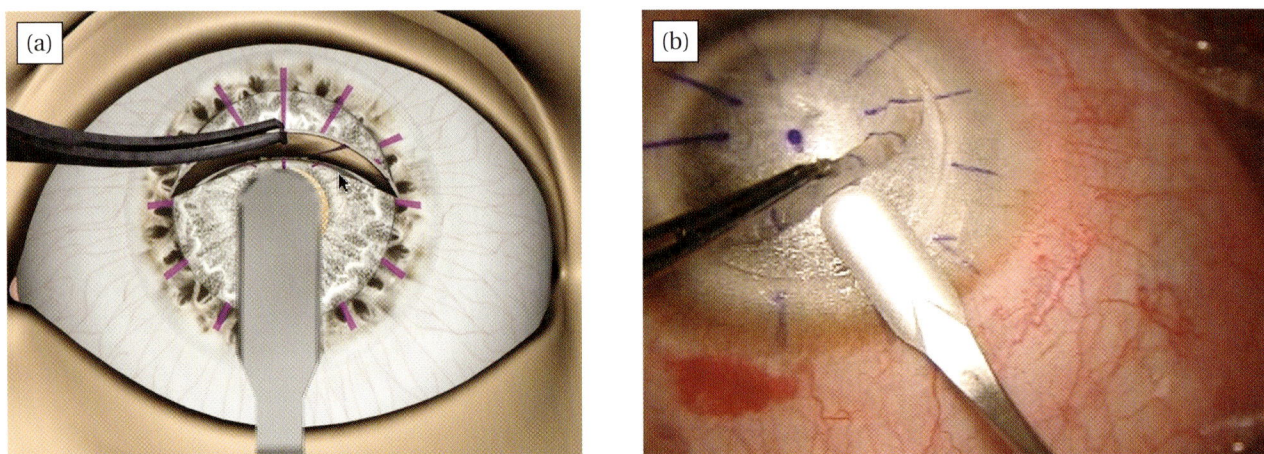

FIGURE 23.4 Lamellar dissection and removal of the anterior stroma with an angled crescent blade. Identify the big bubble in the pre-Descemet's space. If unsure, consider repeat air injection through a different site. This may be preceded by hydration of the posterior stroma by injecting balanced saline solution to increase the thickness of the residual stromal base, thus decreasing the risk of perforation with the repeat insertion of the needle or cannula for injection of air. (Drawing (a) by and courtesy of Eric J. Fleischer, MD.)

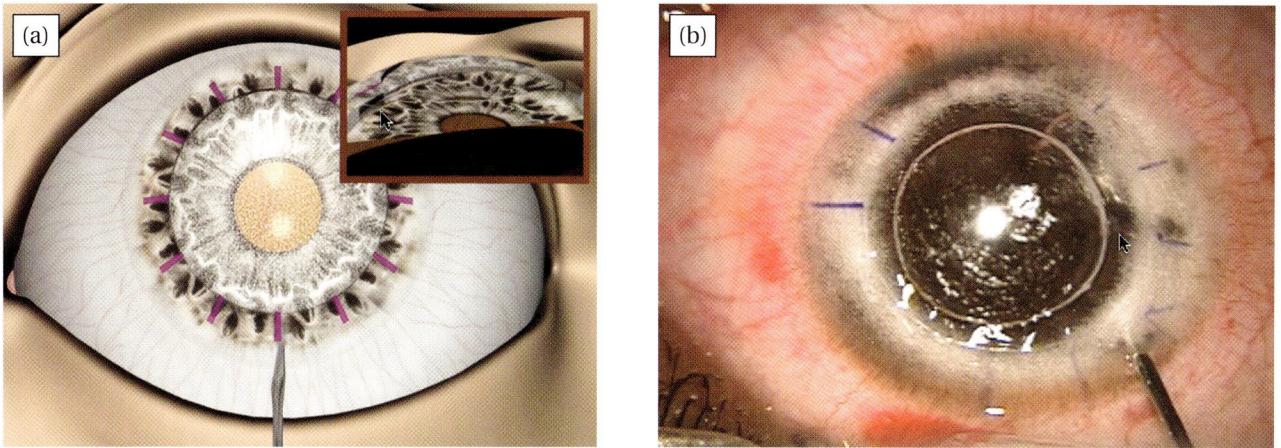

FIGURE 23.5 Placement of a paracentesis into the anterior chamber to decompress the eye, allowing Descemet's membrane to move posteriorly toward the iris. When performing the paracentesis, enter the chamber vertically toward the iris—not horizontally, as is the custom during cataract surgery, since horizontal entry may inadvertently lacerate Descemet's membrane, and prematurely collapse the big bubble, creating unnecessary communication between the pre-Descemet's space and the anterior chamber. Place one or more small air bubbles in the anterior chamber. In the presence of a big bubble in the pre-Descemet's space, these small bubbles will be pushed peripherally in the AC. In the absence of the successful creation of the big bubble, the small bubbles in the anterior chamber will ascend and move centrally (arrow). Also, when the big bubble is entered with a knife in the next step (Fig. 23.6), the small bubble in the anterior chamber will move anteriorly and centrally. (Drawing (a) by and courtesy of Eric J. Fleischer, MD.)

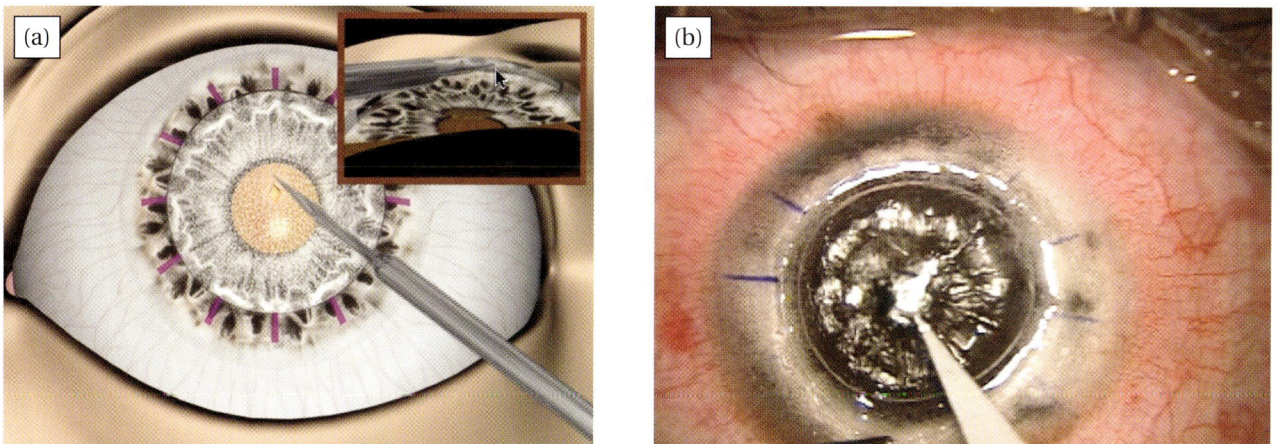

FIGURE 23.6 Entry into the big bubble with a sharp knife. This maneuver should be deliberate and swift, with the sharp side of the blade pointing up to decrease the chance of tearing Descemet's membrane when the bubble collapses and Descemet's membrane moves anteriorly. More controlled entry into the big bubble may be achieved by placing a small bead of cohesive viscoelastic on top of the corneal stroma at the site of entry to slow down the expression of air from the big bubble. (Drawing (a) by and courtesy of Eric J. Fleischer, MD.)

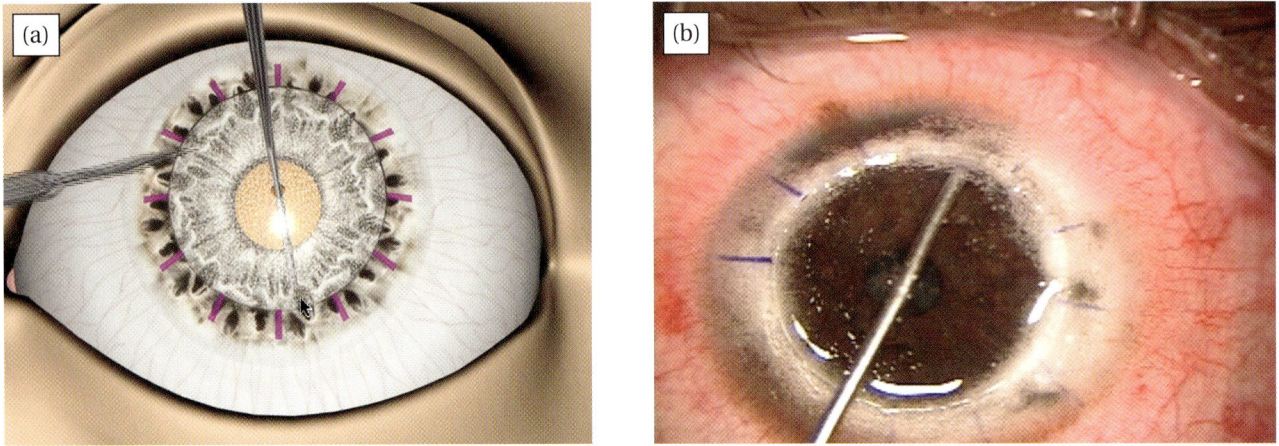

FIGURE 23.7 Placement of an instrument through the posterior stromal fenestration into the pre-Descemet space to confirm that the posterior stroma is separated from Descemet's membrane all the way to the edge of the trephination. (Drawing (a) by and courtesy of Eric J. Fleischer, MD.)

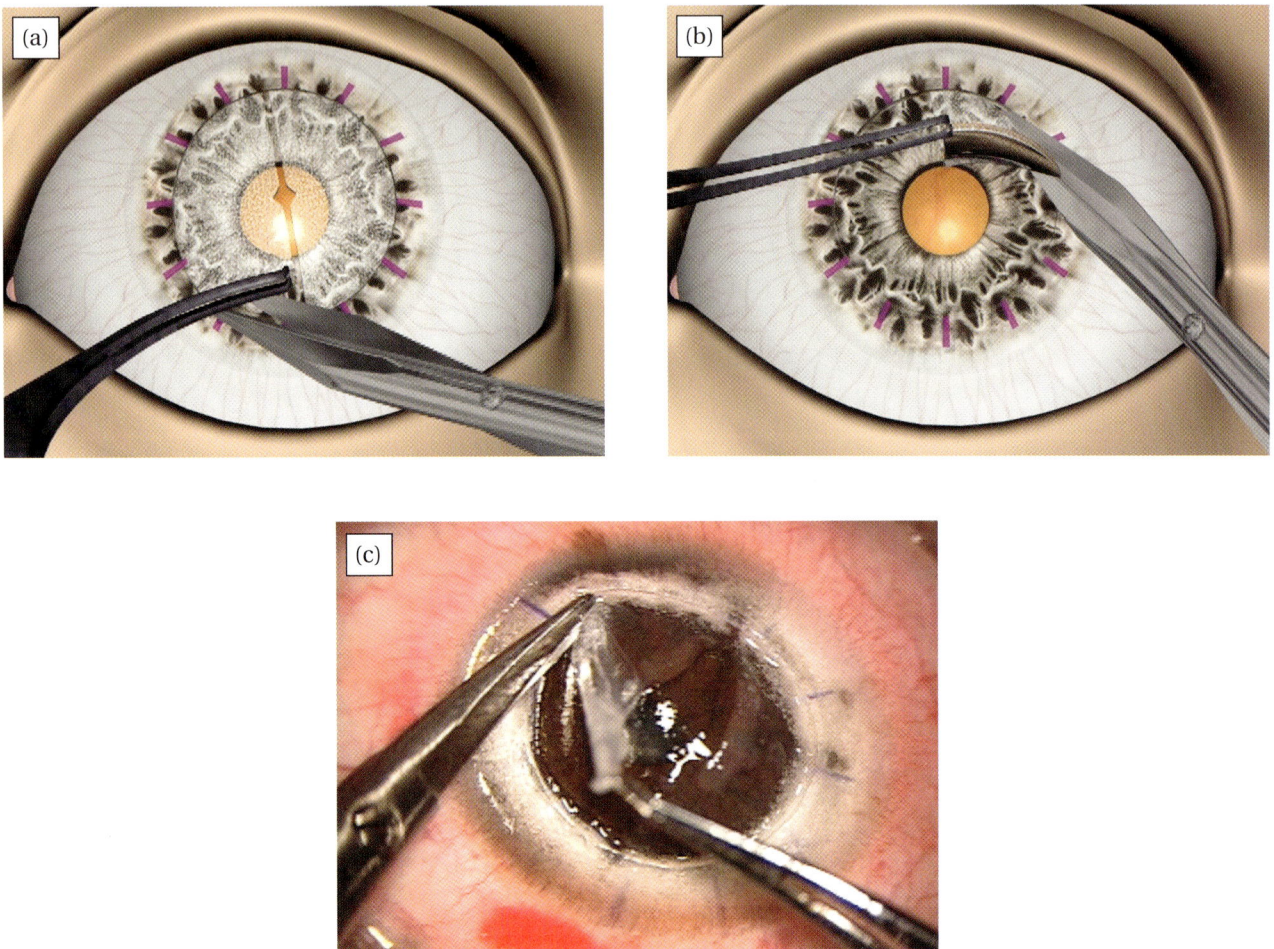

FIGURE 23.8 Creation of radial incisions in the posterior stroma, followed by excision of the posterior stromal lamellae with rounded-tip scissors. Viscodissection with a cohesive agent may be very useful here. Make sure that the posterior stroma is separated from Descemet's membrane out to the edge of the trephinatio n wound, to avoid perforating Descemet's membrane during the resection of the posterior stromal quadrants. (Drawings (a) and (b) by and courtesy of Eric J. Fleischer, MD.)

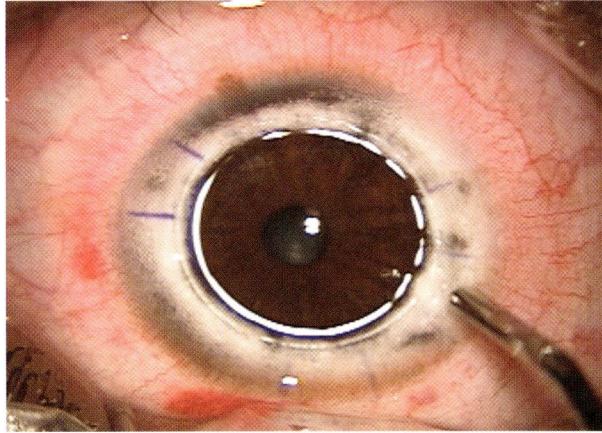

FIGURE 23.9 Irrigation of Descemet's membrane and temporary coverage with a contact lens to protect from operating room debris.

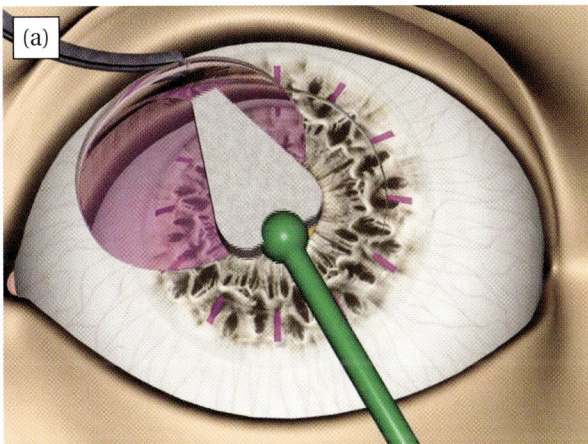

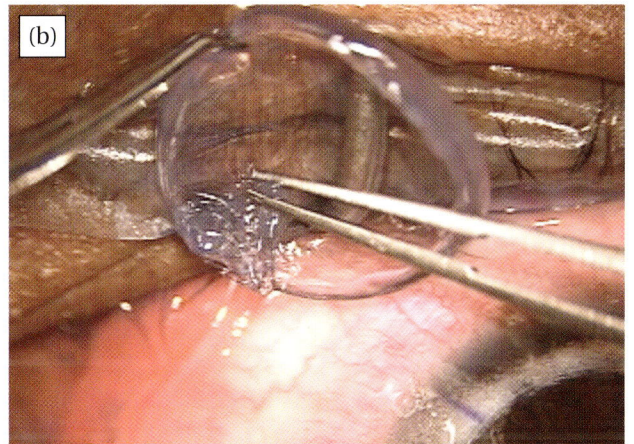

FIGURE 23.10 Preparation of donor tissue and removal of donor Descemet's membrane. Preparation of the donor tissue may be accomplished earlier during the procedure. Depending on the nature of the pathology and the trephination instrument used, a same-sized or a 0.25 mm-oversized donor may be used. If the donor tissue has healthy endothelium, the donor Descemet's membrane should not be removed until the surgeon determines that the host Descemet's membrane is intact for the purpose of lamellar transplantation. Staining the donor Descemet's membrane with trypan blue rubbing off the endothelium facilitates identifying the membrane and removing it successfully. (Drawing (a) by and courtesy of Eric J. Fleischer, MD.)

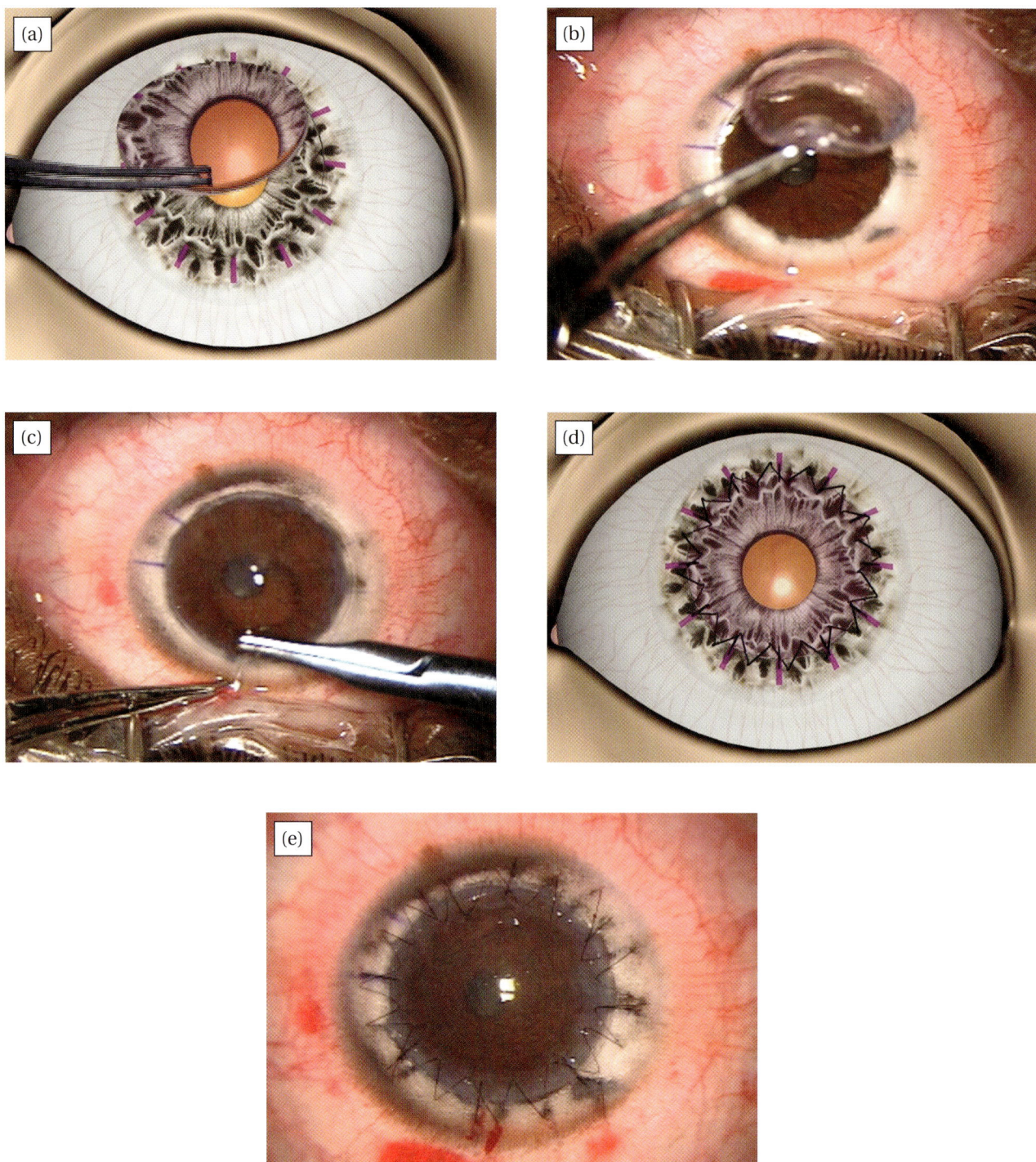

FIGURE 23.11 Suturing the donor graft onto the host Descemet's membrane using the technique of the surgeon's choice. Balanced saline solution is used to pressurize the eye. If a perforation in the host Descemet's membrane is suspected, consider leaving an air bubble in the anterior chamber for tamponade, dilating the pupil and placing the patient in a supine position for approximately one hour before examining them at the slit lamp to ensure that the host Descemet's membrane is apposed to the donor corneal stromal graft. (Drawings (a) and (d) by and courtesy of Eric J. Fleischer, MD.)

TABLE 23.3 *Complications*

A. Intraoperative

1. Problem: Full thickness trephination and perforation into the anterior chamber

   Solution: If the area of perforation is less than 2 clock hours, it may be repaired primarily with interrupted 10-0 nylon sutures, and the DALK procedure resumed using a site 180 degrees away for the injection of air. If, on the other hand, a large perforation results from the initial trephination, the procedure may be converted to a full thickness corneal transplant.

2. Problem: Incomplete resection of the host stroma leaving a thin layer of stroma over Descemet's membrane.

   Solution: Although this is not ideal to create the optically clearest interface, it is indeed the way deep lamellar keratoplasty has been performed for the past 50 years. The procedure may be completed in the same fashion.

3. Problem: Laceration in Descemet's membrane during entry into the big bubble or removal of the posterior stroma.

   Solution: If the laceration is small, the procedure may be completed in the same fashion and an air bubble placed in the anterior chamber for tamponade. If the laceration is large, conversion to a full thickness graft may be considered.

B. Postoperative

1. Problem: Double anterior chamber, which is usually due to an unrecognized perforation of Descemet's membrane resulting in communication between the anterior chamber and pre-Descemet's space.

   Solution: At the slit lamp, an air bubble is placed into the anterior chamber followed by draining the interface, instilling a cycloplegic drug, and positioning the patient appropriately to tamponade the area of separation of Descemet's membrane.

   Draining the interface fluid through the graft-host junction is an important step in allowing the native Descemet's membrane move forward and appose itself to the donor stromal graft tissue.

SELECTED REFERENCES

Anwar M, Teichmann KD. Big Bubble technique to bare Descemet's membrane in anterior lamellar keratoplasty. *J Cataract Refract Surg.* 2002;28:398–403.

Anwar M, Teichmann KD. Deep lamellar keratoplasty. Surgical techniques for anterior lamellar keratoplasty with and without baring of Descemet's membrane. *Cornea.* 2002;21:374–383.

Fontana L, Parente G, Tassinari G. Clinical outcomes after deep anterior lamellar keratoplasty using the Big-bubble technique in patients with keratoconus. *Am J Ophthalmol.* 2007;143:117–124.

Sarnicola V, Toro P, Gentile D, Hannush SB. Descemetic DALK and Predescemetic DALK: Outcomes in 236 Cases of Keratoconus. *Cornea.* 2010;29:53–59.

TABLE 24.1 *Indications for Descemet's Stripping Automated Endothelial Keratoplasty (DSAEK)*

Any condition of endothelial failure without significant stromal scarring:

Fuchs' endothelial dystrophy

Psuedophakic bullous keratopathy

Failed prior penetrating keratoplasty

Endothelial failure from trauma (surgical or environmental)

Endothelial failure from inflammation

Irido-Corneal Endothelial (ICE) syndrome

Posterior polymorphous dystrophy

Congenital hereditary endothelial dystrophy (CHED)

Preoperative Condition

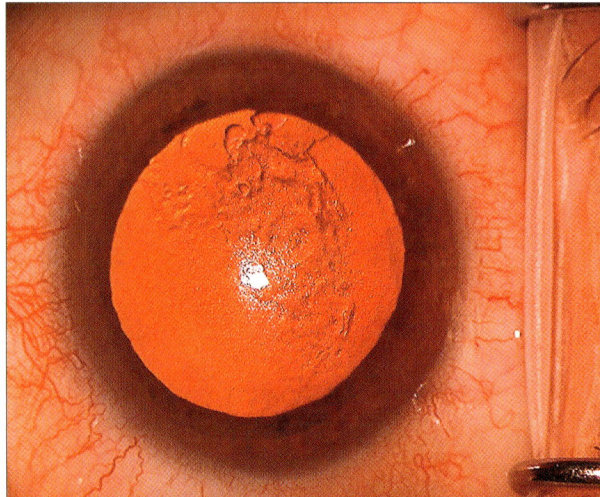

FIGURE 24.1 Patient with corneal edema and guttata from Fuchs' endothelial dystrophy.

Recipient Bed Preparation for DSAEK

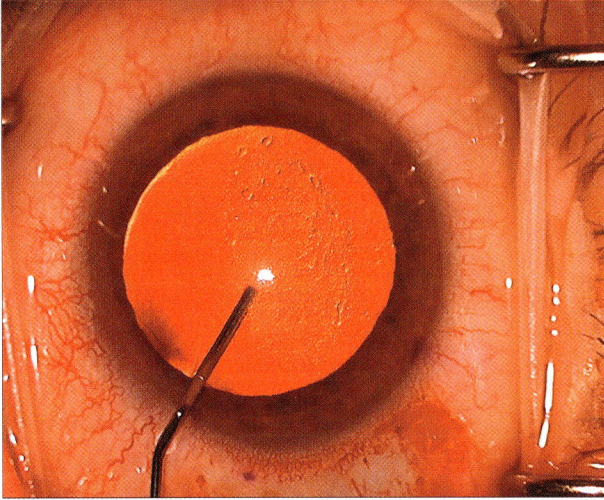

FIGURE 24.2 A temporal approach is commonly utilized, and a scleral access incision provides a stronger wound with less astigmatic shift than a clear corneal access incision. After a conjunctival peritomy, the scleral incision length is marked, two limbal clear corneal 1 mm stab incisions are made, and the anterior chamber is filled with a highly cohesive viscoelastic.

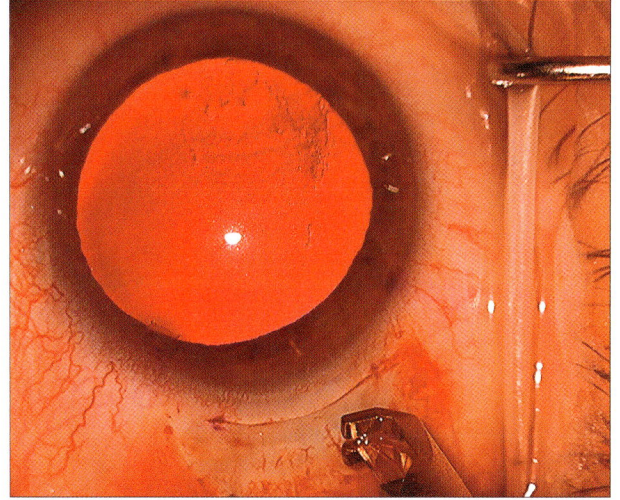

FIGURE 24.3 The 5 mm scleral incision at a depth of about 350 microns is made with a diamond knife or crescent blade, approximately 0.5–1 mm peripheral and concentric with the limbus. Incisions smaller than 5 mm cause significantly higher compression and endothelial cell damage to the donor tissue during insertion.

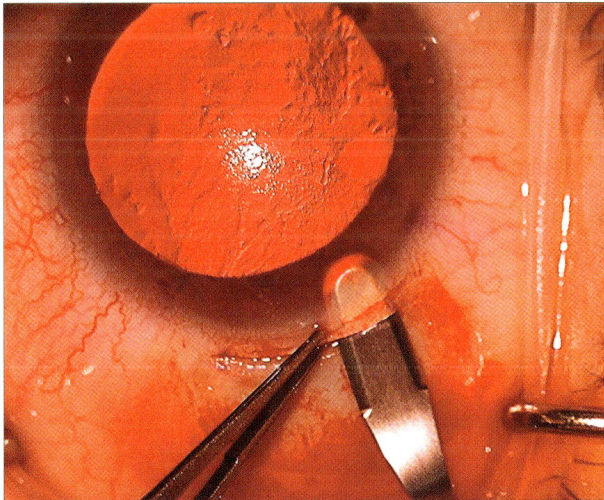

FIGURE 24.4 A scleral-corneal pocket dissection is created with a crescent blade, approximately 2 mm into clear corneal stroma along the entire length of the 5 mm access incision. This beveled wound is self-sealing to air or fluid.

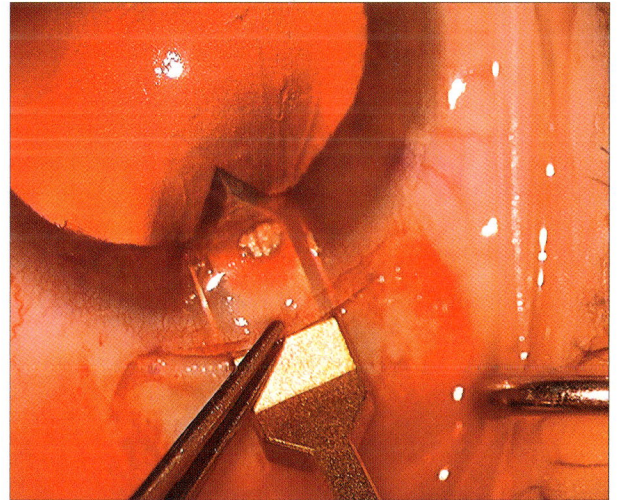

FIGURE 24.5 The anterior chamber is entered with a 2.8 mm diamond or metal keratome, allowing cataract surgery or other intraocular procedures.

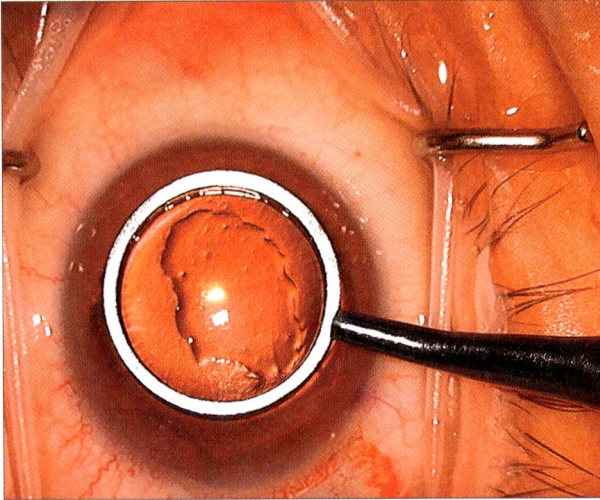

FIGURE 24.6 The surface of the cornea is marked with a circular marker of 8.0–9.0 mm diameter to act as a template for the Descemet's stripping. The largest diameter possible for a given recipient corneal size is chosen, but care is taken to insure that the mark does not overlap the internal opening of the paracentesis sites or the main pocket wound. The epithelial mark is accentuated with ink dots from a marking pen. As shown here, the central epithelial bullous tissue can also be scraped off to improve visualization of the anterior chamber.

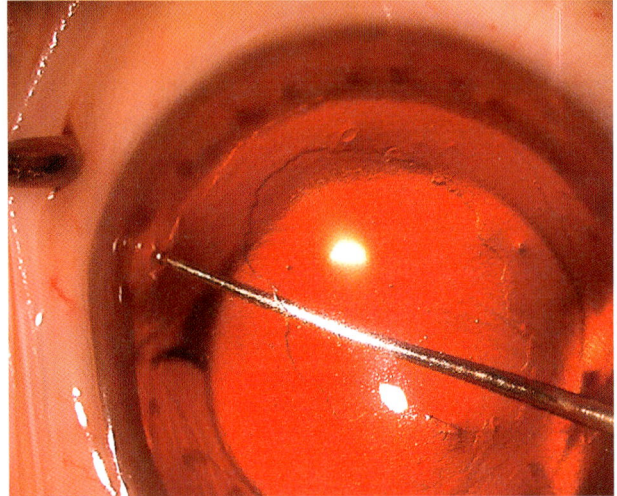

FIGURE 24.7 With Healon stabilizing the chamber, a blunt, reverse Terry-Sinskey hook is used through a paracentesis site to first break through Descemet's membrane and then score Descemet's membrane for 360°, with the scoring made just central to the overlying template circle (e.g., scoring a 7.8 mm circle under an 8.0 mm template).

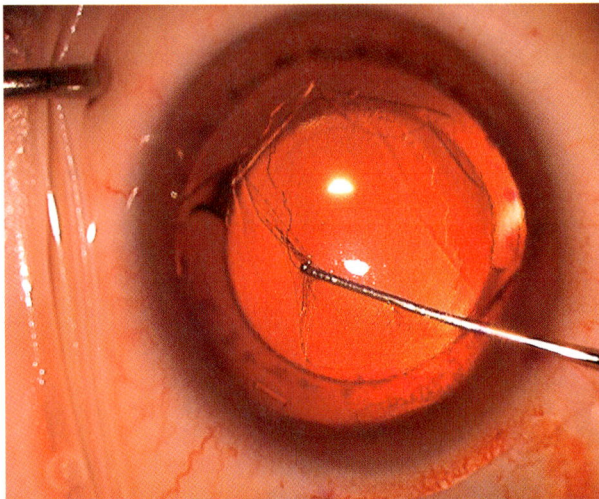

FIGURE 24.8 The same Terry-Sinskey hook is used to strip Descemet's membrane by pulling from the peripheral score to the central area in each quadrant, detaching Descemet's in one piece. The recipient Descemet's membrane is removed from the eye.

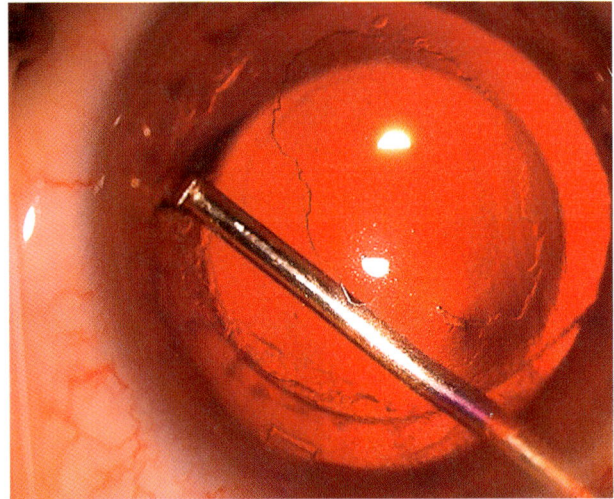

FIGURE 24.9 The Terry Scraper is used to scrape the peripheral recipient bed, creating a 1 mm broad ring of white stromal fibers, which are easily seen against a dilated pupil red reflex. Scraping should be thorough, and the band of scraped white stromal fibers is not subtle.

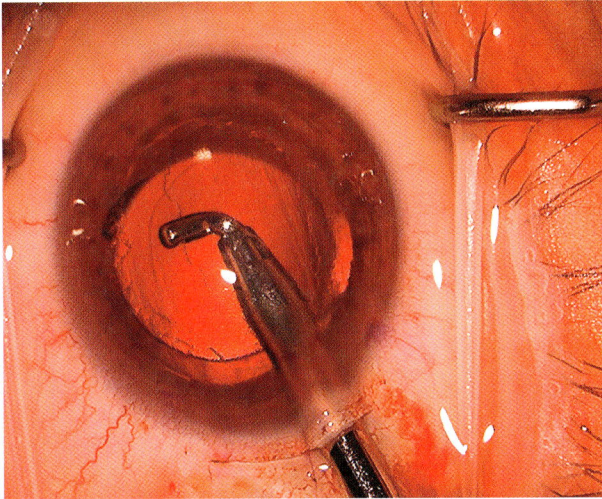

FIGURE 24.10 The main wound opening into the anterior chamber is extended with the crescent blade to the full 5.0 mm length, a temporary suture is placed, and the Healon is completely evacuated from the eye with an irrigation/aspiration tip.

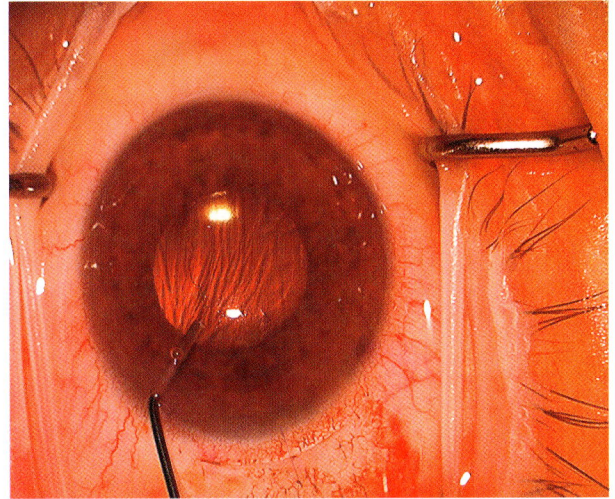

FIGURE 24.11 A short-acting miotic of acetylcholine (Miochol) is used to constrict the pupil to a size of 5 mm or less.

Donor Tissue Preparation

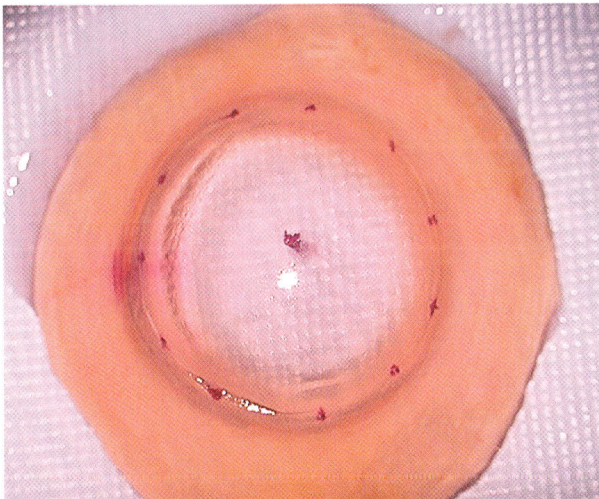

FIGURE 24.12 The microscope should be used for all donor preparation in order to avoid the disaster of an eccentric trephination. The pre-cut donor tissue is placed endothelial side down onto a lint free surface, the surface is dried, and the edges of the microkeratome cut bed are marked with a marking pen. A centering mark based upon the other marks is also placed.

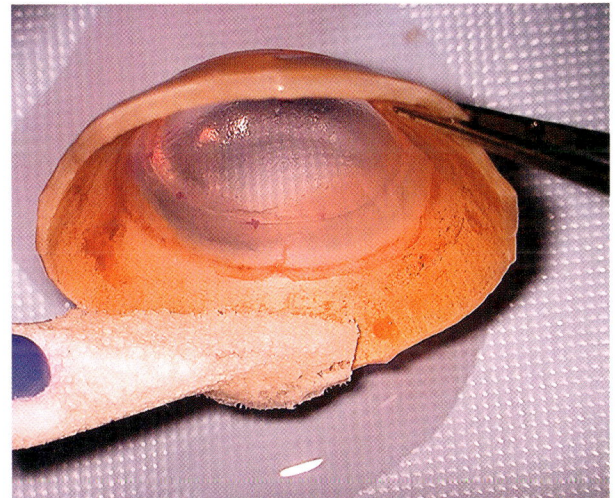

FIGURE 24.13 The donor tissue is picked up by the sclera, and the Optisol solution is wicked off from the endothelium by placing a sponge at the scleral rim.

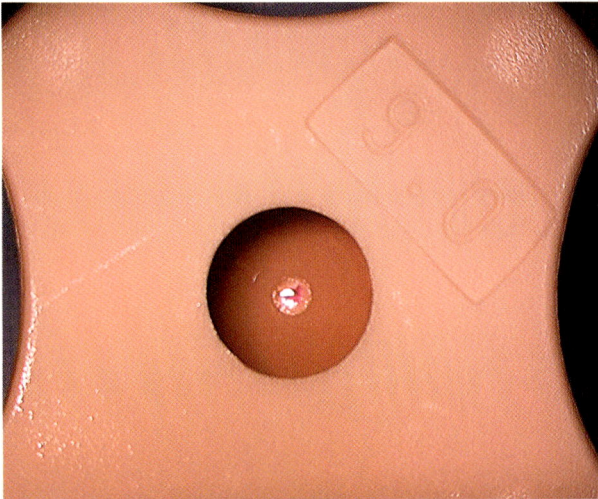

FIGURE 24.14 The donor tissue with the cap still in place is centered over the trephination block, and the donor punch trephine is placed over the tissue while the surgeon looks down the bore of the trephine to insure that no peripheral marks are visible within the trephine area.

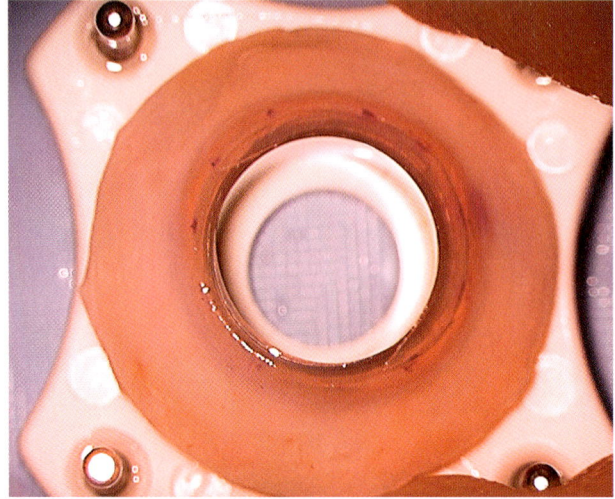

FIGURE 24.15 After trephination, the donor tissue rim is inspected to insure that there has not been an eccentric cut.

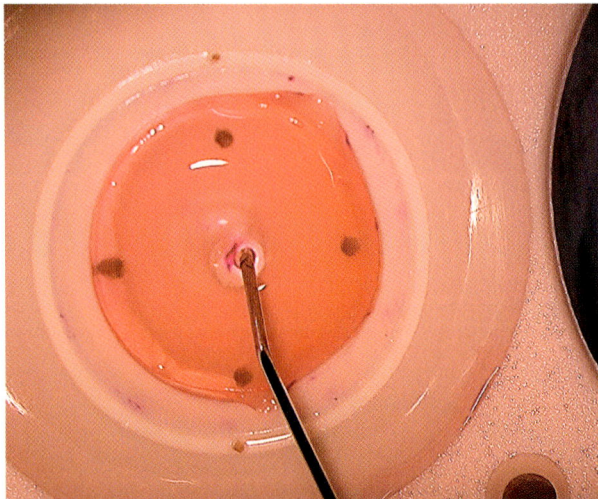

FIGURE 24.16 A thin strip of viscoelastic is placed across the endothelium, prior to folding the tissue.

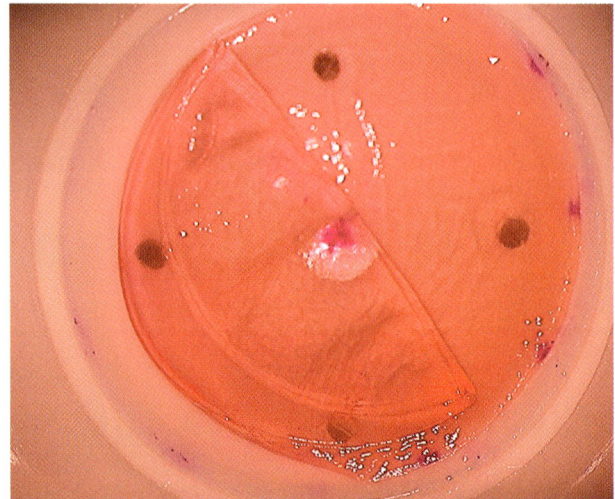

FIGURE 24.17 The relatively dry donor tissue is carefully folded into a 40%/60% "taco" shape, taking care not to stretch the tissue during folding. The donor tissue is lifted to insure separation from the cap. The entire trephine block with the tissue is brought over to the operative field.

Donor Tissue Insertion, Unfolding, and Centration

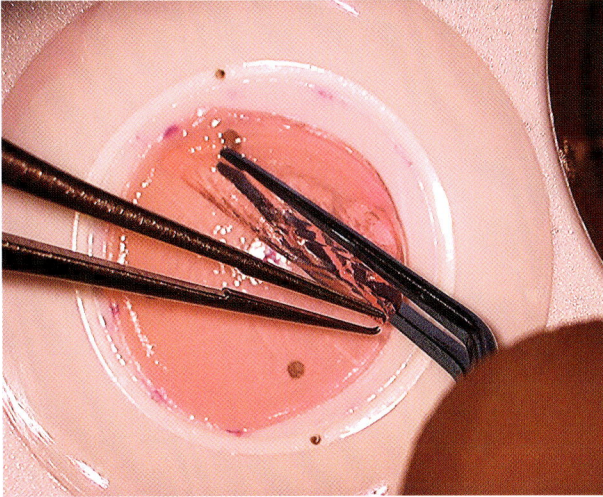

FIGURE 24.18 The "taco" donor tissue is grasped with Charlie insertion forceps (single separated grasp point, non-coapting forceps), placing the tips of the forceps as far distally on the tissue as possible.

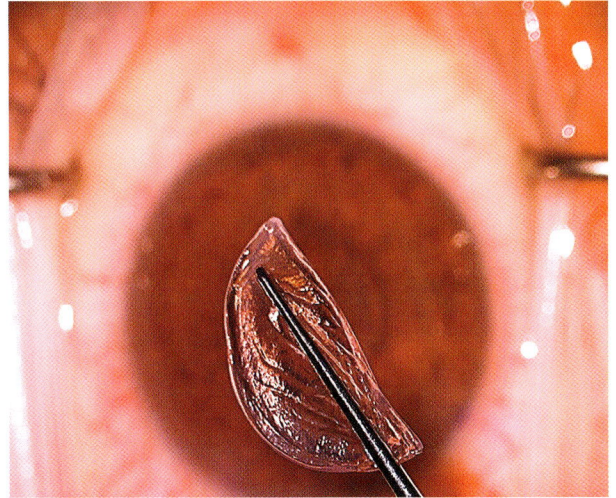

FIGURE 24.19 The surgeon rotates his hand to be absolutely sure that the 60% fold of the taco is anterior prior to insertion of the tissue.

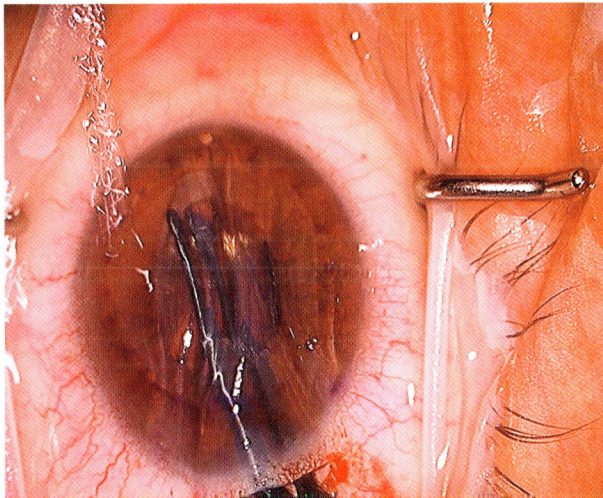

FIGURE 24.20 The tissue is quickly inserted into the anterior chamber, placing the forceps tips as far distally into the chamber as possible, and the tissue is slowly released from the forceps.

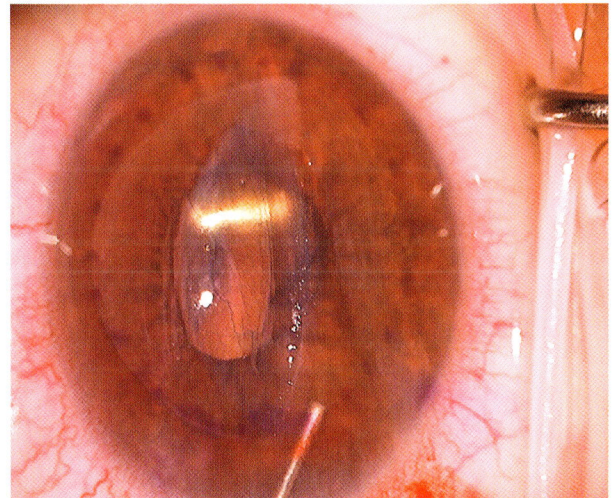

FIGURE 24.21 The tissue is positioned by nudging the proximal stromal edge of the fold with an irrigating cannula through the main wound. The goal is to line up the 60% edge of the taco with the overlying template mark.

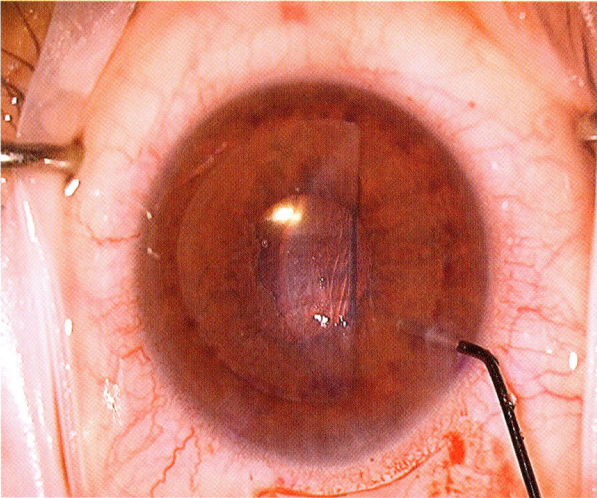

FIGURE 24.22 The anterior chamber is slowly deepened with irrigation through the paracentesis site, which lies on the stromal side of the taco donor. Deepening of the chamber allows opening and unfolding of the tissue.

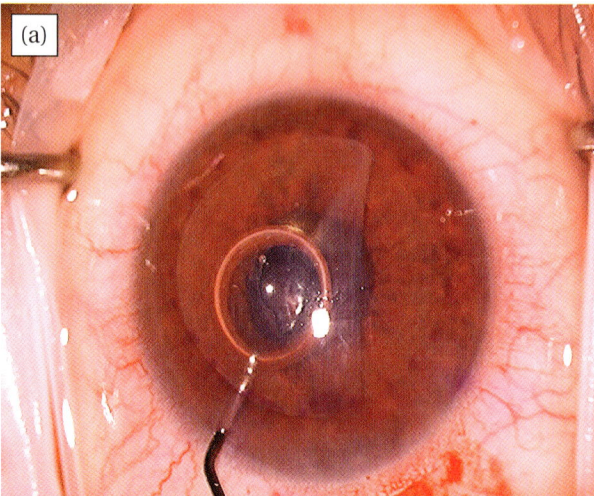

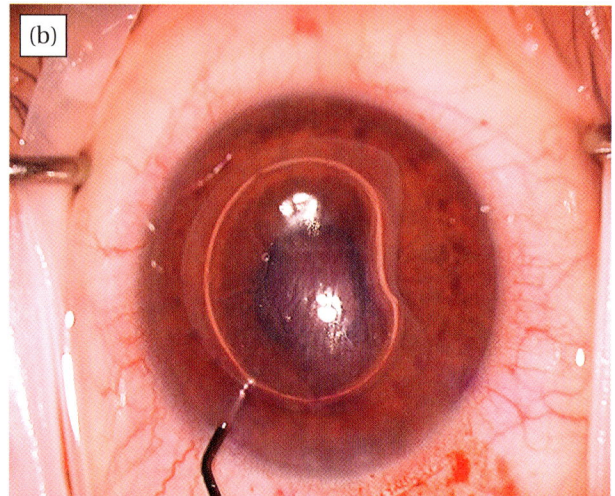

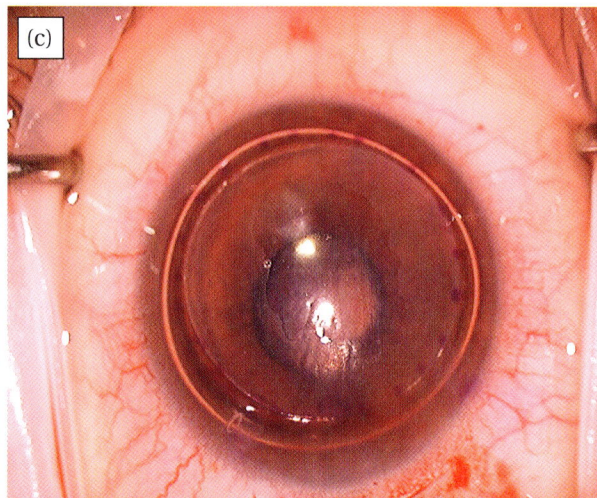

FIGURE 24.23 (a, b, c) An air bubble is VERY slowly injected through the paracentesis site, which lies on the endothelial side of the taco donor. The air bubble slowly completes the unfolding, allowing the 40% side of the taco to coapt onto the recipient bed. Slow injection of air prevents upside-down flipping of the graft.

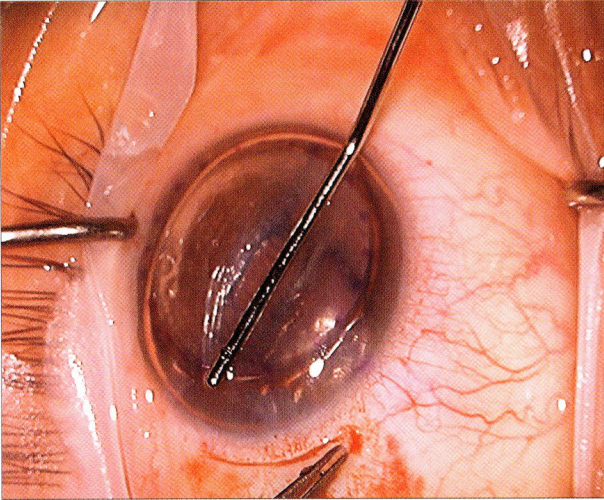

FIGURE 24.24 If the graft is not centered properly, it can be moved into proper position by sweeping the recipient cornea, with compression from limbus to limbus using a Cindy Sweeper. This is facilitated by turning the globe to face the direction that the surgeon wants to move the tissue (i.e., if the tissue is decentered to the temporal side, the eye is abducted and the Cindy Sweeper compresses the cornea from the temporal limbus to the nasal limbus, to move the tissue nasally).

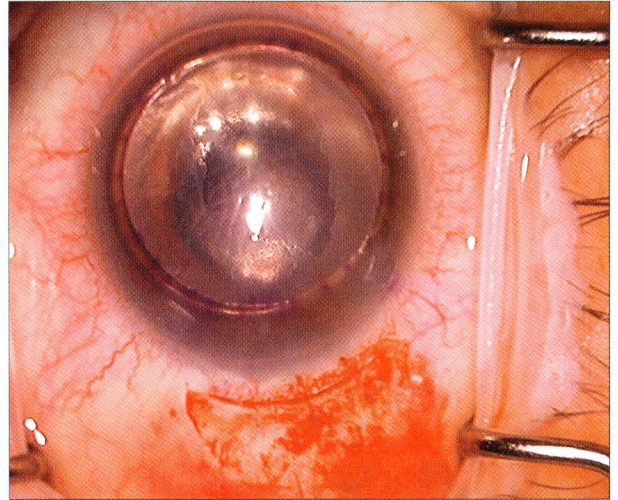

FIGURE 24.25 Once centered, the tissue is locked into position with a full air bubble and the wound is closed with three interrupted absorbable sutures.

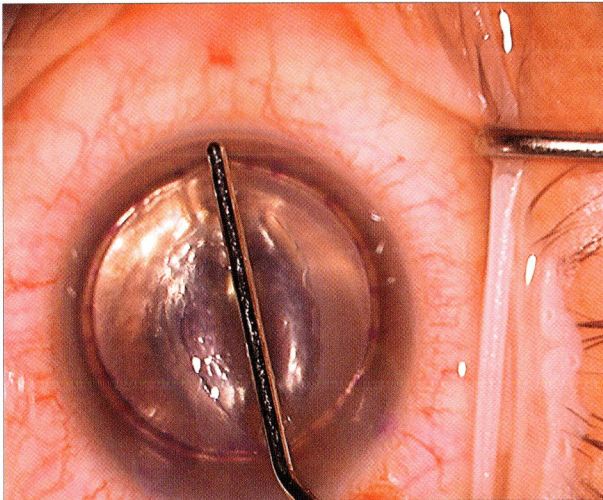

FIGURE 24.26 Interface fluid is removed by injecting more air into the anterior chamber to raise the pressure to 40 mmHg or higher, and then using the Cindy Sweeper to sweep from the central cornea to the limbus in every quadrant. Small air bubbles trapped in the interface which do not move with sweeping indicate that interface fluid has been removed.

Final Steps

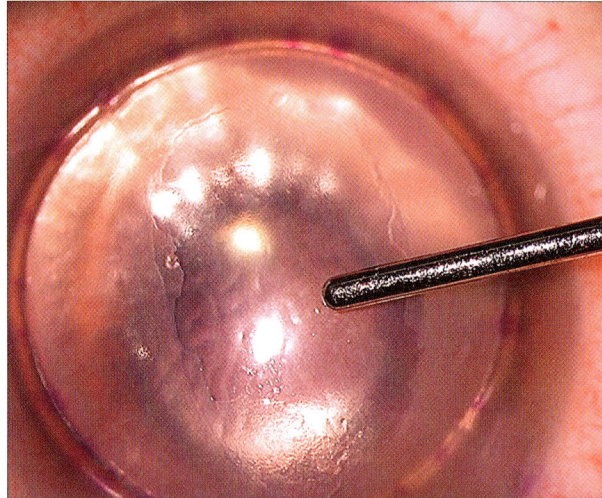

FIGURE 24.27 The ability to visualize donor edema striae, and to see the donor endothelium on high magnification, indicates that no interface fluid is present. Dilating drops are placed (1% cyclopentolate and 5% phenylephrine) to allow postoperative pupillary dilation to prevent postoperative pupillary block. The eye is left without disturbance for 10 minutes, at a normal to slightly high intraocular pressure, with the chamber completely filled with air. The conjunctival peritomy is closed with cautery during this time.

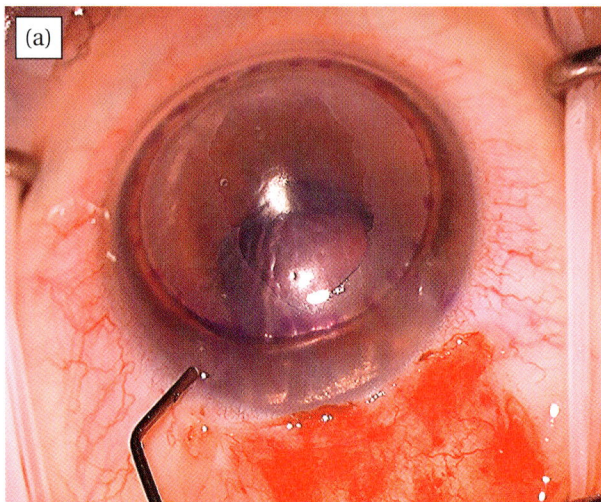

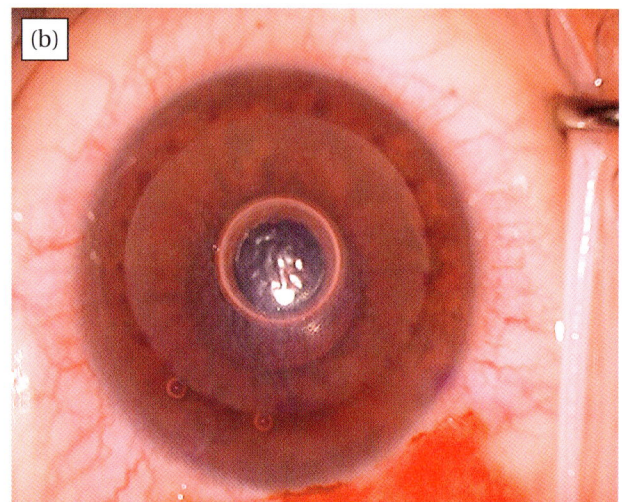

FIGURE 24.28 (a) The anterior chamber air is nearly completely removed by turning the patient's head away from the surgeon (nasally) to allow the temporal paracentesis sites to be positioned up relative to the air bubble. The BSS cannula is placed into the anterior chamber through the paracentesis site and fluid injected, allowing the air to escape through the same paracentesis. (b) All the air is evacuated to leave an air bubble that is smaller than the pupil size.

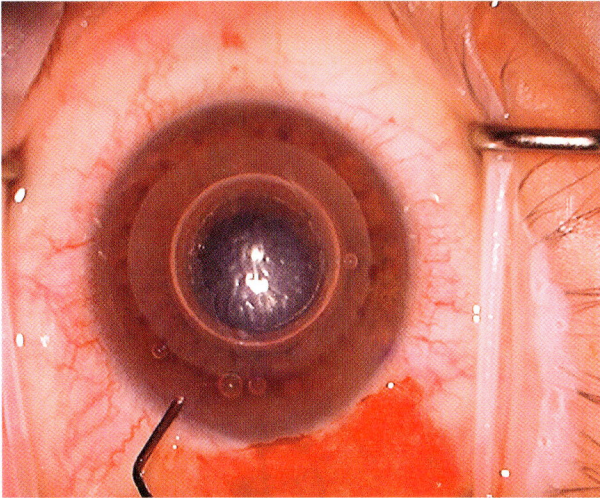

FIGURE 24.29 After the IOP is normalized with BSS, additional air is injected to leave a 5–7 mm freely movable air bubble in the anterior chamber, to support the tissue postoperatively but still prevent pupillary block.

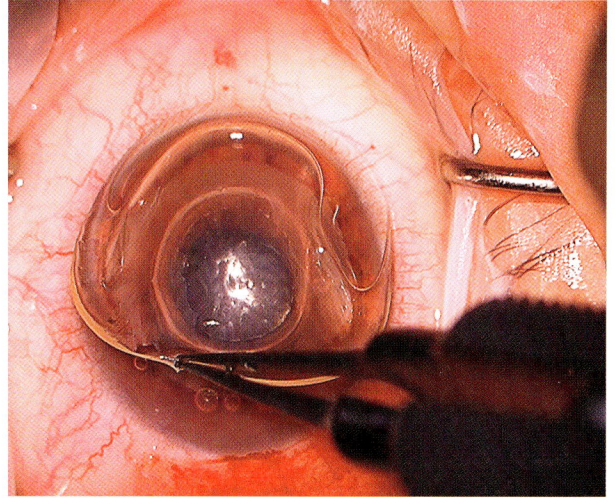

FIGURE 24.30 A collagen shield soaked in antibiotics and steroids is placed on the ocular surface, the lids closed, and a light bandage and shield, *without* pressure is taped into place and not removed until the next day. The patient is positioned supine for one hour postoperatively, and then positioned supine as much as possible until the next day.

TABLE 24.2 *Complications of Descemet's Stripping Endothelial Keratoplasty (DSAEK)*

Incidence using this DSAEK technique in first 500 consecutive cases:

Dislocation of donor tissue requiring second air bubble: 1.8%

Iatrogenic primary graft failure requiring replacement graft: 0%

Pupillary block glaucoma: 0%

Graft rejection (in first 2 years): 6%

Wound leak: 0%

Anterior irido-corneal synechiae: 0%

Epithelial ingrowth into interface or endothelial surface: 0%

Interface infections with bacteria, yeast or fungi: 0%

Upside-down grafts (i.e., endothelium anterior): 0.4%

Endophthalmitis: 0%

Supra-choroidal hemorrhage: 0%

Use of a Tissue Delivery Device in DSAEK Surgery: The NCI Device

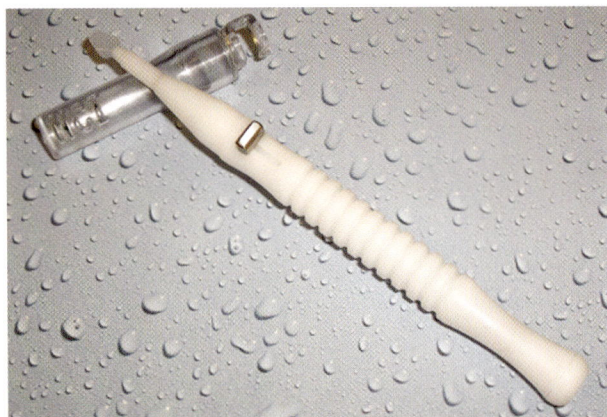

FIGURE 24.31 The Neusidl Corneal Inserter device (Fisher Instruments, St Louis, MO).

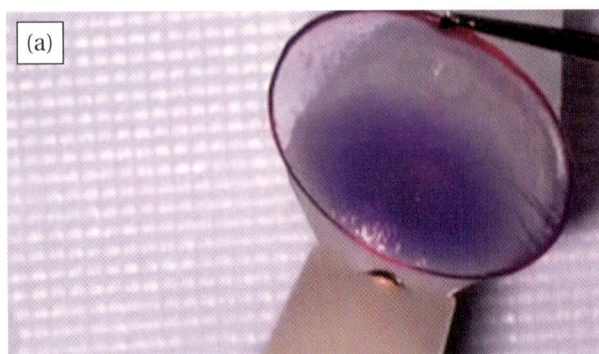

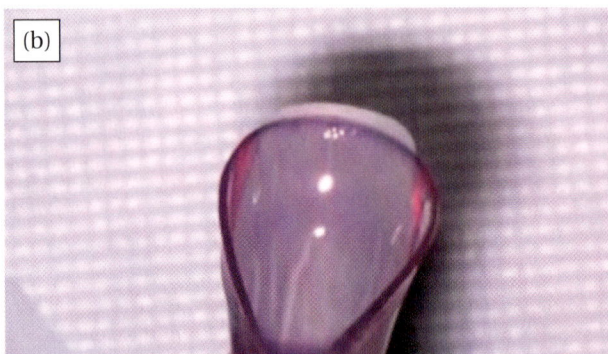

FIGURE 24.32 The trypan blue stained tissue is loaded onto the NCI platform, and the platform is slowly retracted into the tube of the NCI.

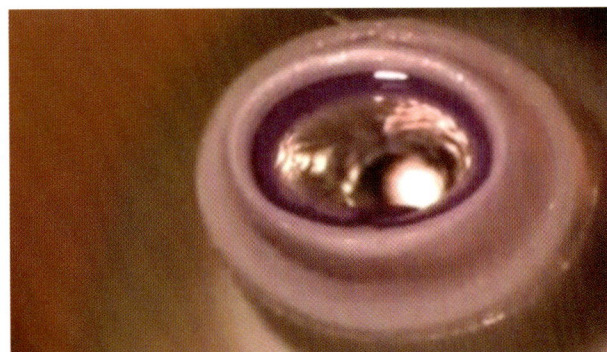

FIGURE 24.33 The tissue is seen rolled without overlap on the retracted NCI platform. Note the blue stained edge delineating the trephinated edge of the graft.

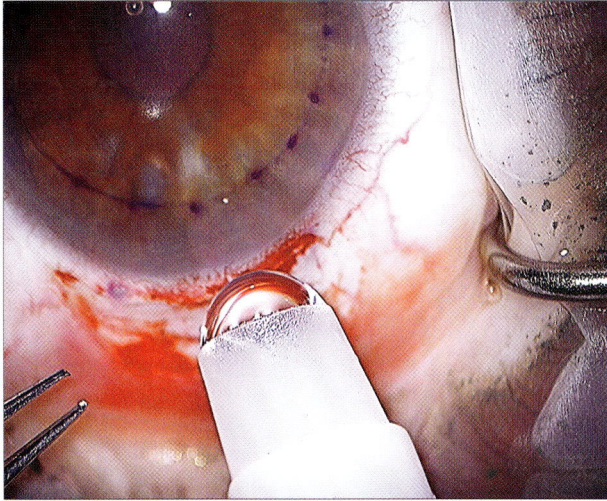

FIGURE 24.34 Low irrigation is activated prior to inserting the distal tip of the tube into the anterior chamber. Note the slow drip of BSS through the tissue on the platform.

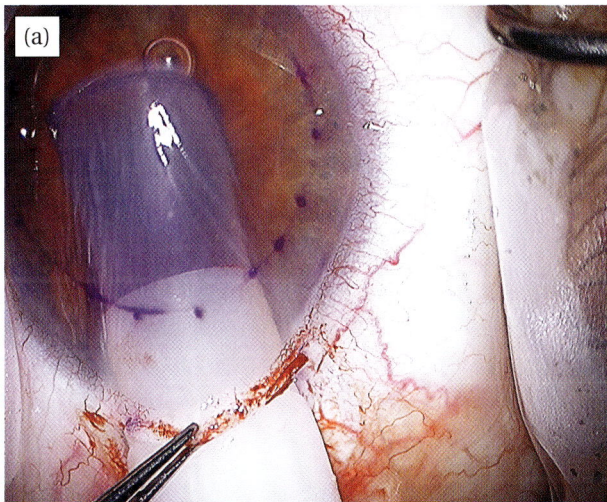

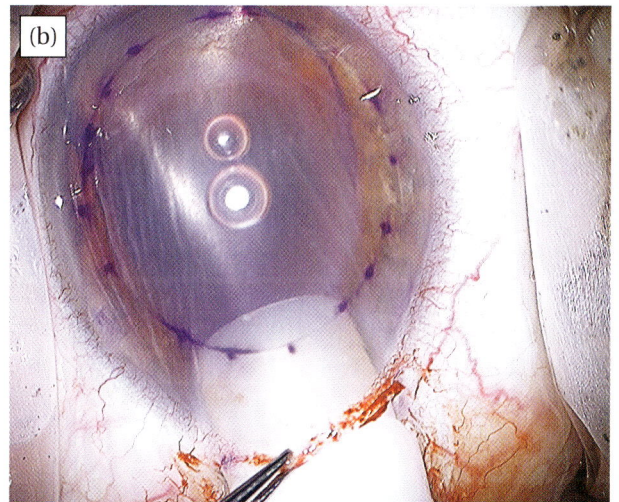

FIGURE 24.35 The platform is extended and unrolled inside the chamber, allowing the tissue to be delivered to the anterior chamber without risk of flipping upside down, and without wound compression trauma. Blue edge of graft seen peripheral to the edge of oval platform.

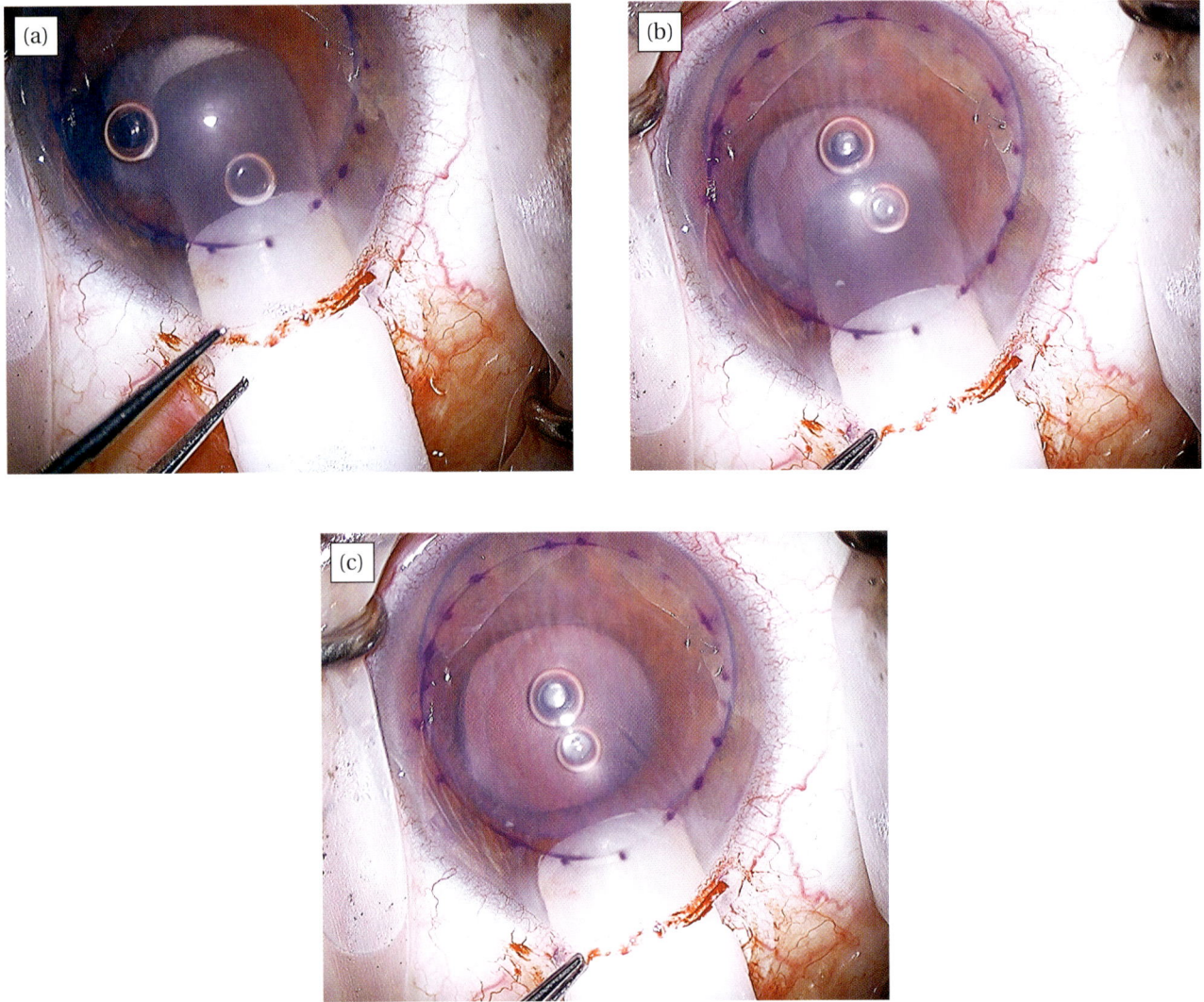

FIGURE 24.36 The platform is slowly retracted back into the tube, allowing the tissue to float off into the anterior chamber, and the distal tube tip is removed from the eye. Blue edge of graft easily seen in anterior chamber as platform fully retracted.

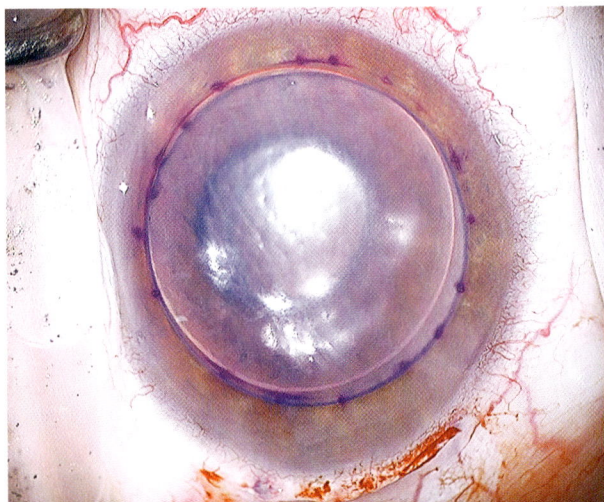

FIGURE 24.37 An air bubble is injected beneath the tissue, securing it into position onto the recipient bed. All further steps of surgery such as interface fluid removal and air bubble management—are the same as in traditional DSAEK techniques.

SELECTED REFERENCES

Terry MA. Endothelial Keratoplasty (EK): History, Current State, and Future Directions. *Cornea.* 2006 (Editorial);25:873–878.

Terry MA, Shamie N, Chen ES, Hoar KL, Friend DF. Endothelial Keratoplasty: A simplified technique to minimize graft dislocation, iatrogenic graft failure and pupillary block. *Ophthalmology.* 2008;115:1179–1186.

Terry MA, Shamie N, Chen ES, Phillips PM, Shah AK, Hoar KL, Friend DJ. Endothelial keratoplasty for Fuchs' dystrophy with cataract: Complications and clinical results with the new Triple Procedure. *Ophthalmology.* 2009;116:631–639.

Price FW, Price MO. Descemet's stripping with endothelial keratoplasty: Comparative outcomes with microkeratome-dissected and manually dissected donor tissue. *Ophthalmology.* 2006;113:1936–1942.

Terry MA. Endothelial keratoplasty: Clinical outcomes in the two years following deep lamellar endothelial keratoplasty (an American Ophthalmological Society thesis). *Trans Am Ophthalmol Soc.* 2007;105:530–563.

25

Boston Keratoprosthesis

Tasha Y. Tanhehco, MD and Kathryn A. Colby, MD, PhD

TABLE 25.1 *Indications for Boston Keratoprosthesis (in order of frequency)*

Corneal graft failure
Chemical injury with corneal scarring*
Aphakic or pseudophakic bullous keratopathy
Herpes simplex virus keratitis
Neurotrophic keratopathy
Corneal dystrophy
Ocular cicatricial pemphigoid*
Stevens-Johnson syndrome*
Corneal scarring
Congenital corneal opacity
Boston keratoprosthesis malfunction
Limbal stem cell deficiency
Corneal neovascularization

* The Boston Keratoprosthesis Type II is used for these conditions in cases with severe dry eye.

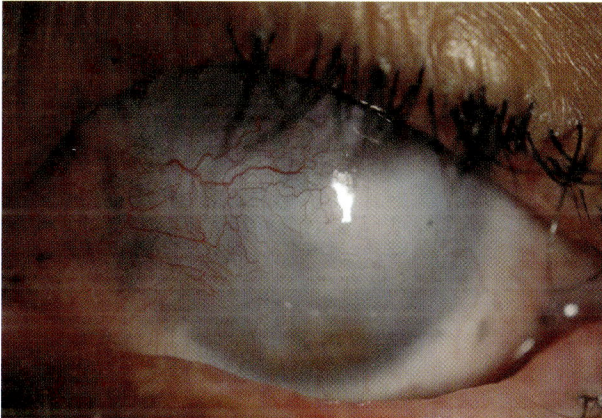

FIGURE 25.1 A bomb explosion resulted in corneal opacification and neovascularization in this patient's left eye. The tear film, blink rate, and eyelid anatomy are adequate for placement of a Boston Keratoprosthesis Type I.

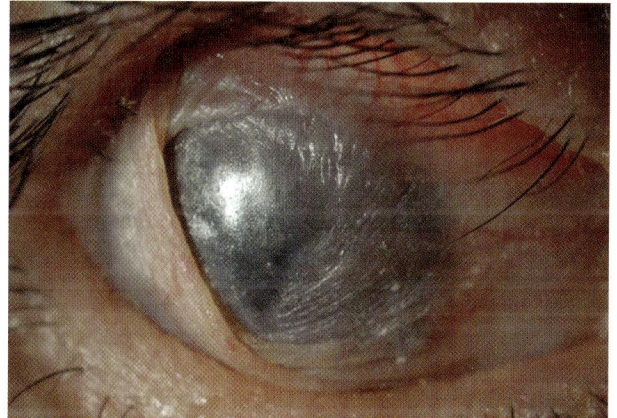

FIGURE 25.2 This patient has a history of Stevens-Johnson syndrome with onset 14 years ago. Severe dry eye, poor tear production, and decreased blink rate all led to keratinization of the ocular surface. This patient is a candidate for the Boston Keratoprosthesis Type II.

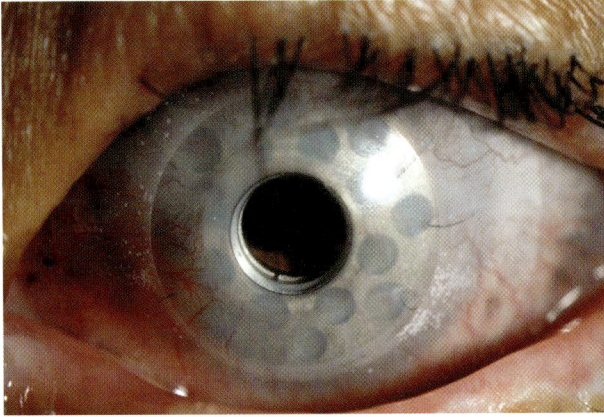

FIGURE 25.3 Picture of eye in Figure 25.1 after placement of the Boston Keratoprosthesis Type I with well-positioned bandage contact lens.

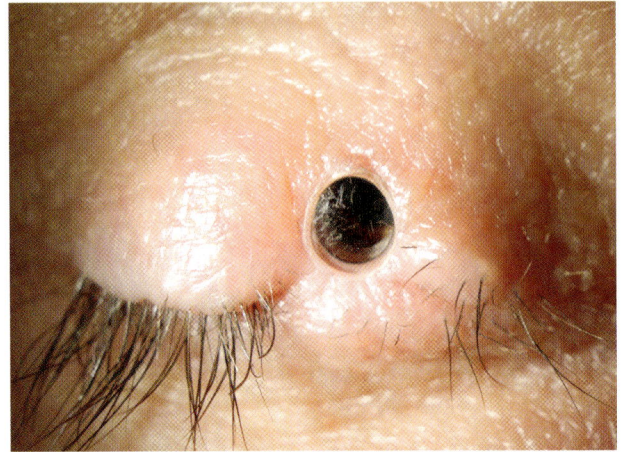

FIGURE 25.4 The same eye from Figure 25.2 after placement of the Boston Keratoprosthesis Type II. Best corrected visual acuity is 20/400 and is limited by mixed mechanism glaucoma.

Boston Keratoprosthesis Type I

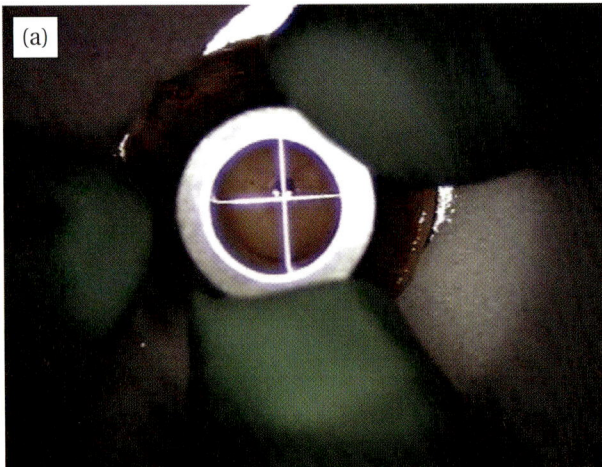

FIGURE 25.5 The donor cornea is trephined on the corneal cutting block. It is oversized by 0.5 mm compared with the recipient bed.

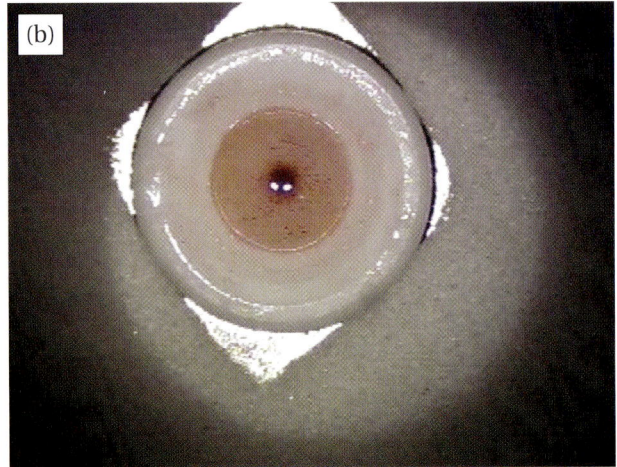

FIGURE 25.6 A dermatologic punch is used to make a 3 mm central trephination in the donor button.

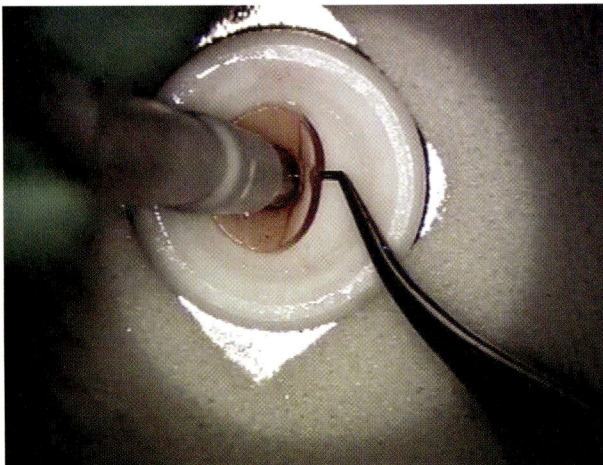

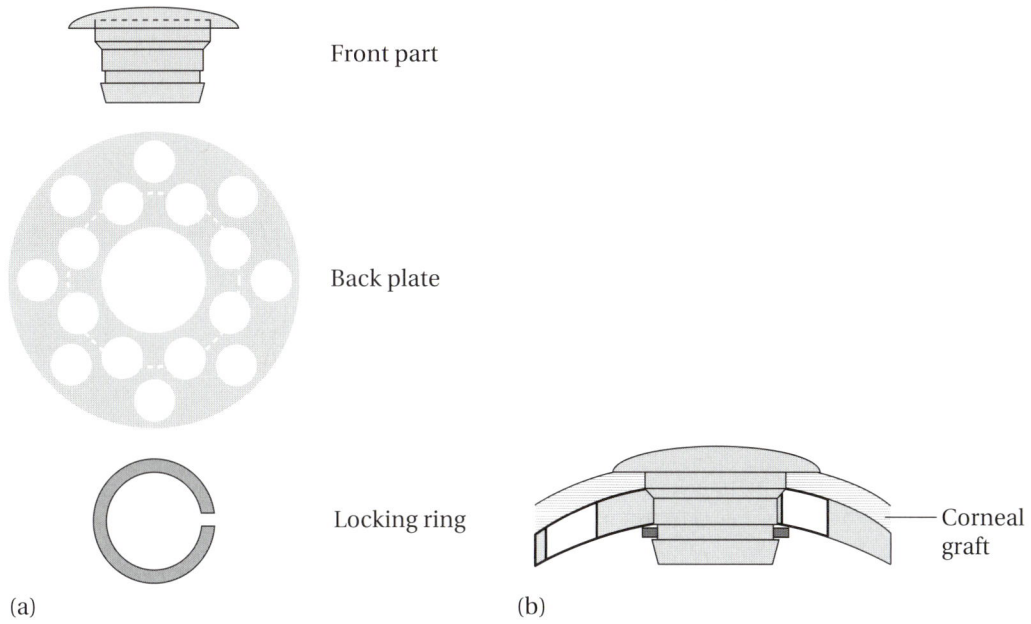

Front part

Back plate

Locking ring

Corneal graft

(a)   (b)

FIGURE 25.7 Attention is then turned to the Boston Keratoprosthesis Type I assembly kit, which includes a front plate, back plate, titanium locking ring, and adhesive stickers. The optical power of the keratoprosthesis is chosen based on the axial length and whether the patient is phakic or pseudophakic. (a) Boston Keratoprosthesis Type I components. (b) Schematic of assembly of the Boston Keratoprosthesis Type I.

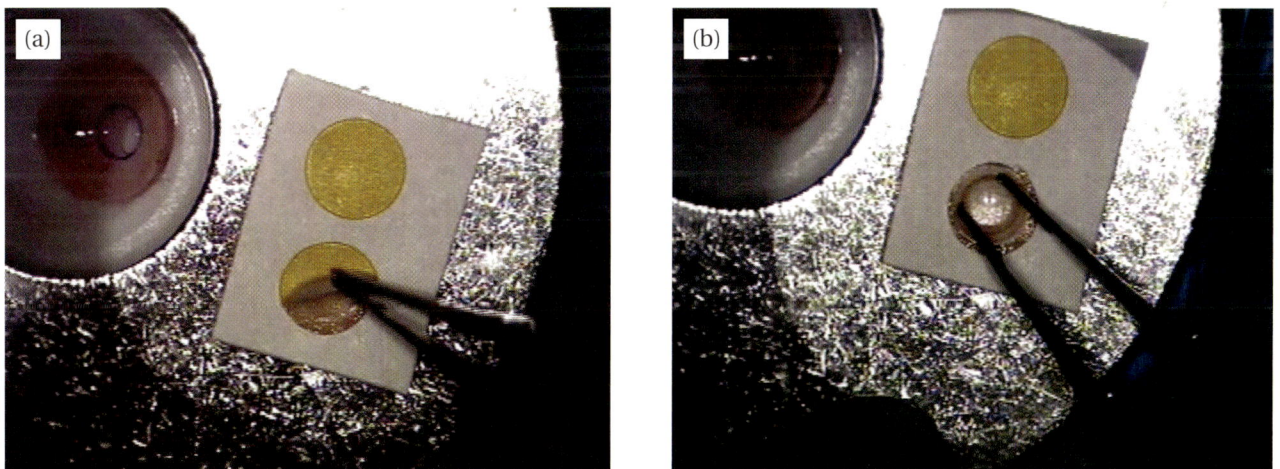

FIGURE 25.8 The keratoprosthesis is assembled on an adhesive sticker for stability. The front plate is placed front side down on the sticker.

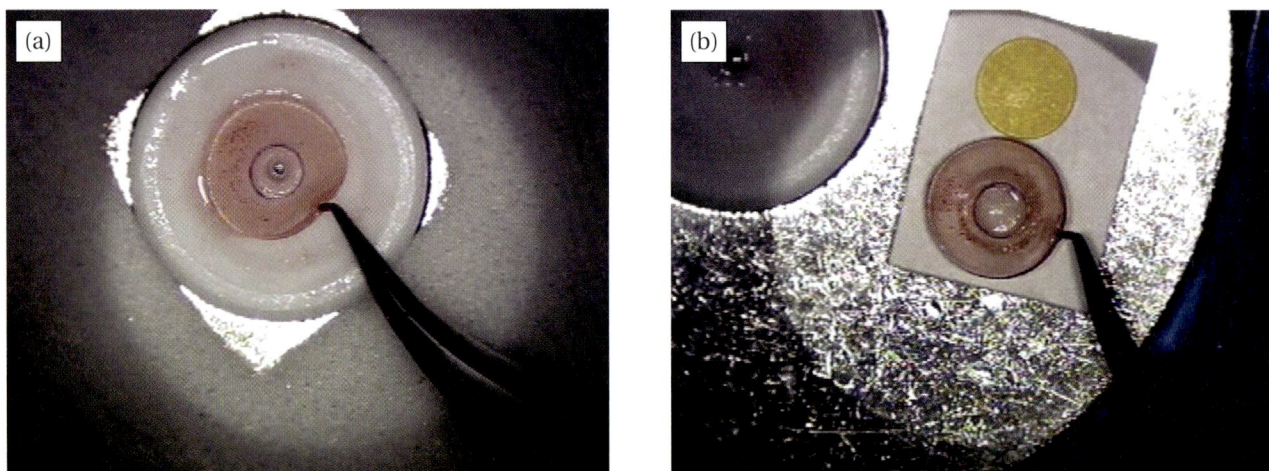

FIGURE 25.9 After viscoelastic is applied to the stem, the corneal graft (a) is slid over the keratoprosthesis stem and gently positioned with forceps (b). Additional viscoelastic is applied to the endothelial surface of the graft.

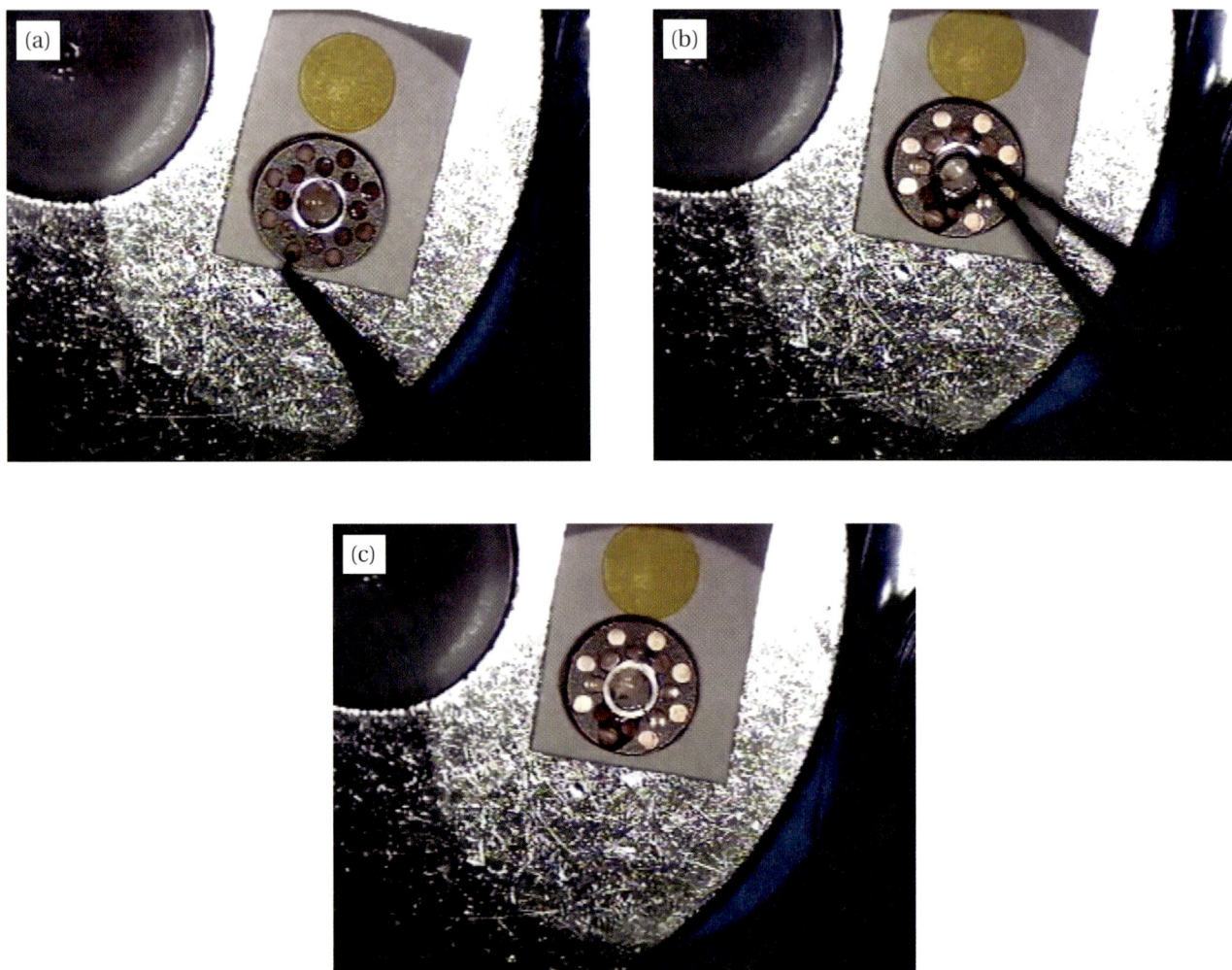

FIGURE 25.10 The back plate (in this case the back plate is made of titanium) is placed over the optic stem and the corneal graft (a), followed by the titanium locking ring (b). The locking ring is pressed down firmly into a groove within the stem with a spanner wrench until an audible snap is heard. Correctly assembled Keratoprosthesis (c).

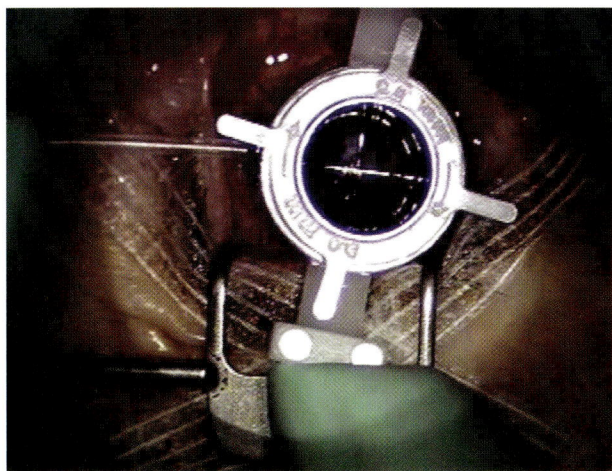

FIGURE 25.11 The host cornea is excised using traditional penetrating keratoplasty techniques. See Chapter 22 for this description.

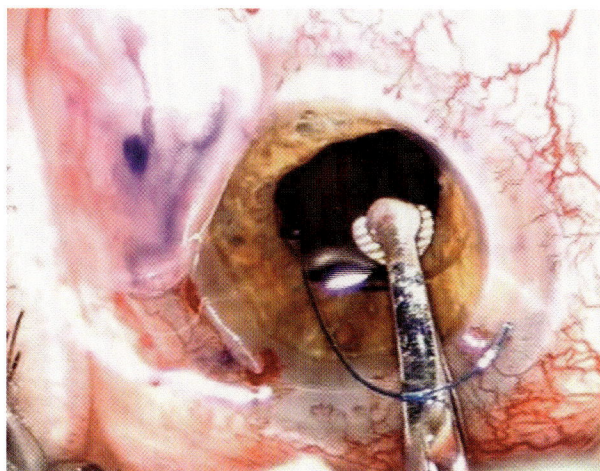

FIGURE 25.12 In aphakic patients, anterior vitrectomy is performed if necessary. Pseudophakic patients usually retain their preexisting intraocular lenses, if the lens is stable. If the patient is phakic, the lens is removed. Several options exist: a plano intraocular lens may be used in combination with an aphakic keratoprosthesis, a powered lens may be placed with a pseudophakic keratoprosthesis, or the patient can be left aphakic and an aphakic keratoprosthesis inserted. Our preference is to insert a plano lens with an aphakic keratoprosthesis, because this combination preserves ocular anatomic relationships and keeps the vitreous in the posterior chamber, an important consideration in cases where glaucoma drainage devices are considered.

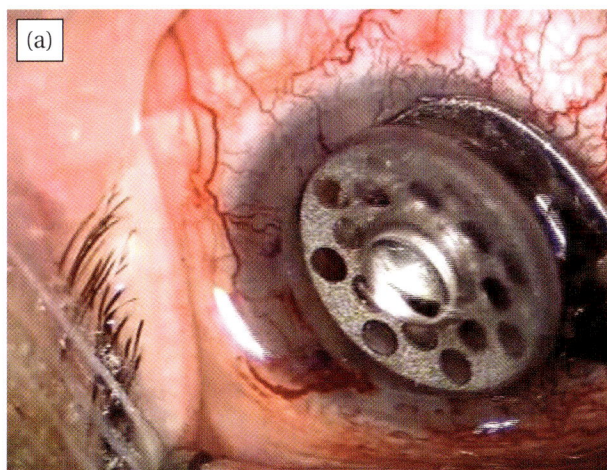

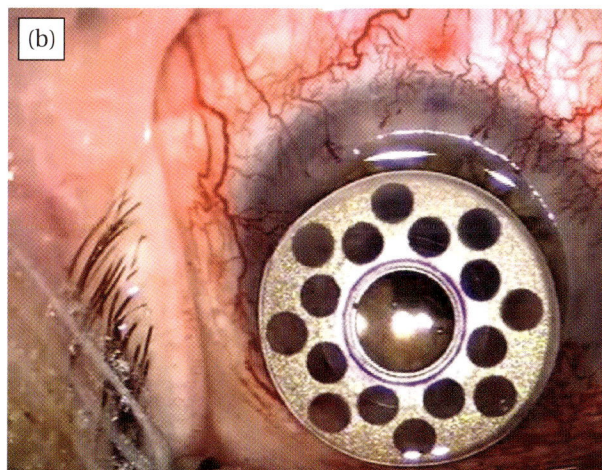

FIGURE 25.13 (a) The keratoprosthesis is positioned over the trephined host cornea, shown here with the titanium back plate facing away from the eye. (b) This is the correct orientation of the keratoprosthesis, with the donor cornea rim and front plate oriented face-up to allow suturing of the donor cornea to the host cornea.

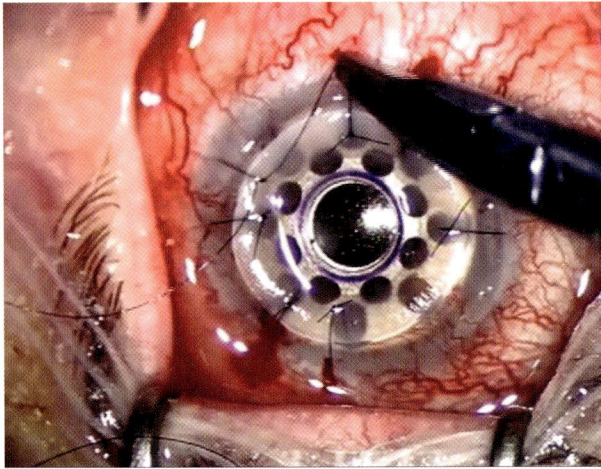

FIGURE 25.14 Interrupted 9-0 nylon sutures secure the donor cornea to the host cornea using the standard technique of traditional penetrating keratoplasty, starting with 4 cardinal sutures. Usually 12 sutures are sufficient to close the wound.

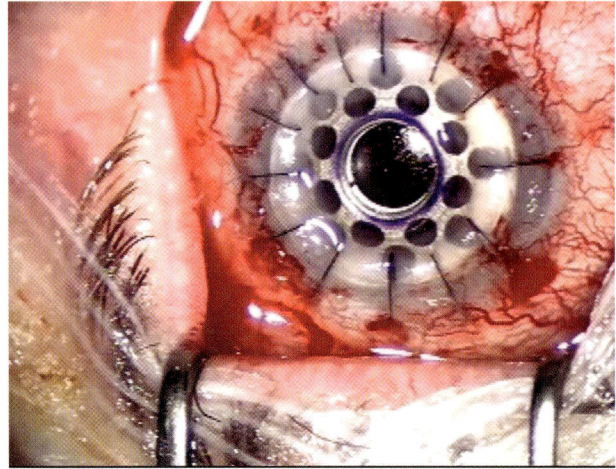

FIGURE 25.15 The keratoprosthesis is secured to the host cornea. A bandage contact lens is placed at the end of the case.

Boston Keratoprosthesis Type II

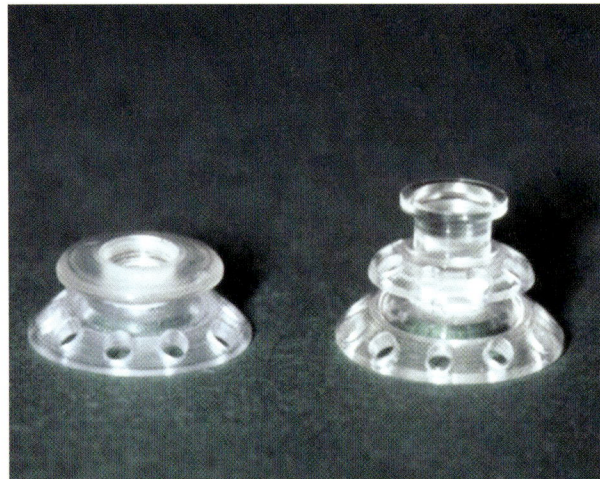

FIGURE 25.16 The Boston Keratoprosthesis Type II assembly kit includes a front plate, back plate, titanium locking ring, spanner wrench, and adhesive stickers. The Type II keratoprosthesis is assembled in the same fashion as the Type I prosthesis (see Figures 25.8–25.10). The assembled Boston Keratoprostheses without donor cornea rim are shown, Type I on the left, Type II on the right.

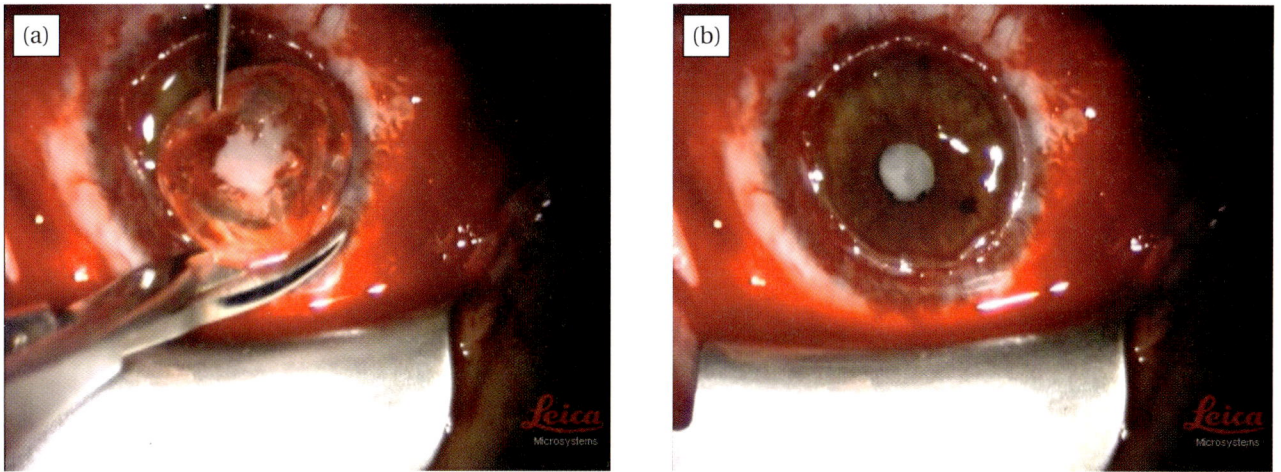

FIGURE 25.17 The host cornea is trephined and removed in a similar fashion to traditional keratoplasty.

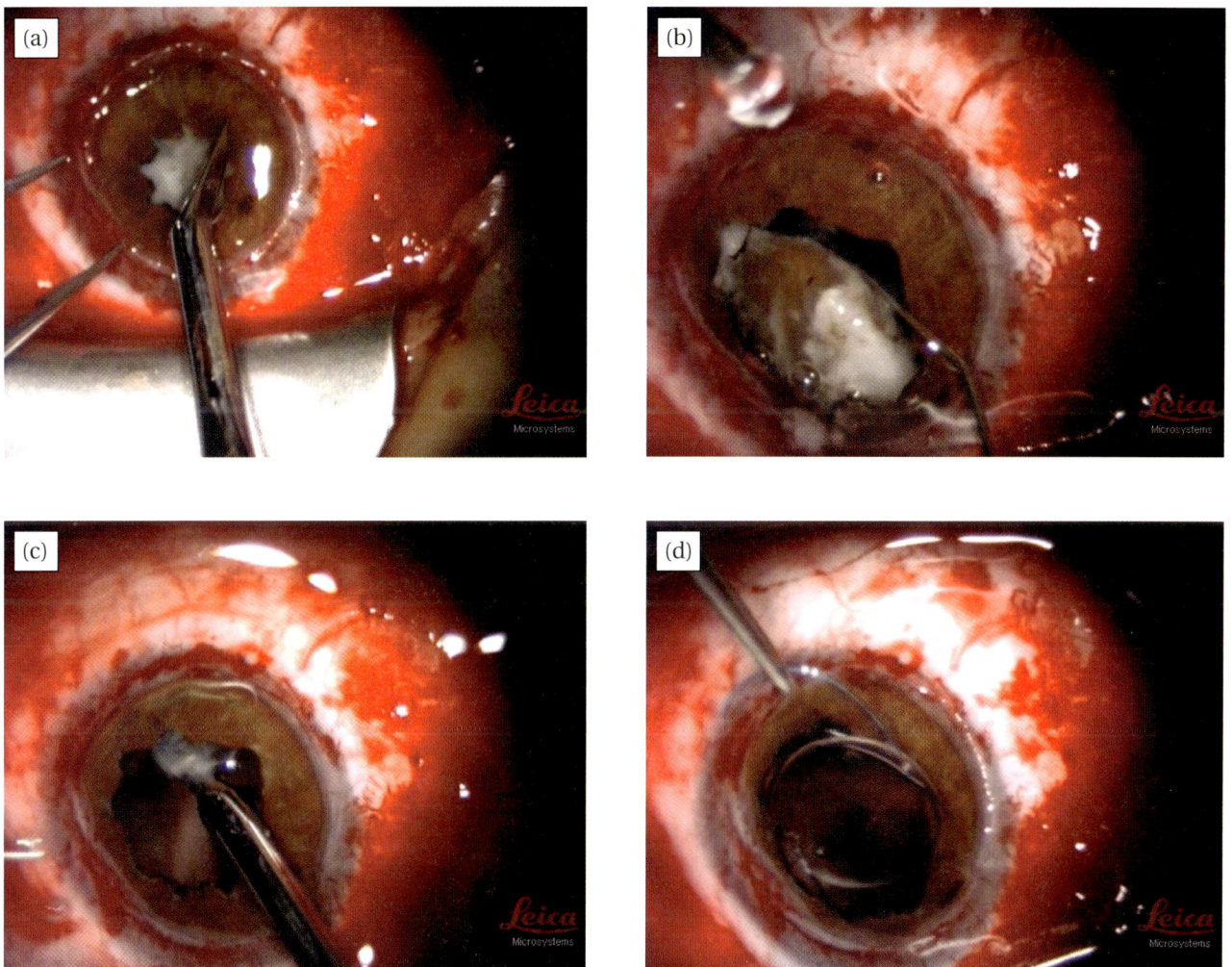

FIGURE 25.18 Open sky extracapsular cataract extraction begins with pupil sphincterotomies using angled Gills scissors (a). The lens is manually expressed (b). Residual lens cortex is removed with the irrigation/aspiration handpiece (c), and a 3-piece lens is placed into either the capsular bag or the sulcus, if possible (d).

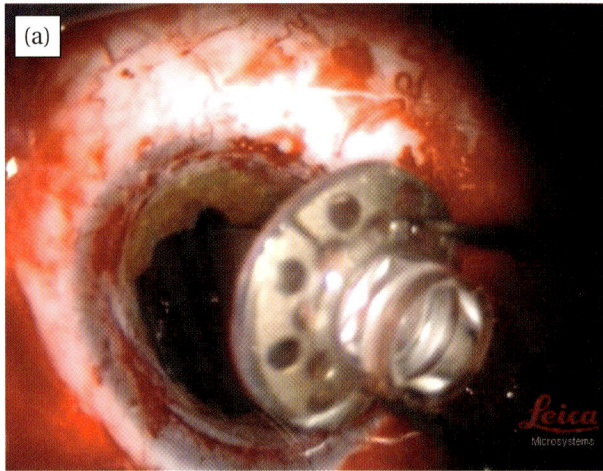

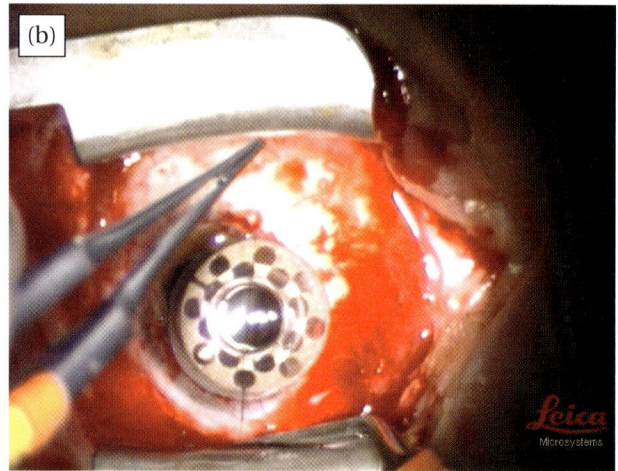

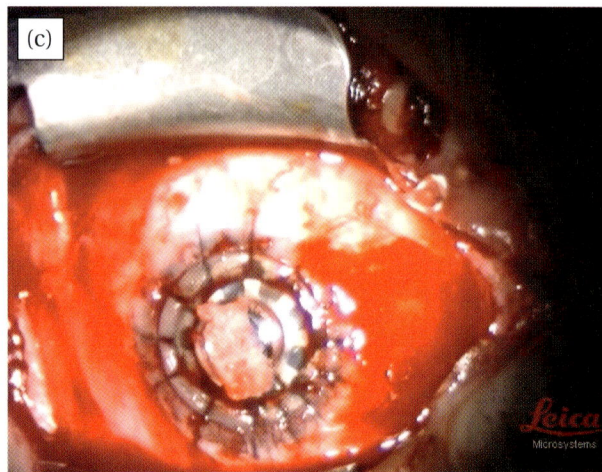

FIGURE 25.19 The keratoprosthesis is positioned (a) and secured with interrupted 9-0 nylon sutures (b). The optically perfect KPro focuses light on the retina as soon as it is in place; therefore, a corneal light shield is used to prevent macular phototoxicity (c).

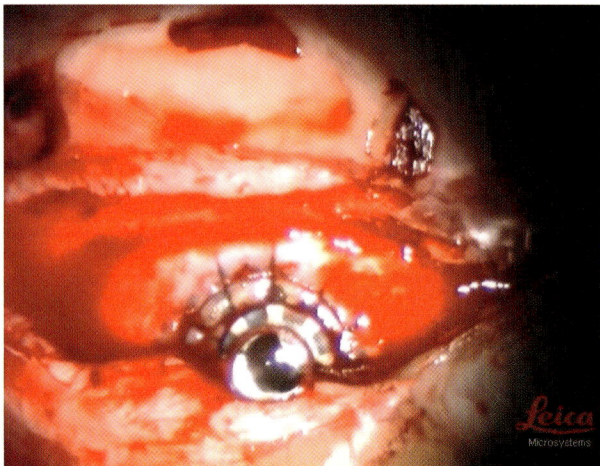

FIGURE 25.20 The eyelid closure begins by excising the eyelid margins with a 15 blade and toothed forceps.

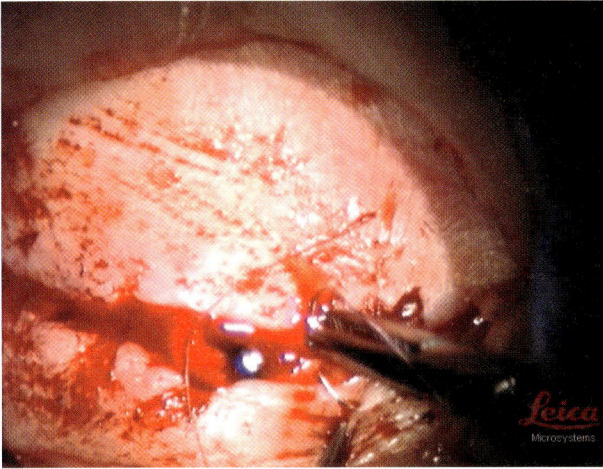

FIGURE 25.21 The orbicularis muscle from the upper and lower eyelids are approximated using 6-0 vicryl sutures, leaving a central opening for the keratoprosthesis front plate.

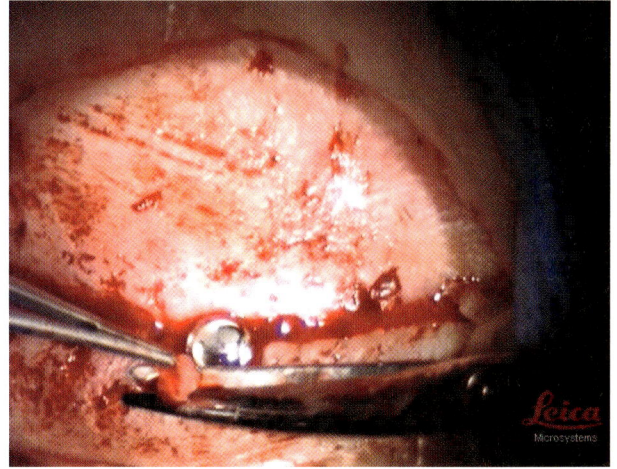

FIGURE 25.22 A central opening in the upper eyelid is created for proper placement of the keratoprosthesis anterior nub.

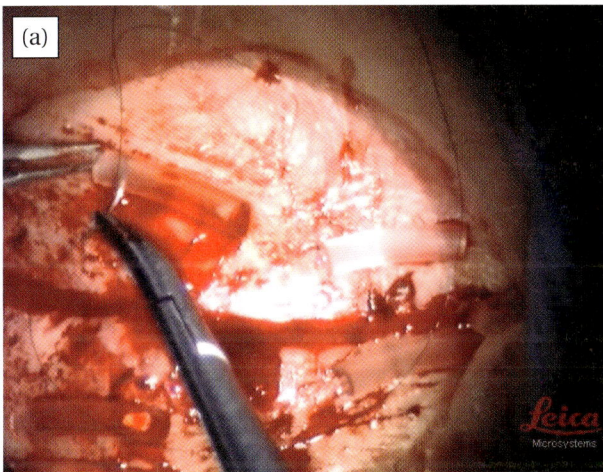

(a)

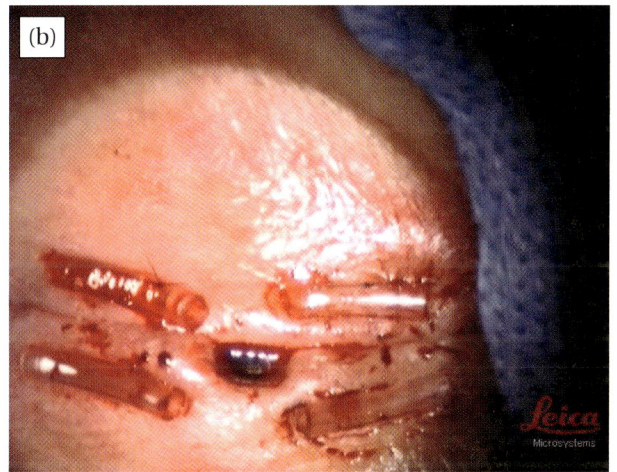

(b)

FIGURE 25.23 A tarsorrhaphy is placed using plastic pegs to protect the delicate periorbital tissue (a). The tarsorrhaphy brings together the upper and lower eyelid epithelia, which will scar together over time (b). Further minor surgical procedures may be necessary to adjust the central eyelid opening around the front plate as the skin heals.

TABLE 25.2   *Potential Complications with the Boston Keratoprosthesis (in order of frequency)*

Retroprosthetic membrane

Elevated intraocular pressure

Sterile vitritis

Vitreous hemorrhage

Retinal detachment

Choroidal hemorrhage or effusion

Posterior capsular opacity

Loss of bandage contact lens

Infectious keratitis*

Peripheral corneal melting*

Keratoprosthesis extrusion*

Wound leak*

High refractive error*

Endophthalmitis*

Cystoid macular edema*

Eyelid skin retraction (Boston Keratoprosthesis Type II)*

* Uncommon complication.

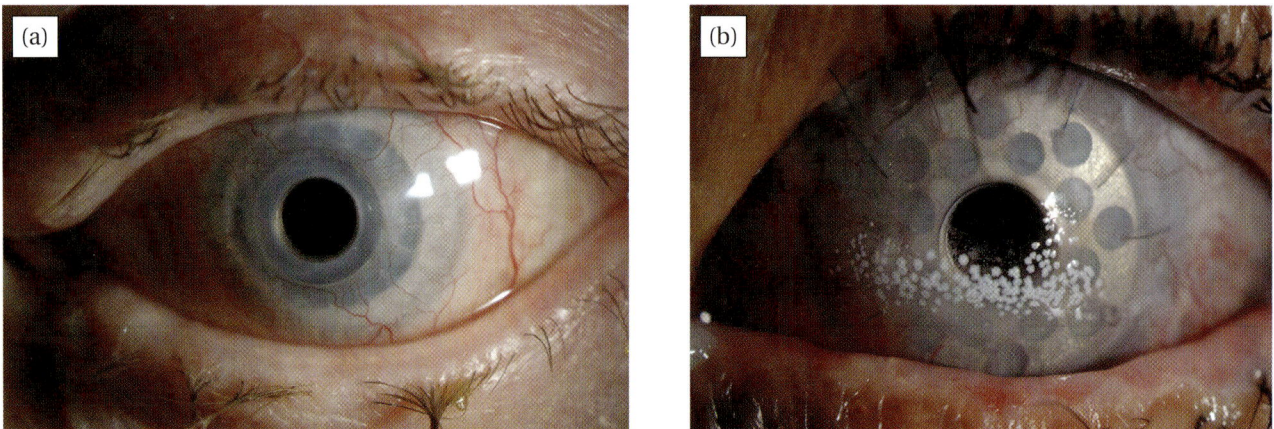

FIGURE 25.24   (a) A bandage soft contact lens is placed over the keratoprosthesis indefinitely in order to keep corneal tissues hydrated and to prevent corneal thinning. The visual axis remains clear despite opacification and neovascularization of the donor corneal rim. (b) Small white deposits on the contact lens are an indication for contact lens replacement. Similar debris is also visible on the contact lens in Figure 25.3.

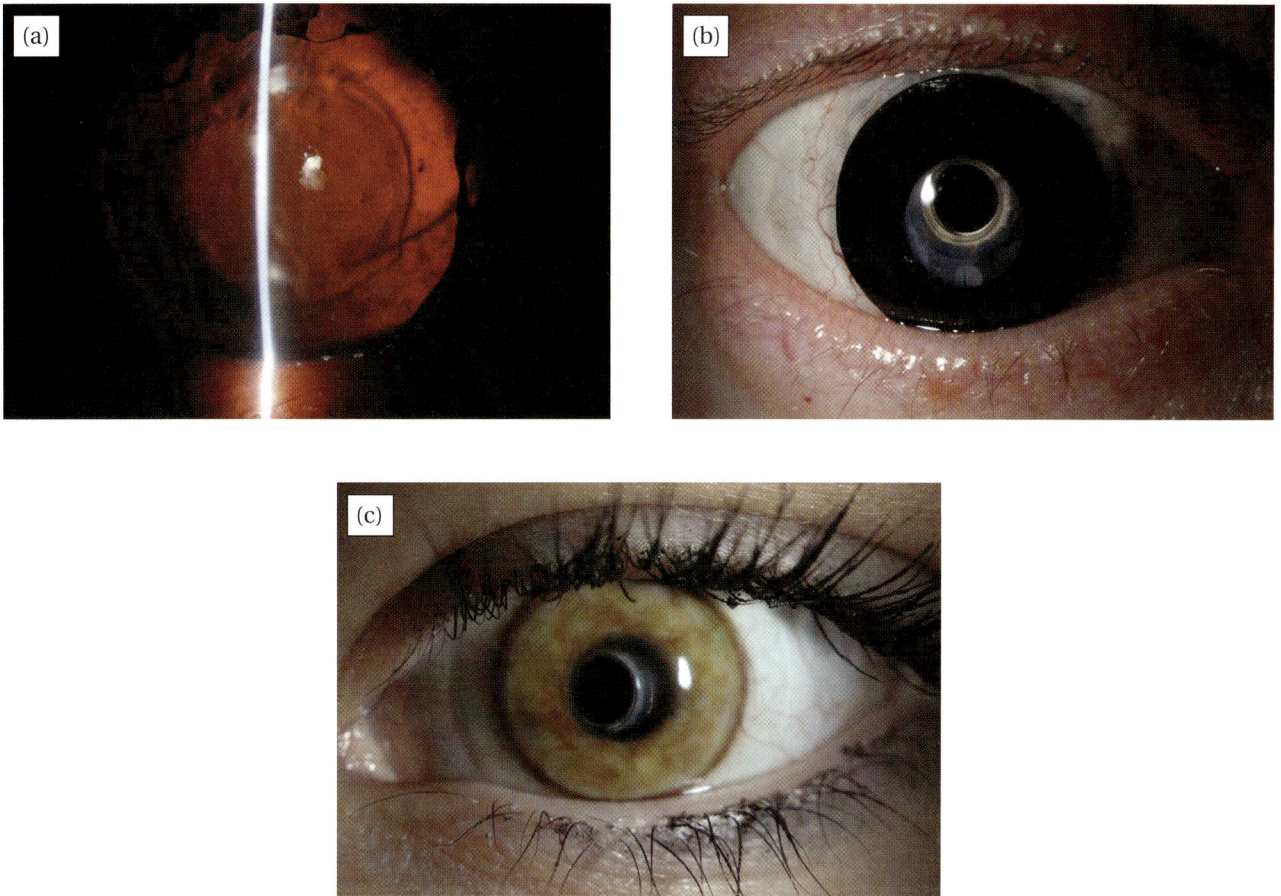

FIGURE 25.25 A tinted bandage contact lens over the keratoprosthesis decreases photophobia in patients with aniridia (a and b), and enhances cosmesis in other cases (c).

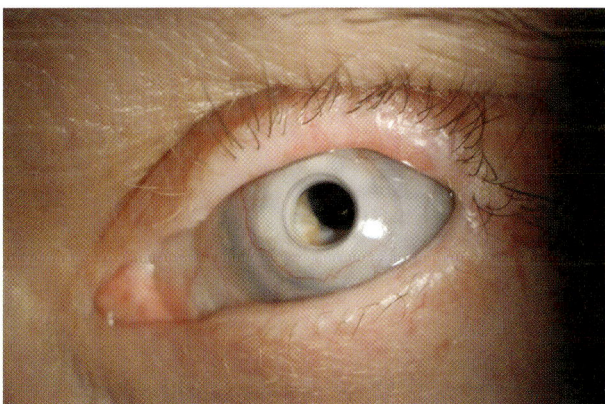

FIGURE 25.26 Lateral tarsorrhaphy can be performed in cases where the bandage contact lens falls out frequently.

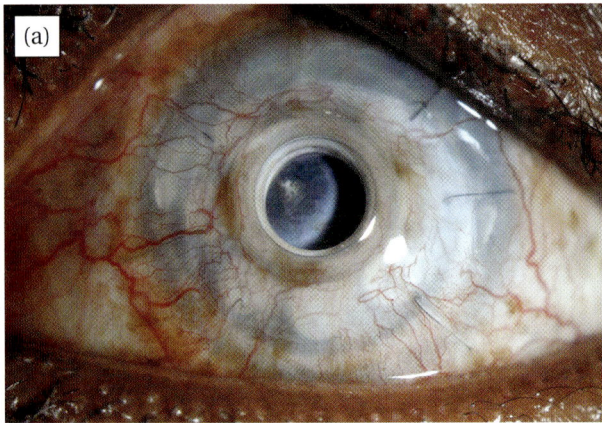

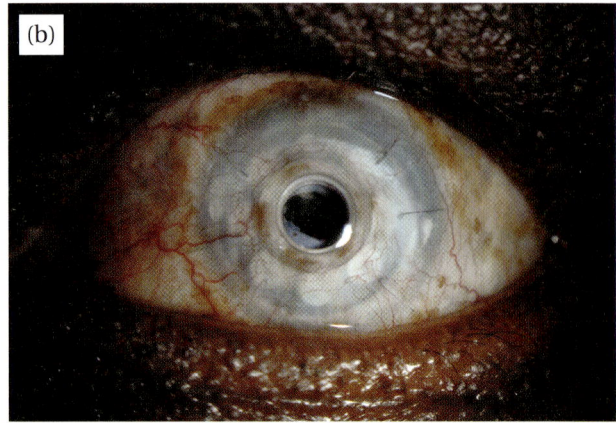

FIGURE 25.27 Postoperative inflammation may lead to elevated intraocular pressure, epiretinal membrane, cystoid macular edema, or a retroprosthetic membrane. Similar to posterior capsular opacification after intraocular lens implantation, YAG laser is often used to open a retroprosthetic membrane. (a) This patient had a retroprosthetic membrane that was too dense to be removed with laser. (b) Surgical removal via a pars plana approach successfully cleared the visual axis.

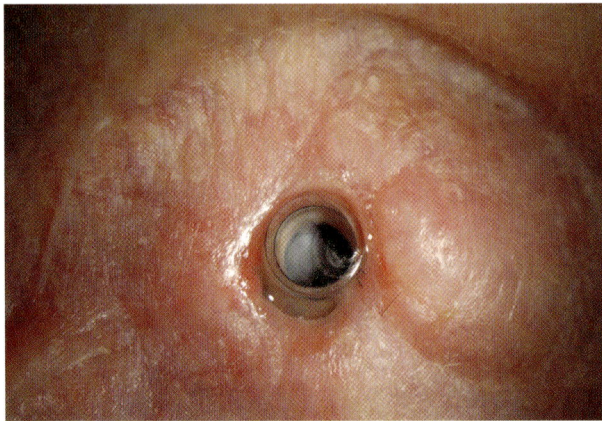

FIGURE 25.28 This patient with Stevens-Johnson syndrome underwent a Type II keratoprosthesis. The fluid collecting below the optic is concerning for aqueous fluid, presumably from a tissue melt.

SELECTED REFERENCES

Aldave AJ, Kamal KM, Vo RC, et al. The Boston type I keratoprosthesis: improving outcomes and expanding indications. *Ophthalmology.* 2009;116:640–651.

Bradley JC, Hernandez EG, Schwab IR, et al. Boston type I keratoprosthesis: The University of California Davis experience. *Cornea.* 2009;28:321–327.

Dohlman CH, Nouri M. Keratoprosthesis Surgery. In: *Smolin and Thoft's The Cornea: Scientific Foundations & Clinical Practice.* New York, NY: Lippincott Williams & Wilkins; 2005:49–51.

Harissi-Dagher M, Beyer J, Dohlman CH. The role of soft contact lenses as an adjunct to the Boston Keratoprosthesis. *Int Ophthalmol Clin.* 2008; 48: 43–51.

Saygh RR, Ang LPK, Foster CS, et al. The Boston Keratoprosthesis in Stevens-Johnson Syndrome. *Am J Ophthalmol.* 2008;145:438–444.

Todani A, Gupta P, Colby K. Type I Boston Keratoprosthesis with cataract extraction and intraocular lens placement for visual rehabilitation of herpes zoster ophthalmicus: the "KPro Triple." *Br J Ophthalmol.* 2009; 93:1191.

Zerbe BL, Belin MW, Ciolino JB, Boston Type I Keratoprosthesis Study Group. Results from the Multicenter Boston Type 1 Keratoprosthesis Study. *Ophthalmology.* 2006;113:1779–1784.

26 Intracorneal Ring Segment Implantation

Bennie H. Jeng, MD and Joseph Colin, MD

TABLE 26.1   *Indications and Contraindications for Intrastromal Ring Segment Implantation*

Indications

Treatment of corneal ectasias where patients have:

- contact lens intolerance
- age 21 years or older
- clear central corneas
- mean keratometry value of <55 D
- corneal thickness >450 microns at incision site
- corneal transplantation as only other remaining option for visual rehabilitation

Contraindications

- mean keratometric value >75 D
- history of corneal hydrops
- central corneal scar
- severe atopy (should be treated previously)
- any local or systemic active infection

Intrastromal Ring Segment Implantation

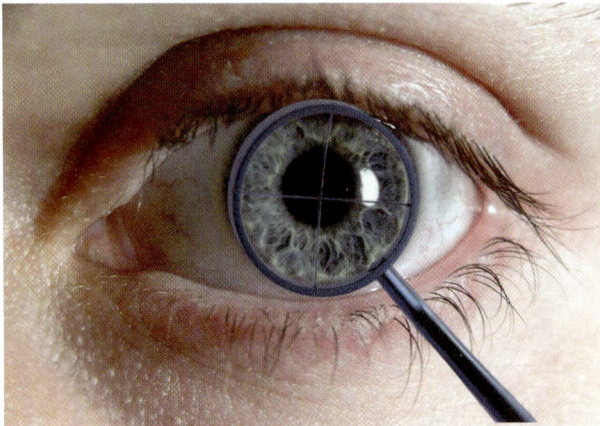

FIGURE 26.1   An impression of the crosshairs of an 11 mm optical zone marker is made to locate the geometric center of the cornea. (Image courtesy of Mark Swanson, MD [Mexico].)

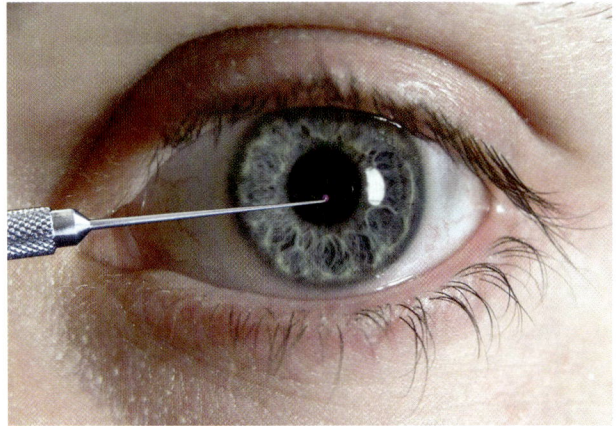

FIGURE 26.2   The geometric center of the cornea is marked using a Sinskey hook marked with alcohol-free gentian violet. (Image courtesy of Mark Swanson, MD [Mexico].)

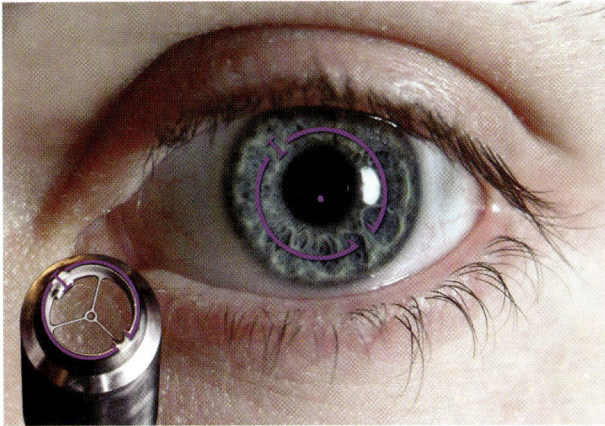

FIGURE 26.3 The incision placement marker is marked with alcohol-free gentian violet. (Image courtesy of Mark Swanson, MD [Mexico].)

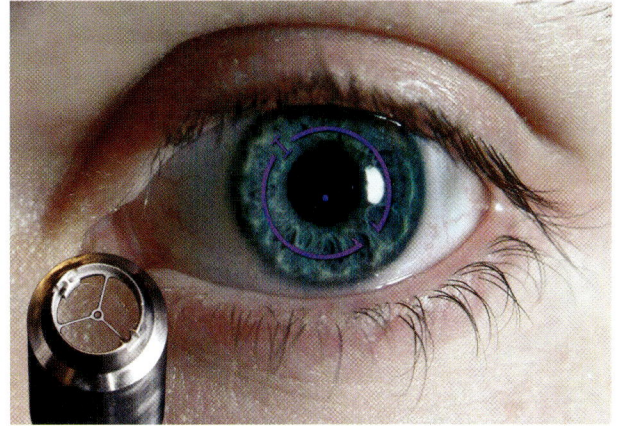

FIGURE 26.4 The cornea is dried, the incision placement marker is aligned with the geometric center of the cornea, and the cornea is marked with the gentian violet ink with the "I" mark at the desired incision site. (Image courtesy of Mark Swanson, MD [Mexico].)

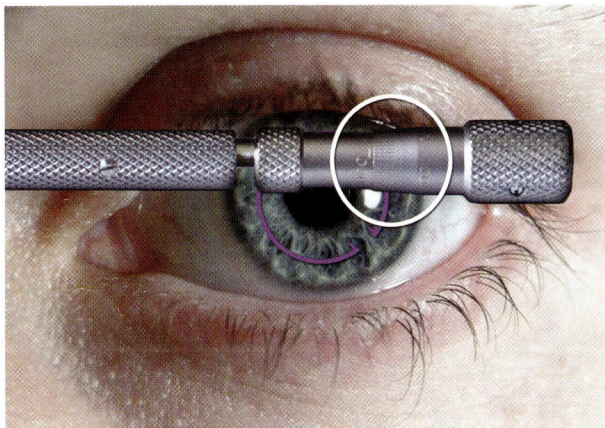

FIGURE 26.5 After checking pachymetry at the incision site, the diamond blade is set at a depth of 70% of the cornea thickness at the incision site. (Image courtesy of Mark Swanson, MD [Mexico].)

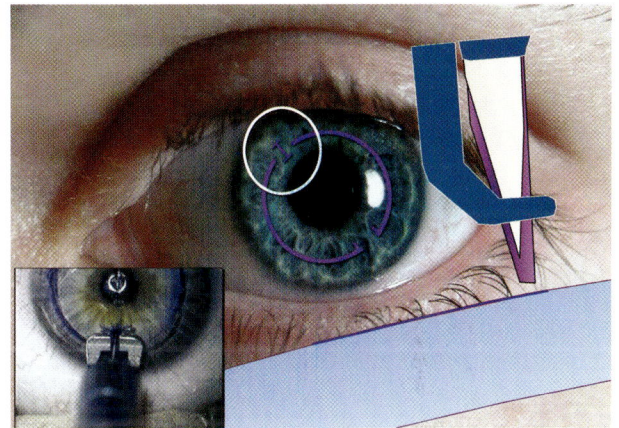

FIGURE 26.6 Schematic of the preparation for the incision. Inset: Preparation for incision at the central edge of the incision mark. (Image courtesy of Addition Technology, Inc. [Des Plaines, IL].)

FIGURE 26.7 Schematic of the incision. Inset: The blade is inserted, and the footplate is seated firmly. (Image courtesy of Addition Technology, Inc. [Des Plaines, IL].)

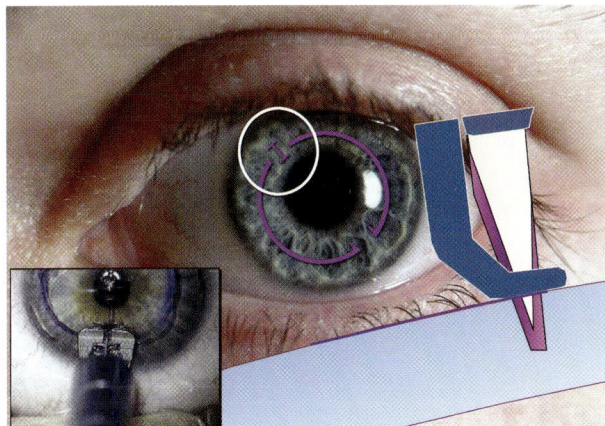

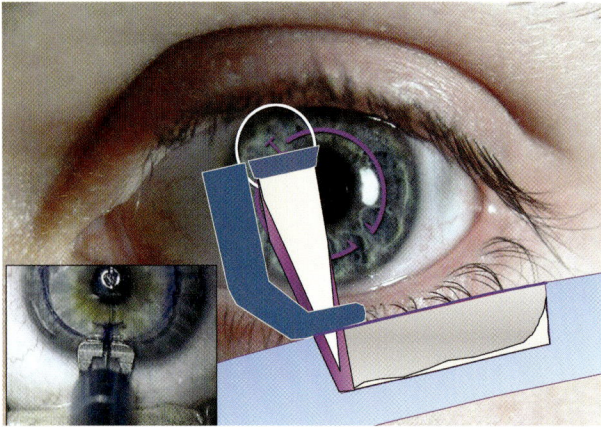

FIGURE 26.8 Schematic of the incision. Inset: Firm footplate contact is maintained, and the blade is pulled to the peripheral edge of the incision mark while maintaining 1 mm distance from the limbus. (Image courtesy of Addition Technology, Inc. [Des Plaines, IL].)

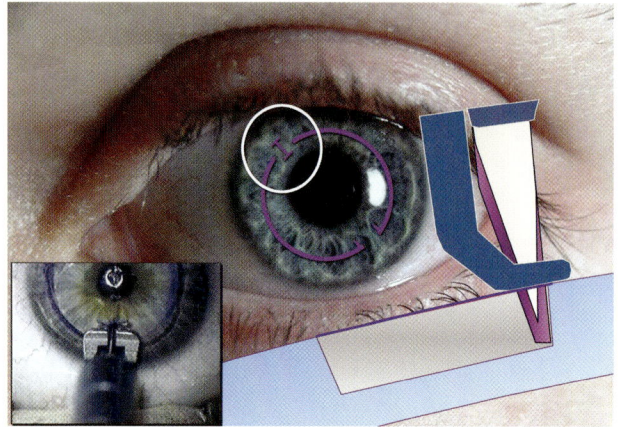

FIGURE 26.9 Schematic demonstrating smooth bed and square incision. Inset: Footplate pressure is maintained on the cornea while the blade is pushed back to entry point. (Image courtesy of Addition Technology, Inc. [Des Plaines, IL].)

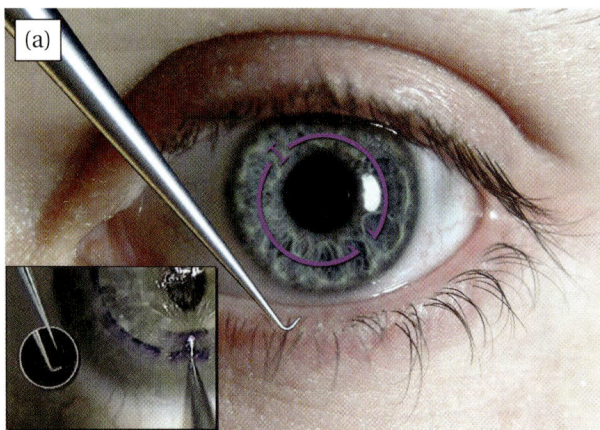

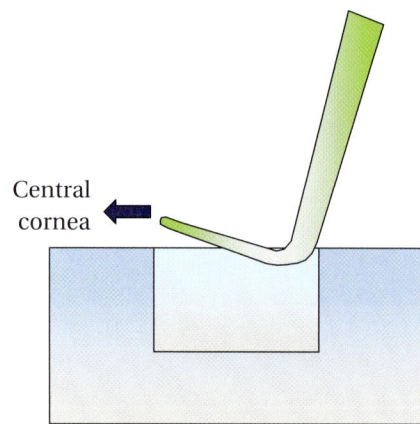

FIGURE 26.10 (a) The pocketing hook (see inset) is used to start the cleavage plane at the base of the incision to create a square stromal pocket. (b) Schematic of placing the pocketing hook in the incision. The pocketing hook should be placed heel down, with the point toward the central cornea. (Image [a] courtesy of Mark Swanson, MD [Mexico]; image [b] courtesy of Addition Technology, Inc. [Des Plaines, IL].)

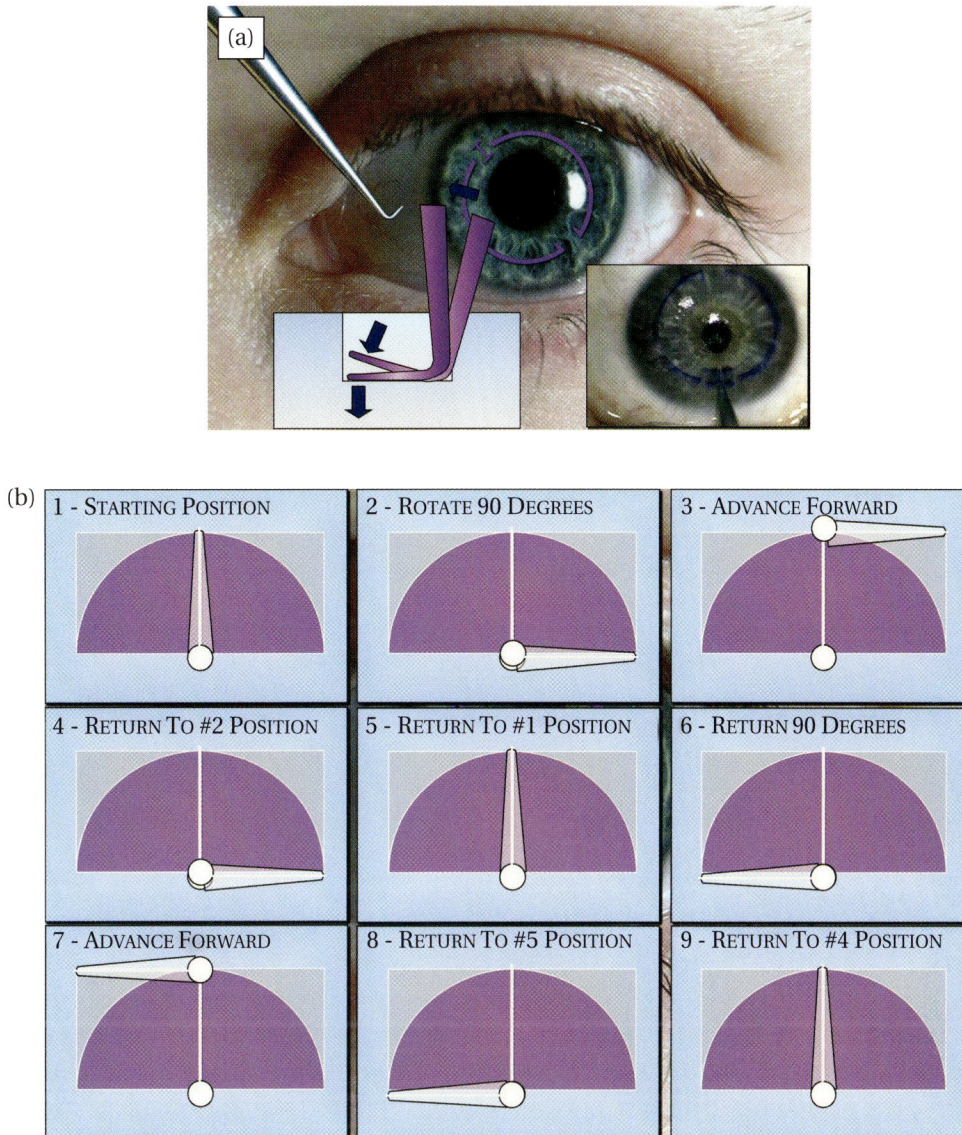

FIGURE 26.11 (a) Once the heel is seated, the hook should be tilted forward to lay the hook flat in the incision. Bottom right: Tip of the pocketing hook is rotated clockwise to create the lamellar pocket. (b) 1: Schematic demonstrating the neutral position of the pocketing hook. 2: Schematic demonstrating the tip of the hook rotated clockwise. 3 and 4: Schematic demonstrating the tip of the hook moved up and down the entire length of the incision on the right. 5 and 6: Schematic demonstrating the tip of the hook rotated counter-clockwise. 7 and 8: Schematic demonstrating the tip of the hook moved up and down the entire length of the incision on the left. 9: Schematic demonstrating return of the hook to the starting position to remove it from the pocket. (Image [a] courtesy of Mark Swanson, MD [Mexico]; image [b] courtesy of Addition Technology, Inc. [Des Plaines, IL].)

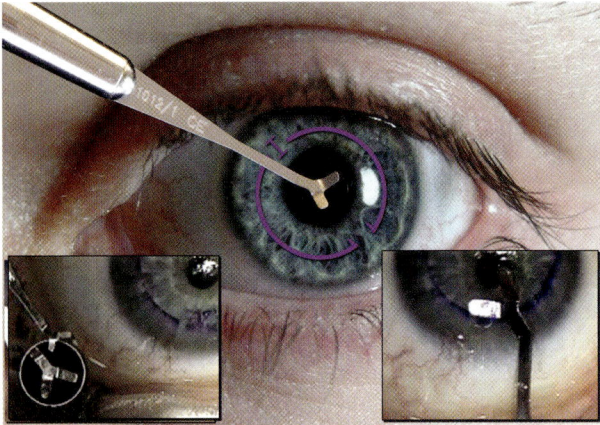

FIGURE 26.12 Bottom left: Inset demonstrating appearance of the symmetric glide instrument. Tip of the symmetric glide is placed vertically into the incision. Bottom right: The instrument is then rotated to the left to enter into the pocket created by the pocketing hook and then pressure is exerted to lengthen the lamellar dissection. The same technique is used to lengthen the lamellar dissection to the right. (Images courtesy of Mark Swanson, MD [Mexico].)

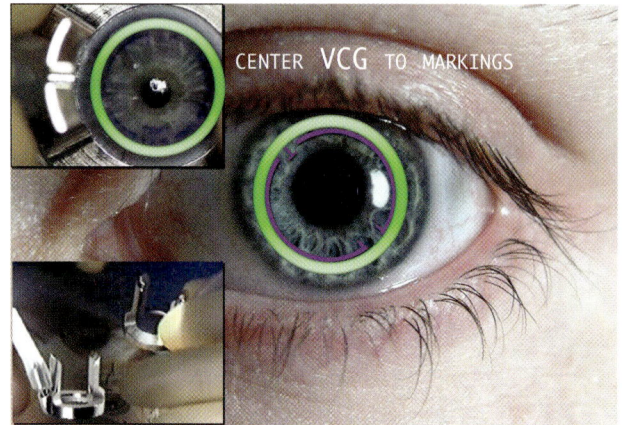

FIGURE 26.13 After vacuum suction ring is placed on the eye under low vacuum (450 mBar), the vacuum centering guide is used to verify centration. (Images courtesy of Mark Swanson, MD [Mexico].)

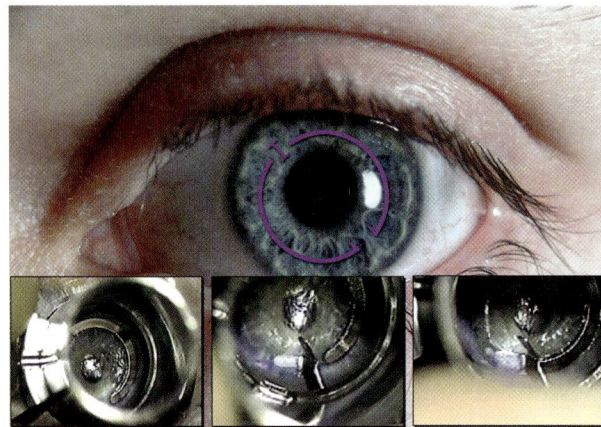

FIGURE 26.14 Bottom left: Once centration is confirmed, high vacuum (630 mBar) is initiated, and the clockwise dissector is placed into the suction ring. Bottom center: The tip of the dissector is rotated 2 clock hours away from the incision, and the symmetric glide is inserted into the lamellar dissection to act as a "shoehorn." Bottom right: The dissector is then rotated under the symmetric glide until the tip is visible. The Symmetric glide is then removed, and the dissector is then rotated 2 clock hours at a time, until the hub of the dissector is at the incision site. The dissector is then rotated out of the channel, and the same procedure is performed in the other direction. The vacuum is the released, and the vacuum suction ring is also removed. (Images courtesy of Mark Swanson, MD [Mexico].)

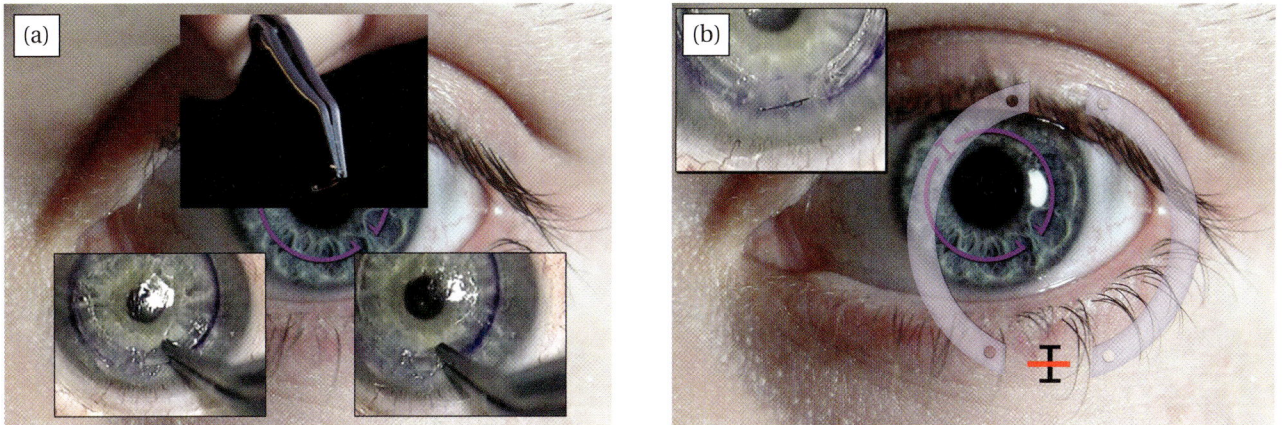

FIGURE 26.15 (a) After a drop of antibiotics is placed on the intracorneal ring segments, one segment is placed in the clockwise channel with forceps. Advance the segment with the forceps until the end of the segment approaches the incision area. Then push the segment fully into the channel with a Sinskey hook. The same procedure is performed in the counterclockwise direction. A single 10-0 nylon suture is then used to close the incision. The knot is buried. (b) Schematic of the correct position of the ring segments. The same procedure is performed in the counterclockwise direction. A single 10-0 nylon suture is then used to close the incision. The knot is buried. (Images courtesy of Addition Technology, Inc. [Des Plaines, IL].)

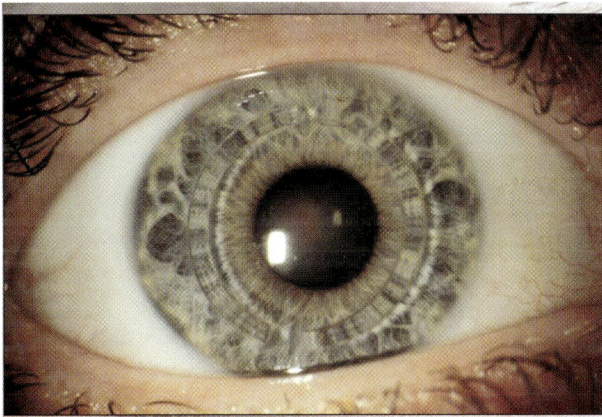

FIGURE 26.16 First-day postoperative image of an eye with intracorneal ring segments implanted. (Image courtesy of Mark Swanson, MD [Mexico].)

TABLE 26.2 *Complications Associated with Intrastromal Ring Segment Implantation*

- Epithelial defects at the keratotomy site
- Anterior and posterior perforations during the incision or while creating the channel
- Extension of the incision toward the central visual axis or toward the limbus
- Shallow, asymmetric, and/or uneven placement and/or uneven placement of the intracorneal ring segments
- Infectious keratitis
- Persisting incisional gap
- Decentration
- Stromal thinning
- Corneal stromal edema around the incision and channel from surgical manipulation
- Sterile keratitis
- Chronic pain after implantation
- Deposition of an extracellular intrastromal substance in the lamellar channel around the segments

SELECTED REFERENCES

Alio JL, Shabayek MH. Intracorneal ring segments (INTACS) for keratoconus correction: long term follow-up. *J Cataract Refract Surg.* 2006;32:978–985.

Chan CC, Sharma M, Wachler BS. Effect of inferior-segment Intacs with and without C3-R on keratoconus. *J Cataract Refract Surg.* 2007 Jan; 33(1):75–80.

Colin J, Cochener B, Savary G, Malet F, Holmes-Higgin D. Intacs Inserts for Treating Keratoconus: One-year results. *Ophthalmology.* 2001;108:1409–1414.

Colin J, Cochner B, Savary G, et al. Correcting keratoconus with intracorneal rings. *J Cataract Refract Surg.* 2000;26:1117–1122.

Colin J. The European clinical evaluation: Use of Intacs prescription inserts for the treatment of keratoconus. *J Cataract Refract Surg.* 2006;32(5):747–755.

Ertan A, J. Colin. Intracorneal rings for keratoconus and keratectasia. *J Cataract Refract Surg.* 2007;33:1303–1314.

Ferrara de A Cunha P. Tecnica cirurgica para correçao de miopia; Anel corneano intra-estromal. *Rev Bras Oftalmol.* 1995;54:577–588.

In Lovisolo CF, Fleming JF, Pesando PM, eds. *Intrastromal Corneal Ring Segments.* Fabiano Editore, 2002;Chapter 2:31–34.

Kanellopoulos AJ, Pe LH, Perry HD, Donnenfeld, ED. Modified intracorneal ring segment implantations (INTACS) for the management of moderate to advanced keratoconus: efficacy and complications. *Cornea.* 2006;25(1):29–33.

McAlister JC, Ardjomand N, Hari L, Mengher LS, et al. Keratitis after intracorneal ring segment insertion for keratoconus. *J Cataract Refract Surg.* 2006; 32:676–678.

Randleman JB, Dawson DG, Larson PM, et al. Chronic pain after Intacs implantation. *J Cataract Refract Surg.* 2006;32: 875–878.

Roberts C. Biomechanics of INTACS in keratoconus. *Intracorneal Ring Segments and Alternative Treatments for Corneal Ectatic Diseases.* ed. Colin J, Ertan A. 159–166, Kudret Göz Yayınları, Ankara, 2007.

Rodriguez-Prats J, Galal A, Garcia-Lledo M, De La Hoz F, Alio JL. Intracorneal rings for correction of pellucid marginal degeneration. *J Cataract Refract Surg.* 2003; 29:1421–1424.

Ruckhofer J, Twa MD, Schanzlin DJ. Clinical characteristics of lamellar channel deposits after implantation of Intacs. *J Cataract Refract Surg.* 2000; 26: 1473–1479.

27 Superficial Keratectomy in the Treatment of Anterior Corneal Pathologies

Neelofar Ghaznawi, MD and Kristin M. Hammersmith, MD

TABLE 27.1 *Indications for Superficial Keratectomy**

Treatment of Elevated Anterior Corneal Lesions
- Salzmann's Nodular Degeneration
- Keratoconus Nodules

Recurrent Erosion Syndrome
- Multiple erosions
- Anterior Basement Membrane Dystrophy
- Loose epithelial sheets

Diagnostic
- Chronic ulceration
- Neoplastic lesions

*Note: Not indicated in corneal pathology involving mid to deep stroma.

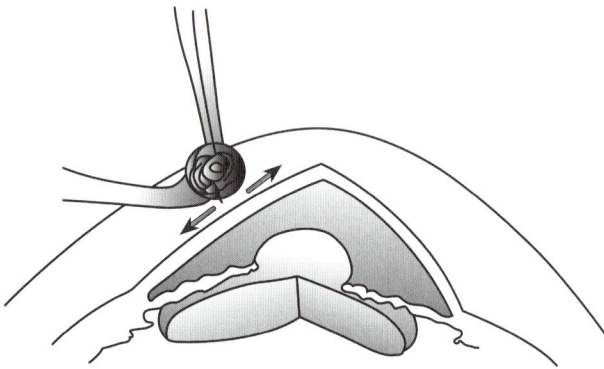

FIGURE 27.1 Superficial keratectomy for Salzmann's nodular degeneration.

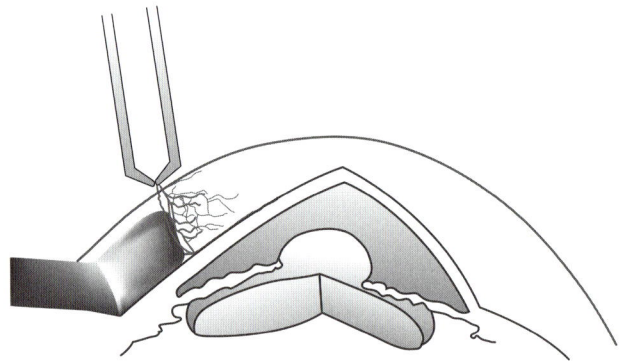

FIGURE 27.2 Superficial keratectomy for pathologic diagnosis.

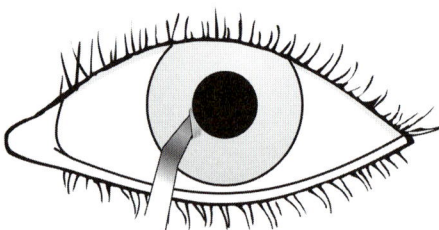

FIGURE 27.3 Epithelial debridement with blade.

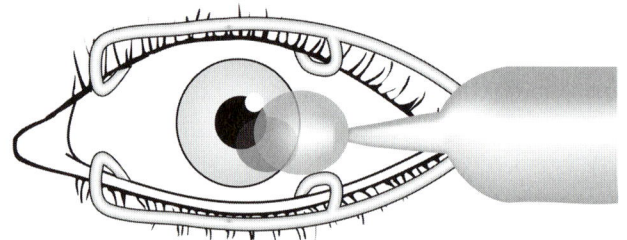

FIGURE 27.4 Diamond burr debridement.

TABLE 27.2 *Surgical Therapies for Recurrent Erosion Syndromes*

Procedure	ASP	Debridement	Diamond Burr Debridement	Excimer PTK
Optimum candidate	Localized erosions outside visual axis	Single area of erosion with localized loose sheet of floppy epithelium	Erosions in multiple areas, moderate to severe ABM dystrophy, loose epithelial sheets	Erosions in multiple areas, moderate to severe ABM dystrophy, loose sheets of epithelium
Debridement required	No	Yes	Yes	Yes
Efficacy	Excellent	Limited	Excellent	Good

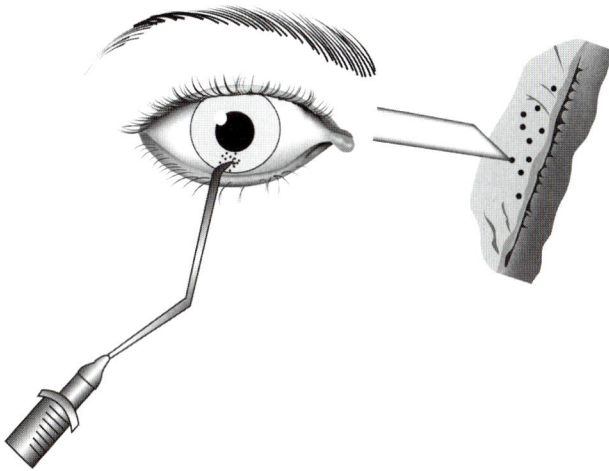

FIGURE 27.5 Anterior stromal puncture with bent 30g needle.

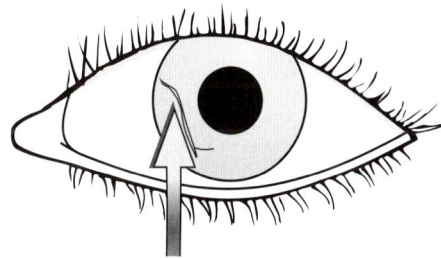

FIGURE 27.3 Epithelial debridement with the Weckcel sponge.

TABLE 27.3 *Complications of Superficial Keratectomy*

Poor healing

Chronic ulceration

Infectious keratitis

Irregular astigmatism

Scarring

SELECTED REFERENCES

Krachmer, JH, Mannis, MJ, Holland, EJ. *Cornea Volume III—Surgery of the Cornea and Conjunctiva.* Mosby 1997; p. 1868.

Krachmer, JH, Mannis, MJ, Holland, EJ. *Cornea Volume II—Cornea and External Disease: Clinical Diagnosis and Management.* Mosby 1997; p. 1320.

Rapuano, CJ, Luchs JI, Kim T. *The Requisites in Ophthalmology: Anterior Segment.* Mosby 2000; p. 148.

28 Femtosecond Laser Keratoplasty (FLK)

Sumit (Sam) Garg, MD, Marjan Farid, MD, and Roger F. Steinert, MD

Preoperative Evaluation

TABLE 28.1 *Preoperative Considerations*

Suitability for full thickness transplant

Corneal diameter (especially vertical) to determine graft diameter

Peripheral pachymetry (to allow for 70 μm posterior bridge)

Informed consent

Healthy endothelium (if considering FLK-Deep Anterior Lamellar Keratoplasty [FLK-DALK])

Patient transfer (if femtosecond laser not in operating room)

FLK incision pattern (see following figures)

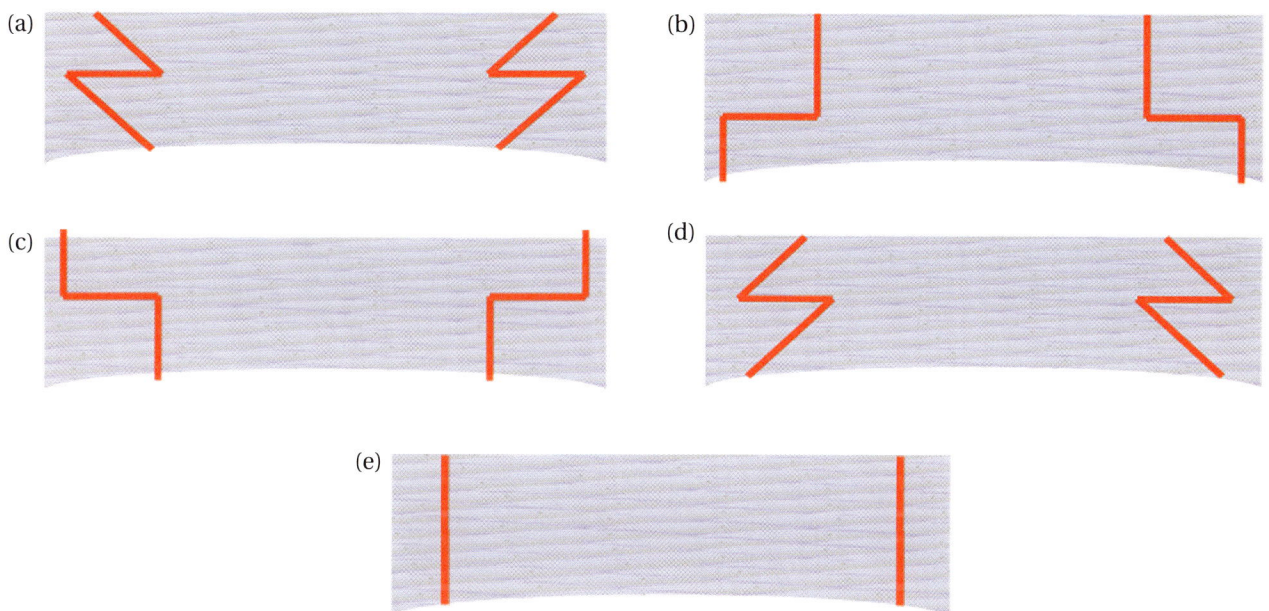

FIGURE 28.1 FLK Incision Patterns. (a) Zigzag. (b) Top-hat. (c) Mushroom. (d) Christmas tree. (e) Traditional.

TABLE 28.2 *Relative Contraindications*

Dense corneal scars (especially peripheral)

Severe peripheral neovascularization

Narrow palpebral fissures (precluding placement of patient interface)

Previous glaucoma implant or active bleb (precluding placement of patient interface)

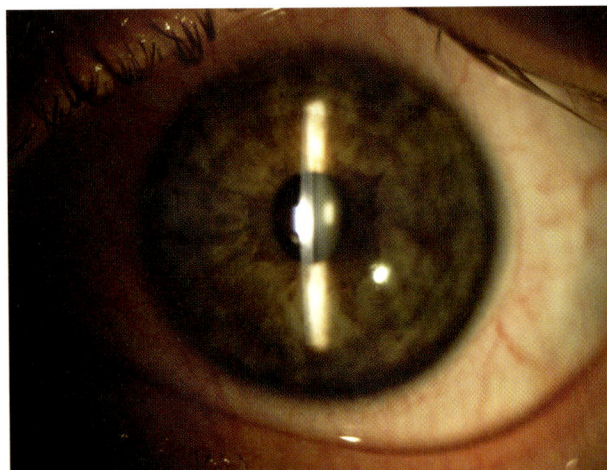

FIGURE 28.2 Slit beam of cornea used to determine diameter. The slit-lamp beam is used to gauge the appropriate graft diameter for the transplant. The largest beam is 8 mm.

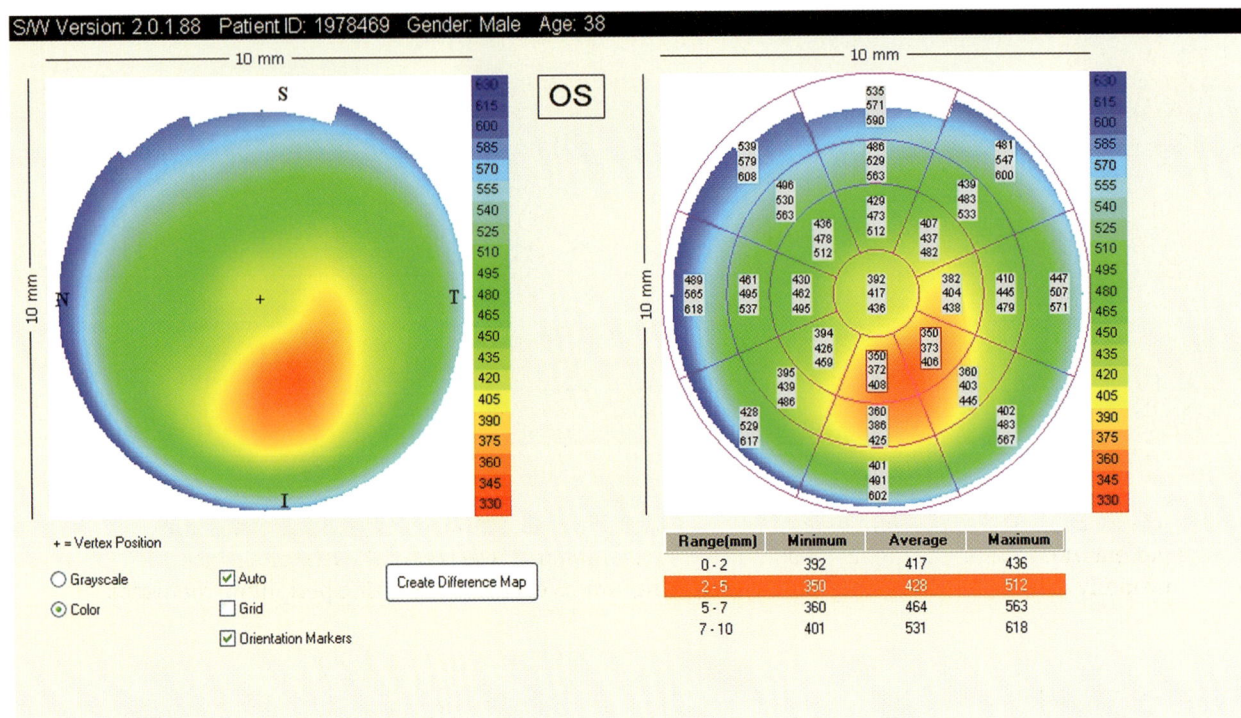

FIGURE 28.3 Pachymetry map. A preoperative pachymetry map either by anterior segment optical coherence tomography (Visante OCT, Carl Zeiss Meditec, Inc., Dublin, California—pictured here), Pentacam (Oculus USA, Lynwood, Washington), Orbscan (Bausch & Lomb, Salt Lake City, UT), or ultrasound is performed to adequately assess and program depth settings for the femtosecond laser incision. Generally, the posterior depth of the FLK incision is set 70 μm anterior to the minimum thickness in the 7–10 mm diameter range.

Operative: FLK

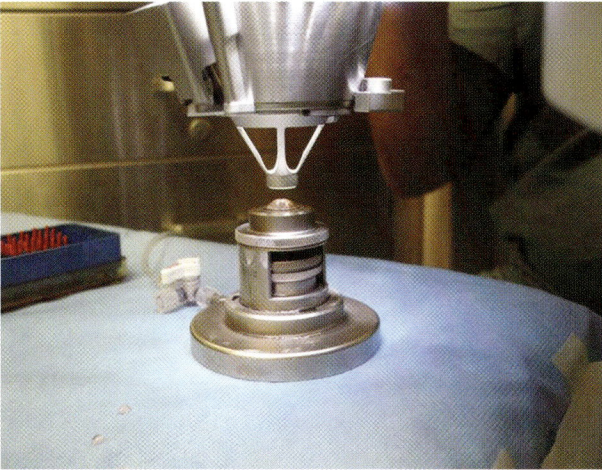

FIGURE 28.4 Donor cornea preparation. Donor corneas can be cut by the femtosecond laser with preprogrammed parameters set by the surgeon. This can be done with the tissue mounted on an artificial anterior chamber or, alternatively, "pre-cut" with the same parameters by the eye bank.

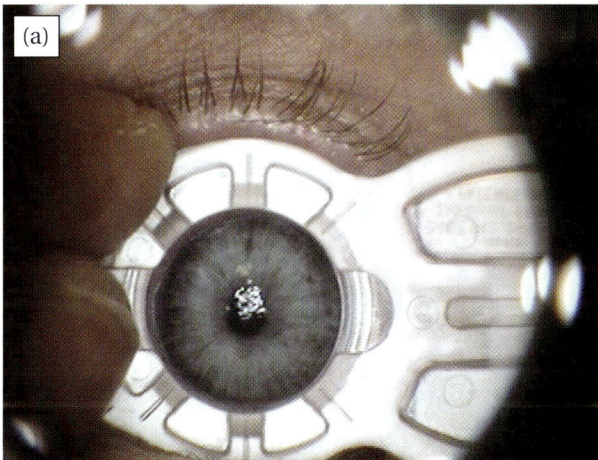

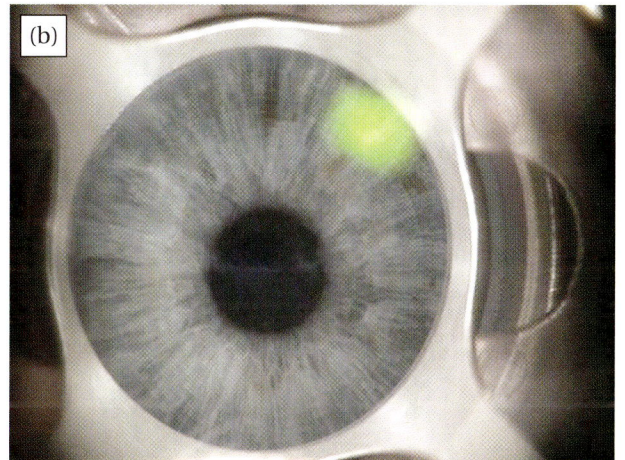

FIGURE 28.5 Docking patient to femtosecond laser. Care must be taken to properly center the patient interface on the globe to allow adequate centration of the graft. (a) Patient interface properly centered. (b) Docking plate applanating cornea evenly, minimizing peripheral meniscus.

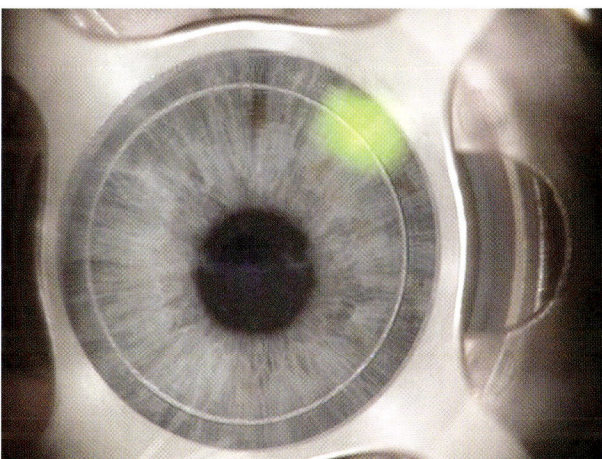

FIGURE 28.6 Posterior side cut. For a "zigzag" incision, a posterior side cut advances from deep stroma at a 30° angle towards the periphery.

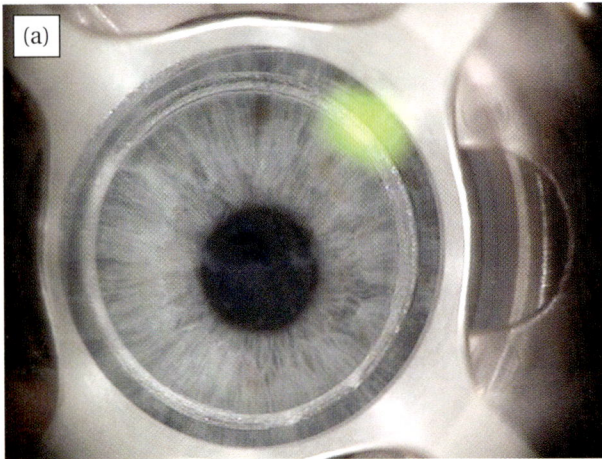

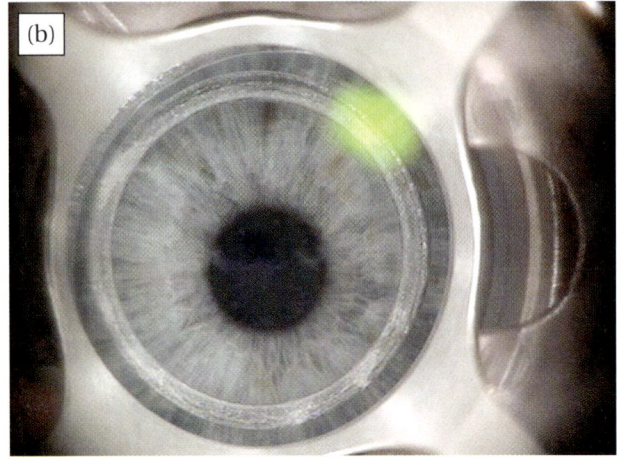

FIGURE 28.7 Ring lamellar cut. For a "zigzag" incision, the posterior side cut intersects the second cut, which is a ring lamellar cut with a width of 0.5 mm at a depth of 300 μm from the anterior corneal surface. The ring cut advances from the periphery (a) toward the center (b).

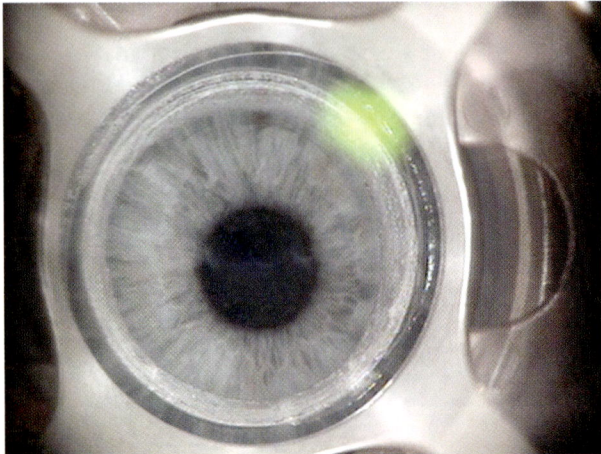

FIGURE 28.8 Anterior side cut. For a "zigzag" incision, after the lamellar ring cut, a third incision, which is the anterior side cut, advances toward the anterior corneal surface angled toward the periphery at 30°.

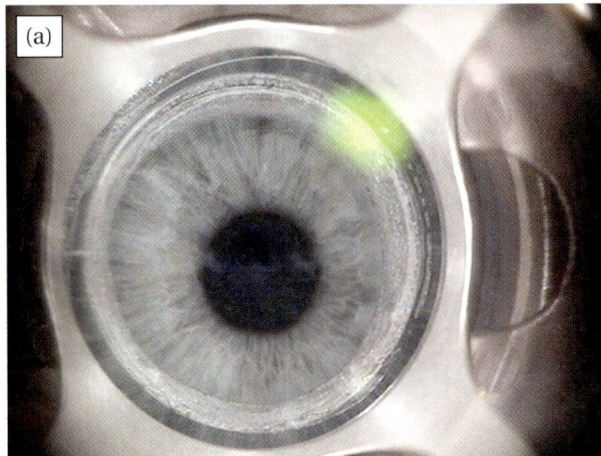

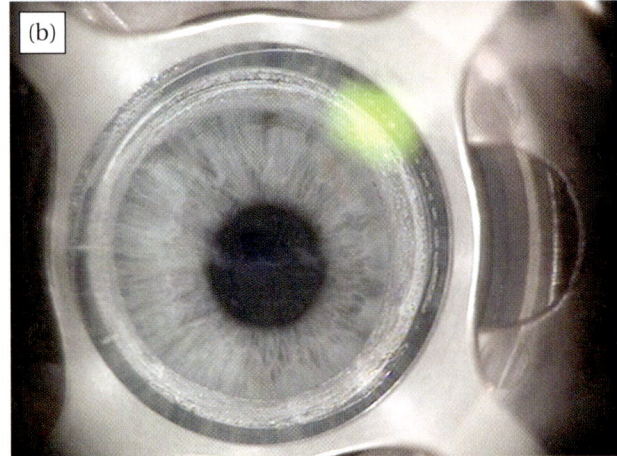

FIGURE 28.9 Radial alignment marks. Radial alignment marks can be placed on recipient and donor to guide suture placement. Note first alignment mark at 3 o'clock (a) and second alignment mark at 2 o'clock (b).

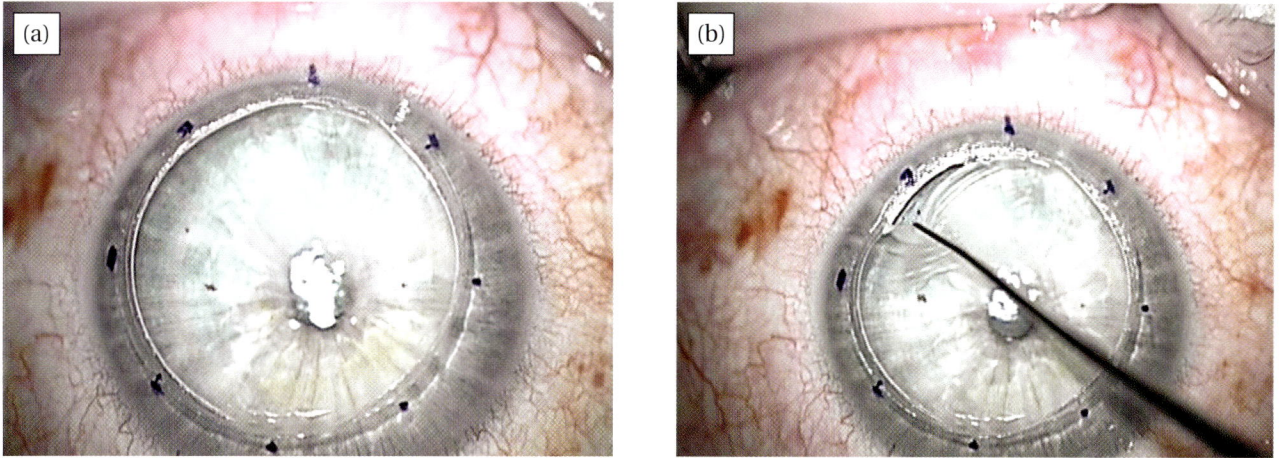

FIGURE 28.10 Teasing apart incision. Once in the operating room, and after either retrobulbar or general anesthesia is administered. The radial alignment marks are then highlighted with a marker (a). The host corneal button is separated by blunt dissection with a Sinskey hook to reveal the incisions made by the laser (b). After the 360° blunt dissection of the laser incision, the anterior chamber is entered with a blade and the posterior cut is completed using corneal scissors.

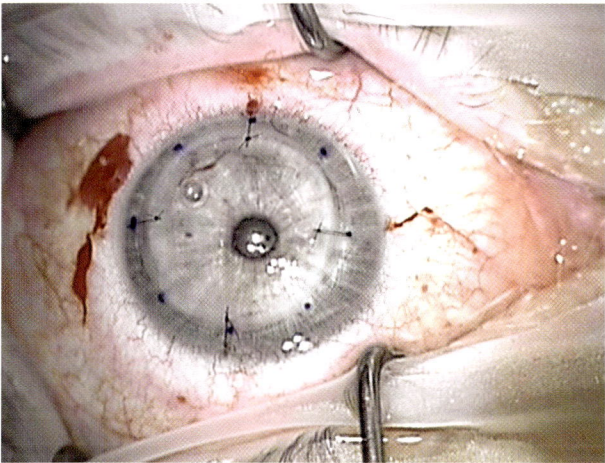

FIGURE 28.11 Cardinal sutures. After removal of the host corneal button, the donor corneal button is secured with four cardinal sutures.

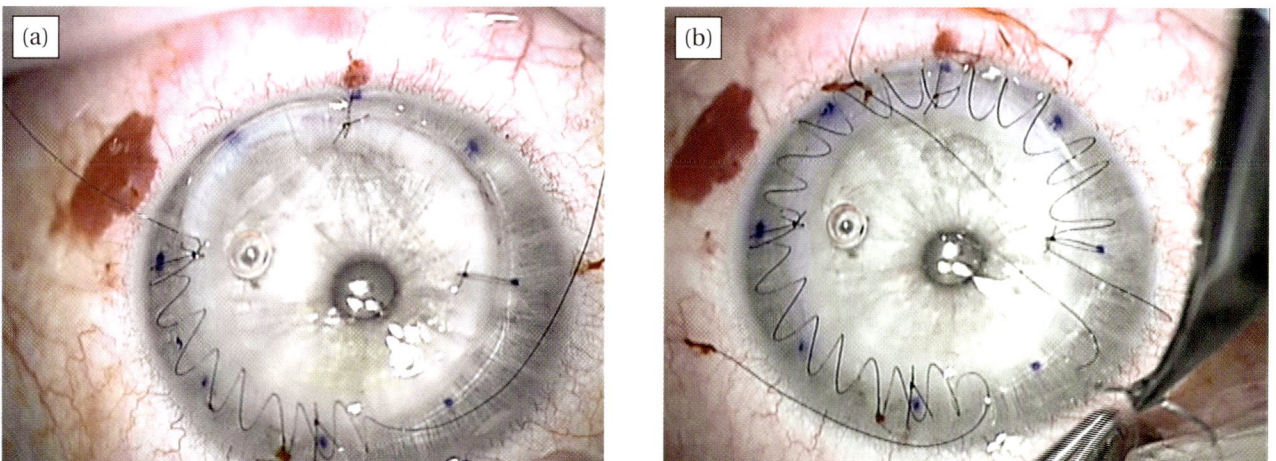

FIGURE 28.12 Suturing of graft. The donor cornea is then sutured into place using whatever suturing style is the surgeon's preference. In this case, a running suture is employed. Note the radial alignment marks (a, b).

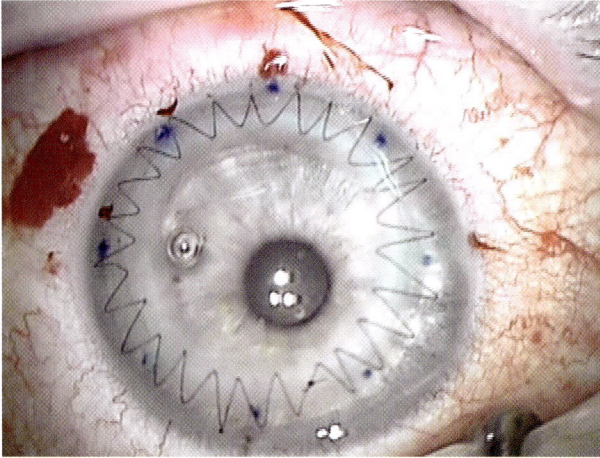

FIGURE 28.13 End of case. At the end of the case, the cardinal sutures are removed and the suture is tightened and tied with care to bury the knot. Subconjunctival injections of steroid and antibiotic are then placed.

Operative: FLK-DALK

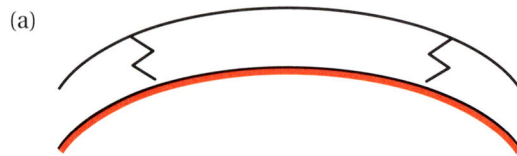

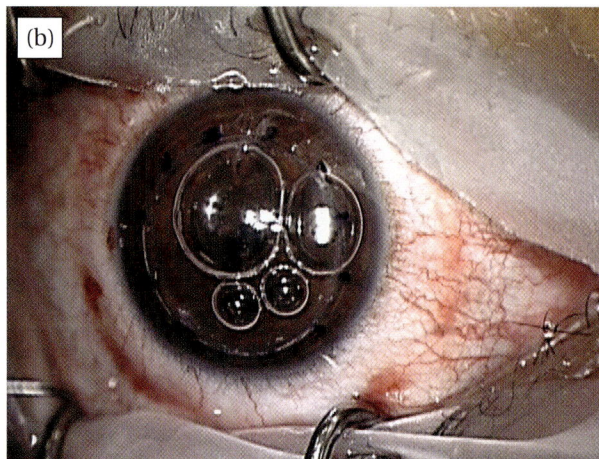

FIGURE 28.14 Femtosecond Laser Keratoplasty—Deep Anterior Lamellar Keratoplasty (FLK-DALK). "Mini-bubble in anterior chamber." Deep Anterior Lamellar Keratoplasty (DALK) can be used to address stromal disease while preserving the patient's non-diseased endothelium. (a) The initial laser cut is carried out in the manner described above. After teasing apart the incision, a paracentesis is made and a "mini-bubble" is placed in the anterior chamber (b).

(a)

(b)

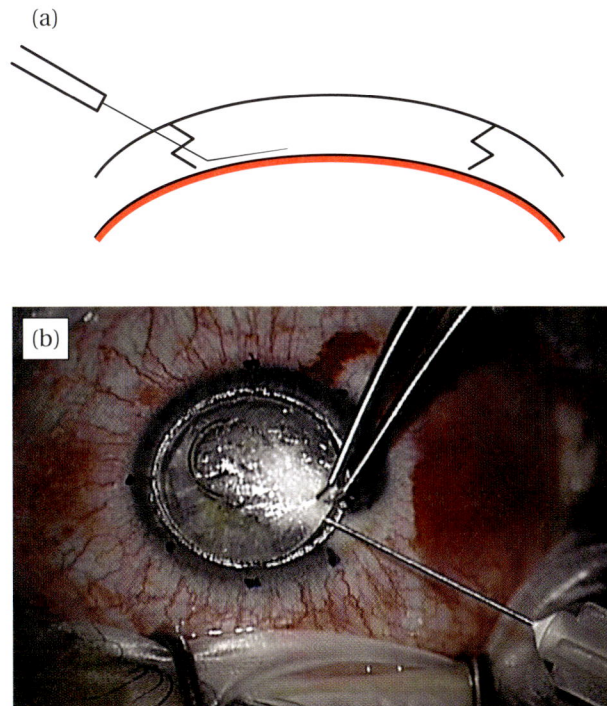

FIGURE 28.15 FLK-DALK—placement of 27g needle. A 27g needle is then placed at the depth of the posterior side cut and advanced centrally, using the "mini-bubble" as a guide to delineate Descemet's membrane (a,b).

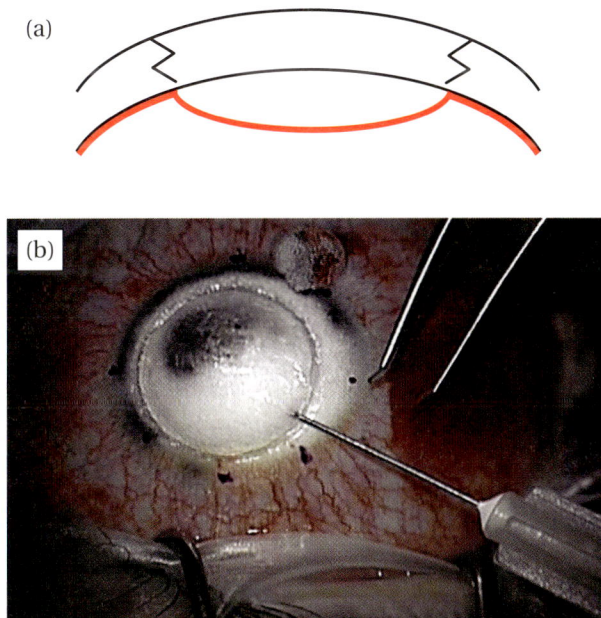

(a)

(b)

FIGURE 28.16 FLK-DALK—insufflation. Once the needle is deemed to be at the appropriate location, air is insufflated to bare Descemet's membrane from the overlying stroma. If this occurs, the "mini-bubble" should be displaced peripherally, signifying a posterior displacement of Descemet's membrane (a, b).

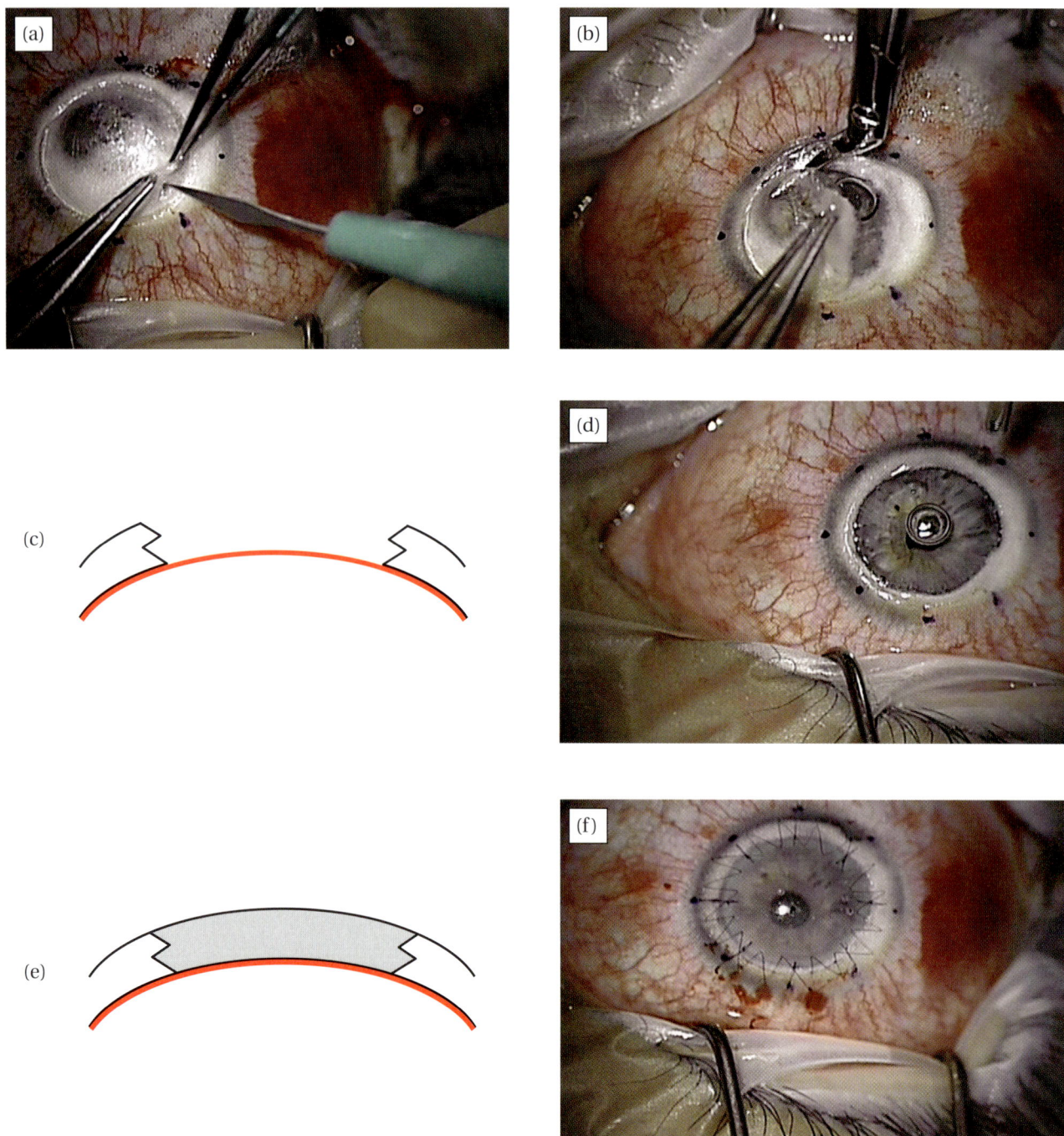

FIGURE 28.17 FLK-DALK—removal of stroma. Once Descemet's membrane is separated from the overlying stroma, viscoelastic is placed in the interface to protect Descemet's membrane, and the stroma is removed (a, b). If done successfully, a clear intact Descemet's membrane remains (c, d). The endothelium from the donor graft is then removed. The graft is then sutured into place (e, f).

Postoperative

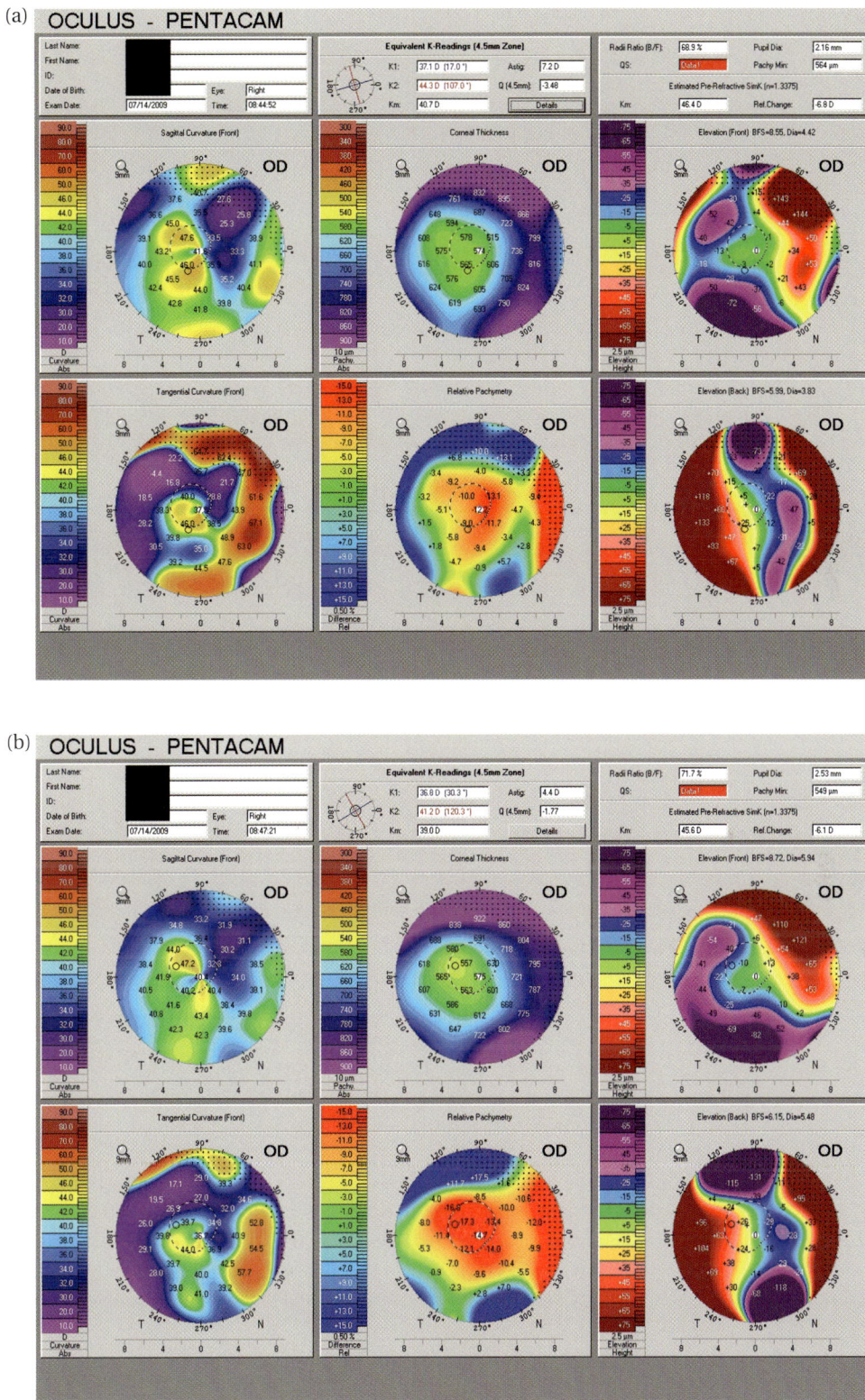

(a)

(b)

FIGURE 28.18 Astigmatism and suture adjustment. If a running suture is employed, astigmatism can be managed at the slit lamp by adjusting the suture distribution. The suture in the flat meridian is fed to the steep meridian to decrease the amount of astigmatism. (a) Pentacam topography prior to adjustment. (b) Pentacam topography immediately after suture adjustment at slit lamp.

(c)

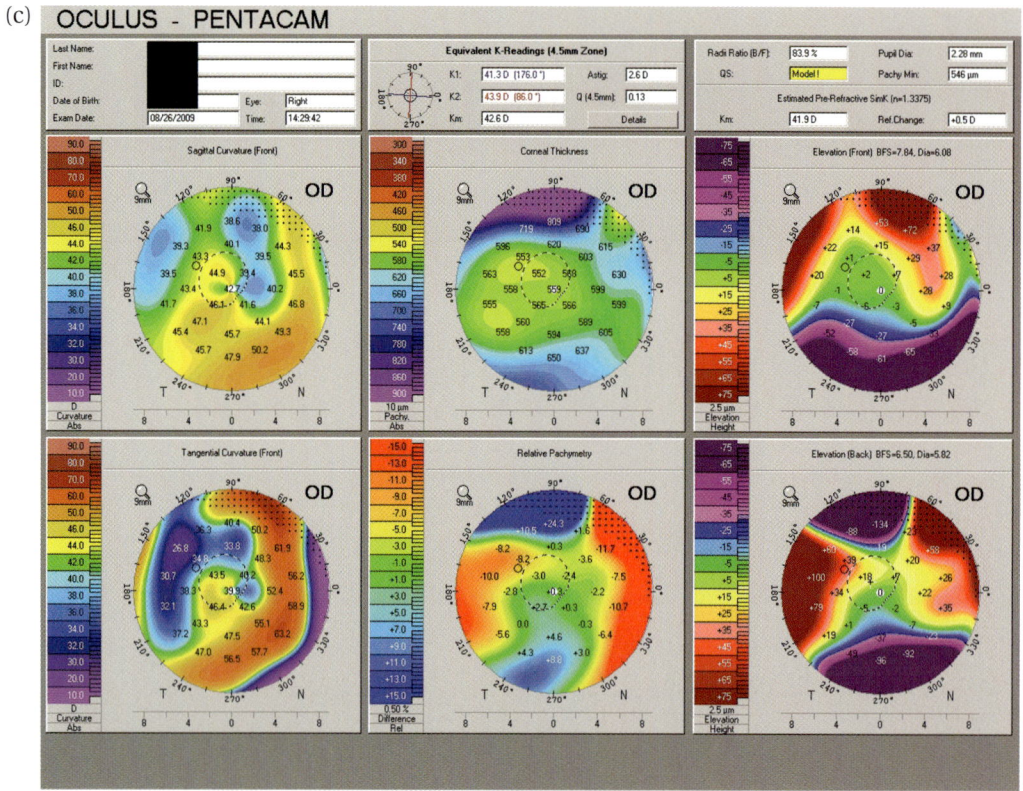

FIGURE 28.18 (*continued*) (c) Six weeks after suture adjustment.

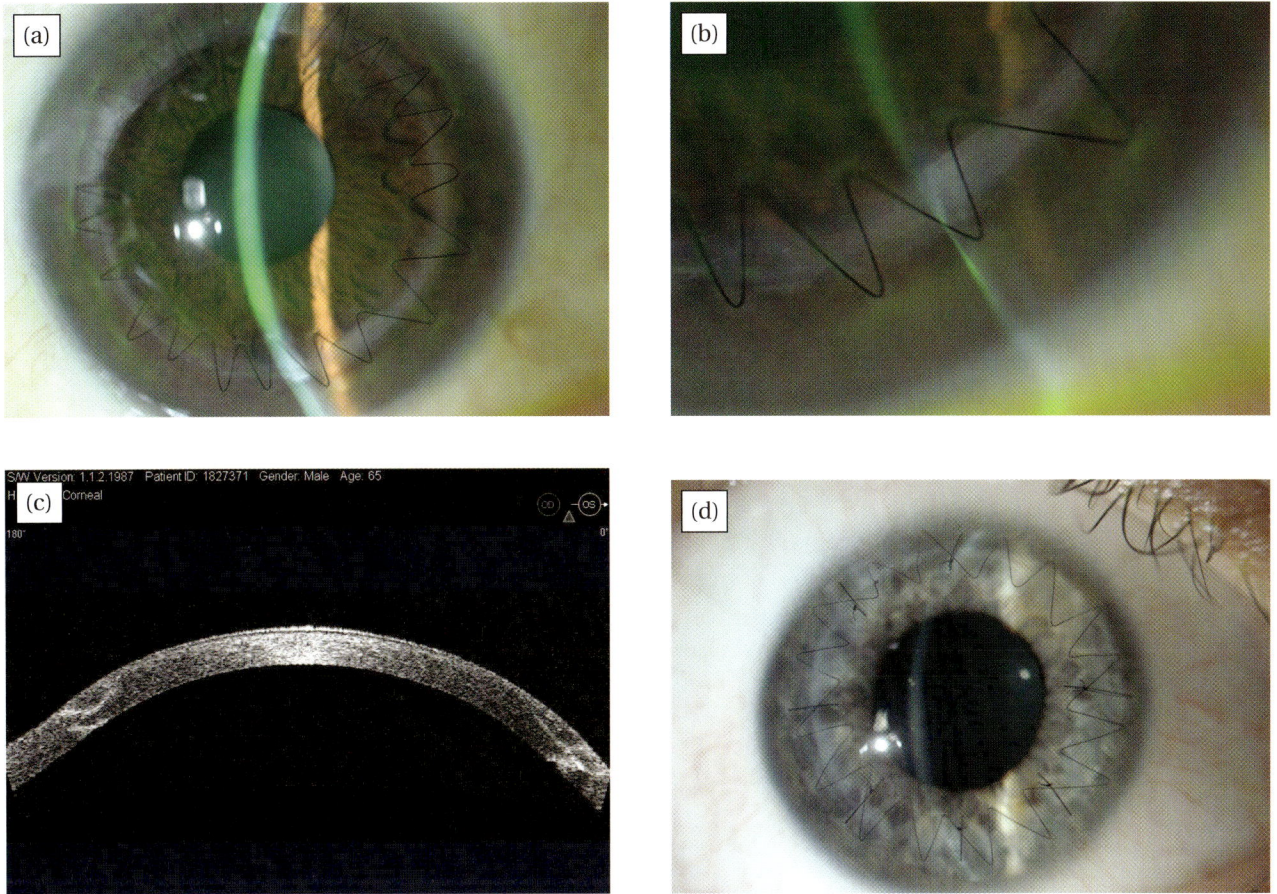

FIGURE 28.19 Wound healing. A femtosecond laser keratoplasty allows for a hermetic wound with smooth anterior and posterior surfaces, as demonstrated in this slit lamp photo (a), high magnification slit lamp photo (b), and anterior segment OCT (c). Similar results are found with the FLK-DALK (d).

TABLE 28.3 *Potential Complications*

Loss of suction during laser cut

Incomplete laser cut

Full thickness penetration during laser cut

Complications common to traditional corneal transplantation

SELECTED REFERENCES

Farid M, Kim M, Steinert RF. Results of penetrating keratoplasty performed with a femtosecond laser zigzag incision initial report. *Ophthalmology.* 2007 Dec;114(12):2208–2212.

Farid M, Steinert RF. Deep anterior lamellar keratoplasty performed with the femtosecond laser zigzag incision for the treatment of stromal corneal pathology and ectatic disease. *J Cataract Refract Surg.* 2009;35(5):809–813.

Farid M, Steinert RF, Gaster RN, Chamberlain W, Lin A. Comparison of penetrating keratoplasty performed with a femtosecond laser zig-zag incision versus conventional blade trephination. *Ophthalmology.* 2009;116(9):1638–1643.

Steinert RF, Ignacio TS, Sarayba MA. "Top hat"-shaped penetrating keratoplasty using the femtosecond laser. *Am J Ophthalmol.* 2007 Apr;143(4):689–691.

Corneal and Scleral Lacerations

Matthew F. Gardiner, MD

TABLE 29.1 *Indications for Surgical Repair of Corneoscleral Lacerations*

Full thickness corneal laceration with:
  (1) Seidel positivity (either spontaneously or with provocation)
  (2) Unformed chamber
  (3) Tissue incarceration

Partial thickness corneal lacerations:
  (1) Not amenable to gluing (i.e., large, displaced/shelved flap)
  (2) Inability to tolerate bandage contact lens

Full thickness scleral lacerations

Partial thickness scleral lacerations with:
  (1) Severe wound gape/scleral thinning
  (2) Disruption of overlying anatomy which is unlikely to stay in apposition

Corneal Sutures—General Principles

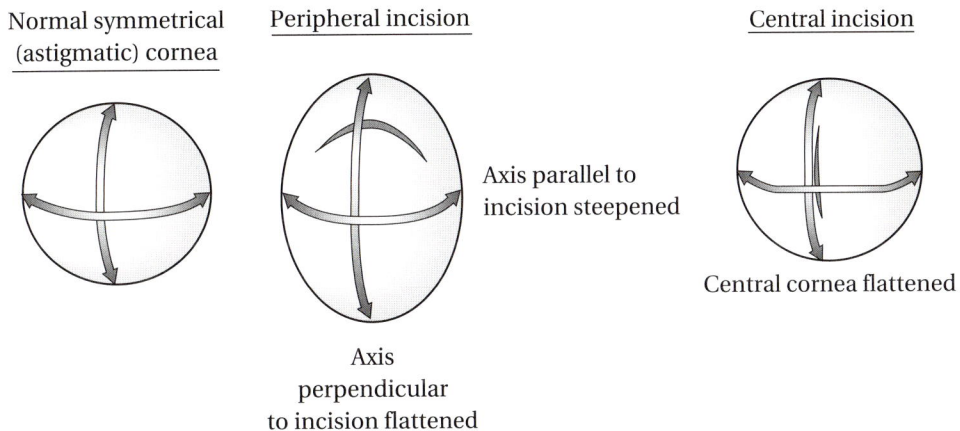

FIGURE 29.1 Effects of peripheral and central corneal incisions on corneal curvature. The cornea tends to flatten over lacerations. Lacerations that are long or close to the visual axis induce greater flattening.

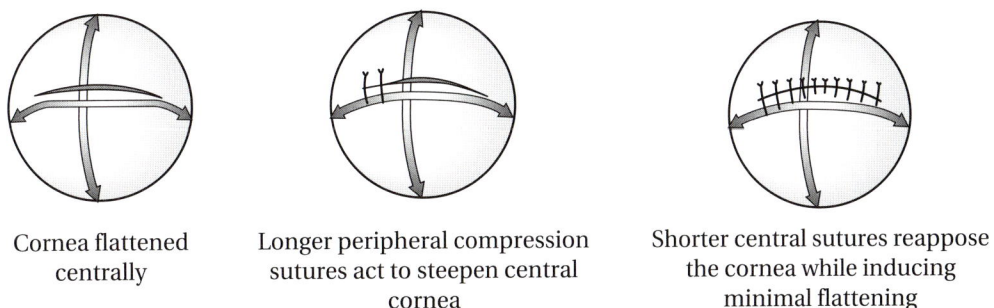

FIGURE 29.2 Suture technique to normalize corneal curvature after lacerations. Large compressive sutures are used to close the peripheral aspects of the corneal laceration that flatten the peripheral cornea and steepen the central cornea. The central aspect of the laceration is then closed using smaller and looser suture bites to approximate the wound edges without causing excessive distortion. Suture passes should be approximately 1.5—2.0 mm total in length. Suture knots should be tied with either 3-1-1 or 2-1-1 throws, and the loose ends cut short with fine scissors or a 15° (super-sharp) blade, then buried if possible.

Full Thickness Corneal Lacerations

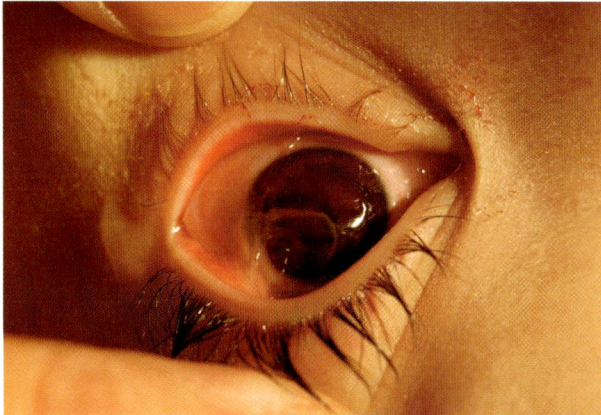

FIGURE 29.3 A full thickness corneal laceration with prolapsing iris resulting in an irregular pupil.

Simple Lacerations

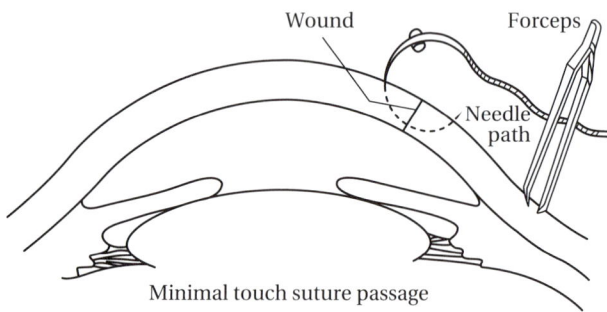

FIGURE 29.4 "Minimal touch" suture passage avoids manipulation of wound edges and flattening of the anterior chamber in wounds with a formed anterior chamber. The needle is directed into the cornea at a 90° angle and passed through the stroma following the curve of the needle.

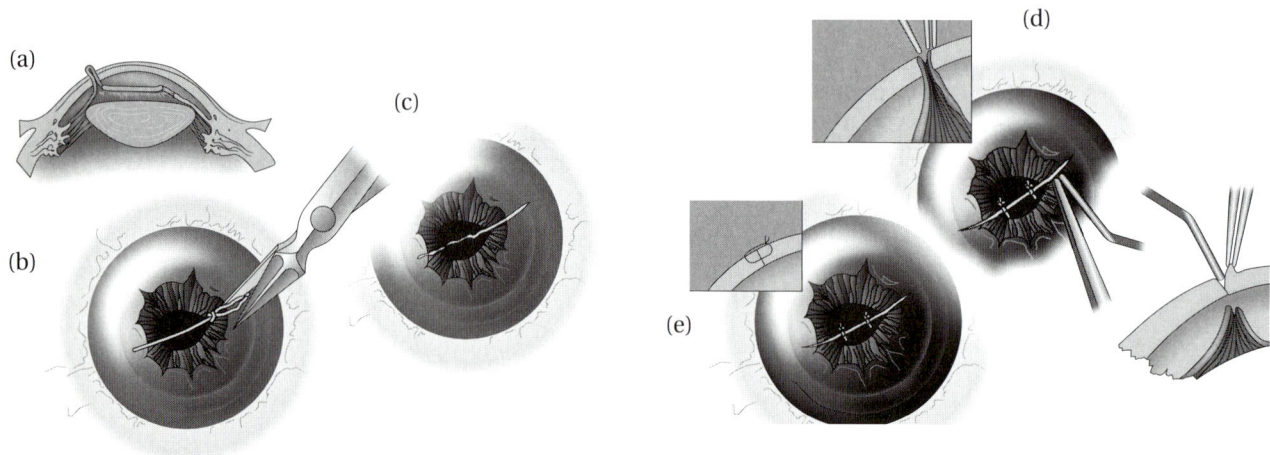

FIGURE 29.5 Prolapsed iris/uvea or other ocular contents should be reposited unless necrotic or infected. (a) Schematic diagram depicting corneal laceration with incarcerated uveal tissue. (b) Tissue is trimmed with scissors at the plane of the corneal surface. (c) Majority of uveal tissue has been freed from the corneal laceration site, although incarcerated tissue may remain at the inner surface of the wound. (d) Residual prolapsed tissue is reposited with a spatula, directly through the wound site. (e) Once residual incarcerated tissue is freed, 10-0 nylon sutures are placed through the corneal laceration, restoring integrity of the globe.

(a)

(b)

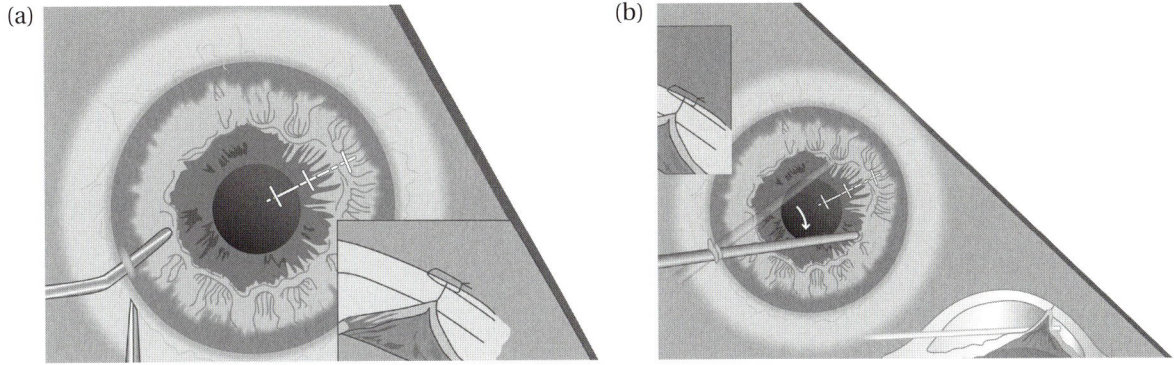

FIGURE 29.6 Uveal tissue may remain entrapped in the inner portion of a corneal laceration following closure of the wound. (a) The anterior chamber is deepened with BSS or viscoelastic. (b) Through the previous paracentesis site, a cyclodialysis spatula or cannula is used to sweep incarcerated tissue from the wound.

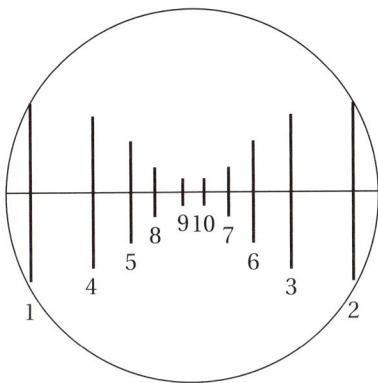

FIGURE 29.7 The order of suture introduction in the cornea. If the wound is long and transects the cornea, the risk of flattening the corneal dome shape by the scar is significant. To counter this effect, suture introduction should start from the two peripheries and with long bites; the bites get progressively shorter as the center is approached. In the apex of the cornea—the visual center—no suture should be placed unless absolutely necessary. The numbers indicate the order of suture placement. (Image courtesy of Springer and Dr. Ferenc Kuhn.)

Stellate Lacerations

"Blow-up" view
Cornea viewed "on edge"

Partial-thickness incisions

Suture

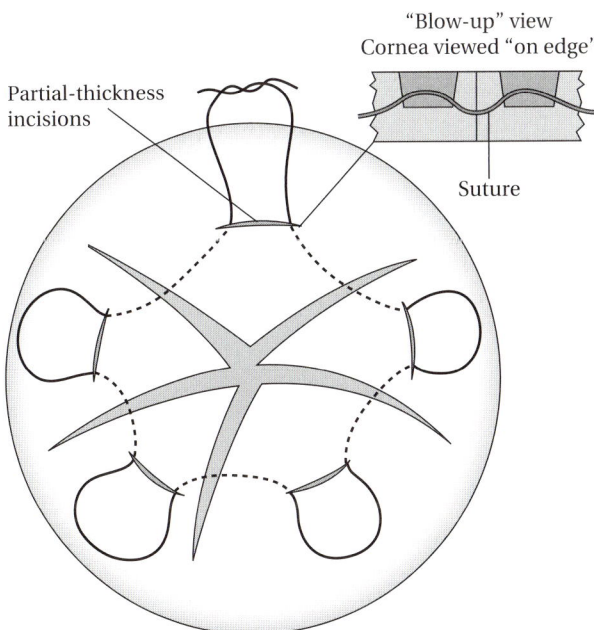

FIGURE 29.8 Stellate laceration repair. Partial-thickness incisions are made in each facet using a guarded (diamond) blade. A deep stromal continuous suture is passed. Additional interrupted sutures are placed to achieve a watertight closure. If there is persistent leakage from the wound, tissue adhesive and a bandage soft contact lens may be used.

Shelved Lacerations

(a)

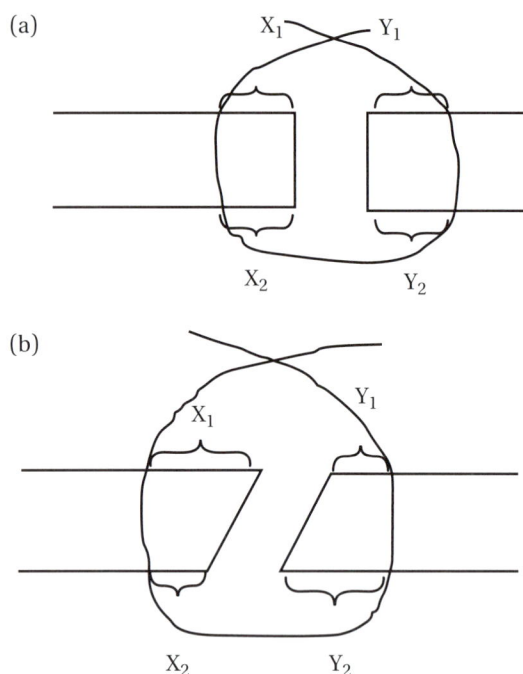

(b)

FIGURE 29.9 Closure of perpendicular vs. oblique (shelved) wounds. (a) If the wound's plane is close to vertical as it relates to the surface, the needle's entry and exit points should be at equal distance from the wound on both the epithelial and endothelial surfaces ($X_1 = Y_1$) and ($X_2 = Y_2$). (b) If the wound's plane is oblique, use of full thickness sutures becomes especially crucial. The distances as measured for needle entry and exit relative to the edge of the wound need to be modified so as to create the same compression on either side. As shown, the epithelial distance on one side is matched up with the endothelial distance on the other side ($X_1 = Y_2$) and ($X_2 = Y_1$). This technique prevents tissue override which is a permanent abnormality. (Image courtesy of Springer and Dr. Ferenc Kuhn.)

Full Thickness vs. Partial Thickness Sutures

There has been debate over the use of partial thickness vs. full thickness suture passes for repair of corneal lacerations. The classic "90%" depth teaching has advocated that the risk of infection (especially endophthalmitis) is reduced by preventing the formation of a pathway for bacteria to enter the anterior chamber via the suture track. The risk of infection during suture removal is also theoretically reduced since externally contaminated suture material is not pulled through into the anterior chamber on cutting and extracting the suture.

Placing full thickness sutures may provide improved closure of the endothelial side of the wound and help to minimize corneal edema. In particular, tissue misalignment may occur as the surgeon attempts to find the 90% depth level on each side, providing a pathway for the entry of fluid into the stroma (Kuhn, page 173). Animal data, however, suggests that full thickness corneal sutures may induce long-term damage to Descemet's and the endothelial cells (Binder PS, Arch Opthalmol. 1978 Oct;96(10):1886–1890).

Corneoscleral Lacerations

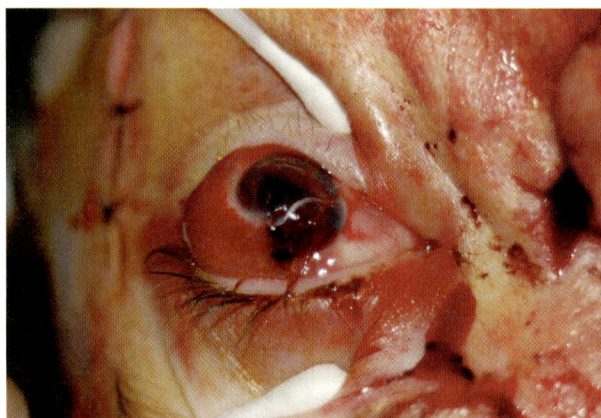

FIGURE 29.10 A full thickness corneoscleral laceration. There is extensive hyphema and clot extrusion with uveal prolapse. The anatomic relationship of the limbus, cornea and sclera has been disrupted.

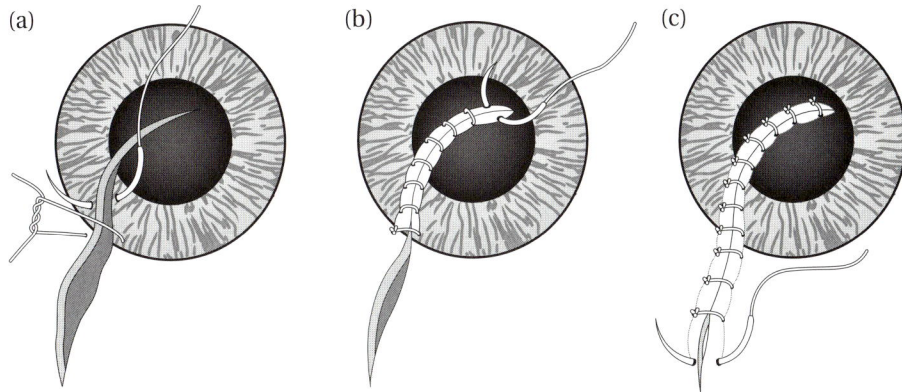

FIGURE 29.11 (a) Schematic diagram showing a corneoscleral laceration. The initial suture is placed at the limbus where the surgeon can precisely reapproximate the proper alignment of the tissue. (b) Corneal portion of wound is closed with interrupted 10-0 nylon sutures. (c) Scleral portion of wound is closed, generally with either 8-0 or 9-0 nylon sutures making certain to fully explore the most posterior extent of the laceration.

Scleral Lacerations

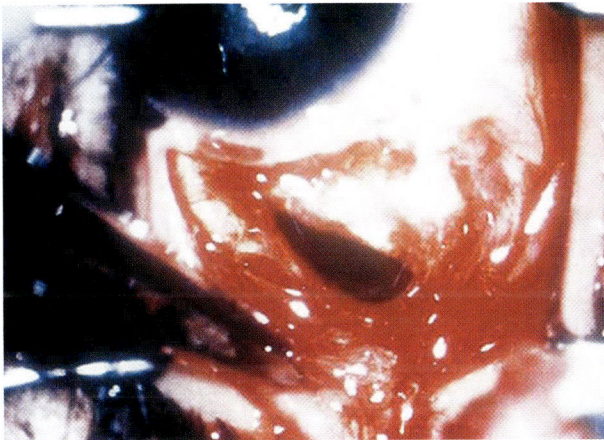

FIGURE 29.12 Open globe injury caused by a sharp object has produced a 6 mm scleral laceration with prolapse of uveal tissue. It is imperative to determine the complete extent of the laceration by performing a careful exploration and examination prior to repair.

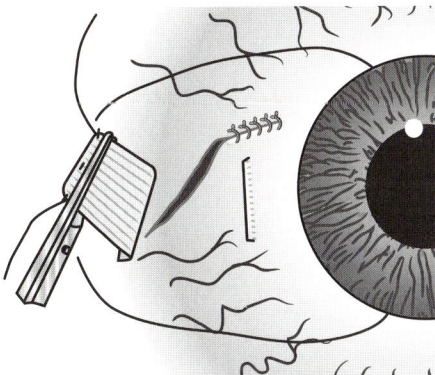

FIGURE 29.13 If exploration of the wound leads the surgeon underneath a rectus muscle, it may be necessary to remove the muscle temporarily from its anterior insertion to complete the repair. During these maneuvers, great care must be taken to avoid undue pressure on the globe. Though it is prudent to attempt to find the posterior termination of a scleral wound, it may be impossible to safely close it completely. If finding the end of the wound requires significant traction on the globe, such that expulsion of intraocular contents is risked, then its remainder should be left open. Sutures for the sclera are generally 8-0 in size and can be nylon, vicryl, prolene, or silk (which can be white for improved cosmesis). Prolapsed uveal tissue should be preserved and reposited, if at all possible. Tissue that is frankly necrotic, infiltrated with debris, or externalized for >24 hours may need to be excised. Excision of choroid or ciliary body should be avoided if at all possible, since severe hemorrhage can result.

TABLE 29.2 *Complications of Repair (by post-op time frame)*

Early (0–2 weeks)

1. Infection
   (a) local
      1. cellulitis
      2. ulcer
      3. scleritis
      4. endophthalmitis
   (b) systemic
      1. sepsis
2. Hemorrhage
   (a) anterior chamber (hyphema)
   (b) vitreous
   (c) choroid (expulsive)
   (d) orbit (compartment syndrome)
3. Wound leak—hypotony/choroidal effusion
4. Hemodynamic instability/death (from ocular manipulation)

Middle (2–8 weeks)

1. Glaucoma
   (a) ghost cell/hyphema
   (b) lens particle
   (c) angle closure/PAS
   (d) angle recession
2. Retinal detachment/PVR

Late (>8 weeks)

1. Refractive
   (a) aphakia
   (b) astigmatism
   (c) corneal scarring
2. Pain—phthisis bulbi
3. Sympathetic ophthalmia
4. Other
   (a) ptosis
   (b) mydriasis
   (c) poor cosmetic appearance of globe

SELECTED REFERENCES

Beatty RF, Beatty RL. The repair of corneal and scleral lacerations. *Semin Ophthalmol*. 1994;9:165–176.

Binder PS. Evaluation of through-and-through corneal sutures. *Arch Ophthalmol*. 1978;96(10):1886–1890.

Hamill MB, Thompson WS. The evaluation and management of corneal lacerations. *Retina*. 1990;10:S1–S7.

Kuhn F. *Ocular Traumatology*. Heidelberg: Springer; 2008.

Rowsey JJ, Hays JC. Refractive reconstruction in acute eye injuries. *Ophthalmic Surg*. 1984; 15:569–574.

Rowsey JJ. Ten caveats in keratorefractive surgery. *Ophthalmology*.1983;90:148–155.

Glaucoma Surgery

Edited by **Peter A. Netland**

30 Laser Iridotomy and Peripheral Iridoplasty

Christopher C. Teng, MD and Jeffrey M. Liebmann, MD

TABLE 30.1　*Indications*

Laser Iridotomy	Peripheral Iridoplasty
Iridotrabecular contact of any cause with or without peripheral anterior synechiae*	Iridotrabecular contact after laser iridotomy**
Acute angle closure glaucoma	Acute angle closure glaucoma
	To facilitate laser trabeculoplasty

* May be due to relative or complete pupillary block, plateau iris, peripheral iris crowding, lens induced (phacomorphic, subluxation, microspherophakia), silicone oil, anterior displacement of lens iris diaphragm, or vitreoretinal etiology

** May be due to plateau iris syndrome, nanophthalmos, lens intumescence.

TABLE 30.2　*Settings*

Laser Iridotomy	Peripheral Iridoplasty
Argon laser	Argon laser
Lens: Abraham lens	Lens: Abraham lens
Duration: 0.02–0.1 seconds	Duration: 0.5–0.7 seconds
Spot size: 50 μm	Spot Size: 500 μm
Power: 300–1500 mW	Power: 200–500 mW
	20–24 spots over 360°
Nd:YAG laser	
Lens: Abraham lens	
Energy: 1–5 mJ	
Pulses per burst: 1–3	

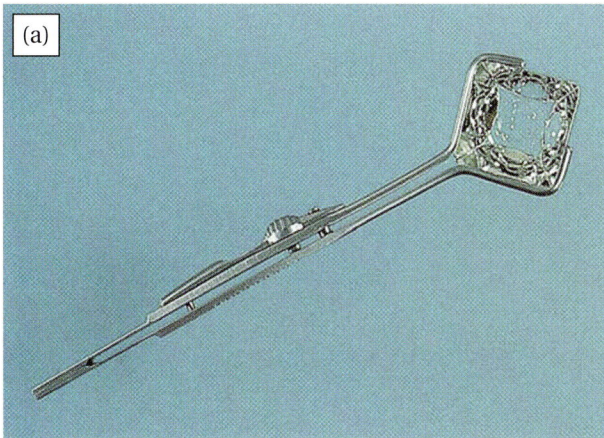

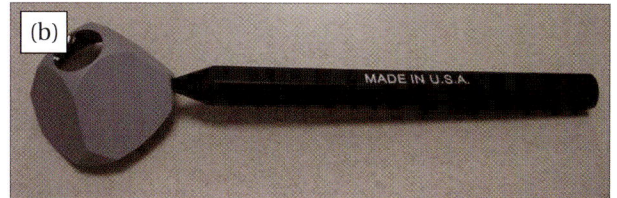

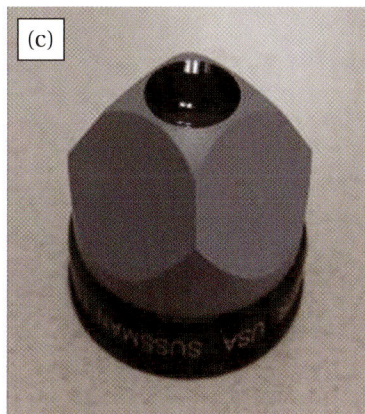

FIGURE 30.1 **(a) Zeiss (b) Posner and (c) Sussman Indentation Gonioprisms.** These lenses have surface area in contact with the cornea that is smaller than the area of the cornea itself, which allows for indentation of the cornea with gentle pressure. Indentation gonioscopy assists in accurately diagnosing narrow or closed anterior chamber angles.

(a)

(b)

Appositional
closure

Synechial
closure

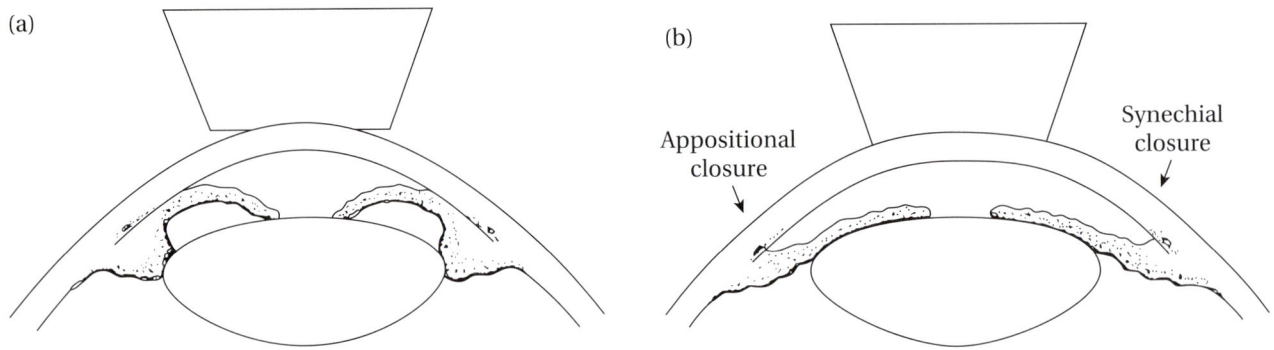

FIGURE 30.2 **Indentation Gonioscopy.** (a) During gonioscopy with the Zeiss, Posner or Sussman gonioprism, the cornea retains its normal configuration. In this drawing, the iris has a convex or "bombé" configuration with a closed angle. (b) During indentation, gentle pressure on the central part of the cornea causes it to flatten posteriorly, shallowing the central part of the anterior chamber. The displaced aqueous is forced into the angle recess and opens areas of appositional angle closure. Regions of synechial angle closure will remain closed. (Drawing by Richi Saito.)

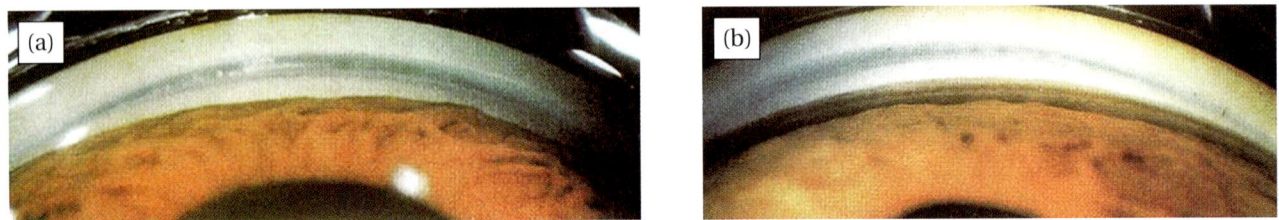

(a)

(b)

FIGURE 30.3 **Indentation Gonioscopy Clinical Appearance.** (a) Goniophotograph of an appositionally closed angle in an eye with relative pupillary block. (b) With gentle pressure during indentation gonioscopy, the angle opens uniformly, revealing the angle structures. (From *Clinical Atlas of Glaucoma*, Van Buskirk, 1986.)

Angle-Closure Glanucoma

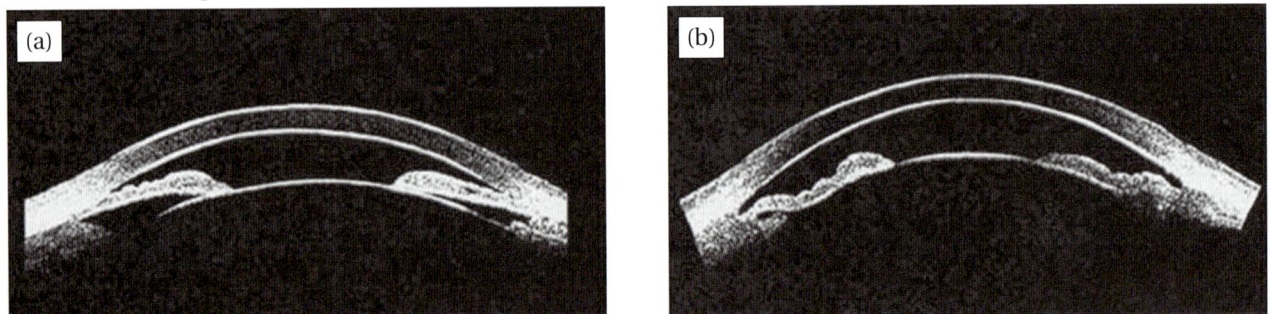

(a)

(b)

FIGURE 30.4 **Ultrasound Biomicrograph before and after Peripheral Iridotomy.** The eye has both relative pupillary block and a shallow anterior chamber. (a) Relative pupillary block angle closure before laser iridotomy. (b) Following laser iridotomy, the iris moves posteriorly and assumes a flat configuration, and the angle opens.

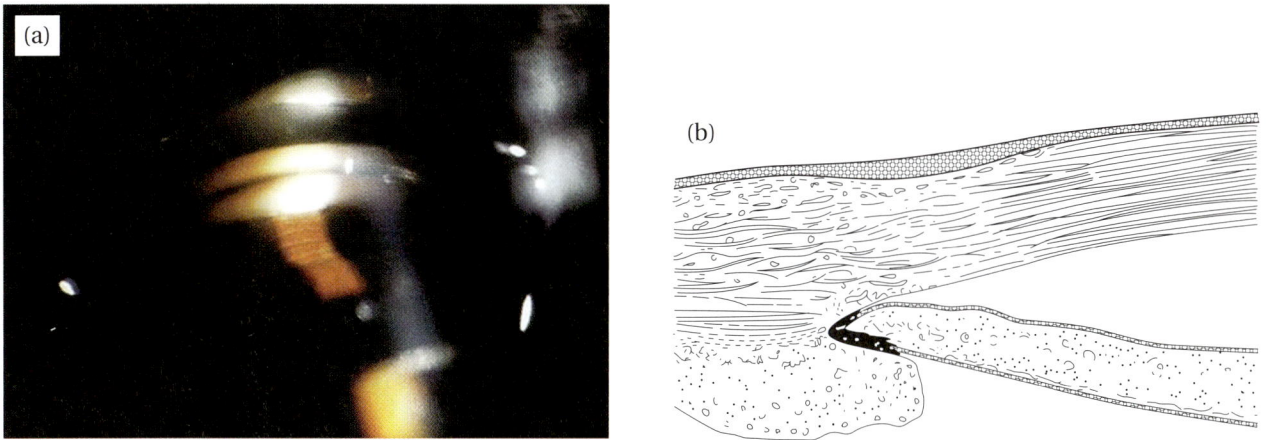

FIGURE 30.5 **Photograph and Line Diagram of Plateau Iris Configuration.** (a) Indentation gonioscopy of plateau iris with a double hump iris configuration. Note that the deepest portion of the anterior chamber is between the lens equator and the ciliary body. (b) Diagram of an eye with plateau iris showing anterior extension of the ciliary body supporting the iris root against the trabecular meshwork.

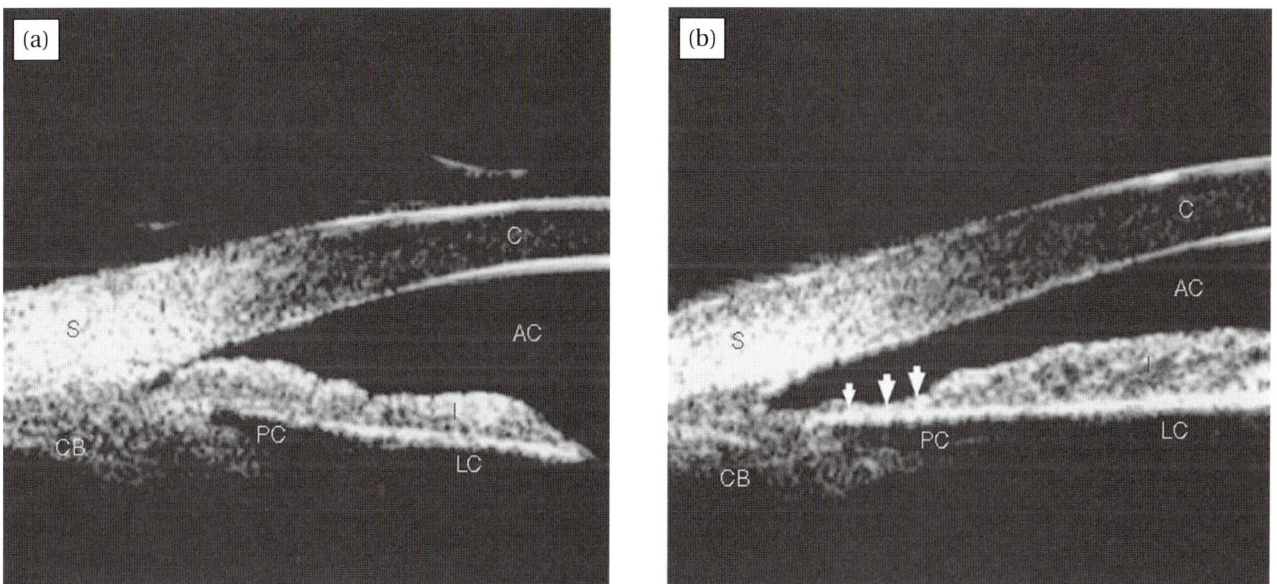

FIGURE 30.6 **Ultrasound Biomicrograph of Plateau Iris.** (a) Ultrasound biomicrograph of plateau iris after laser iridotomy, showing a flat iris without bombé and forward rotation of the ciliary body against peripheral iris. (b) The same eye following peripheral iridoplasty, with the laser spot (arrows) causing contraction and compaction of the iris posteriorly away from the meshwork and angle. S indicates sclera, C = cornea, CB = ciliary body, PC = posterior chamber, AC = anterior chamber, and LC = lens capsule.

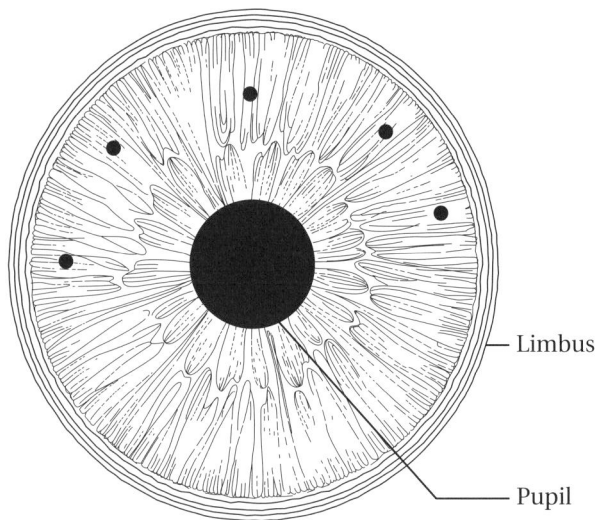

FIGURE 30.7 **Peripheral Iridotomy Technique.** Following pretreatment with pilocarpine and an alpha-2 agonist, the eye is topically anesthetized and the patient seated at the laser slit lamp biomicroscope. An Abraham iridectomy lens may be used. A thin area or large iris crypt is identified in the superior-temporal, superior-nasal, nasal or temporal quadrant. The iridotomy is created in the peripheral third of iris. Treatment is continued until aqueous and pigment is seen to emerge from the posterior to anterior chamber. Potential locations for iridotomy are depicted in the figure.

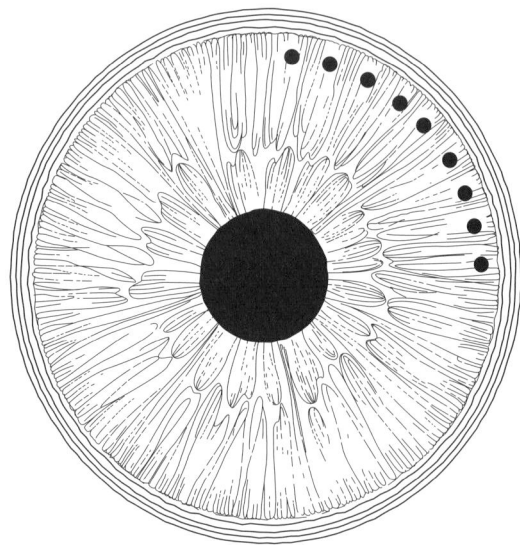

FIGURE 30.8 **Peripheral Iridoplasty Technique.** Following pretreatment with pilocarpine and an alpha-2 agonist, the eye is topically anesthetized and the patient seated at the laser slit lamp biomicroscope. An Abraham iridectomy lens may be used. 20–24 spots are placed over 360°. The laser pedal should be depressed for the entire duration of the burn.

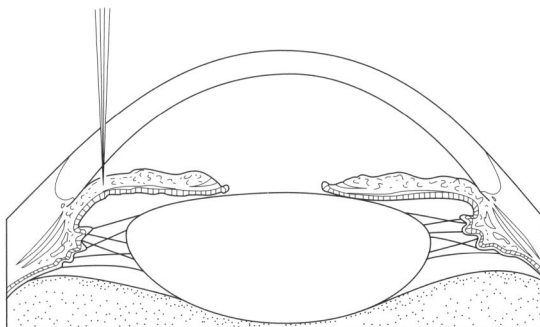

FIGURE 30.9 **Burn Placement for Argon Laser Peripheral Iridoplasty.** Laser spots are placed at the most peripheral portion of the iris, as close to the limbus as possible. One common error is spot placement in the mid-periphery of the iris.

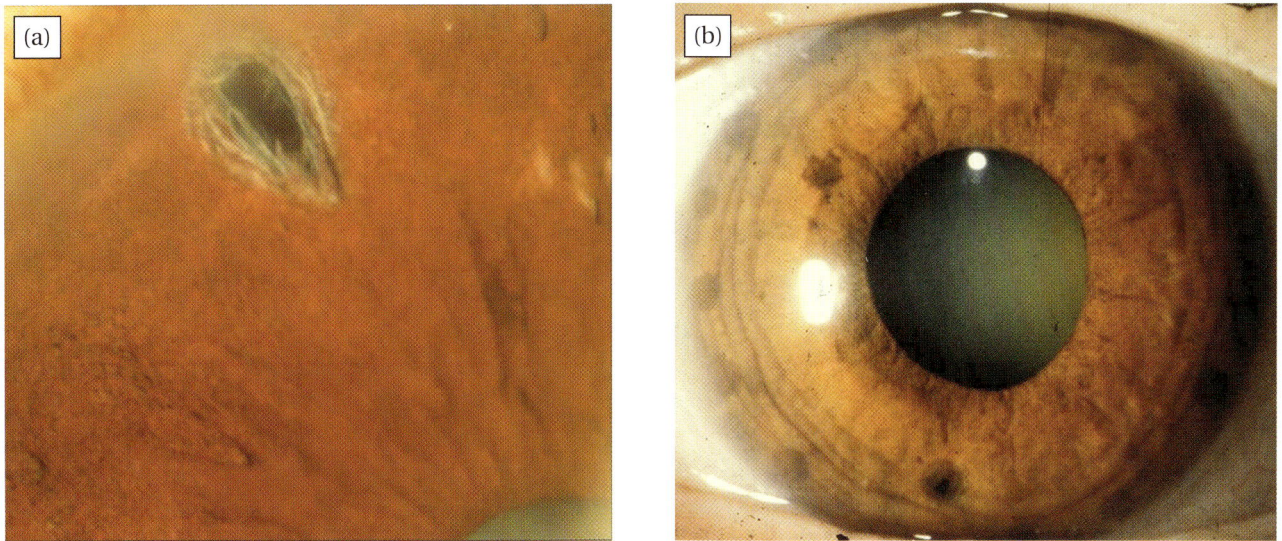

FIGURE 30.10 **Clinical Photographs of Iridotomy and Iridoplasty.** (a) Well placed patent laser iridotomy. (b) Well placed peripheral iridoplasty, with an inferior laser iridotomy.

TABLE 30.3 *Complications*

Laser Iridotomy	Peripheral Iridoplasty
Transient IOP rise	Transient IOP rise
Iritis	Iritis
Corneal damage	Corneal damage
Glare/diplopia	Corectopia/Dilated pupil
Hyphema	Iris atrophy
Focal, localized lens opacity	
Malignant Glaucoma (rare)	
Retina damage (rare)	

SELECTED REFERENCES

Allingham RR, Damji KF, Freedman SF, Moroi SE, Shafranov G. *Shields' Textbook of Glaucoma,* 5th ed. Philadelphia: Lippincott Williams & Wilkins, 2005.

Liebmann JM, Ritch R. Laser surgery for angle closure glaucoma. *Semin Ophthalmol.* 2002;17:84–91.

Ritch R, Shields MB, Krupin T, (eds). *The Glaucomas, Volume 2,* 2nd ed. St. Louis: Mosby-Year Book, 1996.

Ritch R, Tham CC, Lam DS. Argon laser peripheral iridoplasty (ALPI): an update. *Surv Ophthalmol.* 2007;52:279–88.

Shaarawy T, Sherwood MB, Hitchings RA, Crowston JG. *Glaucoma, Volume 2: Surgical Management,* 1st ed. London: W.B. Saunders, 2009.

Tello C, Tran HV, Liebmann J, Ritch R. Angle closure: classification, concepts, and the role of ultrasound biomicroscopy in diagnosis and treatment. *Semin Ophthalmol.* 2002;17:69–78.

Van Buskirk M. *Clinical Atlas of Glaucoma,* 1st ed. Philadelphia: W.B. Saunders, 1986.

31 Laser Trabeculoplasty

Lama A. Al-Aswad, MD and Daniel S. Casper, MD, PhD

TABLE 31.1 *Indications*

Indication *(initial or on maximal medical therapy)*	Contraindication
Chronic open angle glaucoma	Primary or secondary angle closure glaucoma
Pseudoexfoliation glaucoma	Angle-recession glaucoma
Pigmentary glaucoma	Uveitic glaucoma
Secondary open angle glaucoma	Congenital glaucoma

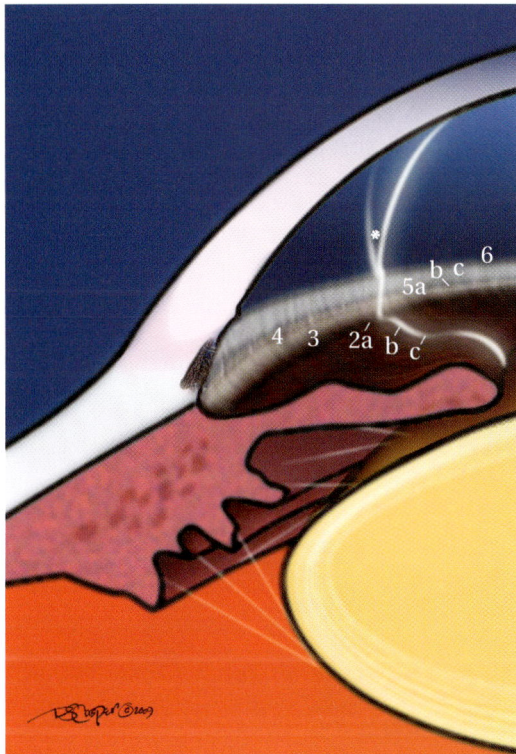

FIGURE 31.1 Gonioscopic appearance of a normal anterior chamber angle. *2a:* Peripheral iris insertion; *b* and *c,* curvature. 3: Ciliary body band. 4: Scleral spur. 5: Trabecular meshwork: *a,* posterior; *b,* mid; *c,* anterior. 6: Schwalbe's line. *Asterisk:* Corneal optical wedge.

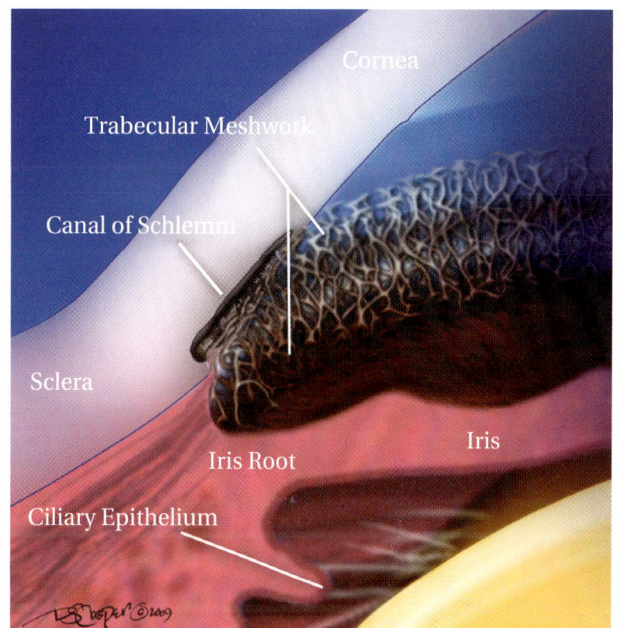

FIGURE 31.2 Schematic diagram of anterior chamber angle, iris root, and corneoscleral junction.

TABLE 31.2 *Settings*

	Argon Laser (ALT)	Diode Laser (DLT)	Selective Laser (SLT)	Micropulse (MLT)
Spot size (µm)	50	75–100	400	300
Duration	0.1–0.2 s	0.1–0.2 s	3 nsec	200 ms (100 laser spot with 300 µs on each separated by 1700 µs off)
Power	700–1200 mW	700–1400 mW	0.5–1.2 mJ	2000 mW
Application (over 180°)	50	50	50–75	50–70

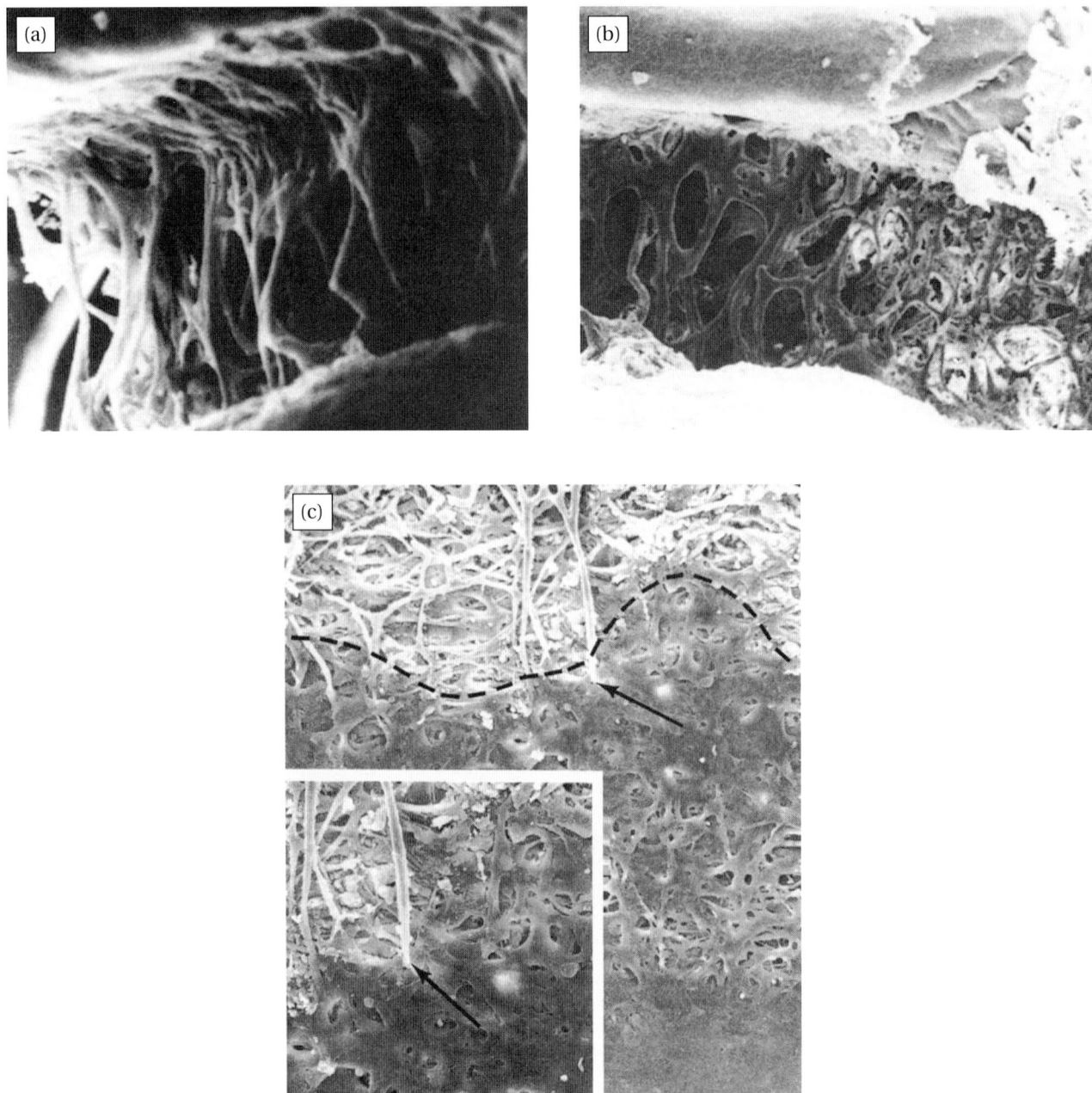

FIGURE 31.3 Scanning electron micrograph (SEM) of monkey anterior chamber angle. (a) Normal SEM Cebus monkey angle. Note the smooth beams of the trabecular meshwork and the even transition into the corneal endothelium. (Reprinted with permission from Warthen DM, Wickam MG, Laser Trabeculectomy in monkeys. *Invest Ophthalmol Vis Sci.* 1973;12:707–711.) (b) SEM Cebus monkey angle immediately after laser trabeculoplasty that received several bursts of 200 mW laser energy for 0.2 seconds and 50 μm spot size. The differential effect between the denuded corneal endothelium above, and the less affected trabeculum below, appears due to the number of individual bursts delivered in each location. The opening is treated trabeculum, which appears smaller than those present in the untreated area. (Reprinted with permission from Warthen DM, Wickam MG, Laser Trabeculectomy in monkeys. *Invest Ophthalmol Vis Sci,* 1973;12:707–711). (c) Eighteen hours after treatment with argon laser energy. The burn area showing coagulative necrosis is the area below the dotted line. Note the fragmented trabecular beam (arrow) at the edge of the lesions. Higher magnification of the same fragment beam (arrow). (Reprinted with permission from Rodrigues MM, Spaeth GL, Donohoo P. Electron microscopy of argon laser therapy in phakic open-angle glaucoma. *Ophthalmology.* 1982;89:198–210.)

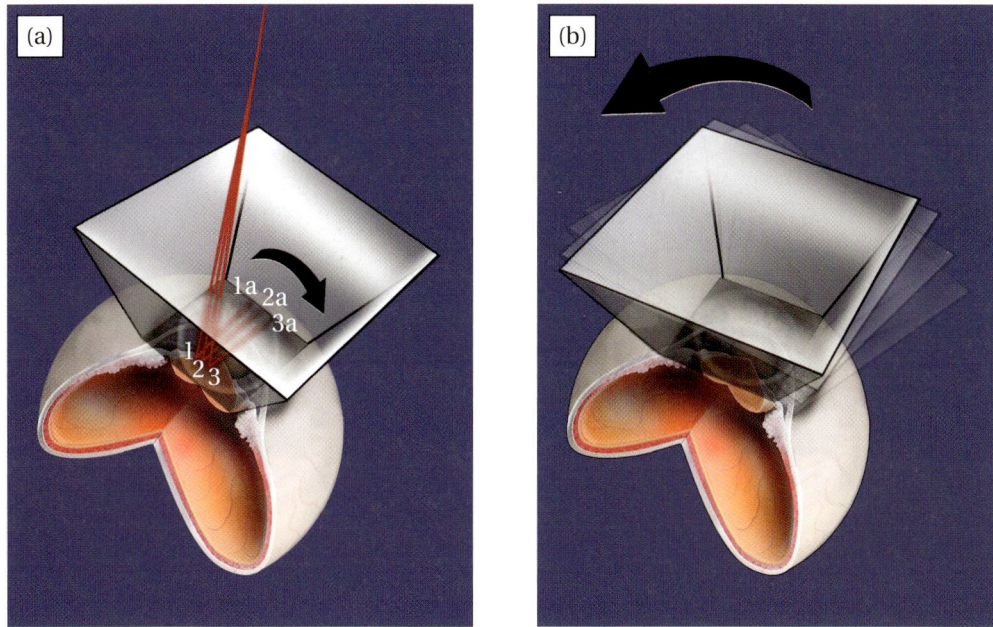

FIGURE 31.4 Trabeculoplasty Technique. In order to treat the superior nasal angle in the right eye, place spots in the inferior mirror from left to right (a). In order to move to an untreated area, move the laser back to the left side of the mirror then rotate lens mirror clockwise to continue adding spots (b).

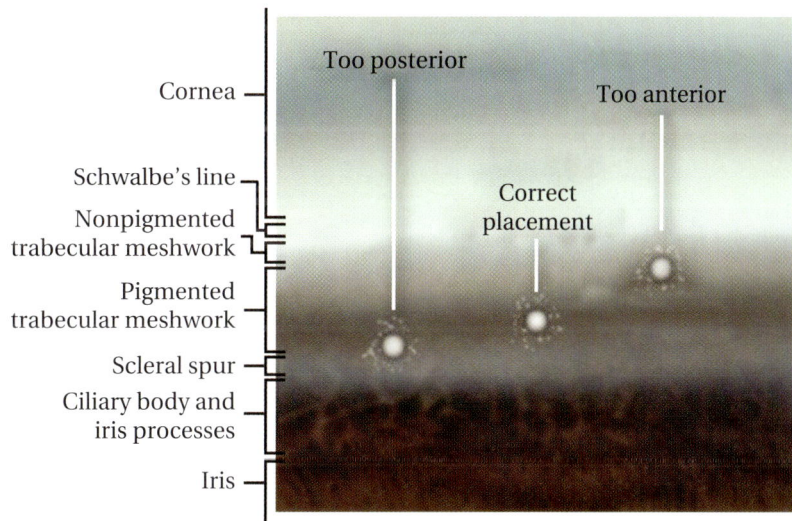

FIGURE 31.5 Placement of Laser Burns. Laser spots are placed in the mid or anterior one-third of the trabecular meshwork after pretreatment with α-2-agonist.

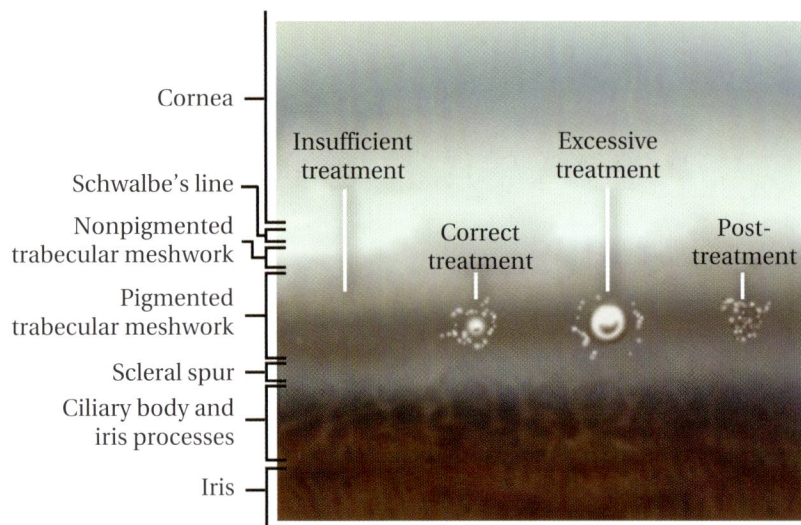

Cornea

Schwalbe's line

Nonpigmented
trabecular meshwork

Pigmented
trabecular meshwork

Scleral spur

Ciliary body and
iris processes

Iris

Insufficient
treatment

Excessive
treatment

Correct
treatment

Post-
treatment

FIGURE 31.6 **Response of the Trabecular Meshwork to Laser Treatment**. The power is adjusted to yield a visible blanching of meshwork pigment with or without a visible bubble in ALT or DLT and champagne bubble in SLT. The spots are spaced to allow delivery of 50 spots per 180°. Treatment may be done in two visits (180° per visit), or as a single treatment (360° in a single visit).

TABLE 31.3 *Complications*

Complication	Mechanism
Transient intraocular pressure elevation	1. Inflammation 2. Contraction of the trabecular meshwork in response to chemical mediators
Peripheral anterior synechiae	Burns located posteriorly (ALT, DLT)

SELECTED REFERENCES

Al-Aswad LA, Netland PA. Laser treatment in glaucoma. In Higginbotham EJ, Lee DA, eds. *Clinical Guide to Glaucoma Management.* Woburn, MA:Butterworth Heinemann, 2004; pp. 391–411.

Chung PY, Schuman JS, Netland PA, et al. Five-year results of a randomized, prospective, clinical trial of diode vs argon laser trabeculoplasty for open-angle glaucoma *Am J Ophthalmol.* 1998;126(2):185–190.

Fea AM, Bosone A, Rolle T, et al. Micropulse diode laser trabeculoplasty (MDLT): A Phase II clinical study with 12 month fellow-up. *Clin Ophthalmol.* 2008;2(2):247–252.

Latin MA, Sibaya SA, Shi DH, et al. Q-switched 532-nm Nd:YAG Laser Trabeculoplasty (Selective Laser Trabeculoplasty) A Multicenter, Pilot, Clinical Study. *Ophthalmology.* 1998;105(11): 2082–2090.

Wise JB, Witter SL. Argon laser therapy for open-angle glaucoma. A pilot study. *Arch Ophthalmol.* 1979;97:319–322.

32 | Cyclophotocoagulation and Cryotherapy

M. Bruce Shields, MD

TABLE 32.1 *Indications*

In general, cases with limited visual potential (rarely in eyes with better than 20/400, especially if that is the better eye)

When other procedures (filtration surgery and drainage implant devices) have repeatedly failed

When filtration surgery or drainage implant devices are felt to have a low chance of success, such as neovascular glaucoma

When the patient is unable (or unwilling) to go to the operating room (transscleral cyclophotocoagulation can be performed in the office in even in a hospital room)

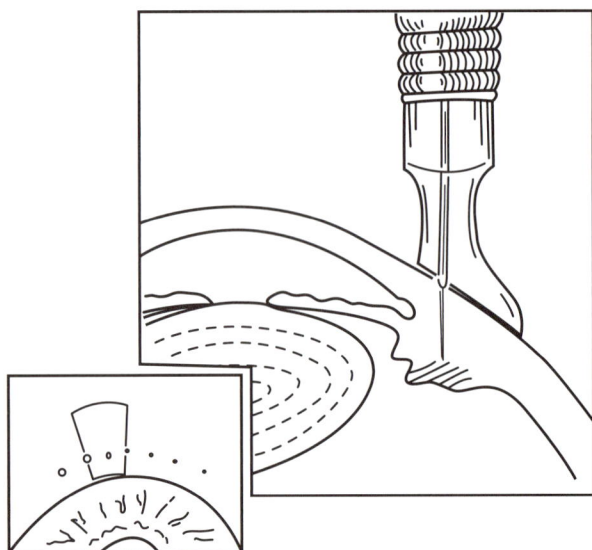

FIGURE 32.1 **Schematic of Transscleral Diode Cyclophotocoagulation.** The most commonly performed cycloablative procedure for control of intraocular pressure is transscleral cyclophotocoagulation with the semiconductor diode laser, using the G-Probe for contact fiberoptic delivery. Placing the anterior edge (closest to fiberoptic tip) of the footplate adjacent to the limbus, positions the fiberoptic approximately 1.2 mm behind the surgical limbus, in line with the pars plicata, the ciliary epithelium of which is the treatment target. The fiberoptic tip extends 0.7 mm from the footplate, which helps to standardize the amount of pressure being applied by the probe. Placing the side of the footplate adjacent to the indentation of the previous fiberoptic application (inset), provides even spacing of the treatments, with six per quadrant. Retrobulbar anesthesia is typically required for this procedure.

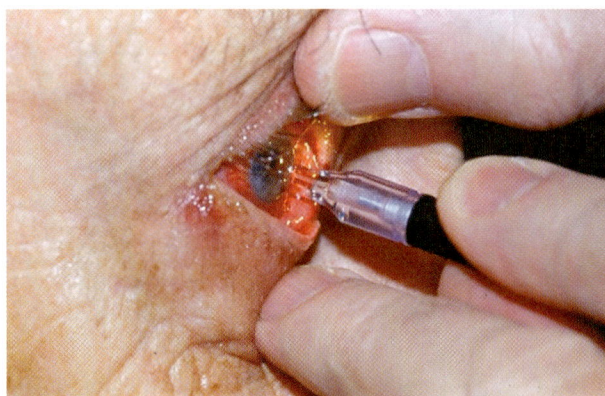

FIGURE 32.2 **Transscleral Diode Cyclophotocoagulation with G-Probe.** The G-Probe is placed at the limbus for transscleral diode cyclophotocoagulation. Typical initial settings are 2 seconds exposure duration and 1,750 mW of power. Some surgeons prefer a longer duration of 3–4 seconds and lower initial power of 1,250–1,500 mW, since longer durations of exposure have been shown to cause less tissue disruption and less inflammation. The duration is kept constant, and the power is increased (or decreased) by increments of 250 mW until a popping sound is heard (or not), and the power is reduced 250 mW below the level at which pops are heard. (The popping sound has been shown by videographic studies to represent excessive tissue disruption; it is not desirable, but signals a threshold, just below which optimum tissue disruption is believed to occur.) In the original protocol, 18 treatments are applied over 270°. However, the author believes this to be insufficient and prefers 24 applications over 360°. (Reprinted with permission from Allingham RR, et al. *Shields' Textbook of Glaucoma*, 5th ed., Fig. 43.6. Philadelphia: Lippincott, Williams & Wilkins, 2005.)

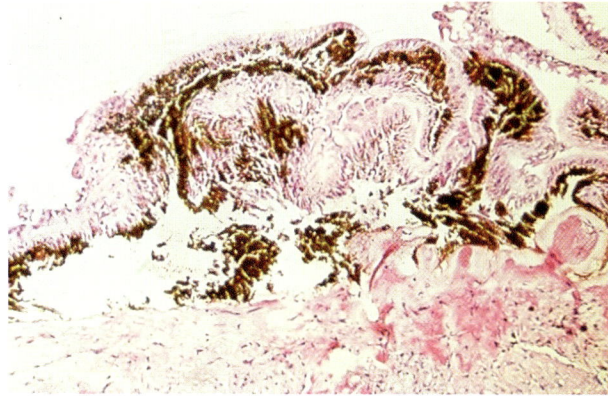

FIGURE 32.3 **Histology of Ciliary Body after Diode Cyclophotocoagulation.** Light microscopic appearance of the coagulative tissue disruption of the ciliary body induced by transscleral diode cyclophotocoagulation. The tissue reaction is typically associated with mild to moderate anterior chamber inflammation, which is treated with prednisolone 1% qid for approximately 10 days. Transient intraocular pressure rise is uncommon, but should be checked for one hour after the procedure and treated as needed. A dull, aching pain is not uncommon after the anesthesia wears off, but can be controlled with mild analgesics and is usually gone by the next day. Glaucoma medications should be continued postoperatively and gradually discontinued as pressure reduction allows.

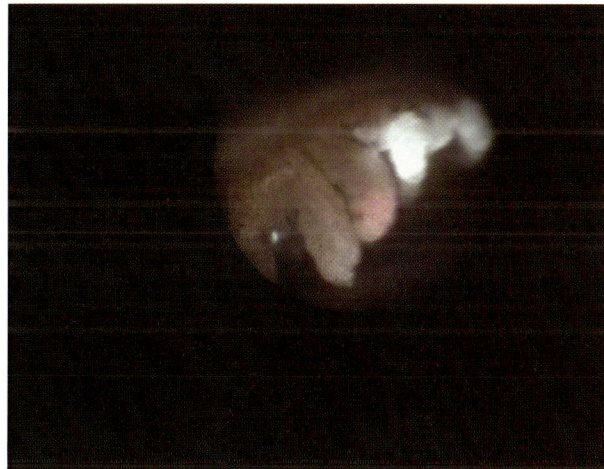

FIGURE 32.4 **Endoscopic View of Intraocular Cyclophotocoagulation**. Endoscopic view of intraocular cyclophotocoagulation, an alternative to transscleral cyclophotocoagulation. A commercial unit houses fiberoptics for a video monitor, diode laser endophotocoagulation, and illumination in a 20-gauge probe. The instrument can be introduced through a self-sealing 2 mm incision either at the level of the pars plana or just inside the limbus. The latter is preferred by most anterior segment surgeons and involves ballooning the iris from the lens with viscoelastic to allow visualization of the ciliary processes. With a power setting of approximately 300 mW, laser energy is applied to individual processes producing a whitening and shrinkage of tissue as shown. About 7–8 clock hours can be treated from a single incision. (Courtesy of Shan Lin, MD.)

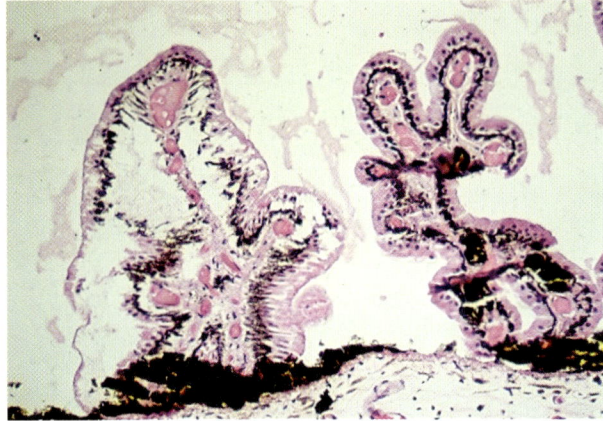

FIGURE 32.5 **Histology of Ciliary Body after Endoscopic Cyclophotocoagulation.** Light microscopic appearance of two ciliary processes of a monkey eye treated with endoscopic cyclophotocoagulation. Note the precision with which one process (left) was extensively disrupted, with minimal damage to adjacent process. This is an advantage of endoscopic over transscleral cyclophotocoagulation. In addition to more precise treatment of individual processes with less collateral damage, the endoscopic approach has the advantage of requiring lower energy levels, with the laser beam directed toward the processes, (rather than posteriorly as with transscleral), all of which may explain why endoscopic cyclophotocoagulation has a lower incidence of visual loss. The disadvantage is that it is an incisional procedure in the operating room, with the potential for intraoperative complications that could affect vision.

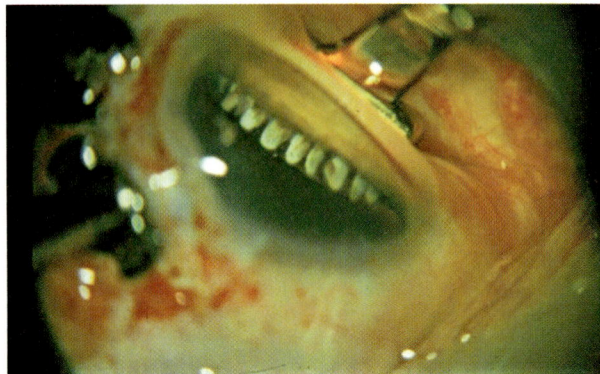

FIGURE 32.6 **Endoscopic Cyclophotocoagulation with Transpupillary Visualization.** Endocyclophotocoagulation can also be performed under direct transpupillary visualization. This is most often performed by the vitreoretinal surgeon in conjunction with pars plana vitrectomy. The endophotocoagulator can be introduced through the same port as the vitrectomy unit, and the intraocular pressure is reduced to allow scleral depression and transpupillary visualization of the ciliary processes for direct treatment. Yet another technique is transpupillary cyclophotocoagulation, in which an argon or diode slit-lamp laser is used for direct treatment of ciliary processes. However, this is only possible when the processes can be visualized gonioscopically, as in aniridia or a large sector iridectomy, and even then the outcome is generally poor. (Reprinted with permission from Allingham RR, et al. *Shields' Textbook of Glaucoma*, 5th ed., Fig. 43.11. Philadelphia: Lippincott, Williams & Wilkins, 2005.)

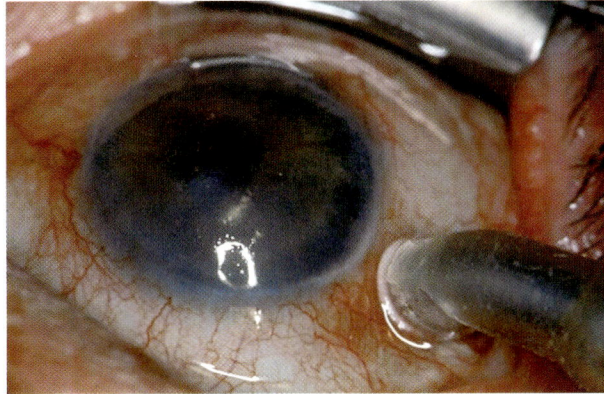

FIGURE 32.7 **Cyclocryotherapy.** Before the advent of laser technology for cyclophotocoagulation, the cyclodestructive procedure of choice was cyclocryotherapy. The cryoprobe is placed just posterior to the limbus and a freeze of –60° to –80° is maintained for 60 seconds, which produces an iceball, as shown, that is then allowed to thaw slowly. A typical treatment is 3–4 applications per quadrant for 2–3 quadrants. In comparison to cyclophotocoagulation, there is a greater risk of significant transient intraocular pressure rise, inflammation, and severe and prolonged pain. Visual loss may also be greater than with transscleral cylophotocoagulation, although it is a major consideration with both techniques. (Reprinted with permission from Shields MB. *Color Atlas of Glaucoma,* Fig. III42c, Baltimore: Williams & Wilkins, 1998, and provided courtesy of A. Robert Bellows, MD.)

TABLE 32.2 *Complications*

Transient intraocular pressure rise (especially with cryotherapy)

Anterior segment inflammation (patients often left with chronic flare due to breakdown of blood-aqueous barrier)

Postoperative pain (mild with cyclophotocoagulation, but can be severe with cryotherapy)

Reduced visual acuity (significant consideration with transscleral cyclophotocoagulation and cryotherapy, but minimal with endoscopic cyclophotocoagulation, unless complications associated with incisional surgery, such as retinal detachment)

SELECTED REFERENCES

Brindley G, Shields MB. Value and limitation of cyclocryotherapy. *Greaefe's Arch Ophthalmol.* 1986;224:545 549.

Chen J, Cohn RA, Lin SC, et al. Endoscopic photocoagulation of the ciliary body for treatment of refractory glaucomas. *Am J Ophthalmol.* 1997; 124:787–796.

Myers JS, Trevisani MG, Imami N,et al. Laser energy reaching the posterior pole during transscleral cyclophotocoagulation. *Arch Ophthalmol.* 1998;116:488–491.

Nasisse, MP, Shields MB, Echelman D, et al. Inflammatory effects of Nd:YAG laser cyclophotocoagulation. *Invest Ophthalmol Vis Sci.* 1992;33:2216–2223.

Simmons RB, Prum BE Jr, Shields SR, et al. Videographic and histologic comparison of Nd:YAG and diode laser contact transscleral cyclophotocoagulation. *Am J Ophthalmol.* 1994;117:337–341.

Youn J, Cox TA, Herndon LW, et al. A clinical comparison of transscleral cyclophotocoagulation with neodymium:YAG and semiconductor diode lasers. *Am J Ophthalmol.* 1998;126:640–647.

33 Surgical Iridectomy and Goniosynechialysis

Robert M. Schertzer, MD, MED, FRCSC and Peter A. Netland, MD, PhD

TABLE 33.1 *Indications*

Surgical iridectomy	Inability to achieve patent iridectomy with a laser
	Corneal edema, flat anterior chamber, insufficient patient cooperation
Goniosynechialysis	Elevated intraocular pressure and angle-closure due to peripheral anterior synechiae

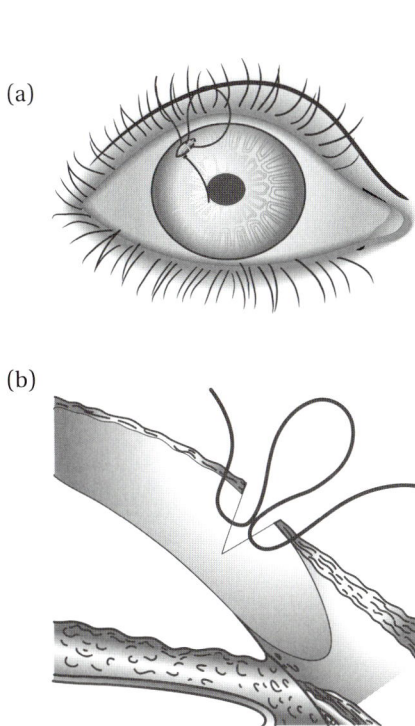

FIGURE 33.1 **Pre-placed Suture.** (a, b) Preplacement of corneal suture. Surgical iridectomy consists of a corneal or scleral incision; exteriorization, excision, and repositioning of the iris; and closure of the corneal incision. Closure of the corneal incision is facilitated by preplacement of a corneal suture at two-thirds depth. (Redrawn with permission from Wilson MR. Peripheral iridectomy and chamber deepening. In: Albert DM, Jakobiec FA, eds. *Principles and Practice of Ophthalmology*. Philadelphia, Pa: WB Saunders; 1994:1618.)

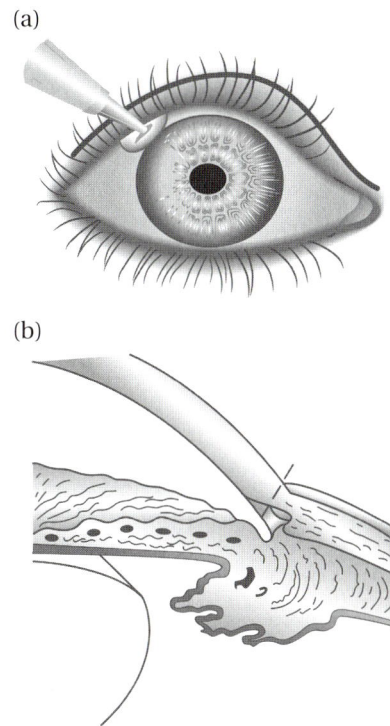

FIGURE 33.2 **Scleral Incision.** A scleral incision 1.0 to 1.5 mm behind the corneolimbal junction. (a) Anterior view. (b) Cross-sectional view. (Redrawn with permission from Spaeth GL. Glaucoma surgery. In Spaeth GL, ed. *Ophthalmic Surgery: Principles and Practice*. Philadelphia, PA: WB Saunders; 1990.)

(a)

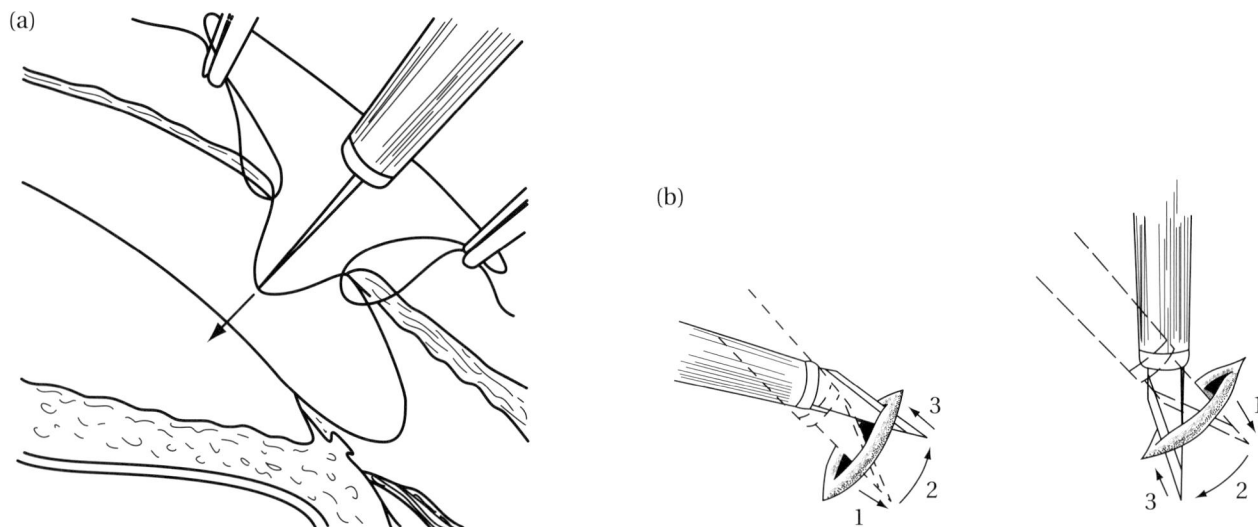

(b)

FIGURE 33.3 **Incision of Inner Cornea.** (a) Preplaced sutures facilitate access to the inner depths of the cornea. (b) Descemet's membrane is penetrated the full length of the corneal wound by entering centrally (1), rotating the blade through an arc (2), and exiting with the cutting edge perpendicular to the wound (3). (Redrawn with permission from Wilson MR. Peripheral iridectomy and chamber deepening. In: Albert DM, Jakobiec FA, eds. *Principles and Practice of Ophthalmology*. Philadelphia, PA: WB Saunders; 1994:1618.)

(a) (b)

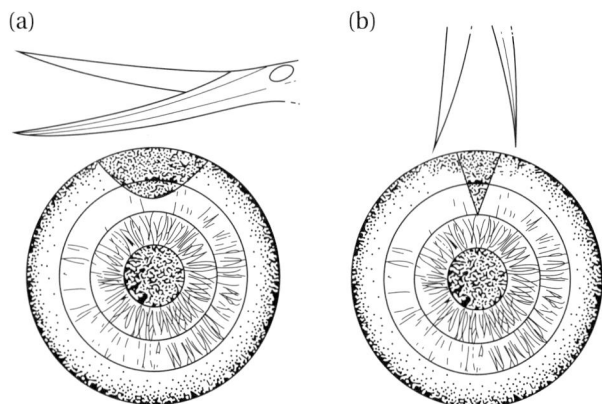

FIGURE 33.4 **Peripheral Iridectomy.** (a) Keeping the scissors parallel to the limbus results in a broad-based iridectomy. (b) With the scissors perpendicular to the limbus, a narrow, sharply peaked iridectomy results.

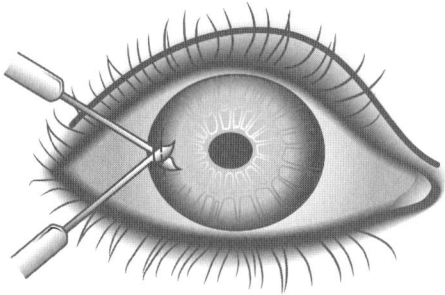

FIGURE 33.5 **Paracentesis for Surgical Goniosynechialysis.** The paracentesis incision may be created wider at its internal aspect than its external aspect. The wide internal aspect allows unhindered rotation of instruments within the anterior chamber, while the narrower external aspect prevents excess loss of viscoelastic substance.

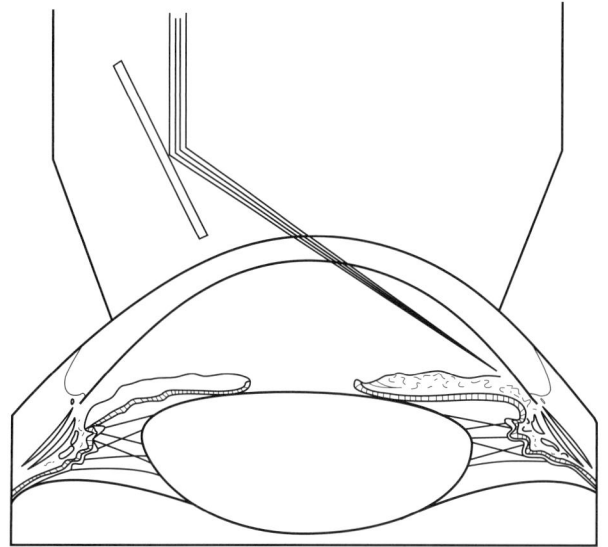

FIGURE 33.6 **Laser Goniosynechialysis.** A gonioscopy lens with a diameter smaller than the corneal diameter may be used, which allows simultaneous compression gonioscopy if necessary. In patients with angle closure of months to even years duration, argon laser gonioplasty may be useful to treat synechial angle closure. A spot size of 100–200 μm is used, but otherwise the settings are similar as for gonioplasty.

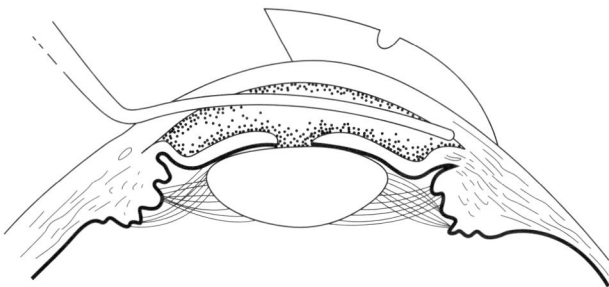

FIGURE 33.7 **Surgical Goniosynechialysis.** Lysis of synechiae is accomplished through a clear-corneal incision and direct mechanical (shown) or viscoelastic cleavage of adhesions in the angle of the opposite quadrant. Multiple paracentesis access ports can be used. The procedure can be viewed through the operating microscope or a prismatic or mirrored goniolens.

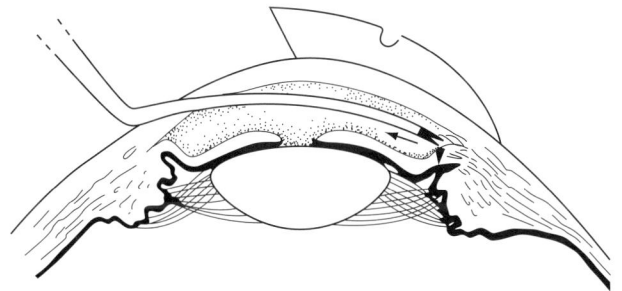

FIGURE 33.8 **Goniosynechialysis, Alternative Surgical Technique.** After injecting viscoelastic into the anterior chamber, vitreous forceps are passed across the anterior chamber through a paracentesis. The peripheral iris is grasped and gently pulled away from the angle, thereby breaking synechia. The direction of traction on the peripheral iris is indicated by the arrow. (Personal communication Ike Ahmed, MD.)

TABLE 33.2 *Complications*

- Hyphema
- Cyclodialysis
- Infection
- Reformation of synechia
- Increased or decreased intraocular pressure
- Cataract

SELECTED REFERENCES

Campbell DG, Vela A. Modern goniosynechialysis for the treatment of synechial angle closure glaucoma. *Ophthalmology.* 1984;91:1052–1060.

Morales J, Ritch R. Incisional surgical iridectomy. In Ritch R, Shields MB, Krupin T, eds. *The Glaucomas,* 2nd ed. St. Louis: Mosby, 1996; pp. 1653–1660.

Shingleton BJ, Chang MA, Bellows AR, et al. Surgical goniosynechialysis for angle-closure glaucoma. *Ophthalmology.* 1990;97:551–556.

Wand M. Argon laser gonioplasty for synechial angle closure. *Arch Ophthalmol.* 1992;110:363–367.

34 Trabeculectomy

Paul F. Palmberg, MD, PhD and Jonathan S. Myers, MD

TABLE 34.1 *Indications and Potential Contraindications for Trabeculectomy*

Indications

Glaucoma diagnosis: primary therapy in selected cases

• Advanced disease

• Poor ability to adhere to medical therapy or monitoring

Failed medical therapy

Failed laser therapy or poor candidate for laser therapy

Progressive loss of optic nerve function or likely loss

Potential Contraindications

Severe conjunctival scarring

• Prior surgery or trauma

• Ocular pemphigoid

• Chemical burns

High risk for infection

• Soft contact lens wear

Uncontrolled inflammation or neovascularization

Inability to return for postoperative care

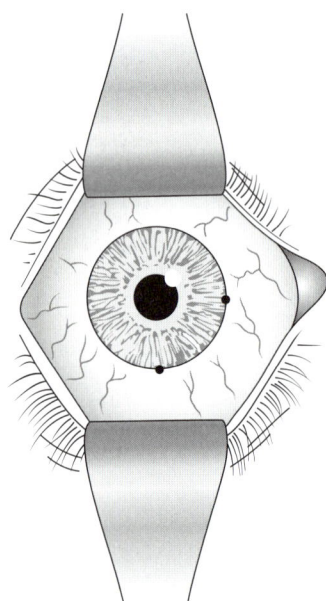

FIGURE 34.1 **Marking the Meridians.** Successful trabeculectomy surgery requires meticulous attention to detail, including marking reference points on the eye before making incisions. Without manipulation of the position of the eye in the orbit, the cardinal meridians of the quadrant are marked. To avoid spread of the surgical ink, careful drying with cellulose sponges is required before marking.

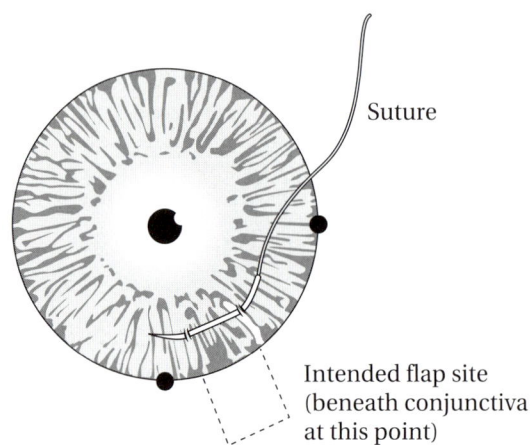

FIGURE 34.2 **Placement of the Corneal Traction Stitch.** With the limits of the quadrant marked at the limbus, a suture is placed into the cornea to provide traction. The track is parallel to the limbus, far enough from the conjunctival insertion to allow creation of the scleral flap. The entry and exit points of the track should correspond to the intended width of the sides of the scleral flap. The track is then used as a guide during creation of the scleral flap.

Traction suture
under tension

Exposed
conjunctiva

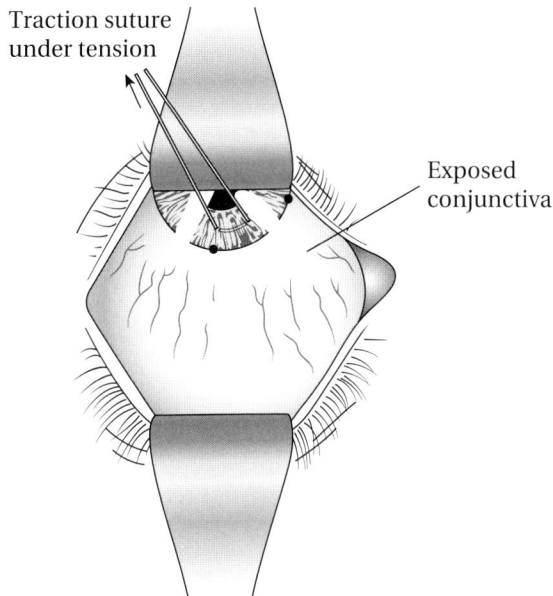

FIGURE 34.3 Infraduction of the Eye, Corneal Traction Stitch. With the track completed, the needle is removed, and the traction suture tied. Force is applied to the stitch to expose the intended quadrant, and the suture is anchored to the drape or speculum. Under topical anesthesia, asking the patient to look down assists in this maneuver.

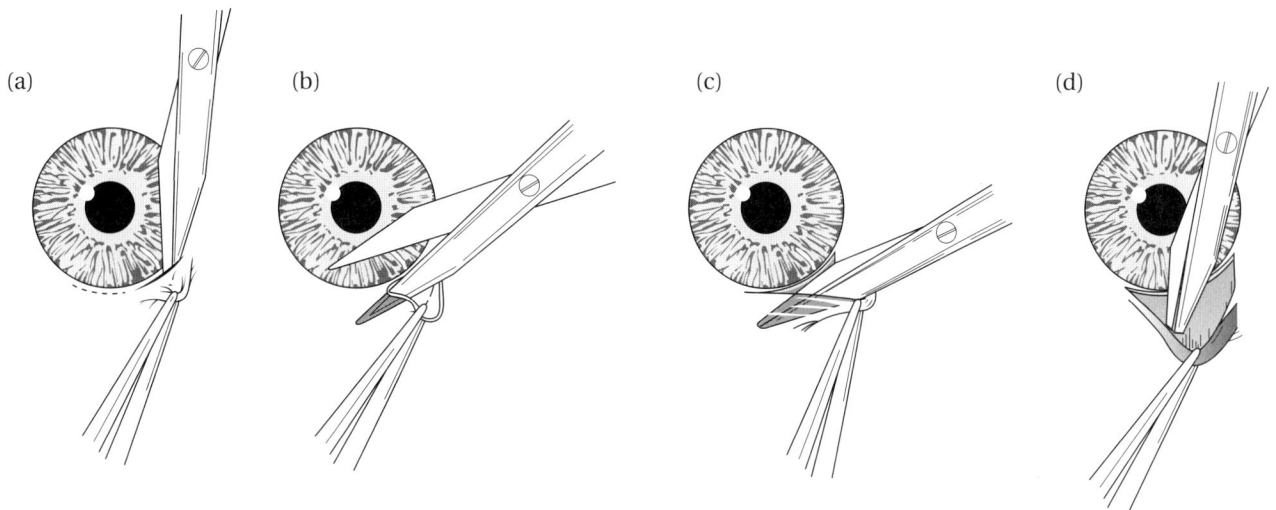

(a)   (b)   (c)   (d)

FIGURE 34.4 Limbal Peritomy, Scissors Technique. Conjunctiva and Tenon capsule tissues are elevated with smooth forceps, and the limbal insertion of each is lysed with rounded-tipped scissors. Care is taken to avoid creation of dog-ear flaps and to completely remove Tenon insertion. The width is appropriate if it barely exposes the sides of the intended flap and allows for placement of flap sutures.

(a)

(b)

Incorrect angle of knife

Correct angle of knife

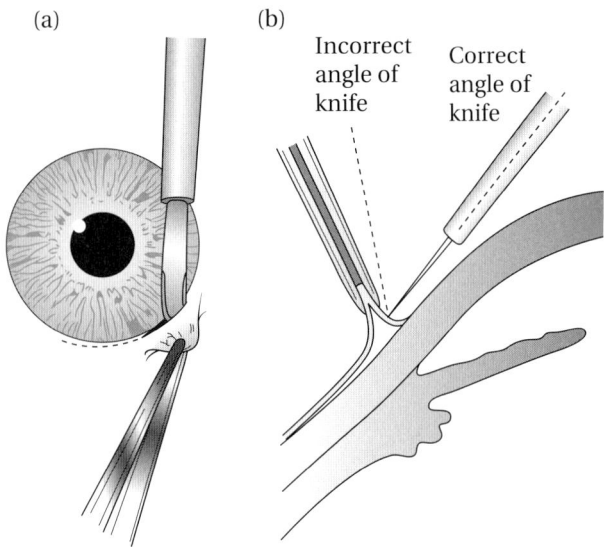

FIGURE 34.5 **Limbal Peritomy, Blade Method.**
(a) While the conjunctiva and Tenon capsule are elevated with smooth forceps, a rounded-tipped blade is used to lyse insertions of each tissue at the limbus. (b) Care is taken to hold the blade parallel to the scleral surface, cutting posteriorly.

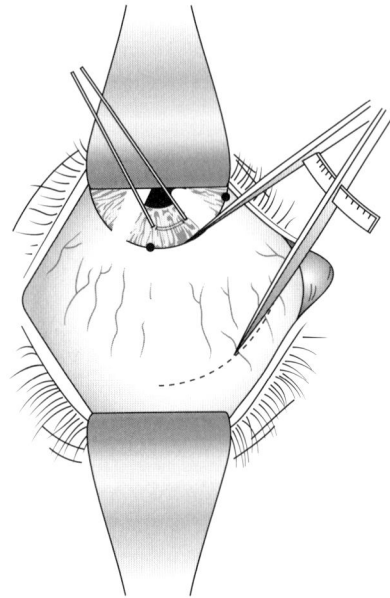

FIGURE 34.6 **Marking for Intended Conjunctival Insertion, with Limbus-based Flap.** As the quadrant is exposed with traction inferiorly, the conjunctival surface is dried completely with cellulose sponges. A surgical marking pen and calipers are used to mark a line 10 mm behind the limbus, extending just beyond the muscles on either side of the quadrant. This line is wide enough to be used as a landmark when the conjunctiva is closed later during the procedure.

(a)

(b)

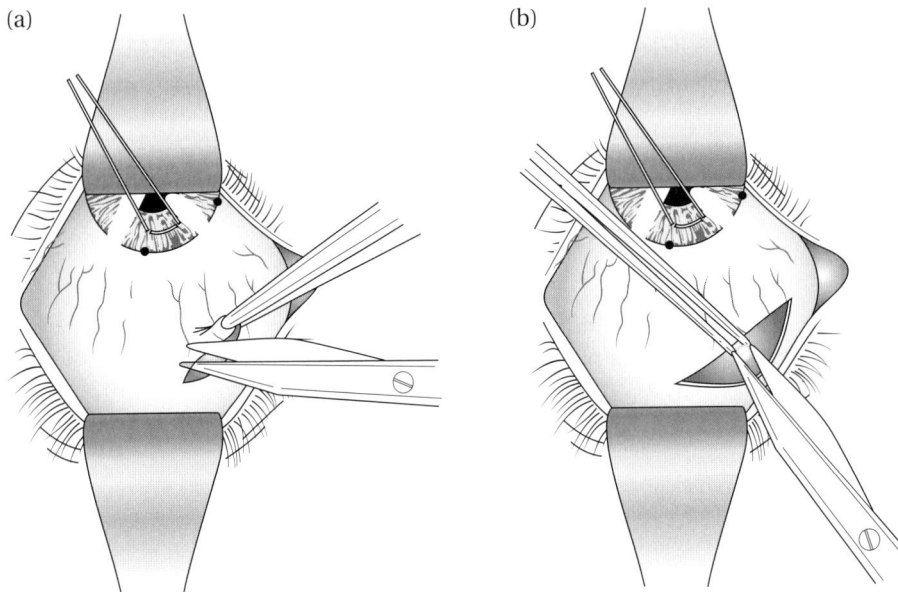

FIGURE 34.7 **Staggering Incisions in Conjunctiva and Tenon Capsule.** (a, b) After opening the conjunctiva along the inked line and undermining in all directions to separate Tenon capsule from conjunctiva, an incision is made into Tenon capsule. The incision should be parallel and 1–2 mm posterior to the conjunctival incision.

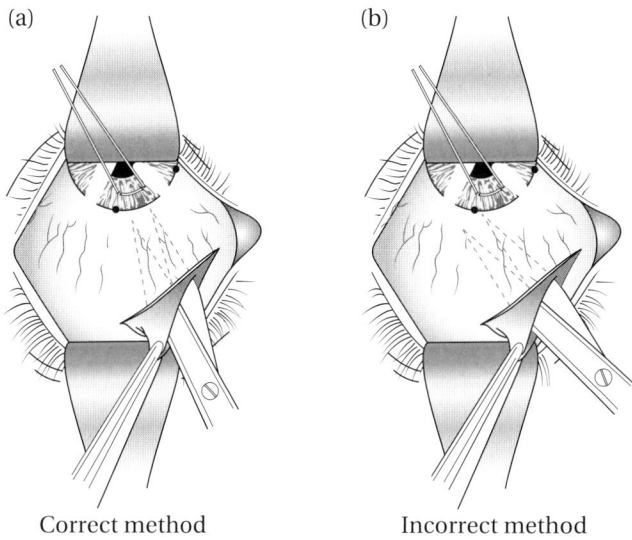

FIGURE 34.8 **Lysing Tenon Insertion at the Corneal Limbus.** As Tenon layer is separated from episclera toward the limbus, care must be taken when Tenon insertion is encountered. The scissors must be rotated, keeping the two blade tips in gentle contact with the limbus before each spreading or cutting action. Spreading the jaws when only one tip is in contact with the insertion may create a limbal buttonhole.

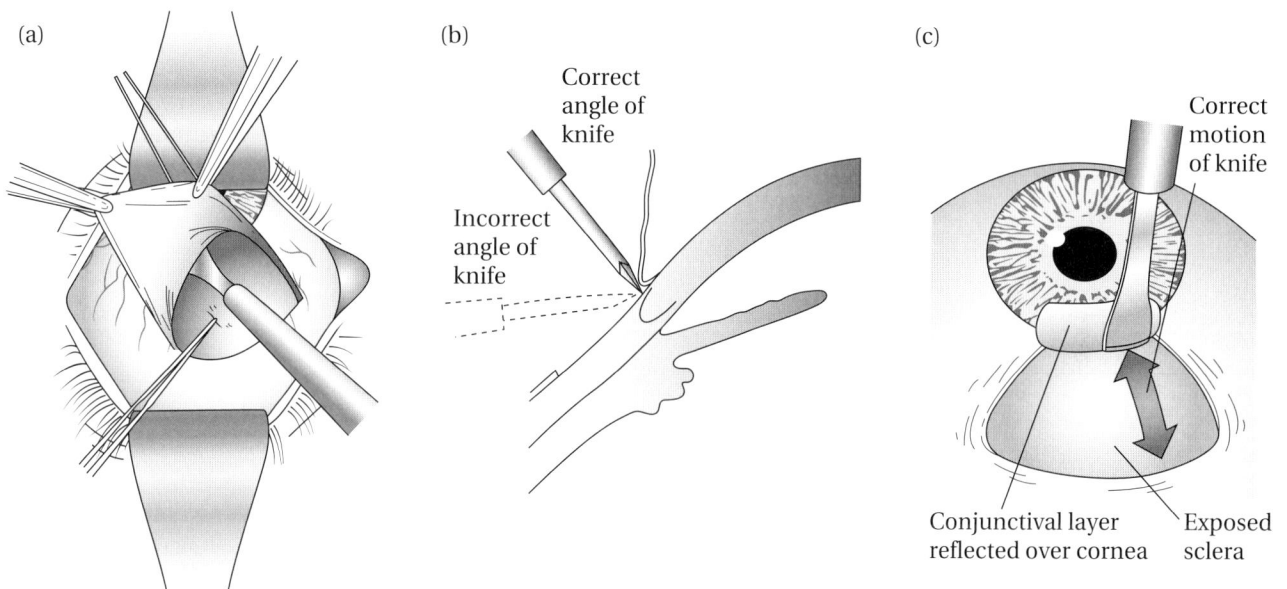

FIGURE 34.9 **Use of a Gill Knife for Tenon Disinsertion.** (a) Lysing the final remnants of the limbal insertion of Tenon capsule may require use of blunt force with a rounded knife. (b, c) The knife is kept perpendicular to the scleral surface, and care is taken to keep a radial motion, not cutting the insertion with circumferential cuts.

(a) (b) (c)

Scleral flap Conjunctiva

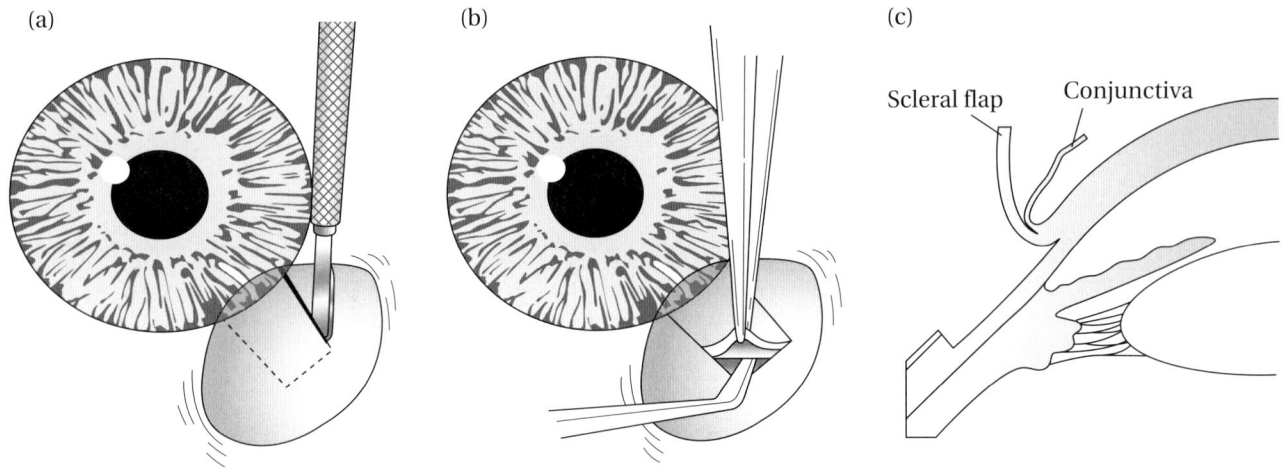

FIGURE 34.10 **Partial-Thickness Scleral Flap.** (a) Cutting the sides of the scleral flap. (b) A sharp knife is used to create perpendicular, half-depth cuts into sclera to outline a flap. (c) The limbal edge of the flap should be as far into cornea as the conjunctival insertion allows.

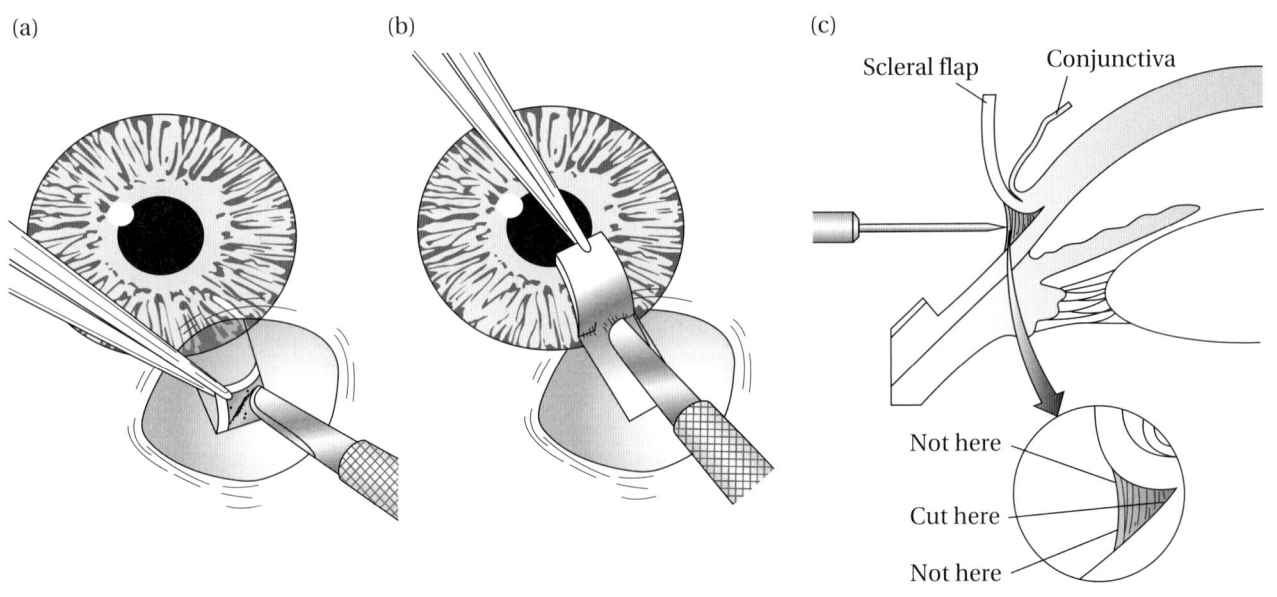

(a) (b) (c)

Scleral flap Conjunctiva

Not here

Cut here

Not here

FIGURE 34.11 **Creation of the Half-thickness Flap.** (a) The scleral flap is cut forward into the limbus. Maintaining a uniform depth is key, and can be accomplished by cutting those fibers "on stretch." (b) As the flap is gently elevated with a toothed forceps, the tissue at the base of the flap creates a curved "meniscus" of tension. (c) Cutting from the middle of the meniscus out to either side allows maintenance of a uniform depth throughout the cut.

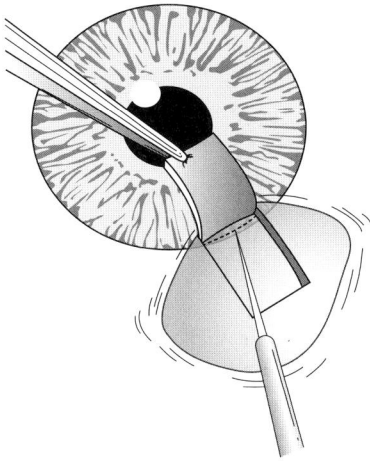

FIGURE 34.12 **Cutting the Sclerostomy.** Once the flap has been dissected into the corneal tissue, a small, sharp blade is used to enter the peripheral region of the cornea. The cut should be slightly beveled, but perpendicular enough to the iris to allow engagement of the posterior edge of the corneal incision by the punch. Care is taken not to extend the excision all the way to the sides of the flap, but to stop 1 mm from each end of the flap.

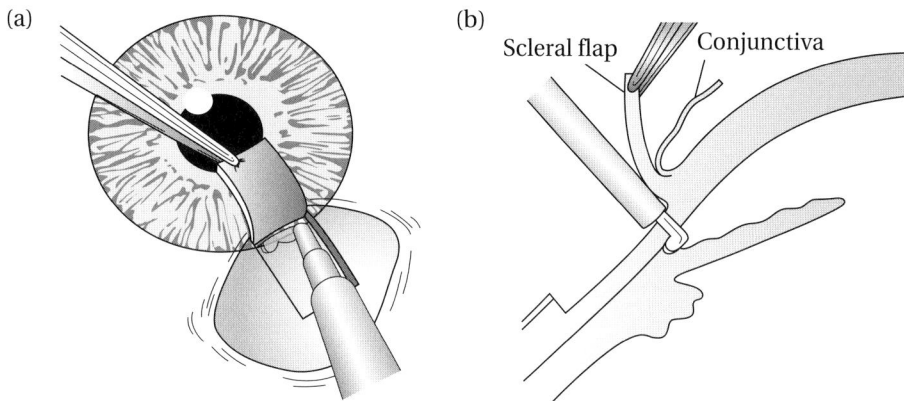

(a)

(b)

Scleral flap   Conjunctiva

FIGURE 34.13 **Completion of the Sclerostomy.** (a) The Kelly Descemet punch is used to widen the corneal ostomy. (b) For most flaps, a final ostomy equal to two full punch bites is adequate to allow sufficient flow of aqueous.

(a)

(b)

Cornea

Cut here

Iris

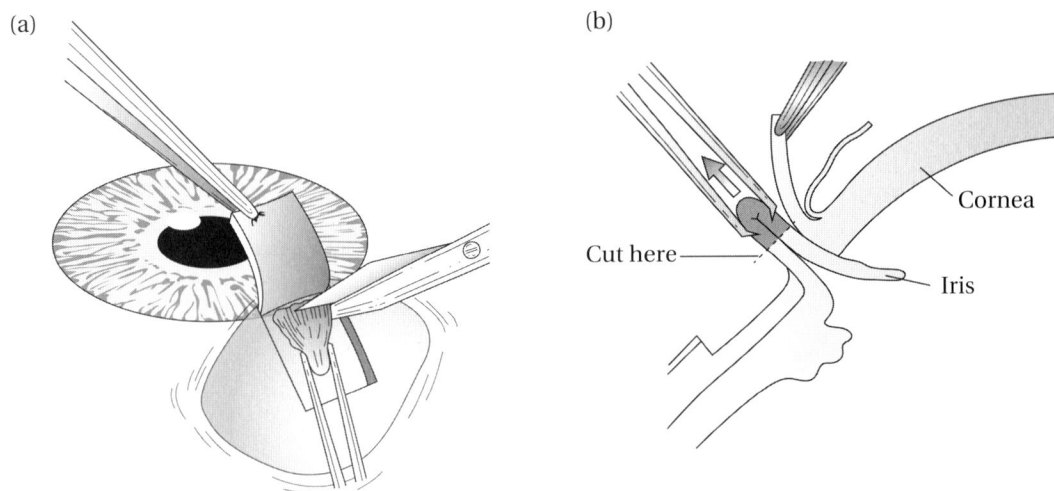

FIGURE 34.14 Iridectomy Technique. (a) The surgical assistant gently elevates the scleral flap. A toothed or serrated iris forceps is used to grasp a pillar of iris. To avoid incorporation of the ciliary body, the jaws should be opened parallel to the limbus, so that a single pillar of iris is grasped. This technique also provides a radially short, but broad based iridectomy. The jaws should be pressed gently against the pupillary margin of the ostomy, to grasp iris well away from the ciliary body and zonules. (b) The iris is gently drawn into the ostomy, and scissors are used to cut both iris stroma and pigment layers. On completion, the scleral flap is released, and the iridectomy inspected for transillumination and direct visualization of ciliary processes.

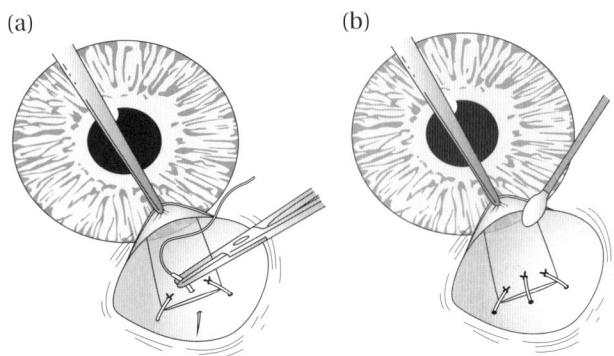

(a)

(b)

FIGURE 34.15 Assessing the Flow of Aqueous. (a) Following closure of the scleral flap with sutures, flow is assessed by refilling the anterior chamber with saline solution through the paracentesis and monitoring the appearance of aqueous at the flap margins. (b) Use of cellulose sponges, gently touched to the flap, can aid in visualization of the rate of flow. More sutures are placed if the flow is excessive, or if the chamber is not maintained.

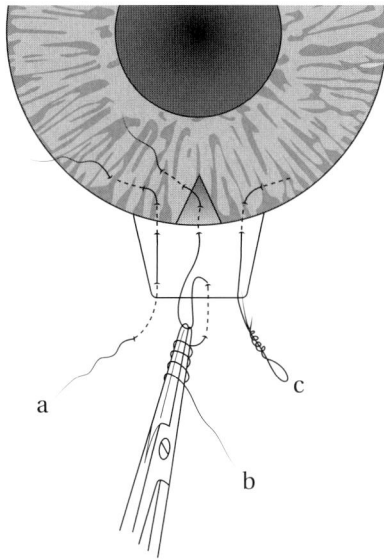

FIGURE 34.16 **Releasable Scleral Flap Sutures.** If the surgeon anticipates difficulty visualizing the sutures for postoperative laser lysis, releasable sutures may be placed. (a) The needle is passed through the posterior sclera and scleral flap. It is then passed through the base of the flap, beneath the conjunctival insertion, and up through peripheral clear cornea. A second, partial-thickness corneal pass is made at an angle to the first, as diagrammed. (b) A slipknot is then tied, pulling the loop of suture overlying the flap through four throws of the free posterior end. (c) After final adjustments have been made, the anterior end of the suture is cut flush with the corneal surface. The suture is released by grasping the exposed portion between the two corneal bites with fine forceps and pulling tangential to the ocular surface and in a direction opposite the site of scleral fixation. The dashed lines indicate buried segments of suture.

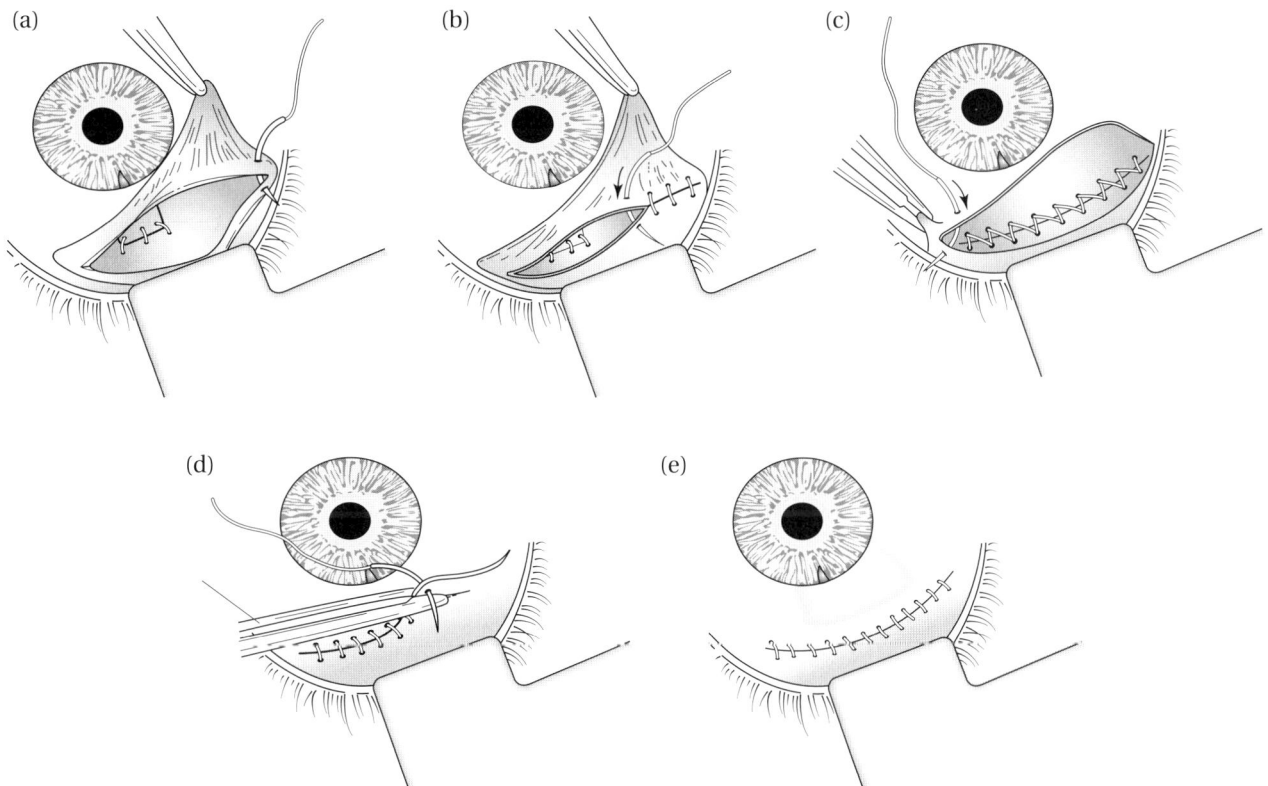

FIGURE 34.17 **Closure of Tenon Capsule and Conjunctiva, Limbus-based Flap.** Running simple or mattress sutures are used. Only enough tissue to create adequate closure is used, allowing as much tissue as possible to form a large bleb. Many surgeons close the two layers separately.

(a)

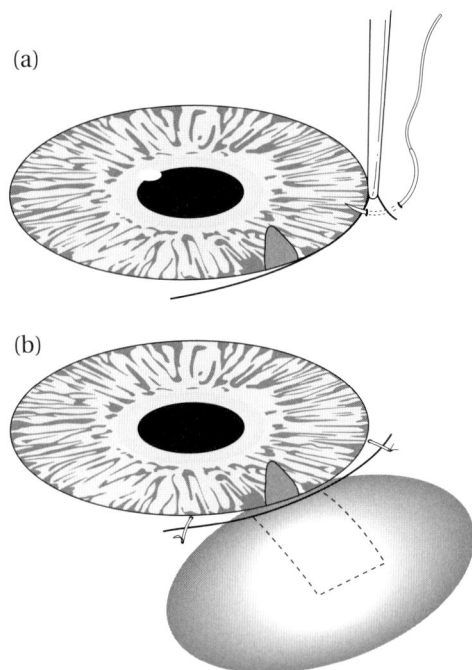

FIGURE 34.18 **Closure of Fornix-based Flap.** (a) The limbal corneal epithelium is scraped away with a rounded blade. (b) The conjunctival flap is secured to cornea on both sides of the scleral flap.

(b)

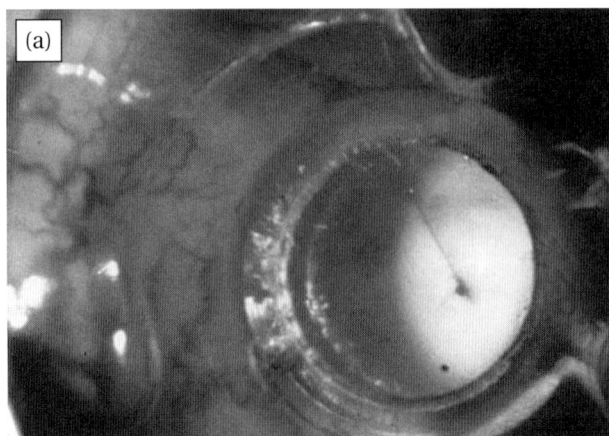

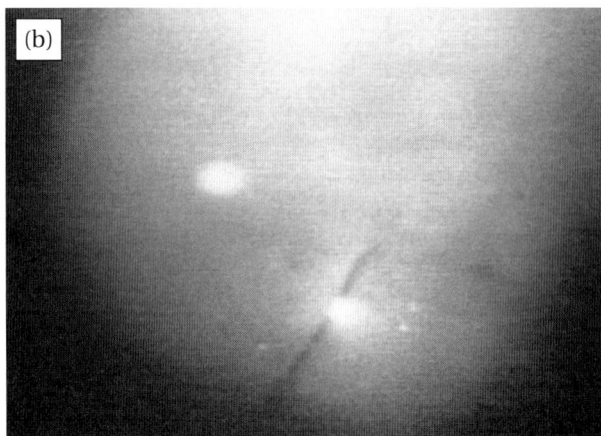

FIGURE 34.19 **Argon Laser Suture Lysis.** If the surgeon has chosen to place nonreleasable sutures to close the scleral flap, laser suture lysis may be performed to allow continued filtration, as scar tissue begins to build postoperatively. The bleb is compressed gently with a Hoskins, Ritch, or Blumenthal suture lysis lens, which presses fluid out of the sponge-like Tenon's capsule. When the suture is visualized, the suture can be melted without damage to the overlying conjunctiva, using an Argon laser set at 0.1 second duration, 50 μm spot size, 200–400 mW power. (Reprinted by permission from Palmberg P. The failing filtering bleb. *Ophthalmol Clin North Am.* 2000;13:520.)

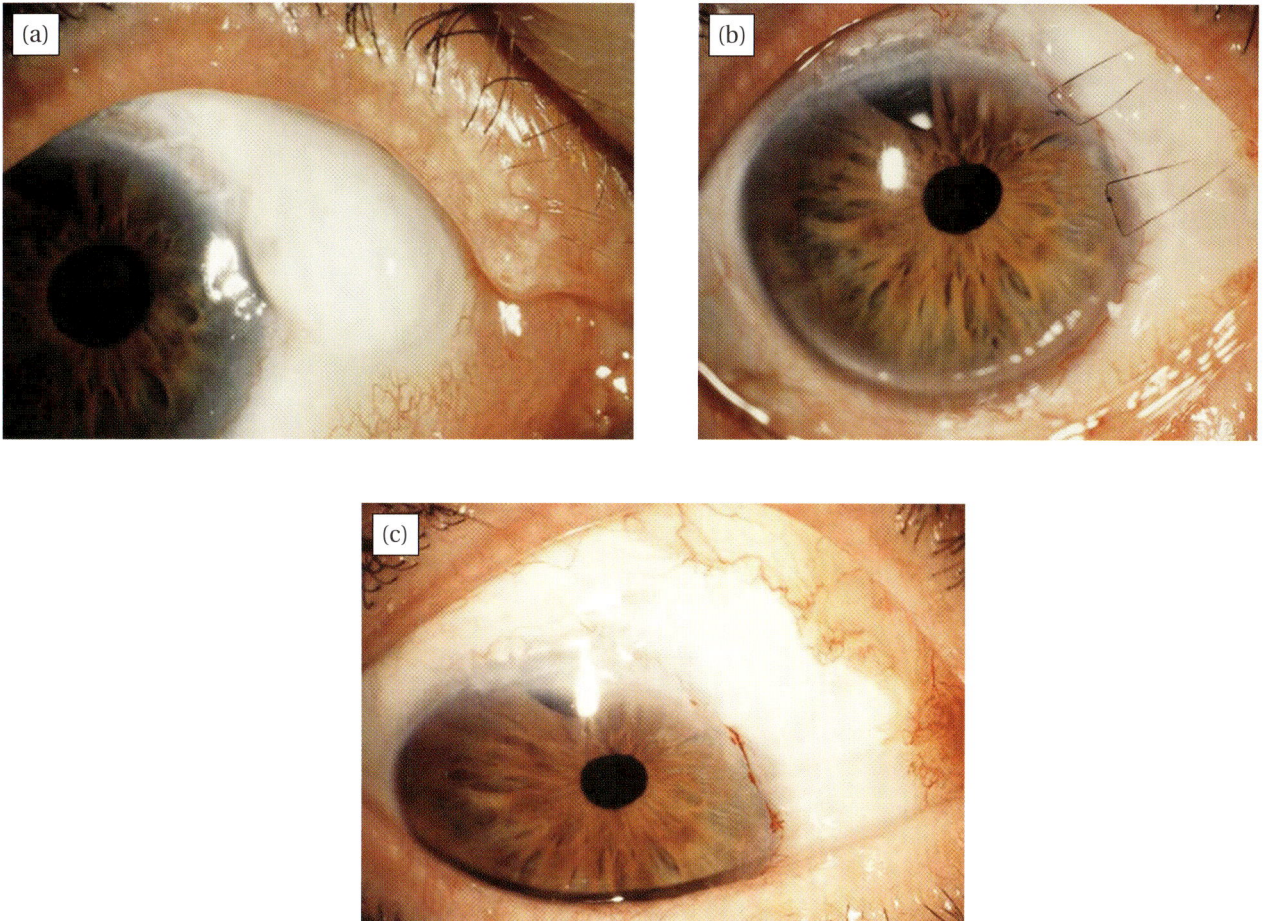

FIGURE 34.20 Compression Sutures for a Bleb causing a Corneal Dellen. (a) A nasal filtering bleb with a high profile near the limbus produced a quite painful dellen. (b) Two 9-0 nylon compression stitches are placed over the bleb, flattening it. Each 9-0 nylon suture is passed in the peripheral part of the cornea at half depth and then back over the bleb to one side of the leak or overly elevated bleb. A bite is taken of conjunctiva and Tenon capsule posterior to the bleb. The stitch is then passed back over the bleb on the other side of the leak and tied tightly. The knot is trimmed and rotated into the peripheral part of the cornea. (c) Final bleb appearance after stitch removal at 2 weeks, with "white suspenders" of apparent connective tissue now present within the bleb, holding it in a lower profile. The dellen healed and did not recur in the remaining 2 years the patient lived. (Reprinted by permission from Fantes FF, Palmberg PF. Late complications of glaucoma surgery. In: Rhee DR, ed. *Glaucoma: Color Atlas & Synopsis of Clinical Ophthalmology.* New York: McGraw-Hill, 2003; pp. 338–362.)

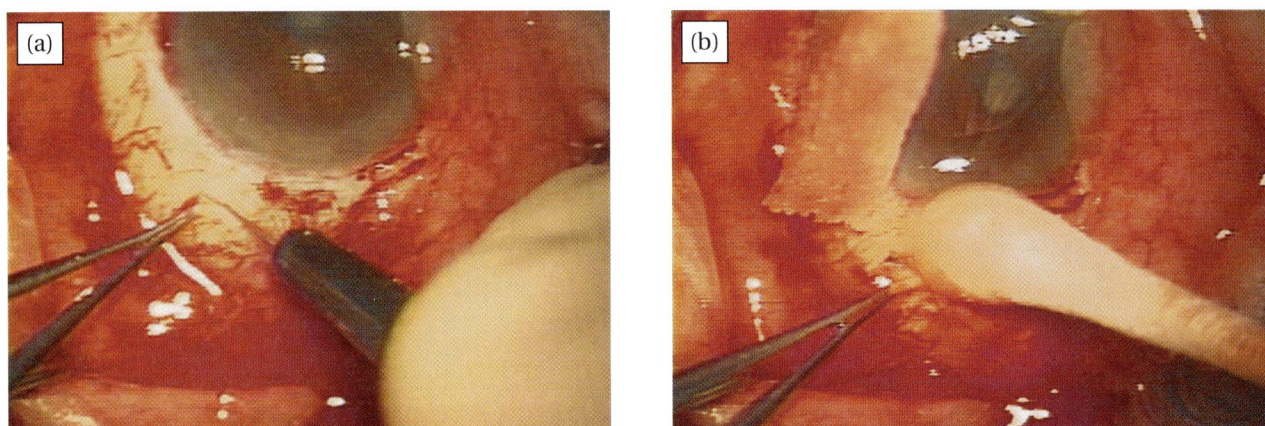

FIGURE 34.21 Drainage of Choroidal Effusions. Prolonged or severe hypotony may result in development of serous choroidal detachments, which require drainage. (a) Cutting an L-shaped sclerotomy, 3–4 mm posterior to the limbus. (b) Milking fluid to the sclerotomy site with the rolling action of a cotton-tipped swab. A self-retaining anterior chamber cannula attached to a hanging bag of balanced salt solution may aid in the egress of the choroidal fluid.

TABLE 34.2 *Complications of Trabeculectomy*

Early Postoperative Complications	Late Postoperative Complications
Wound leak	Leaking bleb
Infection	
Hypotony	Failure of bleb
Shallow or flat anterior chamber	
Choroidal effusions or hemorrhage	
Aqueous misdirection	Cataract
Hyphema	Blebitis
Suprachoroidal hemorrhage	
Uveitis	Endophthalmitis
Dellen formation	Dysthetic bleb
Loss of vision	Hypotony
	Ptosis

SELECTED REFERENCES

de Barros DS, Da Silva RS, Siam GA, Gheith ME, Nunes CM, Lankaranian D, Tittler EH, Myers JS, Spaeth GL. Should an iridectomy be routinely performed as a part of trabeculectomy? Two surgeons' clinical experience. *Eye.* 2009;23:362–367.

Jones LS, Shetty RK, Spaeth GL. Trabeculectomy. In: Chen TC, ed. *Glaucoma Surgery.* Philadelphia, PA: Saunders Elsevier, 2008; pp. 2–28.

Scott IU, Greenfield DS, Schiffman J, Nicolela MT, Rueda JC, Tsai JC, Palmberg PF. Outcomes of primary trabeculectomy with the use of adjunctive mitomycin. *Arch Ophthalmol.* 1998;116:286–291.

Weinreb RN, Mills RP, eds. *Glaucoma Surgery: Principles and Techniques.* 2nd ed. Ophthalmology Monograph 4. San Francisco: American Academy of Ophthalmology; 1998.

Combined Phacoemulsification and Trabeculectomy

Nabeel Farooqui, MD and Peter A. Netland, MD, PhD

Presence of a visually significant cataract requiring extraction in a glaucoma patient, in whom surgery for intraocular pressure control is also indicated*

Cataract surgery planned in a patient with glaucoma, in whom a postoperative pressure spike may lead to substantial loss of visual function

Planned filtration procedure in a patient with a visually insignificant cataract that will likely progress after glaucoma surgery

Chronic angle closure glaucoma uncontrollable either with medication or laser iridotomy, where cataract surgery alone is unlikely to provide successful control of intraocular pressure

*Indications for glaucoma surgery include: uncontrolled or poorly controlled intraocular pressure and/or progressive visual field loss, despite the use of multiple medications; intolerance to medications; noncompliance with medications; and failure of laser trabeculoplasty.

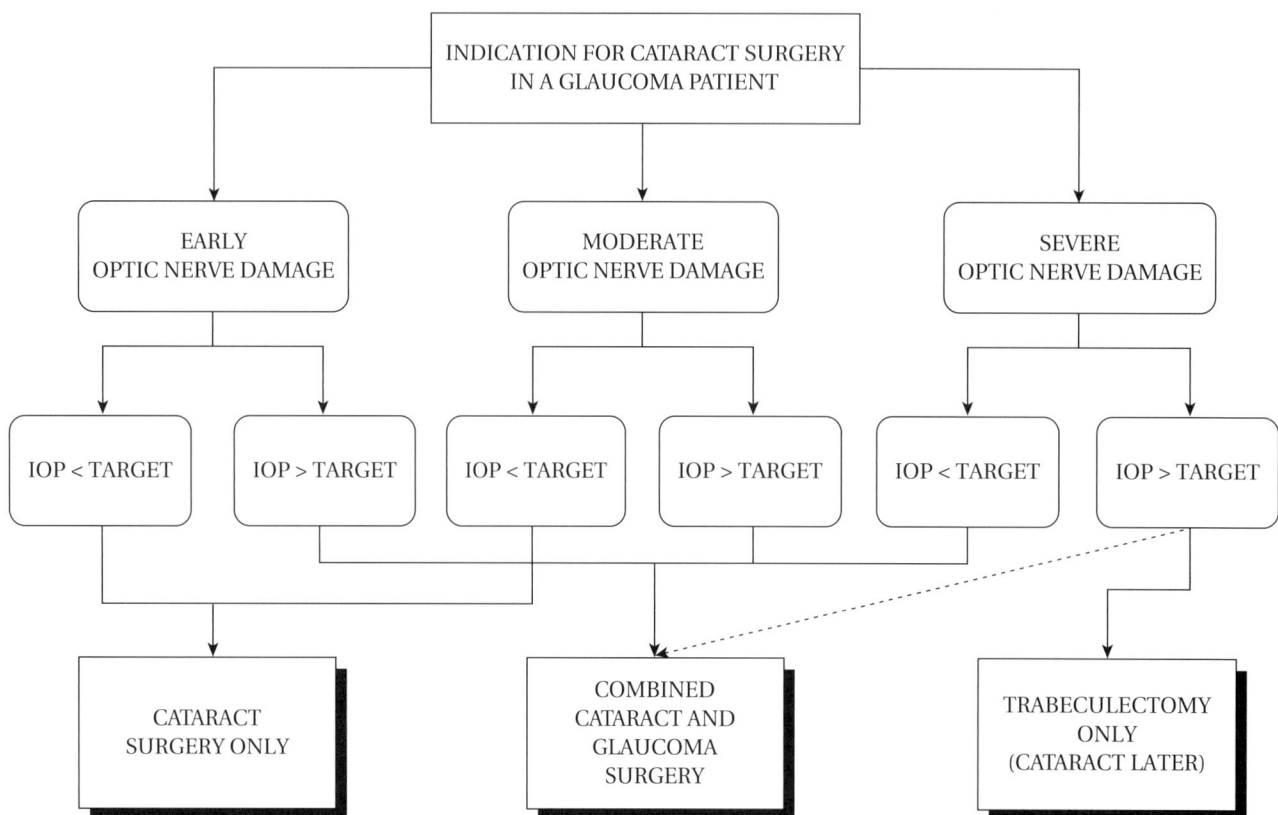

FIGURE 35.1 Algorithm for the selection of cataract surgery alone, trabeculectomy alone, or combined surgery for patients with cataract and glaucoma. This algorithm depends on the severity of optic nerve damage and whether the intraocular pressure has been controlled at or near the target level. Those with early optic nerve damage typically have detectable structural changes to the optic nerve, but little or no visual field loss. Those with moderate optic nerve damage have typical glaucomatous visual field defects in one hemifield only. Those with advanced optic nerve damage have extensive visual field loss involving both hemifields. The dotted line indicates choice of combined surgery for select patients, usually those without marked elevation of intraocular pressure.

(a)

Capsulorrhexis

Pupil

Counter-
incision

Phaco
tip

Conjunctiva
reflected back

Phaco irrigating
handle

(b)

IOL in
the bag

Iridectomy

Trabeculectomy

(c)

9-0
absorbable
suture

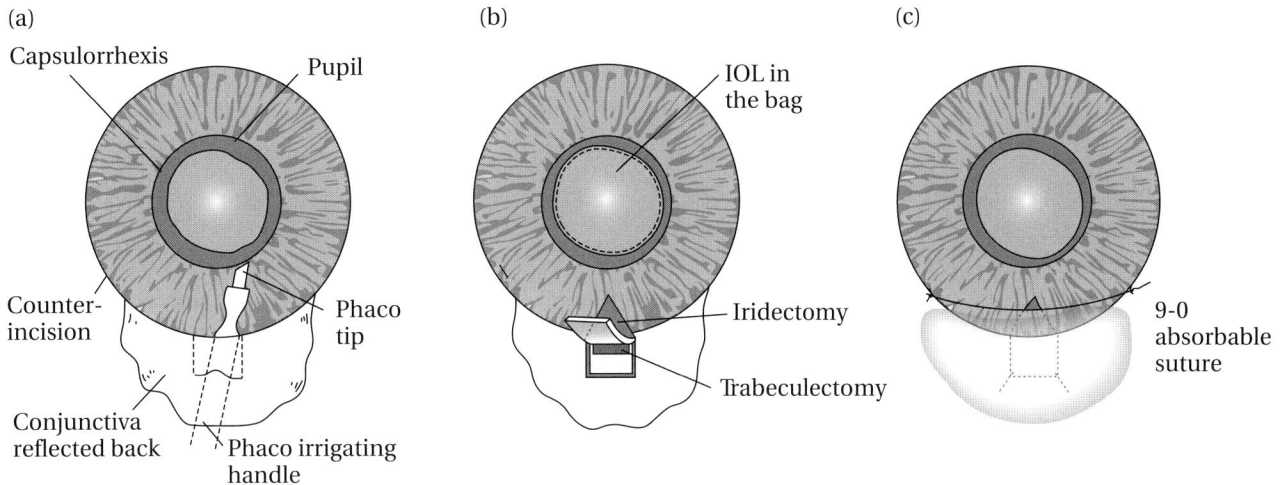

FIGURE 35.2 Technique for combined phacoemulsification and trabeculectomy through the same incision. The conjunctival flap may be fornix or limbus based. A fornix-based flap is shown. (a) Phacoemulsification is performed through a scleral tunnel, and a foldable intraocular lens is inserted through the tunnel. A foldable intraocular lens can be inserted through this incision, or the incision can be extended at the limbus slightly to the left and right to accommodate a rigid intraocular lens. Some surgeons make a short tunnel under a triangular partial-thickness sclera flap. (b) The scleral tunnel is then converted by radial incisions into a rectangular scleral flap. The trabeculectomy and basal iridectomy are then performed. The scleral flap is sutured at each of its corners with interrupted 10-0 nylon sutures. Releasable sutures may be used, according to surgeon preference. (c) The conjunctiva is pulled down toward the limbus and sutured securely at each corner with a 9-0 absorbable suture. The conjunctiva should be held by these sutures taut against the cornea, to reduce possible leakage at the limbus. Alternatively, a running mattress suture using 9-0 absorbable suture may be used to close the conjunctival incision at the limbus. The bleb is raised by injection of balanced salt solution through the clear-corneal paracentesis incision.

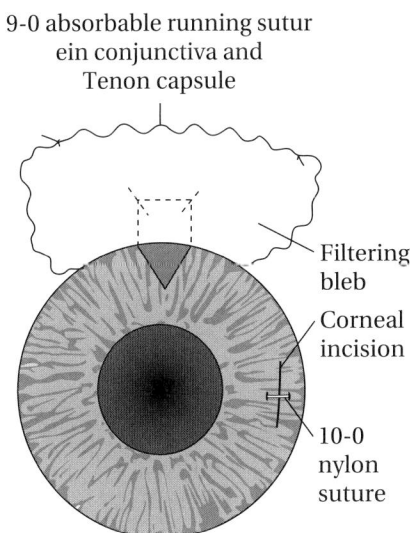

9-0 absorbable running sutur
ein conjunctiva and
Tenon capsule

Filtering
bleb

Corneal
incision

10-0
nylon
suture

FIGURE 35.3 Separate-incision phacoemulsification and trabeculectomy. With use of this technique, clear-corneal phacoemulsification is performed, and a foldable intraocular lens is implanted in the capsular bag. The clear-corneal wound may be sutured with a single 10-0 nylon suture. Next, a standard trabeculectomy is performed superiorly. It is helpful to make sure the eye is firm by instillation of balanced salt or viscoelastic solution through the clear-corneal incision before the scleral flap is dissected. This approach is usually performed with a limbus-based conjunctival flap.

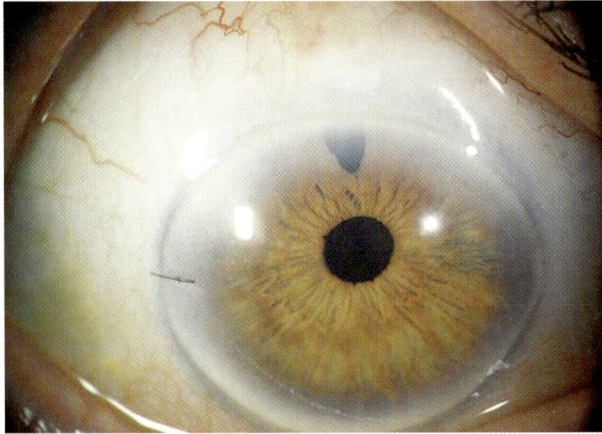

FIGURE 35.4 Postoperative appearance of eye after combined phacoemulsification and trabeculectomy. This slit-lamp photograph was taken 3 weeks postoperatively.

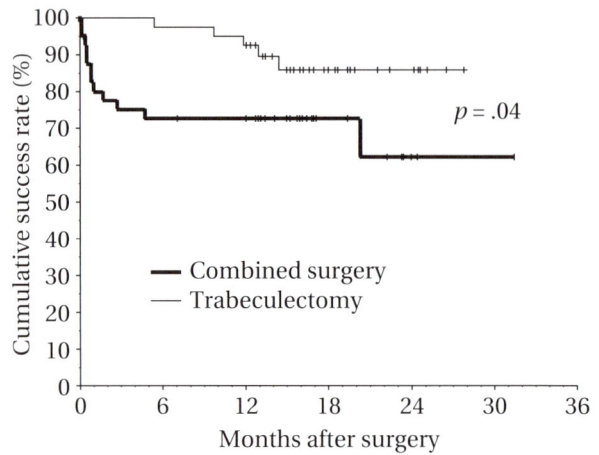

FIGURE 35.5 Survival curves for separate-incision phacoemulsification and trabeculectomy versus trabeculectomy alone. Based on Kaplan-Meier survival analysis, the cumulative intraocular pressure success rate was statistically lower ($p = .04$) in the combined-surgery group than in the trabeculectomy group (log-rank test). (Reprinted with permission from Caprioli J, Park HF, Weitzman M. Temporal corneal phacoemulsification combined with superior trabeculectomy: a controlled study. *Arch Ophthalmol.* 1997;115:318–323. Copyright © 1997, American Medical Association.)

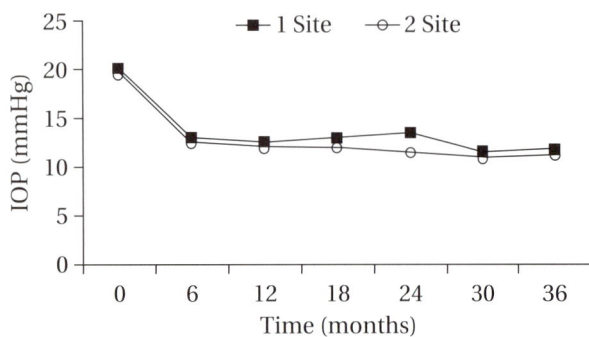

FIGURE 35.6 Average intraocular pressure after 1-site and 2-site phacotrabeculectomy. During a follow-up period of 3 years, no statistically significant difference in pressure was found between the two groups. Although each group had a significant reduction in the requirement of anti-glaucoma medications postoperatively, the average number of medications was the same. (Based on data from Cotran PR, Roh S, McGwin G. Randomized comparison of 1-site and 2-site phacotrabeculectomy with 3-year follow-up. *Ophthalmology.* 2008;115:447–454.)

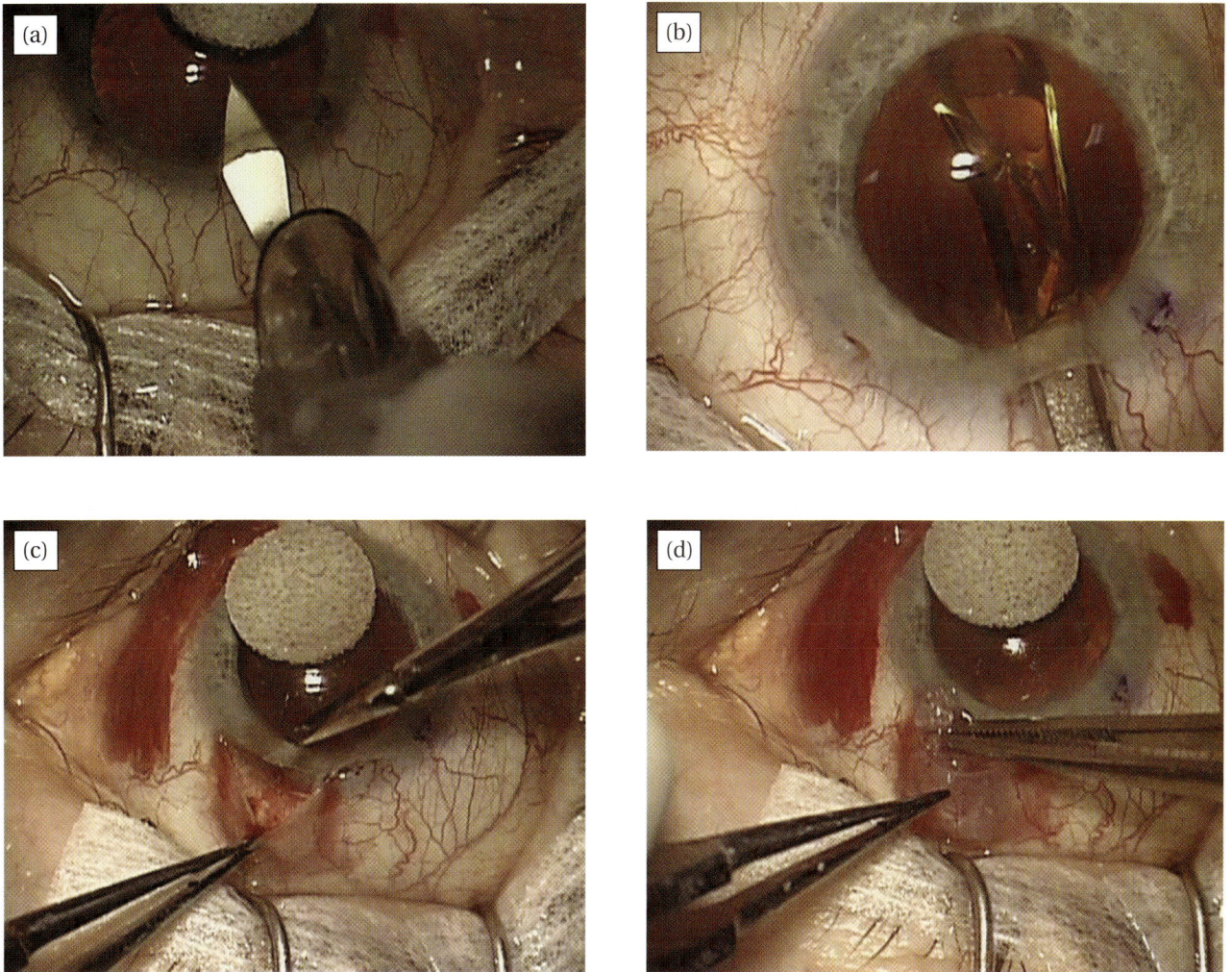

FIGURE 35.7 Separate site, combined phacoemulsification with Ex-PRESS implant. After creation of paracentesis incisions at 10 and 2-o'clock, in preparation for bimanual irrigation and aspiration, the clear-cornea phacoemulsification incision is prepared with a keratome (a). Capsulorhexis is performed, and the lens removed by phacoemulsification, followed by bimanual irrigation and aspiration, after which the foldable intraocular lens is inserted (b). A limbal peritomy is performed, allowing preparation of a fornix-based conjunctival flap (c). After dissection of a partial thickness scleral flap, 0.4 mg/mL of mitomycin C (0.2–0.4 mg/mL) is applied to the surgical area for 1–3 minutes (d).

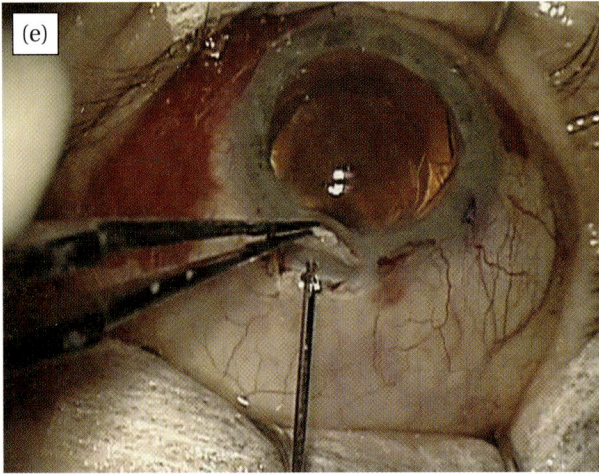

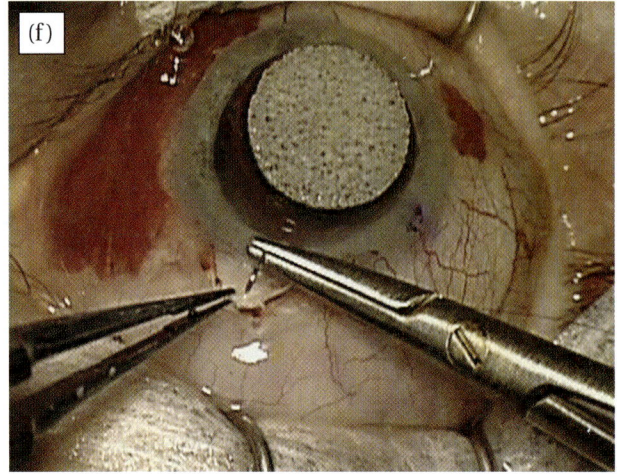

FIGURE 35.7 (*continued*) The Ex-PRESS implant is inserted under the flap at the limbus into the anterior chamber through a 27- or 25 gauge needle track (e). The scleral flap is sutured with 10-0 interrupted nylon sutures (f), followed by closure of the conjunctival incision using a watertight, horizontal mattress technique to minimize wound leakage during the immediate postoperative period. (Photographs courtesy P.A. Netland.)

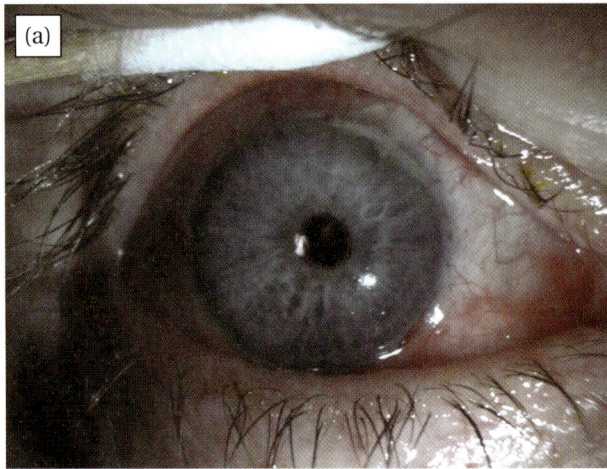

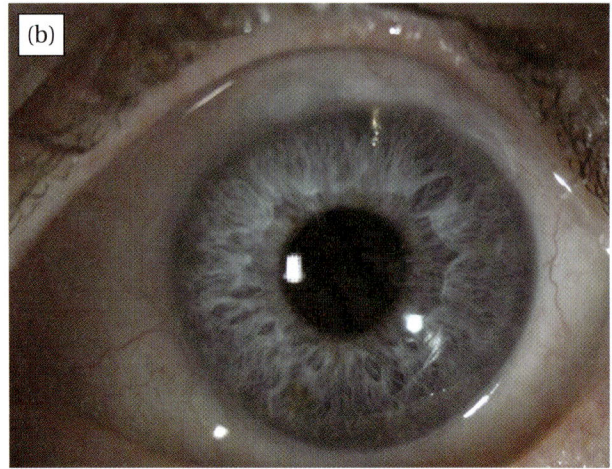

FIGURE 35.8 Postoperative appearance after combined phacoemulsification and Ex-PRESS implant. (a) Appearance of the eye on postoperative day 1. (b) The same patient at 5 months after surgery. At this visit, the vision was 20/20 and the intraocular pressure was in the low teens. (Photographs courtesy P.A. Netland.)

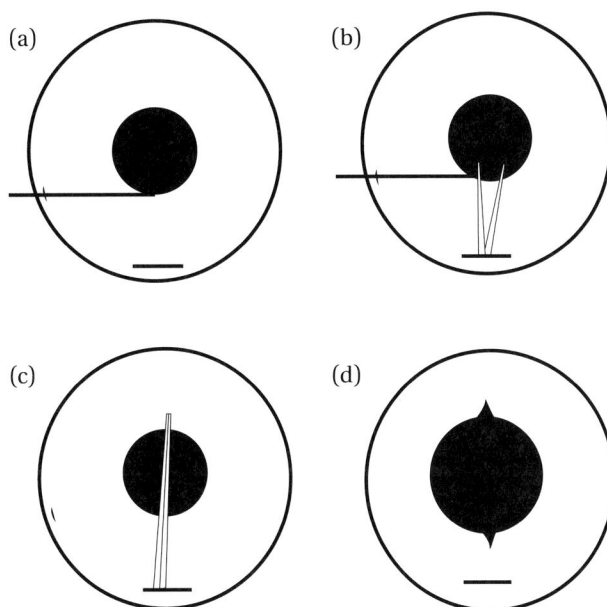

FIGURE 35.9 Management of small pupil. Small pupil despite cycloplegia is a common problem in patients with glaucoma and cataract, and should be addressed in order to minimize the risk of vitreous loss and other intraoperative complications. Multiple approaches are used for enlargement of small pupils to allow for adequate exposure of the lens in preparation for phacoemulsification, including stretch pupilloplasty, multiple sphincterotomies, iris hooks, iris suturing techniques, the Graether pupil expander, the Beehler pupil device, and the Malyugin Ring. In the example shown, posterior synechiae are swept with an iris or Barraquer spatula after instillation of a viscoelastic substance into the anterior chamber (a). After stretching the pupil, small sphincterotomies are made on the temporal (b) and the nasal (c) sides of the pupil using long intraocular scissors. Additional viscoelastic substance is instilled, and the pupil size becomes adequate for continuing phacoemulsification (d).

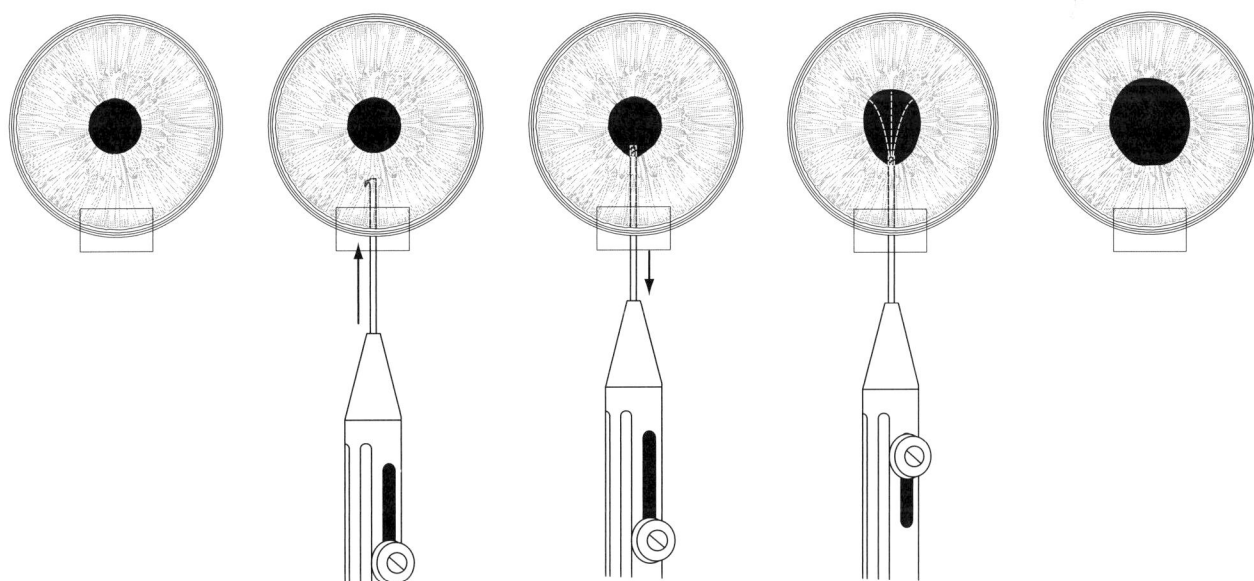

FIGURE 35.10 Beehler pupil stretch. The Beehler device is inserted through the phacoemulsification incision, the barrel hooked onto the subincisional pupil edge, and the three prongs extended to engage the opposite pupillary edge and held dilated for 1 full minute. On careful withdrawal of the barrel, the chamber is reinflated with viscoelastic substance and the pupillary diameter reassessed.

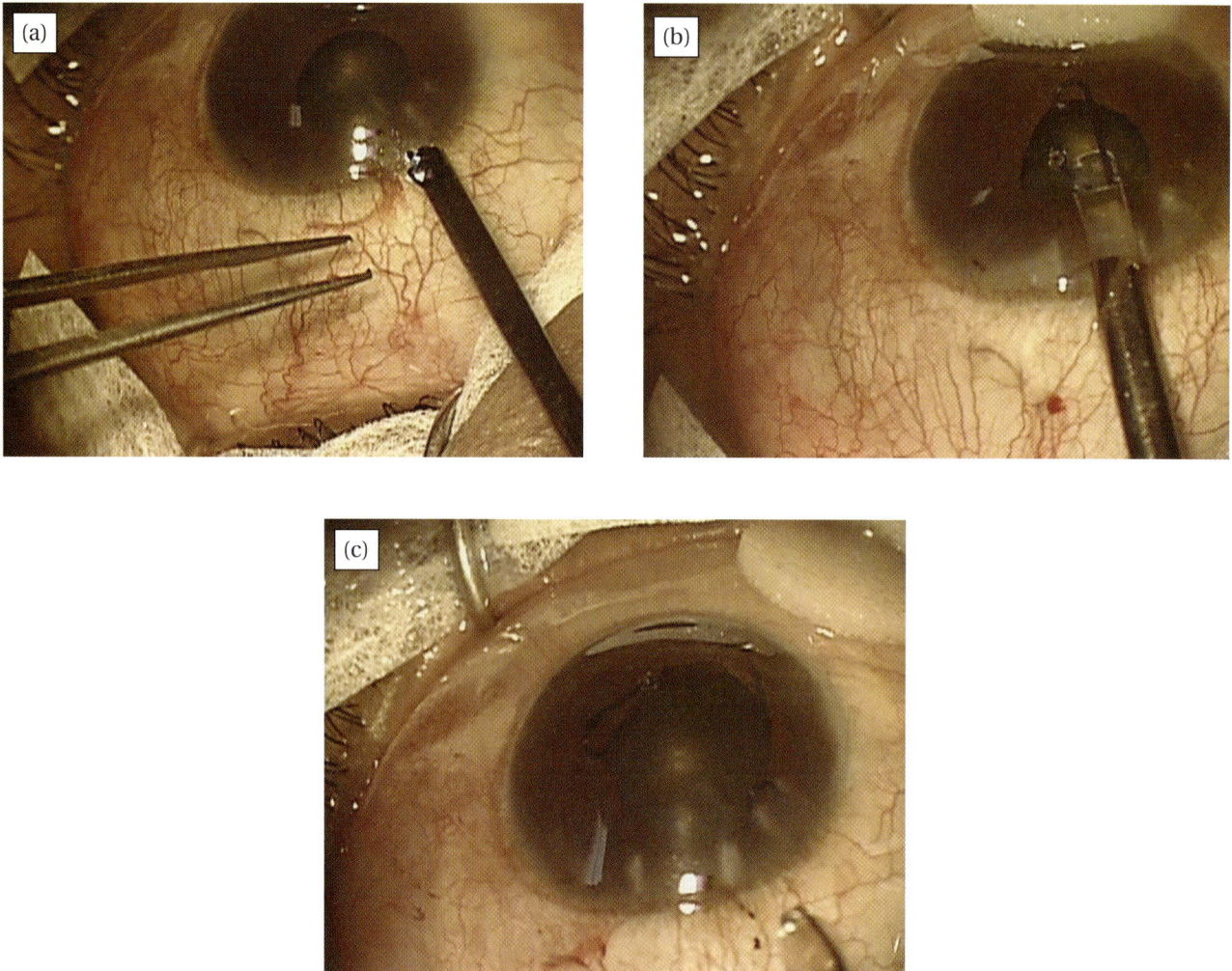

FIGURE 35.11 Malyugin ring. This device is a flexible, square-shaped, temporary implant, with four circular loops that hold the iris open at equidistant points. The ring is loaded in an injector, which is inserted through the primary corneal or scleral incision (a). The distal loop of the Malyugin ring engages the pupillary margin (b). The remaining loops are placed around the iris (c), which expands the pupil to allow for surgical exposure of the lens in preparation for phacoemulsification. (Photographs courtesy P.A. Netland.)

TABLE 35.2 *Complications of Combined Phacoemulsification and Trabeculectomy*

Filtering Procedure Associated	Cataract Removal Associated
Early	*Early*
Infection	Endophthalmitis
Hypotony	Iris trauma/prolapse
Shallow or flat anterior chamber	Anterior chamber hemorrhage
Aqueous misdirection	Hypopyon
Formation or acceleration of cataract	Posterior capsule rupture
Transient IOP elevation	Vitreous loss
Cystoid macular edema	Vitreous hemorrhage
Choroidal effusion	Choroidal hemorrhage
Suprachoroidal hemorrhage	
Persistent uveitis	*Late*
Dellen formation	Bullous keratopathy
Loss of vision	Malposition/dislocation of IOL
	Cystoid macular edema
Late	Retinal detachment
Leakage or failure of the filtering bleb	Uveitis
Blebitis	Increased IOP
Endophthalmitis	Posterior capsular opacification
Bleb migration	
Ptosis	
Eyelid retraction	

SELECTED REFERENCES

Caprioli J, Park HF, Weitzman M. Temporal corneal phacoemulsification combined with superior trabeculectomy: A controlled study. *Arch Ophthalmol.* 1997;115:318–323.

Cioffi GA, Durcan FJ, Girkin CA, et al. Glaucoma. *Basic and Clinical Science Course.* San Francisco, CA: American Academy of Ophthalmology; 2009.

Cotran PR, Roh S, McGwin G. Randomized comparison of 1-Site and 2-Site phacotrabeculectomy with 3-year follow-up. *Ophthalmol.* 2008;115:447–454.

Friedman DS, Jampel HD, Lubomski LH, et al. Surgical strategies for coexisting glaucoma and cataract: An evidence-based update. *Ophthalmol.* 2002;109:1902–1913.

Jampel HD, Friedman DS, Lubomski LH, et al. Effect of technique on intraocular pressure after combined cataract and glaucoma surgery: An evidence-based review. *Ophthalmol.* 2002;109:2215–2224.

Lee RK, Gedde SJ. Surgical management of coexisting cataract and glaucoma. *Int Ophthalmol Clin.* 2004;44:151–166.

Wise JB. Mitomycin-compatible suture technique for fornix-based conjunctival flaps in glaucoma filtration surgery. *Arch Ophthalmol.* 1993;111:992–997.

36 Nonpenetrating Glaucoma Surgery (NPGS)

Vanessa Vera Machado, MD, Graham W. Belovay, BCmp, MD, and Iqbal Ike K. Ahmed, MD, FRCSC

Indications

Initial Steps in Nonpenetrating Glaucoma Surgery

Deep Sclerectomy with or without Collagen Implant

Viscocanalostomy

Indications

TABLE 36.1 *Indications for Nonpenetrating Glaucoma Surgery*

Indications

Primary open-angle glaucoma (POAG), especially if:

Early surgical intervention is required

Monocular patient

Diurnal fluctuations (pigment dispersion/pseudo-exfoliation glaucoma)

Aphakic and pseudophakic glaucoma

High risk of choroidal effusions or hemorrhages (axial myopia, hypertension, history of choroidal effusion or hemorrhages, increased episcleral venous pressure)

High risk of postoperative hypotony (young age, high myopia, male)

Uveitic/traumatic glaucoma without extensive peripheral anterior synechiae

Young patient (juvenile glaucoma)

TABLE 36.2 *Contraindications for Nonpenetrating Glaucoma Surgery*

Contraindications	
Absolute	**Relative**
Primary or secondary angle closure glaucoma	Narrow/occludable angles *
Neovascular glaucoma	Previous laser trabeculoplasty
Altered anatomy (thin sclera, significant limbal scarring from previous sclera tunnel or extracapsular cataract extraction)	

*NPGS can be combined with cataract/lens extraction surgery.

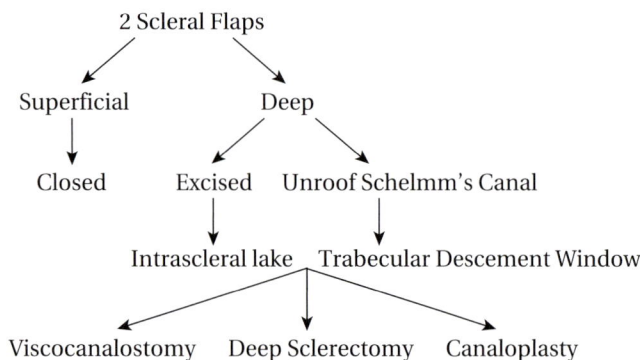

2 Scleral Flaps

Superficial → Closed

Deep → Excised → Intrascleral lake

Deep → Unroof Schelmm's Canal → Trabecular Descement Window

Intrascleral lake / Trabecular Descement Window → Viscocanalostomy, Deep Sclerectomy, Canaloplasty

FIGURE 36.1 **Common Features of Nonpenetrating Glaucoma Surgeries.** Initial Steps in Nonpenetrating Glaucoma Surgery.

Initial Steps in Nonpenetrating Glaucoma Surgery

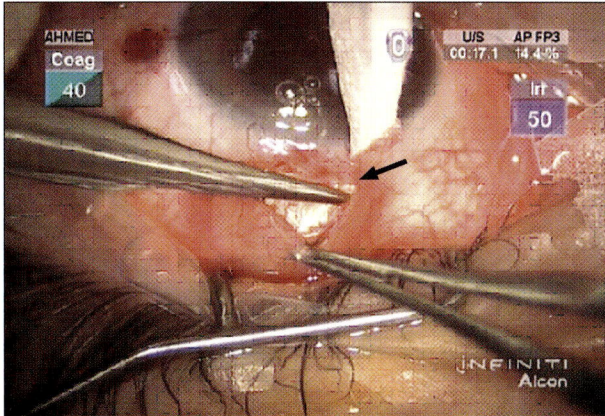

FIGURE 36.2 **Conjunctival Flap.** This varies according to surgeon, with our preference being to create a fornix-based flap in the superior region. We leave a stump (arrow) of conjunctiva to allow for conjunctiva-to-conjunctiva closure at the conclusion of the case. Undermining surrounding conjunctiva should be dissected to allow for proper exposure of the area.

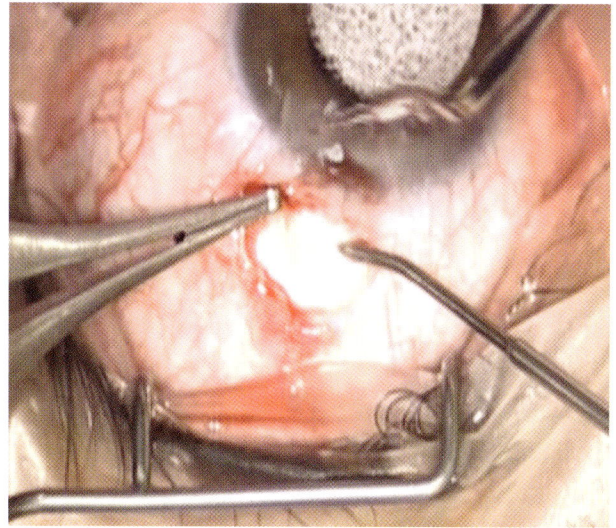

FIGURE 36.3 **Cautery.** Gentle cautery is applied to the bleeding vessels prior to creation of a scleral flap to achieve hemostasis.

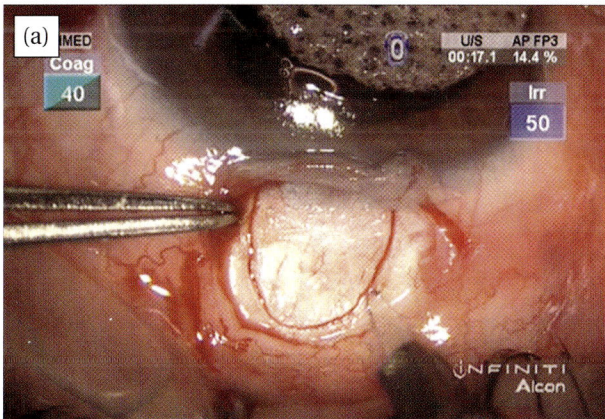

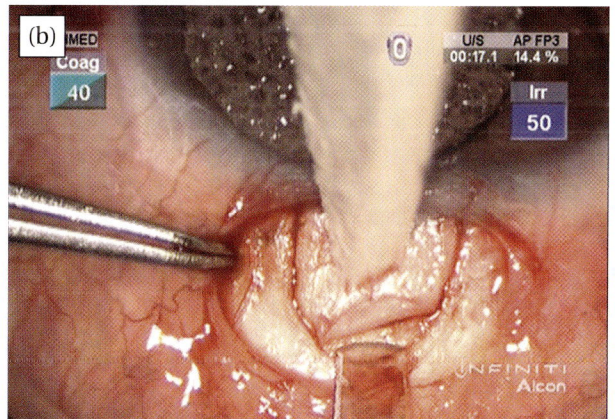

FIGURE 36.4 **Superficial Flap.** A superficial scleral flap is created aiming for one-third to one half of the scleral thickness (approximately 300 μm). The flap is carried 1–2 mm into clear cornea (to be able to reach Descemet's membrane later in the dissection). The shape and size of the flap differs with each type of surgery and will be described in detail later.

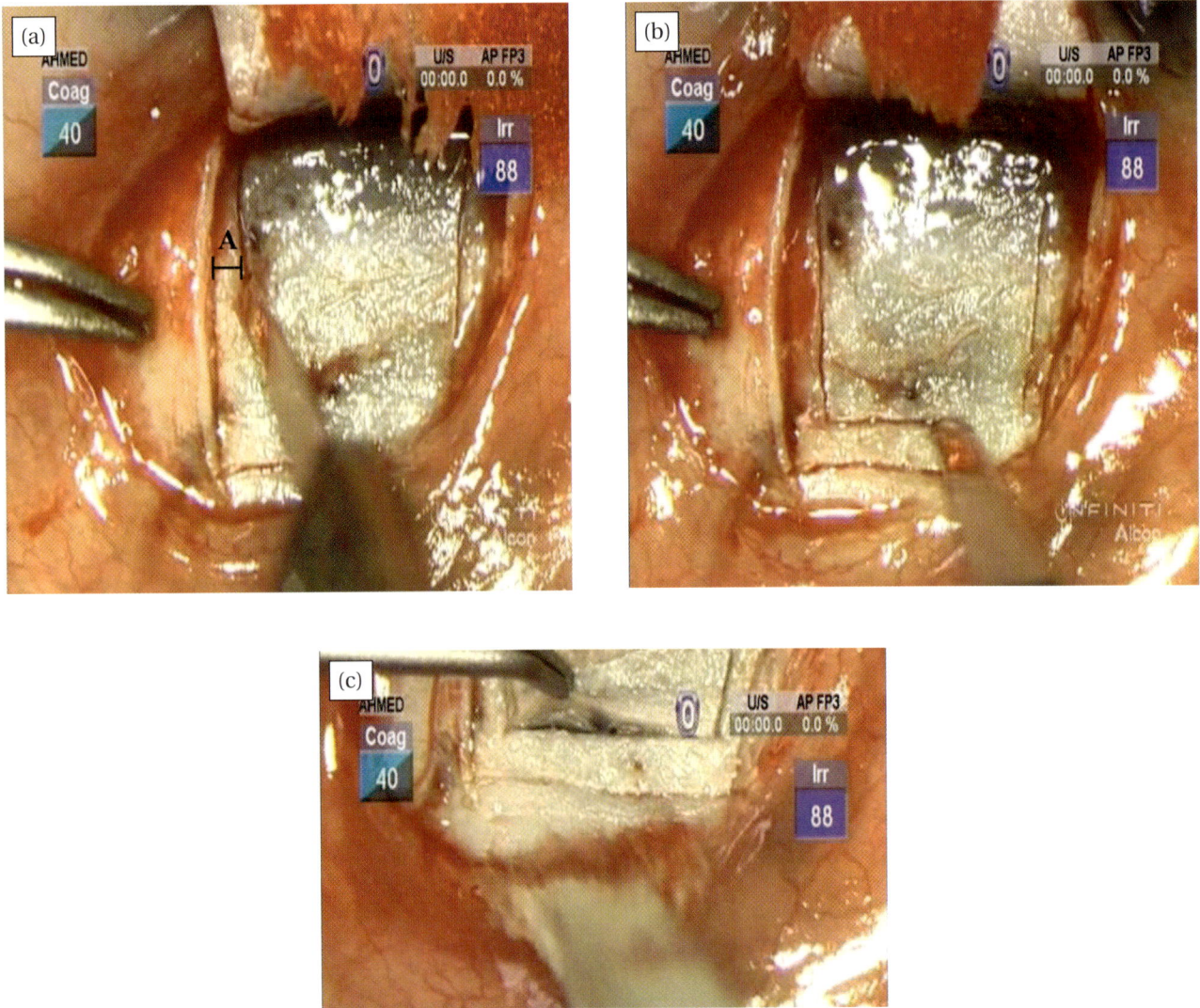

FIGURE 36.5 **Score of the Deep Flap.** This flap is smaller, approximately 0.5–1 mm (a) than the superficial flap, leaving a cuff of scleral base on three sides. It needs to be 90% of the scleral thickness which results in the anterior score been more superficial than the posterior score (should be performed under high magnification).

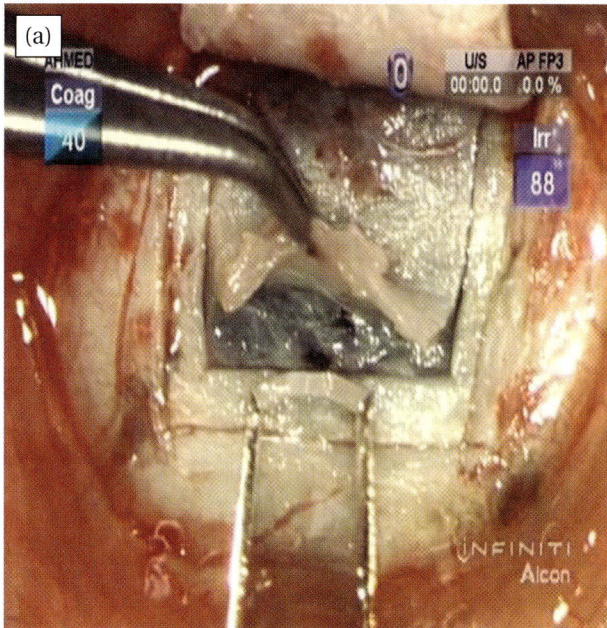

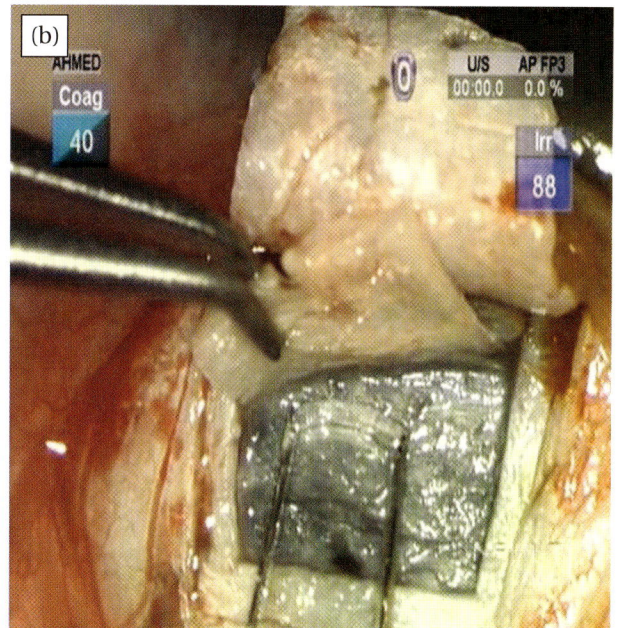

FIGURE 36.6 **Dissection of the Deep Flap**. Only a very thin layer of scleral tissue (approximately 100 μm) should be left covering the choroid. When necessary to assess depth, it is helpful and inconsequential to dissect down to the suprachoroidal space.

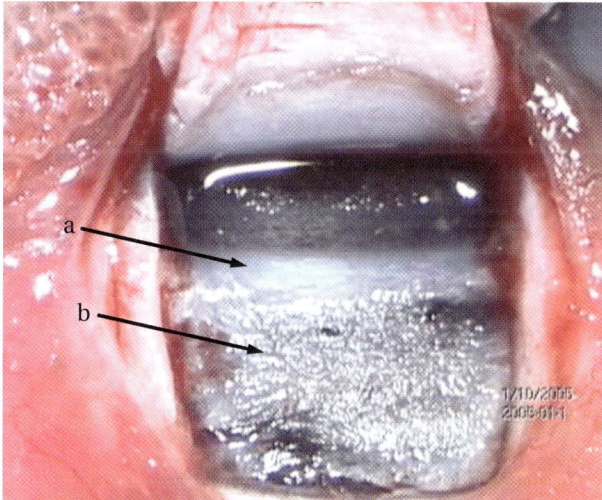

FIGURE 36.7 **Scleral Arrangement.** At the correct depth, the surgeon will notice the irregular arrangement of scleral fibers with the deep purple hue of the choroid. The scleral fibers in the base change from a random arrangement (b) to an organized arrangement circumferential to the limbus; this represents the scleral spur (a). A too-superficial flap will result in difficulty identifying the true anatomic position of Schlemm's canal (SC) or passing over rather than into the canal during dissection.

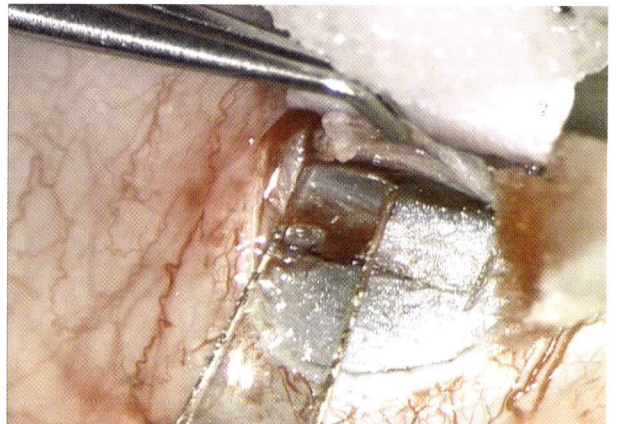

FIGURE 36.8 **Paracentesis and Descemet's Membrane Exposure.** A paracentesis should be created in the temporal clear cornea and aqueous encouraged to egress from the anterior chamber (AC). A low IOP is desired at this point, prior to exposure of Descemet's membrane, to reduce risks of perforation or trauma during this delicate dissection. The deep flap dissection should continue anteriorly approximately 1–2 mm to expose Descemet's membrane.

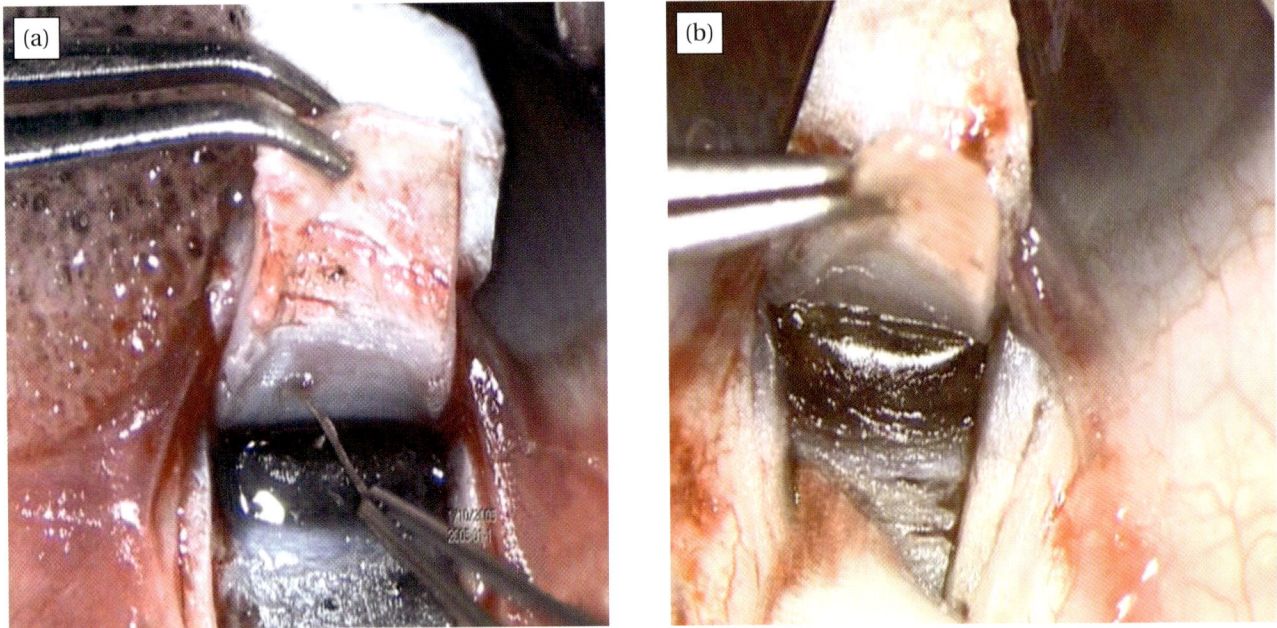

FIGURE 36.9 **Unroof of Schlemm's Canal.** Continuing the dissection forward at the correct level will unroof SC (a), beyond which exists a natural plane between Descemet's membrane and the overlying stroma, which requires little to no force to advance. Aqueous humor may be observed to slowly percolate through Descemet's membrane. This clear window that remains (b) is commonly termed trabeculo-Descemet's window (TDW).

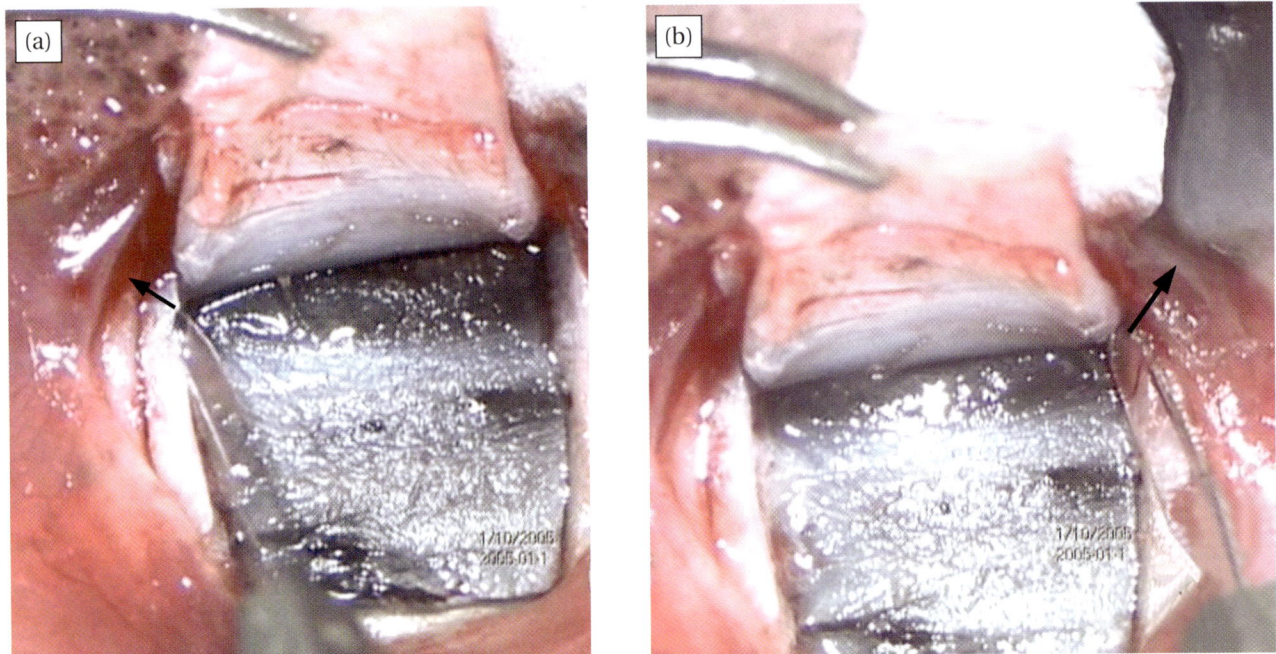

FIGURE 36.10 **Vertical Relaxing Incisions.** These are required on the lateral edges of the flap to carry the flap into the cornea. Great care must be taken to avoid rupturing Descemet's membrane.

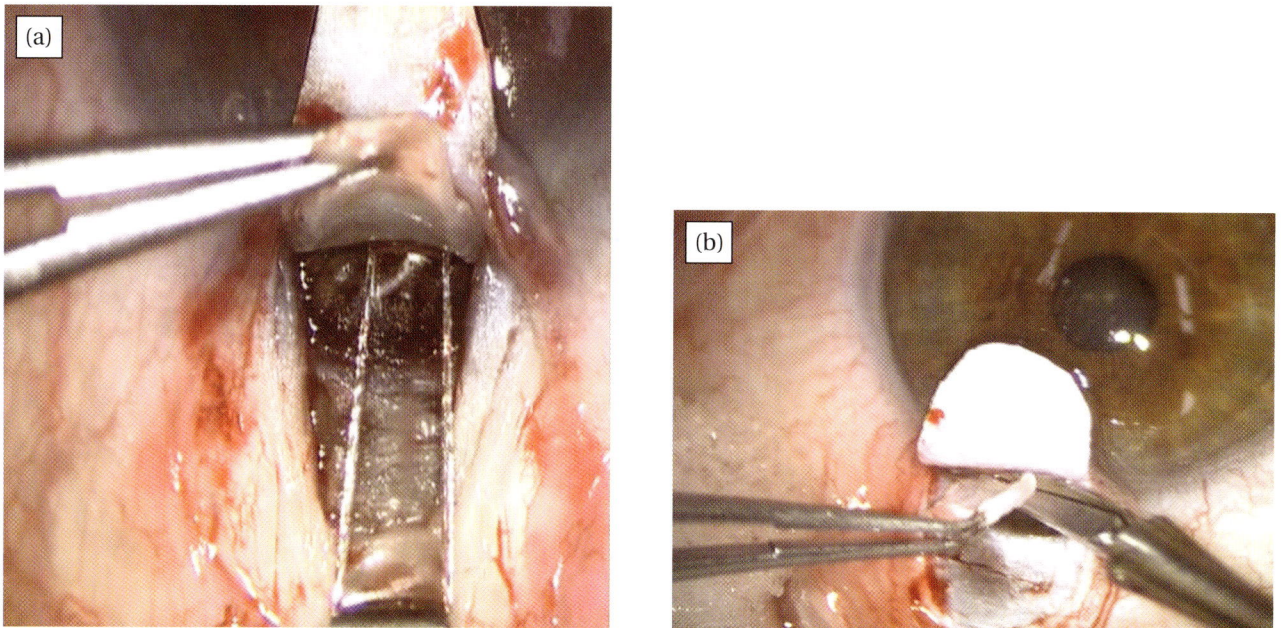

FIGURE 36.11 **Removal of Deep Flap.** This flap must be excised to create space for the scleral lake. First a score is made close to Descement´s membrane (a) and then cut using Vannas scissors (b). Special care must be taken not to leave a large anterior residual lip of tissue; otherwise, it will cover the TDW.

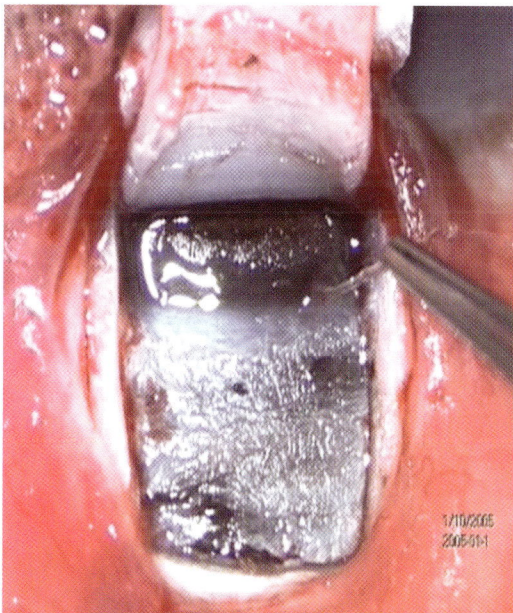

FIGURE 36.12 **Removal of Inner Wall of Schlemm's Canal.** The inner wall is located anterior to the scleral spur. The peeling maneuver is facilitated with the forceps specifically designed for this purpose, Mermoud forceps (Huco Vision SA, Saint-Biaise, Switzerland). Following the removal, the surgeon will notice an immediate increase in the percolation of fluid through the TDW.

Deep Sclerectomy with or without Collagen Implant

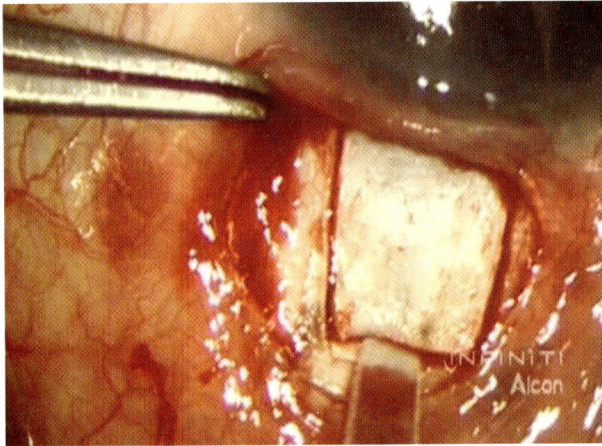

FIGURE 36.13 **Superficial Flap.** Using the technique described in Figure 36.4, a superficial square-shaped scleral flap 5 mm × 5 mm in size is created.

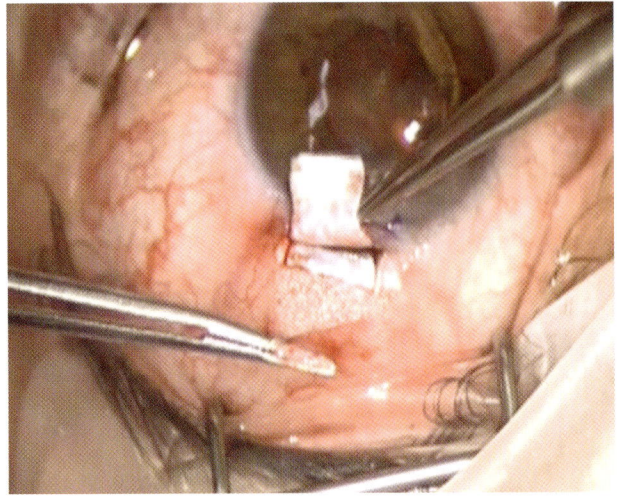

FIGURE 36.14 **Use of Antimetabolites.** Prior to the creation of the deep flap in Figure 36.5, if indicated, mitomycin-C (MMC) soaked sponges are placed under the superficial flap, thereby reducing intrascleral fibrosis that may threaten to obliterate the sclera lake. Note that the edge of the conjunctival flap has been elevated to preclude wound leaks.

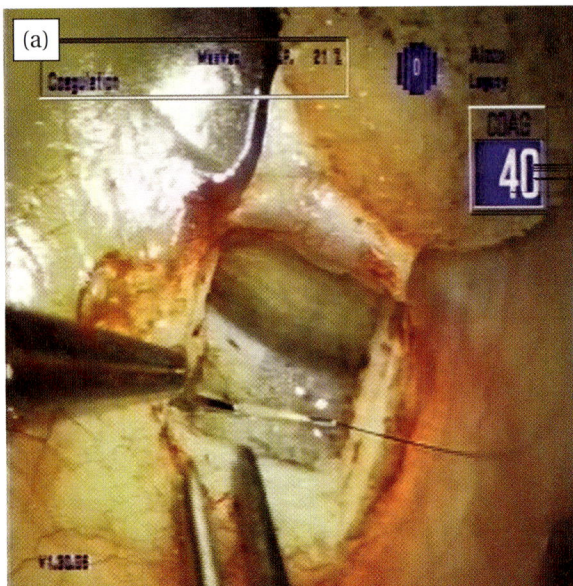

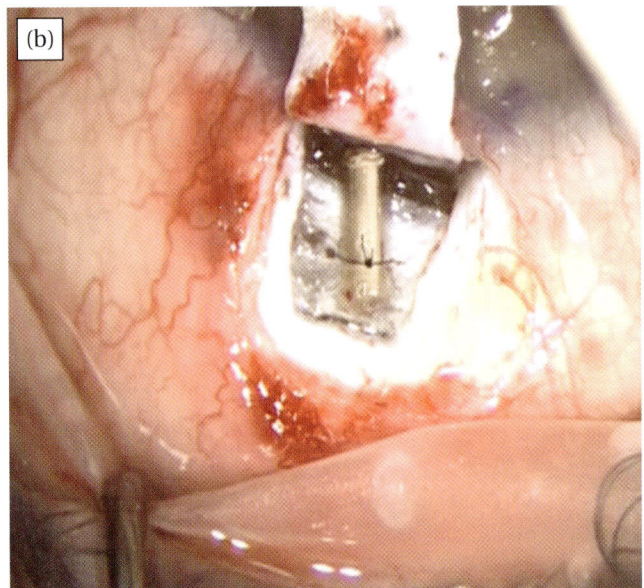

FIGURE 36.15 **Space-maintaining Devices.** Most commonly, a collagen implant (AquaFlow, STAAR Surgical, Manrovia, CA) is employed. A 10-0 nylon suture is placed in the remaining sclera (a). The collagen implant is placed radially in the center (b), as far anterior as possible to be in contact with the remaining trabeculo-Descemet's membrane, and tied into place. These implants are reabsorbed within 6–9 months after surgery.

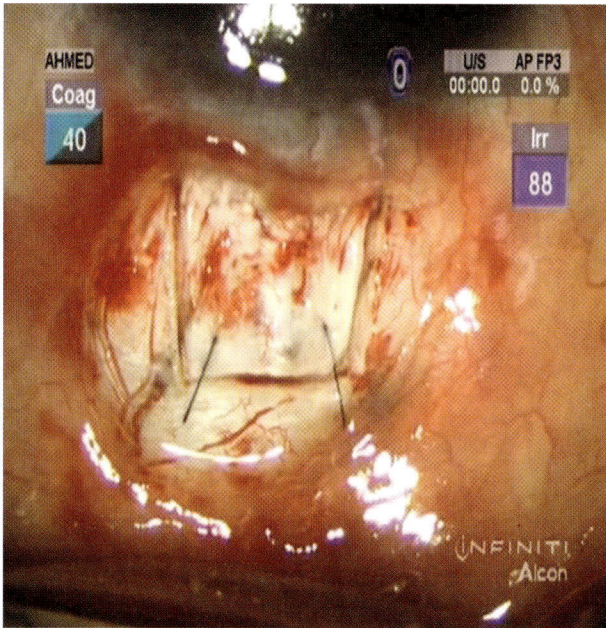

FIGURE 36.16 Closure of the External/Superficial Flap. This flap is then closed loosely, using two 10-0 nylon sutures, to promote bleb formation.

Viscocanalostomy

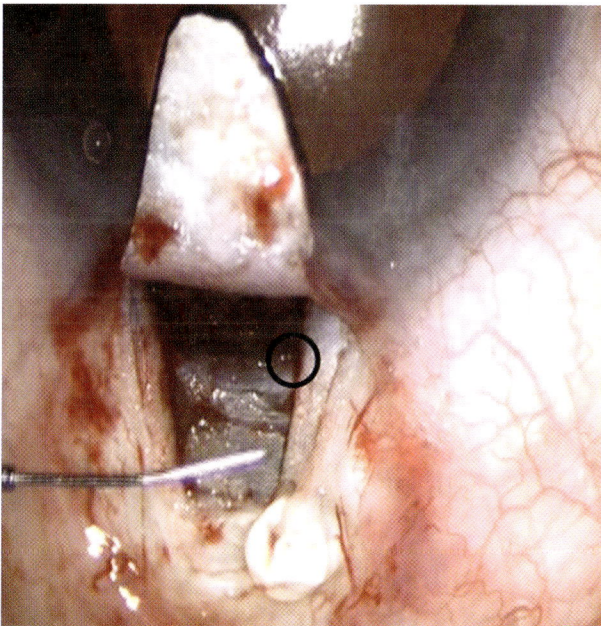

FIGURE 36.17 Decompress the Anterior Chamber. The AC is decompressed again to create a mild degree of hypotony, so that blood refluxes from SC (circle). This helps in localization of the cut ends of SC.

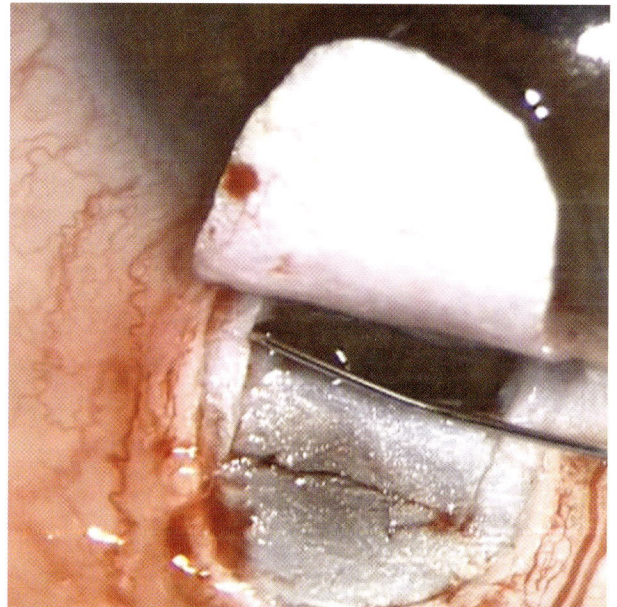

FIGURE 36.18 Intubation of Schlemm´s Canal. The cut ends of SC are intubated with a viscocanalostomy cannula (150 µm diameter, Grieshaber Alcon Laboratories, Fort Worth, TX) and Healon GV (Advanced Medical Optics, Inc., Santa Ana, CA) is injected into each end 5 to 6 times, widening the SC and improving flow through it.

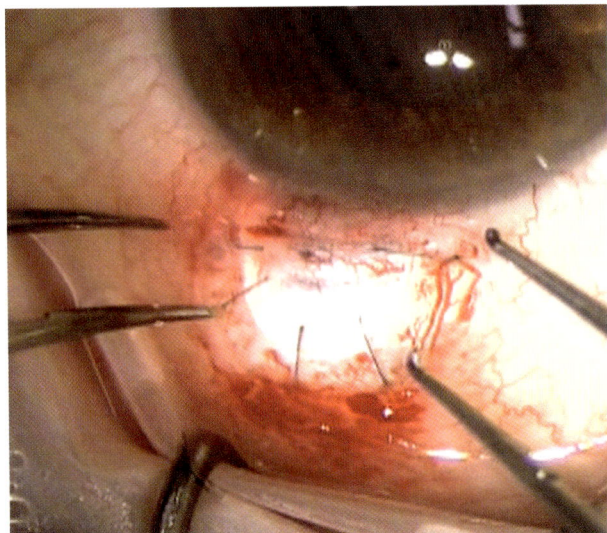

FIGURE 36.19 **Closure of the Superficial Flap.** The superficial parabolic scleral flap is closed in a watertight fashion with 5 interrupted 10-0 nylon sutures.

Canaloplasty

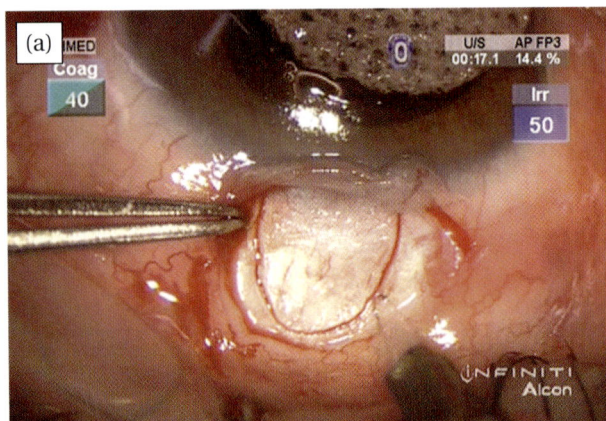

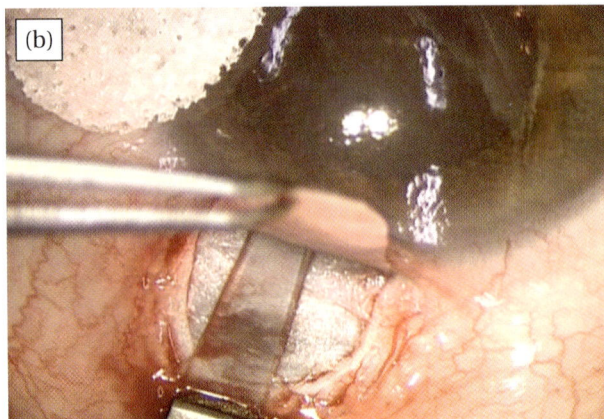

FIGURE 36.20 **Superficial Flap.** Using the technique described in Figure 36.4, a superficial parabolic shaped scleral flap 5 mm × 5 mm in size is created (enhances the watertight closure). This chapter section provides additional surgical detail about canaloplasty, compared with Chapter 37. (Alternative Glaucoma Procedures.)

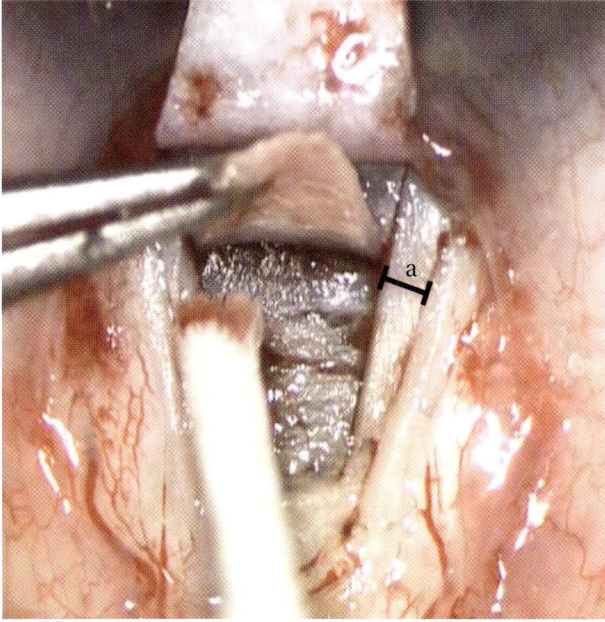

FIGURE 36.21 **Score of the Deep Flap.** This flap is smaller, approximately 0.5–1 mm (a) than the superficial flap, leaving a cuff of scleral base on three sides. It should be 90% of the scleral thickness, which results in the anterior score being more superficial than the posterior score (should be performed under high magnification). Only a very thin layer of scleral tissue (approximately 100 μm) should be left covering the choroid. When necessary to assess depth, it is helpful (and inconsequential) to dissect down to the suprachoroidal space.

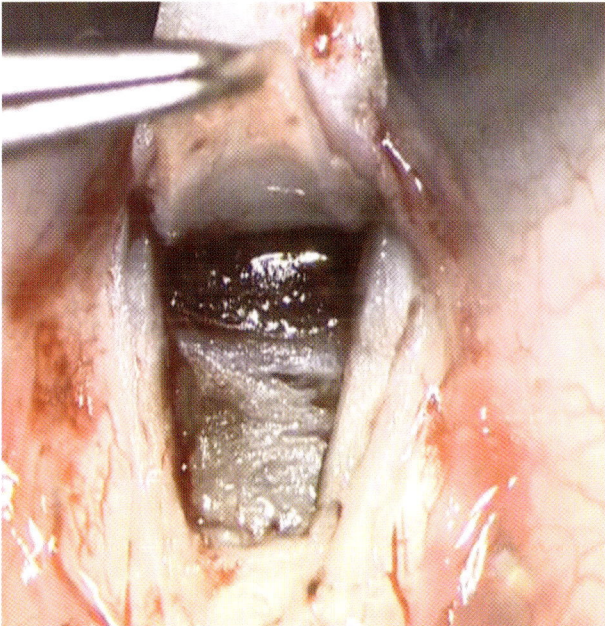

FIGURE 36.22 **Paracentesis and Descemet's Membrane Exposure.** A paracentesis should be created in the temporal clear cornea, and aqueous encouraged to egress from the anterior chamber (AC). A low IOP is desired at this point, prior to exposure of Descemet's membrane, to reduce risks of perforation or trauma during this delicate dissection. The deep flap dissection should continue anteriorly approximately 1–2 mm to expose Descemet's membrane. Continuing the dissection forward at the correct level will unroof SC, beyond which exists a natural plane between Descemet's membrane and the overlying stroma, which requires little to no force to advance. Aqueous humor may be observed to slowly percolate through Descemet's membrane. This clear window that remains is the TDW.

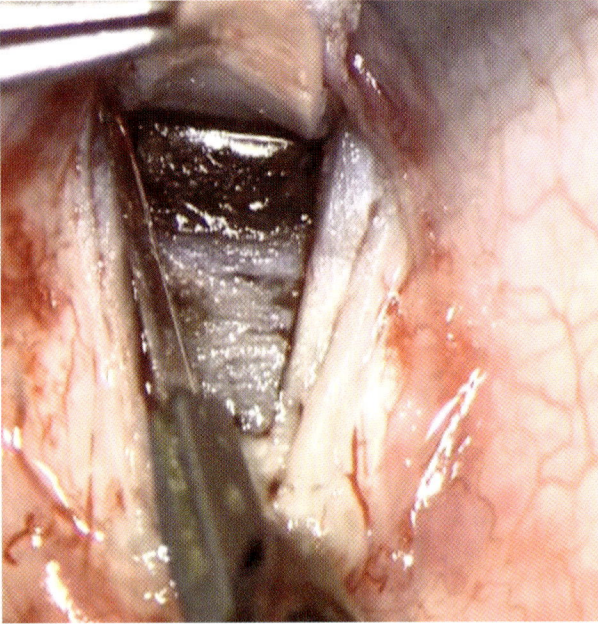

FIGURE 36.23 **Vertical Relaxing Incisions.** These are required on the lateral edges of the flap to carry the flap into the cornea. Great care must be taken to avoid rupturing Descemet's membrane.

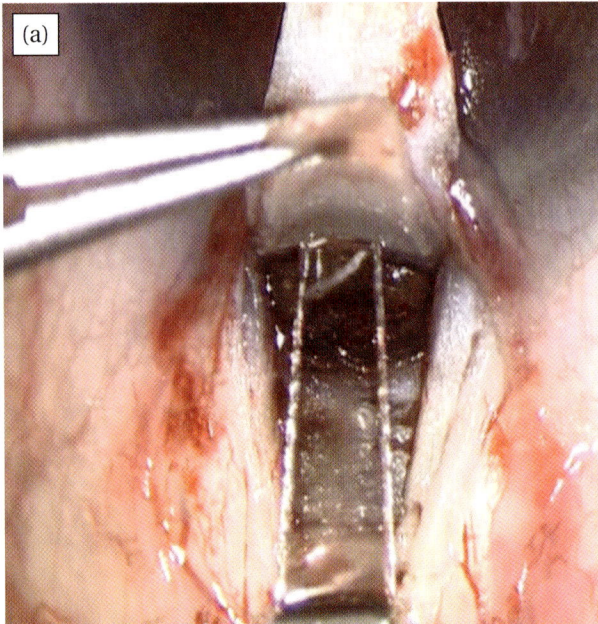

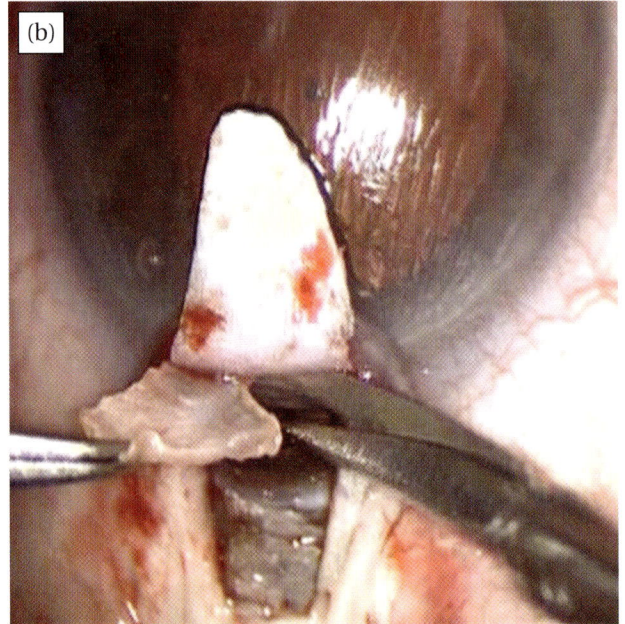

FIGURE 36.24 **Removal of Deep Flap.** This flap must be excised to create space for the scleral lake. First a score is made close to Descemet's membrane (a) and then cut using Vannas scissors (b). Special care must be taken not to leave a large anterior residual lip of tissue; otherwise, it will cover the TDW.

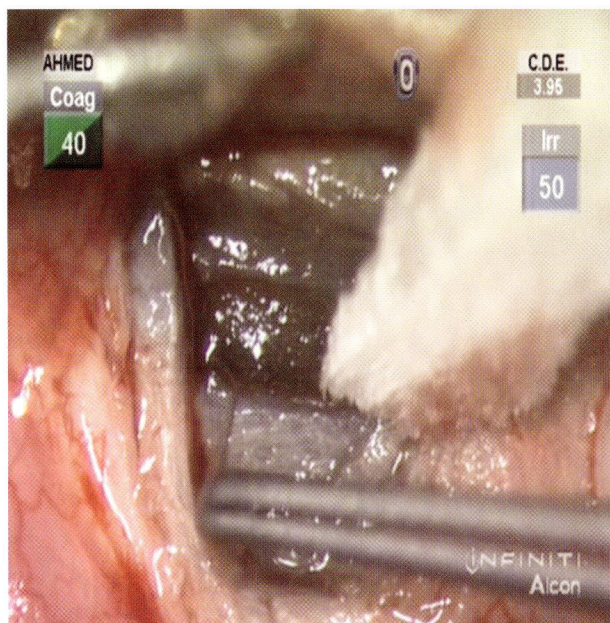

FIGURE 36.25 Removal of Inner Wall of Schlemm's Canal. The inner wall is located anterior to the scleral spur. The peeling maneuver is facilitated with the forceps specifically designed for this purpose, Mermoud forceps. Following the removal, the surgeon will notice an immediate increase in the percolation of fluid through the TDW.

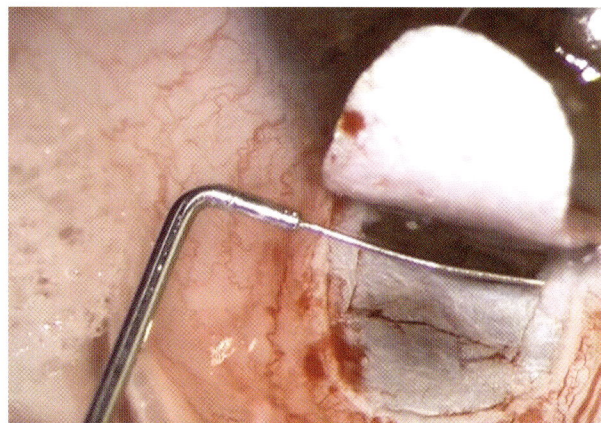

FIGURE 36.26 Intubation of Schlemm´s Canal. The cut ends of SC are intubated with a viscocanalostomy cannula (150 μm diameter) and Healon GV is injected into each.

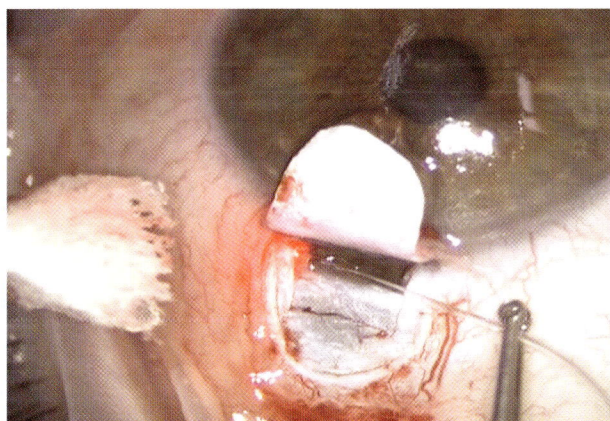

FIGURE 36.27 Catherization of Schlemm´s Canal. A flexible polymer microcatheter (iScience Interventional Inc., Menlo Park, CA), 200 μm shaft diameter, is grasped using two non-toothed forceps, and the rounded atraumatic tip is carefully introduced into one of the cut ends of Schlemm's canal.

(a)

SMA connector for light source

Luer connector for fluid infusion/aspiration

Extension line for light source

Extension line for fluid infusion/aspiration

Hub, attach to drape/patient

(b)

Optical fiber, light transmission

Catheter support wire

Lumen

Polymer shaft and distal atraumatic tip

(c)

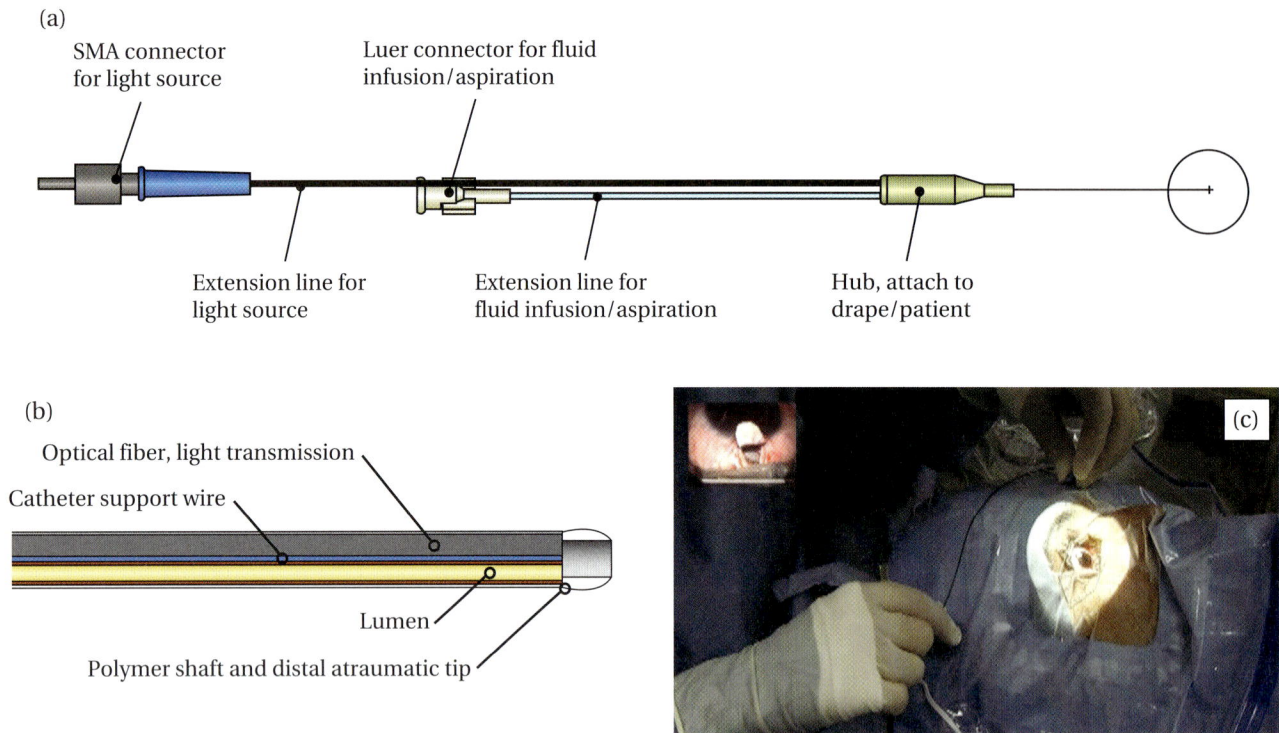

FIGURE 36.28 **Microcatheter.** The microcatheter consists of optical fibers to allow for the transmission of light from a laser-based micro-illumination system to the tip, culminating in a blinking red light. This assists the surgeon in the visualization and localization of the tip within Schlemm's canal. A true lumen exists within the microcatheter to allow for materials such as viscoelastic to be injected into Schlemm's canal.

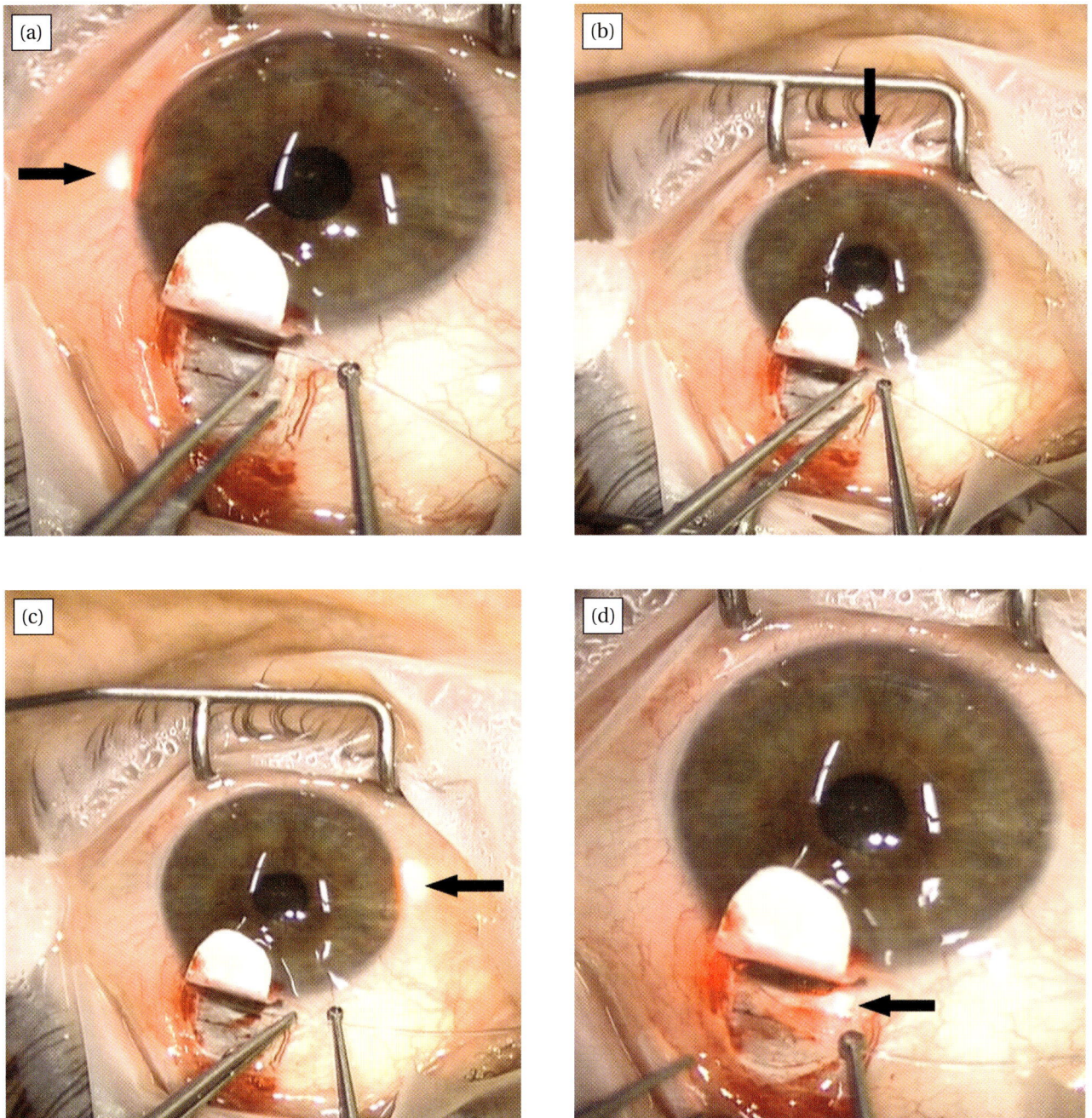

FIGURE 36.29 **360 degrees around the SC.** The microcatheter is slowly advanced using forceps until the entire circumference of Schlemm's canal has been intubated (a—3 clock hours , b—6 clock hours, and c—9 clock hours) and the catheter has emerged from the other cut end of the canal (d).

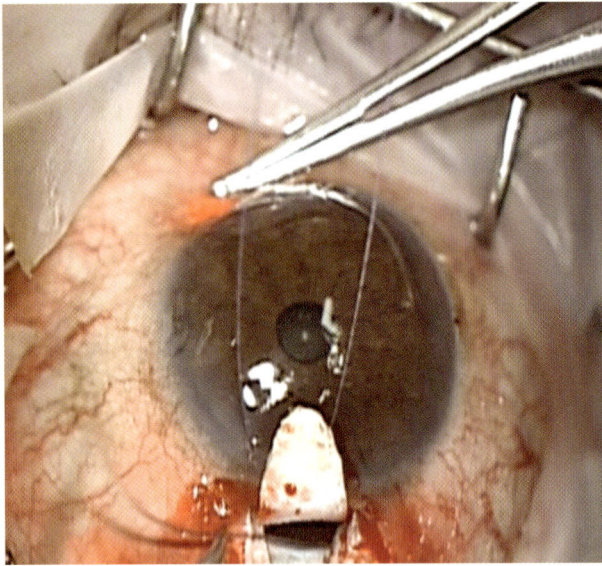

FIGURE 36.30 **Resistance in the Canal.** Possible difficulties passing the microcatheter through the circumference of Schlemm's canal include encountering anatomical variations within the canal or collector channel ostia. Some techniques to assist the microcatheter passage are: focal depression, turning the eye away from the area, injection of viscoelastic, or withdrawal and passage of the microcatheter in the other direction.

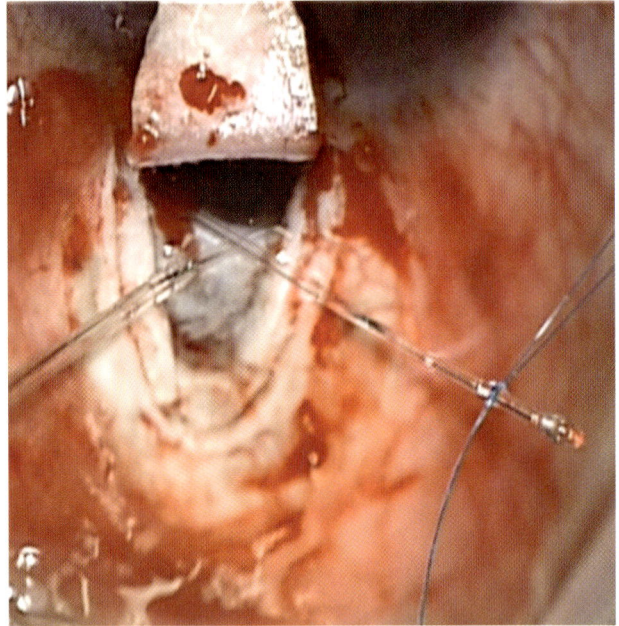

FIGURE 36.31 **Prolene Suture.** A 10-0 needleless prolene suture is tied together, with the loop tied around the just-emerged end of microcatheter (near to the tip, with 2 single throws locked). The procedure is repeated with a second 10-0 prolene suture.

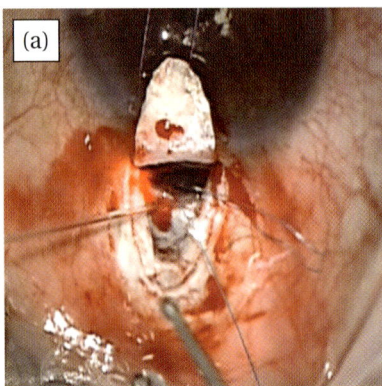

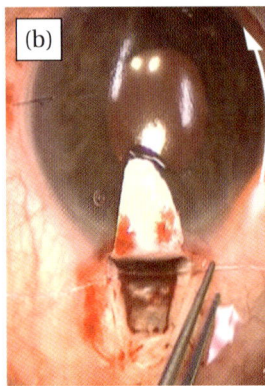

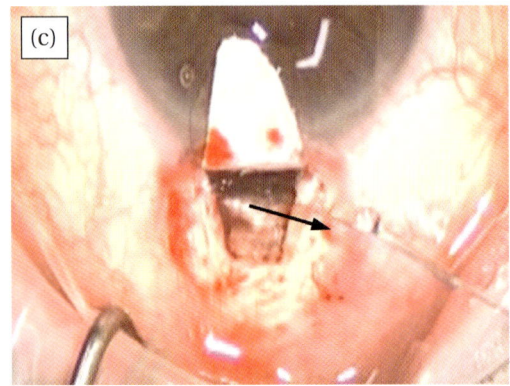

FIGURE 36.32 **Retrieval of Microcatheter Back through SC.** The microcatheter is then withdrawn in the reverse direction of intubation, while an assistant injects viscoelastic (Healon GV). Vigorous injection of viscoelastic may cause Descemet's membrane detachment.

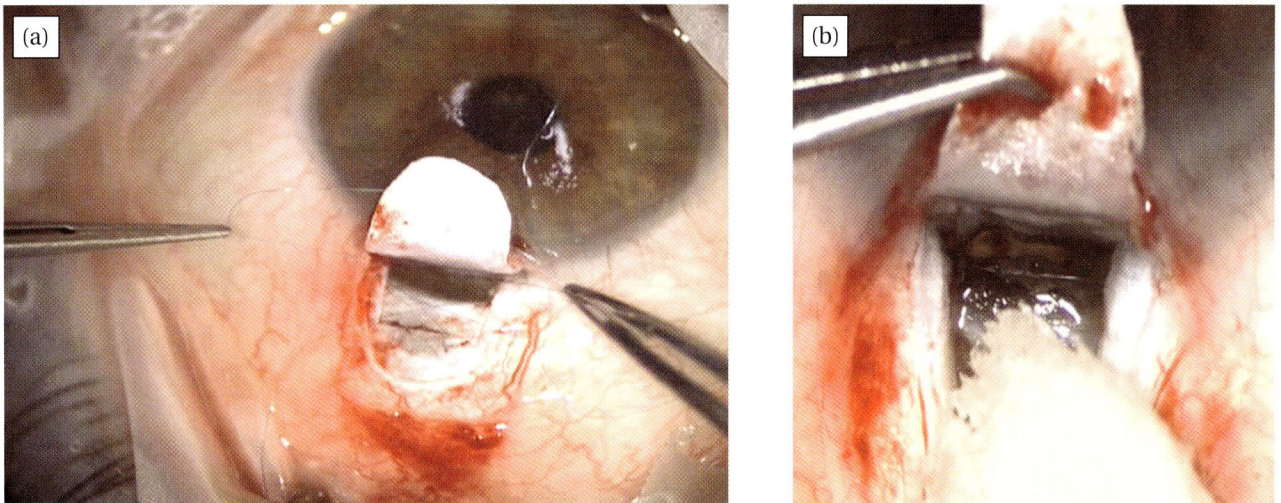

FIGURE 36.33 Tying the Sutures. Once the device has been removed, the 10-0 prolene is cut. Two ends of the 10-0 prolene suture emerge from each cut end of Schlemm's canal. The surgeon should determine which ends correspond (a) and then subsequently tie the sutures in a slipknot fashion in order to allow for the adjustment of suture tension (b).

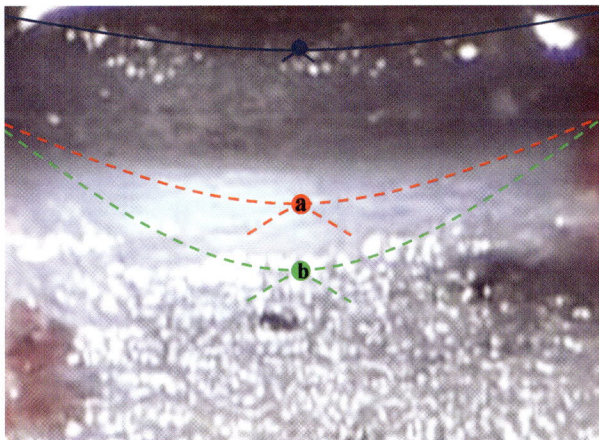

FIGURE 36.34 Suture Tension. This is adjusted by pulling the knot posteriorly until it can just barely reach the scleral spur (a). If suture knot can be pulled past and into the scleral bed (b), then tension should be increased. The same procedure is then carried out with the second suture.

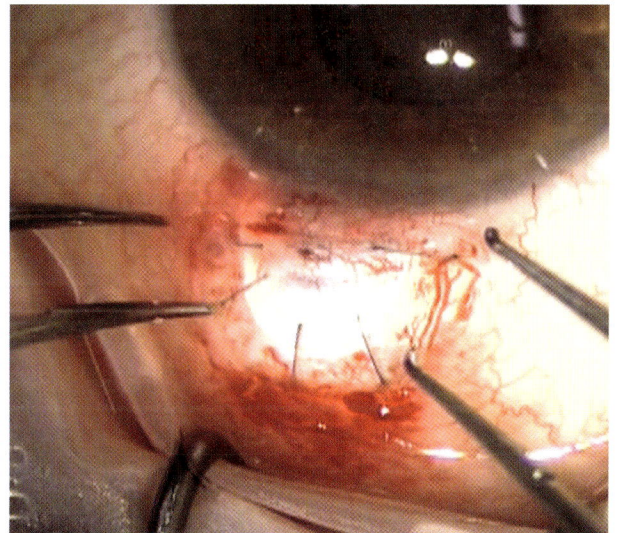

FIGURE 36.35 Closure of the Superficial Flap. The superficial parabolic scleral flap is closed in a watertight fashion with 5 interrupted 10-0 nylon sutures.

Closing Steps in Nonpenetrating Glaucoma Surgery

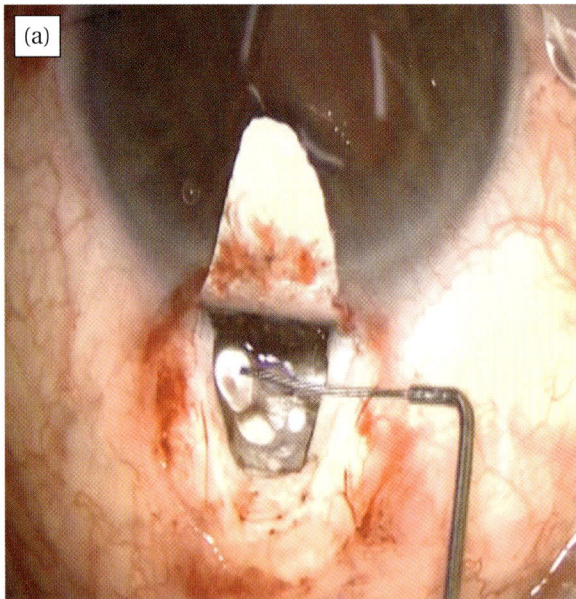

(a)

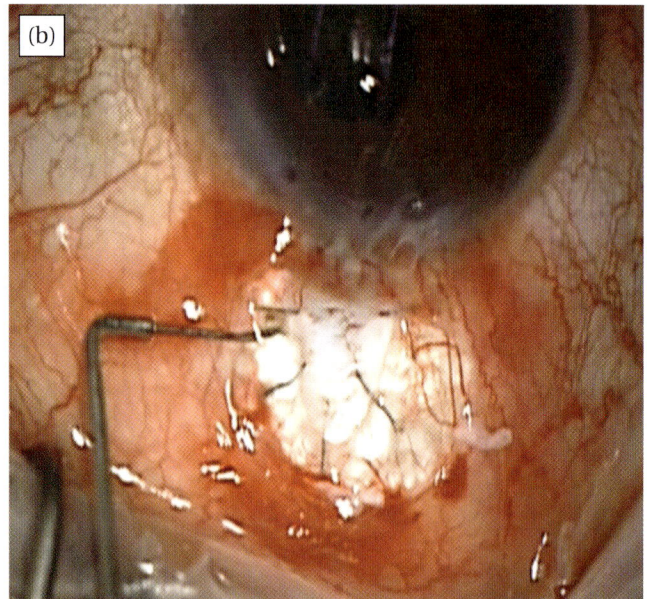

(b)

FIGURE 36.36 **Scleral Lake.** High-viscosity sodium hyaluronate is placed under the superficial scleral flap, using the viscocanalostomy cannula to maintain the scleral lake. The scleral lake is a reservoir for aqueous humor percolating through the TDW to ultimately be absorbed into circulation through scleral, episcleral, or choroidal vasculature, or the cut ends of Schlemm's canal.

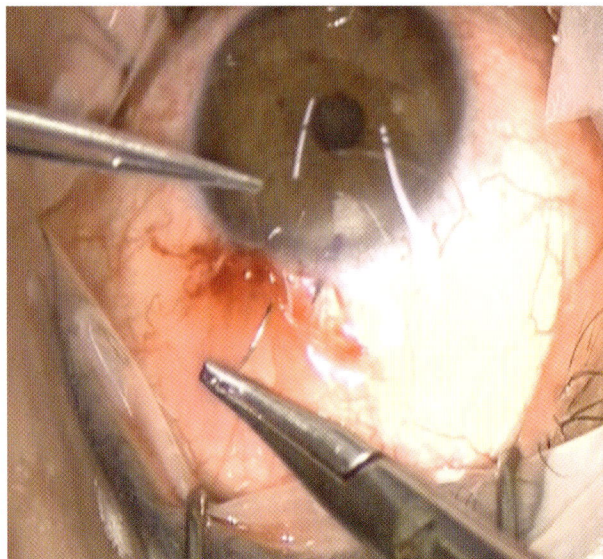

FIGURE 36.37 **Closure of the Conjunctiva.** The conjunctiva is closed using 10-0 vicryl suture on a vascular needle in horizontal mattress fashion across the extent of the incision. Suturing the conjunctiva to the deeper perilimbal tissue risks inadvertent damage and/ or perforation of the superficial flap of sclera.

Postoperatively after Nonpenetrating Glaucoma Surgery

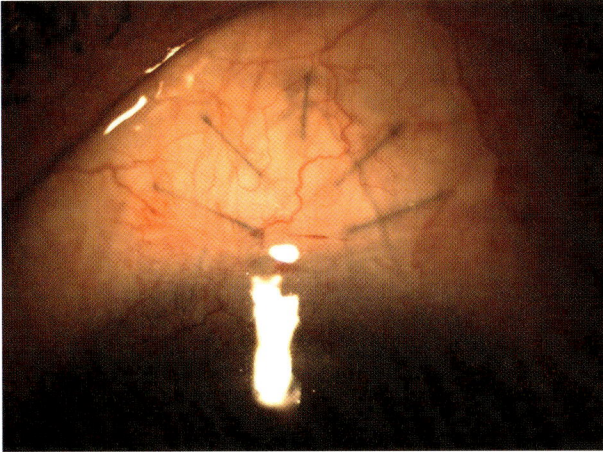

FIGURE 36.38 Slit lamp picture of the flap postoperatively in canaloplasty. Note the absence of a bleb.

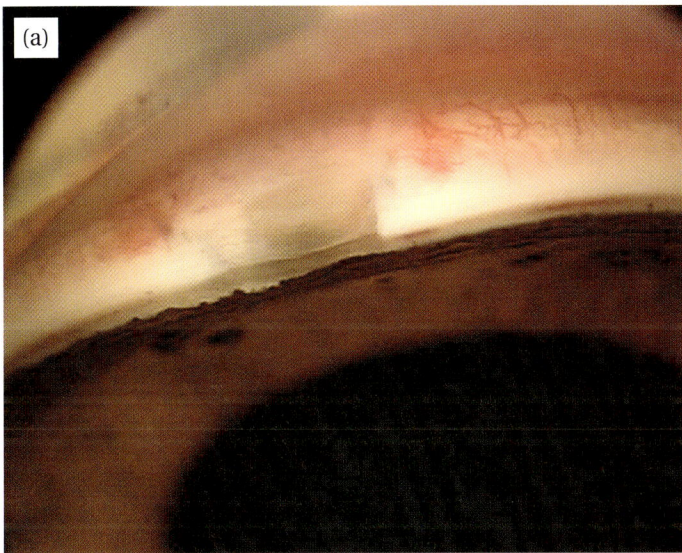

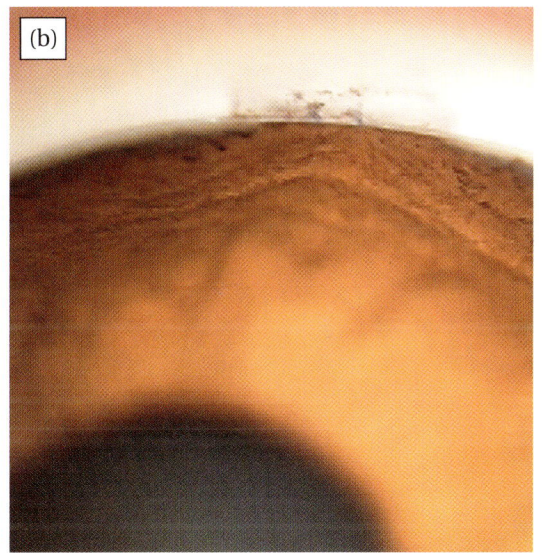

FIGURE 36.39 RetCam images showing the TDW postoperatively in deep sclerectomy.

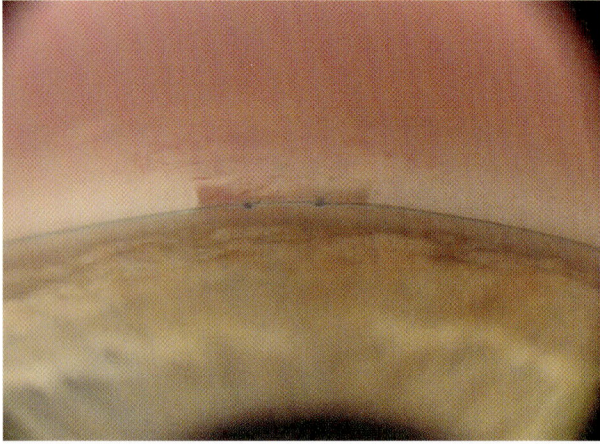

FIGURE 36.40 RetCam image of the TDW postoperatively in canaloplasty.

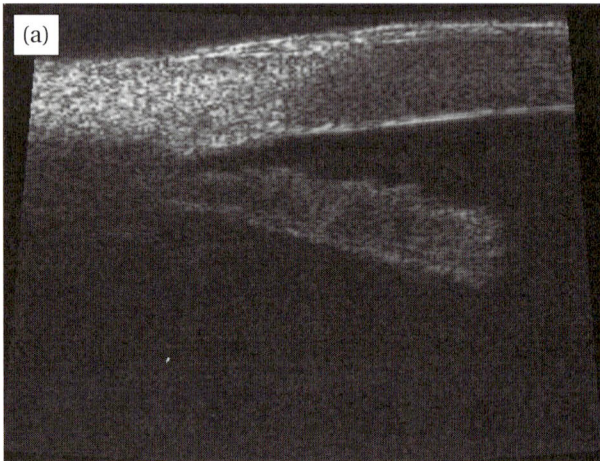

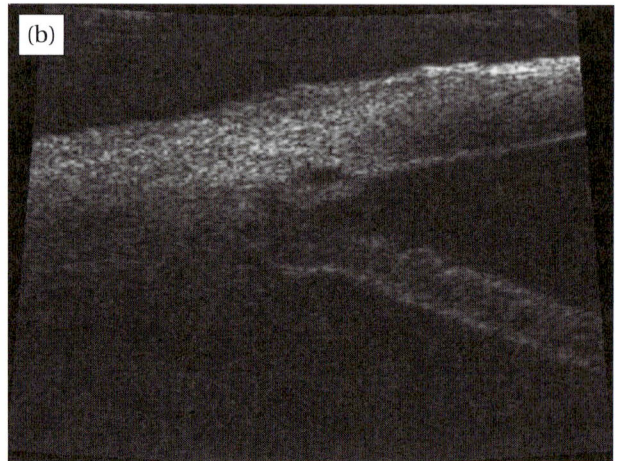

FIGURE 36.41 Visante OCT image of Schlemm's canal, preoperatively (a) and postoperatively (b) after canaloplasty.

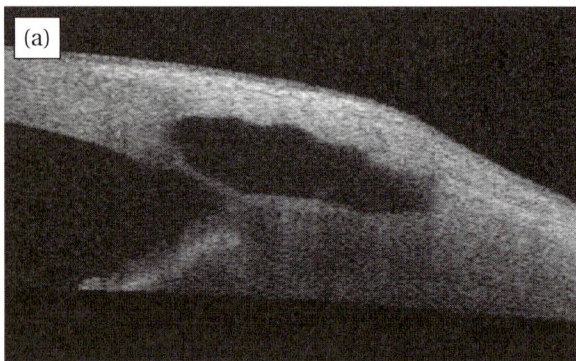

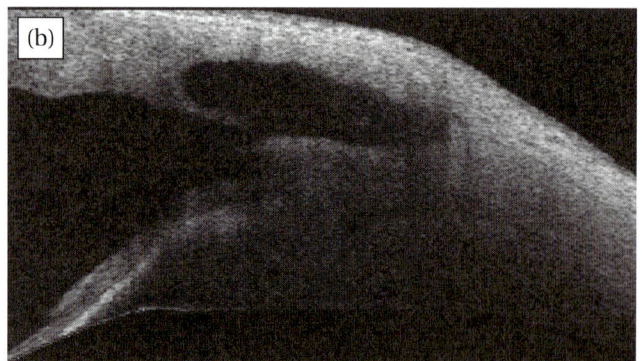

FIGURE 36.42 Visante OCT image showing the scleral lake before YAG laser treatment (a) and after YAG laser treatment (b) to open the TDW.

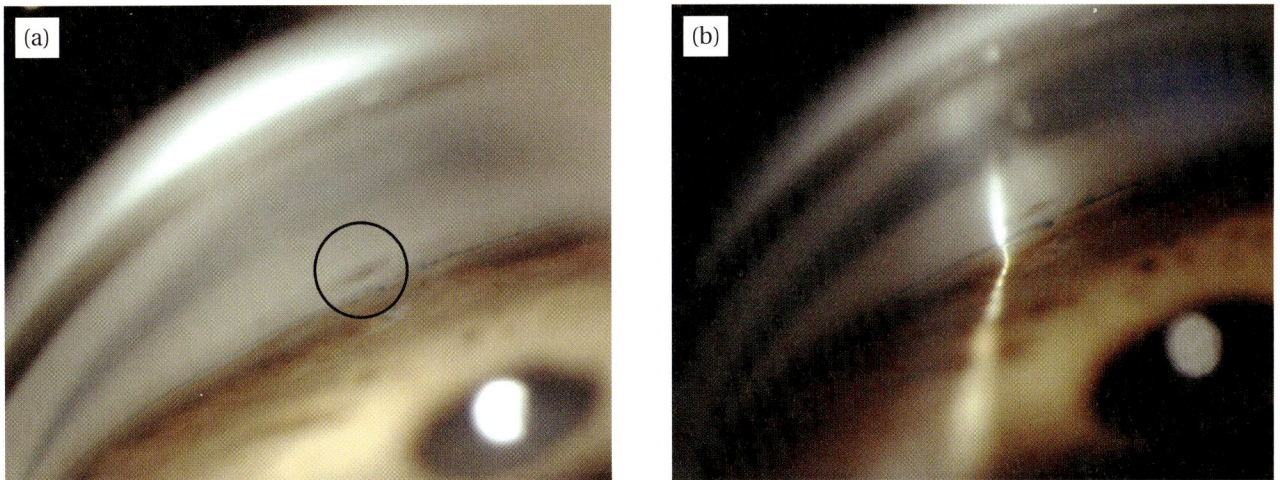

FIGURE 36.43 Slit lamp pictures of an open (circle) TDW following YAG laser treatment.

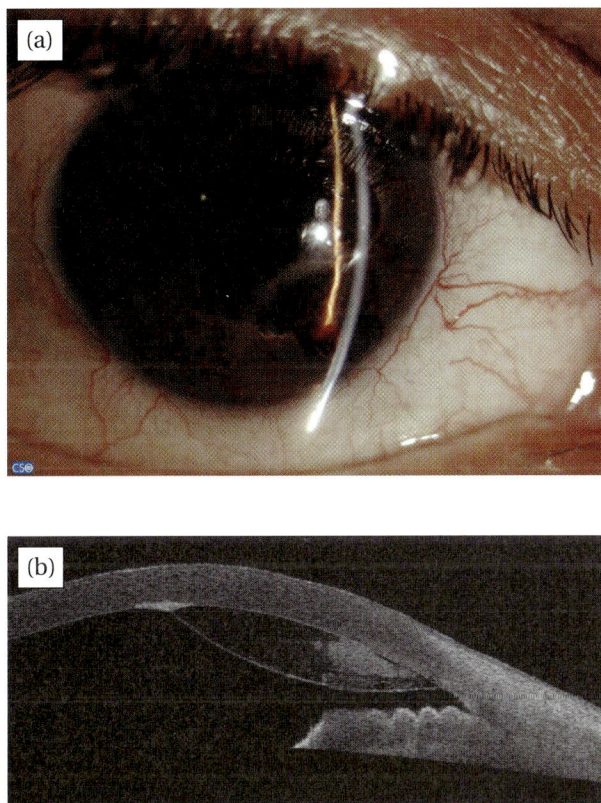

FIGURE 36.44 Slit lamp picture (a) and Visante-OCT (b) showing a Descemet's membrane hemorrhage.

TABLE 36.3 *The Most Common Complications after Nonpenetrating Glaucoma Surgery*

Complications

Perforation of trabeculo-Descemet´s membrane (intraoperative)

Surgically induced cataract

Inflammation

Hyphema

Hypotony and associated conditions

Descemet´s membrane detachment/hemorrhage

Flat/shallow anterior chamber

Choroidal detachment

Bleb fibrosis (deep sclerectomy)*

Bleb encapsulation (deep sclerectomy)*

Elevated IOP**

Suture cheesewire

PAS/iris prolapsed

Late cataract progression

*Postoperative needling with mitomycin-C or 5-fluorouracil can also be performed with similar indications following trabeculectomy.

**YAG goniopuncture of the trabeculo-Descemet's window.

SELECTED REFERENCES

Goldsmith JA, Ahmed IK, Crandall AS. Nonpenetrating glaucoma surgery. *Ophthalmol Clin North Am.* 2005;18(3):443–460, vii.

Lachkar Y, Hamard P. Nonpenetrating filtering surgery. *Curr Opin Ophthalmol.* Apr 2002;13(2):110–115.

Lewis RA, von Wolff K, Tetz M, et al. Canaloplasty: Circumferential viscodilation and tensioning of Schlemm canal using a flexible microcatheter for the treatment of open-angle glaucoma in adults: Two-year interim clinical study results. *J Cataract Refract Surg.* May 2009;35(5):814–824.

Netland PA., Ophthalmic Technology Assessment Committee Glaucoma Panel, AAO. Nonpenetrating glaucoma surgery. *Ophthalmology.* Feb 2001; 108(2):416–421.

END NOTES

Financial Interests: Dr. Ahmed is a consultant for iScience Interventional Inc.

37 Alternative Glaucoma Procedures

Scott D. Lawrence, MD and Peter A. Netland, MD, PhD

TABLE 37.1 *Indications*

Procedure	Indications
Ex-PRESS Miniature Glaucoma Shunt*	Alternative to trabeculectomy in adults with open-angle glaucoma[†] when target IOP cannot be reached by medical or laser management alone. Decreased rates of early postoperative hypotony and inflammation compared with trabeculectomy. May be combined with cataract surgery.
Trabectome*	Alternative to angle surgery in children, and filtering surgery and laser trabeculoplasty in adults with open-angle glaucoma[†] who require a moderate reduction in IOP. Spares conjunctiva and does not preclude subsequent filtering procedures. May be combined with cataract surgery.
Canaloplasty: iTrack microcatheter*	Adult patients with open-angle glaucoma[†] when target IOP cannot be reached by medical or laser management alone. May be combined with cataract surgery.
iStent Trabecular Bypass Microstent	Alternative to filtering surgery in adult patients with open-angle glaucoma[†] and a target IOP in the mid-teens, with or without adjunctive medical treatment. Stents may be placed successively in refractory cases or to titrate IOP. May be combined with cataract surgery.
SOLX Gold Shunt	Adults with open-angle glaucomas[†] unresponsive to medical and laser therapy (primary surgery), or in patients refractory to other glaucoma surgery.

IOP indicates intraocular pressure, OAG = open-angle glaucoma.

* FDA-approved.

† Primary open angle glaucoma, exfoliative glaucoma, pigmentary glaucoma.

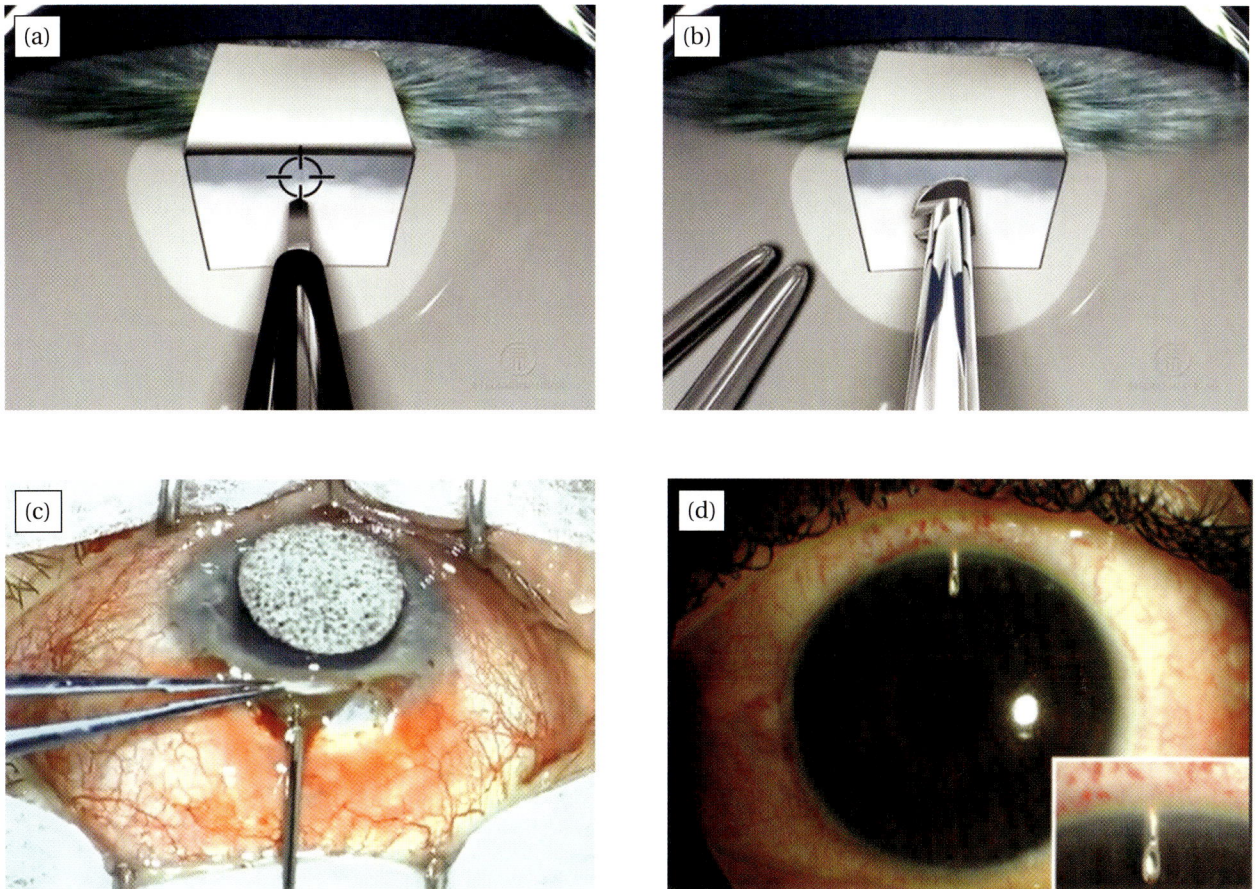

FIGURE 37.1 **Variation of Filtration Surgery: Ex-PRESS Miniature Glaucoma Shunt.** The Ex-PRESS mini glaucoma shunt (Alcon, Inc., Fort Worth, TX) is a small, non-valved device designed to shunt aqueous from the anterior chamber to the subconjunctival space near the limbus. It has demonstrated good biocompatibility and is considered safe with MRI scanning. This stainless steel device is prepackaged on a disposable inserter, and has a restricted internal lumen of either 50 or 200 μm. A limbal or fornix-based peritomy is followed by the creation of a partial-thickness scleral flap with or without adjunctive mitomycin-C. Anterior dissection of the flap is made to the surgical limbus, and a 25- or 27-gauge needle is used to create a tunnel into the anterior chamber, beginning at the limbus and angling slightly toward the iris (a). The implant is inserted on the injector through the scleral tunnel—rotation of the device 90 degrees upon entry into the anterior chamber facilitates insertion (b). Once implanted, the device is rotated so that its base is flush with the sclera. Placement of the implant above the iris and without corneal touch is identified by direct visualization or by goniolens. A cellulose sponge is used to test flow at the base of the shunt. The scleral flap is then sutured with interrupted 10-0 nylon sutures, and the conjunctiva is closed with 9-0 polyglactin suture. (c) Intraoperative photo demonstrating implant insertion under a scleral flap. (d) Slit lamp photograph (postoperative day 1) of the Ex-PRESS implant in proper position above the iris, bevel up. (Images **a** and **b** provided by Alcon, Inc./Optonol Ltd.; **c** and **d** provided by P.A. Netland.)

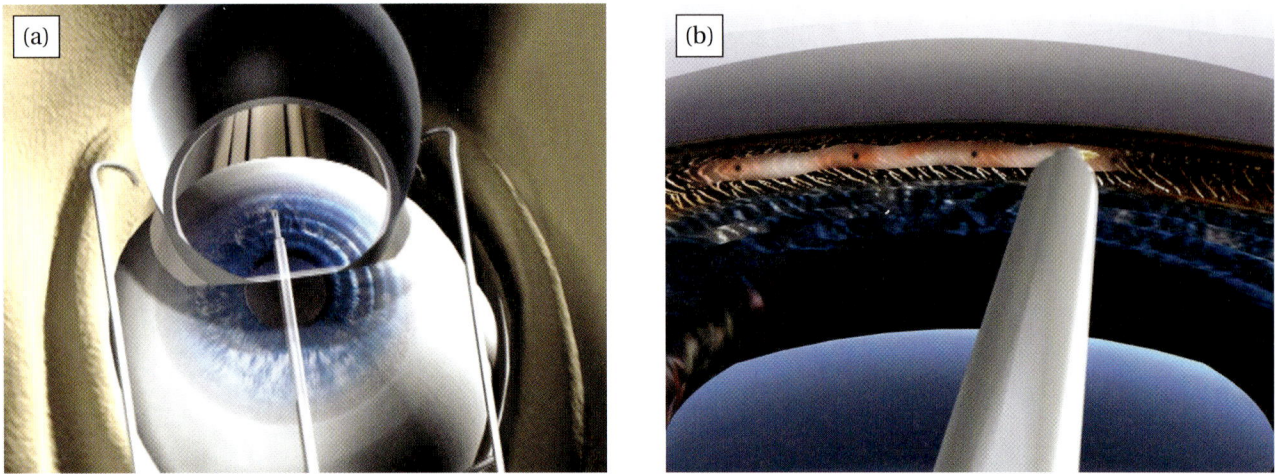

FIGURE 37.2 **Variations of Angle Surgery: Trabectome.** The Trabectome (NeoMedix Corp., Tustin, CA) is a 19-gauge microelectrosurgical device designed to ablate the trabecular meshwork and inner wall of Schlemm's canal ab interno. Following a 1.6 mm temporal, clear corneal incision and injection of viscoelastic, the Trabectome handpiece (containing an irrigation port) is inserted into the anterior chamber, and the nasal trabecular meshwork and angle structures are identified using a goniolens (a). The tip of the handpiece is inserted into nasal or inferonasal trabecular meshwork: aspiration and electrocautery are commenced via a foot pedal. The tip of the unit is gradually rotated along trabecular meshwork in order to achieve circumferential ablation of approximately 60–120 degrees (b). Irrigation and aspiration of viscoelastic is achieved prior to exiting the eye. A single, interrupted 10-0 nylon suture may be placed at the corneal wound. (Images provided by Neomedix Corp.)

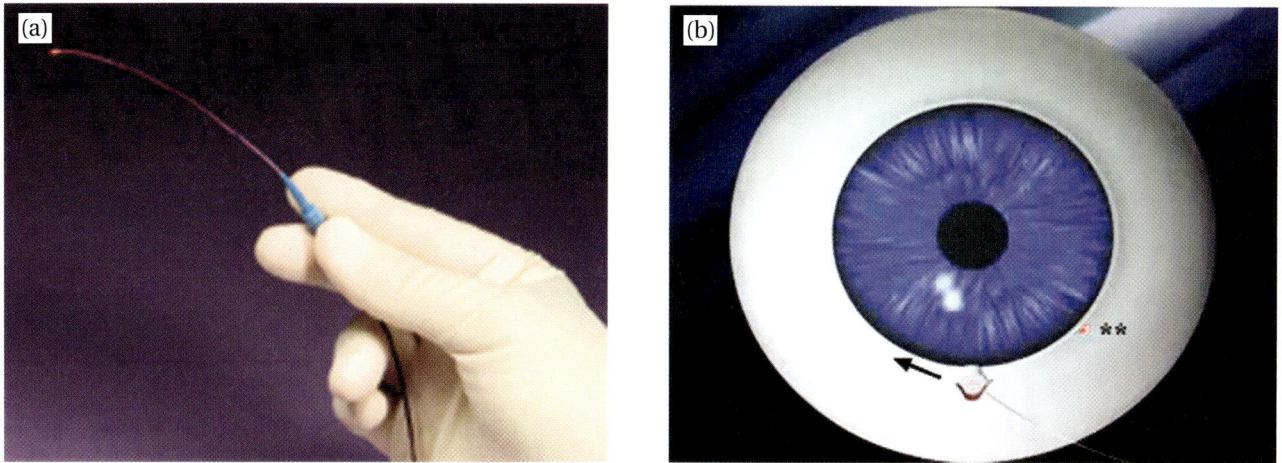

FIGURE 37.3 Canaloplasty: iTrack 250A Canaloplasty Microcatheter. The iTrack microcatheter (iScience Interventional, Menlo Park, CA) is a small, flexible stent (250 microns in diameter) that contains an infusion port and a support wire, as well as a fiber optic for illuminating the tip (a). A 5.0 mm partial-thickness scleral flap is created at the limbus. A smaller, full-thickness flap (0.5 mm inside the initial flap) is created and advanced into Schlemm's canal, extending approximately 1.0 mm into clear cornea, creating a Descemet's-trabecular window. (b) The catheter is advanced stepwise along the complete circumference of the canal (arrow). During advancement of the catheter, the illuminated tip can be visualized through the sclera (double asterisk). A viscoelastic (i.e. Healon GV) is injected during insertion of the catheter or, alternatively, during withdrawal. This achieves a dilation of Schlemm's canal to a width of approximately 300 µm. Prior to retracting the instrument, a 10-0 prolene suture is attached to the tip of the microcatheter, and the catheter is subsequently withdrawn in a direction opposite from insertion. The suture is then cut and tied at a tension force necessary to apply permanent traction on the trabecular meshwork. The superficial scleral flap is sutured with interrupted 8-0 nylon sutures. Treatment effect can be monitored intraoperatively with a high-resolution ultrasound system. (Images provided by iScience Interventional.)

(a)

(b)

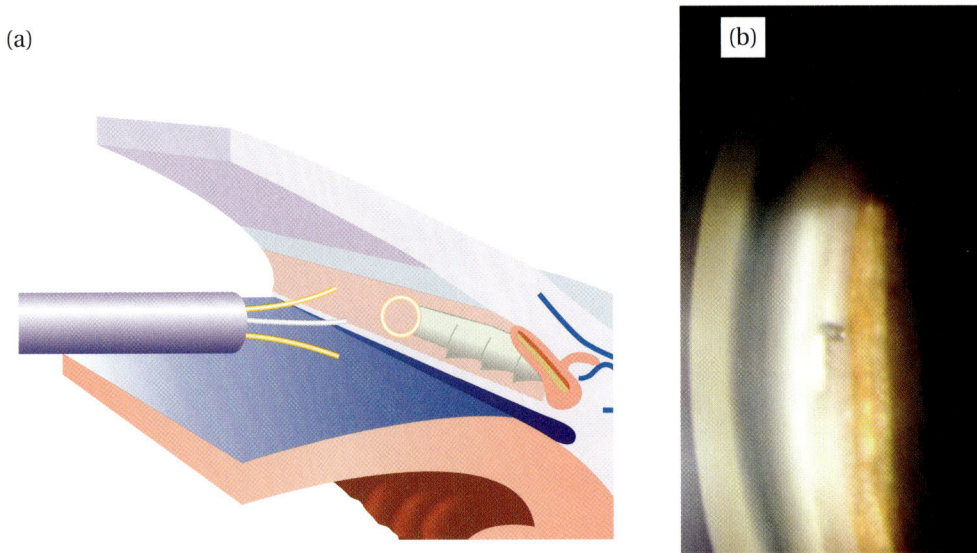

FIGURE 37.4 iStent Trabecular Micro-Bypass Stent. The iStent (Glaukos Corp., Laguna Hills, CA) is a 0.5 mm × 1.0 mm titanium device (heparin-coated) on a single-use, 26-gauge inserter that is designed to overcome trabecular resistance to aqueous drainage. The inserter permits retrieval of the device if dislodged into the anterior chamber. The stent has an internal lumen of 80 μm that creates a direct pathway from the anterior chamber to Schlemm's canal. The device is inserted through a 1.5 mm clear corneal incision at the temporal limbus. A gonioscope is placed on the cornea to visualize the angle structures and to guide entry of the device across the anterior chamber. The iStent is then inserted into the trabecular meshwork and released with the push of a button on the inserter (a). At the time of surgery, reflux of blood from Schlemm's canal may be evident. (b) Gonioscopic view demonstrates proper placement of the iStent implant. The body of the device is in Schlemm's canal, while the neck traverses trabecular meshwork and the lumen is in the anterior chamber. (**Images** provided by Glaukos Corp.)

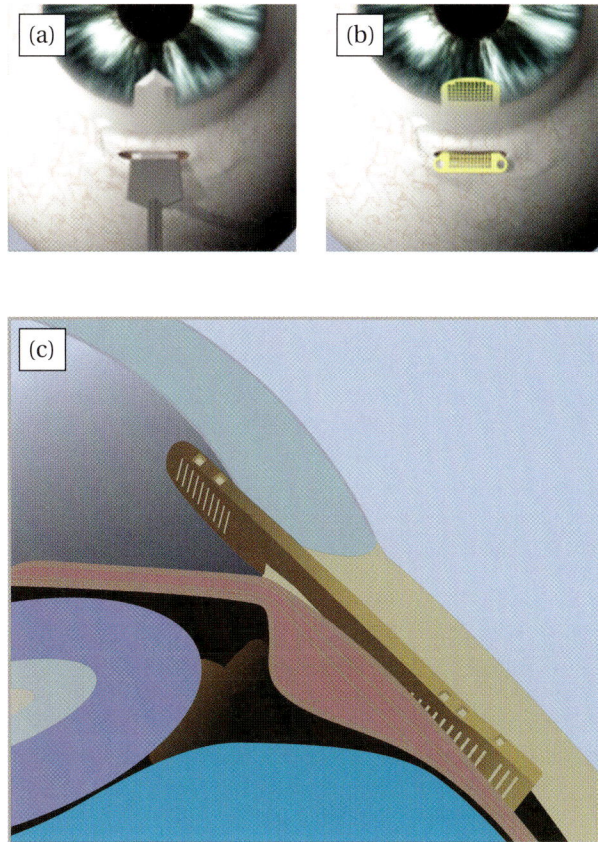

FIGURE 37.5 **Choroidal shunting of aqueous: SOLX Gold Micro Shunt.** The Gold Micro Shunt (SOLX, Ltd, Boston, Massachusetts) is a non-valved, flat-plate made from medical-grade 24-karat gold. The drainage device transmits aqueous fluid from the anterior chamber into the suprachoroidal space. Following creation of a fornix-based conjunctival flap, an initial 4.0 mm incision is made 2.0 to 2.5 mm posterior to the limbus. A scleral tunnel is created, and a crescent knife is advanced into the anterior chamber (a). A full-thickness scleral incision is made at the original incision site into the suprachoroidal space. This incision is then swept with a blunt spatula to insure good access into the suprachoroidal space. The anterior segment of the Gold Micro Shunt is advanced through the scleral tunnel and into the anterior chamber (b). The posterior tabs of the shunt are tucked into the suprachoroidal space and moved posteriorly until approximately 0.5–1.0 mm of the shunt remains visible in the anterior chamber. The scleral incision should be sutured to prevent wound leakage. (c). Schematic cross-sectional view demonstrates proper anatomic placement of the device. (Images provided by SOLX, Ltd.)

TABLE 37.2 *Complications*

Procedure	Complications
Ex-PRESS Miniature Glaucoma Implant	*Common*: Transient postoperative hypotony; transient choroidal effusion.
	Rare: Blocked shunt; early or late bleb leak; hypotony maculopathy; hyphema; intraoperative shallowing of anterior chamber; endophthalmitis.
Trabectome	*Common*: Intraoperative bleeding from Schlemm's canal; transient postoperative hyphema; early IOP spike.
	Rare: Intraoperative cyclodialysis; corneal epithelial defect; Descemet's detachment; postoperative focal peripheral anterior synechiae; iris injury.
Canaloplasty: iTrack microcatheter	*Common*: Hyphema; failure of 360-degree cannulation; failure of tensioning suture; postoperative elevated intraocular pressure.
	Rare: Descemet's detachment.
iStent Trabecular Bypass Microstent	*Common:* Intraoperative reflux bleeding from Schlemm's canal.
	Rare: Stent lumen obstruction; stent malpositioning.
SOLX Gold Micro Shunt	*Common*: Mild to moderate transient hyphema.
	Rare: Shunt exposure; synechia formation, exudative retinal detachment (data limited).

SELECTED REFERENCES

Dahan E, Carmichael TR. Implantation of a miniature glaucoma device under a scleral flap. *J Glaucoma.* 2005;14:98–102.

Francis BA, See RF, Rao NA, Minckler DS, Baerveldt G. Ab interno trabeculectomy: Development of a novel device (Trabectome) and surgery for open-angle glaucoma. *J Glaucoma.* 2006;15:68–73.

Kanner EM, Netland PA, Sarkisian SR Du H. Ex-PRESS miniature glaucoma device implanted under a scleral flap alone or combined with phacoemulsification cataract surgery. *J Glaucoma.* 2009;18:488–491.

Lewis RA, von Wolff K, Tetz M, Korber N, Kearney JR, Shingleton B, *et al.* Canaloplasty: Circumferential viscodilation and tensioning of Schlemm's canal using a flexible microcatheter for the treatment of open-angle glaucoma in adults: Two-year interim clinical study results. *J Cataract Refract Surg.* 2009;35:814–824.

Maris PJ Jr, Ishida K, and Netland PA. Comparison of trabeculectomy with Ex-PRESS miniature glaucoma device implanted under scleral flap. *J Glaucoma.* 2007;16:14–19.

Melamed S, Ben Simon GJ, Goldenfeld M, Simon G. Efficacy and safety of gold micro shunt implantation to the supraciliary space in patients with glaucoma: a pilot study. *Arch Ophthalmol.* 2009;127:264–269.

Minckler DS, Mosaed S, Dustin L, Francis BA and the Trabectome Study Group. Trabectome (Trabeculotomy—internal approach): Additional experience and extended follow up. *Trans Am Ophthalmol Soc.* 2008;106:149–160

Netland PA. What other new surgical techniques are available for glaucoma? In: Heuer DK, Gedde SJ, Lewis RA, eds. *Curbside Consultation in Glaucoma.* Thorofare, NJ: Slack, Inc., 2008, pp. 223–228.

Spiegel D, Wetzel W, Neuhann T, Stuermer J, Hoeh H, Garcia-Feijoo J, *et al.* Coexistent primary open-angle glaucoma and cataract: Interim analysis of a trabecular micro-bypass stent and concurrent cataract surgery. *Eur J Ophthalmol.* 2009;19:393–399.

38 | Non-Flow-Resistive Glaucoma Drainage Device Implantation

James C. Robinson, MD

TABLE 38.1 *Indications*

Failure of trabeculectomy, with or without antifibrosis drugs

Active uveitis

Neovascular glaucoma

Inadequate conjunctiva (ocular surface disease, previous ocular surgery and other causes)

Poor candidate for trabeculectomy (includes post-keratoplasty, traumatic glaucoma, epithelial downgrowth, previous retinal surgery, irido-corneal-endothelial syndromes and other poor prognosis glaucomas)

Primary glaucoma surgery (under investigation)

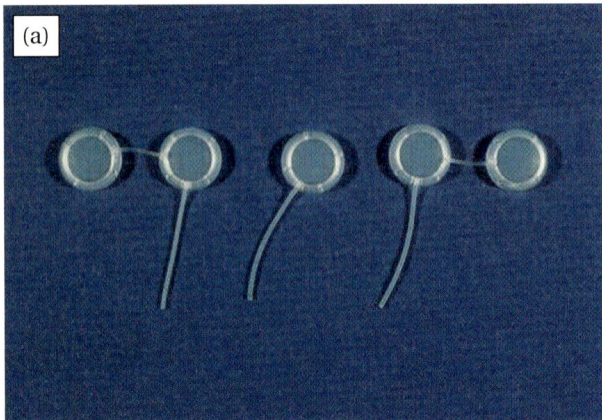

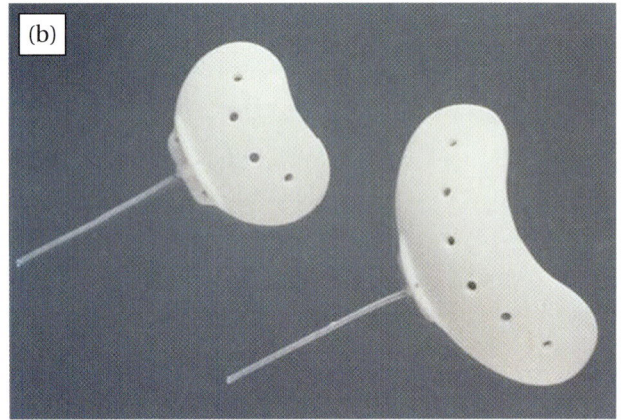

FIGURE 38.1 Non-flow-resistive glaucoma drainage implants. (a) Molteno implants: left double plate, single plate, and right double plate, with pressure ridge on primary plate. (Courtesy IOP, Inc., Costa Mesa, CA.) (b) Baerveldt implant with fenestrations.

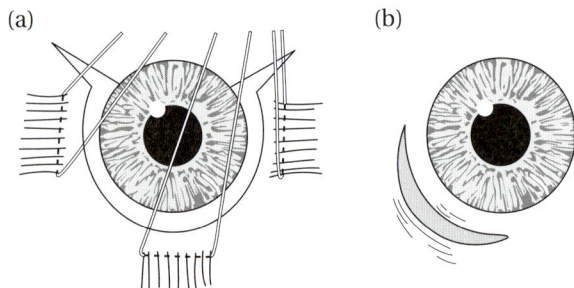

FIGURE 38.2 Conjunctival incision. (a) Conjunctival opening for the double-plate Molteno implant. (b) Dissection of quadrant for the single-quadrant device.

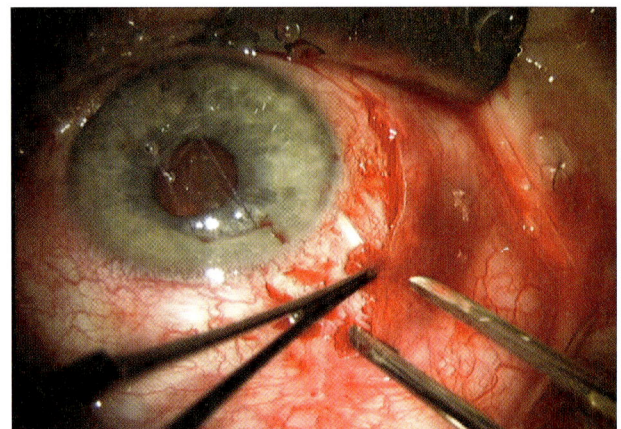

FIGURE 38.3 Conjunctival opening for the Baerveldt implant.

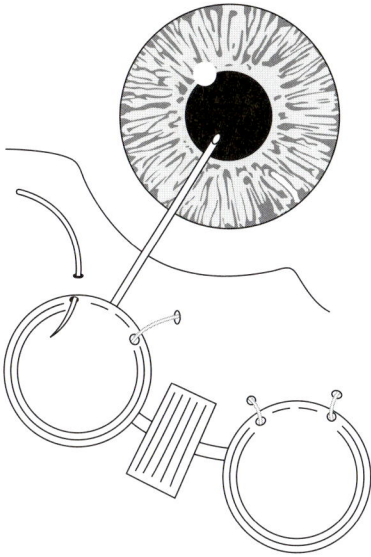

FIGURE 38.4 The episcleral plate is sutured to the sclera.

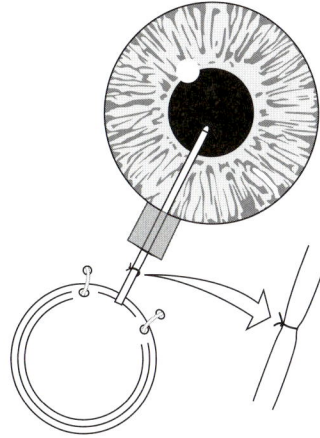

FIGURE 38.5 Free-flow tube occluded with an absorbable suture (polyglactin) ligature in association with a venting slit.

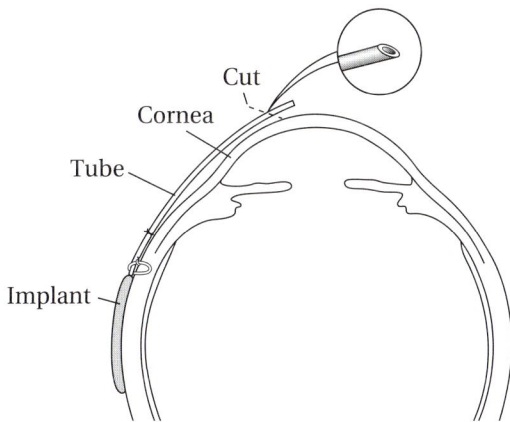

FIGURE 38.6 Implant tube trimmed to the appropriate length with the bevel facing anteriorly.

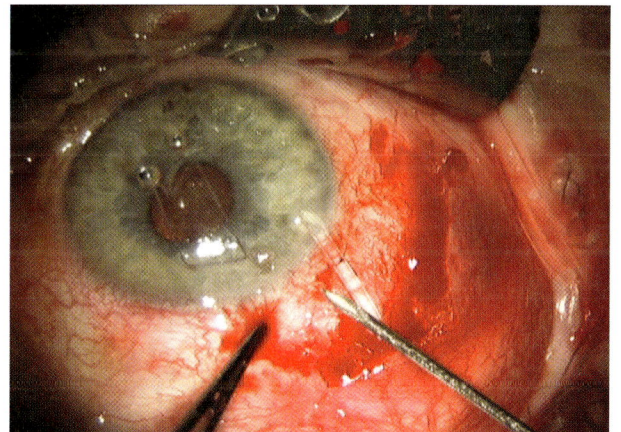

FIGURE 38.7 Implant tube trimmed to the appropriate length with bevel facing anteriorly.

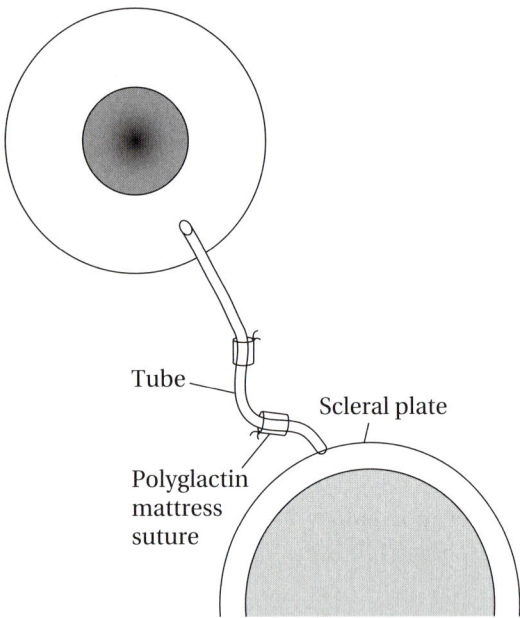

FIGURE 38.8 If the surgeon anticipates difficulty orienting the tube, or the need for later repositioning, excess tubing can be stored by directing the tube into an S shape with mattress sutures. This can be done before or after inserting the tube into the anterior chamber.

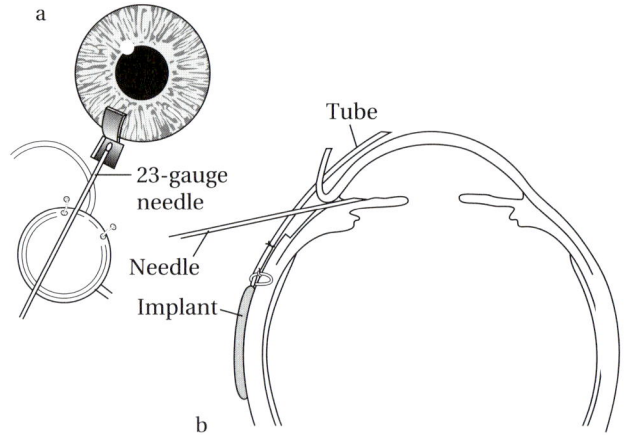

FIGURE 38.9 Insertion of a 23-gauge needle into the anterior chamber just anterior to and parallel to the iris.

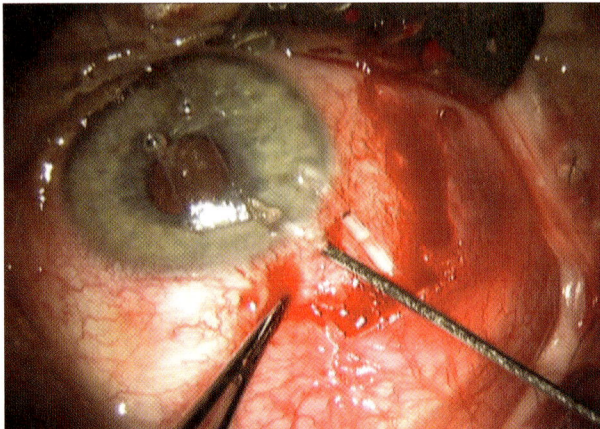

FIGURE 38.10 A 23 gauge needle is placed into the anterior chamber parallel to the iris plane.

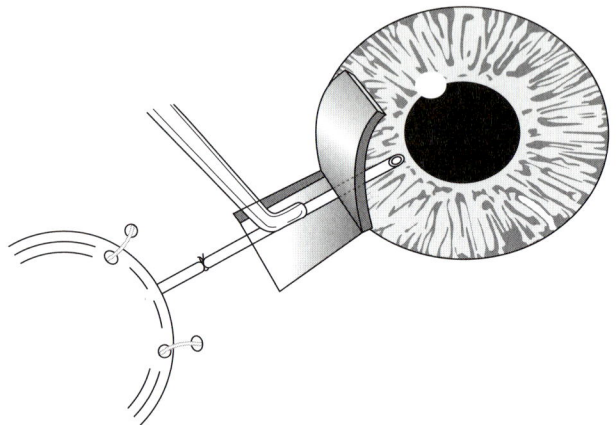

FIGURE 38.11 Introduction of the tube into the anterior chamber with introducer forceps.

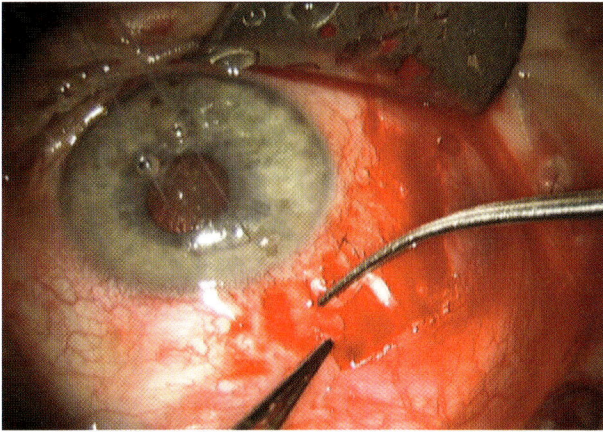

FIGURE 38.12 Placement of the tube into the anterior chamber with curved tying forceps.

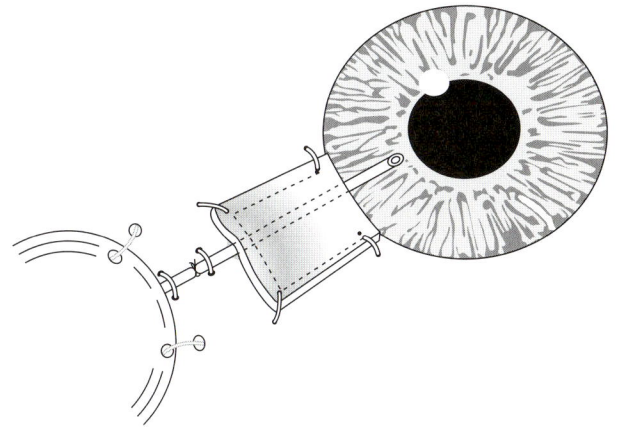

FIGURE 38.13 The scleral flap is reapproximated with the edges inset, and donor sclera or banked material is placed over the tube.

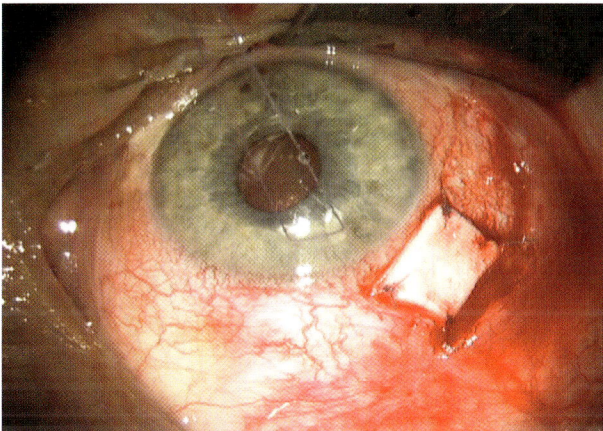

FIGURE 38.14 Scleral patch graft sutured on top of implant tube with polyglactin (7-0 to 9-0) or nylon (9-0 to 10-0) suture.

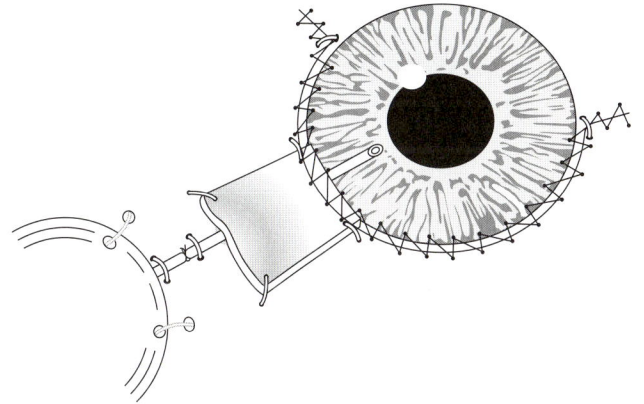

FIGURE 38.15 Conjunctival closure. The edge of the conjunctival flap will be positioned anterior to the graft during final wound closure.

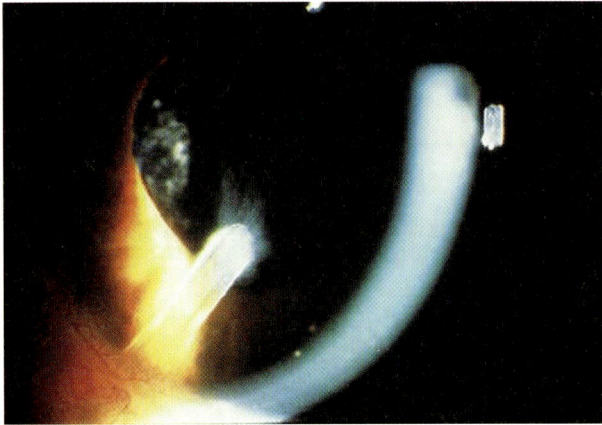

FIGURE 38.16 Obstruction of tube. Vitreous may follow the flow of aqueous into the tube tip, requiring YAG laser vitreolysis or vitrectomy.

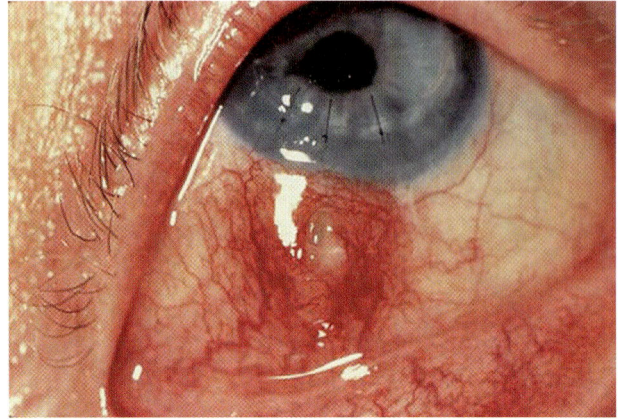

FIGURE 38.17 Exposure of the tube due to wound dehiscence. With the constant rubbing of the upper lid, the tube may erode through the conjunctiva and scleral patch graft. An emergency, this finding must quickly be remedied with conjunctivoplasty and scleral patch replacement to avoid endophthalmitis.

TABLE 38.2 *Complications*

Overfiltration/hypotony	Shallow anterior chamber
Choroidal detachment	Suprachoroidal hemorrhage
Visual loss	Hyphema
Hypertensive phase	Tube-cornea touch
Tube lens touch	Tube occlusion by vitreous/fibrin/blood/iris
Corneal decompensation	Conjunctival dehiscence/leakage
Tube extrusion	Tube exposure post melting of the patch
Tube migration	Endophthalmitis
Motility disorders	Ocular perforation during implant fixation

SELECTED REFERENCES

Ancker E, Molteno ACB. Molteno drainage implant for neovascular glaucoma. *Trans Ophthalmol Soc UK.* 1982;102:122–124.

Christmann LM, Wilson ME. Motility disturbances after Molteno implants. *J Pediatr Ophthalmol Strabismus.* 1992;29:44–48.

Costa VP, Katz LJ, Cohen EJ, Raber IM. Glaucoma associated with epithelial downgrowth controlled with Molteno tube shunts. *Ophthalmic Surg.* 1992;23:797–800.

Ellis BD, Varley GA, Kalenak JW, Meisler DM, Huang SS. Bacterial endophthalmitis following cataract surgery in an eye with a preexisting Molteno implant. *Ophthalmic Surg.* 1993;24:117–118.

Heuer DK, Lloyd MA, Abrams DA, Baerveldt G, Minckler DS, Lee MB, Martone JF. Which is better? One or two? A randomized clinical trial of single-plate versus double-plate Molteno implantation for glaucomas in aphakia and pseudophakia. *Ophthalmology.* 1992;99:1512–1519.

Hodkin MJ, Goldblatt WS, Burgoyne CF, Ball SF, Insler MS. Early clinical experience with the Baerveldt implant in complicated glaucomas. *Am J Ophthalmol.* 1995;120:32–40.

Lloyd ME, Baerveldt G, Heuer DK, Minckler DS, Martone JF. Initial clinical experience with the Baerveldt implant in complicated glaucomas. *Ophthalmology.* 1994;101:640–650.

Mermoud A, Salmon JF, Alexander P, Straker C, Murray AD. Molteno tube implantation for neovascular glaucoma. Long-term results and factors influencing the outcome. *Ophthalmology.* 1993;100:897–902.

Siegner SW, Netland PA, Urban RC Jr, Williams AS, Richards DW, Latina MA, Brandt JD: Clinical experience with the Baerveldt glaucoma drainage implant. *Ophthalmology.* 1995;102:1298–1307.

Smith SL, Starita RJ, Fellman RL, Lynn JR. Early clinical experience with the Baerveldt 350 mm² implant and associated extraocular muscle imbalance. *Ophthalmology.* 1993;100:914–918.

Flow-Resistive Glaucoma Drainage Device Implantation

Kleyton Barella, MD and Vital Paulino Costa, MD

TABLE 39.1 *Indications*

Failure of trabeculectomy, with or without antifibrosis drugs

Active uveitis

Neovascular glaucoma

Inadequate conjunctiva (ocular surface disease, previous ocular surgery and other causes)

Poor candidate for trabeculectomy (includes post-keratoplasty, traumatic glaucoma, epithelial downgrowth, previous retinal surgery, irido-corneal-endothelial syndromes and other poor prognosis glaucomas)

Primary glaucoma surgery (under investigation)

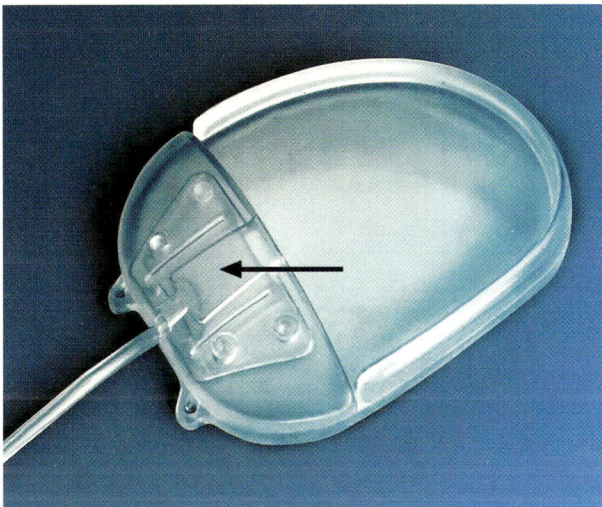

FIGURE 39.1 **Flow-resistive Glaucoma Drainage Implant.** Presently available glaucoma drainage implants can be characterized as resistance (flow-restrictive or valved) devices or nonresistance (non-valved) devices. An early flow-resistive device was the slit "valve" used on the Krupin Valve. The device shown is the Ahmed Glaucoma Valve (New World Medical, Rancho Cucamonga, CA), which is currently the most frequently implanted resistance glaucoma drainage device. The arrow indicates the valve mechanism. (Image courtesy of New World Medical.)

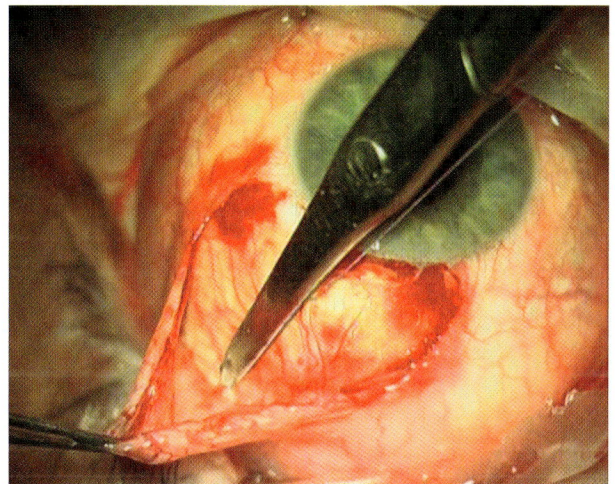

FIGURE 39.2 **Initial Steps for Implantation of Device.** The earlier stages of implantation are similar for both flow-resistive and non-flow-resistive glaucoma drainage devices. In order to achieve adequate exposure, a 6-0 or 7-0 silk or polyglactin traction suture on a spatulated (side-cutting) needle is placed through the cornea near the limbus or in the sclera. Maximal exposure for suturing the plate is achieved by placing the bridle suture adjacent to the quadrant chosen for implantation. In the quadrant chosen for implantation of the Ahmed Glaucoma Valve, a fornix-based incision is made through the conjunctiva and Tenon's capsule. Blunt Westcott scissors are used to dissect between the episclera and Tenon's capsule. The closed blades of Stevens tenotomy scissors (curved or straight) are inserted posteriorly and spread, creating a pocket between the rectus muscles.

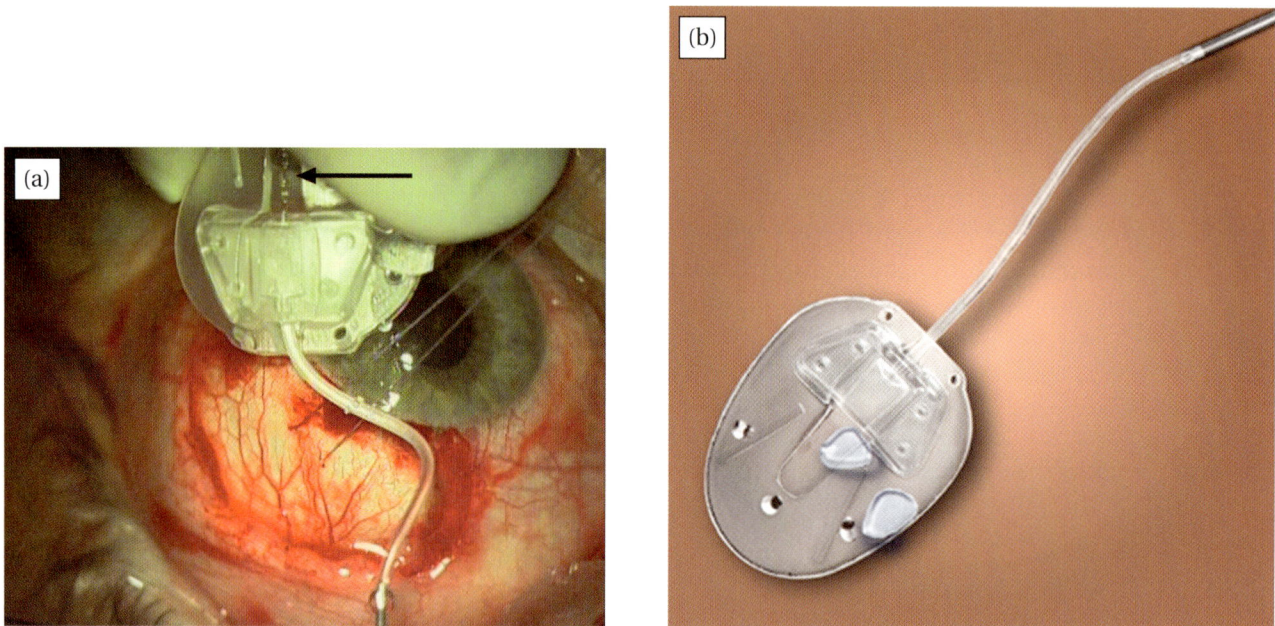

FIGURE 39.3 Opening of the Ahmed Glaucoma Valve (Model FP-7). The implant is "primed" before use with balanced salt solution, in order to open the valve mechanism. (a) Intraoperative priming of the valve is performed by using a 27- or 30-gauge cannula to irrigate balanced salt solution (BSS) through the tube, ensuring patency of the valve mechanism. Note the flow of balanced salt solution at the top of the picture (arrow). (b) A diagram shows the cannula attached to the tube, after successful priming of the Ahmed Glaucoma Valve. (Image b courtesy of New World Medical.)

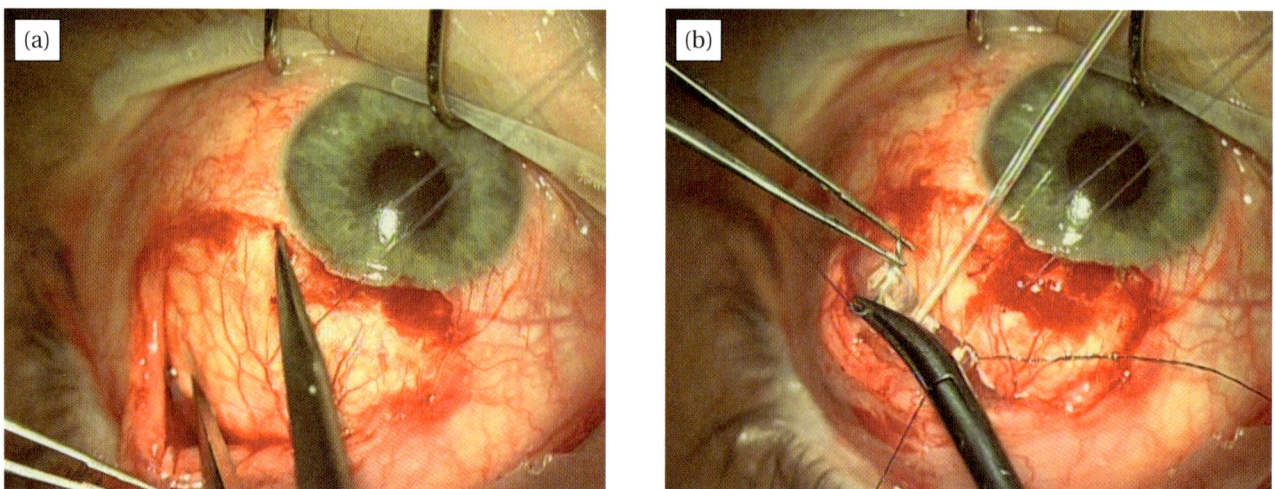

FIGURE 39.4 Fixing the Plate to the Sclera. (a) The plate is anchored 8–10 mm posterior to the limbus, measured by calipers. (b) The plate is then anchored to the sclera with two interrupted 8-0 or 9-0 silk, nylon, or prolene sutures placed through holes on the anterior edge of the plate. During placement of the plate, the anterior edge of the plate may be grasped using non-toothed forceps, or the surgeon's fingers may be used to hold the anterior part of the plate for insertion of the device into the pocket. The valve mechanism should not be grasped with forceps when inserting the plate into the sub-Tenon pocket, because this may damage the device. Although some surgeons apply mitomycin-C to the area around the plate during surgery (similar to the approach for trabeculectomy), this approach has shown little or no benefit in clinical trials.

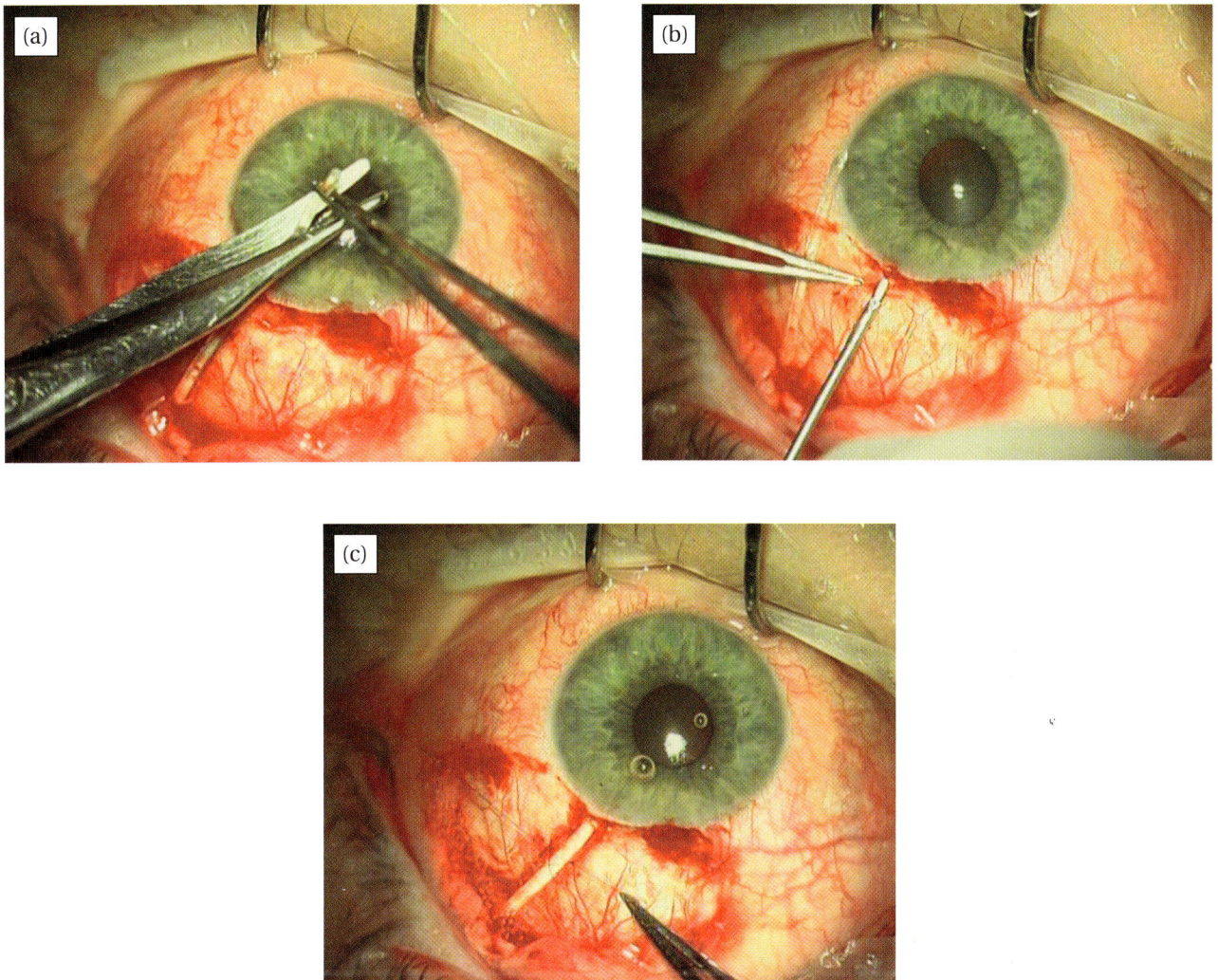

FIGURE 39.5 Insertion of the Tube into the Anterior Chamber. (a) The tube tip is cut obliquely (bevel up) to protect the tube lumen from occlusion by the iris. The tube is cut to the appropriate length, to extend approximately 2–4 mm into the anterior chamber. (b) A 23 gauge needle is used to enter the anterior chamber approximately 0.5–2 mm posterior to the limbus. The 23 gauge needle tract allows tube insertion, with minimal leakage around the tube. (c) The tube is inserted into the anterior chamber, anterior to the iris and posterior to the corneal endothelium. The tube is secured to the sclera with a 9-0 or 10-0 nylon suture. Viscoelastic is not required for routine cases; however, in certain patients, surgeons may use viscoelastic. This can be placed through the 23 gauge needle tract or through a separate paracentesis. Use of viscoelastic is not recommended in non-valved devices, although it can be helpful with valved-device implantation intraoperatively (e.g., to avoid shallowing of the anterior chamber or loss of silicone oil) or postoperatively (e.g., in patients at risk for hypotony during the early postoperative period). In certain patients who are pseudophakic or aphakic, and who have had a vitrectomy performed previously, it may be preferable to place the tube into the vitreous cavity rather than the anterior chamber. This can be done with pars plana placement of the tube using a pars plana clip (New World Medical).

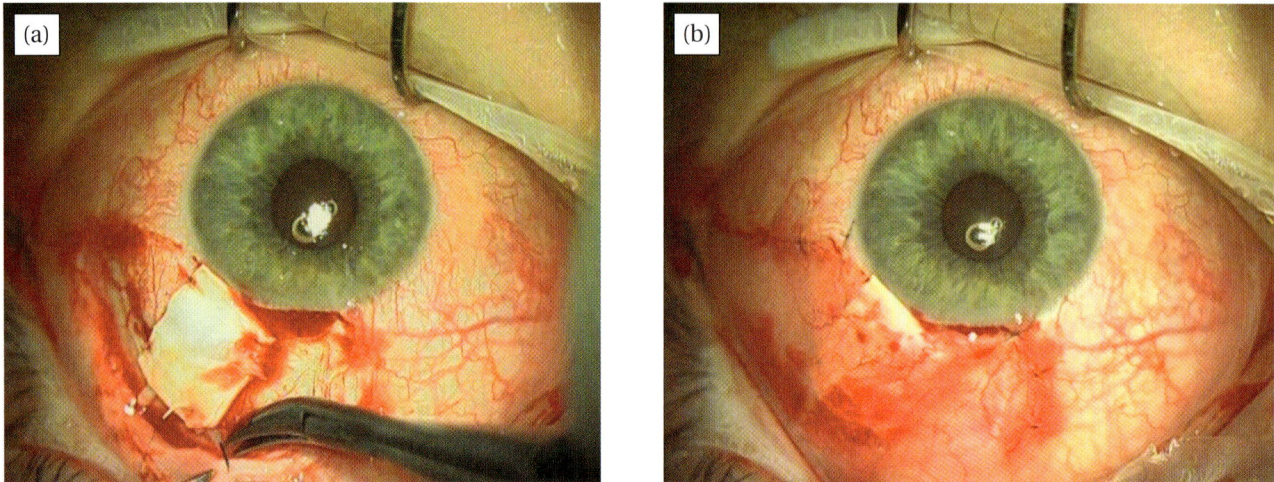

FIGURE 39.6 **Coverage of the Tube.** (a) To prevent erosion of the tube through the conjunctiva near the limbus, a rectangular flap of sclera (shown) or processed pericardium (Tutoplast, New World Medical, Rancho Cucamonga, CA; or IOP, Inc., Costa Mesa, CA) is sutured over the tube using interrupted 9-0 or 10-0 nylon sutures. Other suitable patch graft materials may be used, such as fascia lata, dura, or cornea. (b) The conjunctiva is reapproximated using 10-0 nylon suture, or 9-0 or 8-0 polyglactin suture on a tapered needle. Subconjunctival steroids and antibiotics are injected intraoperatively, and topical steroid and antibiotics are started during the postoperative period.

TABLE 39.2 *Complications*

Overfiltration/hypotony	Shallow anterior chamber
Choroidal detachment	Suprachoroidal hemorrhage
Visual loss	Hyphema
Hypertensive phase	Tube-cornea touch
Tube lens touch	Tube occlusion by vitreous/fibrin/blood/iris
Corneal decompensation	Conjunctival dehiscence/leakage
Tube extrusion	Tube exposure post melting of the patch
Tube migration	Endophthalmitis
Motility disorders	Ocular perforation during implant fixation

SELECTED REFERENCES

Boyle JW IV, Netland PA. Ahmed Glaucoma Valve drainage implant. In: Shaarawy TM, Sherwood MB, Hitchings RA, Crowston JG, eds. *Glaucoma,* 1st ed. *Volume Two, Surgical Management.* Edinburgh: Saunders Elsevier, 2009; pp. 425–435.

Costa VP, Azuara-Blanco A, Netland PA, Lesk MR, Arcieri ES. Efficacy and safety of adjunctive mitomycin C during Ahmed Glaucoma Valve implantation: A prospective randomized clinical trial. *Ophthalmology.* 2004;111:1071–1076.

Ishida K, Netland PA, Costa VP, Shiroma L, Khan B, Ahmed II. Comparison of polypropylene and silicone Ahmed Glaucoma Valves. *Ophthalmology.* 2006;113:1320–1326.

Gedde SJ, Herndon LW, Brandt JD, Budenz DL, Feuer WJ, Schiffman JC. Surgical complications in the Tube Versus Trabeculectomy Study during the first year of follow-up. *Am J Ophthalmol.* 2007;143:23–31.

Gedde SJ, Schiffman JC, Feuer WJ, Herndon LW, Brandt JD, Budenz DL. Treatment outcomes in the tube versus trabeculectomy study after one year of follow-up. *Am J Ophthalmol.* 2007;143:9–22.

Minckler DS, Francis BA, Hodapp EA, Jampel HD, Lin SC, Samples JR, Smith SD, Singh K. Aqueous shunts in glaucoma: A report by the American Academy of Ophthalmology. *Ophthalmology.* 2008;115: 1089–1098.

Minckler DS, Vedula SS, Li TJ, Mathew MC, Ayyala RS, Francis BA. Aqueous shunts for glaucoma. *Cochrane Database Syst Rev.* 2006;(2):CD004918. Review.

Schwartz KS, Lee RK, Gedde SJ. Glaucoma drainage implants: A critical comparison of types. *Curr Opin Ophthalmol.* 2006 Apr;17(2):181–189. Review.

Topouzis F, Coleman AL, Choplin N, Bethlem MM, Hill R, Yu F, Panek WC, Wilson MR. Follow-up of the original cohort with the Ahmed glaucoma valve implant. *Am J Ophthalmol.* 1999;128: 198–204.

Tsai JC, Johnson CC, Dietrich MS. The Ahmed shunt versus the Baerveldt shunt for refractory glaucoma: A single-surgeon comparison of outcome. *Ophthalmology.* 2003;110:1814–1821.

Wilson MR, Mendis U, Smith SD, Paliwal A. Ahmed glaucoma valve implant vs trabeculectomy in the surgical treatment of glaucoma: A randomized clinical trial. *Am J Ophthalmol.* 2000;130:267–273.

40   Pediatric Glaucoma

Anil K. Mandal, MD and Peter A. Netland, MD, PhD

SELECTED REFERENCES

Goniotomy or trabeculotomy are the most commonly performed primary surgical procedures for developmental glaucoma in the United States. These procedures are covered in the Pediatric Section (Freedman and co-authors, Section 6, Chapter 64). This chapter highlights the surgical procedure of combined trabeculotomy-trabeculectomy in the management of developmental glaucoma. Combined trabeculotomy-trabeculectomy is primarily used as a primary surgical procedure for patients with a poor prognosis for goniotomy or trabeculotomy. Patients who fail primary surgical treatment may be candidates for other secondary surgical procedures such as trabeculectomy with antifibrosis drugs, glaucoma drainage implants, or cyclophotocoagulation, which are covered in other Chapters in the Glaucoma Section.

TABLE 40.1 *Indications for Combined Trabeculotomy–Trabeculectomy*

1. Infantile glaucoma, with a poor prognosis for goniotomy or trabeculotomy (e.g., Arab or Indian descent)
2. Congenital glaucoma with significant corneal edema
3. Developmental glaucoma with severe degree of corneal edema and/or corneal scar
4. Developmental glaucoma when goniotomy or trabeculotomy has failed

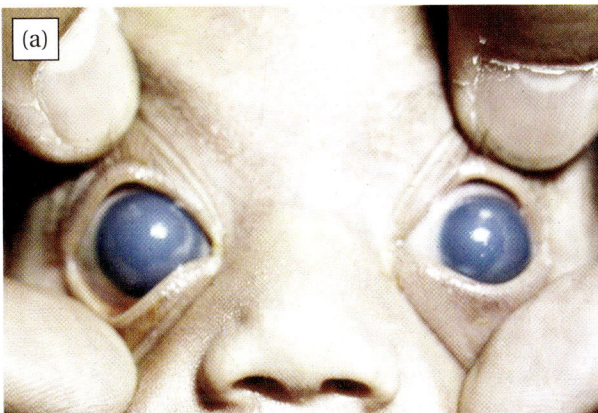

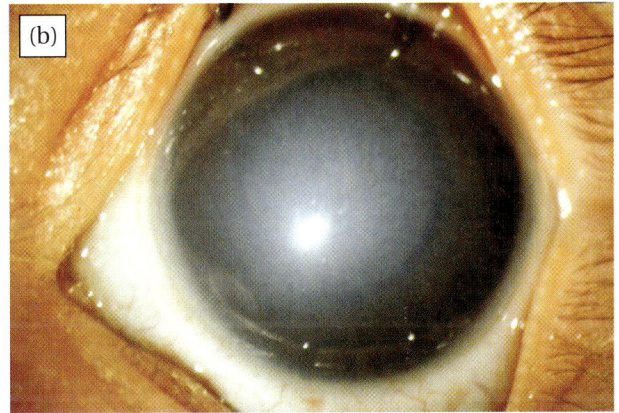

FIGURE 40.1 **Infantile Glaucoma.** (a) Clinical appearance of a patient with newborn glaucoma showing bilateral opaque enlarged corneas. (b) Slit lamp biomicroscope view, showing megalocornea and corneal edema.

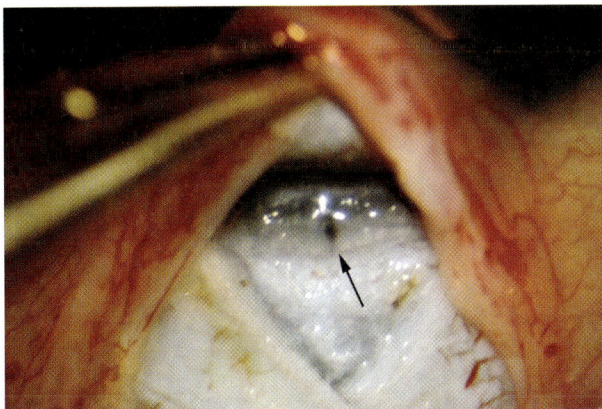

FIGURE 40.2 **Combined Trabeculotomy–Trabeculectomy.** After preparing a limbus- or fornix-based conjunctival flap (limbus-based flap shown in the photograph), a partial thickness sclera flap is created, either in a rectangular or triangular configuration, depending on surgeon preference. The surgeon may use an antifibrosis drug such as mitomycin-C at this time. A radial incision is made under the flap, in order to identify and create an opening into Schlemm's canal. The intraoperative microphotograph shows the anatomy of the limbal region under a partial thickness of scleral flap, with an opening into Schlemm's canal in the center (arrow).

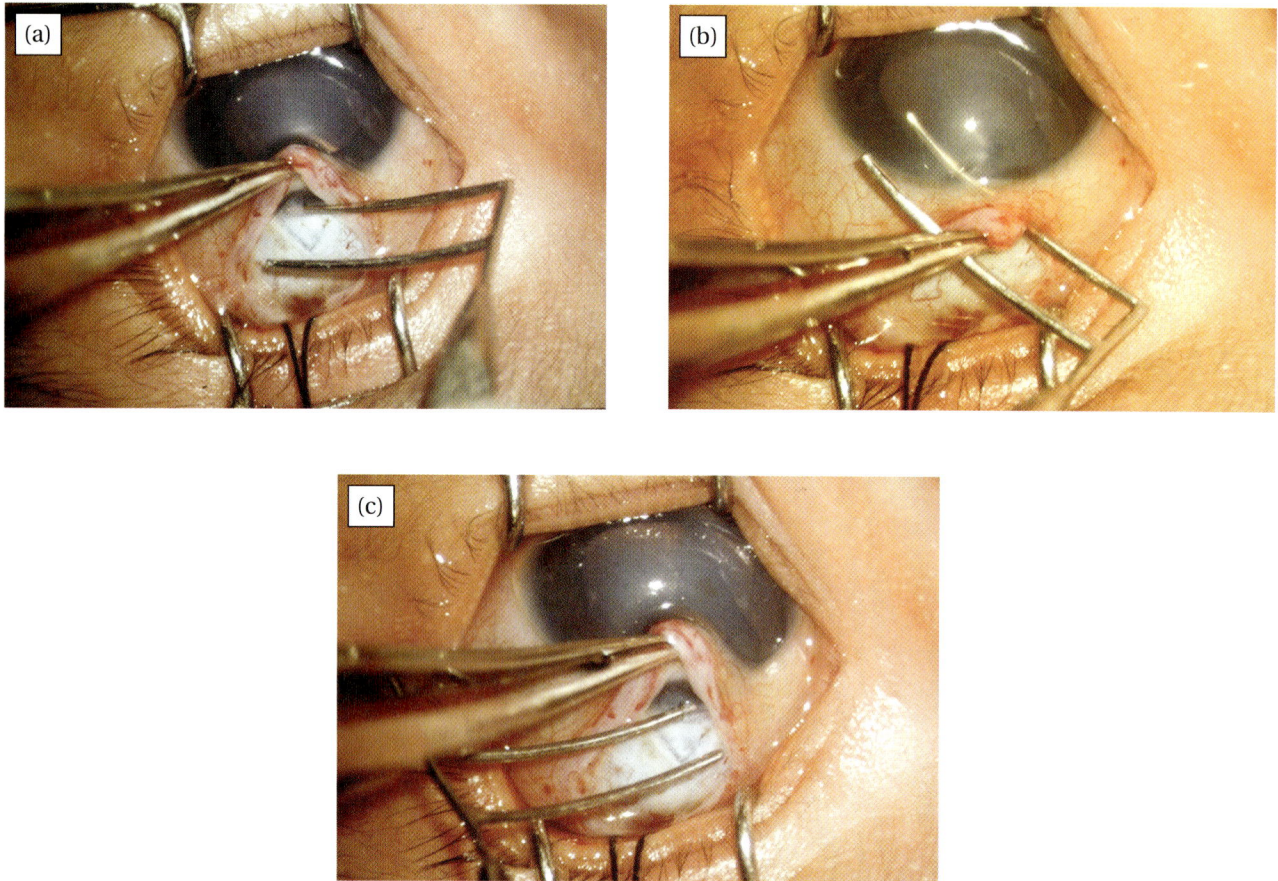

FIGURE 40.3 Trabeculotomy Step of the Procedure. (a) The internal arm of the trabeculotome is inserted into Schlemm's canal in one direction. The outer arm serves as an external guide for positioning the instrument. In the illustration, the internal arm is inserted to the left of the radial incision. (b) The probe is rotated into the anterior chamber, opening the trabecular meshwork. (c) The internal arm of the trabeculotome is then inserted into Schlemm's canal in the opposite direction. In the illustration, the internal arm is inserted to the right of the radial incision.

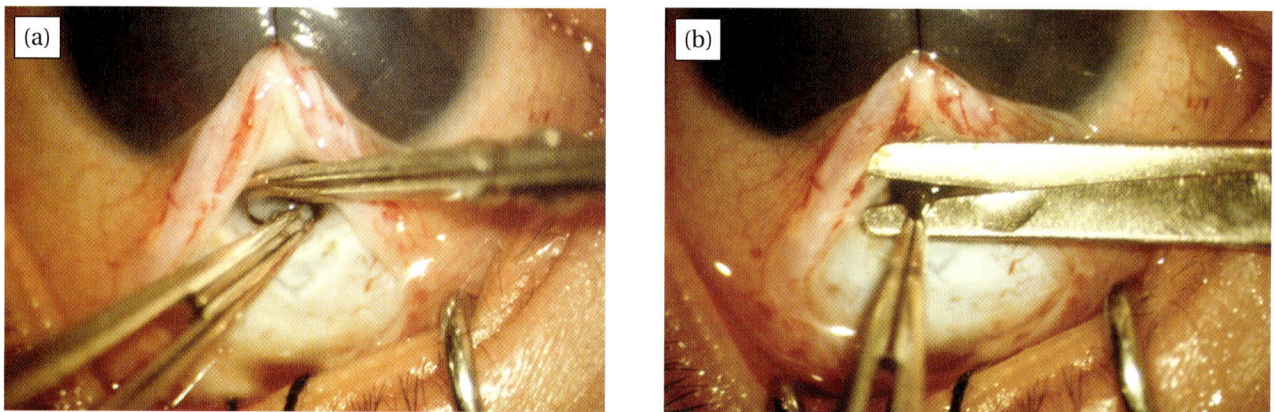

FIGURE 40.4 Trabeculectomy Step of the Procedure. (a) Using a Descemet's punch or sharp knife and scissors, the trabecular block is removed to complete the trabeculectomy part of the surgery. (b) A peripheral iridectomy is performed.

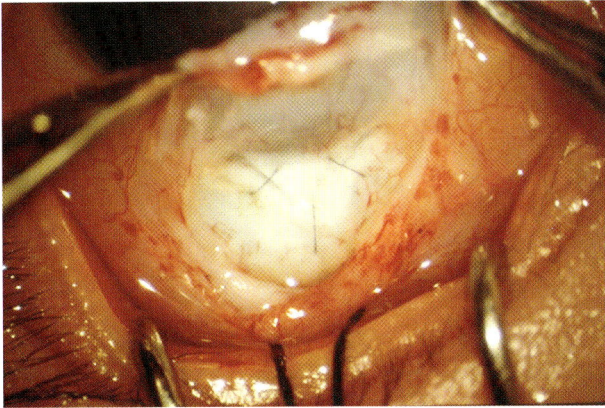

FIGURE 40.5 **Completion of the Procedure.** The scleral flap is sutured with 10-0 nylon or 10-0 absorbable suture. With a triangular flap, one suture is placed at the apex and one suture on each lateral side of the scleral flap. The conjunctival incision is closed with 8-0 or 9-0 polyglactin suture with a round (tapered) needle.

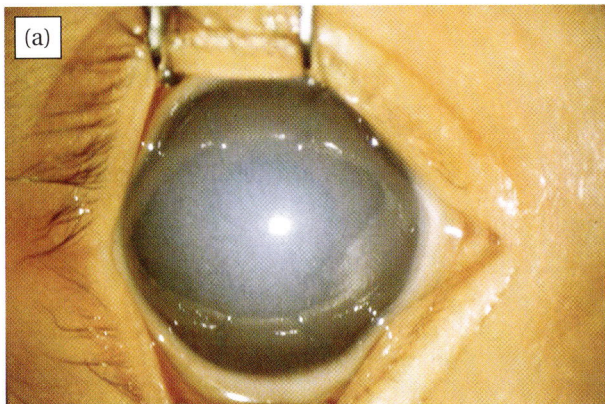

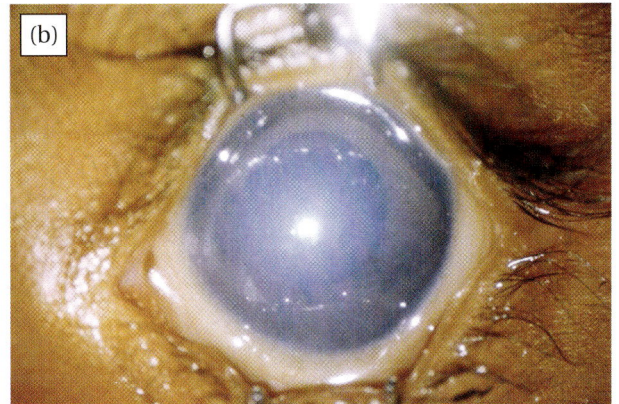

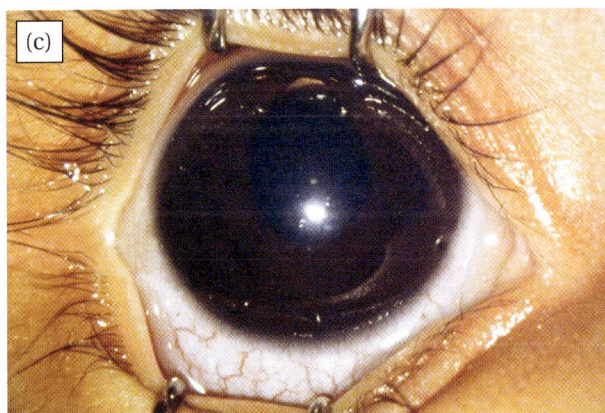

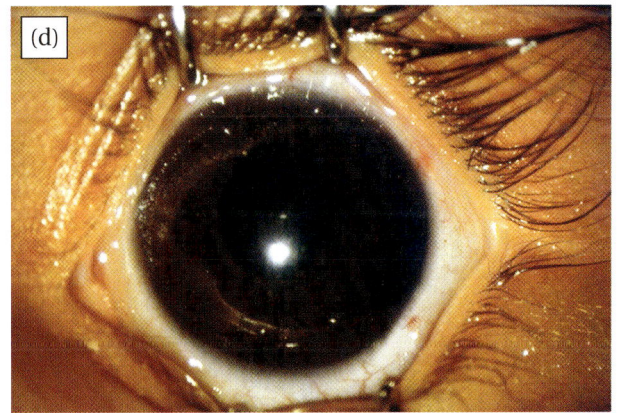

FIGURE 40.6 **Preoperative and Postoperative Appearance of the Eye.** Preoperative appearance of the right (a) and left (b) eyes of a child treated with combined trabeculotomy–trabeculectomy at the age of two weeks. Postoperative appearance of the right (c) and left (d) eyes of the same child at 6 months after surgery, showing complete clearing of the corneal edema.

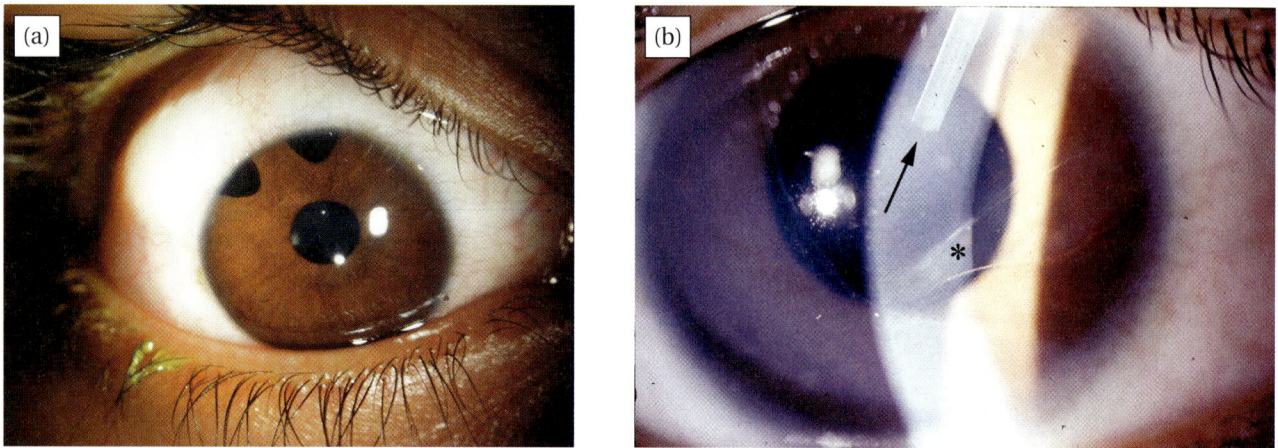

FIGURE 40.7 **Secondary Surgical Procedures for Refractory Pediatric Glaucoma.** Patients refractory to primary surgical treatment with goniotomy, trabeculotomy, or combined trabeculotomy–trabeculectomy may be treated with trabeculectomy with antifibrosis drugs, glaucoma drainage implant, cyclophotocoagulation, or other procedures. These procedures are shown in detail in other chapters in the glaucoma section. (a) Trabeculectomy with mitomycin-C. This child had been treated previously with trabeculectomy, which had failed to control the intraocular pressure. (b) Glaucoma drainage implant. The tube (arrow) is shown in the anterior chamber of an 11-year-old with a history of congenital glaucoma. The child had failed primary surgery and had significant conjunctival scarring. There are Haab's striae in the cornea (asterisk). (Modified with permission from Mandal AK, Netland PA. *The Pediatric Glaucomas.* New York, NY: Elsevier, Inc., 2006, pp. 81, 83.)

TABLE 40.2 *Complications of Combined Trabeculotomy-Trabeculectomy*

Intraoperative

Hyphema
False passage during introduction of trabeculotome
Descemet's tear, Descemet's detachment
Iridodialysis
Injury to the lens

Postoperative

Hyphema
Shallow or flat anterior chamber
Wound leak
Overfiltration
Choroidal detachment
Bleb failure
Blebitis, bleb infection and endophthalmitis

SELECTED REFERENCES

Elder MJ. Combined trabeculotomy–trabeculectomy compared with primary trabeculectomy for congenital glaucoma. *Br J Ophthalmol.* 1994;78:745–748.

Ishida K, Mandal AK, Netland PA. Glaucoma drainage implants in pediatric patients. *Ophthalmol Clin N Am.* 2005;18:431–442.

Mandal AK, Bhatia PG, Bhaskar A, Nutheti R. Long-term surgical and visual outcomes in Indian children with developmental glaucoma operated on within 6 months of birth. *Ophthalmology.* 2004;111:283–290.

Mandal AK, Naduvilath TJ, Jayagandan A. Surgical results of combined trabeculotomy–trabeculectomy for developmental glaucoma. *Ophthalmol.* 1998;105:974–982.

Mandal AK, Netland PA, Gothwal VK. Advances in the management of developmental glaucoma. Nema HV, Nema N, eds. *Recent Advances in Ophthalmology-8.* New Delhi: Jaypee Brothers, 2006, pp. 83–129.

Mandal AK, Netland PA. *The Pediatric Glaucomas.* New York, NY: Elsevier, Inc., 2006.

Mullaney PB, Selleck C, Al-Awad A, et al. Combined trabeculotomy and trabeculectomy as an initial procedure in uncomplicated congenital glaucoma. *Arch Ophthalmol.* 1999;117:457–460.

Retina Surgery

Edited by **Jay S. Duker**

Scleral Buckling and Pneumatic Retinopexy

Daniel P. Joseph, MD, PhD

Preoperative Considerations

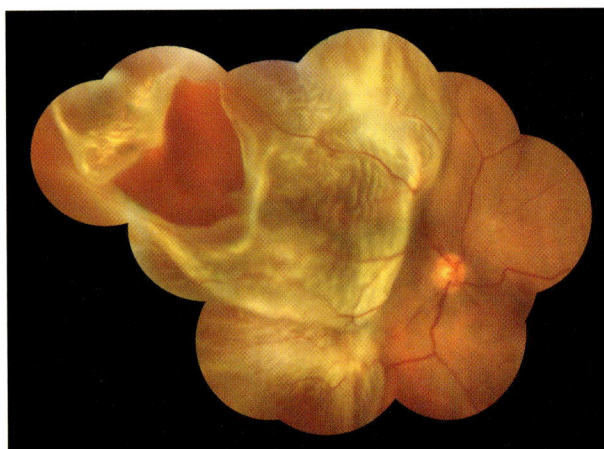

FIGURE 41.1   Retinal detachment due to a horseshoe tear.

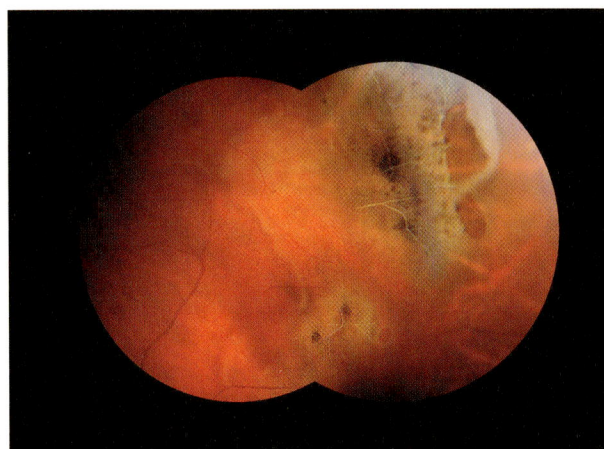

FIGURE 41.2   Retinal tears and holes in an eye with lattice degeneration. Multiple zones of pathology may occur in attached and detached retina.

TABLE 41.1   *General Principles of Scleral Buckle*

Localize all breaks

Treatment of breaks

• Cryotherapy

• Laser

Close breaks on the buckle

Relieve vitreous traction

Drainage of subretinal fluid

Intravitreal gas

TABLE 41.2   *Types of Buckles and Elements*

Encircling (circumferential) versus radial

Solid versus sponge

Encircling Bands—may be used with other circumferential or radial elements

• 240 (2.0 mm) supports most pathology

• 41 (2.5 mm) slightly larger

Added elements

• Tires—circumferential

• Segmental wedges—radial

• Plates—radial

Sponges can be radial or encircling

Bands

42   41   240   40

{1.25   {0.75   {0.6   {0.75

4.0   3.5   2.5   2.0

Sponges

5.5   3.0

7.5   5.0

Tires

287   277   276

9.0   9.0   9.0
7.0   7.0   7.0

Meridionals   106

10.5   6.0

Accessories

22
5.0   5.0

112

12.0   12.0

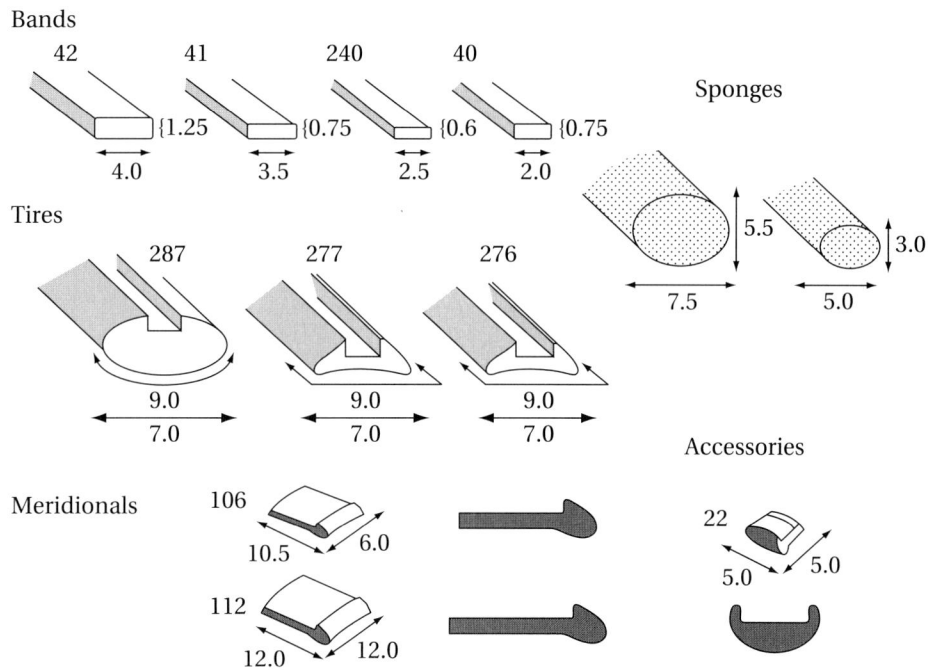

FIGURE 41.3 *Types of Buckles and Elements.* Encircling bands and elements come in a variety of sizes and shapes constructed of solid silicon rubber. Encircling and radial compressible silicon sponges can be cut to fit need.

TABLE 41.3 *Choosing a Buckle*

Encircling
- Multiple tears
- Tears plus lattice
- Multiple zones of pathology (wider elements)
- Phakic eyes
- Vitreous changes/traction (PVR)

Radial
- Single tear
- Radially oriented tear
- "Fishmouthed" open tear after placement of a band
- Posterior tear

TABLE 41.4 *Contraindications and Concerns of Scleral Buckles*

Thin or weakened sclera
Posterior pathology
Previous muscle surgery
Previous filtration surgery
Orbital tumors or other implants
Orbital trauma

Surgical Procedures

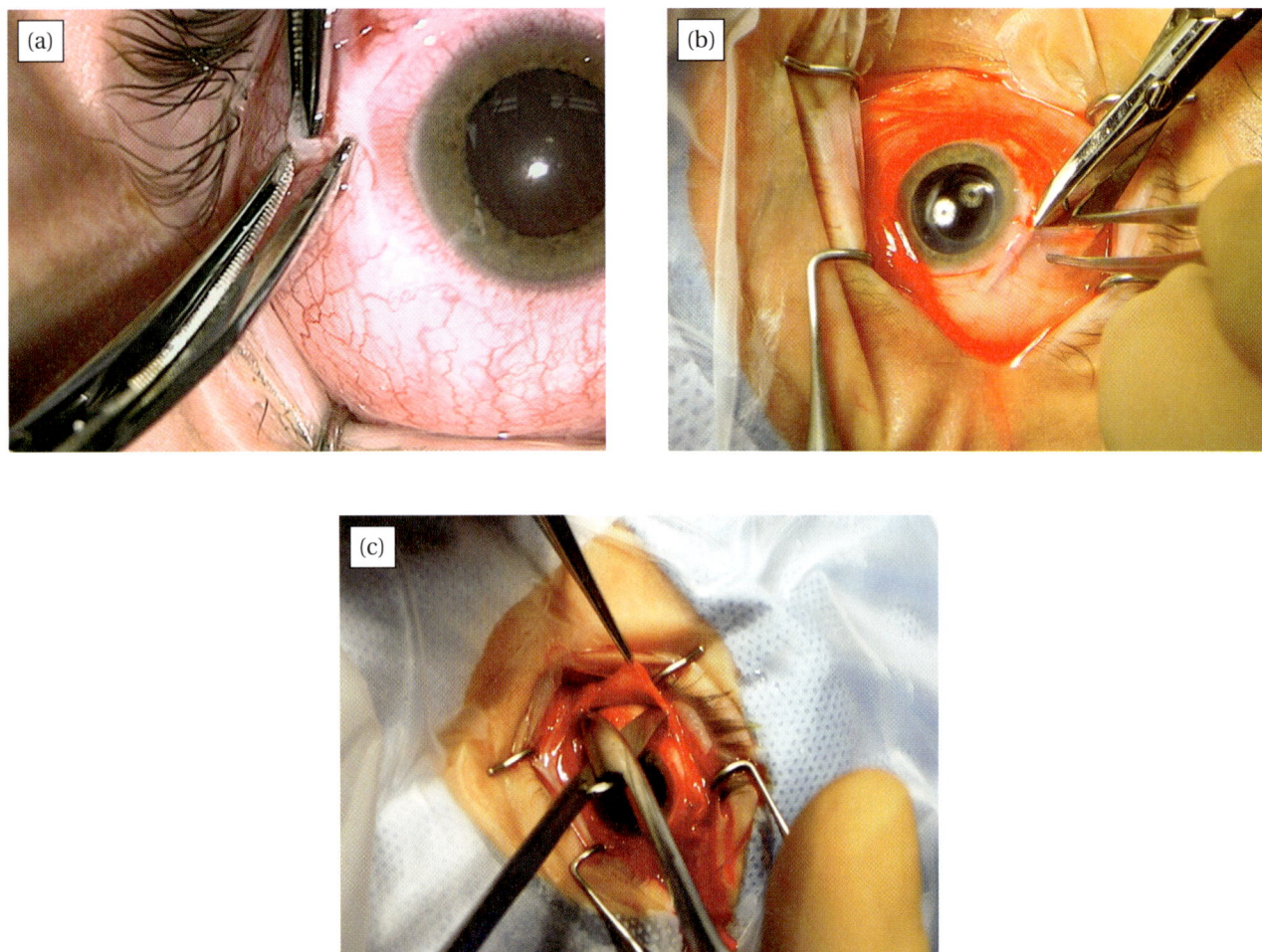

FIGURE 41.4 Opening conjunctiva and Tenon's. (a) To place an encircling element in one or more quadrants conjunctiva and Tenon's capsule are opened by tenting up the conjunctiva with toothed forceps and incising both layers with Wescott scissors. The incision is extended along the limbus. (b) Tenon's and conjunctiva are separated from the globe by blunt dissection with Wescott scissors. Radial relaxing incisions made at the 3 and 9 o'clock positions prevent tearing of the conjunctiva when placing encircling elements. (c) Curved Stevens or tenotomy scissors are used to dissect Tenon's capsule from the globe in all quadrants.

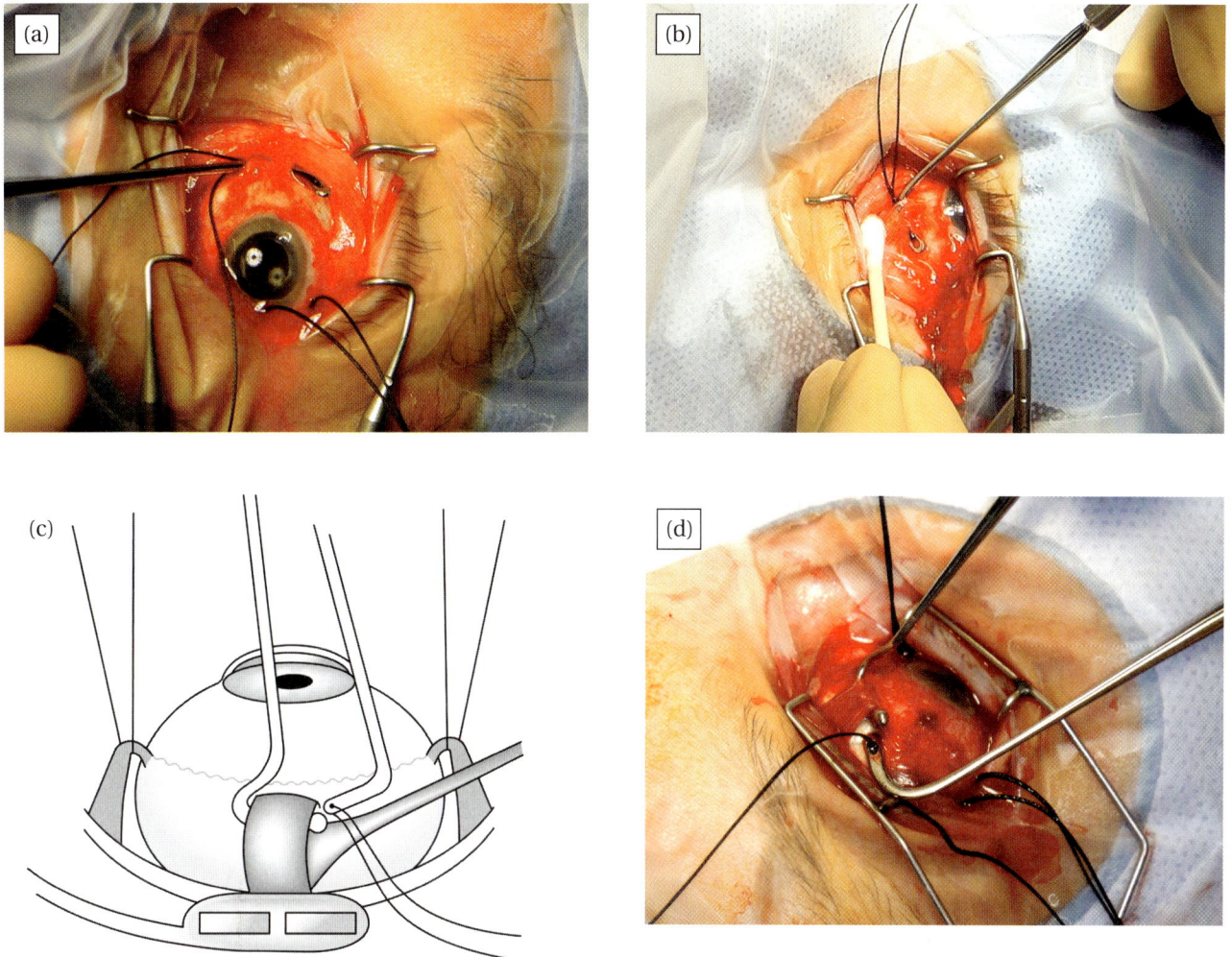

FIGURE 41.5 Isolating and looping muscles on suture. (a) The rectus muscles are isolated and looped with 2.0 silk suture by passing a Gass or fenestrated muscle hook preloaded with 2.0 silk suture. (b) Adherent Tenon's capsule is reflected away from muscle insertions using forceps or cotton-tip applicator to expose the muscle and the sclera around the muscle insertion. (c, d) Isolating the superior rectus from the globe and from the superior oblique can be facilitated by first passing a Jameson muscle hook to elevate the superior rectus as the globe is rotated inferiorly. A second muscle hook with suture is then passed in the opposite direction, between the first muscle hook and the insertion of the superior rectus muscle.

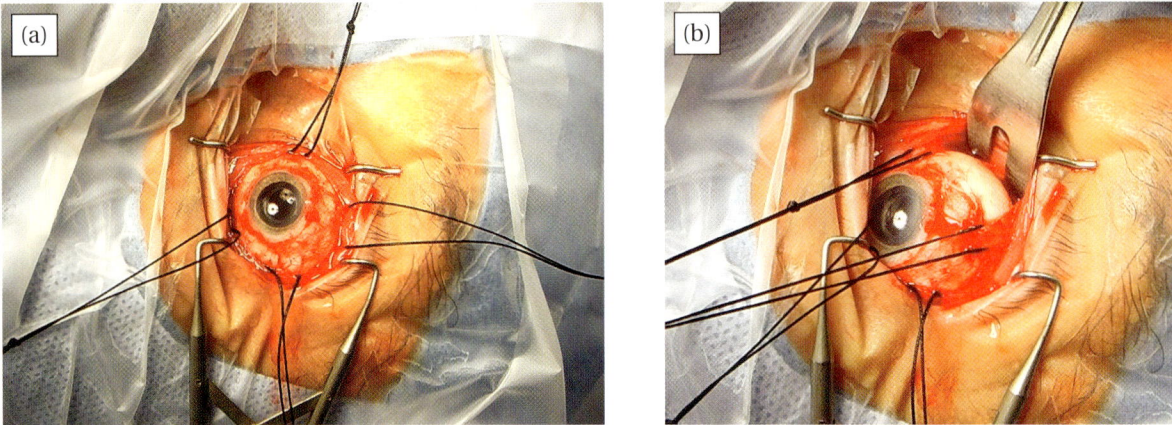

FIGURE 41.6 Inspection the external globe. (a, b) Once the vertical and horizontal rectus muscles are looped on 2.0 silk suture, a Schepens retractor is used to inspect the sclera in each quadrant for thinning, or out-pouching, and to insure that the entire muscle is looped.

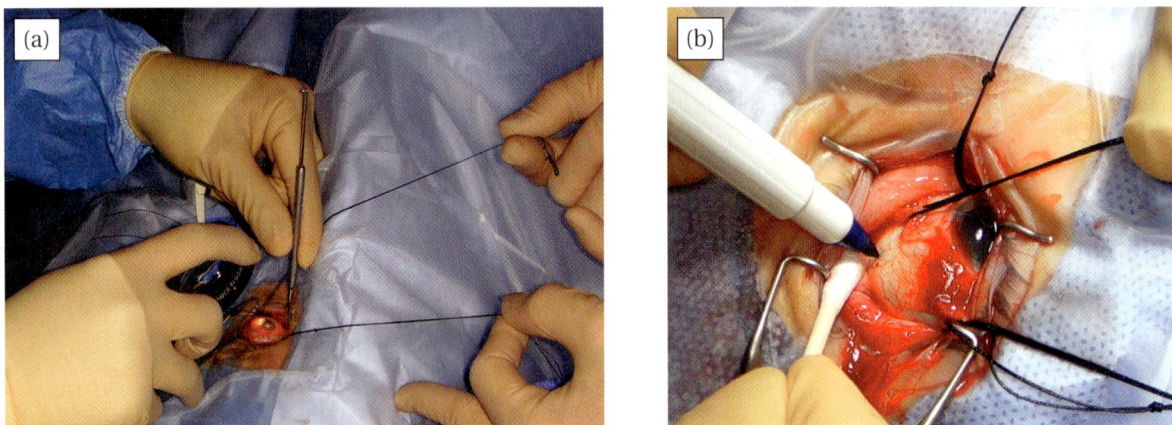

FIGURE 41.7 Identify breaks and mark peripheral pathology. (a) The surgeon inspects the peripheral retina by performing indirect ophthalmoscopy using a 28 or 20 diopter lens, depressing peripheral retina while an assistant uses the muscle sutures to help orient the globe. An O'Connell depressor (or other marking depressor) is used to mark the posterior edge and extent of all tears and pathology. (b) A permanent mark can be made with diathermy or a marking pen. Marking the anterior aspect of the breaks facilitates placement of radial or encircling elements for tears that cannot be supported by a band.

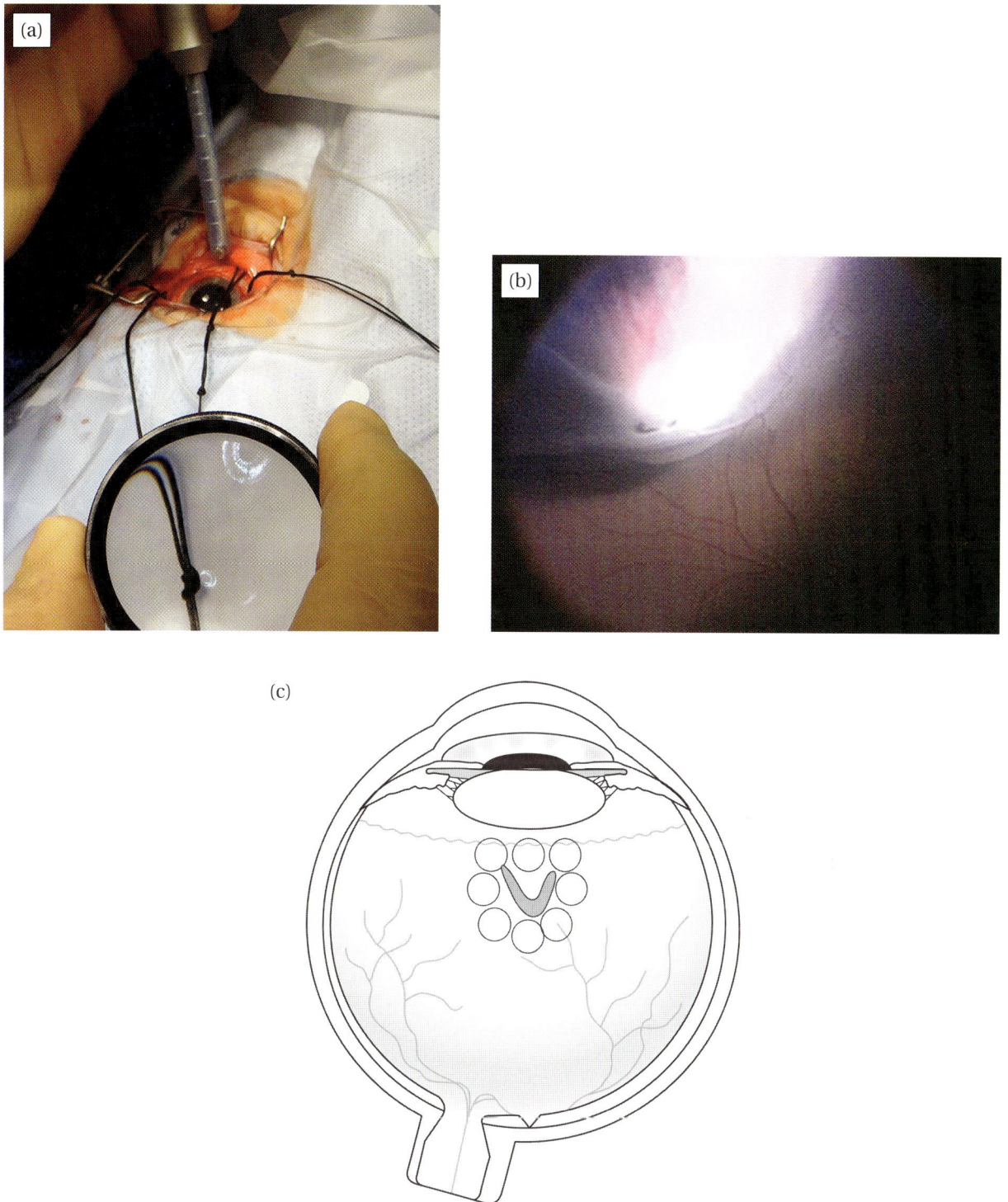

FIGURE 41.8 Treating the tears. (a) The retinal tears and other pathology are treated with cryotherapy prior to placement of the buckle. (b) Small tears may "light up" when treated, confirming full-thickness tear. (c) The tears are surrounded by cryotherapy (circles). One advantage of cryotherapy is that tears can be treated in detached retina. Alternatively, tears can be treated with laser photocoagulation once the retina is reattached.

(a)

(b)

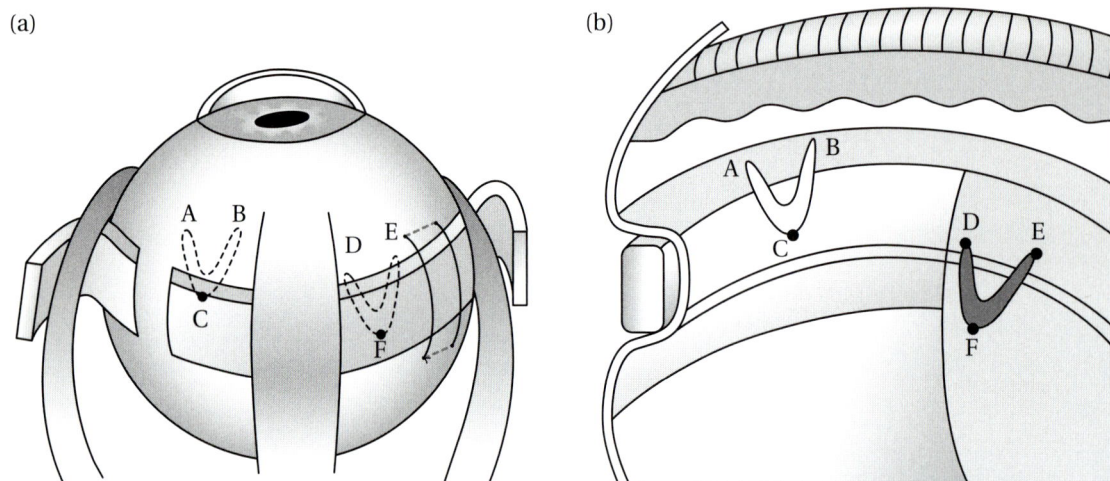

FIGURE 41.9 Location of tears on the buckle. (a) Tears and other pathology are supported by an encircling band (e.g., 240 or 41); the posterior edge of the break is aligned with the anterior edge of the band. The band can be attached to the globe with lamellar belt loops or suture. (b) Failure to place the tear on the anterior crest of the buckle results in an open break. Open breaks may be closed by revising the buckle position, adding other elements (tires, radial or meridional), performing external drainage, using gas tamponade, or a combination of these procedures.

TABLE 41.5 *Attachment of the Buckle to the Globe*

Suture
- Non-absorbable material (5.0 nylon)
- Spatulated needle
- Partial thickness passes
- Length: 3–5 mm passes
- Width: 2 mm greater than width of element
- Posterior pass should be 3 mm posterior to edge of break

Lamellar Belt Loops
- Vertical incision perpendicular to limbus partial thickness: 64 blade
- Horizontal scleral tunnel: 66 blade

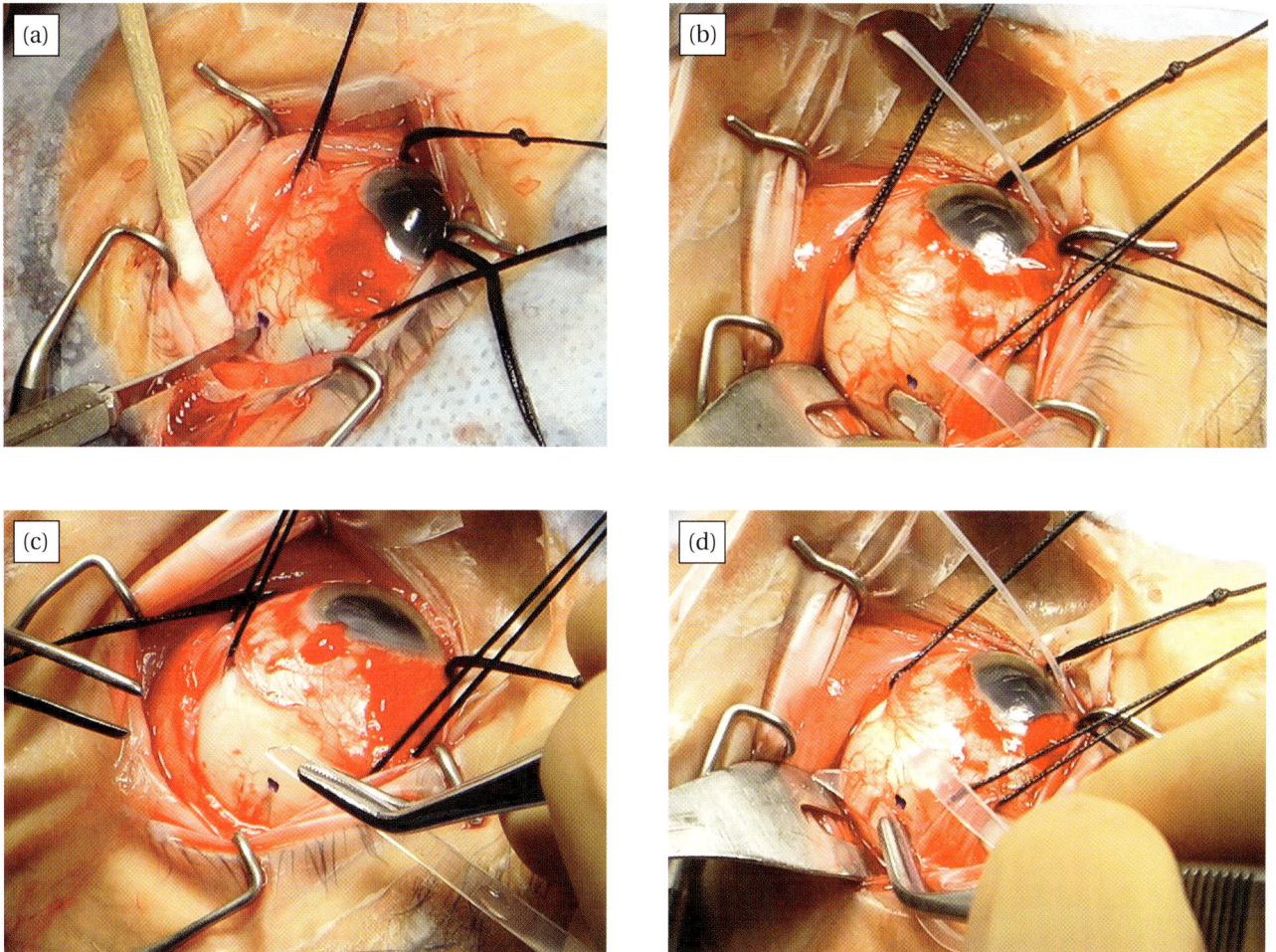

FIGURE 41.10 Fixation to the globe with scleral belt loops. Creating scleral belt loops. (a) The 64 blade is used to create two parallel partial-thickness radial scleral incisions 3–4 mm apart, perpendicular to the limbus. (b) The 66 blade is used to create the scleral tunnel connecting vertical incisions. (c, d) The band is passed as belt loops are created.

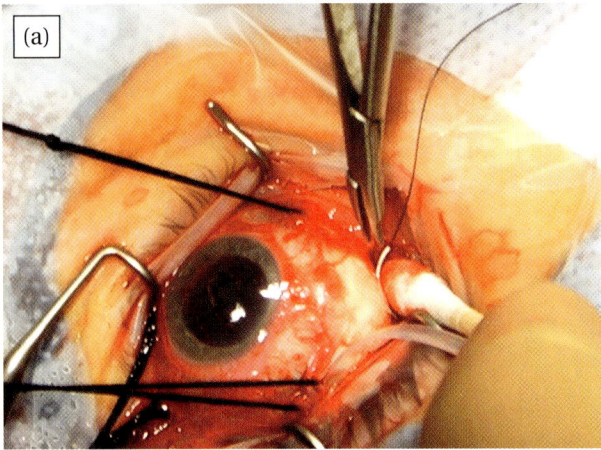

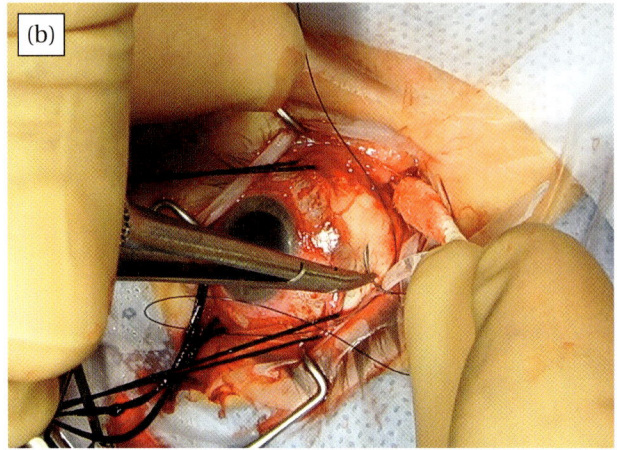

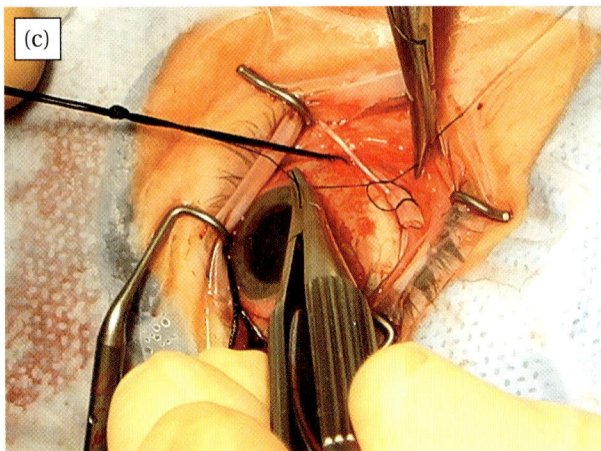

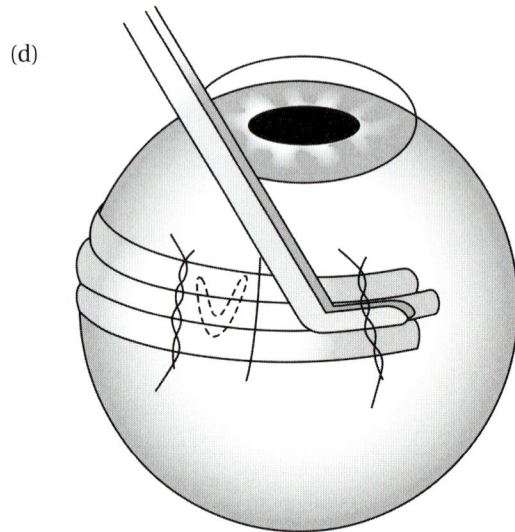

FIGURE 41.11 Fixation to the globe with sutures. Mattress sutures are used for wider encircling elements, or in quadrants with sclera too thin to create belt loops. The posterior and anterior location of the suture is 1 mm posterior (a) and 1 mm anterior (b) to the edge of the band, or tire. (c) The last suture is tied after the Watzke sleeve has been placed. (d) Encircling elements too wide for belt loops are passed through preplaced mattress sutures.

(a)

(b)

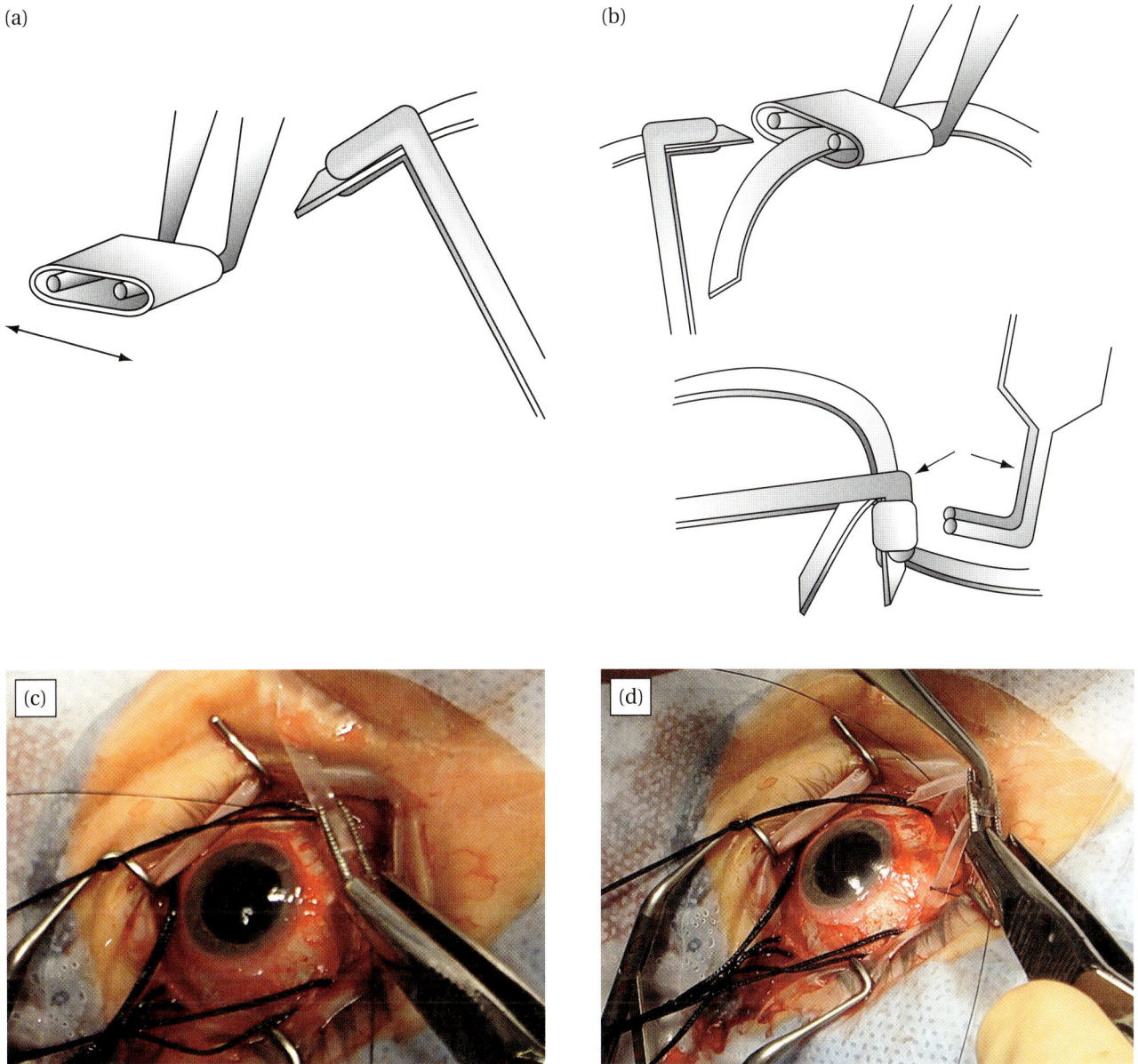

(c)

(d)

FIGURE 41.12 Placing of a sleeve to connect the band. (a, b) The sleeve is backed over the end of the band closest to the belt loop (or suture). (c, d) The other end of the band is grasped with forceps and passed through the sleeve on top of the band. The forceps is rotated and used to pull the sleeve off the sleeve spreader.

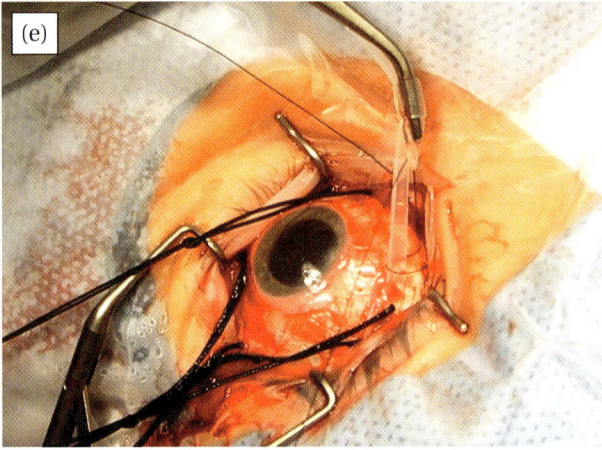

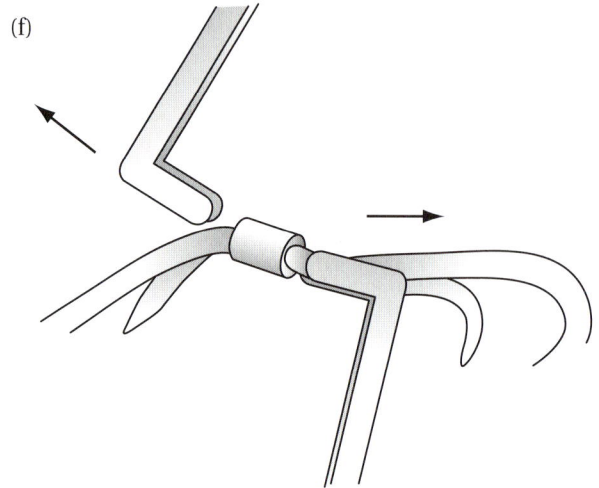

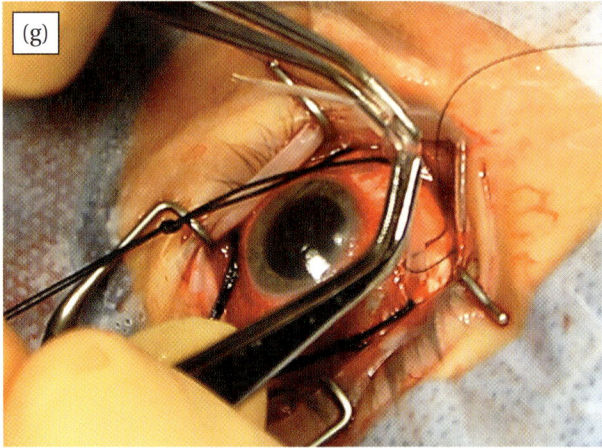

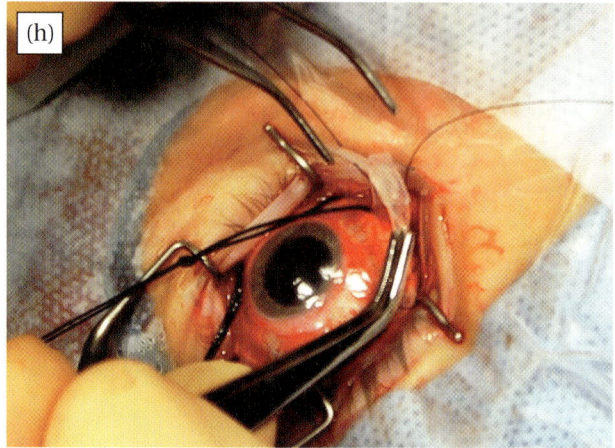

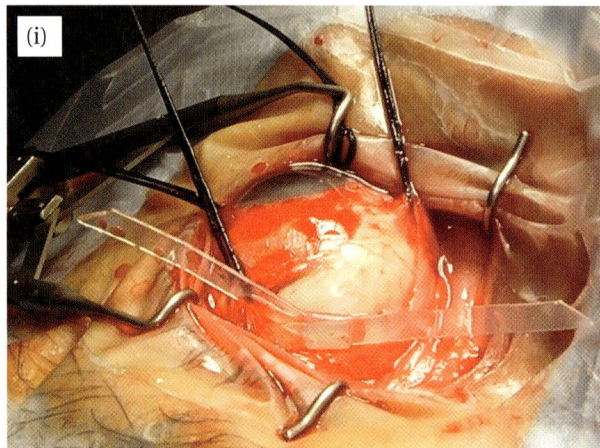

FIGURE 41.12 (*continued*) (e) The sleeve is transferred from the sleeve spreader to the forceps. (f, g, h) A second forceps is used to pull the band and sleeve off the forceps. (i) The Watske sleeve and overlapping ends of the band. The buckle is inspected for twists. Excess silicone is trimmed after adjustment of the buckle height. This technique does not require help from an assistant. Alternatively, the ends of the band can be attached with suture or clips, but adjustment of buckle height is easier with a silicone sleeve.

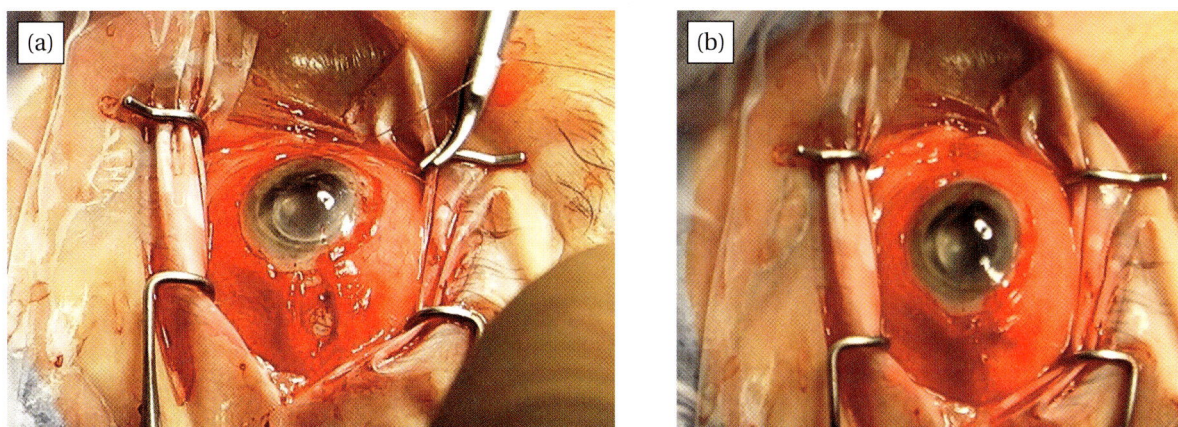

FIGURE 41.13 Closing conjunctiva. After adjustment of the buckle height, the retina is inspected for proper location and closure of tear(s) on the buckle. Depending on the location, a tear that remains open or is not properly supported by the buckle may be treated by external drainage, addition of elements, gas tamponade, or buckle revision. (a) The conjunctiva is closed with buried running or interrupted absorbable suture (vicryl or gut). (b) Care is taken to approximate and evert edges.

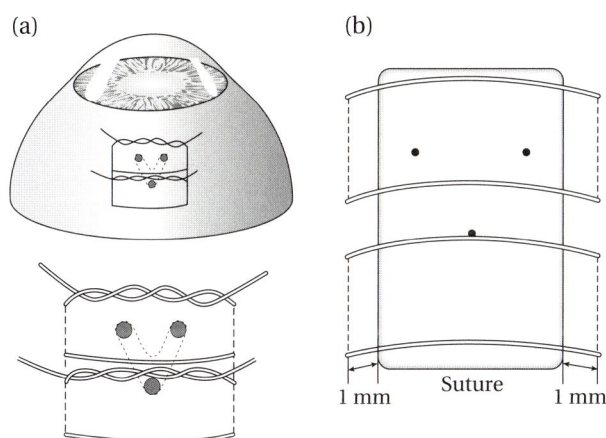

FIGURE 41.14 Use of radial elements. Radial elements may be used alone or in combination with encircling elements. They help to avoid radial folds and "fishmouthing" of large tears that may occur with an encircling element. Proper suture placement to support a tear on a radial element does not require the suture pass to be as far posterior as is required for encircling elements. (a) Place anterior suture about 1 mm anterior to anterior edge of break, and posterior suture about 2 mm posterior to posterior edge of break to be supported on radial element. (b) Use one or two mattress sutures. Depending on length of element, each mattress suture extends about 3–4 mm in length.

TABLE 41.6 *Complications of Scleral Buckle*

Complication	Frequency	Treatment
Open break	Common	Modify buckle position, add elements, drain, inject gas, vitrectomy
Infection	Rare	Antibiotics, anti-inflammatory agents, remove buckle
Perforation	Rare	Treat breaks
Strabismus	Occasional	Observe, prisms, surgery
Cataract	Rare	Surgery
Refractive change	Common	Refract
Extrusion	Rare	Remove or cover exposed piece
Choroidals	Rare	Loosen buckle if observed during surgery
		Observe for improvement

TABLE 41.7 *Indications for External Drainage of Subretinal Fluid*

Breaks not closed by the buckle

High bullous detachments

Inferior detachments

Chronic detachments

PVR

Inferior breaks

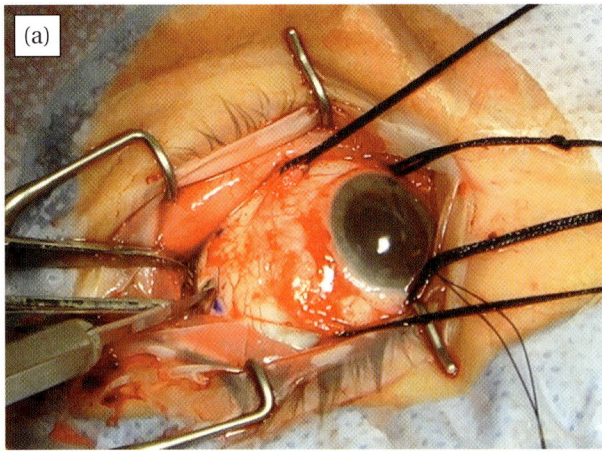

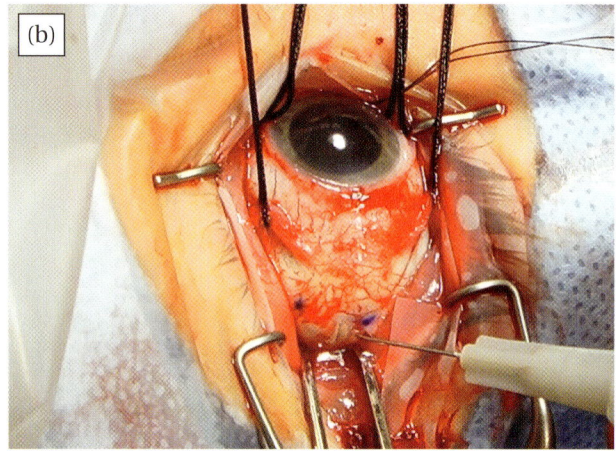

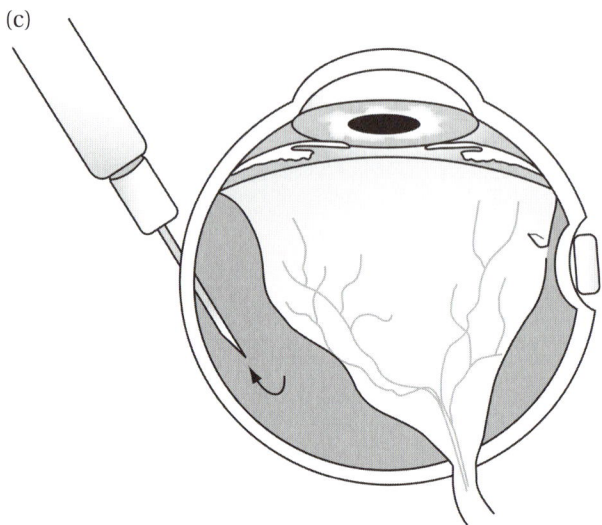

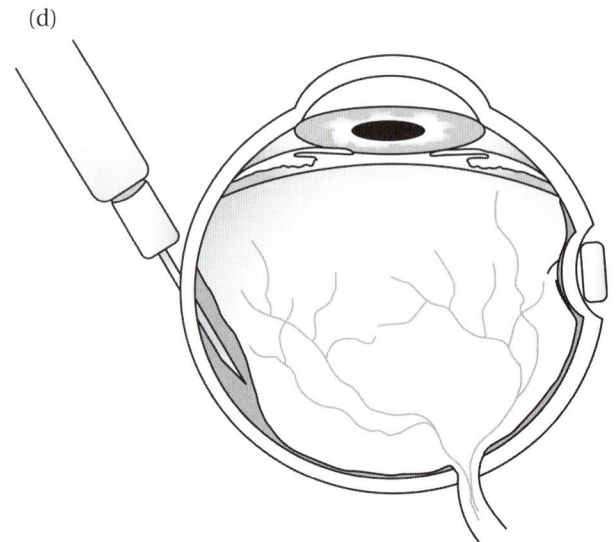

FIGURE 41.15 External Drainage: Two Techniques. (a) The drainage site is chosen to avoid vortex veins and to be located away from the retinal breaks or tears. A radial scleral incision is made to expose the choroid. The buckle is pulled inferiorly away from the sclerotomy with forceps. (b) Choroid is punctured with a sharp 27-gauge needle or (diathermy tip). Placement of cotton swabs in opposite quadrants facilitates drainage of subretinal fluid. Pigment efflux often indicates cessation of drainage. If a lot of fluid is drained, volume replacement can be accomplished by "pulling up the buckle," injecting saline or gas after the buckle is tightened. Placement of the drainage site in bed of the buckle avoids need to suture sclerotomy. Indirect ophthalmoscopy is used to check for complications such as retinal incarceration, and subretinal hemorrhage. (c) Alternatively, a 27- or 25-gauge needle on a 1 cc syringe with plunger removed may be inserted bevel down, directly into the subretinal space under ophthalmoscopic visualization. (d) Drainage is complete when retina is seen to drape over the needle.

TABLE 41.8 *Complications of External Drainage*

Complication	Treatment
Subretinal Hemorrhage (day of)	Position patient with hemorrhage site lower than macula over night
Thin (next day)	Observe regardless of location
Thick (next day)	Consider pneumatic displacement or extraction ±TPA if subfoveal, watch if extrafoveal
Retinal incarceration	Treat with laser or cryo, vitrectomy if severe
Suprachoroidal hemorrhage	Close drain site, observe, consider drainage if severe pain, or very large (give time for clot to lyse)

TABLE 41.9 *Indications for Pneumatic Retinopexy*

Single superior tear preferred

Break(s) limited to 1 or 2 clock hours

Break(s) located in superior hemisphere

Small to modest sized breaks

Lack of extensive inferior pathology (lattice, atrophic holes, tears)

Compliant patient—able to maintain position to keep bubble on break(s)

TABLE 41.10 *Choice of Gas*

Gas–Air mix	Expansile	Duration
20%–24% SF6	No	3–4 weeks
14% C3F8	No	6–8 weeks
Air	No	1–2 weeks
100% C3F8	4X	6–8 weeks
100% SF6	2X	3–4 weeks

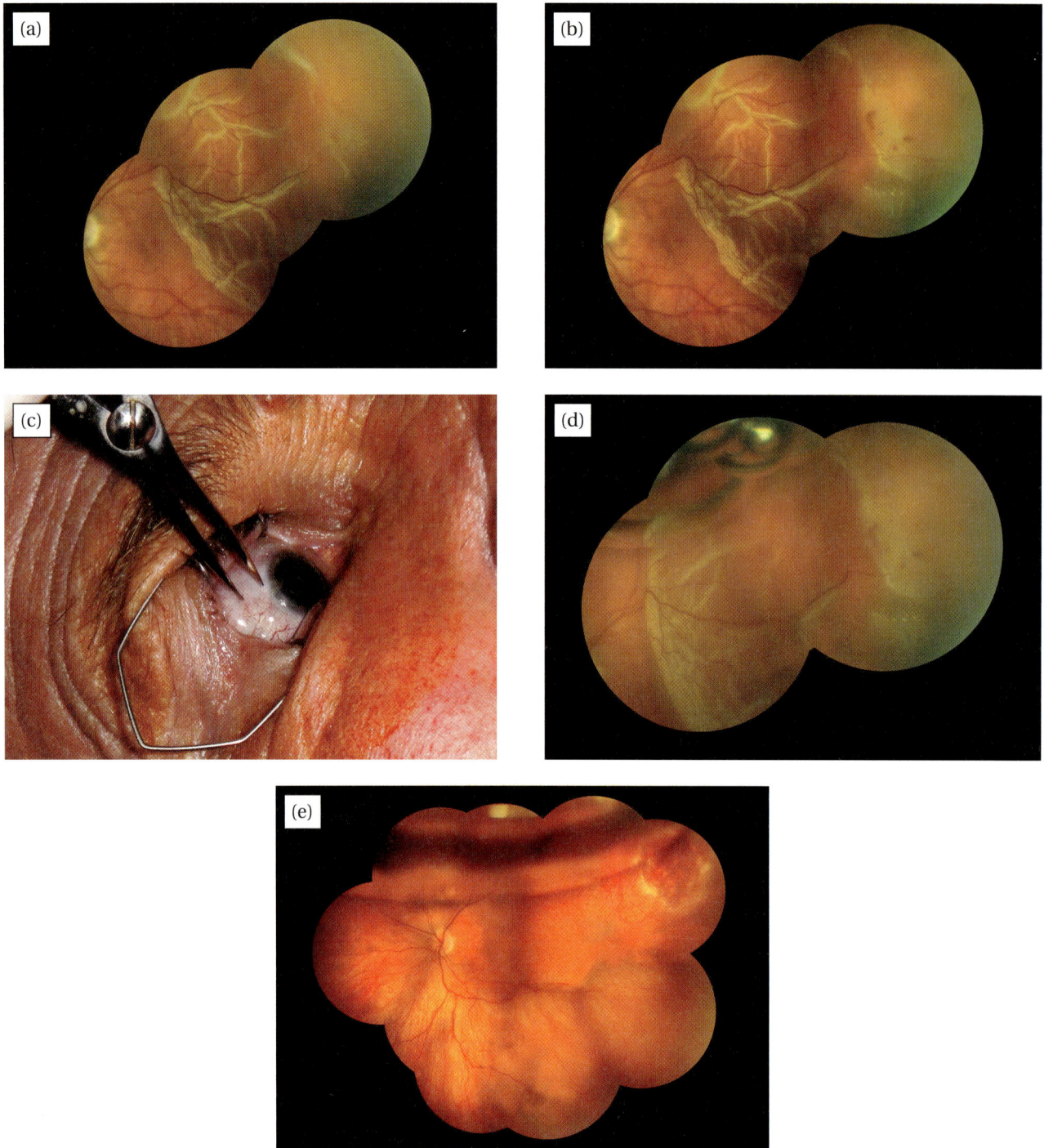

FIGURE 41.16 Pneumatic retinopexy and gas tamponade may be used to treat tears located in the superior 180 degrees of the retina. Injection of gas may be done before or after treatment of the tear. Choice of gas depends on desired volume and length of tamponade. (a) Macular off-retinal detachment with horseshoe tear located superotemporally. (b) Tear is easier to visualize after treatment with cryotherapy. (c) Subconjunctival lidocaine is given for anesthesia prior to cryotherapy and injection of gas. The eye is prepared for injection with betadine. 0.3 cc of 100% C3F8 is injected 3.5 mm posterior to the limbus. (d) Indirect ophthalmoscopy is used to visualize gas in the vitreous cavity. Small bubbles will coalesce as the bubble expands. The patient is positioned so that the gas bubble will close the hole. IOP and arterial perfusion are checked after injecting gas. Medicines and anterior chamber paracentesis are used to treat high pressures if needed after injection of gas. (e) Appearance of bubble and treated tear 5 days after pneumatic. A chorioretinal adhesion is forming, the bubble has expanded, the macula and superior retina is reattached, and a small amount of fluid persists in the inferotemporal quadrant.

TABLE 41.11 *Complications of Pneumatic Retinopexy*

Complication	Treatment
Infection	Antibiotics
Elevated IOP	Medicines
Subretinal gas	Position, observation for resolution
Hemorrhage	Observation if mild, vitrectomy if severe
Persistent fluid	No new breaks—observe
	New breaks—treat new breaks, reposition, buckle, vitrectomy
Central artery occlusion	Anterior chamber paracentesis, medicines

SELECTED REFERENCES

Brazitikos PD, Androudi S, Christen WG, Stangos NT. Primary pars plana vitrectomy versus scleral buckle surgery for the treatment of pseudophakic retinal detachment: A randomized clinical trial. *Retina.* 2005;25(8):957–964.

Brinton DA, Hilton GF. Pneumatic retinopexy and alternative retinal detachment techniques. In Ryan SJ, ed. *Retina* (pp. 2047–2062). St. Louis: Mosby; 2001.

Brinton DA, Wilkinson CP. *Retinal detachments: Principles and practice,* 3rd ed. New York: Oxford University Press; 2009.

Kreissig I, ed. *Primary retinal detachment: options for repair.* Berlin: Springer Verlag; 2005.

Schepens CL, Okamura ID, Brockhurst RJ. The scleral buckling procedures. I: Surgical techniques and management. *AMA Arch Opthalmol.* 1957;58(6):797–811.

Schwartz SG, Kuhl DP, McPherson AR, Holz ER, Mieler WF. Twenty-year follow-up for scleral buckling. *Arch Ophthalmol.* 2002;120(3):325–329.

Williams GA, Aaberg TM Sr. Techniques of scleral buckling. In Ryan SJ, ed. *Retina* (pp. 2010–2046). St. Louis: Mosby; 2001.

42 | Basic Vitreoretinal Surgery Techniques

Schonmei Wu, MD, Ron Margolis, MD, and Stanley Chang, MD

TABLE 42.1 *Indications for Vitrectomy*

Vitreous Opacity
    Vitreous hemorrhage
    Amyloidosis
    Inflammatory debris
Vitreoretinal Interface Disorders
    Macular hole
    Macular pucker
    Vitreomacular traction syndrome
    Myopic traction maculopathy
Retinal Detachment
    Rhegmatogenous retinal detachment
    Giant retinal tear
    Traction retinal detachment
    Retinoschisis
Proliferative Diabetic Retinopathy
    Traction detachment or distortion
    Macular edema
Submacular Hemorrhage
    Age-related macular degeneration
    Retinal macroaneurysm
Posterior segment trauma
Retinal vascular occlusion
Retained lens fragments following cataract surgery
Dislocated posterior chamber intraocular lens
Aqueous misdirection syndrome (malignant glaucoma)
Endophthalmitis

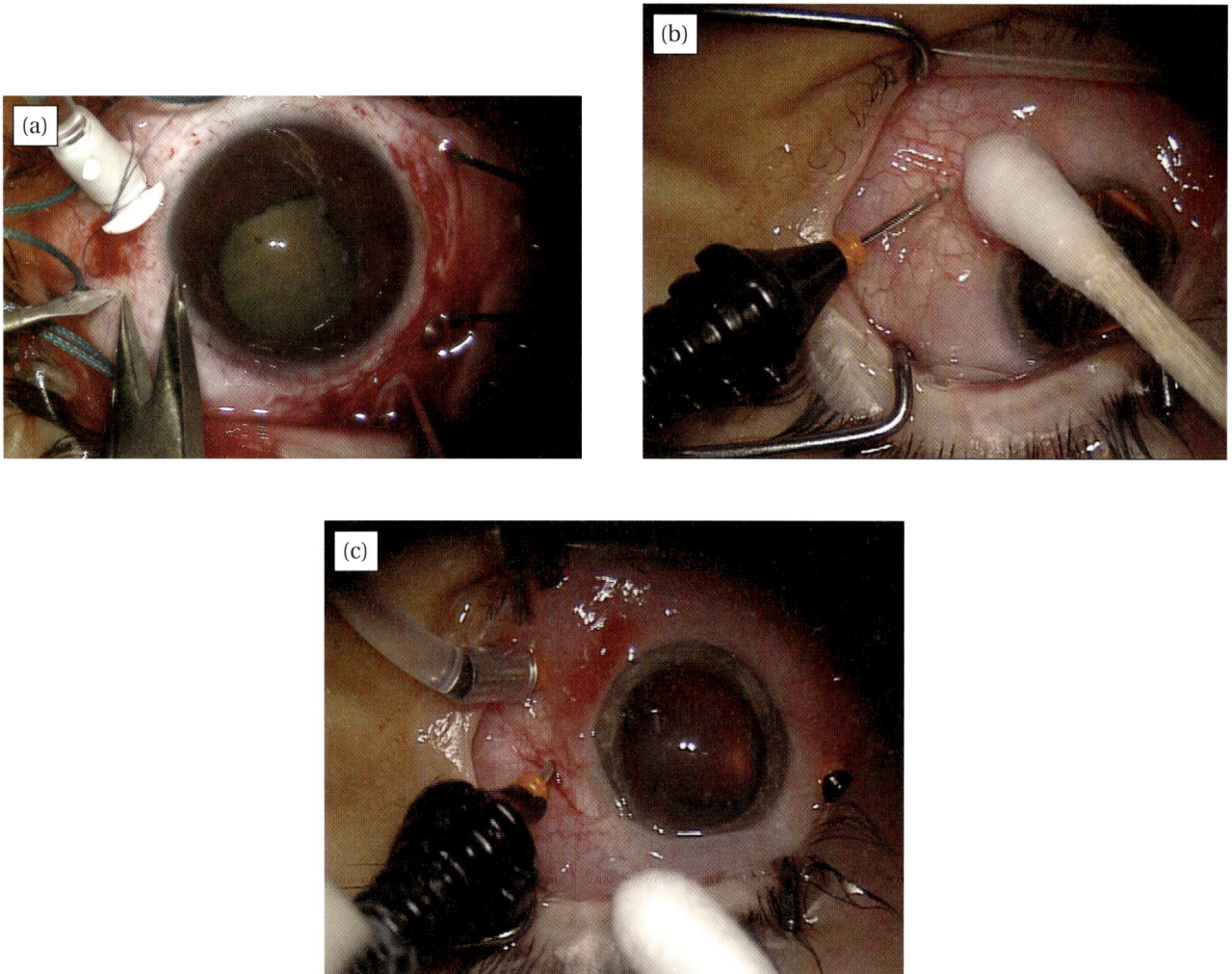

FIGURE 42.1 (a) Standard three-port 20 gauge vitrectomy. Limited conjunctival peritomies or a 360 degree conjunctival peritomy to place an encircling band (as shown) is created, and bleeding is controlled with diathermy. A microvitreoretinal (MVR) blade is used to make an inferotemporal sclerotomy 3–3.5 mm posterior to the limbus if the crystalline lens is absent or to be removed, and 4 mm posterior to the limbus if the eye is to remain phakic. The infusion cannula is inserted, secured with a polyglactin suture, and inspected to ensure it is properly positioned in the vitreous cavity before being turned on. The superior sclerotomies are similarly performed via stab incision with the MVR blade. (b) Microincisional (23 gauge) vitrectomy. The conjunctiva is displaced using a cotton-tipped applicator, and sclerotomies are created by inserting the blade of the trocar into the eye parallel to the limbus, at an approximately 45-degree bevel to the sclera. Once the blade is through the sclera, the trocar is rotated so that it is perpendicular to the eye wall, and inserted into the vitreous cavity (c). The self-retaining cannula (orange) is kept in place with the forceps while the trocar is removed. Instruments are introduced into the eye through the cannulas.

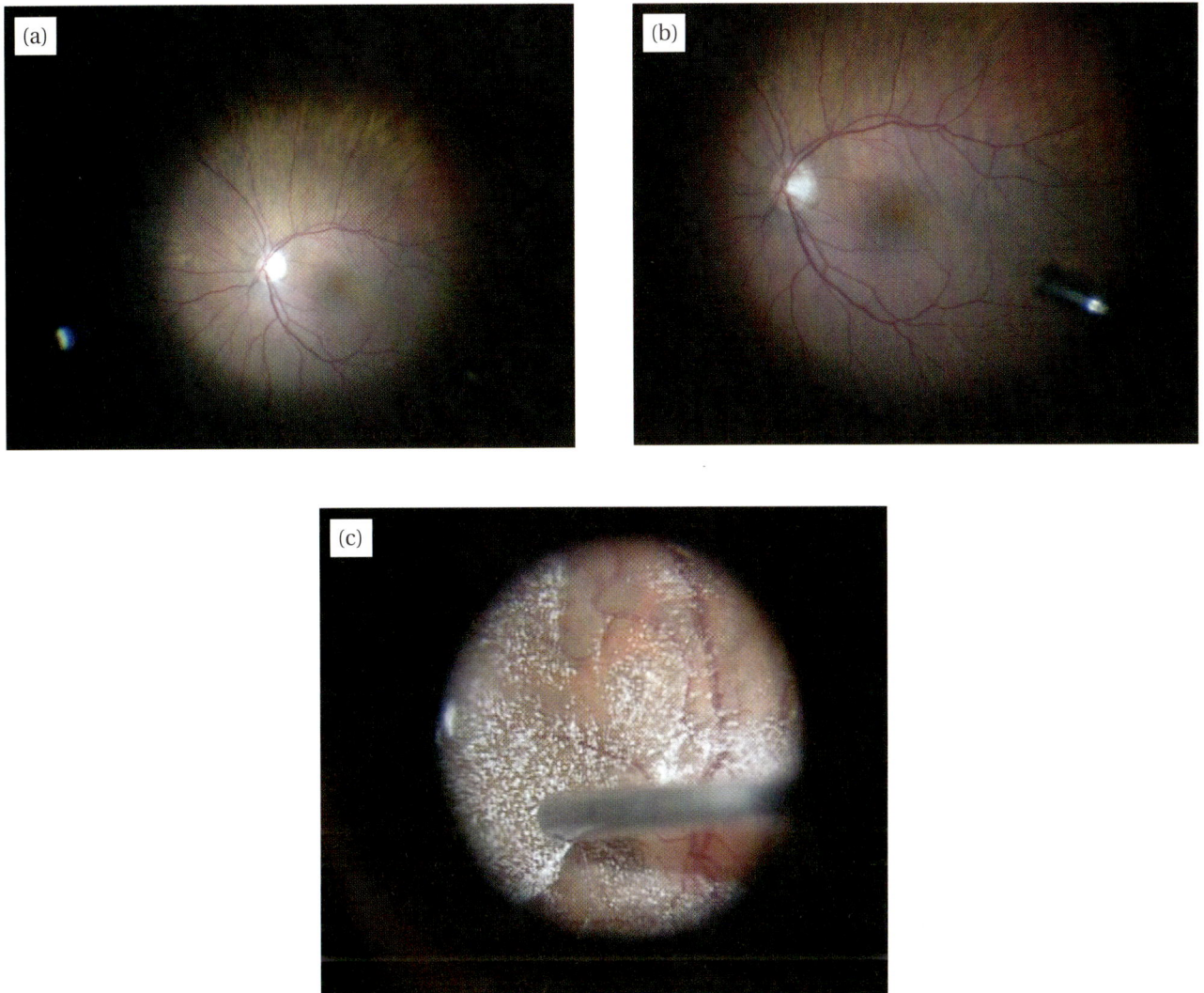

FIGURE 42.2 Wide-angle viewing systems provide panoramic viewing of the fundus, and are particularly useful for peripheral vitreous removal, injection of heavy liquid, fluid–air exchange, internal drainage of subretinal fluid through anterior breaks, and endophotocoagulation of peripheral breaks. The non-contact variety, such as the BIOM, requires no assistant, but increases the need to rotate the eye to view the far periphery. Handheld contact lenses eliminate corneal asphericity, but require a trained assistant. The 130 diopter lens (a) provides the widest possible field of view, whereas the 68 diopter lens (b) provides improved stereopsis and resolution. Plano-concave lenses (c) are used for macular surgery and provide the most detailed view of posterior pole structures.

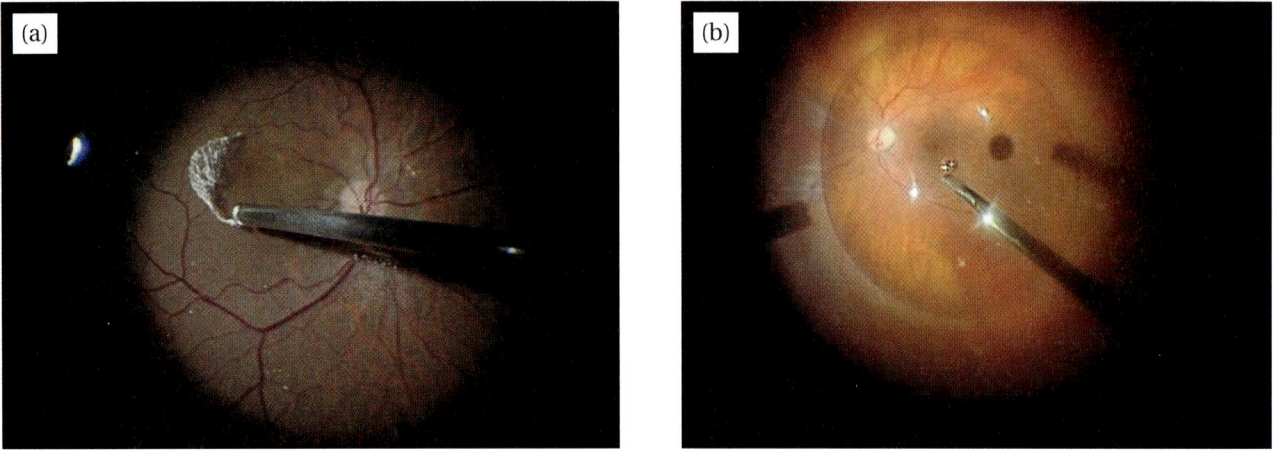

FIGURE 42.3 Endoillumination with a fiberoptic probe is used bimanually with other instruments, and allows illumination of any area of interest (a). Retro, focal, and specular illumination with the endoilluminator allows visualization of clear vitreous. Wide-angle illumination probes (b) make visualization of clear vitreous more difficult but, together with wide-angle visualization systems, are useful for viewing peripheral pathology.

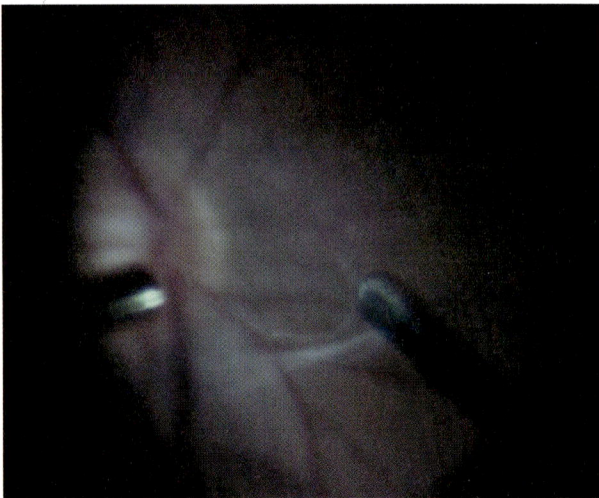

FIGURE 42.4 After a limited core vitrectomy is performed using the vitreous cutter and the endoilluminator, a posterior vitreous detachment (PVD) is induced, using active aspiration by the vitrectomy probe, and a Weiss ring is seen over the optic disc.

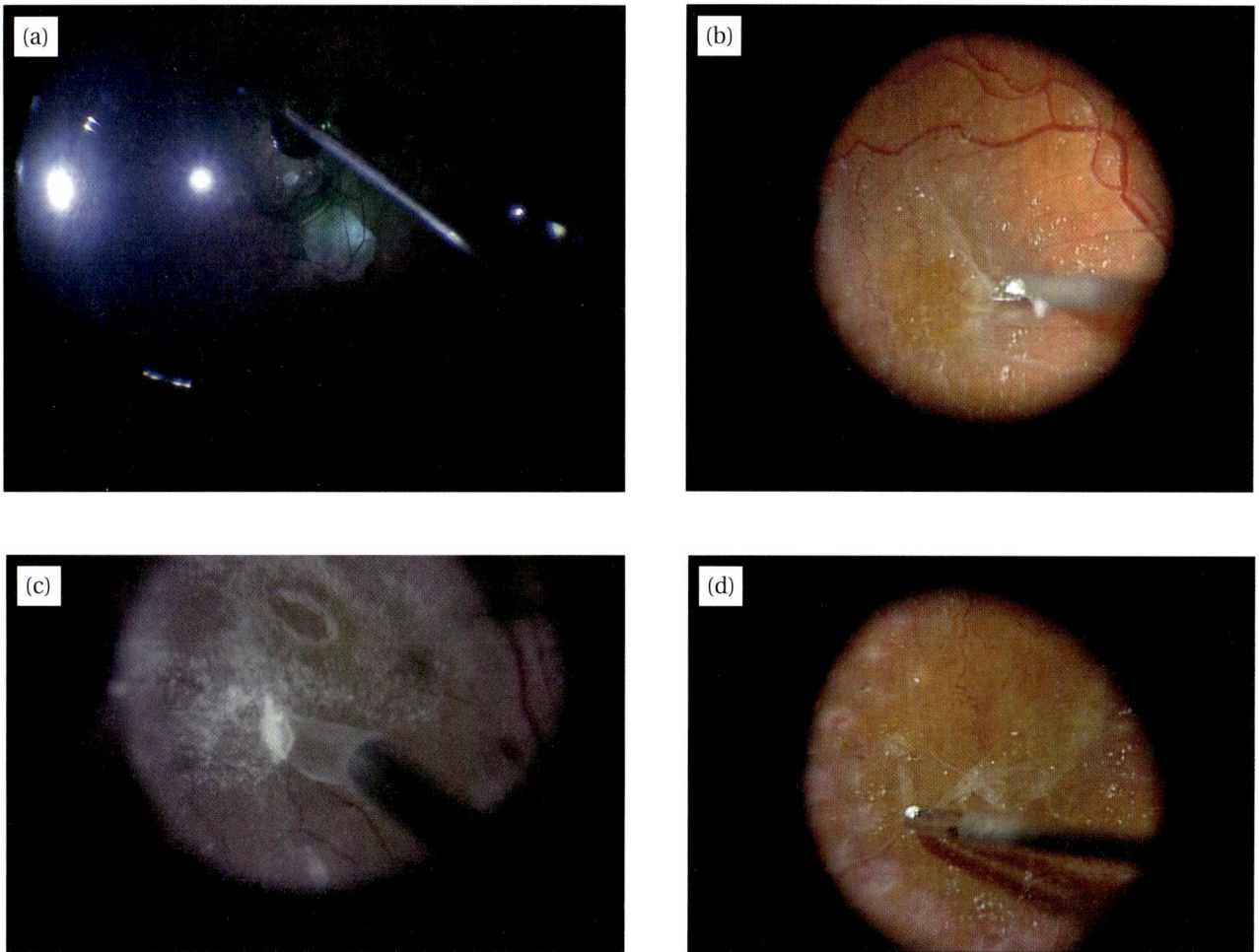

FIGURE 42.5 Epiretinal membrane is removed after a vitrectomy is performed. The membrane may be stained with a dye such as indocyanine green (a) or triamcinolone suspension for better visualization. The peeling may be started by either elevating an edge with a bent needle (b) or diamond-dusted brush (c), or by directly pinching the membrane with end-grasping forceps. Membrane peeling is accomplished by moving the forceps tangentially along the surface of the retina (d). Internal limiting membrane may be peeled in a similar fashion.

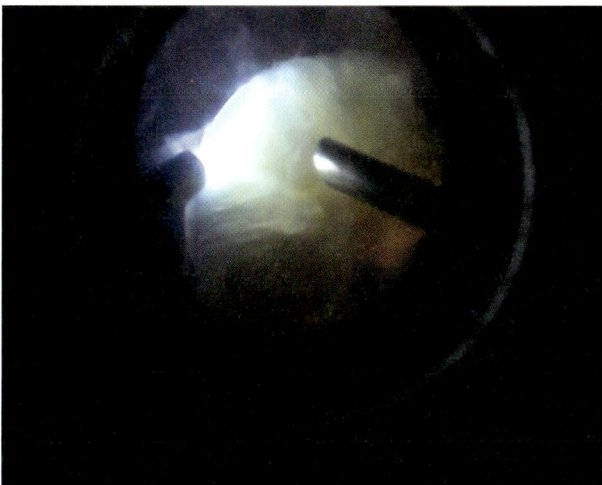

FIGURE 42.6 Lensectomy is performed in combination with pars plana vitrectomy in selected cases of complicated retinal detachment, and in eyes with retained lens fragments after complicated cataract surgery. In primary lensectomy, the lens equator is incised using an MVR blade, and hydrodissection is performed. Lens removal is performed with the phacofragmatome probe, which uses continuous aspiration with sonification. Active aspiration keeps the lens fragment at the tip of the probe while the fragmenter sculpts the nucleus. Epinucleus and cortex may be aspirated with either the fragmenter or the vitreous cutter. If the lens dislocates posteriorly, the endoilluminator may be used to direct and rotate the lens fragments as needed.

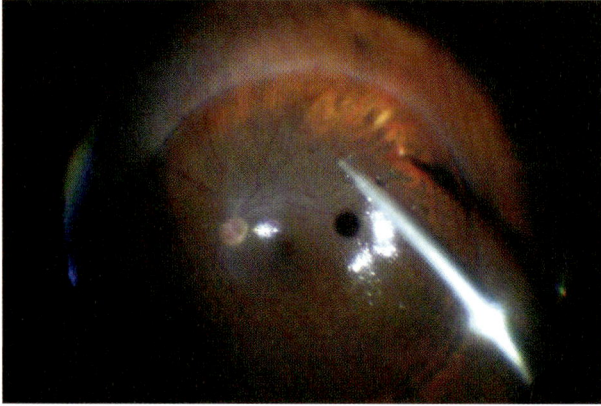

FIGURE 42.7 Retinal detachment repair with perfluorocarbon liquid (PFCL). PFCL is injected over the optic disc to stabilize the macula, and to displace subretinal fluid anteriorly and avoid a posterior drainage retinotomy. In complicated retinal detachments, PFCL can unroll a giant retinal tear, and facilitate dissection of peripheral adherent tractional membranes.

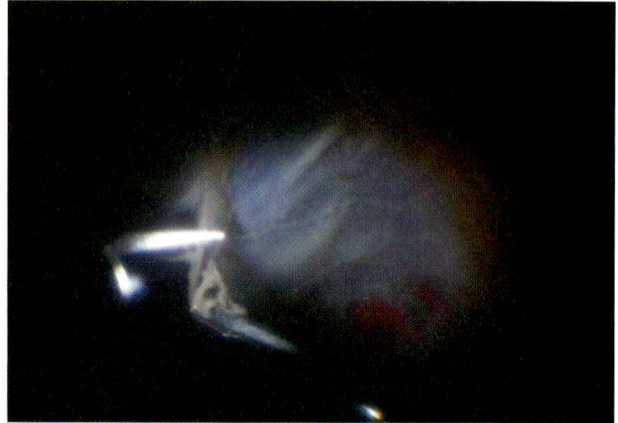

FIGURE 42.8 Adherent proliferative membranes are removed by a bimanual dissection technique using a lighted pick and intraocular forceps. The pick provides countertraction to be placed on the retina, and keeps the retina in the desired position while the forceps is used to peel membranes from the retinal surface.

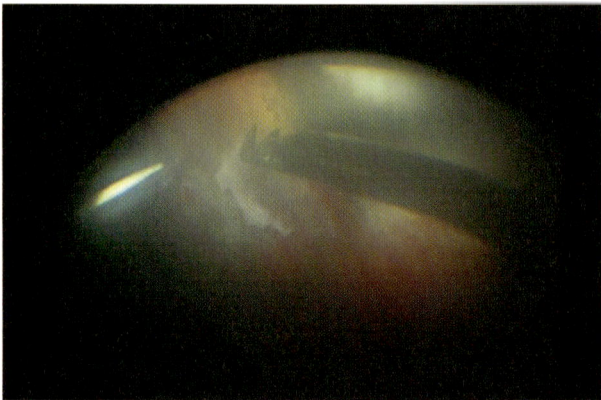

FIGURE 42.9 Removal of fibrovascular membranes is performed by scissor segmentation and delamination. Tractional forces are eliminated by isolating tractional fibrovascular membranes and removing their connections to other areas of traction. Delamination involves separation the fibrovascular tissue from the surface of the retina.

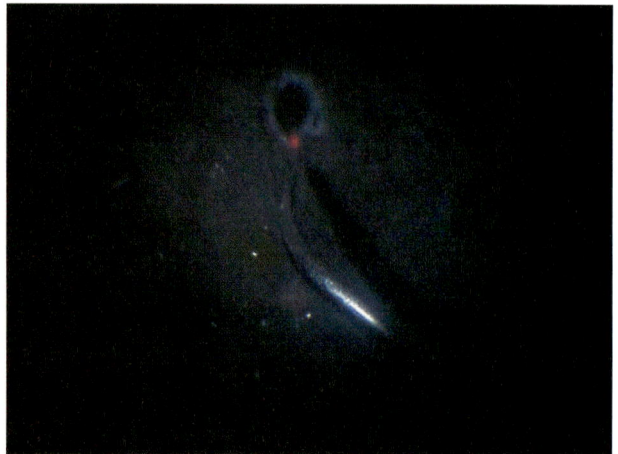

FIGURE 42.10 Endophotocoagulation is used to surround retinal breaks, or to treat retinal vascular occlusive disease with panretinal photocoagulation. Lesion size is dependent on the distance of the tip of the probe from the retinal surface, the beam divergence, and the power setting. After the retina is flattened, laser of retinal breaks is performed by discrete photocoagulation spots in rows, and may be done under fluid, PFCL, air, or silicone oil.

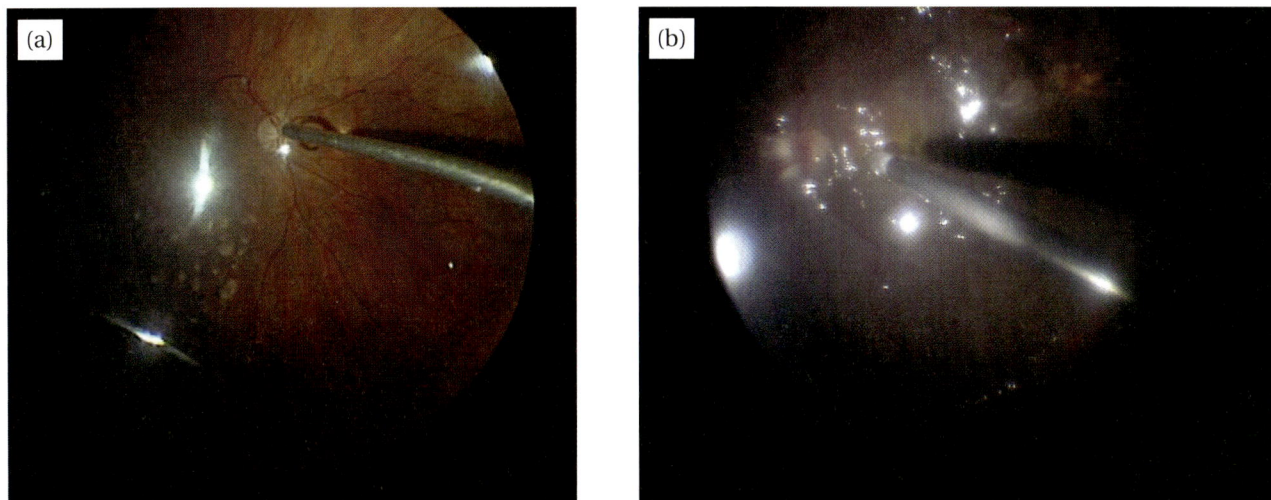

FIGURE 42.11 (a) In air–fluid exchange, air is pumped into the eye through the infusion cannula while fluid is removed passively through a regular or silicone-tipped fluted needle or by active aspiration. Endophotocoagulation of retinal breaks may be performed at this time. The eye is then flushed with a long-acting gas. (b) When long-acting tamponade with silicone oil is indicated, it may be exchanged directly with PFCL.

TABLE 42.2 *Complications of Vitrectomy*

Cataract

Retinal tears

Retinal detachment

Endophthalmitis

Suprachoroidal hemorrhage

Open angle glaucoma

SELECTED REFERENCES

Chalam KV, Shah VA. Optics of wide-angle panoramic viewing system-assisted vitreous surgery. *Surv Ophthalmol.* 2004 Jul–Aug;49(4):437–445.

Chang S, Lincoff HA, Coleman DJ, Fuchs W, Farber ME.Perfluorocarbon gases in vitreous surgery. *Ophthalmology.* 1985 May;92(5):651–656.

Chang S, Reppucci V, Zimmerman NJ, Heinemann MH, Coleman DJ. Perfluorocarbon liquids in the management of traumatic retinal detachments. *Ophthalmology.* 1989 Jun;96(6):785–791;

Chang S. Low viscosity liquid fluorochemicals in vitreous surgery. *Am J Ophthalmol.* 1987 Jan 15;103(1):38–43.

Charles S. Endophotocoagulation. *Retina.* 1981;1(2):117–120.

Eckardt C. Transconjunctival sutureless 23-gauge vitrectomy. *Retina.* 2005 Feb–Mar;25(2):208–211.

Farah ME, Maia M, Rodrigues EB. Dyes in ocular surgery: principles for use in chromovitrectomy. *Am J Ophthalmol.* 2009 Sep;148(3):332–340.

Fujii GY, De Juan E Jr, Humayun MS, Chang TS, Pieramici DJ, Barnes A, Kent D. Initial experience using the transconjunctival sutureless vitrectomy system for vitreoretinal surgery. *Ophthalmology.* 2002 Oct;109(10):1814–1820.

Machemer R, Buettner H, Norton EW, Parel JM. Vitrectomy: A pars plana approach. *Trans Am Acad Ophthalmol Otolaryngol.* 1971 Jul–Aug;75(4):813–820.

McCuen BW 2nd, Bessler M, Hickingbotham D, Isbey E 3rd. Automated fluid-gas exchange. *Am J Ophthalmol.* 1983 May;95(5):717.

Management of Complicated Retinal Detachments

Tamer H. Mahmoud, MD, PhD, Jamin S. Brown, MD, and Gary W. Abrams, MD

Etiology of PVR

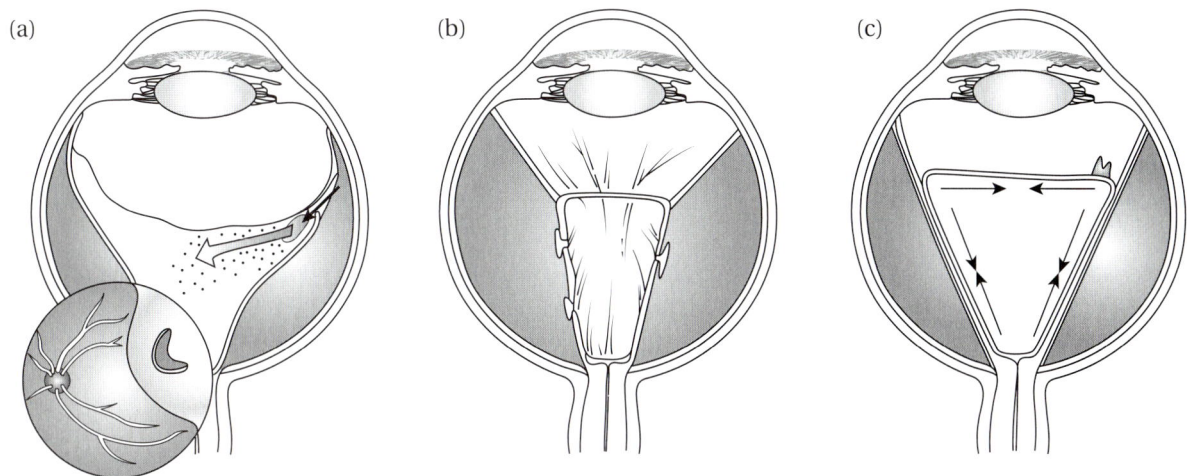

FIGURE 43.1 **Pathogenesis of PVR.** Proliferative vitreoretinopathy (PVR) is the leading cause of failure in retinal detachment surgery. It is characterized by the formation of cellular membranes on retinal surface, undersurface, and vitreous cavity. (a) Migration of pigment epithelial and other cells into vitreous cavity and subretinal space. (b) Proliferation and contraction of cells on retinal and vitreous interfaces. (c) Fixed folds due to contraction of cellular membranes. (Adapted from Abrams GW, Aaberg TM. Posterior segment vitrectomy. In: Waltman SR, ed. *Surgery of the Eye.* New York, NY: Churchill-Livingstone; 1988, pp. 903–1012.)

(a)   (b)

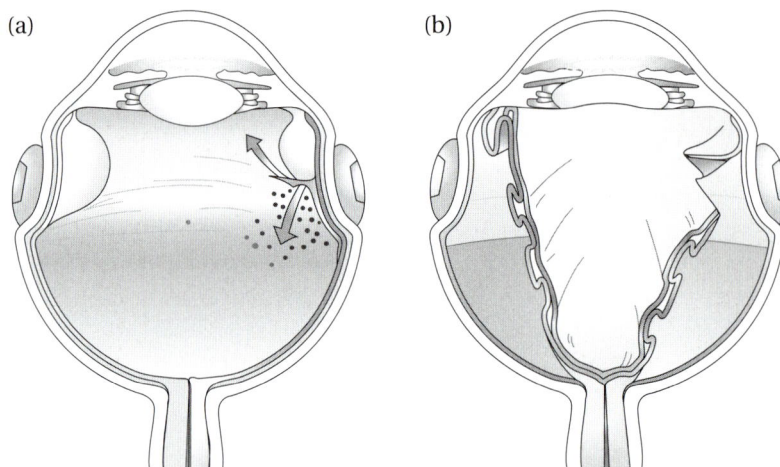

FIGURE 43.2 (a, b) Anterior retinal displacement in PVR occurs when proliferating cells form a membrane on the surface of the peripheral vitreous and contract and pull the peripheral retina anteriorly toward the pars plana.

Clinical Pictures of PVR

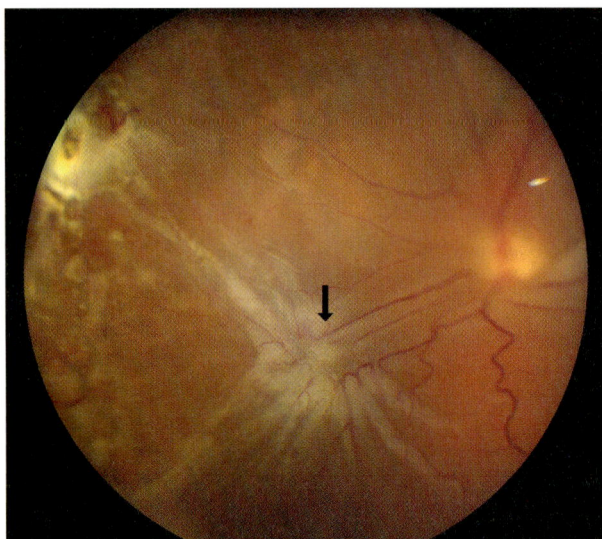

FIGURE 43.3 An example of posterior PVR with diffuse contraction (arrow).

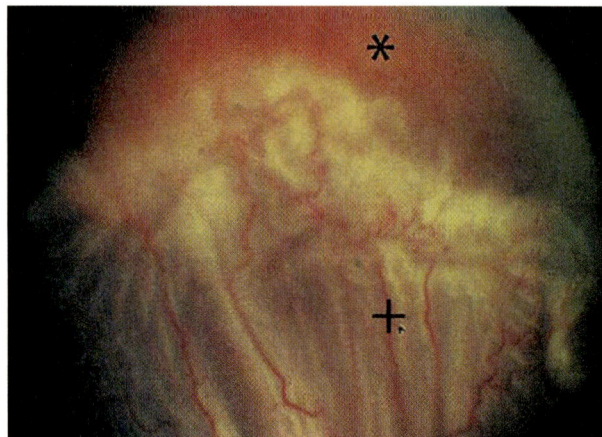

FIGURE 43.4 An example of anterior PV R. Contraction occurs along the posterior edge of the vitreous base with central displacement of retina. Peripheral retina is stretched (*); posterior retina is in radial folds (+). (Reprinted with permission from Machemer R, Aaberg TM, Freeman HM, et al. An updated classification of retinal detachment with proliferative vitreoretinopathy. *Am J Ophthalmol.* 1991;112:159–165.)

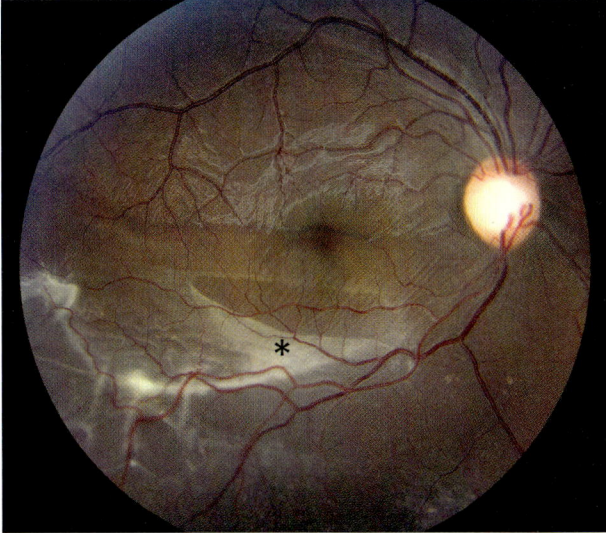

FIGURE 43.5 An example of subretinal PVR (*) in a case of chronic long-term retinal detachment.

Steps in Repairing Complicated Retinal Detachments

TABLE 43.2 *Steps in Repairing Complicated Retinal Detachments*

Shaving the vitreous base

Remove epiretinal membranes (posterior first and then anterior)

Flatten retina (PFCL, air)

Decision: remove subretinal membranes, relaxing retinectomy

Create long-term chorioretinal adhesion (endolaser)

Provide long-term tamponade while chorioretinal adhesions form (gas vs. silicone oil)

Shaving the Vitreous Base

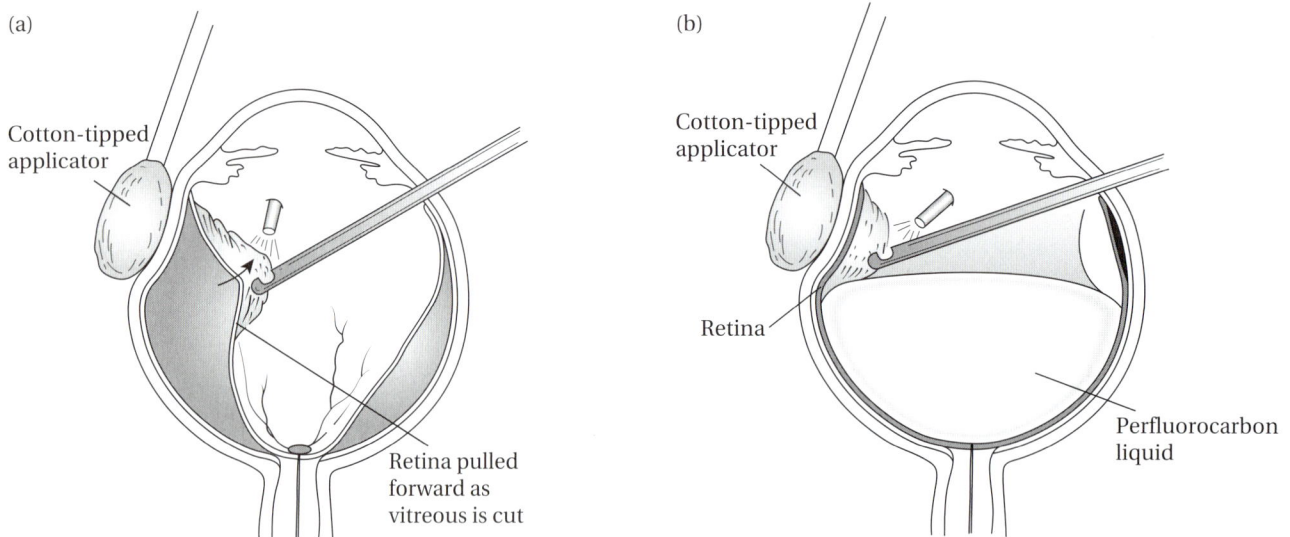

FIGURE 43.6 Perfluorocarbon liquid (PFCL) can be used to stabilize mobile retina during removal of anterior vitreous or anterior membranes. (a) In this eye with a bullous retinal detachment, the mobile retina is drawn toward the vitreous-cutting instrument, risking anterior retinal breaks. (b) Liquid PFCL is injected to flatten and stabilize the posterior retina and facilitate anterior vitrectomy.

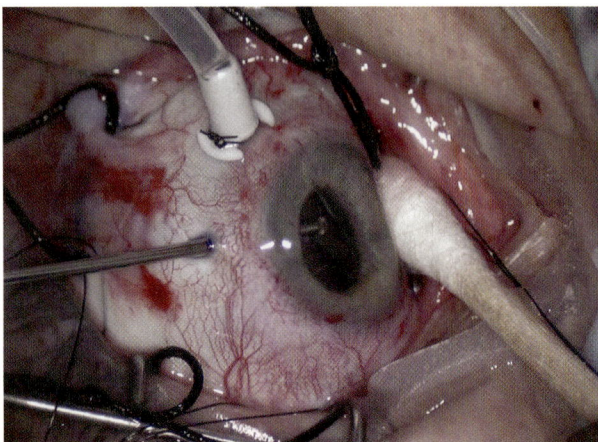

FIGURE 43.7 Scleral depression can be used to assist in visualization and stabilization of the peripheral retina during anterior vitreous and/or membrane removal.

Remove Epiretinal Membranes

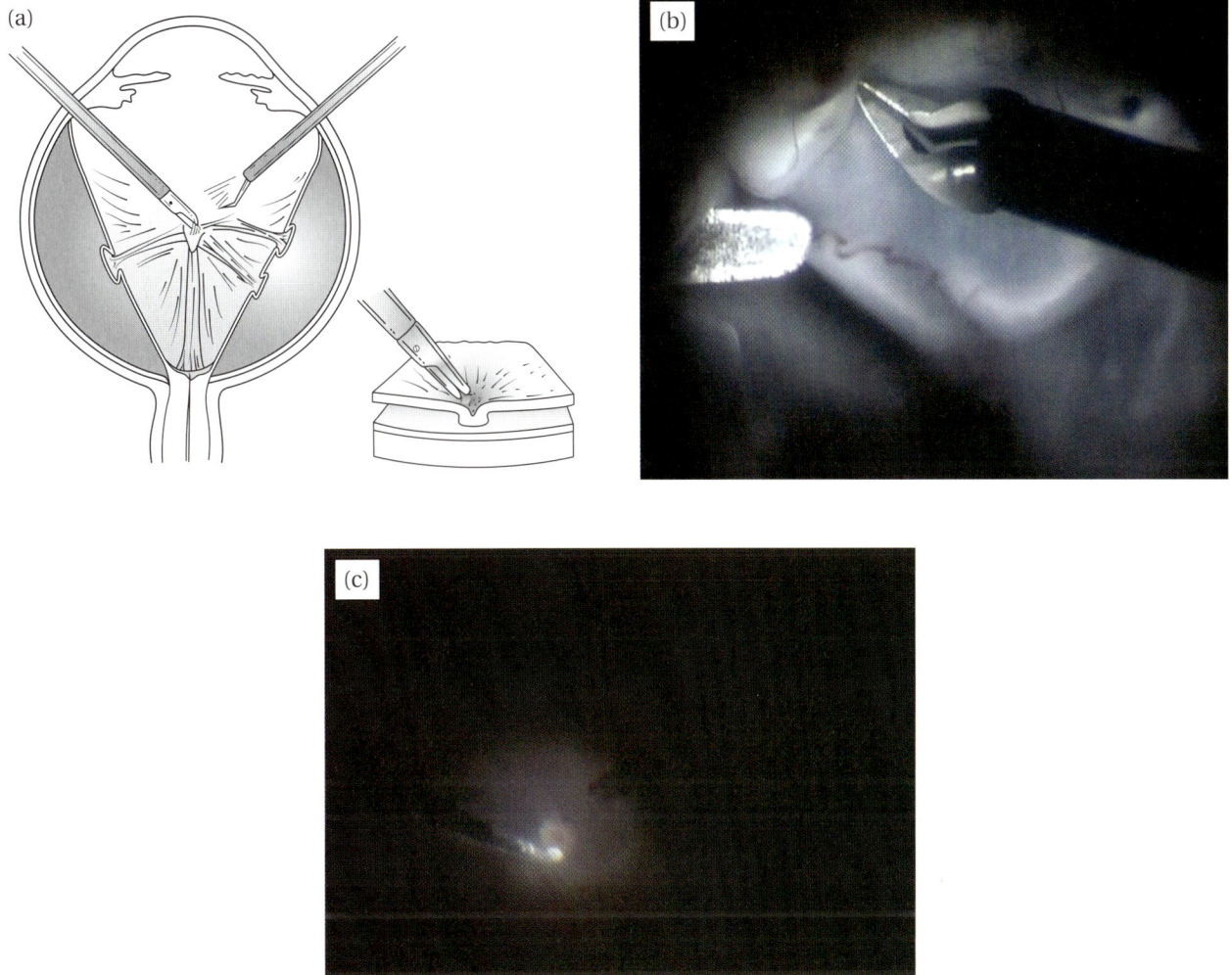

FIGURE 43.8 (a) Thick membranes with prominent edges may be engaged with end-grasping forceps. Once grasped, the membranes may be peeled, while an illuminated pick is used to apply countertraction on the retina. The shaft of the illuminated pick is bent 30° from the light axis to give broader illumination and reduce shadows cast by the pick. (b) Intraocular image of bent illuminated pick applying countertraction while a forceps is used to engage a membrane. (c) A diamond dusted membrane scraper may be used to help find membranes and create an edge initially prior to the bimanual peel. Alternatively, an illuminated pick or a sharp pick might be used to engage the membrane and vertical forceps used to remove it. Two forceps along with chandelier illumination or a lighted infusion can be used to identify, engage, and remove membranes. We prefer 20-gauge instrumentation because of the large number of available instruments, but newer generation 23- and 25-gauge can achieve similar outcomes.

(a)

Vitreous

Retina

(b)

Vitreous

Retina

(c)

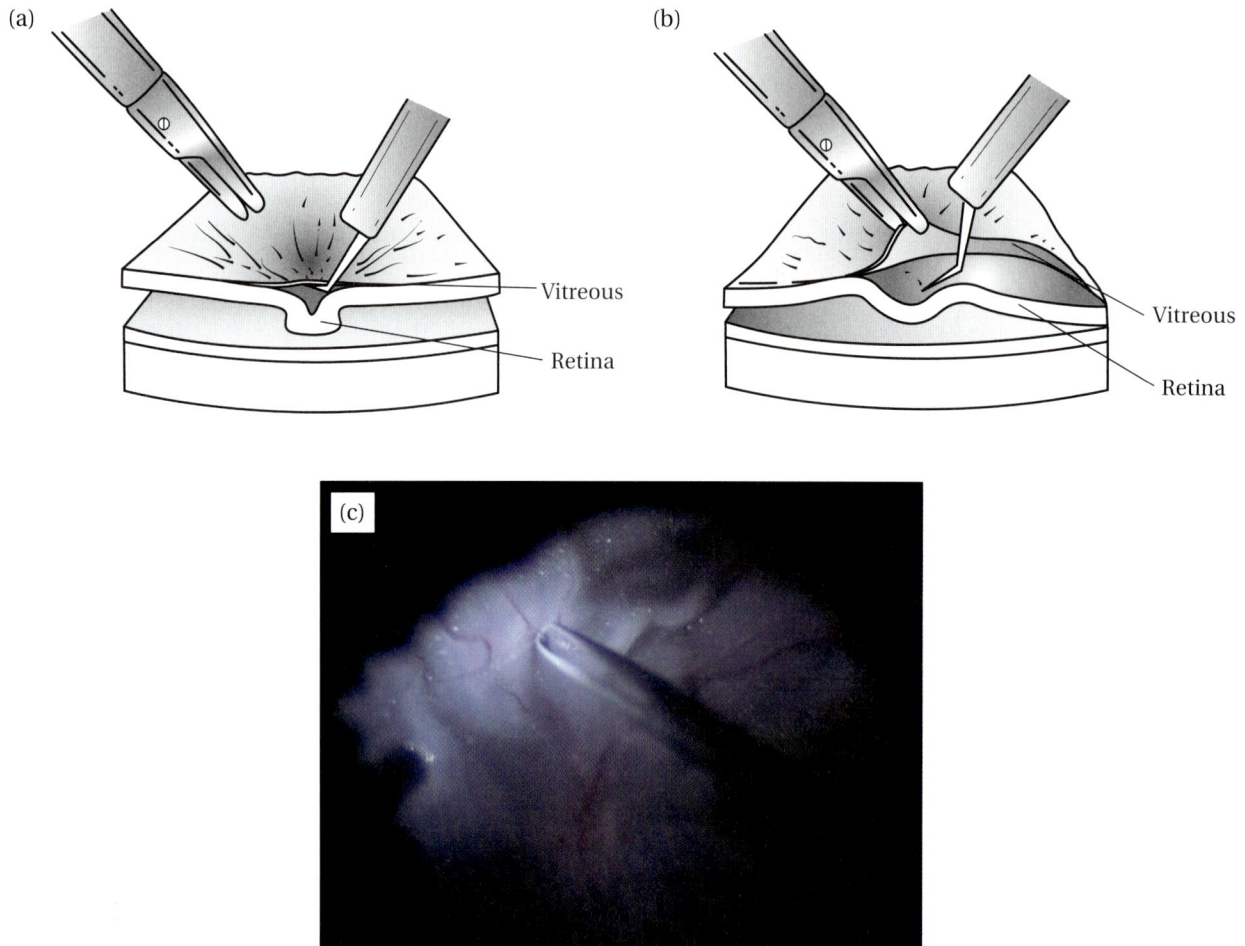

FIGURE 43.9 Broad, thin membranes may cross and obscure a retinal fold. (a) Such membranes may be elevated by passing a pick into a fold or by using a Tano brush and gently pulling the membrane toward the center of the fold. (b) The engaged membrane may then be grasped with forceps and peeled, while the pick is then used to hold back the retina during membrane peeling. (c) Intraocular image of end-grasping forceps peeling a broad thin membrane (note that dilute triamcinolone acetate has been used to "stain" the vitreous to assist with membrane removal). Alternatively, trypan blue may be used as a membrane stain.

(a)

Vessel tortuous
under membrane

Stripping in
fold with MVR
blade

Retinal
vessels

Epiretinal
membrane

Retina

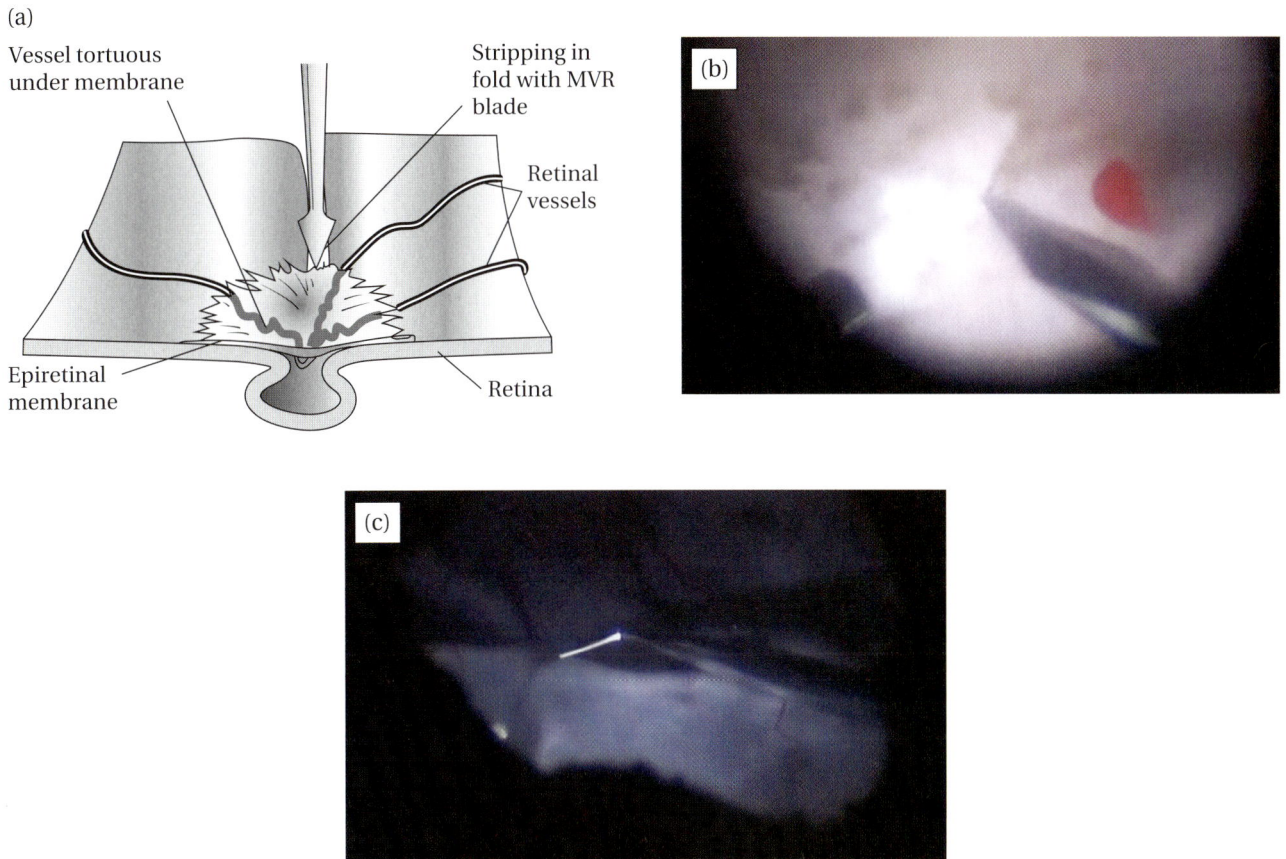

FIGURE 43.10 (a) Thin, "tight" membranes may be difficult to engage with the blunt illuminated pick, so these membranes are sometimes best engaged for peeling with a sharp pick. A barbed microvitreoretinal (MVR) blade is placed in a fold adjacent to the membrane and gently passed beneath the membrane edge. (b) Here, a barbed MVR is used to elevate a "tight" membrane from the surface of the retina. (c) In a similar fashion to the MVR blade, a small pick may be used to elevate a "tight" membrane as shown here.

(a)

(b)   Extraction of
subretinal strand
through retinotomy

Subretinal
strand

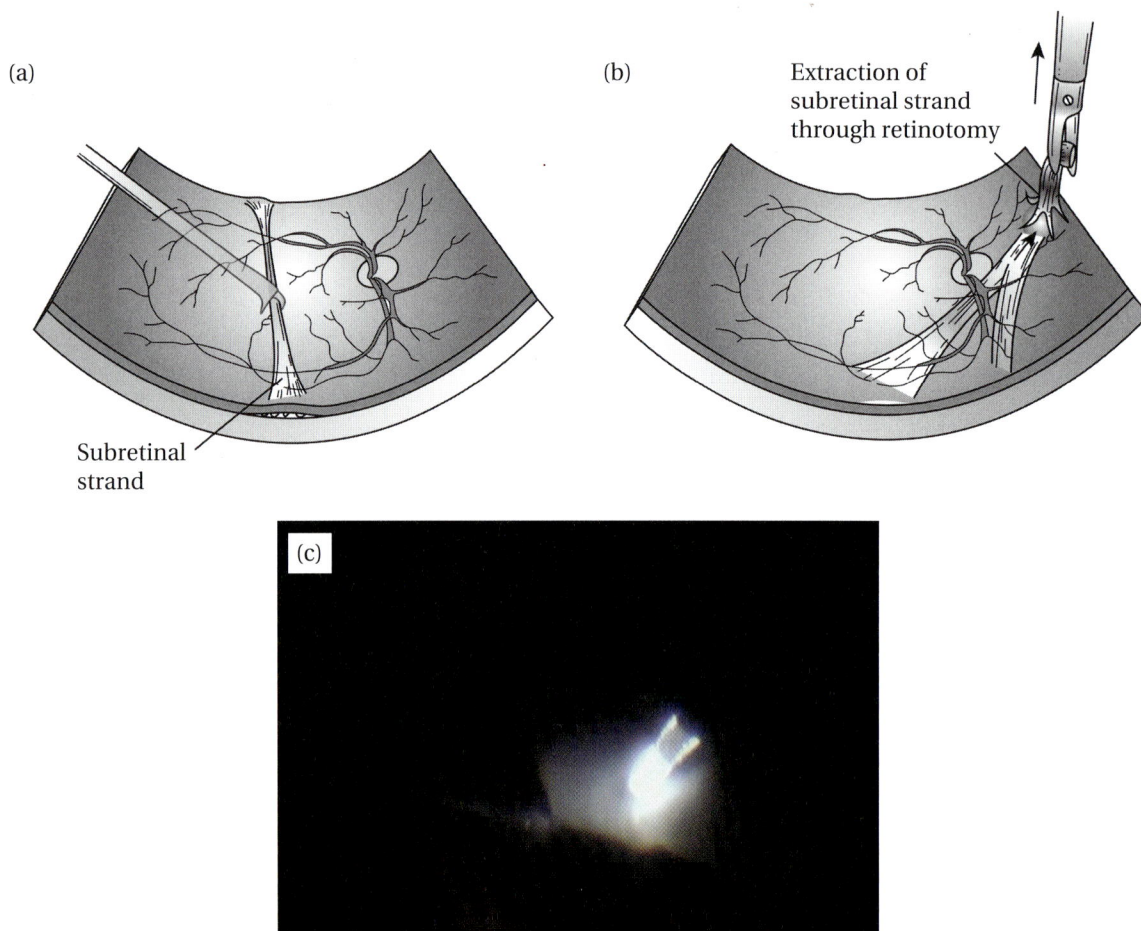

(c)

FIGURE 43.11 Eyes with severe PVR may develop subretinal membranes, preventing reattachment due to taut subretinal traction. The following alternatives are used to relieve traction. (a) Sectioning of the subretinal strand with scissors placed through a retinotomy. If the membrane is not adherent to the retina or choroid, the membranes will retract after sectioning. (b) Extraction of the strand through a retinotomy with intraocular forceps. (c) Removing the strands from the under surface of the retina following the creation of a large relaxing retinotomy, as shown in the photo (Adapted from Abrams GW. Retinotomies and retinectomies. In: Ryan SJ, ed. *Retina*. Vol. 3. St Louis, MO: Mosby; 1989, pp. 317–346.)

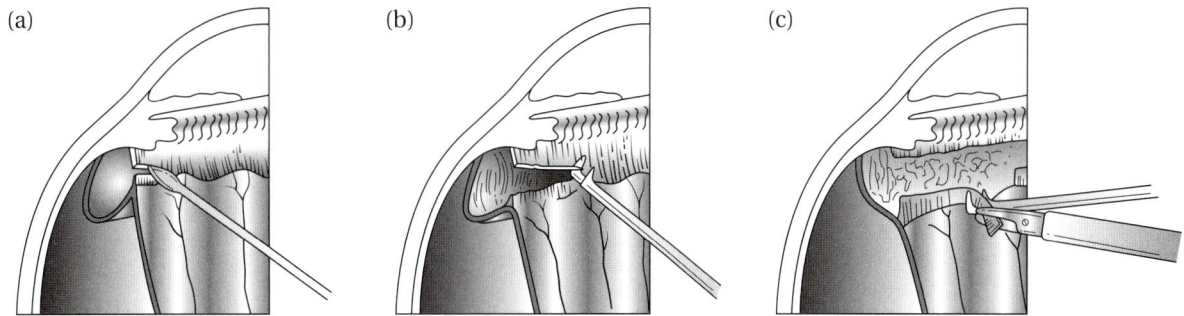

FIGURE 43.12 Management of anterior retinal displacement in PVR. A circumferential membrane has formed on the peripheral vitreous and, with contraction, has pulled the retina at the posterior aspect of the vitreous base anteriorly to the anterior pars plana. The membrane obscures a "trough" of redundant retina created by the anterior displacement of the retina. (a) The membrane is sectioned circumferentially with a microvitreoretinal blade. (b) Once an opening is made in the membrane with the blade, vertically-cutting vitreoretinal scissors are used to section the membrane throughout its extent. (c) The trough has opened up, and the retina has relaxed posteriorly. If a circumferential membrane remains on the posterior aspect of the vitreous base, it should be removed or radially sectioned.

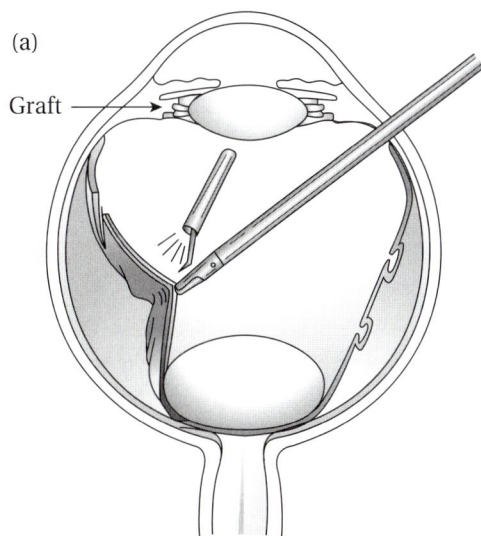

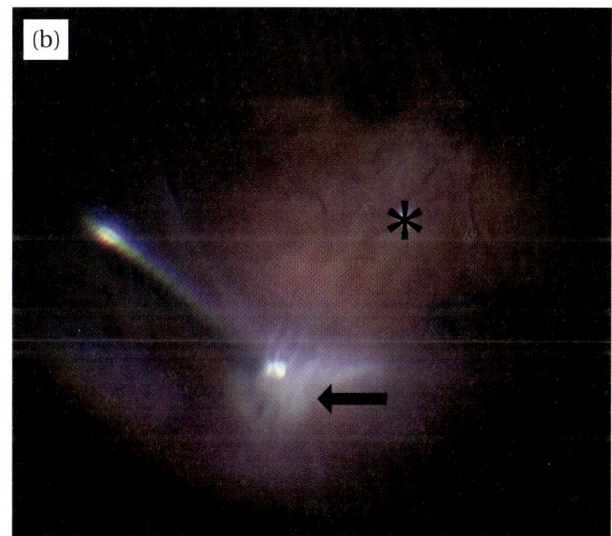

FIGURE 43.13 (a) Following removal of posterior membranes, a small volume of PFC is injected over the posterior retina. The liquid acts as an additional surgical device in the eye by providing retinal stability during removal of peripheral membranes. (b) Removal of this membrane (arrow) is assisted by the retinal stability provided through the use of PFC over the posterior pole (*).

Flattening the Retinal Detachment

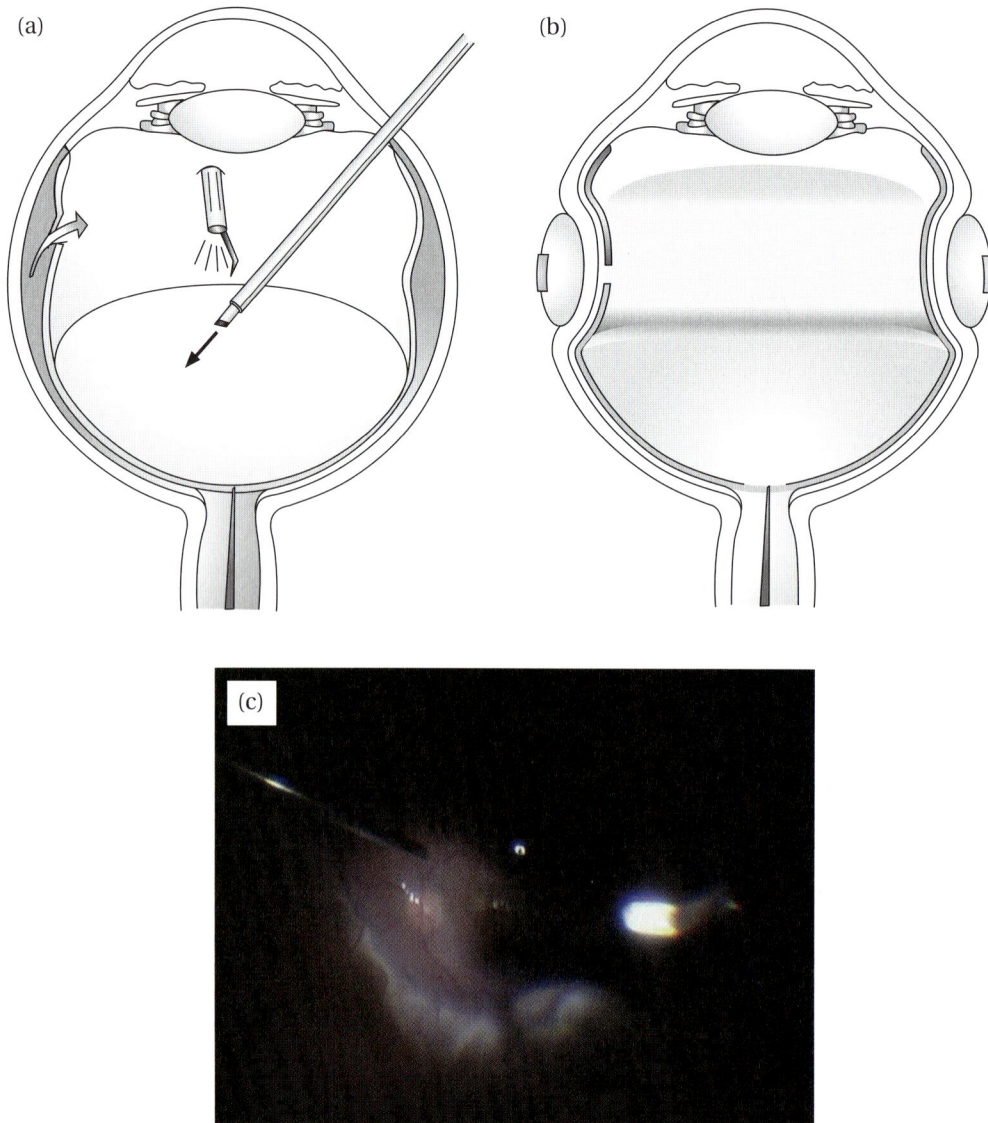

FIGURE 43.14 After all membranes have been removed, the retina can be reattached by injecting PFCL. (a) In this case, subretinal fluid drains into the vitreous cavity from an anterior retinal break. If there is no anterior retinal break, an anterior retinotomy must be created. (b) More PFCL has been injected to reattach the retina. An encircling scleral buckle has been placed to support the vitreous base and decrease traction on the retinal tear. If an encircling scleral buckle is already present, revision or replacement is rarely done. However, if no scleral buckle is present, placement of a #42 band as the buckling element is recommended because it has less overall volume in comparison to a tire or sponge. The scleral buckle can be placed prior to the vitrectomy, but tightening the buckle should wait until the retina is flattened by PFCL. (c) PFCL is being injected over the posterior pole to flatten the retina.

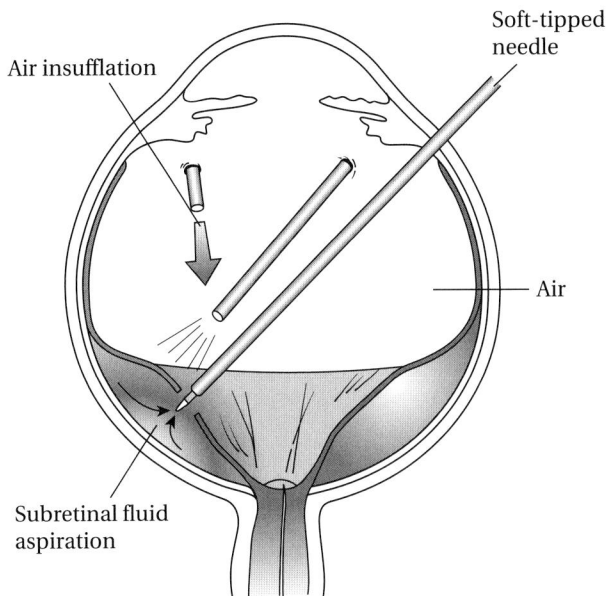

FIGURE 43.15 Flattening the retina through a posterior retinal break. While PFCL is a useful adjunct for stabilization of bullous retina during membrane removal or flattening giant retinal tears, fluid–air exchange may be used for many cases to reattach the retina after vitrectomy. If there is an existing posterior break, subretinal fluid is aspirated through the retinal break as the eye is simultaneously filled by the air pump. However, because of the complications of posterior retinotomies, creation of a posterior retinotomy to facilitate reattachment of the retina with fluid–air exchange should be avoided if possible. (Adapted from Abrams GW. Retinotomies and retinectomies. In: Ryan SJ, ed. *Retina.* Vol 3. St Louis, MO: Mosby; 1989, pp. 317–346.)

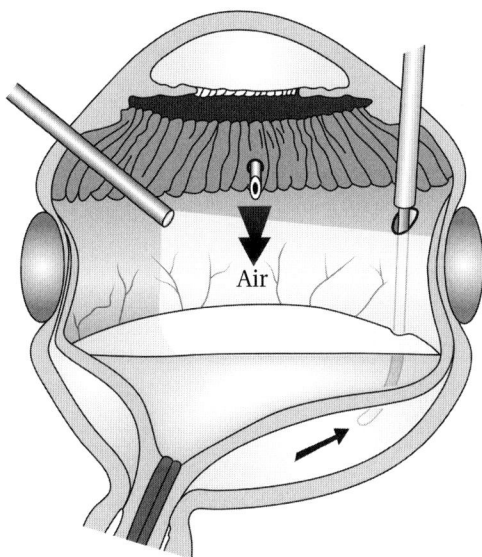

FIGURE 43.16 As an alternative to using PFCL to reattach the retina, fluid–air exchange can be done using a peripheral retinal break. An existing retinal break or a drainage retinotomy is created anteriorly over the scleral buckle. The extendable soft silicone tubing of the Cannulated Extrusion Needle (Alcon, Ft Worth, TX) is passed through the retinotomy into the posterior subretinal space for fluid–air exchange. (Adapted from Abrams GW, Glazer LC. Proliferative Vitreoretinopathy. In: Freeman WR, ed. *Practical Atlas of Retinal Disease and Therapy.* 2nd ed. Philadelphia, PA: Lippincott-Raven; 1997, pp. 303–323.)

Decision for Relaxing Retinectomy

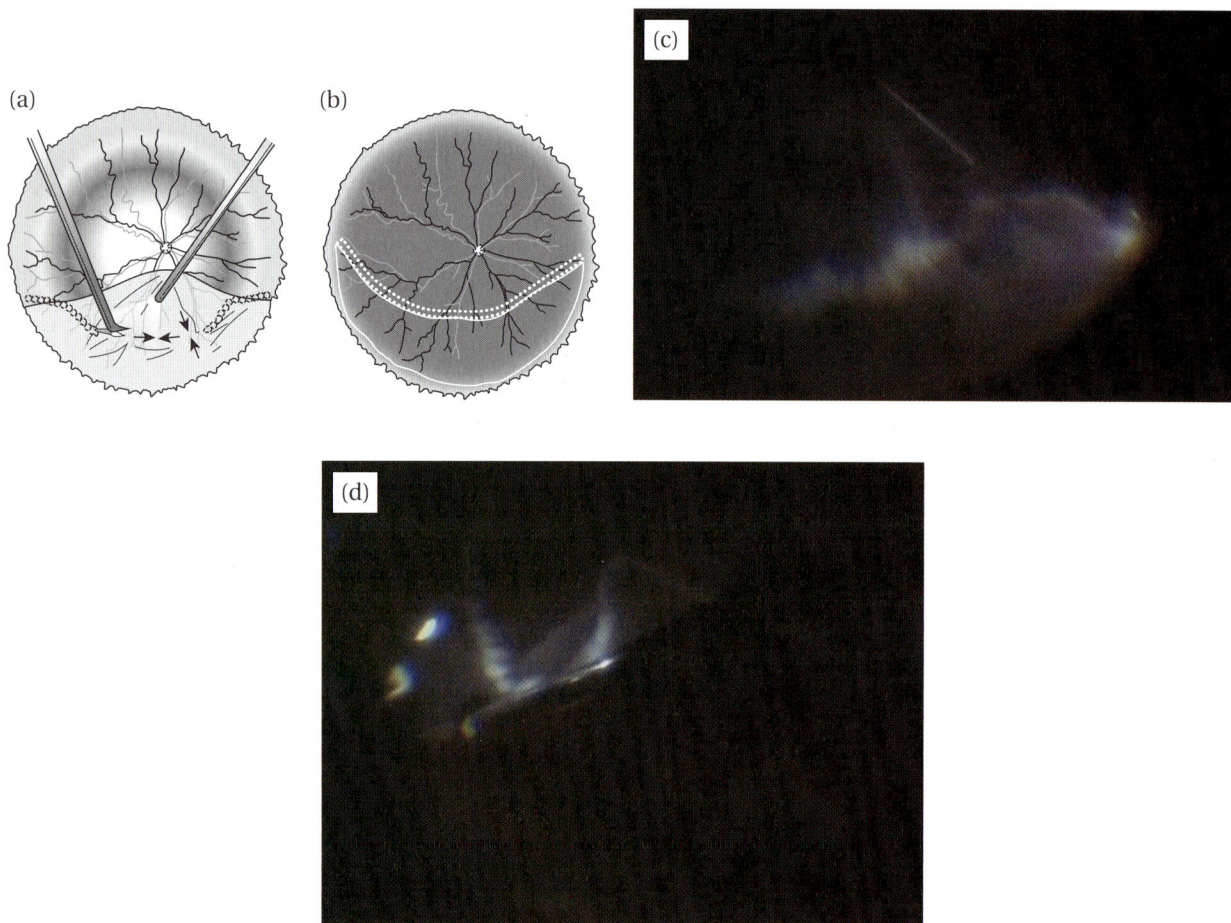

FIGURE 43.17 (a) Some eyes with severe anterior PVR may develop retinal shortening that makes reattachment impossible, in spite of removal of membranes. In such cases, a relaxing retinotomy with retinectomy is necessary. PFCL is placed over the posterior pole, then diathermy is applied to the retina to be cut, extending into normal retina on each end of contracted retina. Retinal blood vessels in particular should be well treated with diathermy before cutting. Vertically cutting scissors or the vitrectomy cutter is used to cut along the posterior edge of contracted retina at and anterior to the line of diathermy. (b) Retina is reattached with PFCL following relaxing retinotomy. Retinotomy is extended anteriorly to ora serrata or pars plana (if involved). (c) Diathermy applied to area of planned retinotomy to minimize bleeding during the retinotomy. (d) The anterior retina is excised using the vitrectomy cutter. (Adapted from Abrams GW. Retinotomies and retinectomies. In: Ryan SJ, ed. *Retina*. Vol. 3. St Louis, MO: Mosby; 1989, pp. 317–346.)

Creating Long-term Chorioretinal Adhesions

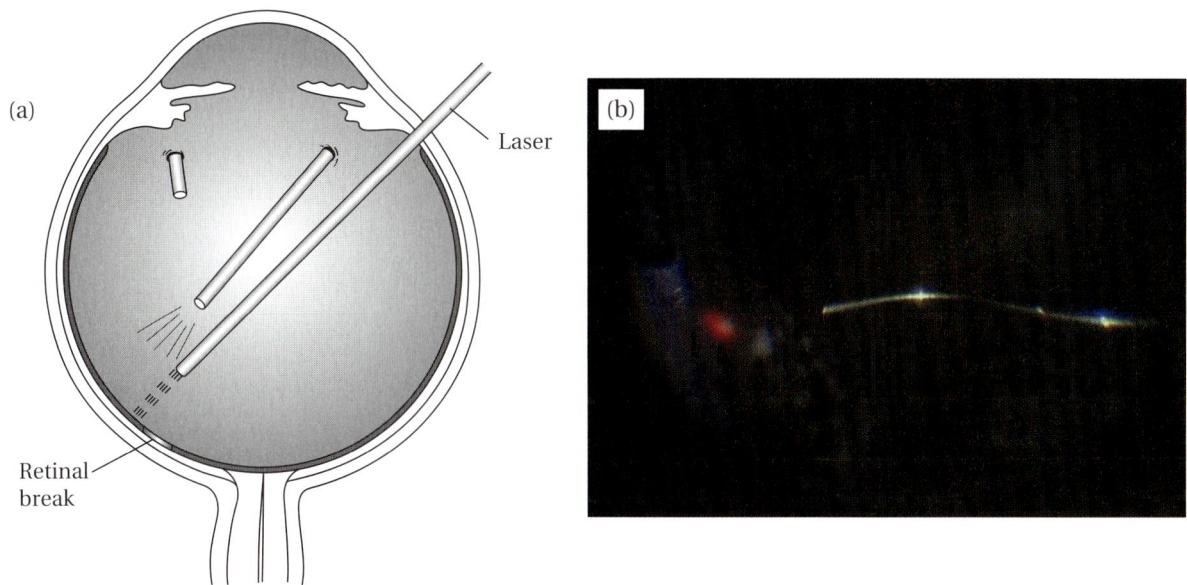

FIGURE 43.18 (a) After reattachment of the retina under PFCL or air, 2 or 3 rows of confluent laser endophotocoagulation is applied around the retinal breaks and along the posterior margin of a retinectomy. We apply scatter laser treatment (usually one burn width between laser burns) over the entire surface of any buckled retina. (b) Laser being applied to the surface of buckled retina under PFCL using the curved endolaser probe. The curved probe has the advantage of reaching the anterior retina near the ora settata, especially in phakic patients. (Adapted from Abrams GW. Retinotomies and retinectomies. In: Ryan SJ, ed. *Retina*. Vol. 3. St Louis, MO: Mosby; 1989, pp. 317–346.)

Providing Long-term Retinal Tamponade

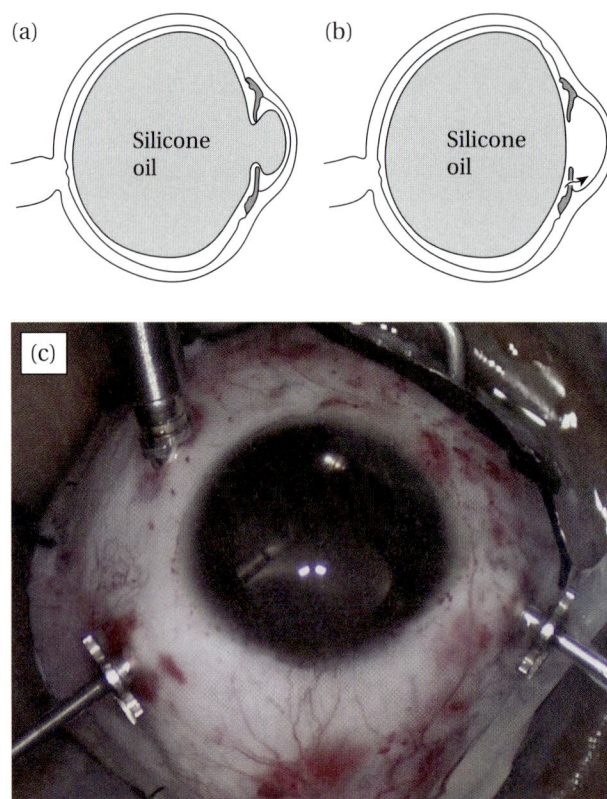

FIGURE 43.19   Once the retina is attached and endolaser photocoagulation has been applied, long-term tamponade must be used to maximize a successful outcome. The two main choices are C3F8 gas or silicone oil. C3F8 gas may have an overall better chance of success in eyes undergoing their first operation for PVR. Silicone oil may be the preferred long-term tamponade in patients who cannot maintain a prone position, cases with large retinectomies, cases with high risk of postoperative hypotony, and cases that have had multiple operations for PVR. In aphakic eyes, an inferior iridectomy is required (make iridectomy prior to fluid–air exchange). (a) Without inferior iridectomy, silicone oil may herniate into the anterior chamber, causing pupillary block and elevated intraocular pressure. (b) Inferior iridectomy allows access of aqueous into the anterior chamber, relieving pupillary block so that aqueous no longer forces silicone oil into the anterior chamber. (c) Creation of an interior PI with the vitreous cutter; iris stretched by forceps in an aphakic patient. Silicone oil can be injected after a fluid–air exchange, or via a direct perfluorocarbon–silicone oil exchange using a flute needle. A high-viscosity infusion line needs to be used to withstand the silicone oil injection in the latter situation. (Adapted from Abrams GW, Glazer LC. Proliferative vitreoretinopathy. In: Freeman WR, ed. *Practical Atlas of Retinal Disease and Therapy.* 2nd ed. Philadelphia, PA: Lippincott-Raven; 1997, pp. 303–323.)

Nondiabetic Traction Retinal Detachment

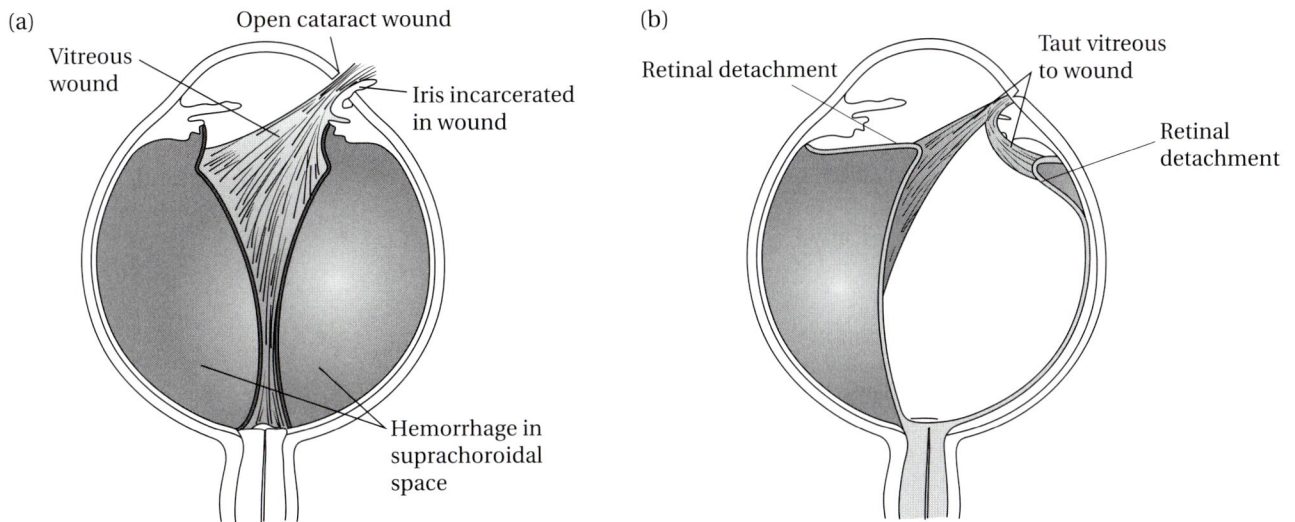

FIGURE 43.20 Complex traction retinal detachments may occur following intraoperative choroidal hemorrhage or trauma. (a) An eye with an intraoperative choroidal hemorrhage during cataract surgery. The mass effect of the choroidal hemorrhage displaces vitreous into the open cataract wound. (b) With resolution of the choroidal hemorrhage, the band of incarcerated vitreous applies tractional force to the retina, leading to traction retinal detachment. Vitrectomy can be particularly difficult in these eyes because the pars plana is often detached, and it may be difficult to place the infusion port properly into the vitreous cavity and retinal breaks may occur at the sclerotomy sites. It may be useful to enter the eye through a limbal approach and a limbal infusion. After the vitreous is released from the wound, then it is usually possible to safely place the infusion port and instruments through the pars plana.

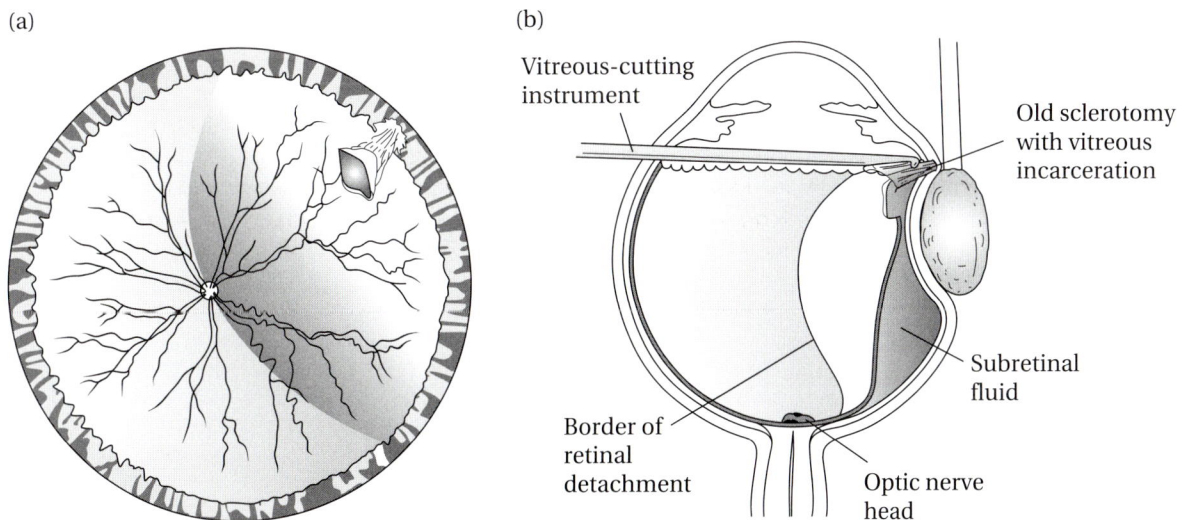

FIGURE 43.21 Vitreous incarceration in a sclerotomy wound after pars plana vitrectomy may lead to a retinal detachment. (a) Vitreous streams from the sclerotomy site in the pars plana to the vitreous base, producing peripheral traction on the retina, with a resultant retinal break formation and a traction/rhegmatogenous retinal detachment. (b) Release of vitreous traction with vitrectomy.

(a)　　　　　　　　　　　(b)

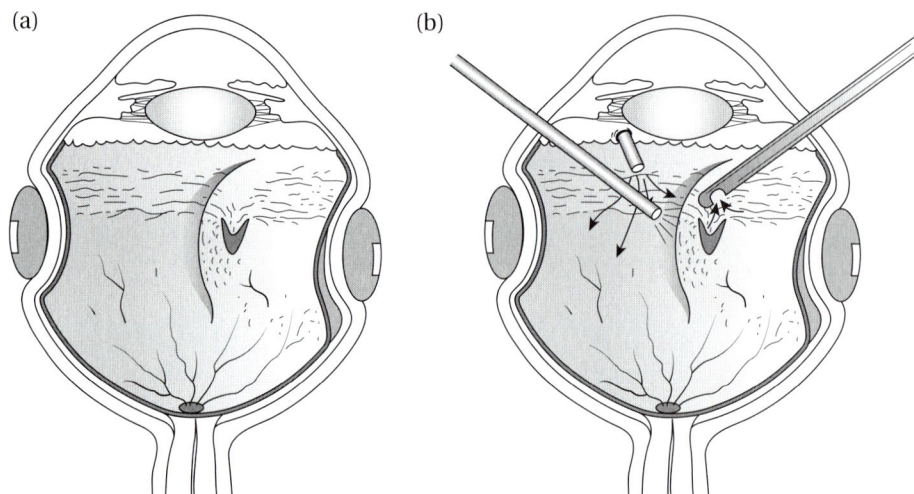

FIGURE 43.22 Recurrent rhegmatogenous retinal detachment may occur after scleral buckling surgery due to persistent vitreous traction on the retinal tear. (a) A band of vitreous elevates the inferior retinal break, causing the subretinal fluid overlying the buckle and extending posteriorly to involve the macula. (b) Release of vitreous traction with vitrectomy allows the retina to reattach.

TABLE 43.3 *Potential Complications in Repairing Complicated Retinal Detachments*

Cataract

Recurrent rhegmatogenous retinal detachment/ Proliferative vitreoretinopathy

Complications of intraocular gas or silicone oil

Keratopathy

Increased intraocular pressure/Hypotony

SELECTED REFERENCES

Abrams GW, Glazer LC. Proliferative vitreoretinopathy. In: Freeman WR, ed. *Practical Atlas of Retinal Disease and Therapy.* 2nd ed. Philadelphia, PA: Lippincott-Raven; 1997, pp. 303–323.

Abrams GW. Retinotomies and retinectomies. In: Ryan SJ, ed. *Retina.* Vol. 3. St Louis, MO: Mosby; 2006, pp. 2312–2343.

Lewis JM, Abrams GW, Werner JC. Management of Complicated Retinal Detachment. In: Albert DM, ed. *Ophthalmic Surgery: Principles and Practice.* Malden, MA: Blackwell Science; 1999, pp. 531–566.

44 Adjuncts to Vitreoretinal Surgery

Janet R. Sparrow, PhD, Stanley Chang, MD, and Jay S. Duker, MD

TABLE 44.1   *Indications for Adjuncts to Vitreous Surgery*

a. Perfluorocarbon liquid

    (i)   Giant retinal tear

    (ii)   Proliferative vitreoretinopathy without posterior break

    (iii) Dislocated lens material

    (iv)   Dislocated intraocular lens

    (v)   Choroidal hemorrhage

b. Silicone oil

    (i)   Recurrent retinal detachment

    (ii)   Proliferative vitreoretinopathy

    (iii) Retinal detachment associated with viral retinitis

    (iv)   Retinal detachment with multiple, posterior breaks

    (v)   Recurrent diabetic vitreous hemorrhage

    (vi)   Retinal tamponade in patients who must fly or cannot position

c. Intraocular gas

    (i)   Retinal break

    (ii)   Macular hole

Perfluorocarbon Liquid

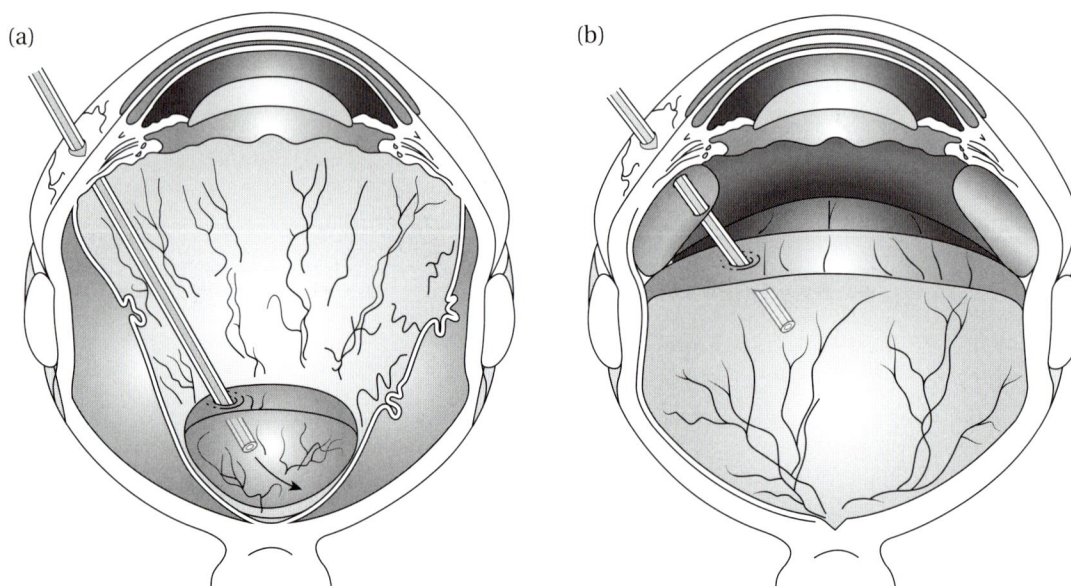

FIGURE 44.1   Perfluorocarbon liquid density is almost twice that of water. This high density makes it especially useful to manipulate the retina during vitrectomy. The PFC liquid is useful in the management of complicated retinal detachment with PVR. (a) The PFC liquid is used to open the funnel of the detachment and flatten the retina. (b) As epiretinal membranes are removed in a posterior-to-anterior direction, additional PFC liquid can be injected with the tip of the cannula positioned within the liquid.

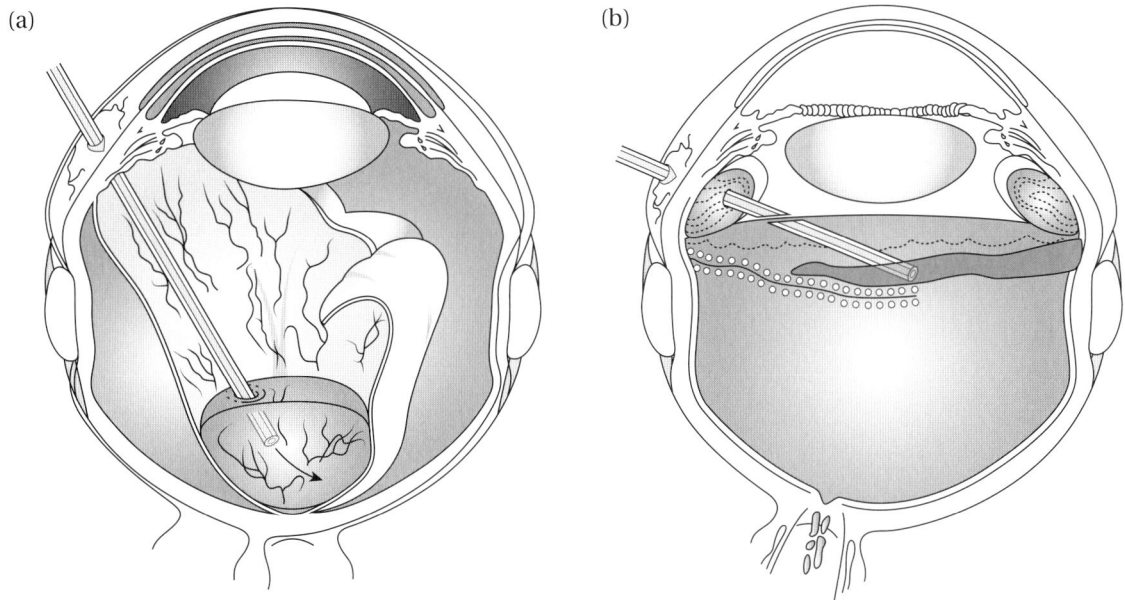

FIGURE 44.2 Perfluorocarbon liquid has proved invaluable in the management of giant retinal tears. (a) The PFC liquid may be used to manipulate and unfold a retinal tear and stabilize the retina during membrane dissection. (b) The PFC liquid remains stable when exposed to argon laser and does not absorb radiation at wavelengths used for photocoagulation. The PFC supports the repositioned retina while endophotocoagulation is applied through the liquid.

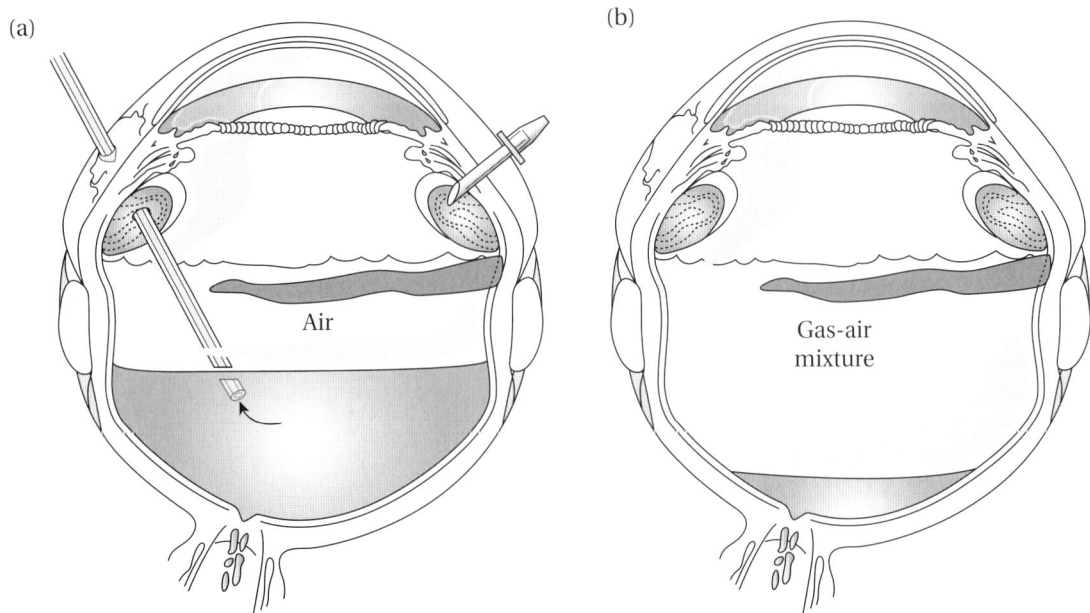

FIGURE 44.3 (a) When PFC gas is to be used for postoperative tamponade, the PFC liquid is removed by fluid–air exchange. Aspiration of PFC liquid is started anteriorly as air enters through the infusion line. (b) After complete removal of the PFC liquid, a gas–air mixture is substituted for the air.

Intraocular Gas

TABLE 44.2 *Features of Some Intraocular Gases Used in Vitreoretinal Surgery*

	Expansion	Nonexpanding Concentration, %	Minimally Expanding Concentration, %
Sulfur hexafluoride	1.9–2.0	18	20–25
Perfluoromethane	1.9	—	—
Perfluoroethane	3.3	16	20
Perfluoropropane	4	12	17

Silicone Oil

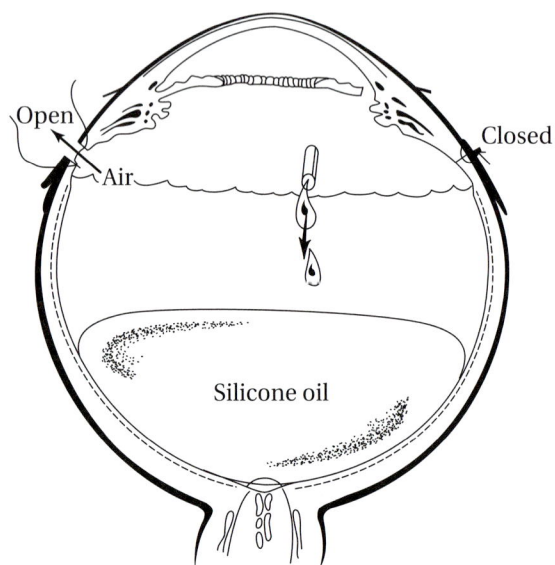

FIGURE 44.4 Silicone oil is most frequently indicated when long-term support and tamponade are needed in cases complicated by PVR, giant retinal tears, retinal detachment due to proliferative diabetic retinopathy, or ocular trauma. It also may be used in primary surgeries when patients are unable to comply with postoperative positioning, or air travel is necessary. Silicone oil is infused into the air-filled eye through the infusion line or a superior sclerotomy, as air is vented through a second sclerotomy.

TABLE 44.3 *Complications of Adjuncts to Vitreoretinal Surgery*

I.   Perfluorocarbon liquid
   a.   Large volume retained intravitreal perfluorocarbon
      i.   Inflammation
      ii. Elevated intraocular pressure
   b.   Small volume retained intravitreal perfluorocarbon
      i.   Floaters
II.   Silicone oil
   a.   Elevated intraocular pressure
      i.   Pupillary block
      ii. Emulsification of oil blocking trabecular meshwork
   b.   Corneal opacification
      i.   Corneal decompensation
      ii. Band keratopathy
   c.   Cataract formation
III. Intraocular gas
   a.   Cataract
   b.   Elevated intraocular pressure

SELECTED REFERENCES

Abrams GW, Azen SP, McCuen BW 2nd, Flynn HW Jr, Lai MY, Ryan SJ. Vitrectomy with silicone oil or long-acting gas in eyes with severe proliferative vitreoretinopathy: Results of additional and long-term follow-up. Silicone Study Report 11. *Arch Ophthalmol.* 1997;115(3):335–344.

Chang S, Lincoff H, Zimmerman NJ, *Fuchs W*. Giant retinal tears. Surgical techniques and results using perfluorocarbon liquids. *Arch Ophthalmol.* 1989;107(5):761–766.

Chang S, Ozmert E, Zimmerman NJ. Intraoperative perfluorocarbon liquids in the management of proliferative vitreoretinopathy. *Am J Ophthalmol.* 1988;106(6):668–674.

Da Mata AP, Burk SE, Riemann CD, Rosa RH Jr, Snyder ME, Petersen MR, Foster RE. Indocyanine green-assisted peeling of the retinal internal limiting membrane during vitrectomy surgery for macular hole repair. *Opthalmology.* 2001;108(7):1187–1192.

45

Principles and Treatment of Giant Retinal Tears

Leon D. Charkoudian, MD and Timothy W. Olsen, MD

TABLE 45.1 *Indications for the Treatment of Giant Retinal Tears*

Rhegmatogenous retinal tears greater than 90 degrees in circumference

Retinal dialyses

Visual potential (chronicity of a giant tear may limit surgical outcomes)

Definitions of Giant Retinal Tears

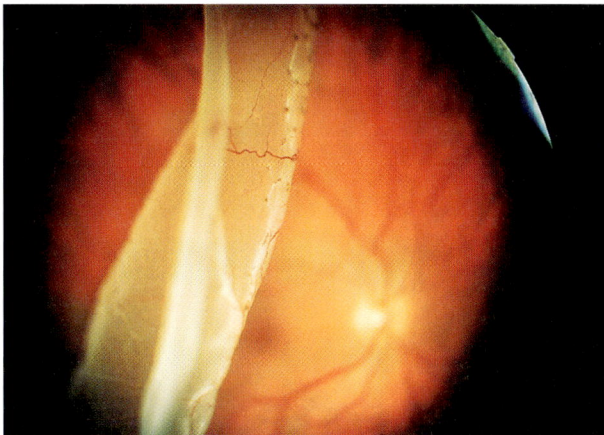

FIGURE 45.1 A giant retinal tear is defined as a full-thickness retinal break that extends 90° or more circumferentially (more than three contiguous clock hours). A broad tear posterior to the vitreous base results in an unsupported posterior edge, which frequently folds or rolls posteriorly. Note the folded, inverted edge of the torn retina that extends into the vitreous cavity. The dark spots at the folded border of the tear represent aggregates of pigmented cells and indicate early proliferative vitreoretinopathy (PVR), a frequent complication of giant retinal breaks. *(Reprinted with permission from Olsen TW, Chang TS, Sternberg P Jr. Retinal detachments associated with blunt trauma. Semin Ophthalmol. 1995;10:17–27.)*

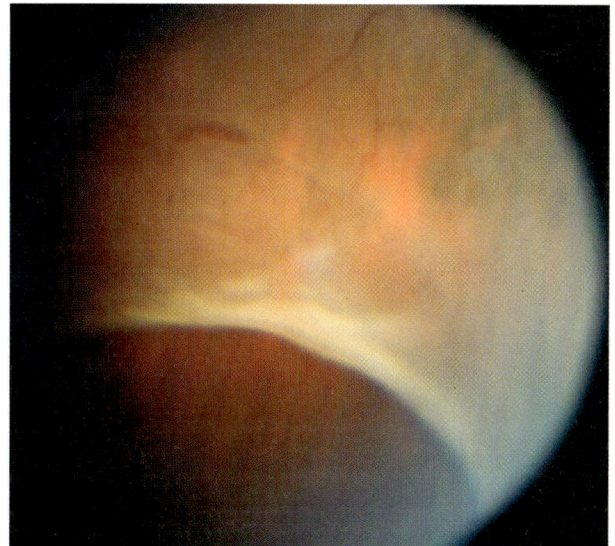

FIGURE 45.2 A retinal dialysis is a type of giant retinal tear. Tractional forces cause an avulsion at the vitreous base resulting in a dialysis, or tearing, of the retina at the ora serrate, or in a region of retina under the vitreous base insertion. As opposed to the classical giant retinal tear, in a dialysis the vitreous is attached at the posterior retinal edge at the break. Trauma is a frequent etiology. Although retinal dialyses carry some risk of PVR, the risk is significantly lower than that of conventional giant retinal tears; it is likely that pigment cells are dispersed in the classic giant retinal tear, whereas in a dialysis, the RPE cells remain localized by the vitreous base barrier.

Operative Approach to Giant Retinal Tears

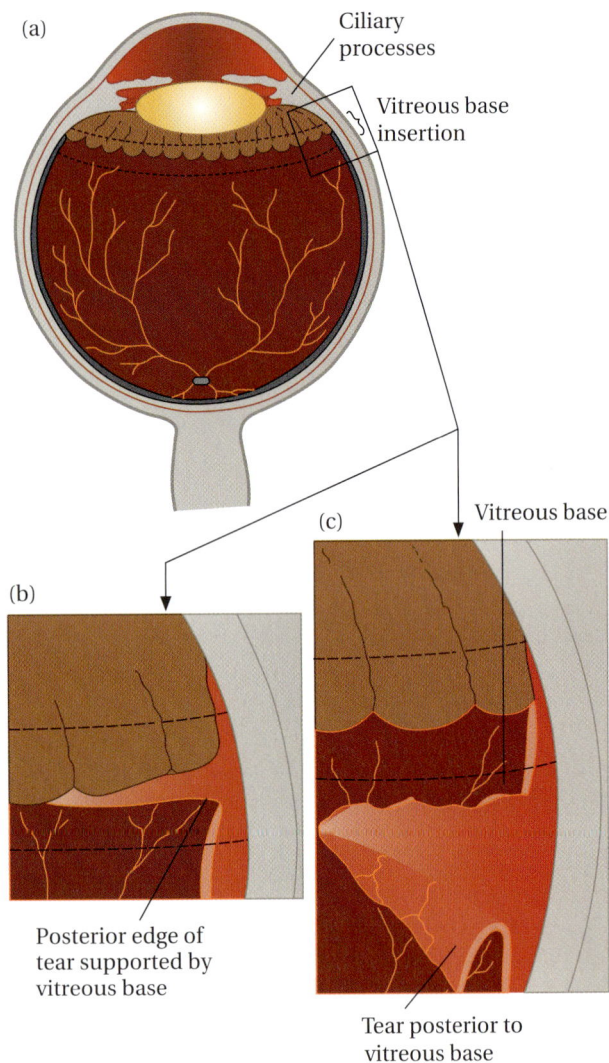

(a)

Ciliary processes

Vitreous base insertion

Vitreous base

(c)

(b)

Posterior edge of tear supported by vitreous base

Tear posterior to vitreous base

FIGURE 45.3   Preoperative localization of a giant retinal tear relative to the vitreous base is essential. A broad retinal tear occurring within the vitreous base such as a dialysis is associated with an excellent reattachment rate and visual prognosis, while a giant retinal tear posterior to the vitreous base with a scrolled posterior edge is a more challenging surgical repair. (a) Normal anatomy of the vitreous base. (b) Magnified diagram shows the location of a dialysis (under the vitreous base), with the posterior torn edge supported by the vitreous. (c) Magnified diagram of the torn, folded posterior edge of a giant retinal tear. The vitreous base inserts into the anterior flap of the tear.

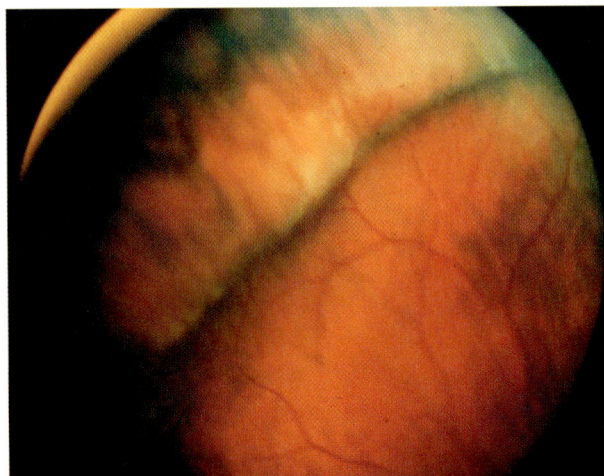

FIGURE 45.4   The use of a scleral buckle as an adjunct for giant retinal tears is controversial but there has been some support in the literature (see references). A buckle may be used to support the retina that is still connected anteriorly and to prevent extension of the tear, or in cases of giant retinal tear with PVR and retinal shortening. Theoretic risks of buckling include posterior retinal slippage and radial folds.

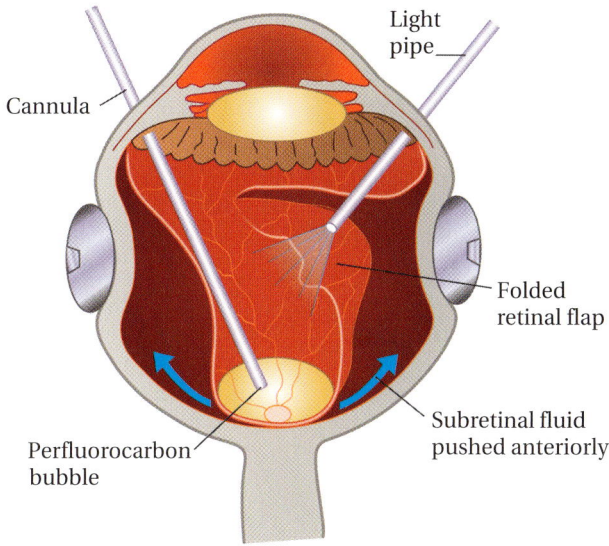

FIGURE 45.5 The surgical principles in repair of a giant retinal tear are (1) re-apposition of the retina; (2) relief of internal vitreous traction; and (3) establishment of a firm chorioretinal adhesion. Following core pars plana vitrectomy and removal of posterior or subretinal proliferative tissue, perfluorocarbon (PFC) liquid is injected over the optic nerve. This maneuver forces the subretinal fluid anteriorly and unrolls the inverted retinal edge. Most subretinal fluid is forced into the vitreous cavity through the tear; the remainder migrates into the anterior subretinal space. Please note that while a tire buckling element is shown, a silicone band (such as a 42-style) may be used and appears to be equally effective.

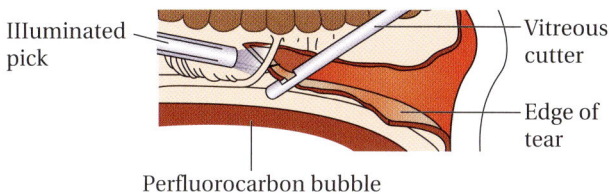

FIGURE 45.6 Bimanual dissection technique of the vitreous base. An illuminated pick and the vitreous-cutting instrument are used to dissect vitreous from the torn edge of the retina. The vitreous base should be carefully dissected to prevent further vitreous contraction and extension of the retinal tear. Special attention is directed to the ends of the giant retinal tear; specifically, the 'corners of the mouth', where tears could extend if improperly addressed.

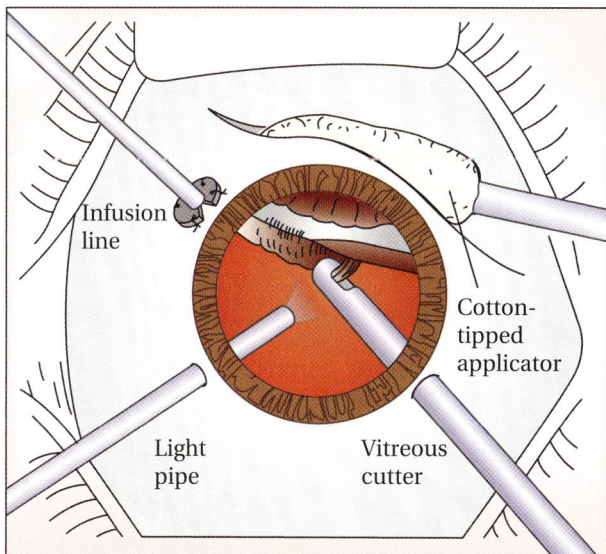

FIGURE 45.7 In order to facilitate meticulous dissection of the vitreous base and the edges of the tear, scleral depression is required. External depression by either the assistant, or the surgeon facilitates maximal vitreous dissection. The vitreous base is "shaved" as closely as possible to prevent future contraction with extension of the tear. In some instances, it may be necessary to remove the crystalline lens to ensure a thorough peripheral retinal examination. High myopes may be more accessible near the vitreous base. If the crystalline lens is preserved, the surgeon must be careful to avoid lens touch.

(a)

(b)

Cautery marks

Proliferative tissue may prevent unrolling the retinal flap

Retina lies flat

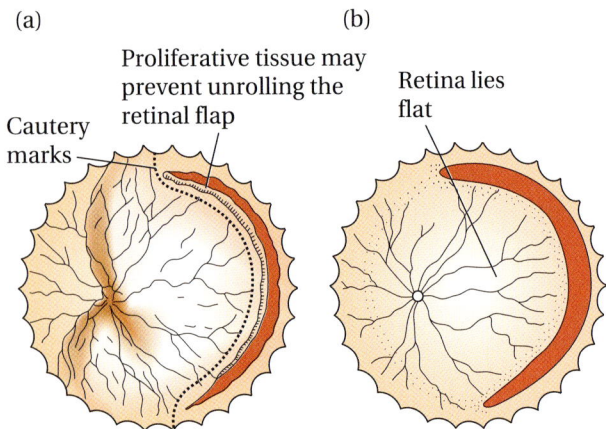

FIGURE 45.8 (a) If the edges of the tear cannot be unfolded and do not lie flat because of PVR, a retinectomy may be performed. This procedure will also provide a more stable configuration to the apices of the tear. A border of normal retina just posterior to the rolled edge is cauterized as shown. A high-speed vitreous-cutting instrument is then used to excise the demarcated retina. (b) Post-retinectomy diagram shows laser treatment at the border. The posterior edge of the tear is supported by an encircling scleral buckle.

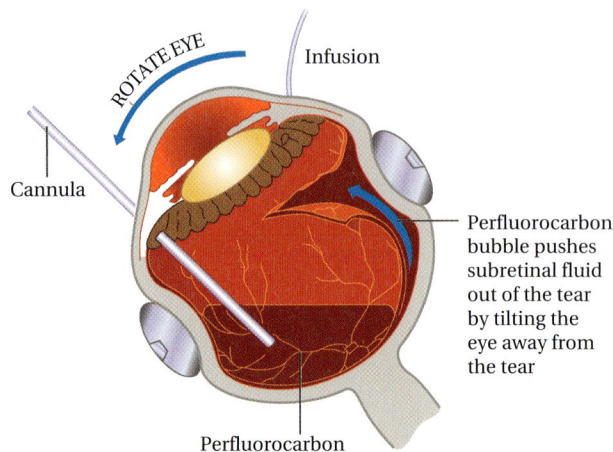

ROTATE EYE

Infusion

Cannula

Perfluorocarbon bubble pushes subretinal fluid out of the tear by tilting the eye away from the tear

Perfluorocarbon

FIGURE 45.9 Perfluorocarbon (PFC) liquid is added, with the tear in the nondependent (uppermost) position. This approach forces subretinal fluid anteriorly, with a majority of the fluid passing through the tear. Some subretinal fluid still remains anterior to the PFC liquid away from the retinal tear.

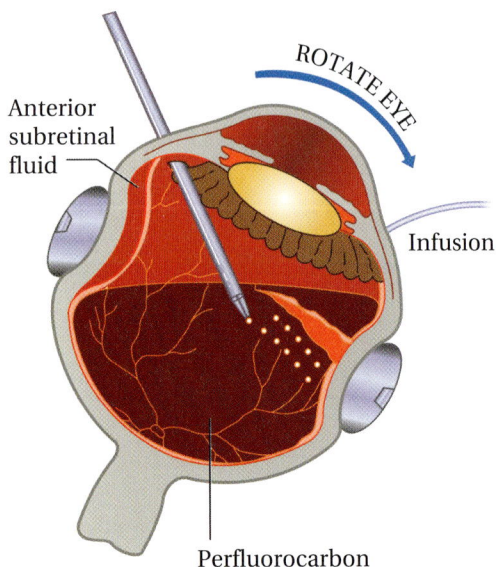

Anterior subretinal fluid

ROTATE EYE

Infusion

Perfluorocarbon

FIGURE 45.10 The globe is rotated so that the tear is covered by PFC liquid. This action allows for retinal apposition to the retinal pigment epithelium and endophotocoagulation along the posterior border of the tear. The remaining anterior retinal flap is retinectomized. The treatment is usually extended for 360° along the scleral buckle. Several rows of laser burns are usually sufficient. Cryotherapy should be avoided as it increases the risk of subsequent PVR.

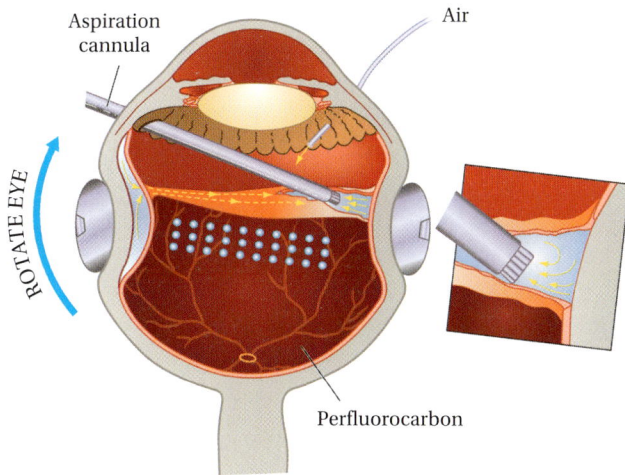

FIGURE 45.11 Following re-apposition of the retina and endophotocoagulation, some residual subretinal fluid is often still present anterior to the PFC liquid. This anterior fluid must be addressed during the fluid–gas exchange. The fluid–gas exchange requires meticulous attention to the eye position, fluid meniscus, and PFC liquid level. An air–fluid exchange will force the anterior subretinal fluid posterior in a circumferential manner. The fluid is removed at the posterior edge of the giant tear. The PFC liquid restricts the fluid from the posterior subretinal space. The PFC liquid and air menisci create a triangular area of fluid, which is slowly and meticulously aspirated using a soft-tipped extrusion cannula. The passage of time is necessary to ensure that all anterior fluid is aspirated. Failure to spend adequate attention during this stage may lead to posterior retinal slippage, a frequent error for beginning surgeons.

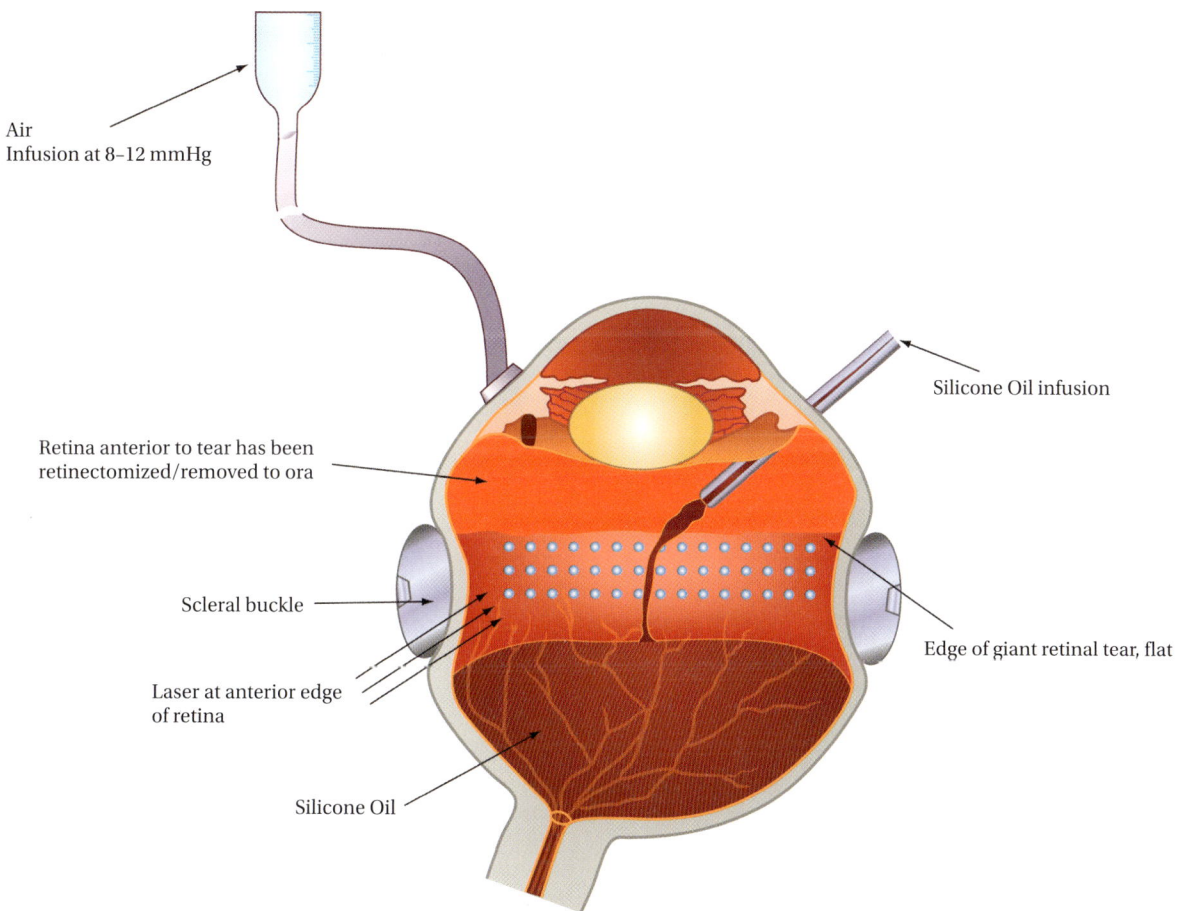

FIGURE 45.12 Postoperative retinal tamponade may be performed to reduce the risk of retinal redetachment. Long-term tamponade with silicone oil (above) is effective but requires a second procedure for oil removal. For superior or smaller breaks (i.e., <180 degrees), a shorter-term tamponade may be considered with perfluoro-propane (C_3F_8) gas.

TABLE 45.2 *Selected Complications of Treatment for Giant Retinal Tears*

Complication type		Potential corrective measure(s)
Vitrectomy-related	Endophthalmitis	Tap and inject as appropriate
	Suprachoroidal hemorrhage	Immediate closure and discontinuation of surgery if severe; raise intraocular pressure and consider continuation if minor
	Retinal redetachment	Reoperation
	Iatrogenic retinal breaks	Laser retinopexy (ideally intraoperatively)
	Proliferative vitreoretinopathy	Reoperation
	Lens touch/postoperative cataract formation	Cataract removal
	Postoperative hypotony	Ensure adequate wound closure
	Visual field loss	Avoid prolonged drying of retina during air–fluid exchange
	Central visual loss	Avoid overexposure of light to macula during vitrectomy
Gas-specific	Gas overfill/ocular hypertension	IOP-lowering medications; paracentesis
Silicone oil-specific	Band keratopathy	Silicone oil removal if indicated; penetrating keratoplasty if severe
	Retinal toxicity	Silicone oil removal
	Late glaucoma	Glaucoma surgery often indicated
Perfluoro-octane-specific	Subretinal perfluoro-octane	Surgical removal if near the fovea
Scleral buckle-specific	Perforation	Laser retinopexy if retinal break occurs
	Induced myopia	Refraction
	Implant exposure	Removal of buckle
	Implant infection	Removal of buckle
	Ptosis	Ptosis repair
	Diplopia	Prism correction or strabismus repair

SELECTED REFERENCES

Alexander P, Prasad R, Ang A, Poulson AV, Scott JD, Snead MP. Prevention and control of proliferative vitreoretinopathy: Primary retinal detachment surgery using silicone oil as a planned two-stage procedure in high-risk cases. *Eye.* 2008 Jun;22(6):815–818.

Campochiaro PA, Kaden IH, Vidaurri-Leal J, Glaser BM. Cryotherapy enhances intravitreal dispersion of viable retinal pigment epithelial cells. *Arch Ophthalmol.* 1985 Mar;103(3):434–436.

Chang S, Lincoff H, Zimmerman NJ, Fuchs W. Giant retinal tears. Surgical techniques and results using perfluorocarbon liquids. *Arch Ophthalmol.* 1989 May;107(5):761–766.

Glaser BM, Carter JB, Kuppermann BD, Michels RG. Perfluoro-octane in the treatment of giant retinal tears with proliferative vitreoretinopathy. *Ophthalmology.* 1991 Nov;98(11):1613–1621.

Goezinne F, LA Heij EC, Berendschot TT, Gast ST, Liem AT, Lundqvist IL, Hendrikse F. Low redetachment rate due to encircling scleral buckle in giant retinal tears treated with vitrectomy and silicone oil. *Retina.* 2008 Mar;28(3):485–492.

Irvine AR, Lahey JM. Pneumatic retinopexy for giant retinal tears. *Ophthalmology.* 1994 Mar;101(3):524–528.

Joondeph BC, Flynn HW Jr, Blankenship GW, Glaser BM, Stern WH. The surgical management of giant retinal tears with the cannulated extrusion needle. *Am J Ophthalmol.* 1989 Nov 15;108(5):548–553.

Kanski JJ. Giant retinal tears. *Am J Ophthalmol.* 1975 May;79(5):846–852.

Kreiger AE, Lewis H. Management of giant retinal tears without scleral buckling. Use of radical dissection of the vitreous base and perfluoro-octane and intraocular tamponade. *Ophthalmology.* 1992 Apr;99(4):491–497.

Leaver PK, Cooling RJ, Feretis EB, Lean JS, McLeod D. Vitrectomy and fluid/silicone-oil exchange for giant retinal tears: Results at six months. *Br J Ophthalmol.* 1984 Jun;68(6):432–438.

Lee SY, Ong SG, Wong DW, Ang CL. Giant retinal tear management: An Asian experience. *Eye.* 2009 Mar;23(3):601–605. Epub 2008 Feb 29.

Machemer R, Allen AW. Retinal tears 180 degrees and greater. Management with vitrectomy and intravitreal gas. *Arch Ophthalmol.* 1976 Aug;94(8):1340–1346.

Norton EW, Aaberg T, Fung W, Curtin VT. Giant retinal tears. I. Clinical management with intravitreal air. Trans *Am Ophthalmol Soc.* 1969;67:374–393.

Rofail M, Lee LR. Perfluoro-n-octane as a postoperative vitreoretinal tamponade in the management of giant retinal tears. *Retina.* 2005 Oct–Nov;25(7):897–901.

Schepens CL, Freeman HM. Current management of giant retinal breaks. *Trans Am Acad Ophthalmol Otolaryngol.* 1967 May–Jun;71(3):474–487.

Scott JD. Giant retinal tears. *Mod Probl Ophthalmol.* 1979;20:275–278.

Smiddy WE, Green WR. Retinal dialysis: Pathology and pathogenesis. *Retina.* 1982;2(2):94–116.

Diabetic Retinopathy

Stephen G. Schwartz, MD, MBA and Harry W. Flynn, Jr., MD

SELECTED REFERENCES

TABLE 46.1 *Indications for Diabetic Vitrectomy*

Media opacity
   Non-clearing vitreous hemorrhage
   Non-clearing subhyaloid (premacular) hemorrhage
   Anterior segment neovascularization with posterior segment media opacity
   Cataract preventing treatment of severe proliferative diabetic retinopathy
Tractional pathology
   Progressive fibrovascular proliferation
   Traction retinal detachment involving the macula
   Combined traction-rhegmatogenous retinal detachment
   Macular edema associated with taut and thickened posterior hyaloid face
Other indications
   Ghost cell glaucoma
   Anterior hyaloid fibrovascular proliferation
   Fibrinoid syndrome
   Epiretinal membrane
   Macular heterotopia
   Macular hole
   Macular edema not associated with traction

Adapted from Smiddy WE, Flynn HW Jr. Vitrectomy for Diabetic Retinopathy. In: Scott IU, Flynn HW Jr, and Smiddy WE (eds.), *Diabetes and Ocular Disease: Past, Present and Future Therapies.* New York: Oxford University Press, 2010.

TABLE 46.2 *Preoperative Considerations*

Consider improved metabolic control, if surgery can be delayed.

Consider panretinal photocoagulation prior to surgery, if media are clear.

Consider preoperative intravitreal bevacizumab, if active neovascularization is present.

Consider concomitant cataract surgery, if visually significant cataract.

Consider concomitant scleral buckling, if significant peripheral traction or concomitant rhegmatogenous retinal detachment.

Case 1: Non-clearing Vitreous Hemorrhage

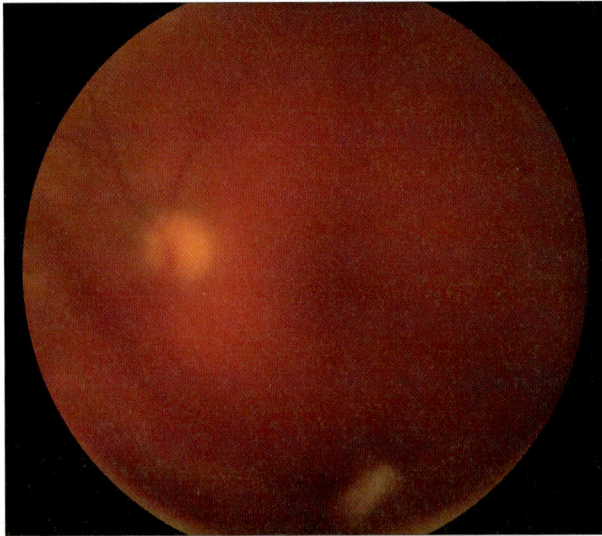

FIGURE 46.1 Preoperative fundus photograph. Note the vitreous hemorrhage obscuring fundus details.

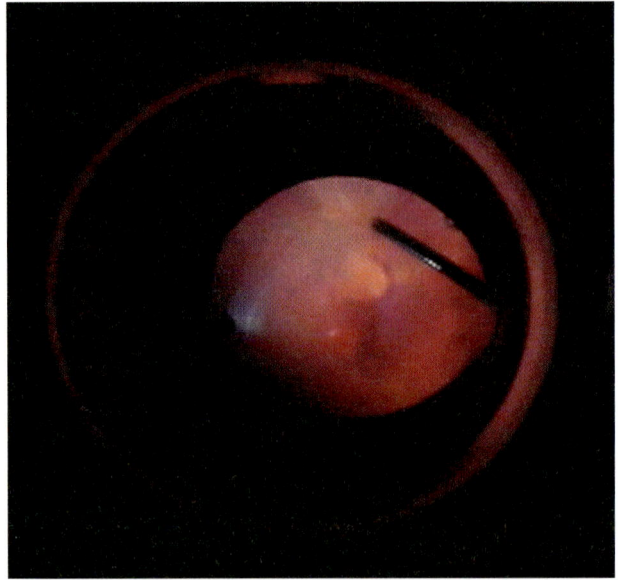

FIGURE 46.2 Intraoperative photograph. Note removal of vitreous hemorrhage and posterior cortical vitreous with vitreous cutter.

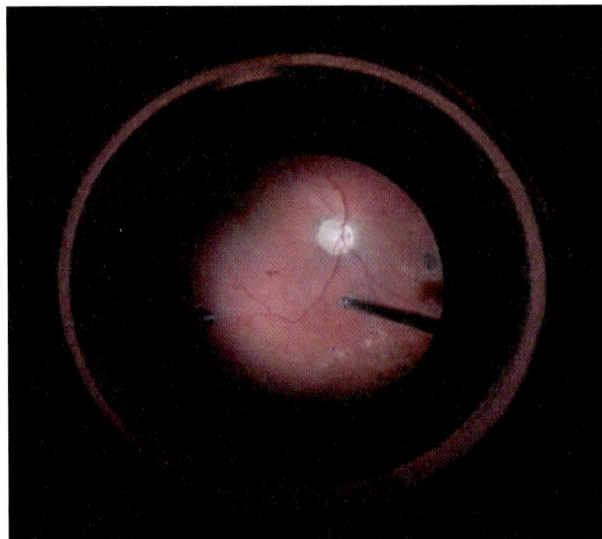

FIGURE 46.3 Intraoperative photograph. Note clear media, with view of fundus details after removal of hemorrhage.

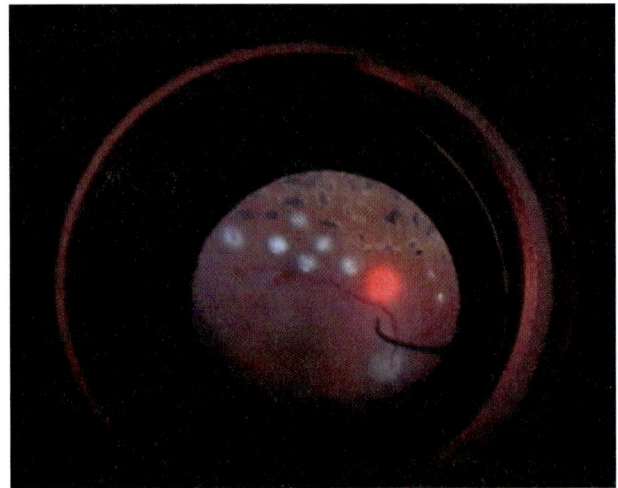

FIGURE 46.4 Intraoperative photograph. Note placement of panretinal photocoagulation with endolaser probe.

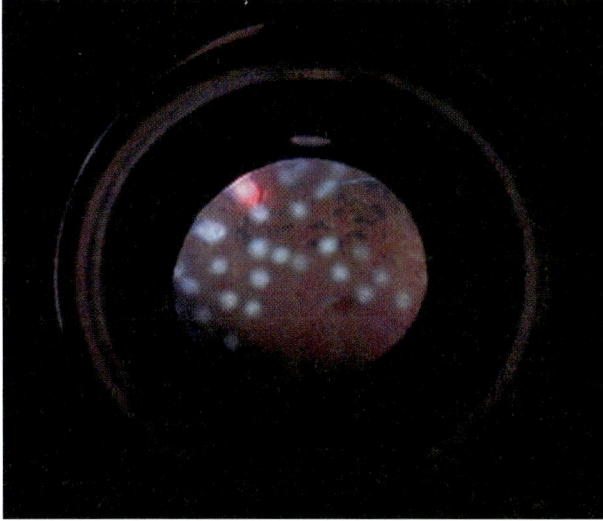

FIGURE 46.5 Intraoperative photograph. Note fresh panretinal photocoagulation burns.

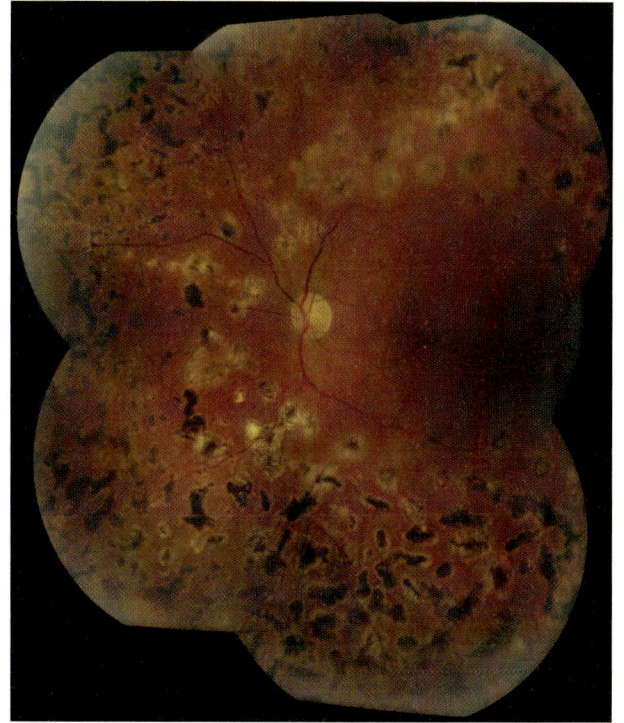

FIGURE 46.6 Postoperative montage photograph. Note the clear media, and the panretinal photocoagulation. The visual acuity returned to 20/30 in the left eye.

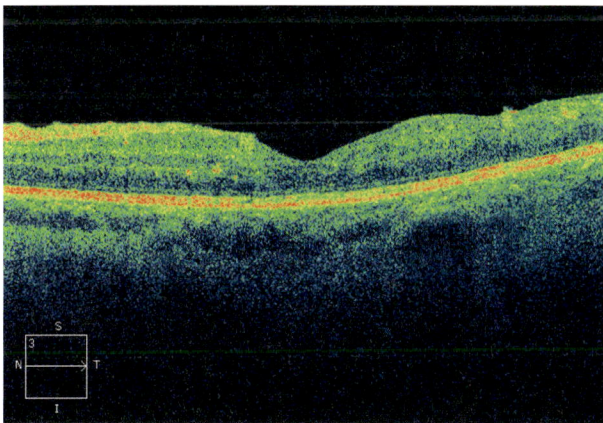

FIGURE 46.7 Postoperative optical coherence tomograph. Note the relatively normal foveal contour.

Case 2: Severe Proliferative Diabetic Retinopathy with Intermittent Vitreous Hemorrhage

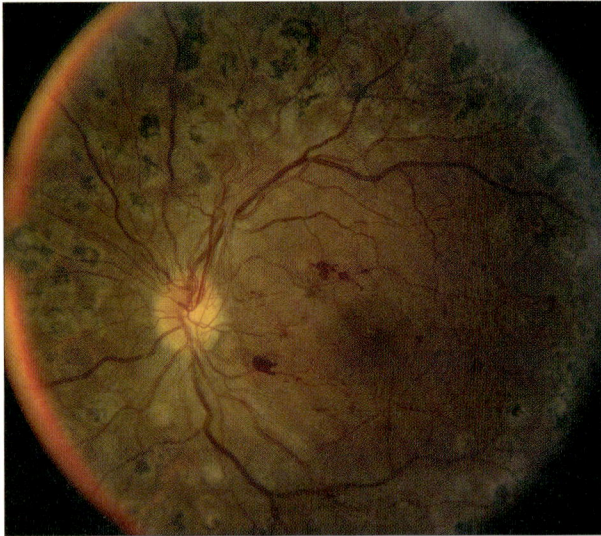

FIGURE 46.8 Preoperative photograph. Note persistent neovascularization of the disc despite full panretinal photocoagulation.

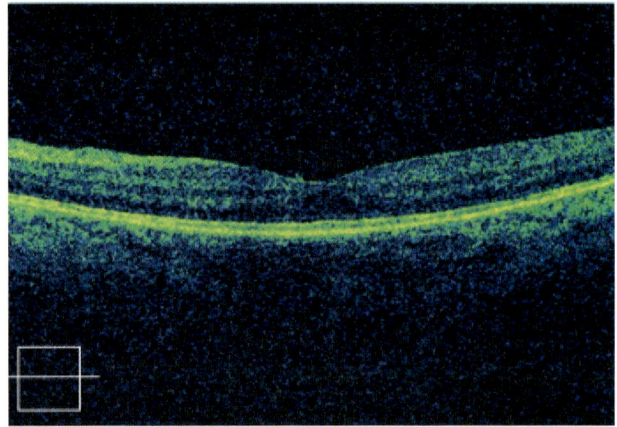

FIGURE 46.9 Preoperative optical coherence tomograph. Note the normal foveal contour.

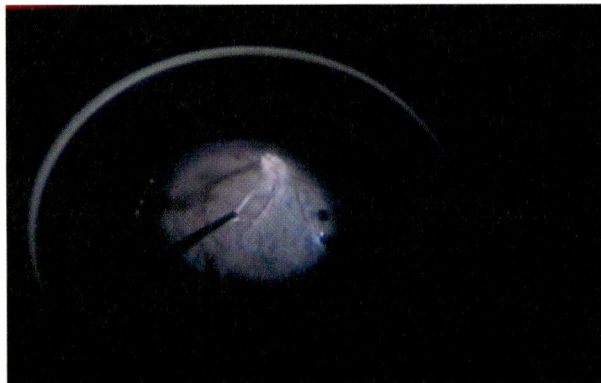

FIGURE 46.10 Intraoperative photograph. Peeling the posterior hyaloid face with the vitreous cutter.

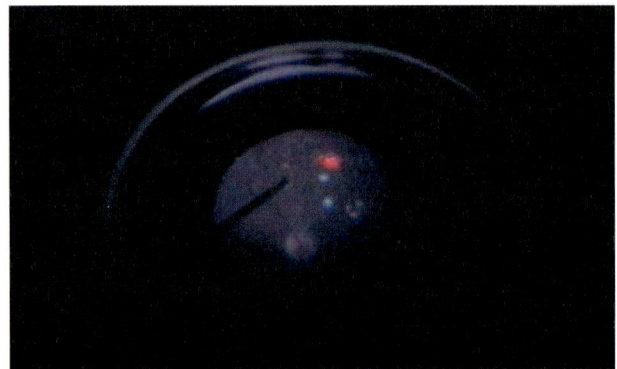

FIGURE 46.11 Intraoperative photograph. Note placement of panretinal photocoagulation with endolaser probe.

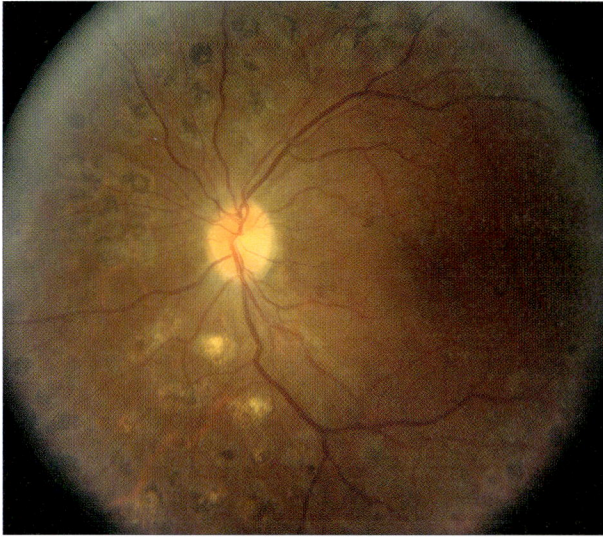

FIGURE 46.12 Postoperative photograph. Note the absence of neovascularization of the disc and additional panretinal photocoagulation.

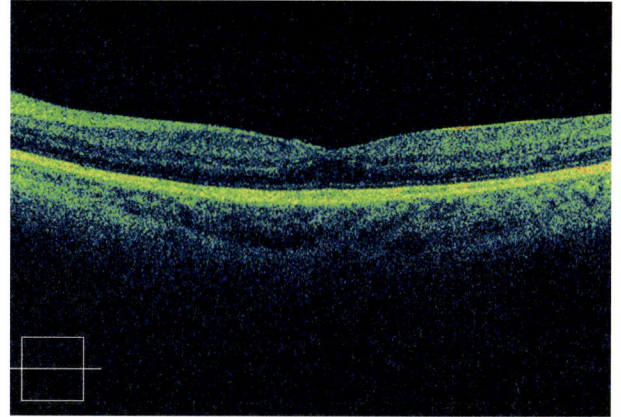

FIGURE 46.13 Postoperative optical coherence tomograph. Note the normal foveal contour.

Case 3: Taut and Thickened Posterior Hyaloid Face

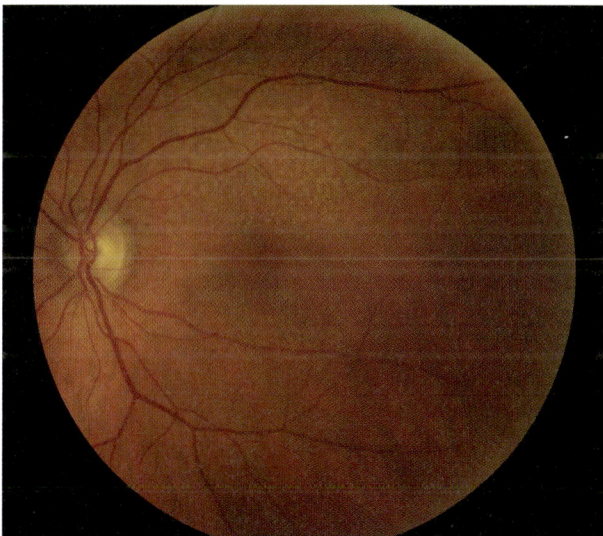

FIGURE 46.14 Preoperative photograph. The taut and thickened posterior hyaloid face is poorly visualized.

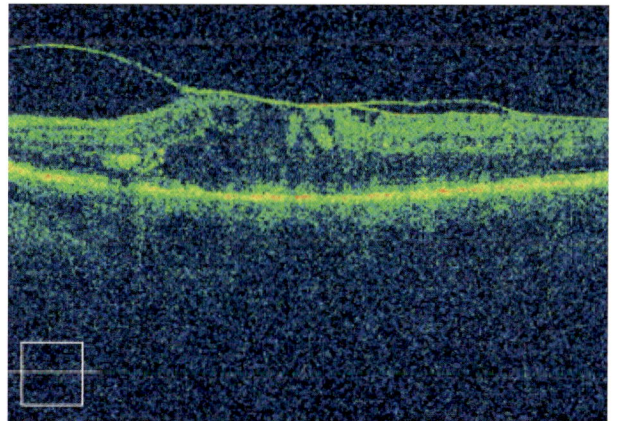

FIGURE 46.15 Preoperative optical coherence tomograph. The taut and thickened posterior hyaloid face is well visualized.

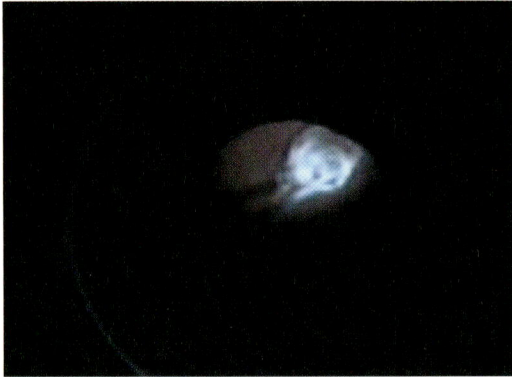

FIGURE 46.16 Intraoperative photograph. Using triamcinolone acetonide to stain the posterior hyaloid face.

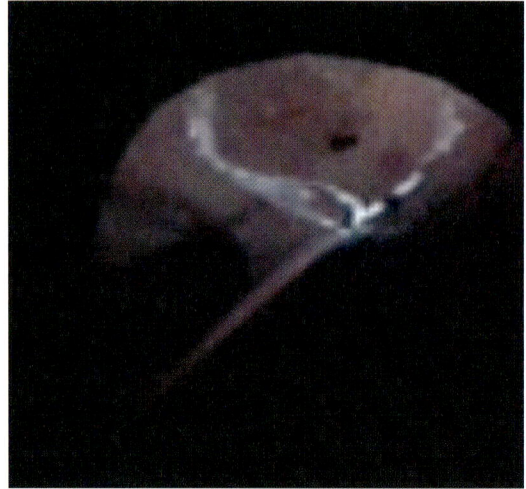

FIGURE 46.17 Intraoperative photograph. Using the vitreous cutter to peel the posterior hyaloid face.

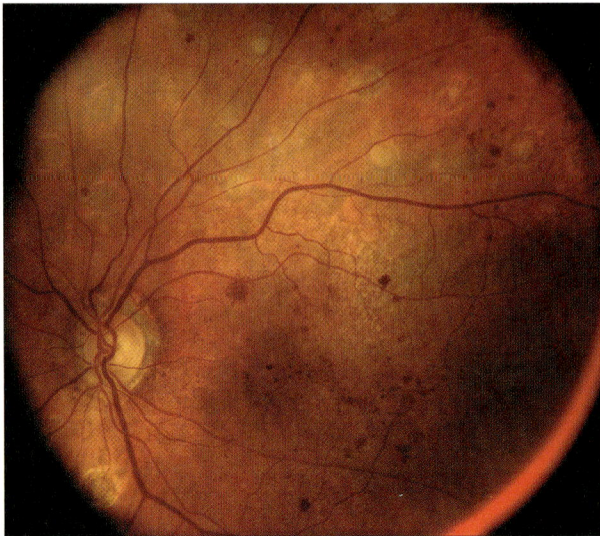

FIGURE 46.18 Postoperative photograph. Note the more normal macular appearance and the panretinal photocoagulation burns.

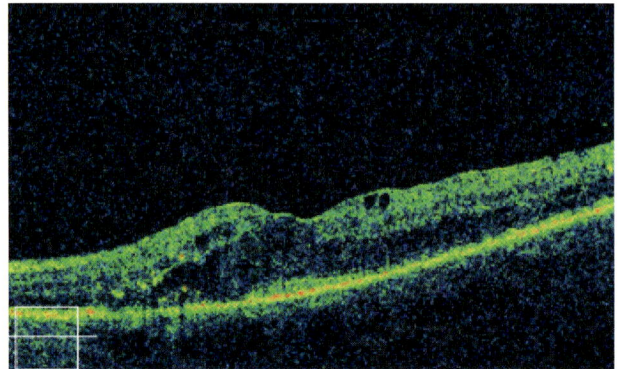

FIGURE 46.19 Postoperative optical coherence tomograph. Note the improved macular contour but persistent diabetic macular edema.

TABLE 46.3 *Potential Complications of Diabetic Vitrectomy*

Complications related to pars plana vitrectomy

    Peripheral retinal breaks

    Rhegmatogenous retinal detachment

Complications related to membrane peeling

    Posterior retinal breaks

    Other retinal trauma (e.g., macular hole)

Complications related to photocoagulation

    Choroidal effusion

    Macular photocoagulation

Complications related to fluid-gas exchange

    Cataract formation

    Increased intraocular pressure

Other complications

    Endophthalmitis

    Optic atrophy

    Neovascular glaucoma

SELECTED REFERENCES

Flynn HW Jr, Chew EY, Simons BD, Barton FB, Remaley NA, Ferris FL 3rd. Pars plana vitrectomy in the Early Treatment Diabetic Retinopathy Study: ETDRS report number 17: The Early Treatment Diabetic Retinopathy Study Research Group. *Ophthalmology.* 1992;99(9):1351–1357.

Harbour JW, Smiddy WE, Flynn HW Jr, Rubsamen PE. Vitrectomy for diabetic macular edema associated with a thickened and taut posterior hyaloid membrane. *Am J Ophthalmol.* 1996;121(4):405–413.

Hartley KL, Smiddy WE, Flynn HW Jr, Murray TG. Pars plana vitrectomy with internal limiting membrane peeling for diabetic macular edema. *Retina.* 2008;28(3):410–419.

Scott IU, Flynn HW Jr, Smiddy WE (eds.), *Diabetes and Ocular Disease: Past, Present and Future Therapies.* Oxford University Press, 2009.

Smiddy WE, Feuer W, Irvine WD, Flynn HW Jr, Blankenship GW. Vitrectomy for complications of proliferative diabetic retinopathy: Functional outcomes. *Ophthalmology.* 1995;102(11): 1688–1695.

Smiddy WE, Flynn HW Jr. Vitrectomy in the management of diabetic retinopathy. *Surv Ophthalmol.* 1999;43(6):491–507.

47

Surgical Management of Open Globe Injuries

Stephen S. Couvillion, MD and Dante J. Pieramici, MD

SELECTED REFERENCES

TABLE 47.1 *Indications for the Repair of Open Globe Injuries*

Blunt, perforating or penetrating injuries resulting in rupture of the cornea or sclera

Prolapse of uveal tissue

Violation of lens capsule or development of a traumatic cataract

Vitreous incarceration and resulting retinal detachment

Intraocular foreign body

Traumatic endophthalmitis

TABLE 47.2 *Preoperative Considerations*

Penetrating and perforating injuries should be evaluated by ultrasound or CT scan to identify foreign bodies.

Lens capsule violation increases the risk of traumatic endophthalmitis.

Consider staged repair of complex open globe injuries. Initial surgery should focus on closure of the wound and reestablishing the integrity of the globe.

Management of Penetrating and Perforating Ocular Injury

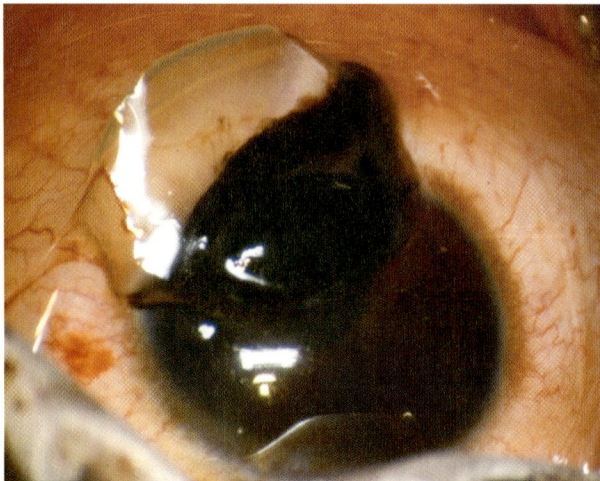

FIGURE 47.1 Open globe injury caused by a sharp object produced an approximately 6-mm corneal laceration with prolapse of uveal tissue and the crystalline lens. The primary goal guiding repair of such lacerations or ruptures of the globe is restoration of the integrity of the globe. It is imperative to determine the extent of injury prior to repair of any laceration, taking care not to exacerbate the extent of the injury. Preoperative evaluation by CT scan or ocular ultrasound may aid in surgical decision making.

(a)

(b)

30 g

Needle

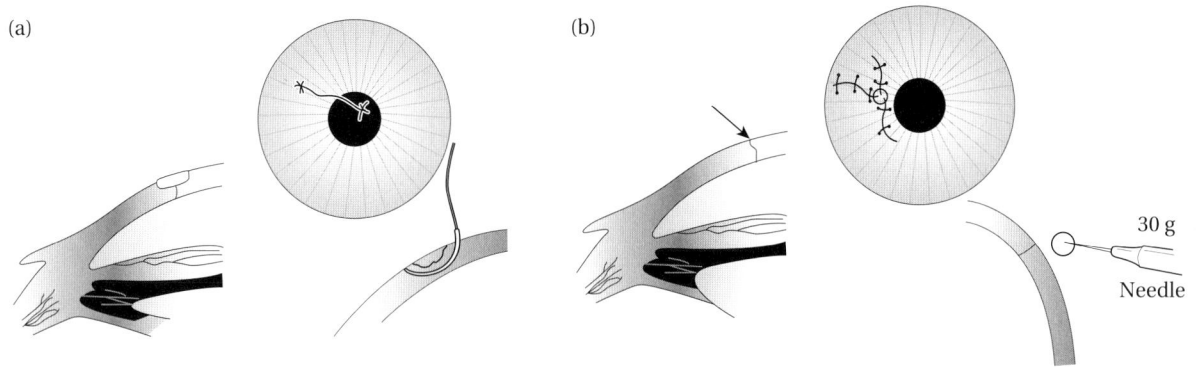

FIGURE 47.2 (a) Schematic diagram of clean, straight corneal laceration. The initial 10-0 nylon suture is placed in the center of the wound. All sutures should be approximately two-thirds corneal depth and about 1 mm apart. Once the wound is reapproximated, and the eye repressured, the wound should be checked for leakage with the Seidel test. (b) Schematic diagram of stellate corneal laceration at risk for poor wound apposition with potential post-operative wound leakage. Wound edges are reapproximated using 10-0 nylon. The remaining stellate edges are sealed with cyanoacrylate tissue glue. The cornea surface is thoroughly dried with a Weck cell prior to application of a disk of sterile filter paper saturated with glue. A bandage contact lens is placed at the end of the procedure.

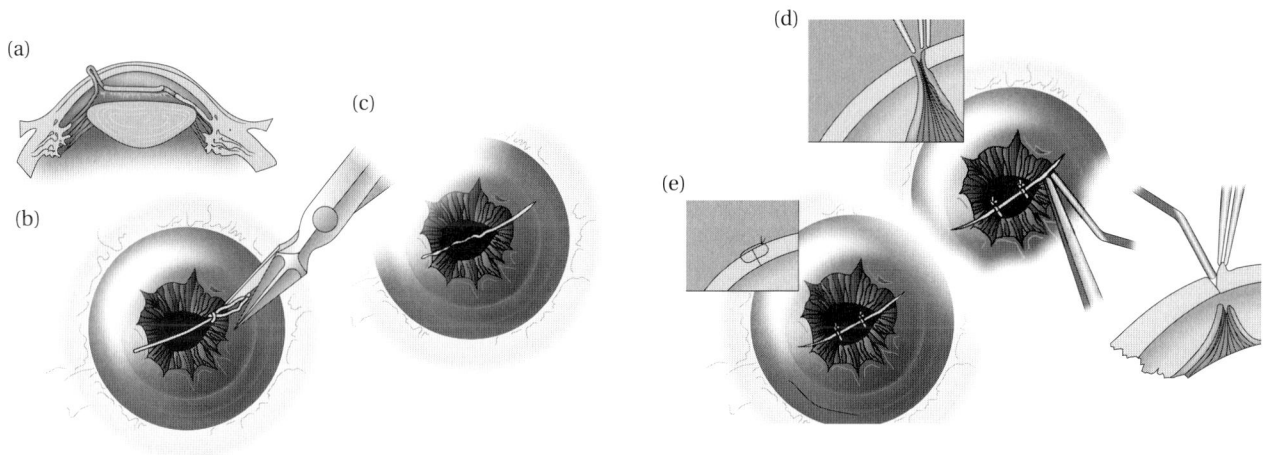

(a)

(b)

(c)

(d)

(e)

FIGURE 47.3 Prolapsed iris, uvea or other ocular contents (with the exception of lens material) should be reposited unless obviously necrotic or infected. (a) Schematic diagram depicting corneal laceration with incarcerated uveal tissue. (b) Tissue is trimmed with scissors at the plane of the corneal surface only when necessary. (c) Majority of uveal tissue has been freed from the corneal laceration site, although incarcerated tissue may remain at the inner surface of the wound. (d) Residual prolapsed tissue is reposited with the assistance of a viscoelastic cannula directly through the wound site. Further prolapse is prevented by viscoelastic tamponade. (e) Once residual incarcerated tissue is freed, 10-0 nylon sutures are placed through the corneal laceration, restoring integrity of the globe.

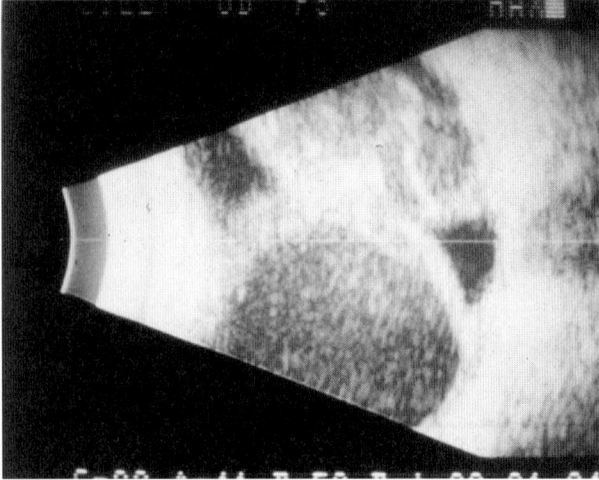

FIGURE 47.4 A preoperative evaluation with ocular ultrasound may aid in surgical management of complex trauma. This patient had dense choroidal hemorrhage from the initial injury. Repair was staged with vitrectomy and drainage of choroidal hemorrhage ten days following the primary globe closure.

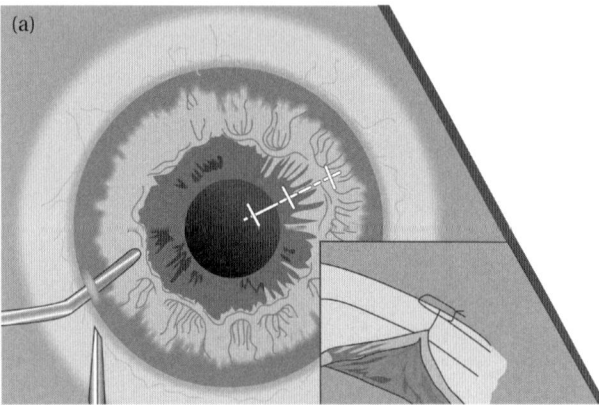

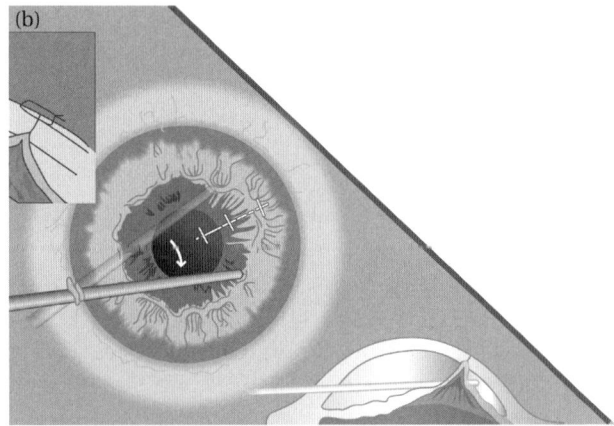

FIGURE 47.5 Uveal tissue may remain entrapped in the inner portion of a corneal laceration following closure of the wound. (a) Maintaining low posterior pressure prior to infusion placement allows viscoelastic or an infusion cannula, placed through the limbus, to deepen the anterior chamber. As the iris incarceration is reduced, the wound is sutured. (b) Through the previous infusion cannula site, a cyclodialysis spatula is used to sweep incarcerated tissue from the wound. Small amounts of viscoelastic may be left between the iris and wound to prevent reincarceration.

(a)

(b)

(c)

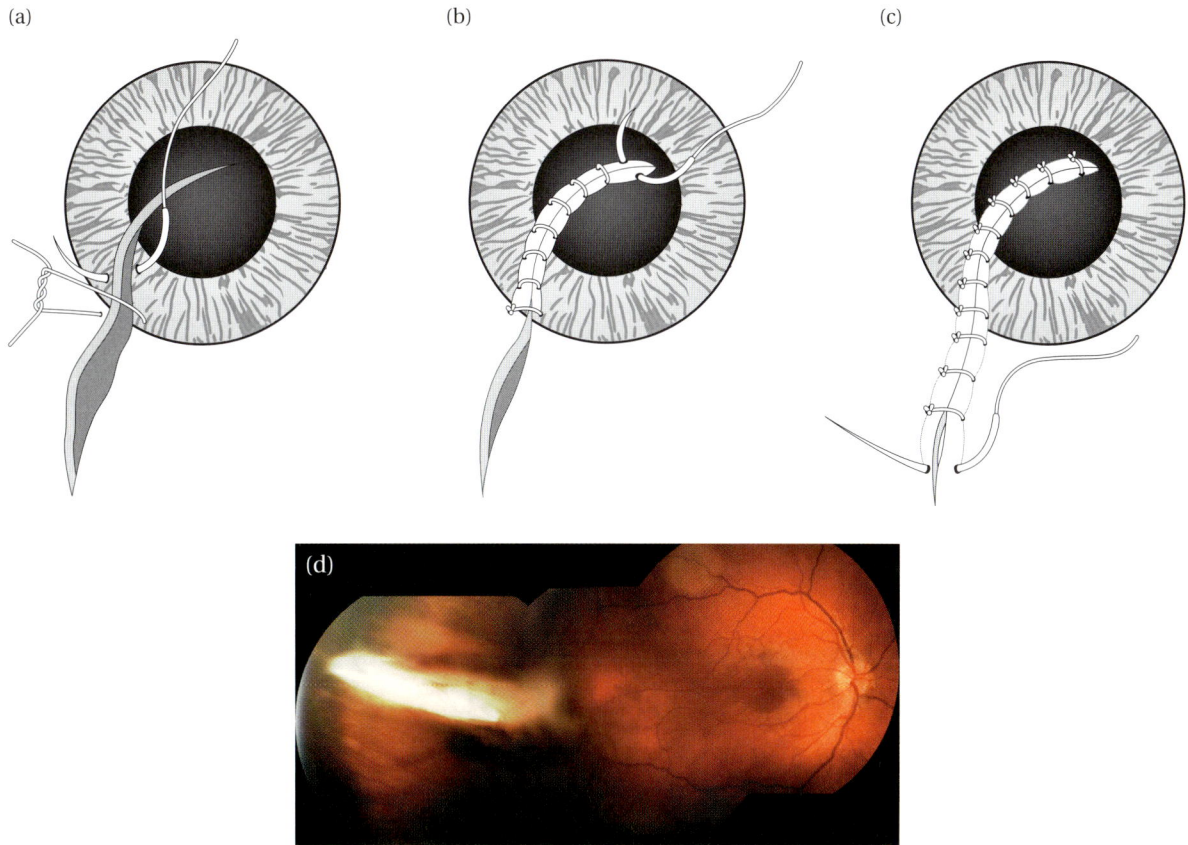

(d)

FIGURE 47.6 (a) Schematic diagram showing corneoscleral laceration. The initial suture is placed at the limbus, making it simpler to precisely re-approximate the proper alignment of the tissue. (b) Corneal portion of wound is closed with interrupted 10-0 nylon sutures. (c) Then, scleral portion of wound is closed, generally with either 8-0 or 9-0 nylon sutures, making certain to fully explore most posterior extent of laceration. A complete peritomy should be performed with gentle dissection to expose all quadrants of the globe. Special attention should be paid to the visualization of region of the muscle insertions to rule out further posterior rupture extension. (d) A full thickness posterior laceration involving the lateral rectus muscle. Repair required the isolation and removal of the lateral rectus muscle. The sclera was closed with 8-0 nylon visible intraocularly. A prophylactic scleral buckle was placed at the time of repair.

Cataract, Subluxation, and Dislocation of Lenses

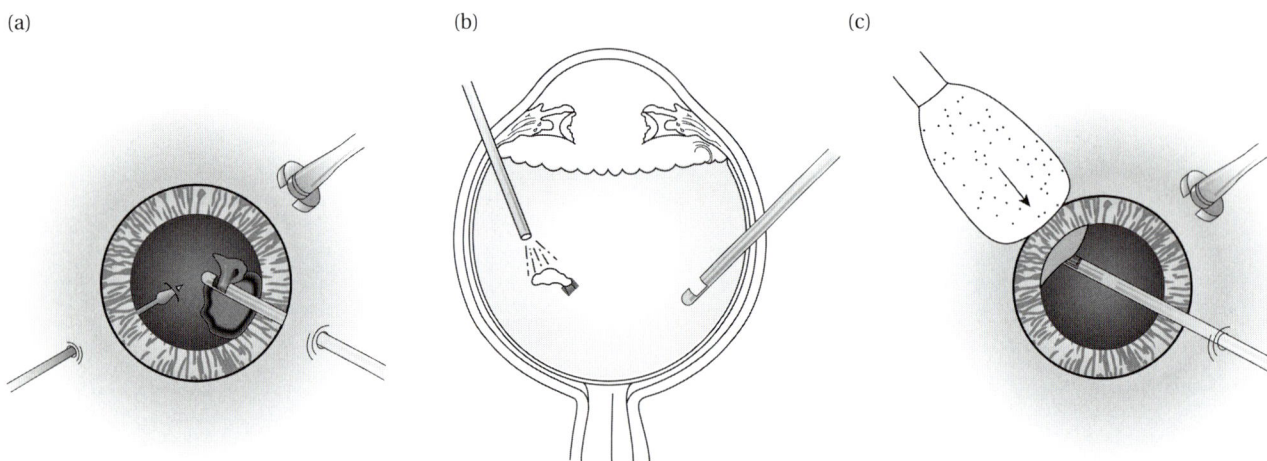

(a)

(b)

(c)

FIGURE 47.7 Contusive ocular injury may cause opacification, subluxation, or dislocation of the crystalline lens. A pars plana approach to remove the subluxed or dislocated lens is recommended. Violation of the lens capsule puts patients at increased risk for traumatic endophthalmitis. (a) Schematic diagram shows 3-port pars plana vitrectomy setup. A myringotomy blade or secondary irrigation needle may be placed into subluxated lens to help secure its position. Irrigation may also help to soften the lens. (b) If lens remnants fall posteriorly, they may be removed with combination vitrectomy and phacofragmentation. (c) Remnants of lens capsule can be removed with a vitreous-cutting instrument. Gentle scleral indentation aids in removal of peripheral capsular remnants.

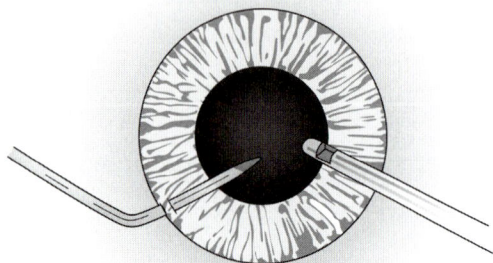

FIGURE 47.8 When surgery is performed to clear vitreous hemorrhage, preoperative assessment for hemorrhagic choroidal detachment, lens status, and possible retinal detachment is mandatory. For surgery, a standard 3-port pars plana vitrectomy is performed. If hyphema or vitreous hemorrhage precludes visualization of the pars plana infusion cannula, temporary infusion in the anterior segment through the limbus should be employed.

Retinal Detachment

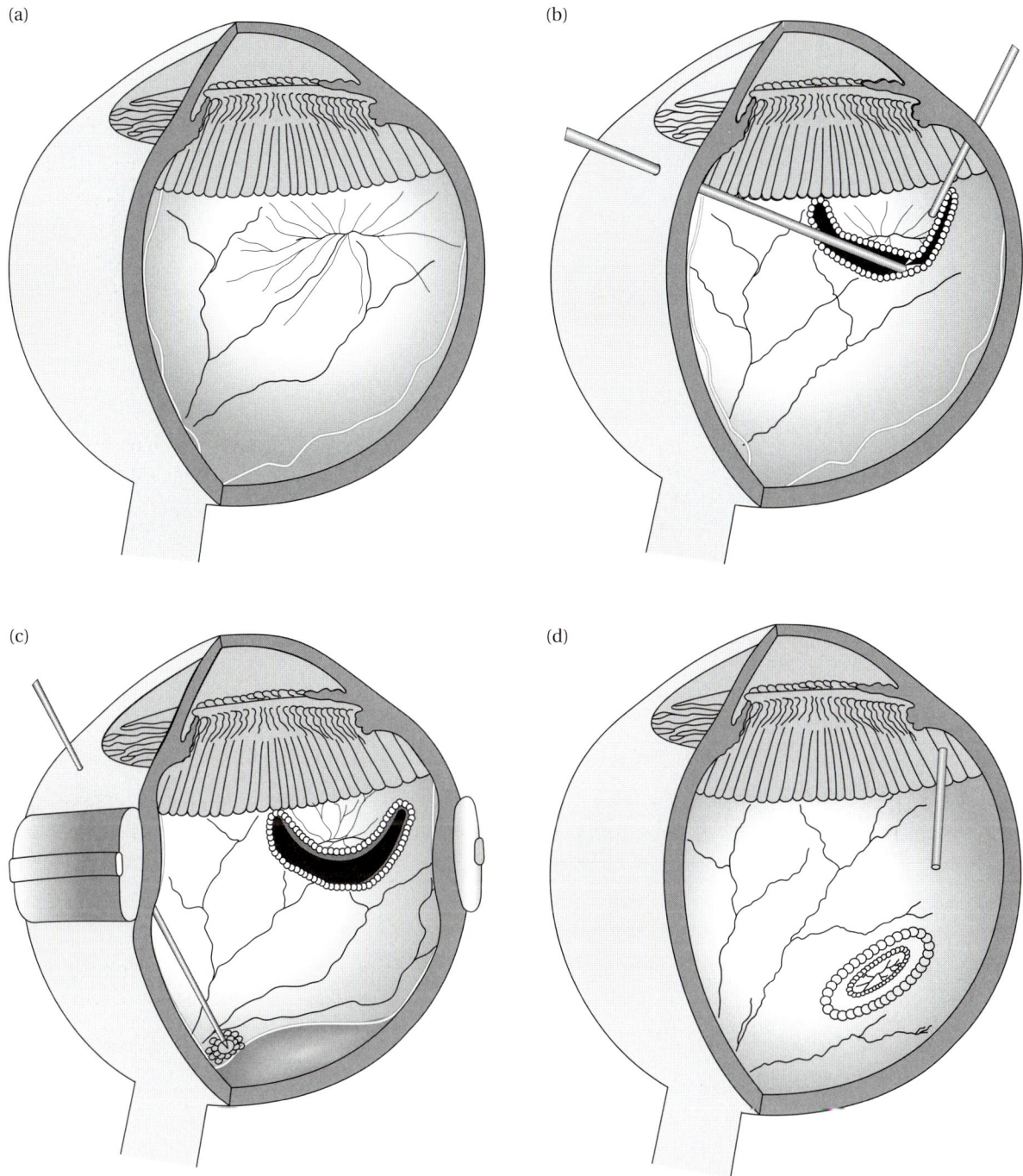

FIGURE 47.9 A particular problem seen with posterior segment penetrating ocular injuries is retinal or vitreous incarceration in the scleral laceration site. This condition can complicate the management of subsequent retinal detachment. Vitreous surgery may be performed at the time of injury or during the early postoperative period. (a) Schematic diagram of anterior retinal incarceration site. (b) Vitrectomy surgery has been performed, and photocoagulation placed along margins of incarceration site. A retinotomy is performed to excise incarcerated tissue. (c) The region is then supported by a scleral buckle. (d) Posterior retinal incarceration site. Retinotomy has been performed, to be followed by placement of either long-acting gas or silicone oil to provide tamponade of this region.

Surgical Management of Retained Intraocular Foreign Body

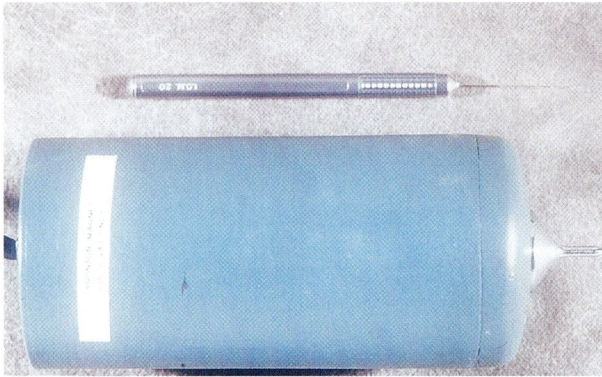

FIGURE 47.10 Bronson electromagnet and intraocular rare earth magnet. An external electromagnet or internal rare earth magnet may be used to remove magnetic foreign bodies from the posterior segment.

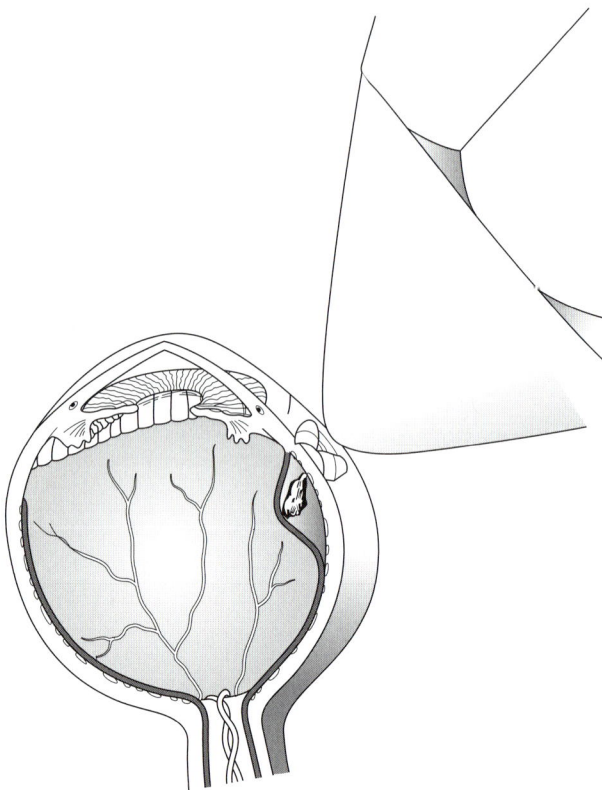

FIGURE 47.11 Schematic diagram depicting removal of anteriorly located subretinal magnetic intraocular foreign body (IOFB). The external electromagnet is placed over a scleral cutdown incision adjacent to the magnetic IOFB. Visualization and localization by indirect ophthalmoscopy are essential. The external magnet brings the IOFB through the uvea.

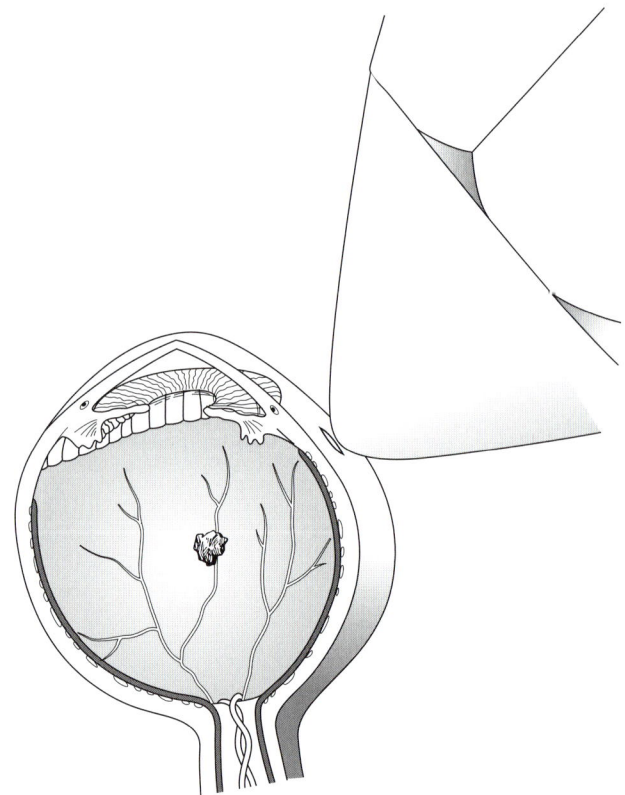

FIGURE 47.12 Schematic diagram showing removal of magnetic intravitreal foreign body through sclerotomy site at pars plana with external electromagnet. This method is used primarily for small magnetic intravitreal IOFBs, or when pars plana vitrectomy is not available.

(a)

(b)

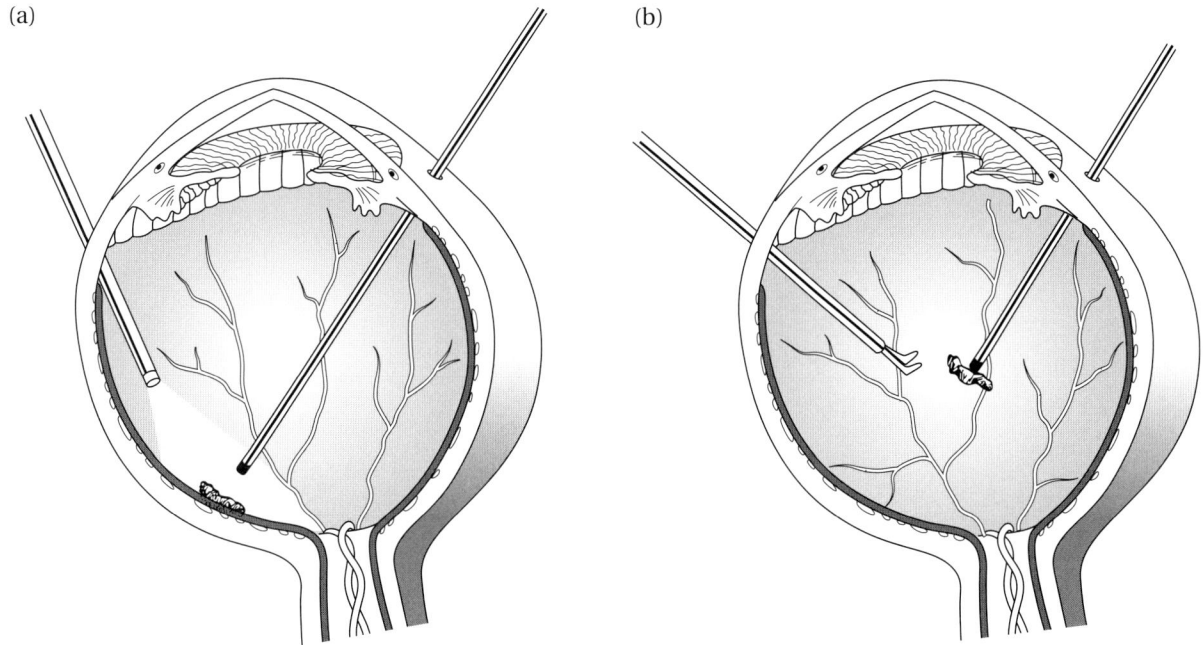

FIGURE 47.13 Intraocular rare earth magnets are used in conjunction with pars plana vitrectomy when there is tissue incarceration, associated intraocular damage, or media opacities precluding adequate initial visualization of a magnetic IOFB. (a) Schematic diagram showing magnetic IOFB lying on retinal surface. Vitrectomy has been performed. The IOFB is then freed of any encapsulated tissue before being raised off the retinal surface with an intraocular rare earth magnet. (b) Before the IOFB is removed from eye, it is passed off to intraocular forcep in the midvitreous cavity.

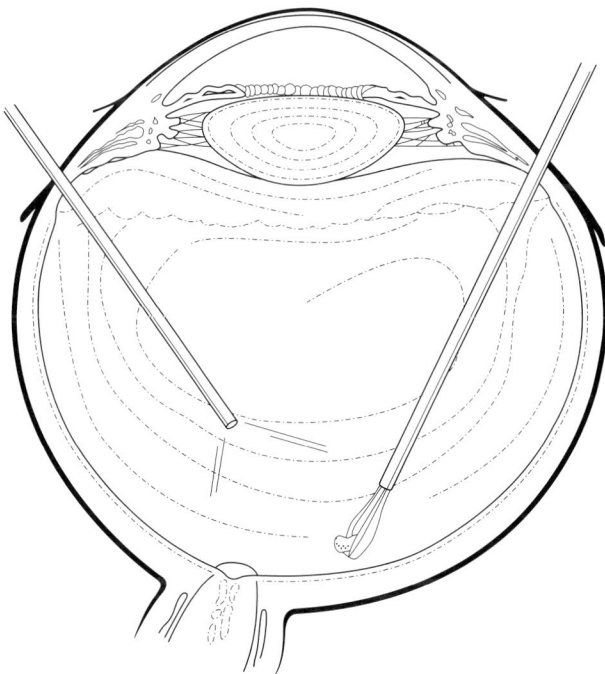

FIGURE 47.14 Pars plana vitrectomy with forcep removal of the IOFB should be used in all cases of nonmagnetic foreign bodies; posterior, incarcerated foreign bodies; media opacities precluding view of the IOFB or fundus; associated ocular injuries requiring vitrectomy, lensectomy, or other manipulation; and with signs and symptoms of endophthalmitis. Schematic diagram depicting nonmagnetic IOFB lying near retinal surface. Following pars plana vitrectomy to clear media opacities, the IOFB is grasped with intraocular forcep and removed from the eye.

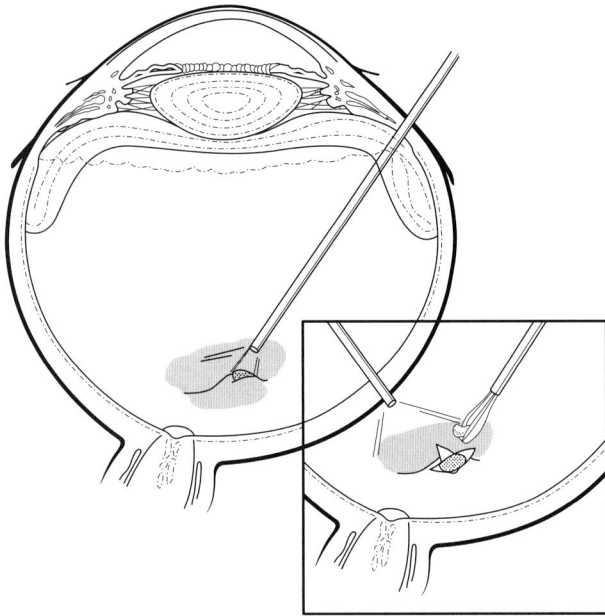

FIGURE 47.15 Schematic diagram showing incarcerated intraretinal foreign body. The foreign body is freed of all incarcerated tissue and any encapsulated material before removal with intraocular forcep. Endophotocoagulation may be applied around the base of the IOFB either before or after removal.

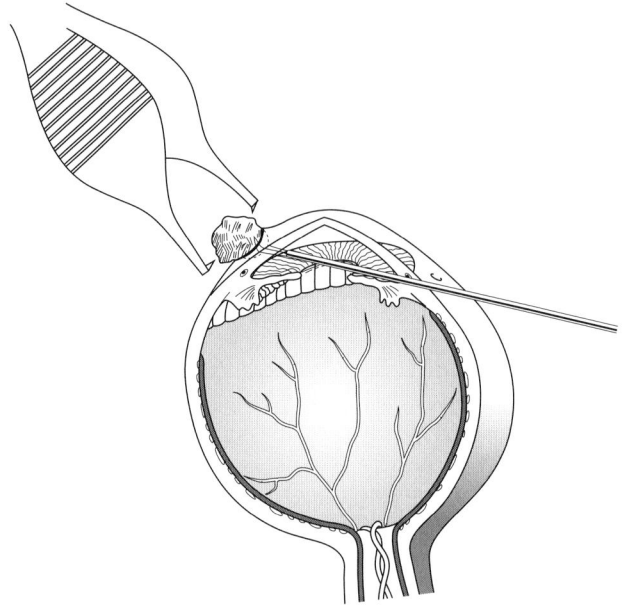

FIGURE 47.16 If an IOFB is too large to be safely removed through the pars plana, it may be brought into the anterior chamber and removed via a limbal wound. Intraocular forcep passes the IOFB through the pupil into the anterior chamber, where it may be grasped externally with forcep.

FIGURE 47.17 Antibiotic prophylaxis is placed intracamerally following penetrating trauma when the status of the posterior pole is unknown, or choroidals prevent safe entry of the posterior pole.

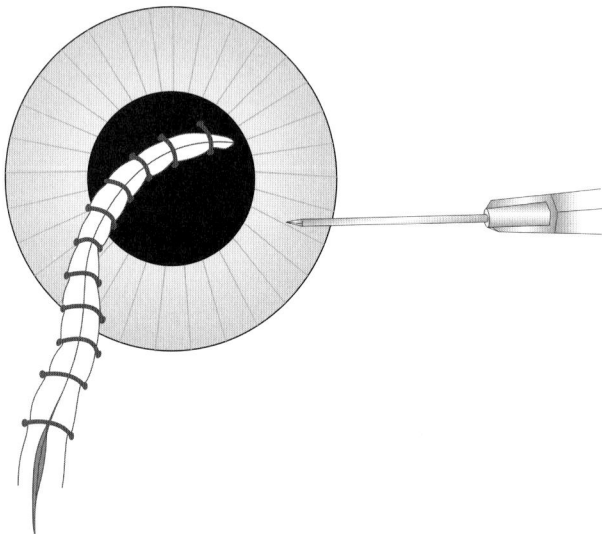

TABLE 47.3 *Potential Complications of Open Globe Injuries*

Traumatic endophthalmitis
Choroidal hemorrhage
Retinal detachment
Proliferative vitreoretinopathy

SELECTED REFERENCES

Albert DM, Lucarelli MJ. *The Clinical Atlas of Procedures in Ophthalmic Surgery*, Chicago: American Medical Association; 2003.

Cebulla CM, Flynn HW Jr. Endophthalmitis after open globe injuries. *Am J Ophthalmol.* 2009;147(4):567–568.

Kuhn F, Pieramici DJ. *Ocular Trauma: Principles and Practice.* New York: Thieme Medical Publishers; 2002, p. 277.

Lieb DF, Scott IU, Flynn HW, Miller D, Feuer WJ. Open globe injuries with positive intraocular cultures Factors influencing final visual acuity outcomes. *Ophthalmology.* 2003 Aug;110(8):1560–1566.

Pieramici DJ, Au Eong KG, Sternberg P Jr, Marsh MJ. The prognostic significance of a system for classifying mechanical injuries of the eye (globe) in open-globe injuries. *J Trauma.* 2003;54 (4):750–754.

48

Endophthalmitis

Dennis P. Han, MD

TABLE 48.1 *Table of Indications*

Procedure	Indication (for all procedures listed)
Intraocular sampling techniques and dosages for intravitreal antimicrobial agents Vitreous biopsy and vitreous needle tap Diagnostic anterior chamber tap Pars plana vitrectomy techniques for severe infectious endophthalmitis, ancillary techniques	Presumed infectious endophthalmitis

Intraocular Sampling Techniques and Dosages for Intravitreal Antimicrobial Agents

*Procedure: Vitreous Biopsy and Vitreous Needle Tap For presumed Infectious Endophthalmitis**

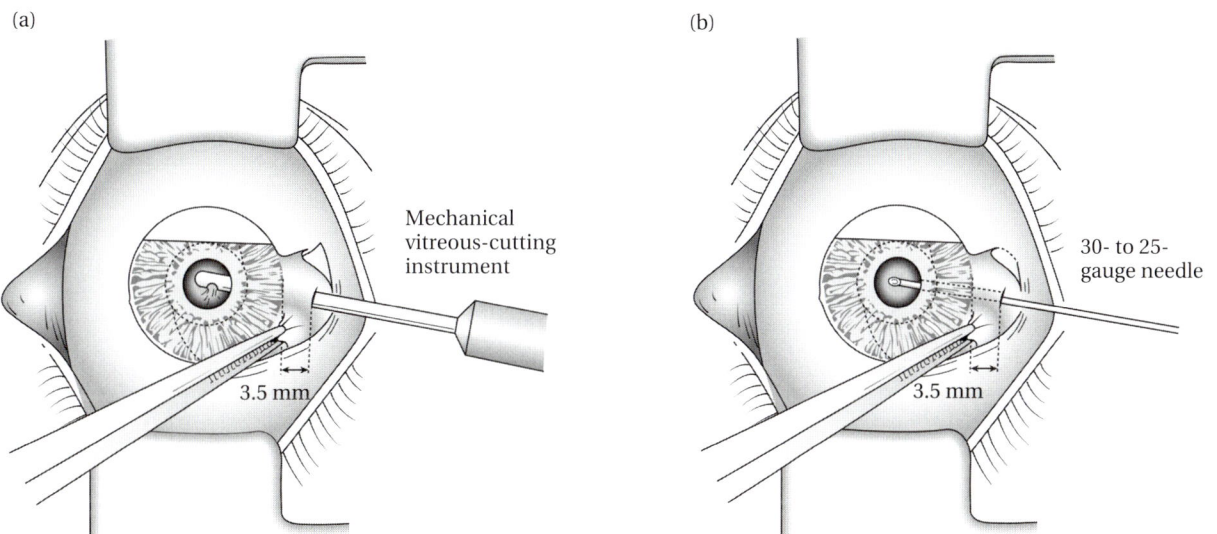

FIGURE 48.1 **Vitreous Biopsy and Vitreous Tap** Vitreous samples may be obtained by vitreous biopsy using a vitreous-cutting instrument or by needle tap. (a) Vitreous biopsy. After topical anesthesia and proper antisepsis, a subconjunctival injection of anesthetic is first administered in a temporal quadrant 4 mm posterior to limbus. A T-shaped conjunctival incision is made and the vitreous-cutting instrument is inserted into the vitreous cavity through a sclerotomy incision placed 3.5 mm posterior to the limbus. Approximately 0.2–0.3 mL of vitreous is removed from the anterior vitreous cavity using the automated cutting mechanism of the probe and slow, manual aspiration of vitreous fluid. If 20-gauge instrumentation is used, conjunctival suture closure is usually required. (b) Vitreous needle tap. A 30- to 25-gauge needle attached to a 1 mL tuberculin syringe is inserted into the vitreous cavity 3.0–3.5 mm posterior to the limbus. Approximately 0.2–0.3 mL is gently aspirated. If resistance is met and no fluid vitreous can be obtained, a vitreous biopsy must be performed instead, to avoid aspirating formed vitreous. Following acquisition of a vitreous specimen, intravitreal injections of appropriate antibiotics are given via the pars plana in phakic or pseudophakic eyes, or via the limbus in aphakic eyes. See Table 48.2 for dosage of commonly used antibiotics. (Reprinted with permission from Albert D, Lucarelli M. *Clinical Atlas of Procedures in Ophthalmic Surgery,* 1st ed. American Medical Association Press, 2003.)

*If pars plana vitrectomy is not planned or possible, a vitreous biopsy or needle tap is performed to obtain microbiological specimens and permit injections of intraocular antibiotics without severe intraocular pressure elevation. In cases of endogenous endophthalmitis, in which identification of a systemically infecting agent may be a high priority, a mechanized vitreous biopsy may be preferred over a needle tap, the latter of which may not always be successful in obtaining a specimen due to formed vitreous occluding the needle.

TABLE 48.2 *Dosages of Commonly Used Intravitreal Antimicrobial Agents for Treatment of Infectious Endophthalmitis*

Antimicrobial agent	Intravitreal dose (usually given in 0.1 mL volume)
Vancomycin	1 mg
Ceftazidime	2.25 mg
Amikacin	400 mcg
Clindamycin	250 mcg
Amphotericin	5–10 mcg
Voriconazole	100 mcg

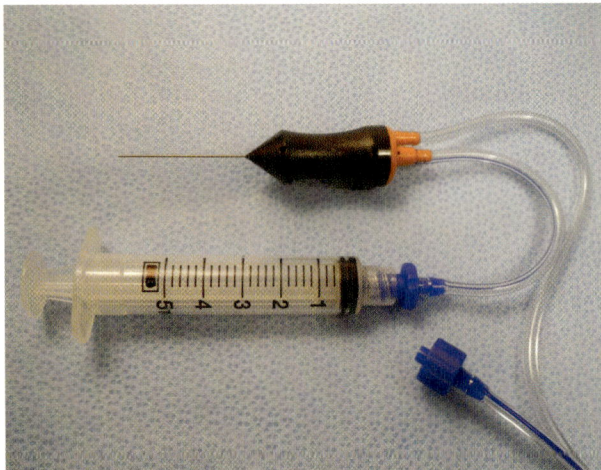

FIGURE 48.2 Modification of the vitreous-cutting instrument to allow vitreous biopsy. A 1–5 mL syringe is attached to the aspiration tubing of the vitreous-cutting instrument via a female Luer lock microadapter or connector supplied commercially with the cutter. To minimize dead space, the tubing is kept short. Volume of the syringe must exceed dead space by at least the amount of specimen desired. During activation of cutting mechanism, manual aspiration of 0.2–0.4 mL of vitreous fluid into the tubing is performed. Once the vitreous cutter is removed from the eye, the fluid can be aspirated into the syringe and submitted for microbiological studies. If proceeding to subsequent vitrectomy, care must be taken to reconnect tubing to proper configuration to avoid dangerous intraocular pressure elevation from pneumatic drive mechanism.

Anterior Chamber Tap for Presumed Infectious Endophthalmitis*

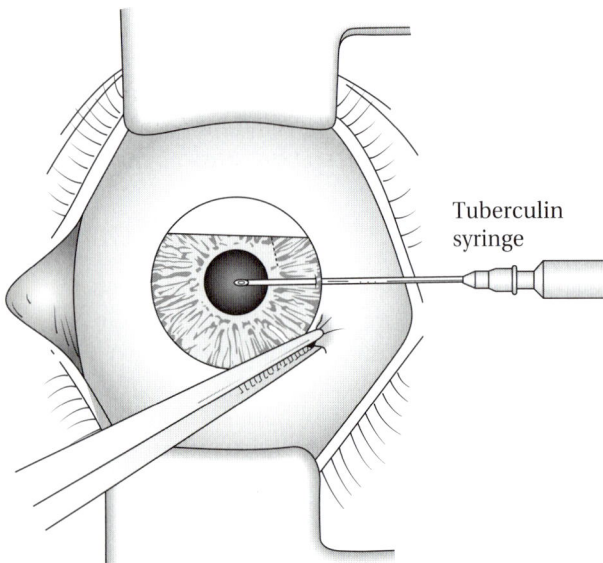

Tuberculin syringe

FIGURE 48.3 Anterior chamber tap (surgeon's view). The episclera is first grasped near the limbal insertion site with 0.12 mm toothed forceps, followed by insertion of a 27- to 30-gauge needle attached to a 1 mL (tuberculin) syringe into the anterior chamber. Aspiration of 0.1–0.2 mL of aqueous fluid into the syringe is performed manually. The limbal entry wound is usually self-sealing. (Reprinted with permission from Albert D, Lucarelli M. *Clinical Atlas of Procedures in Ophthalmic Surgery,* 1st ed. American Medical Association Press, 2003.)

*Indicated for cases in which insufficient vitreous specimen is acquired from vitreous tap (less than 0.1–0.2 ml), and severe intraocular pressure elevation is expected following injection of intravitreal antibiotics; may also be performed optionally in addition to vitreous tap/biopsy to increase specimen for microbiological studies.

Pars Plana Vitrectomy Techniques for Acute Postoperative Endophthalmitis following cataract surgery* and for Severe Infectious Endophthalmitis of Various Etiologies, Ancillary Techniques

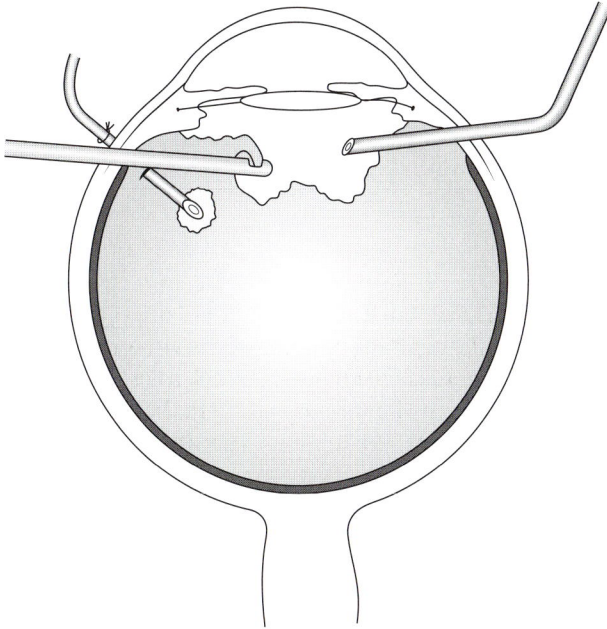

FIGURE 48.4 Initial approach to three port vitrectomy when pars plan infusion cannula cannot be visualized due to severe media opacity. A pars plana vitrectomy can be carried out as either a 2-port or 3-port procedure. In the 3-port procedure, an infusion cannula is secured through a sclerotomy 3.5 mm posterior to the limbus. If the sutured infusion cannula is obscured by media opacity, an angled 20-gauge cannula or bent needle can be inserted through the pars plana into the retropupillary space as a secondary infusion, until the sutured cannula tip can be seen within the vitreous cavity. Microscope illumination is used. Subsequently, an endoilluminator may be substituted for the secondary infusion to allow a three port vitrectomy and more posterior viewing without microscope illumination. (Reprinted with permission from Albert D, Lucarelli M. *Clinical Atlas of Procedures in Ophthalmic Surgery,* 1st ed. American Medical Association Press, 2003.)

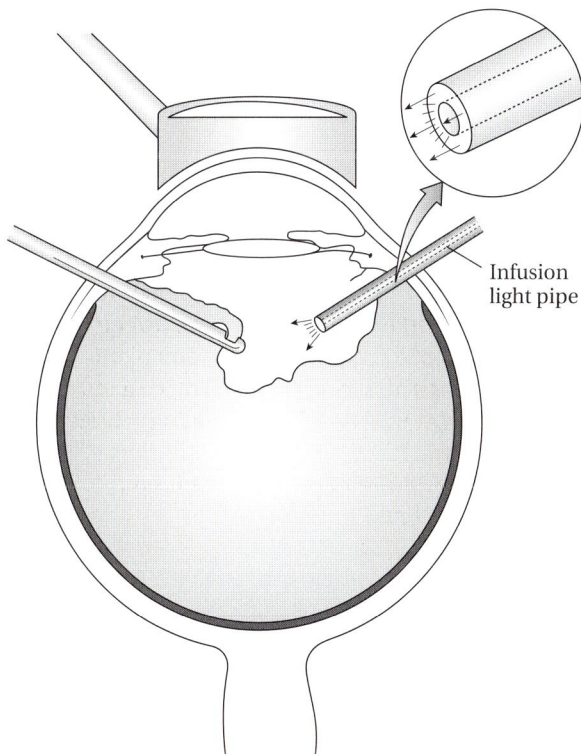

Infusion light pipe

FIGURE 48.5 Two-port vitrectomy using hand-held infusion-endoilluminator. In the 2-port vitrectomy procedure, a handheld infusion-endoilluminator ("irrigating light pipe") is inserted through one of the superior sclerotomies and is used in place of a presutured infusion cannula throughout the procedure. Fluid-air exchange, if needed, can also be performed by injecting air or gas through the infusion-endoilluminator during evacuation of vitreous fluid with an aspirating cannula. (Reprinted with permission from Albert D, Lucarelli M. *Clinical Atlas of Procedures in Ophthalmic Surgery,* 1st ed. American Medical Association Press, 2003.)

* The Endophthalmitis Vitrectomy Study found that pars plana vitrectomy was beneficial for patients with acute postoperative endophthalmitis wvho presented with severe visual loss to the level of light perception only.

(a)

(b)

(c)

(d)

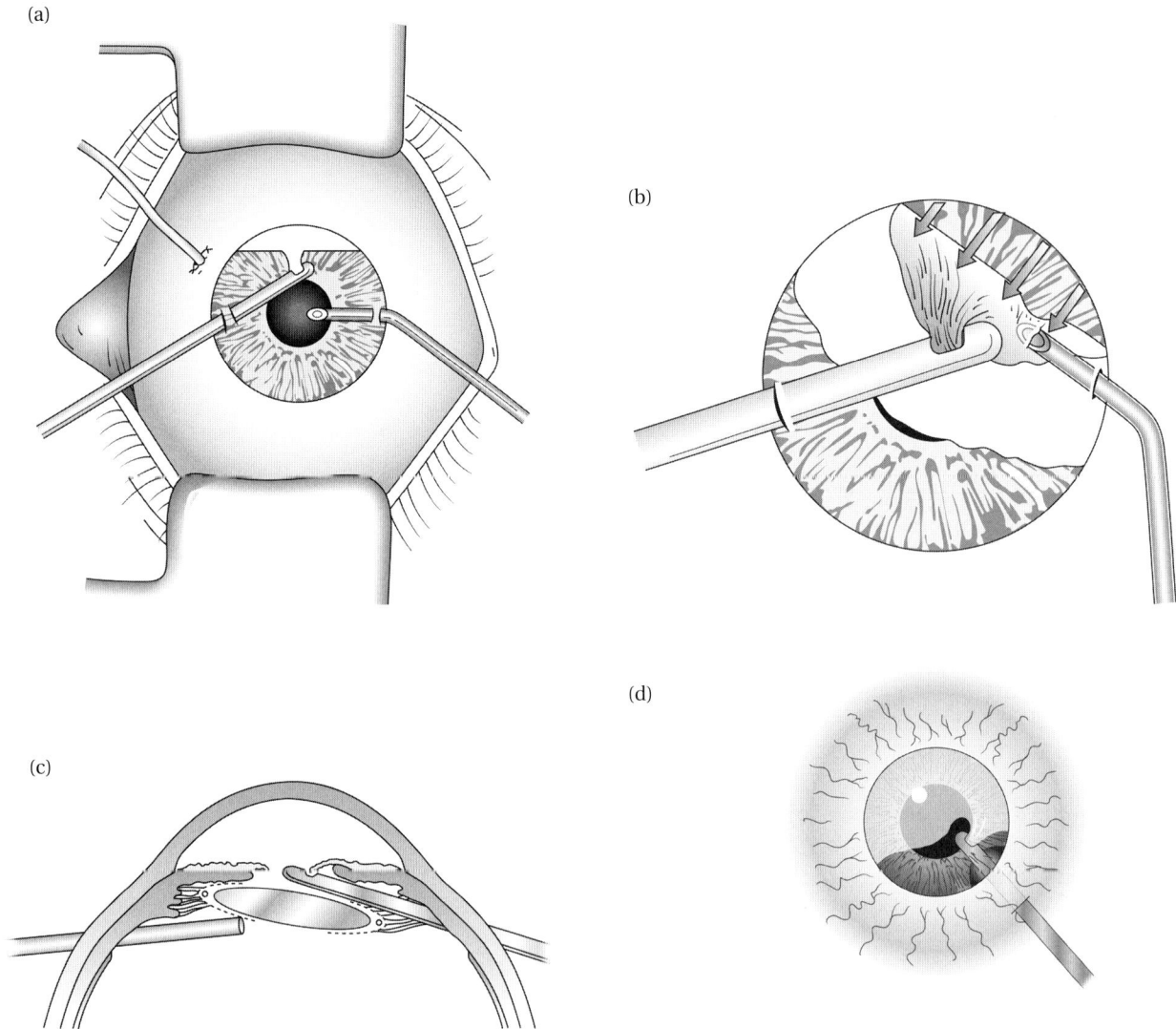

FIGURE 48.6 Technique: Removal of inflammatory membranes on iris and intraocular lens. Inflammatory membranes are commonly adherent to the iris and intraocular lens and may obscure the posterior segment. Removal of these membranes may be required for adequate visualization during pars plana vitrectomy. (a) Removal of anterior chamber opacities with a bimanual, limbal technique. A 20- to 23-gauge bent needle attached to an infusion cannula and a 20- to 23-gauge vitreous-cutting instrument are inserted through the limbus into the anterior chamber at approximately the 2:30 and 9:30 meridians. If present, any layered, purulent material is removed, followed by mobilization of adherent membranes. (b) Removal of adherent membranes in the anterior chamber. Membranes can be engaged initially with the needle or vitreous-cutting instrument, stripped from the surface of the iris, and subsequently excised with the cutting instrument. (c) Posterior approach to inflammatory pupillary membranes, without iridectomy. Vitreous cutter can be inserted behind iris and anterior to posterior intraocular lens optic to gain access to pupillary membranes on anterior IOL surface. High suction should be avoided to reduce risk of anterior chamber collapse. Secondary infusion may be inserted into anterior chamber via pars plana in similar fashion, or via limbus. Surgeon must monitor IOL stability during this approach to reduce risk of IOL dislocation. (d) Posterior approach to inflammatory pupillary membranes, with iridectomy (surgeon's view). Access to anterior chamber is created by performing peripheral iridectomy with vitreous cutter through which it may be inserted to remove membranes anterior to IOL and iris. Iridectomy should be placed as superior as possible to reduce risk of postoperative monocular diplopia. (Parts (a) and (b) Reprinted with permission from Albert D, Lucarelli M. *Clinical Atlas of Procedures in Ophthalmic Surgery,* 1st ed. American Medical Association Press, 2003.)

(a)

(b)

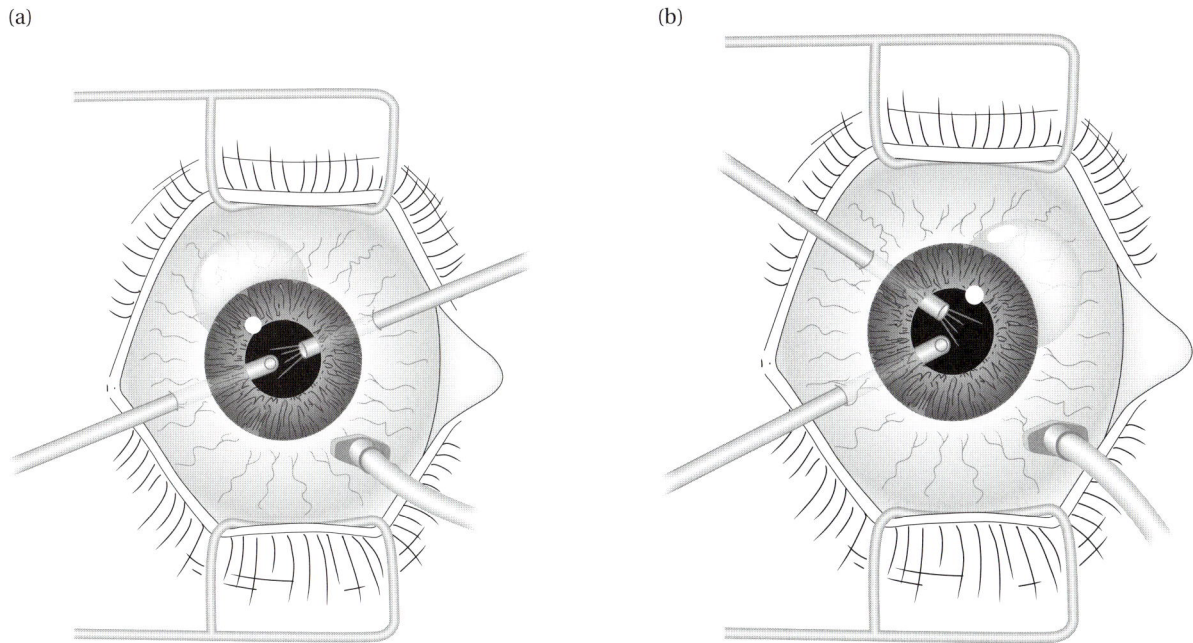

FIGURE 48.7 Technique: Three port pars plana vitrectomy approach in eyes with filtration bleb-related endophthalmitis. In eyes with filtration bleb-related endophthalmitis, in which continued bleb function is desired , the bleb should not be tapped and sclerotomies should be placed away from the bleb, so as to avoid subsequent bleb leak or failure. A pre-existent glaucoma implant tube should similarly be avoided to avoid exposure or extrusion. (a) Configuration of sclerotomy sites for three port vitrectomy in a right eye with bleb precluding superotemporal sclerotomy (upright view). Infusion cannula can be placed inferonasally, allowing inferotemporal sclerotomy to serve as site for vitreous cutter and other hand-held instruments. (b) Configuration of sclerotomy sites if bleb precludes superonasal sclerotomy (upright view). Infusion cannula is placed inferonasally and sites for hand-held instruments are placed superotemporally and inferotemporally. Surgeon is positioned temporally and should be prepared for a smaller degree of separation of hand-held instruments with this approach.

SELECTED REFERENCES

Doft BH, Lobes LA, Jr., and Rinkoff JS. A technique to clear the anterior chamber media to allow pars plana vitrectomy in endophthalmitis. *Ophthalmology.* 1991;98:412–413.

The Endophthalmitis Vitrectomy Study Group. Results of the Endophthalmitis Vitrectomy Study: a randomized trial of vitrectomy and intravenous antibiotics for the treatment of post-operative bacterial endophthalmitis. *Arch Ophthalmol.* 1995;113:1479–1496.

Frambach DA, Ma C, Liggett PE. Modified tubing connections for vitrectomy can be dangerous. *Arch Ophthalmol.* 1990;108:781.

Han DP. Endophthalmitis. In: Albert, D. M. *Ophthalmic Surgery: Principles and Techniques. Volume 1* (pp. 650–662). Malden, MA: Blackwell Science; 1999.

49 Surgical Management of Inflammatory Diseases

Pouya N. Dayani, MD and Glenn J. Jaffe, MD

Fluocinolone Acetonide Implantation

Surgical Treatment of Cytomegalovirus Retinitis with Ganciclovir Implantation

Ganciclovir implantation

SELECTED REFERENCES

Diagnostic Procedures for Inflammatory Eye Disease

TABLE 49.1 *Indications for Vitreous and Transvitreal Chorioretinal Biopsy*

Suspected intraocular malignancy (such as primary intraocular lymphoma)

Uveitis with atypical course

Suspect infection (such as fungal or viral) unresponsive to standard therapy

Suspected intraocular foreign body

Tailor a poorly tolerated therapeutic regimen

Diagnostic Pars Plana Vitrectomy

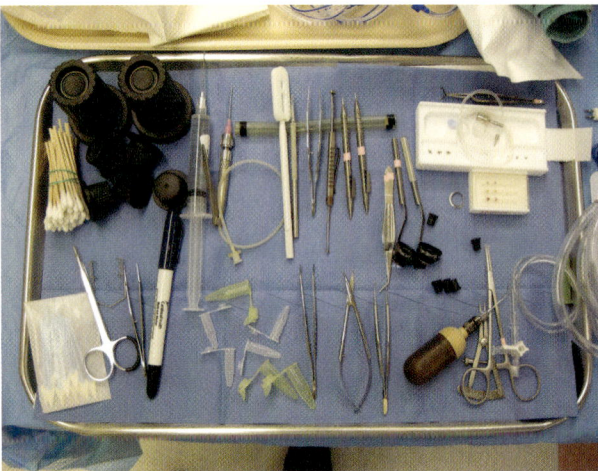

FIGURE 49.1 **Surgical Tray for 20-Gauge Pars Plana Vitrectomy.** A complete setup of all required instruments is essential prior to surgery in order to avoid vitreous loss or delays in specimen handling.

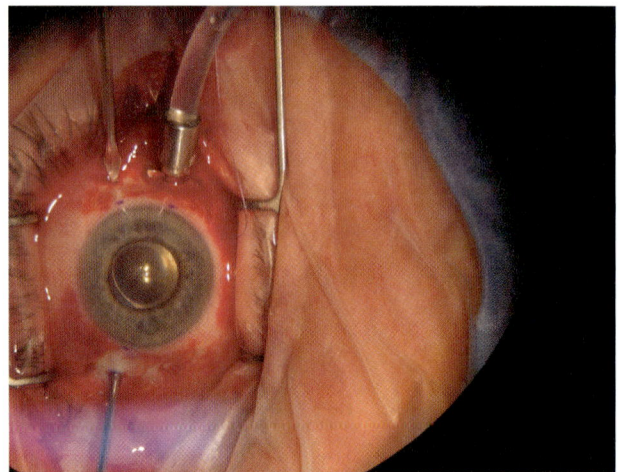

FIGURE 49.2 **20-Gauge Diagnostic Pars Plana Vitrectomy Setup.** 7-0 vicryl sutures are preplaced in the inferotemporal quadrant. An MVR blade is used to create a circumferential sclerotomy 3.5 mm posterior to the surgical limbus. A transscleral cannula is placed, and an infusion line assembled. Two additional sclerotomies are made at the 2:30 and 9:30 position. The light pipe and vitreous cutter are immediately placed in midvitreous cavity to avoid vitreous loss.

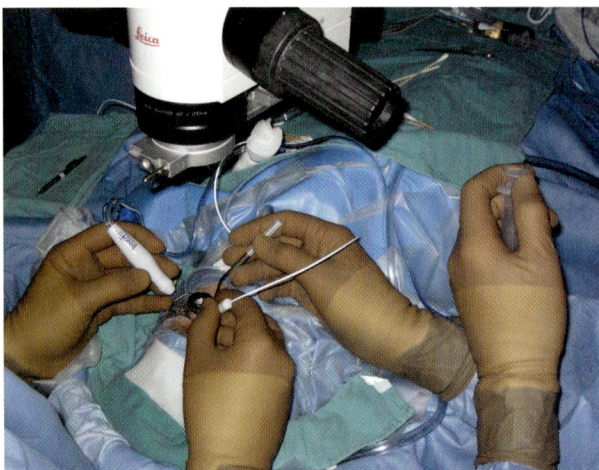

FIGURE 49.3 **Obtaining Vitreous Samples.** To obtain the samples, the vitreous cutter is connected to a 10 mL syringe and the vitrectomy machine is left unprimed. Under direct visualization, an undiluted vitreous sample is first obtained with mechanical cutting and simultaneous manual aspiration by the surgical assistant. The infusion is then begun, and additional diluted samples are obtained in an identical manner. Care must be taken to avoid lenticular or retinal damage as the eye softens.

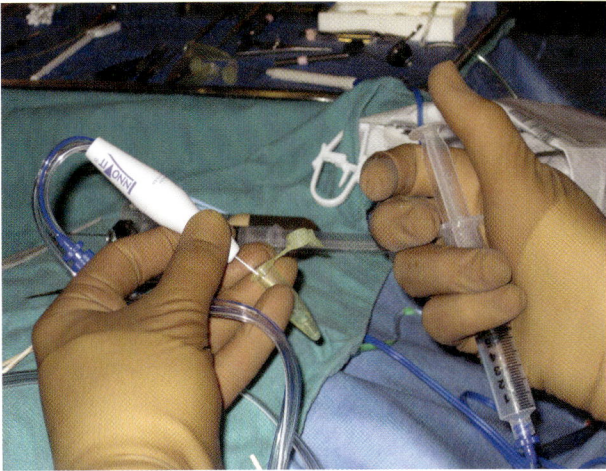

FIGURE 49.4 **Specimen Handling.** Once adequate specimens are obtained, the undiluted and diluted samples are placed in Eppendorf tubes and immediately sent for appropriate laboratory testing, including culture, cytopathologic, flow cytometric, and PCR analysis.

Transvitreal Chorioretinal Biopsy

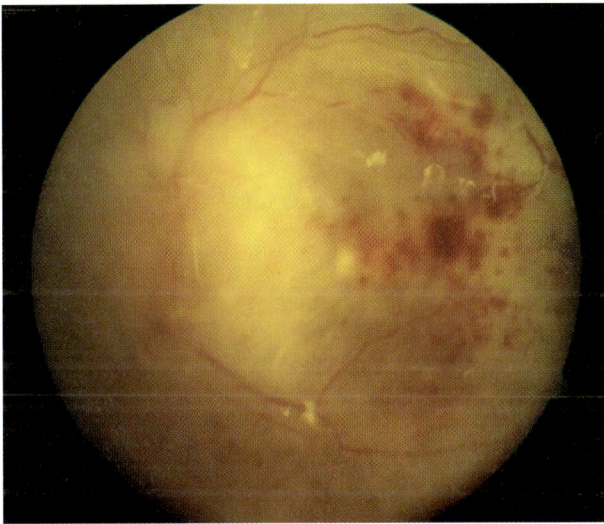

FIGURE 49.5 **Case Presentation—Preoperative Fundus Photo.** Fundus photo of a 57-year-old African-American male with a history of HIV infection and non-Hodgkin's lymphoma, status post-chemotherapy. There is significant optic nerve whitening and obscured disc margins. The veins appear engorged, and there is retinal whitening with scattered intraretinal hemorrhages. (Photo courtesy of Dr. Prithvi Mruthyunjaya.)

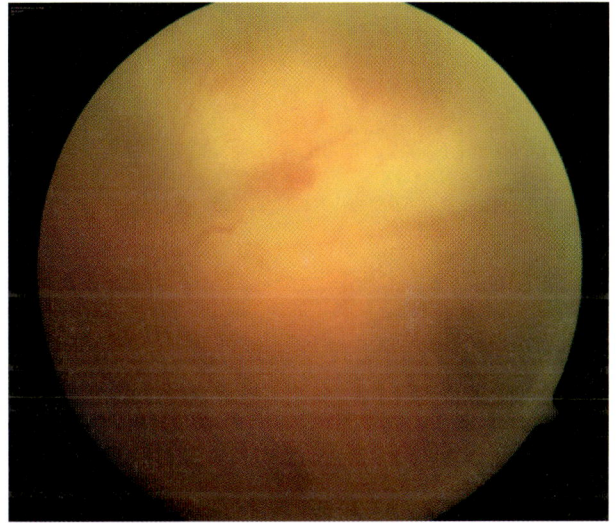

FIGURE 49.6 **Case Presentation—Preoperative Fundus Photo.** Area of planned retinochoroidal biopsy showing active vitreous and vascular inflammation, retinal whitening and hemorrhage. (Photo courtesy of Dr. Prithvi Mruthyunjaya.)

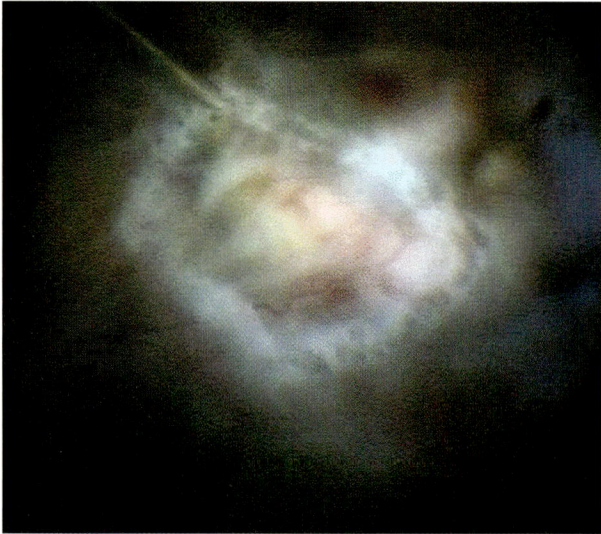

FIGURE 49.7 **Endodiathermy for Hemostasis.**
Following complete 20 gauge pars plana vitrectomy,
generous endodiathermy is used to surround the
area of planned biopsy. (Photo courtesy of Dr. Prithvi
Mruthyunjaya.)

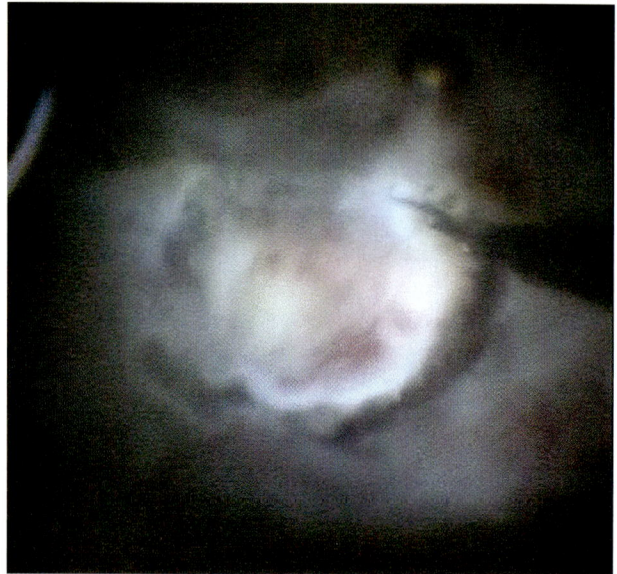

FIGURE 49.8 **Obtaining a Full-Thickness
Chorioretinal Sample.** Using a combination
of intraocular scissors (curved horizontal or
automated MPC scissors) and the vitreous cutter, an
incision is created and extended within the area of
endodiathermy. A small hinge of tissue is left to keep
the specimen attached. (Photo courtesy of Dr. Prithvi
Mruthyunjaya.)

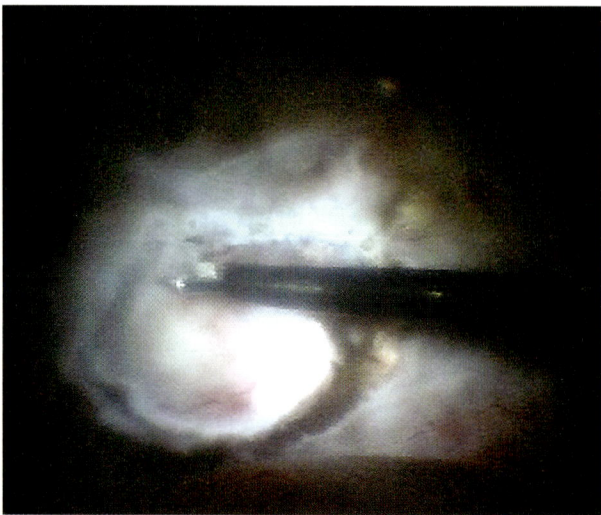

FIGURE 49.9 **Removal of Tissue Specimen.** One
sclerotomy is enlarged in preparation for the removal
of the specimen. Diamond-dusted end-grasping
intraocular forceps are used to grasp the tissue and
remove it from the enlarged incision. The specimen
is then placed on filter paper and sent to pathology
for review. Fluid-air exchange is performed,
endolaser photocoagulation applied, and the eye is
left with silicone oil. (Photo courtesy of Dr. Prithvi
Mruthyunjaya.)

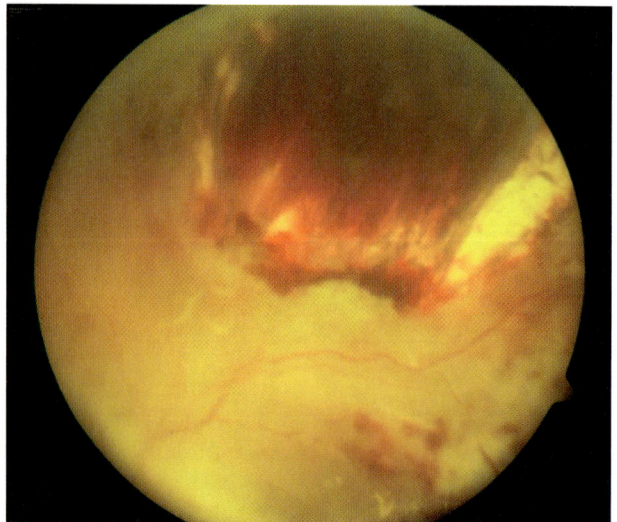

FIGURE 49.10 **Case Presentation—Postoperative
Fundus Photo.** The area of retinochoroidal biopsy
with healed borders and resolving hemorrhage
following surgery. The specimen was diagnostic for
large B-cell lymphoma. (Photo courtesy of Dr. Prithvi
Mruthyunjaya.)

TABLE 49.2 *Complications of Diagnostic Vitrectomy and Transvitreal Chorioretinal Biopsy*

Retinal Detachment

Infection
Vitreous or subretinal hemorrhage
Tumor Seeding
Cataract
Exacerbation of inflammation

Surgical Treatment of Inflammatory Eye Disease

TABLE 49.3 *Indications for Ocular Steroid Administration*

Routes of Ocular Steroid Administration	Indications
Topical	Anterior segment inflammation
SubTenon (anterior or posterior)/Intravitreal injection	Anterior and posterior segment inflammation, macular edema, and retinal vein occlusion
Retisert implantation (triamcinolone acetonide)/Ozurdex injection (dexamethasone)	Chronic, refractory, posterior segment inflammation, diabetic macular edema, and retinal vein occlusion

Sub-Tenon Steroid Injection

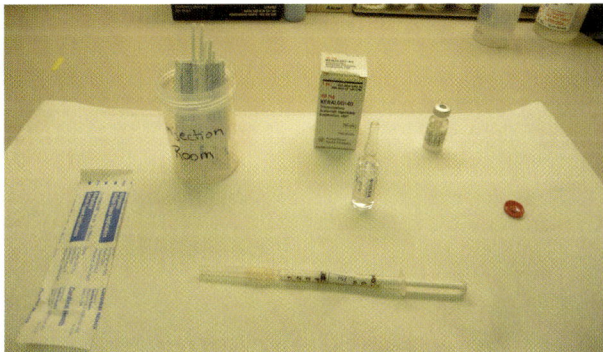

FIGURE 49.11 **Setup for Posterior Sub-Tenon Steroid Injection.** Cotton tip applicators soaked in 2% lidocaine are used to anesthetize the superior fornix. 40 mg of triamcinolone acetonide is injected with a 25 gauge, 5/8-inch needle on 1 mL tuberculin or 3 mL syringe.

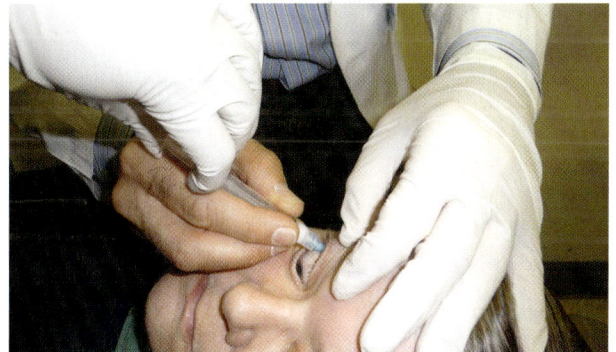

FIGURE 49.12 **Technique for Posterior Sub-Tenon Steroid Injection.** With the patient looking down and in, the needle is advanced along the superotemporal quadrant posteriorly with the bevel toward the globe. The syringe is moved side to side while advancing along the contour of the globe, to ensure that the sclera is not engaged. Once the hub is reached, the steroid is slowly injected.

Intravitreal Injection

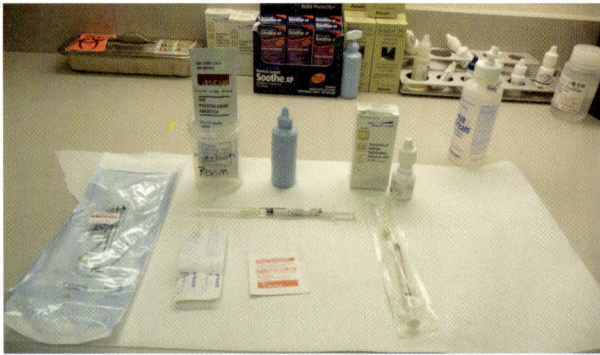

FIGURE 49.13 **Setup for an Intravitreal Injection.**
For an intravitreal injection, a sterile lid speculum,
betadine, cotton-tip applicators, 1 mL tuberculin
syringe, 30- or 32-gauge needle, and topical
antibiotics are required. The site of injection (typically
inferotemporal) is anesthetized with lidocaine-soaked
cotton-tip applicators or ophthalmic gel anesthetic.

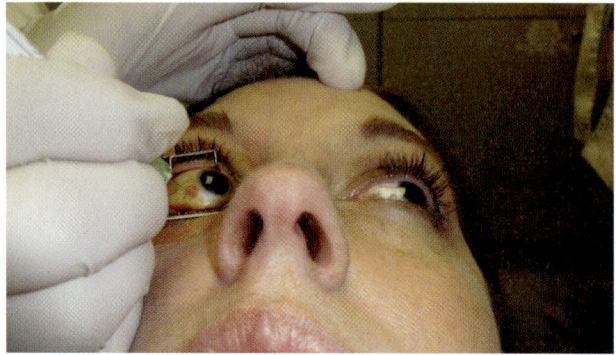

FIGURE 49.14 **Technique for an Intravitreal Injection.**
Once the eye is anesthetized, betadine is applied to
the lid area and a lid speculum is placed. Calipers
are used to mark 3.0 mm from the surgical limbus in
pseudophakic patients (3.5 mm in phakic patients),
and additional betadine is applied to the injection
site. With the patient looking away, the injection
is performed by directing the needle toward the
midvitreous cavity. The needle is slowly withdrawn,
and antibiotic drops are placed. The eye pressure is
measured and the eye irrigated.

Fluocinolone Acetonide Implantation

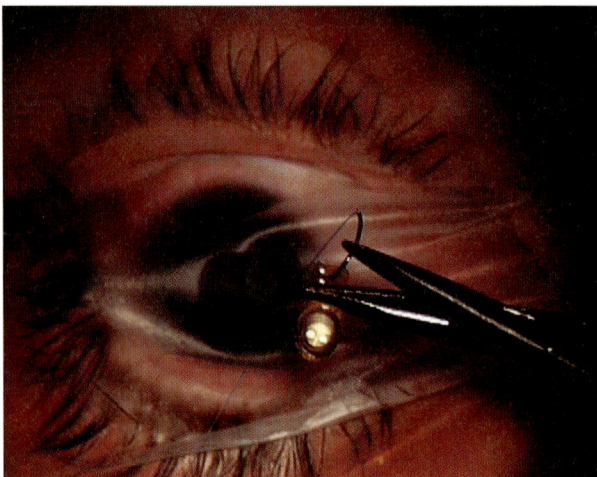

FIGURE 49.15 **Preparing the Retisert Implant.** The
Retisert implant is first prepared by passing an 8-0
double-armed prolene suture through the hole in the
strut. A single suture throw is then placed over the strut
and the implant set aside.

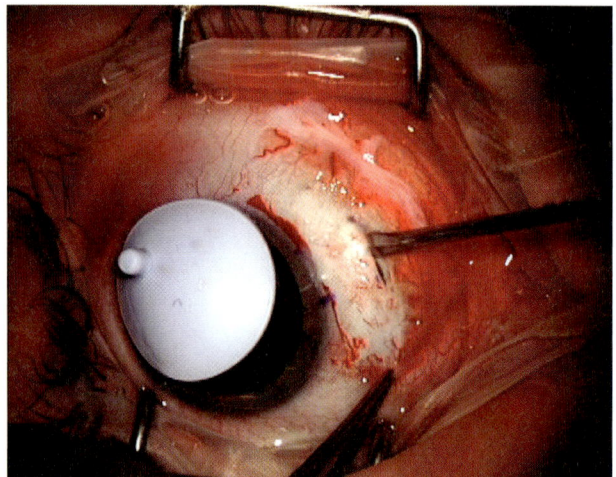

FIGURE 49.16 **Creating a Sclerotomy.** A fornix-based
limbal peritomy is performed in the inferotemporal or
inferonasal quadrant, and diathermy applied. Calipers
are used to make two marks 3.5 mm apart, 3.75–4.0 mm
posterior to the surgical limbus. An MVR blade is used
to create a sclerotomy, ensuring complete penetration
of the pars plana tissue.

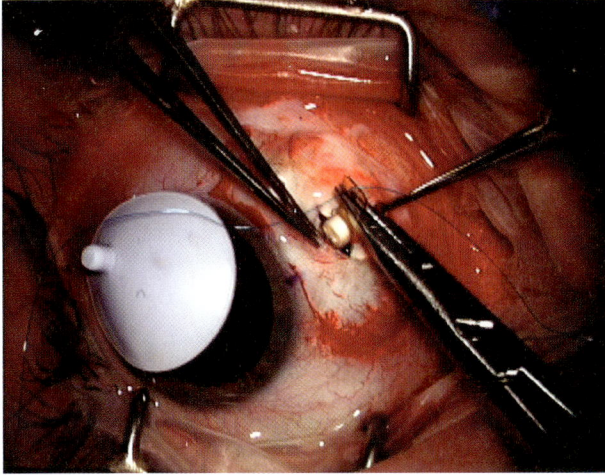

FIGURE 49.17 **Inserting the Implant.** The incision is gaped on both sides with toothed forceps. Prolapsed vitreous is excised with either the vitreous cutter or cellulose sponge and scissors. Using a needle holder to grasp the implant strut, the implant is gently inserted through the scleral incision.

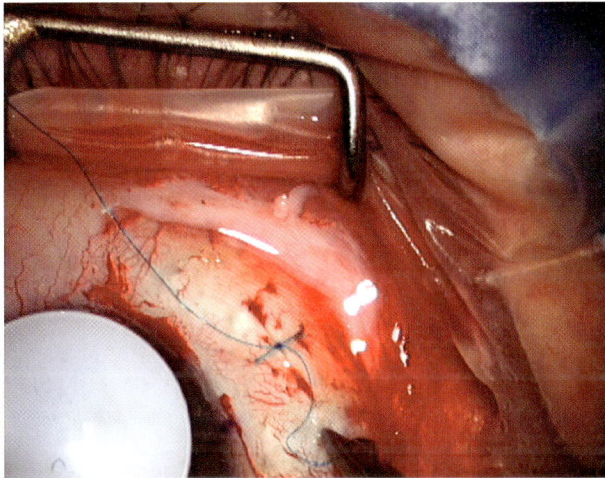

FIGURE 49.18 **Placing the Anchoring Suture.** Using the previously placed 8-0 prolene anchoring suture, full thickness bites are taken on either side of the scleral incision and tied down tightly. The suture ends are temporarily left long. Indirect ophthalmoscopy is performed to confirm correct placement of the implant.

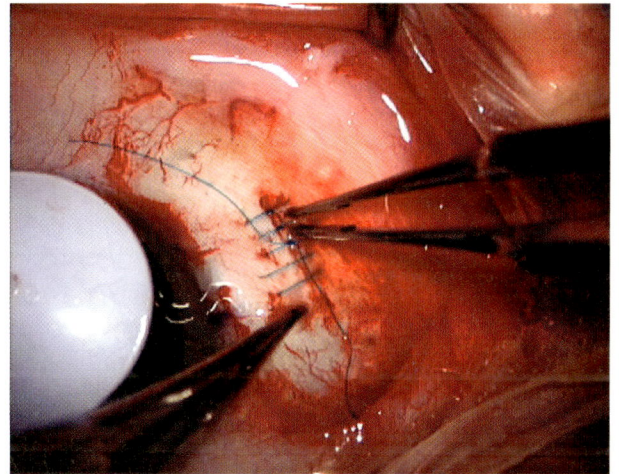

FIGURE 49.19 **Suturing the Sclerotomy.** Using 9-0 prolene, multiple interrupted, partial-thickness sutures are placed and tied over the tails of the anchoring suture. The knots are then buried. The Tenon's and conjunctiva tissue are closed separately with interrupted, 6-0 plain gut sutures.

TABLE 49.4 *Routes of Ocular Steroid Administration and Associated Complications*

Routes of Ocular Steroid Administration	Complications
Topical	Ocular hypertension, cataract and corneal complications
SubTenon (anterior or posterior)	Same as topical, ptosis, subdermal fat atrophy, and inadvertent globe penetration
Intravitreal injection	Same as topical, sterile or infectious endophthalmitis, hemorrhage, and retinal detachment
Ozurdex injection (dexamethasone)	Same as intravitreal injection
Retisert implantation (triamcinolone acetonide)	Same as intravitreal injection, suprachoroidal placement and dislocation
Systemic steroids (oral prednisone)	Acute: Elevation in blood sugar and blood pressure, dyspepsia, electrolyte imbalance, and aseptic necrosis of the femoral head.
	Chronic: Osteoporosis, Cushinoid state, growth retardation, and reactivation of infections.

Surgical Treatment of Cytomegalovirus Retinitis with Ganciclovir Implantation

TABLE 49.5 *Indications for Ganciclovir Implantation*

Vision-threatening CMV retinitis (zone 1) or monocular patient

Unable to tolerate systemic therapy due to adverse effects (i.e., neutropenia, renal disease)

Poor potential for immune reconstitution

Unreliable compliance with therapeutic regimen

CMV = cytomegalovirus virus.

Ganciclovir implantation

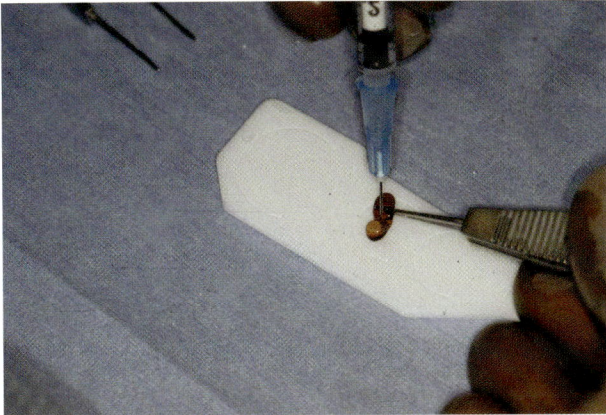

FIGURE 49.20 **Preparing the Ganciclovir Implant.** The implant is first prepared by puncturing a hole in the center of the strut with a 30-gauge needle, 2.0 mm from the edge of the pellet. Wescott scissors are then used to trim the strut 0.5 mm distal to the edge of the previously created hole. An 8-0 double-armed nylon suture is placed through the hole in the strut. (Photo courtesy of Dr. Jay S. Duker.)

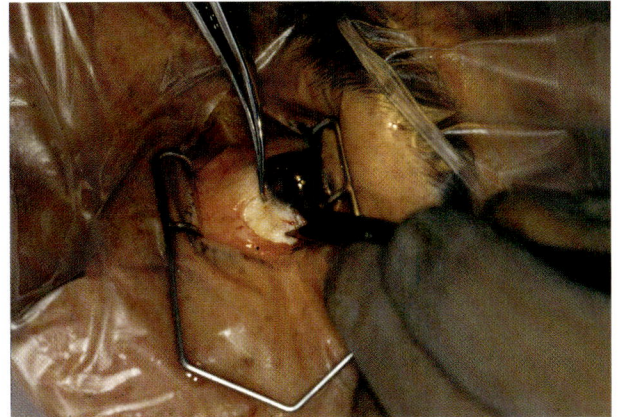

FIGURE 49.21 **Preparing the Site for Implantation.** Once the implant is prepared, a fornix-based limbal conjunctival peritomy is performed in the inferotemporal quadrant and diathermy applied. Calipers are used to create two marks 3.75–4 mm posterior to the surgical limbus and 5–6 mm apart. (Photo courtesy of Dr. Jay S. Duker.)

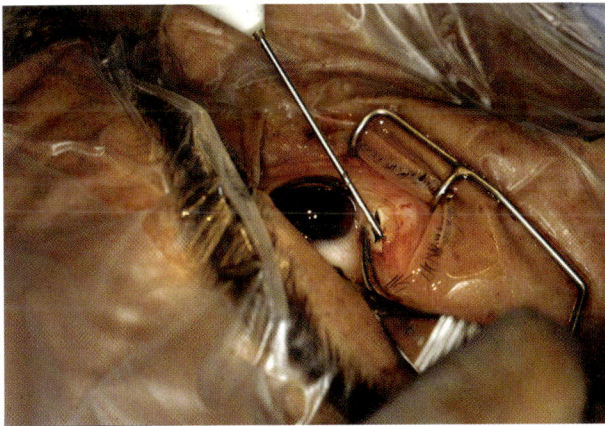

FIGURE 49.22 **Creating the Sclerotomy.** Using forceps to stabilize the globe, an MVR blade is utilized to create a 5–6 mm circumferential sclerotomy while ensuring complete penetration of ciliary tissue. A limited external vitrectomy is performed to remove prolapsed vitreous. (Photo courtesy of Dr. Jay S. Duker.)

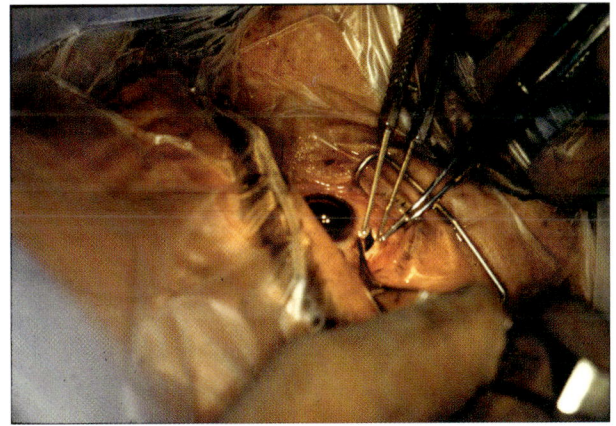

FIGURE 49.23 **Inserting the Ganciclovir Implant.** Toothed forceps are used to grasp the anterior lip of the sclera incision. The implant strut is grasped with smooth forceps and is carefully placed into the vitreous cavity so that the pellet is facing anteriorly (toward the cornea). (Photo courtesy of Dr. Jay S. Duker.)

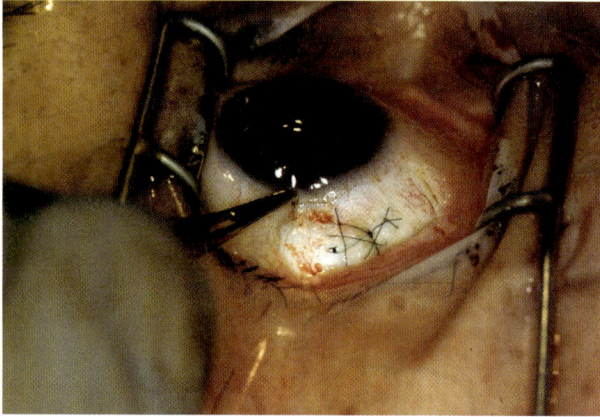

FIGURE 49.24 Suturing of the Sclerotomy. The implant is anchored at the center of the incision using the preplaced 8-0 nylon suture, by taking full thickness bites of the anterior and posterior sclerotomy edges. The suture ends are left long so that they can be tucked under the remaining sutures that are used to close the sclerotomy. (Photo courtesy of Dr. Jay S. Duker.)

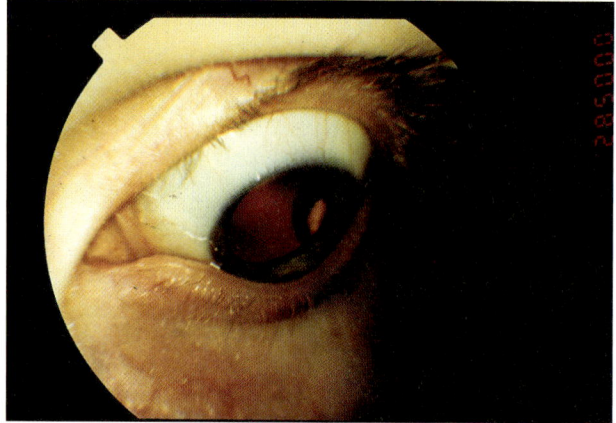

FIGURE 49.25 Confirming Implant Placement. The intraocular pressure is then checked, followed by indirect ophthalmoscopy to ensure proper positioning of the implant. The implant should be in the vitreous cavity with the pellet facing anteriorly. (Photo courtesy of Dr. Jay S. Duker.)

TABLE 49.6 *Complications Associated with Ganciclovir Implantation*

Endophthalmitis

Vitreous hemorrhage

Hypotony

Cataract

Retinal detachment

Astigmatism (typically temporary)

Misplacement (i.e., suprachoroidal space)

SELECTED REFERENCES

Jaffe GJ, Martin D, Callanan D, Pearson PA, Levy B, Comstock T; Fluocinolone Acetonide Uveitis Study Group. Fluocinolone acetonide implant (Retisert) for noninfectious posterior uveitis: thirty-four-week results of a multicenter randomized clinical study. *Ophthalmology.* 2006 Jun;113(6):1020-1027.

Lim LL, Suhler EB, Rosenbaum JT, Wilson DJ. The role of choroidal and retinal biopsies in the diagnosis and management of atypical presentations of uveitis. *Trans Am Ophthalmol Soc.* 2005;103:84-91; discussion 91.

Martin DF, Chan CC, de Smet MD, Palestine AG, Davis JL, Whitcup SM, Burnier MN Jr, Nussenblatt RB. The role of chorioretinal biopsy in the management of posterior uveitis. *Ophthalmology.* 1993 May;100(5):705-714.

Mruthyunjaya P, Jumper JM, McCallum R, Patel DJ, Cox TA, Jaffe GJ. Diagnostic yield of vitrectomy in eyes with suspected posterior segment infection or malignancy. *Ophthalmology.* 2002 Jun;109(6):1123-1129.

Musch DC, Martin DF, Gordon JF, Davis MD, Kuppermann BD. Treatment of cytomegalovirus retinitis with a sustained-release ganciclovir implant. The Ganciclovir Implant Study Group. *N Engl J Med.* 1997 Jul 10;337(2):83-90.

50

Management of Intraocular Tumors

Charles C. Wykoff, MD, PhD and Timothy G. Murray, MD, MBA, FACS

Uveal Melanoma

TABLE 50.1 *Uveal Melanoma Associated Mortality is Related to Tumor Size*

Tumor Size Category	Apical Height (mm)	Longest Basal Diameter (mm)	5-Year Melanoma-Specific Mortality
Small	<2.5	<16	<4%
Medium	2.5–10	<16	10%
Large	>10	>16	30%

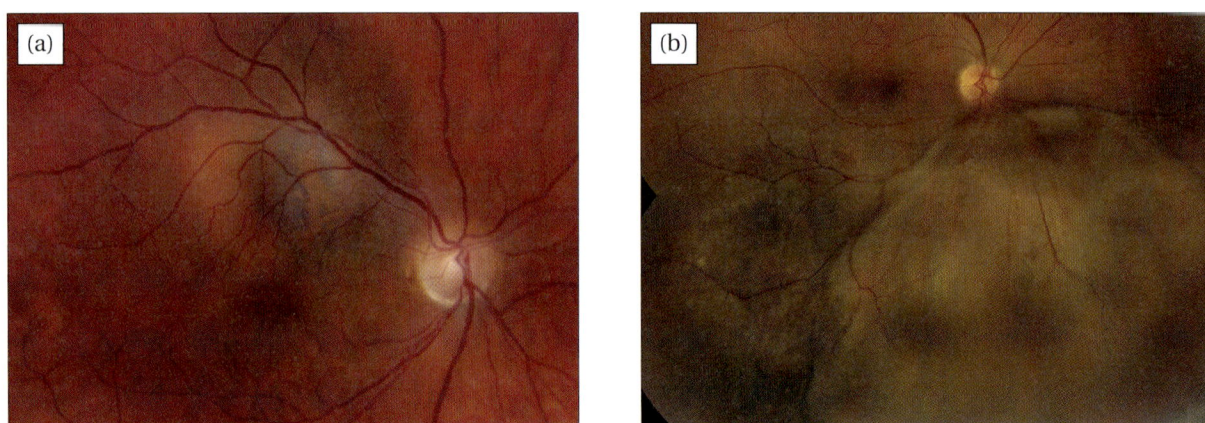

FIGURE 50.1 (a) Small posterior uveal melanoma involving the superior macula with orange pigmentation. (b) Large posterior uveal melanoma with associated serous retinal detachment. (Images courtesy of Ditte Hess, Bascom Palmer Eye Institute Miami, Florida.)

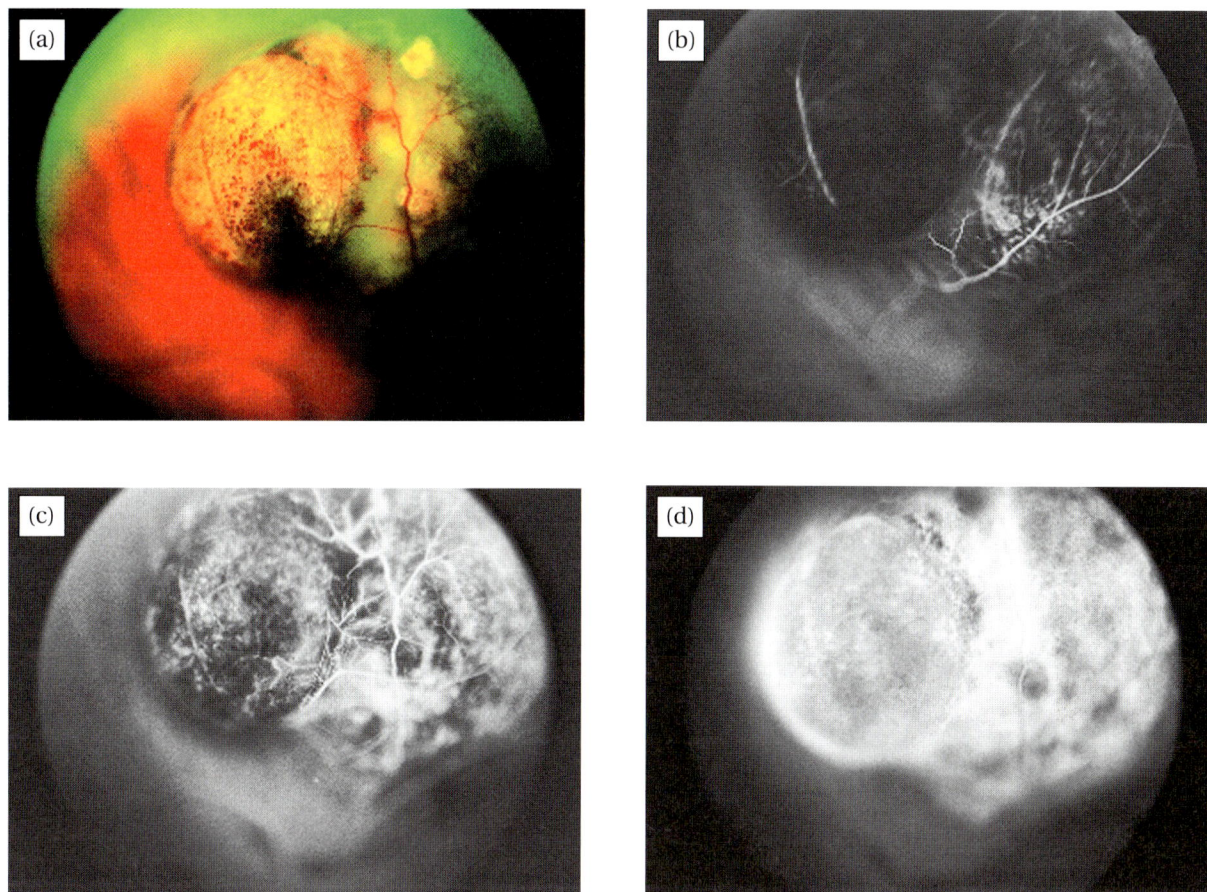

FIGURE 50.2 Uveal melanomas are about 60 times less common than cutaneous melanomas, and are the most common primary intraocular malignancy in adults, with an annual incidence of 6 per 1 million. These tumors originate from the choroid (84%), the ciliary body (10%), or the iris or trabecular meshwork (6%). (a) Pigmented choroidal mass with "collar button" configuration suggesting that it has broken through Bruch's membrane and extended into the subretinal space. (b) Fluorescein angiography of choroidal melanoma. Early frames demonstrate hypofluorescence of the lesion with focal areas of hyperfluorescence. (c) Intrinsic tumor vessels are visualized in addition to the normal choroidal vasculature. (d) Late frames demonstrate diffuse leakage of fluorescein from the tumor vasculature. (Images from Murray T. Management of Intraocular Tumors. In: Albert, D. M. *Ophthalmic Surgery: Principles and Techniques.* Malden, MA: Blackwell Science; 1999, p. 165.)

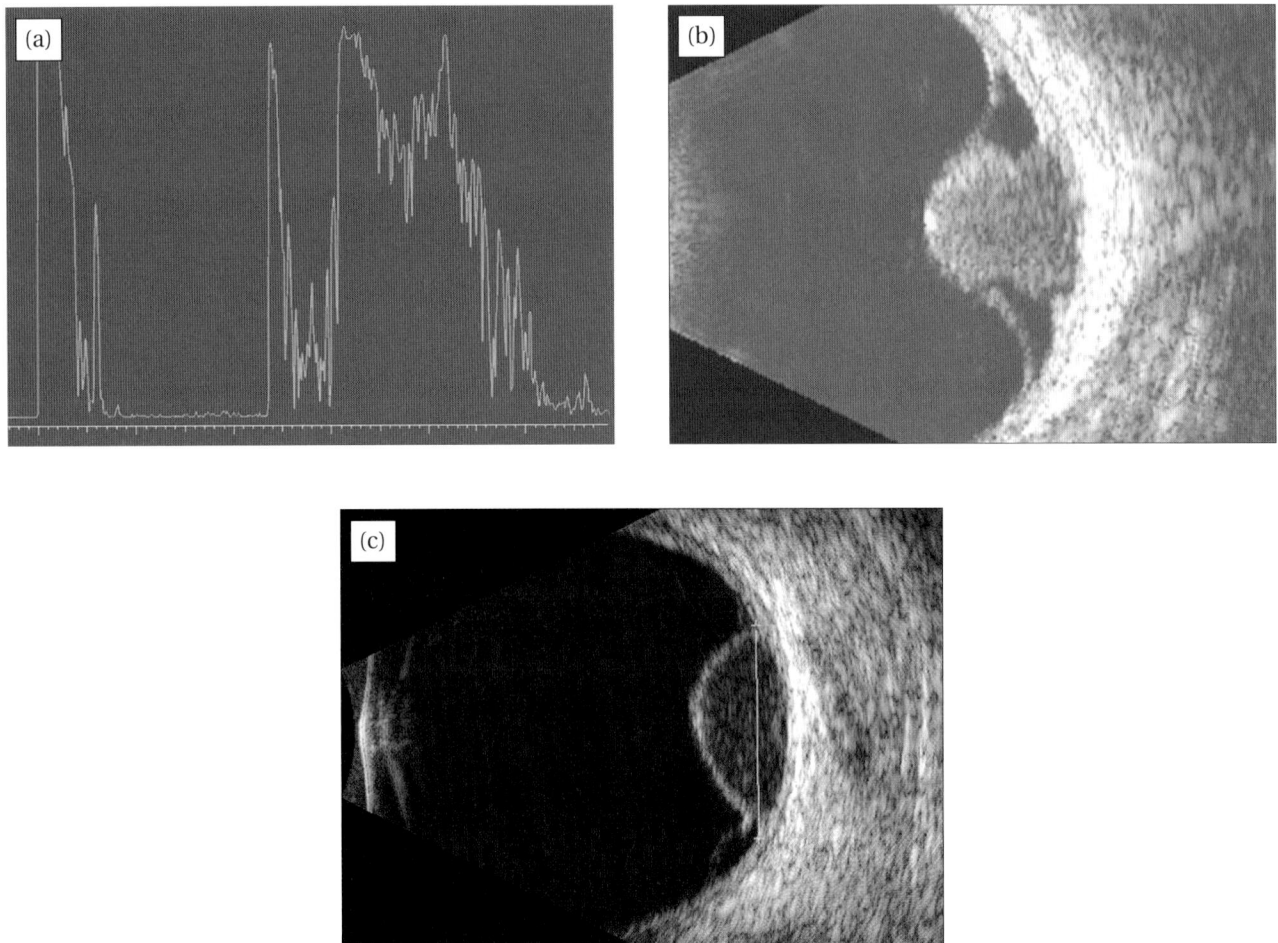

FIGURE 50.3 Echography is the most useful ancillary test for characterizing uveal melanomas with diagnostic accuracy > 95% for tumors with thickness > 2.5 mm in expert hands. (a) A-scan shows regular structure with medium to low internal reflectivity, classically with marked vascularity seen with dynamic evaluation. B-scan imaging of melanomas showing the classic collar button, or mushroom shape with adjacent serous retinal detachment (b), and an internal acoustic quiet zone likely due to attenuation of the signal by the homogenous, dense cellularity of the tumor (c). Choroidal excavation and orbital acoustic shadowing can also be seen.

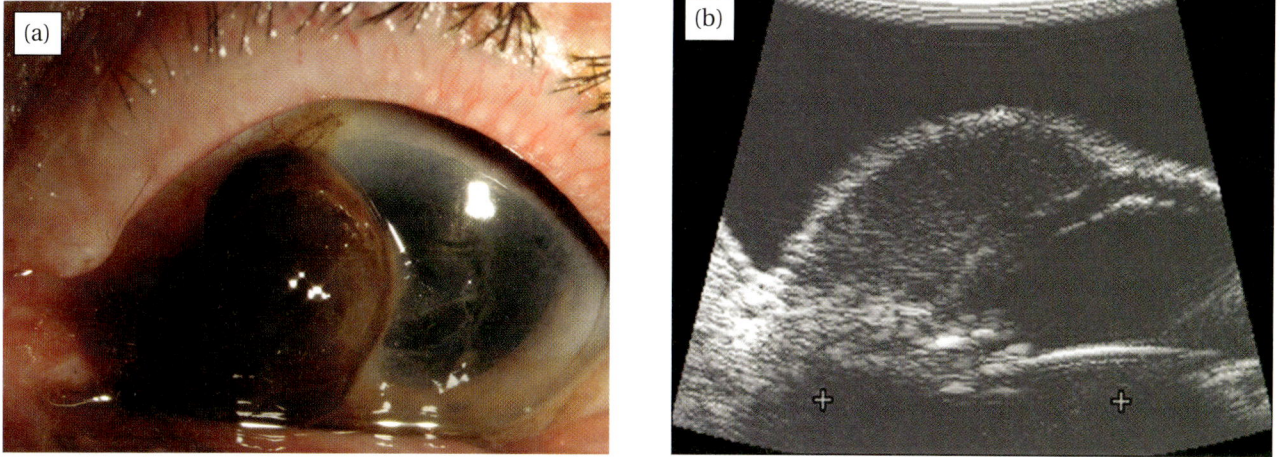

FIGURE 50.4 Uveal melanoma arising from the ciliary body. Melanomas arising from the ciliary body are often not appreciated until they are larger than more posteriorly located uveal melanomas. (a) Ciliary body melanoma with extrascleral extension. Direct extrascleral extension is identified histologically in <5% of eyes with small or medium tumors, and in about 15% of eyes with large melanomas, increasing to 20% when Bruch's membrane is disrupted and >50% if there is invasion into the vitreous cavity. (b) High resolution (20 Hz) anterior segment echogram showing tumor involving the ciliary body and extending onto the ocular surface.

Localizing Intraocular Tumors

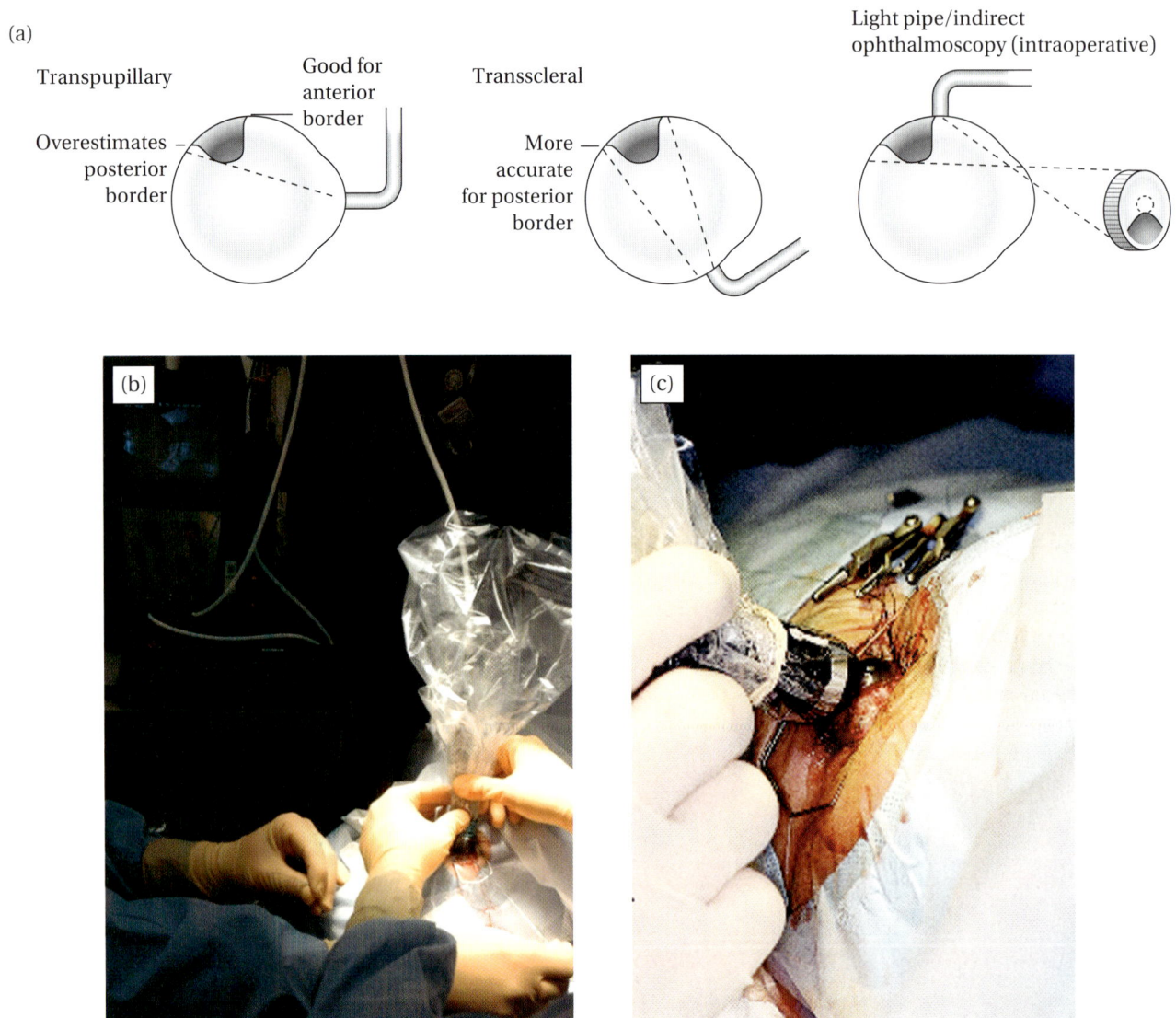

FIGURE 50.5 (a) Transillumination: transpupillary and transscleral transillumination are best for identifying the anterior and posterior tumor margins respectively. Indirect ophthalmoscopy and scleral indentation with fiberoptic light pipe can also be used. (b, c) Intraoperative echography: the probe tip is covered with a sterile sleeve and brought into the surgical field. (Images (a) and (c) from Murray T. Management of Intraocular Tumors. In: Albert, D. M. *Ophthalmic Surgery: Principles and Techniques.* Malden, MA: Blackwell Science; 1999, pp. 166–167.)

Uveal Tumor Biopsy

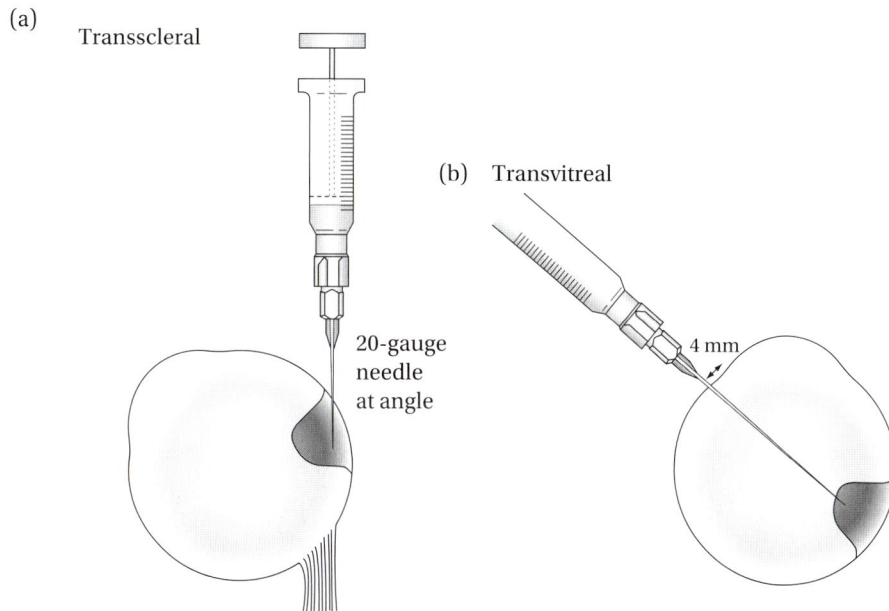

(a)
Transscleral

20-gauge
needle
at angle

(b)   Transvitreal

4 mm

FIGURE 50.6 Fine-needle biopsy of a posterior segment mass is indicated when noninvasive measures cannot reliably establish a diagnosis and when the results of biopsy will affect management. (a) Transscleral biopsy employs a 25- or 27-gauge needle passed through the sclera after localization of the tumor as described above. Moderate aspiration is applied while moving the needle tip along the scleral track. (b) Transvitreal approach employs a long 25- or 27-gauge needle and is guided into the tumor. The scleral entry site is via the pars plana 180° from the lesion. (Images from Murray T. Management of Intraocular Tumors. In: Albert, D. M. *Ophthalmic Surgery: Principles and Techniques*. Malden, MA: Blackwell Science; 1999, p. 166.)

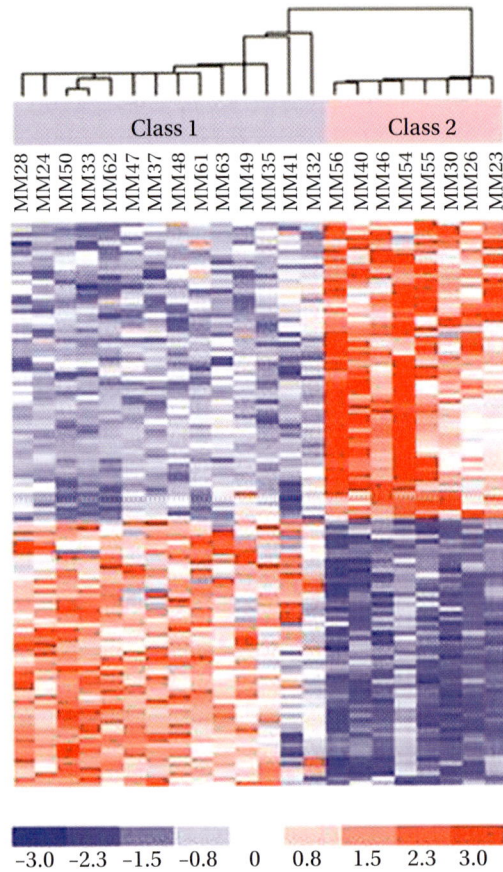

FIGURE 50.7 Gene Array. Uveal melanoma can be highly aggressive, with a strong predilection for hematogenous metastasis, particularly to the liver. By quantifying the amount of specific mRNAs produced by different tumors, mRNA expression profiling has identified two distinct subtypes of uveal melanomas (Class 1 and Class 2), each with a unique phenotype associated with the development of metastatic disease. Tumors with a Class 1 signature are associated with a low metastatic potential, whereas those with a Class 2 signature have a high metastatic potential. Such predictive testing of which patients are at greatest risk for metastatic disease may allow customized therapy and systemic prophylaxis in high-risk patients. Here shown is a hierarchical clustering heat map of gene expression from 22 uveal melanomas, each from a different patient. (Image courtesy of Castle Biosciences Inc., Friendswood, TX.)

Radioactive Plaque Therapy

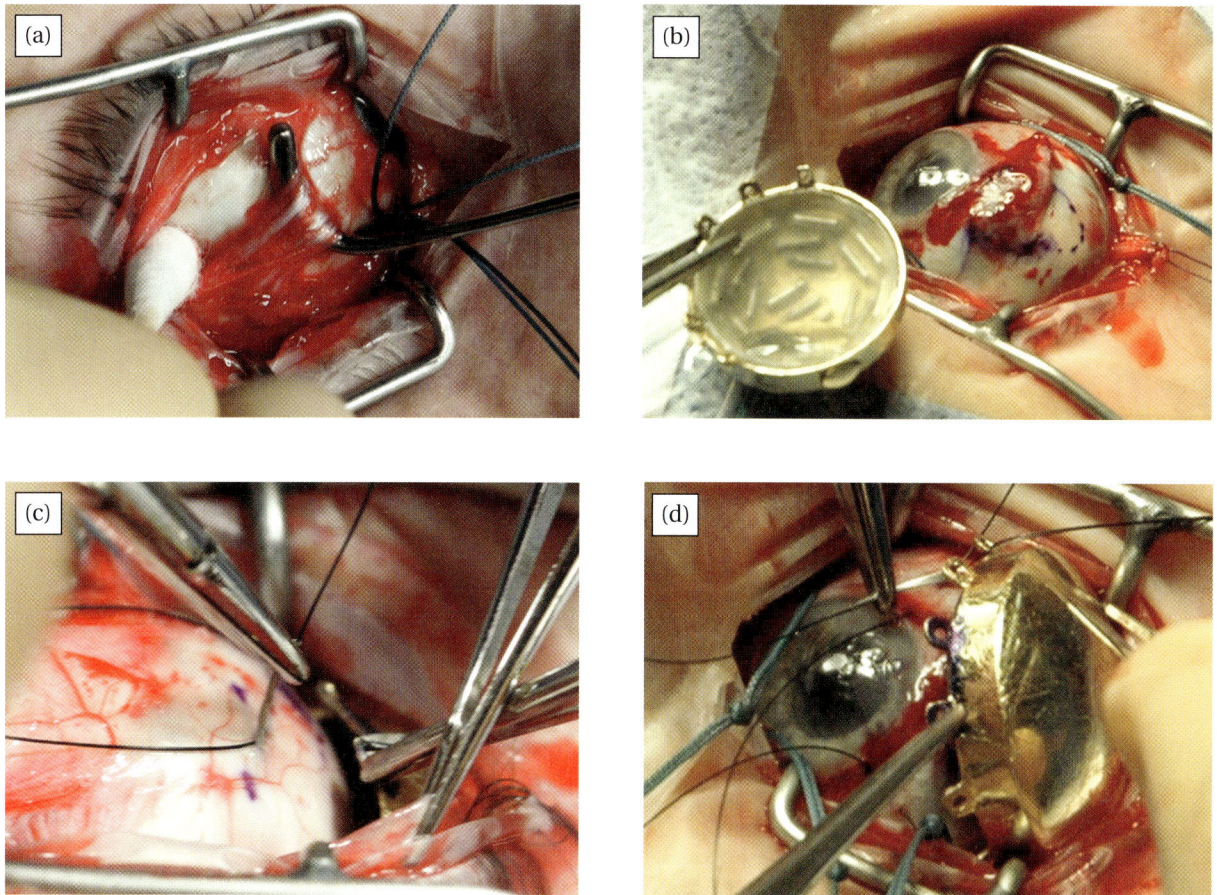

FIGURE 50.8 Episcleral radioactive plaque bracytherapy is the most common treatment for medium-sized choroidal melanomas. Surgical technique for application of episcleral plaque: (a) After conjunctival peritomy, the rectus muscles are isolated with sutures. The tumor is localized with transillumination or direct visualization, the margins are marked with a sterile pen, and the pre-constructed plaque is brought into the surgical field. (b) Here shown is a Collaborative Ocular Melanoma Study (COMS)-type gold plaque with iodine-125 seeds. Any rectus muscle blocking access to the tumor is secured with double-armed polyglactin 910 (Vicryl) suture and temporarily disinserted. (c, d) The radioactive plaque is secured to the sclera with three 5-0 nylon sutures, each passed in a lamellar fashion through sclera and then through a plaque islet. Accurate plaque localization is then confirmed with intraoperative echography, confirming ≥ 2 mm plaque margin beyond the extent of the tumor in all directions. The overlying conjunctiva is re-approximated, and the eye is then covered with a lead shield. The radioactive plaque is removed 3 days later.

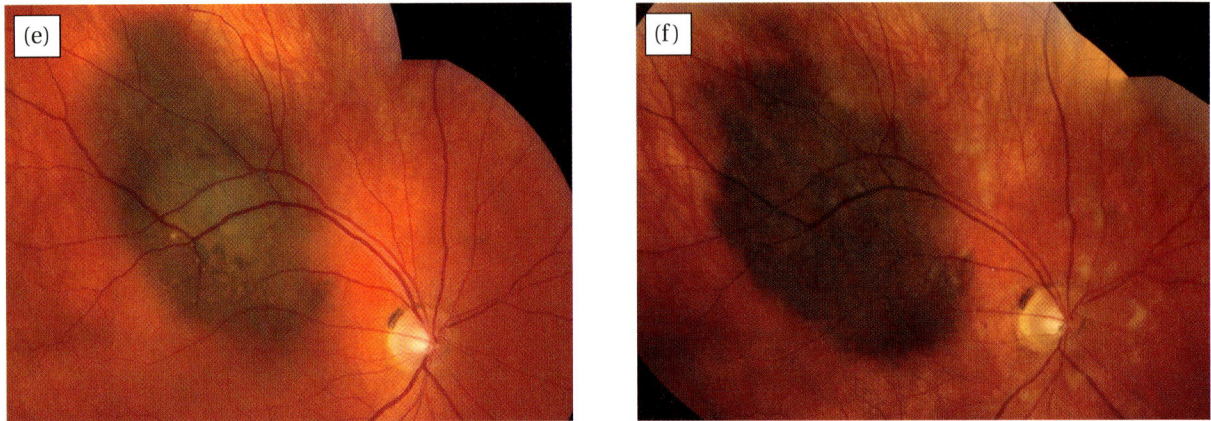

FIGURE 50.8 (*continued*) (e) Choroidal melanoma with orange pigment and serous detachment of the macula. (f) Same choroidal melanoma as in (e), status post radioactive iodine 125 brachytherapy; nerve fiber layer infarcts are noted adjacent to the optic nerve head consistent with radiation retinopathy. (Images (e) and (f) courtesy of Ditte Hess, Bascom Palmer Eye Institute, Miami, Florida.)

Local Resection of Uveal Melanoma: Choroidectomy

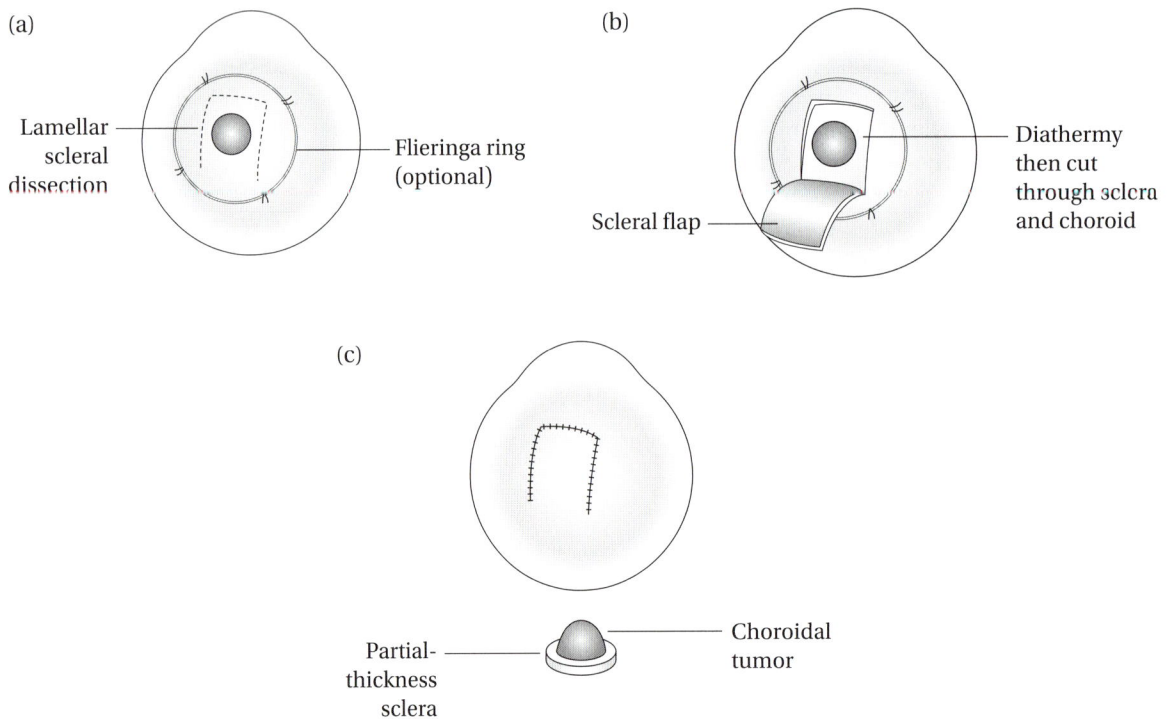

FIGURE 50.9 Local resection of posterior uveal tumors is rarely employed because of technical difficulties of the surgery, and potential complications including local recurrence, hemorrhage, and retinal detachment. (a) Tumor is localized and the margins are marked. (b) Scleral flap (80% depth) with posterior hinge is developed. Scleral bed is treated with three rows of diathermy. Vitreous (1.0–1.5 mL) is removed from midvitreous cavity with vitreous-cutting instrument. (c) Sclera and uvea are incised with No. 75 blade and Vannas scissors. Tumor block is removed. Scleral wound is secured with nylon sutures. Prophylactic encircling scleral buckle can be placed. (Images from Murray T. Management of Intraocular Tumors. In: Albert, D. M. *Ophthalmic Surgery: Principles and Techniques*. Malden, Mass: Blackwell Science; 1999, p. 169.)

Enucleation with Snare Technique to Maximize Stump Length

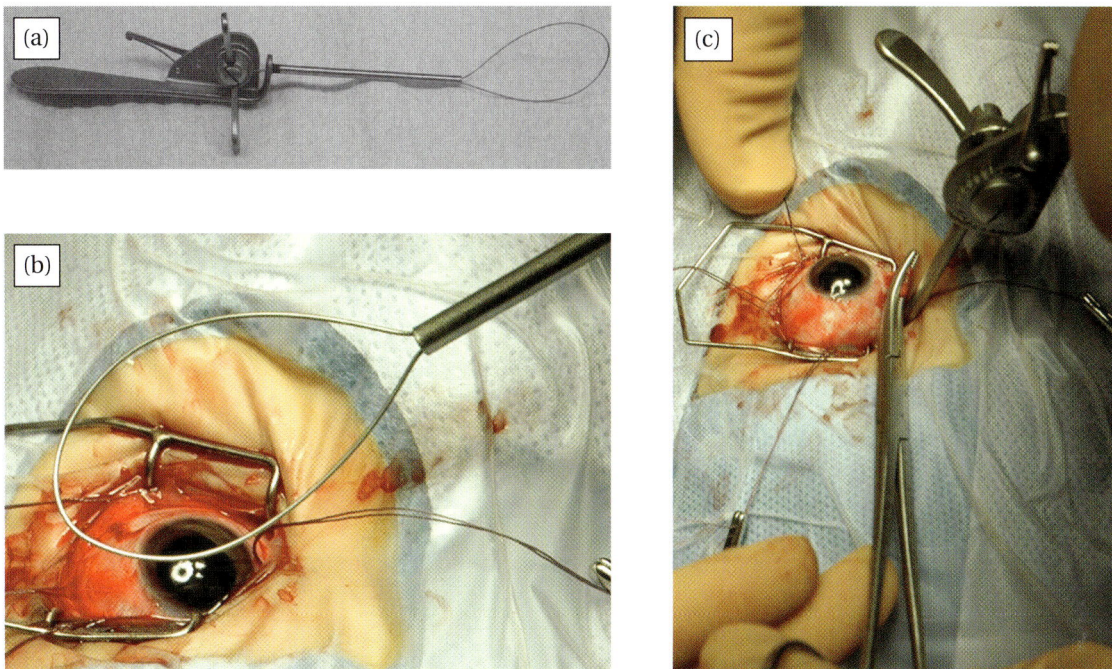

FIGURE 50.10 Enucleation for intraocular tumors using a snare. (a) Conjunctival peritomy is performed. The four rectus muscles are secured. The two oblique muscles are identified and severed. (b) Enucleation snare is placed over the globe and directed posteriorly. (c) Hemostat clamp is used to grasp the medial rectus stump, and firm anterior traction is exerted. The snare is directed posteriorly within in the orbit, and the optic nerve is cut as far posteriorly as possible to obtain a long optic nerve stump. After hemostasis is achieved, an implant is placed and the rectus muscles are attached. Tenons layer is closed in two layers to minimize the risk of implant extrusion: (1) deep Tenons closure with interrupted horizontal mattress sutures using polyglactin (Vicryl); (2) superficial Tenons closure with vertical mattress sutures using polyglactin (Vicryl). Conjunctiva is then closed without tension using a running plain gut suture.

Retinoblastoma

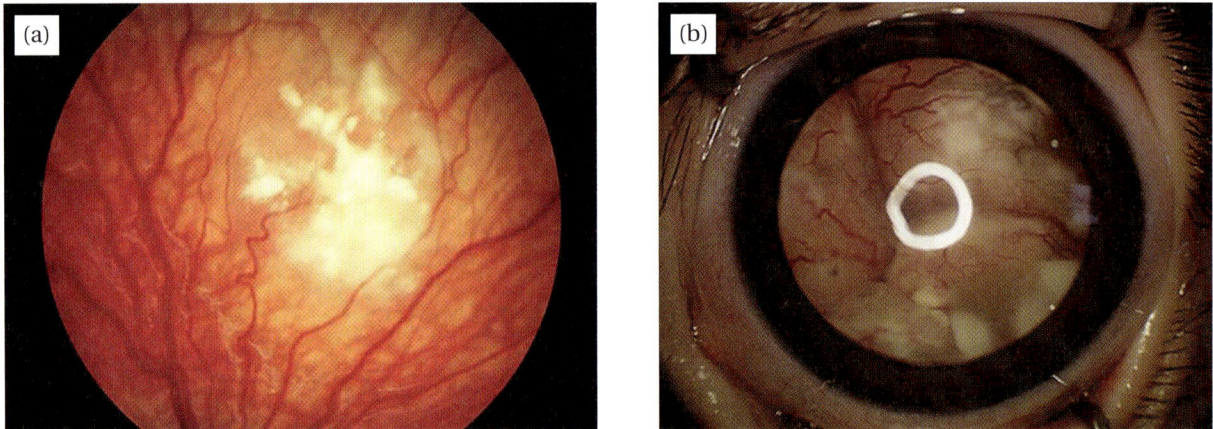

FIGURE 50.11 Retinoblastoma (RB) is the most common primary intraocular tumor in children, affecting approximately 1 in 15,000 live births. Retinoblastoma begins as a focus within the neural retina, and is bilateral and related to a germinal mutation in the RB1 gene on chromosome 13q14 in 35% of cases, and unilateral and related to a somatic mutation in 65% of cases. (a) Small intraretinal RB is associated with calcified intratumoral flecks. (b) Very large tumor filling the vitreous cavity, which required enucleation. Current treatment regimens afford patients with this disease a 99% survival rate and a 90% rate of normal vision retention in at least one eye.

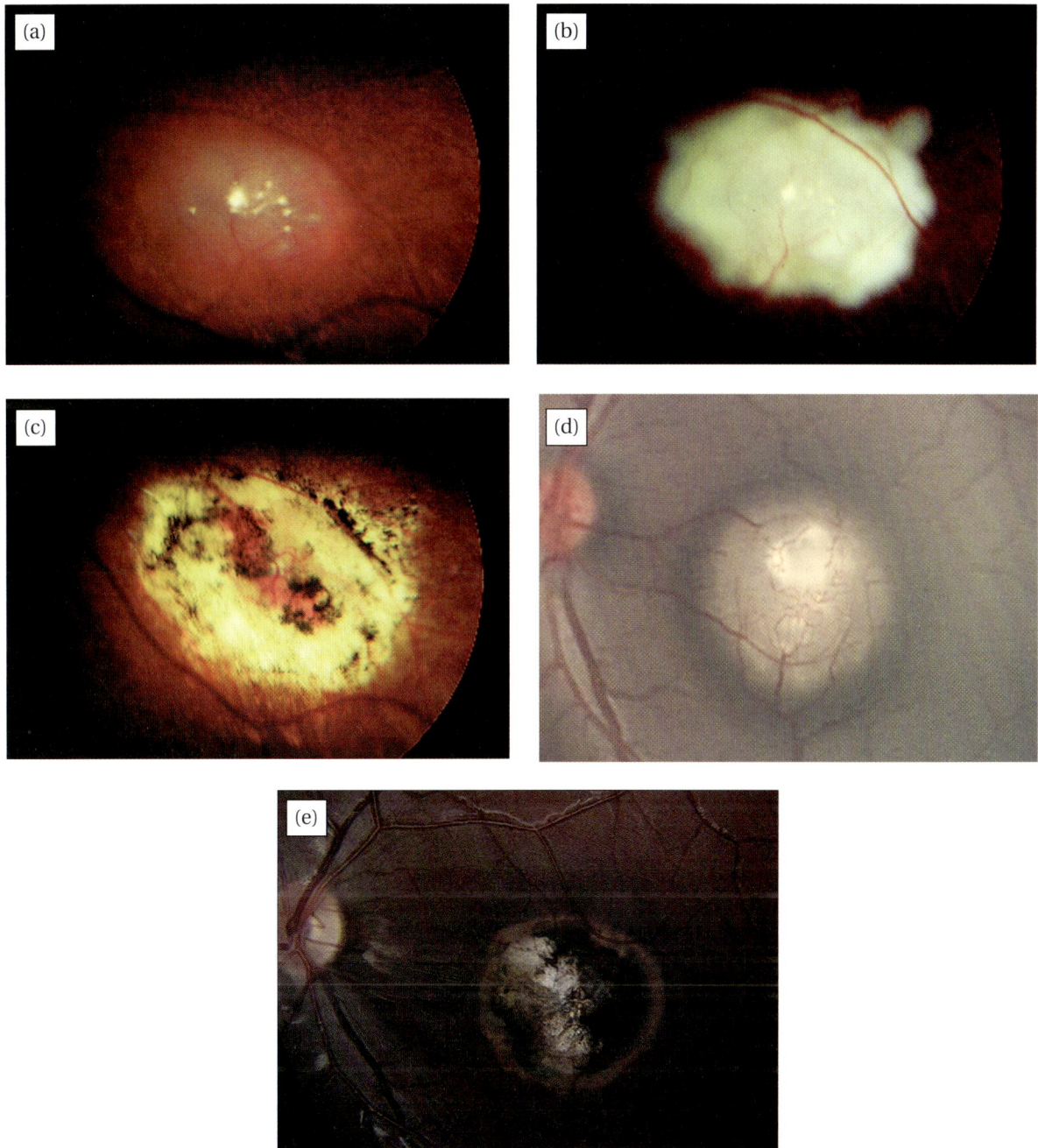

FIGURE 50.12 Laser photoablation is often used in the management of retinoblastoma, most commonly in combination with other treatment modalities such as chemoreduction. If the retinoblastoma tumors are small (<3 mm height), have no vitreous seeds, and are not associated with the optic nerve head, focal therapy may be sufficient for complete treatment. (a) Small tumors easily visualized are well suited for laser photoablation. (b) Confluent laser burns over the tumor with one row surrounding the tumor margin (imaged immediately after treatment). Many times, repeated laser treatment is necessary. (c) Chorioretinal scar with no tumor activity 2 months after laser ablation. (d) Small macular RB. (e) Same eye as (d) 10 years after treatment with systemic chemotherapy and focal laser photoablation. (Images (a), (b), and (c) from Murray T. Management of Intraocular Tumors. In: Albert, D. M. *Ophthalmic Surgery: Principles and Techniques.* Malden, MA: Blackwell Science; 1999, p. 171. Images (d) and (e) courtesy of Ditte Hess, Bascom Palmer Eye Institute Miami, Florida.)

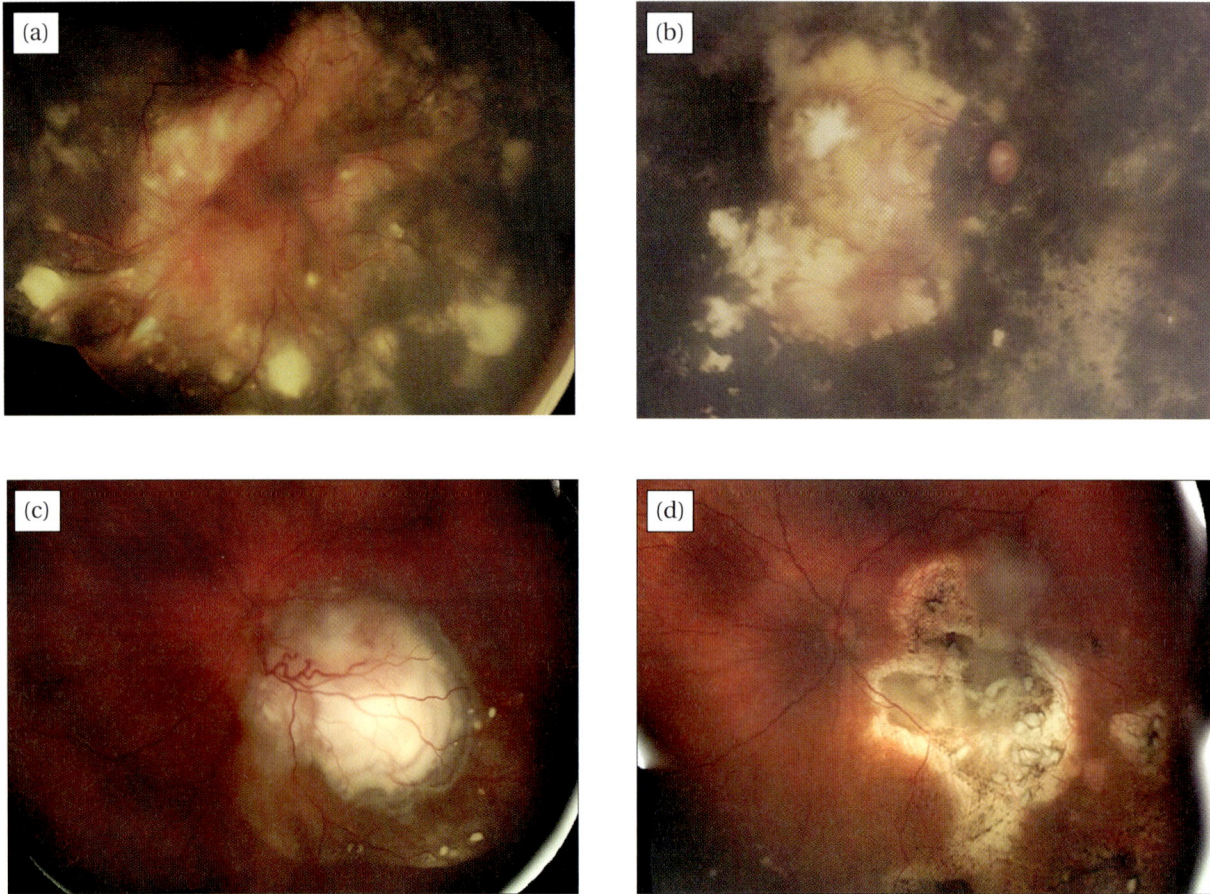

FIGURE 50.13 If a retinoblastoma tumor is large with vitreous and/or subretinal seeding, focal ablative therapy can be used in combination with systemic chemotherapy (2- or 3-drug combinations of carboplatin, etoposide, and vincristine,) and/or locally administered chemotherapy (sub-Tenon carboplatin or intra-ophthalmic artery melphalan). (a) Large RB tumor with extensive subretinal and vitreous seeding and areas of calcification. (b) Same eye as (a), showing regressed tumor after systemic chemotherapy, focal ablative laser therapy and local chemotherapy. (c) Macular RB tumor with serous retinal detachment and subretinal seeding. (d) Same eye as (c) 7 months later, showing regression of the tumor after systemic chemotherapy and focal ablative laser therapy; note the presence of active tumor temporally, adjacent to the macular scarring. (Images (c) and (d) courtesy of Ditte Hess, Bascom Palmer Eye Institute, Miami, Florida.)

Choroidal Metastases

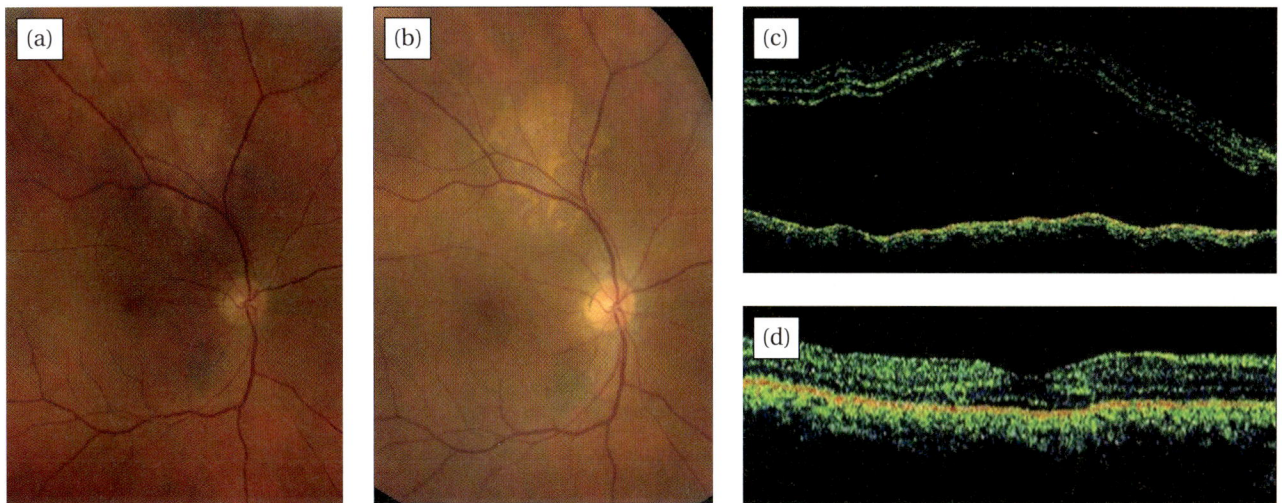

FIGURE 50.14 Metastatic tumors to the eye most commonly involve the choroid and most commonly derive from breast cancer in women and lung cancer in men. Other, less common primary sites include prostate, kidney, thyroid, and gastrointestinal tract cancers. A careful medical history and a thorough examination of both eyes is crucial, as metastases are often bilateral (30%) and multifocal within the involved eye (20%). Ancillary evaluation often shows associated serous retinal detachment and medium to high reflectivity by echography. Patients require co-management with a medical oncologist and systemic evaluation. Treatment often includes a combination of systemic chemotherapy and radiation therapy (either external beam radiation or plaque brachytherapy). (a) Metastatic thyroid carcinoma superiorly, with associated serous retinal detachment involving the macula as shown by the horizontally oriented ocular coherence tomography (OCT) image through the fovea (c). (b) After external beam radiation treatment, the lesion has become inactive and the subretinal fluid is nearly completely resolved, as shown by the horizontally oriented OCT image through the fovea (d).

Iris Melanocytic Tumors

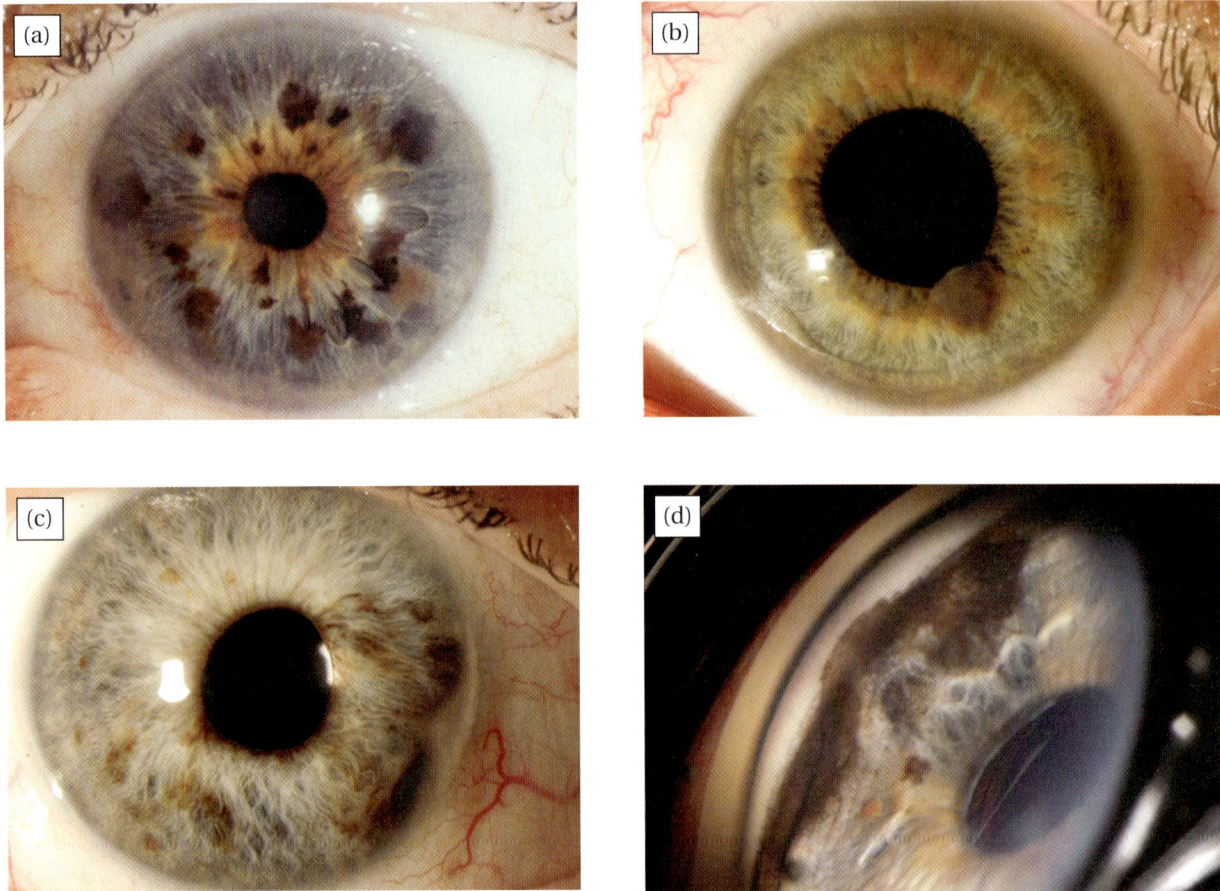

FIGURE 50.15 Iris melanocytic tumors include a spectrum of lesions ranging from benign nevi to malignant melanomas. (a) Multifocal, uniformly pigmented melanocytic iris nevi preserving normal iris architecture have low probability of malignancy. (b) Small iris melanoma disrupting normal iris architecture and pupillary margin. (c) Irregularly pigmented iris melanoma with variable thickness. (d) Gonioscopic image of same melanoma in (c); broad peripheral anterior synechiae are visible, with tumor involvement and heavy pigmentation of the angle.

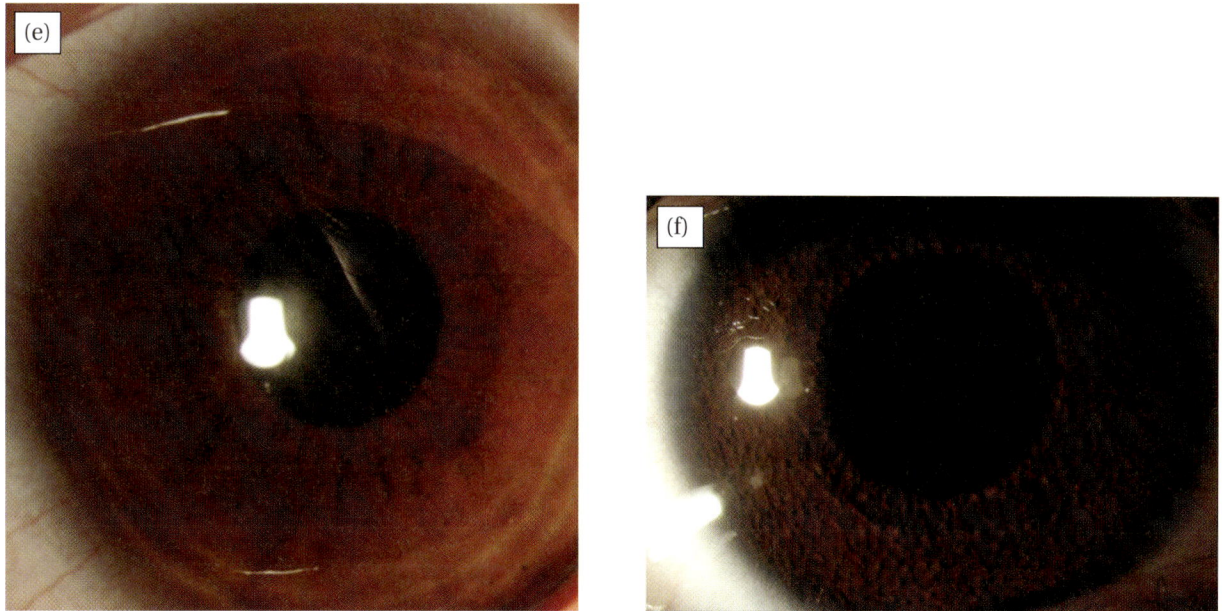

FIGURE 50.15 (*continued*) (e) Normal iris; (f) contralateral iris with oculodermal melanocytosis (also known as Nevus of Ota), a congenital melanocytic hyperpigmentation of the face and ocular tissues, most commonly unilateral and distributed along the course of the trigeminal nerve; ocular pigment most frequently involves the choroid and episcleral, but can also involve the iris as shown here; this condition is important to recognize clinically because it is associated with an increased risk of uveal melanoma, up to 1 out of 400 patients in some populations. (Images (a–d) courtesy of Ditte Hess, Bascom Palmer Eye Institute Miami, Florida.)

Iridocyclectomy

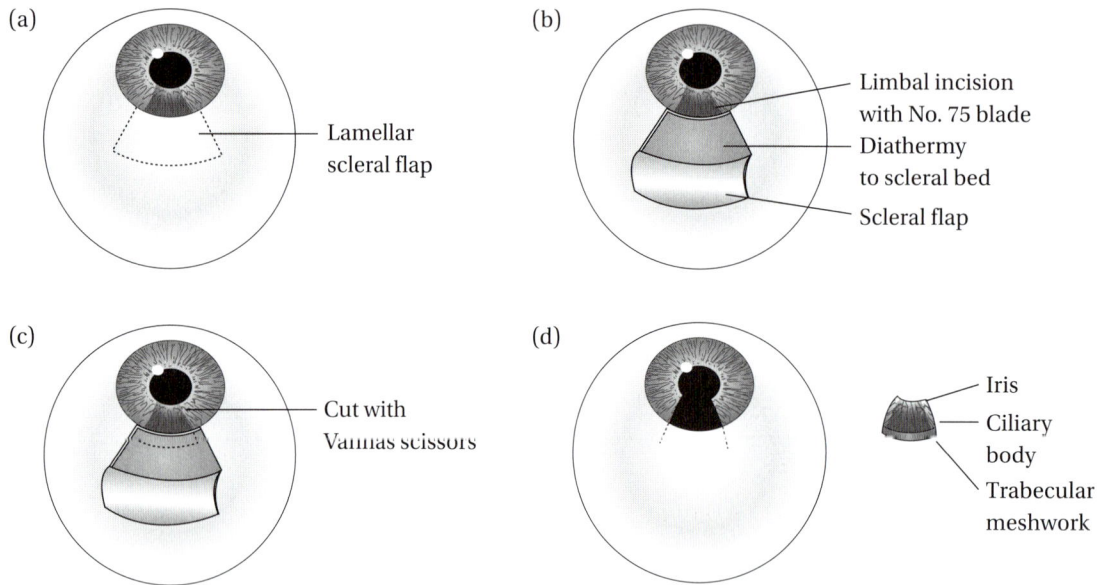

(a)

Lamellar
scleral flap

(b)

Limbal incision
with No. 75 blade

Diathermy
to scleral bed

Scleral flap

(c)

Cut with
Vannas scissors

(d)

Iris

Ciliary
body

Trabecular
meshwork

FIGURE 50.16 If a clinically suspicious iris lesion is isolated to the iris, surgical biopsy can many times be performed through a clear corneal incision similar to that created during routine cataract surgery. If the tumor involves the ciliary body, however, iridocyclectomy may be indicated; this technically challenging procedure is generally reserved for tumors involving less than 3 clock hours. (a) 80% scleral thickness lamellar flap is created. (b) Scleral bed is treated with 2–3 rows of diathermy. (c) Anterior chamber is entered, and viscoelastic material is injected into the anterior chamber. Sclera and iris are incised with No. 75 blade and Vannas scissors. Tumor block is removed. (d) Scleral wound is secured with nylon sutures. (Images from Murray T. Management of Intraocular Tumors. In: Albert, D. M. *Ophthalmic Surgery: Principles and Techniques*. Malden, MA: Blackwell Science; 1999, p. 172.)

SELECTED REFERENCES

Christmas NJ, Van Quill K, Murray TG, Gordon CD, Garonzik S, Tse D, Johnson T, Schiffman J, O'Brien JM. Evaluation of efficacy and complications: Primary pediatric orbital implants after enucleation. *Arch Ophthalmol.* 2000;118(4):503–506.

Onken MD, Worley LA, Tuscan MD, Harbour JW. An accurate, clinically feasible multi-gene expression assay for predicting metastasis in uveal melanoma. *J Mol Diagn.* 2010;12(4):461–468.

Schefler AC, Cicciarelli N, Feuer W, Toledano S, Murray TG. Macular retinoblastoma: Evaluation of tumor control, local complications, and visual outcomes for eyes treated with chemotherapy and repetitive foveal laser ablation. *Ophthalmology.* 2007;114(1):162–169.

Schiedler V, Dubovy SR, Murray TG. Snare technique for enucleation of eyes with advanced retinoblastoma. *Arch Ophthalmol.* 2007;125(5):680–683.

Tabandeh H, Chaudhry NA, Murray TG, Ehlies F, Hughes R, Scott IU, Markoe AM. Intraoperative echographic localization of iodine-125 episcleral plaque for brachytherapy of choroidal melanoma. *Am J Ophthalmol.* 2000;129(2):199–204.

51

Macular Surgery

William E. Smiddy, MD

TABLE 51.1 *Indications for Surgery*

Macular Pucker and Vitreomacular Traction:

- visual loss to the range of 20/50
- if visual acuity is >20/50, but subjective symptoms such as metamorphopsia or macropsia are functionally debilitating
- about 1–2 years of onset of symptoms

Macular Hole

- definitive full-thickness defect in macula
- duration of about 1 year or less (longer if smaller)

Subretinal Hemorrhage

- under macula, especially if more inferior
- occurrence within 2–3 days
- generally, diagnosis not due to wet age-related macular degeneration

Macular Pucker

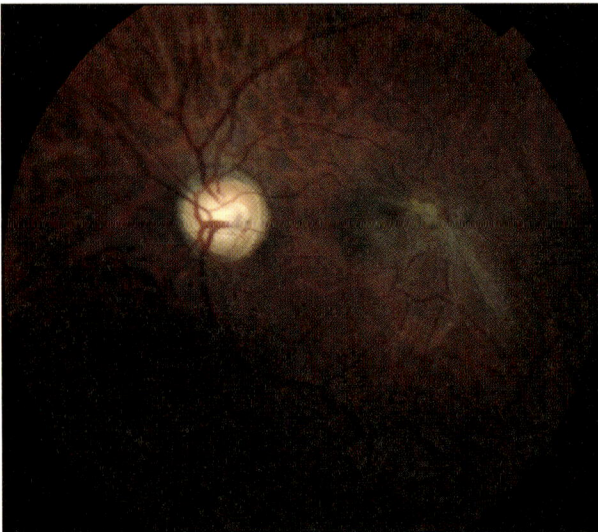

FIGURE 51.1 An epiretinal membrane may appear discrete with fibrous components emanating from an epicenter, configured in a stellate pattern. Visual loss may be through one or more of the following effects: distortion of retinal cells (manifested as metamorphopsia); induction of macular edema; some degree of media opacity from thick or more opaque membranes; or interference with axoplasmic flow (sometimes visible by a cotton-wool type opacity). Visual loss or symptoms sufficient to interfere with activities of daily living may constitute an indication for surgical intervention.

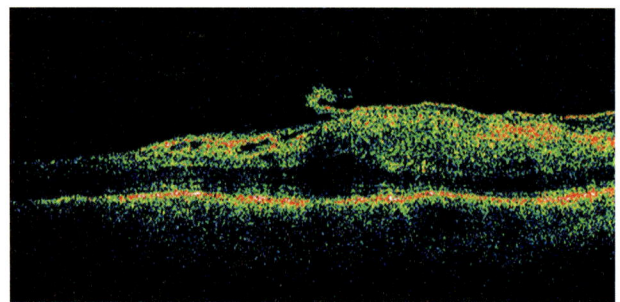

FIGURE 51.2 Optical coherence tomography (OCT) shows an irregularly thickened, sometimes elevated profile on the retinal surface. The convolutions of the retinal surface may be prominent and the normal pattern of the retinal layers may be distorted, either from edema or mechanical traction effects.

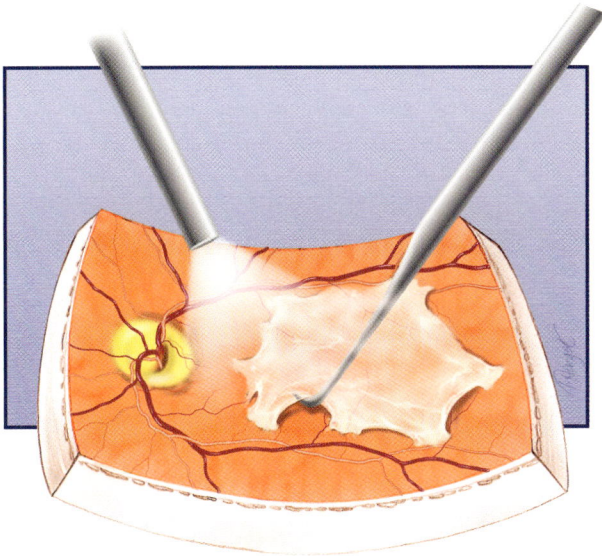

FIGURE 51.3 Fibrotic epiretinal membrane may be engaged with a pick or a fine needle at the preexisting edge. Alternating a side-to-side motion with a gentle lifting motion releases the membrane from the surface with a minimum of retinal trauma. Generally, the attachments at the center should be released early in the course of the peeling.

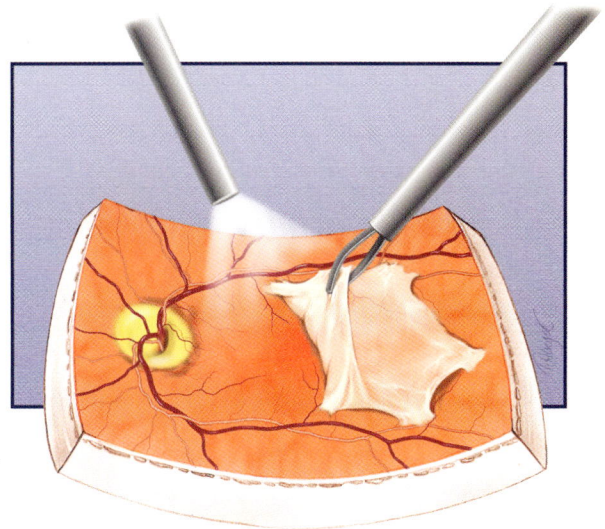

FIGURE 51.4 Once the membrane is lifted over about one-half of its extent, it is most expeditious to use the forceps to remove the membrane the rest of the way from the surface and out of the eye, usually in one large, confluent piece.

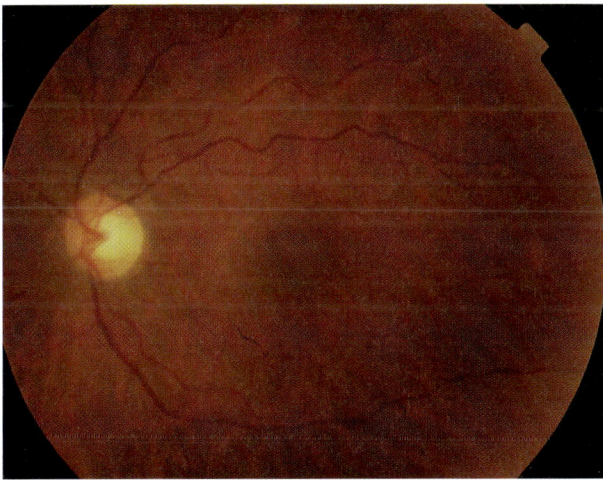

FIGURE 51.5 Some epiretinal membranes have a shiny, cellophane-like appearance. The tissue may be nearly transparent and, characteristically, is more broadly distributed. Although not clearly established as fact, the cellophane morphology seems more common with idiopathic ERMs, whereas the fibrotic appearance may be more common in association with a retinal tear.

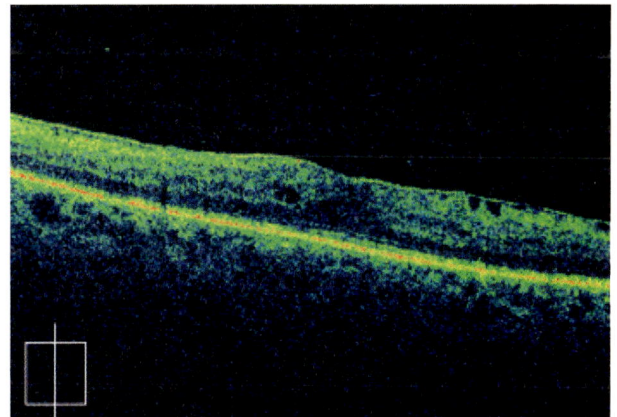

FIGURE 51.6 The OCT appearance may be more subtle, since the epiretinal membrane is thinner and more homogenous. However, the convolutions of the retinal surface, though more subtle, are frequently still present, betraying the presence of the membrane. As in the fibrotic membrane, intraretinal edema spaces and distorted retinal layers are also common.

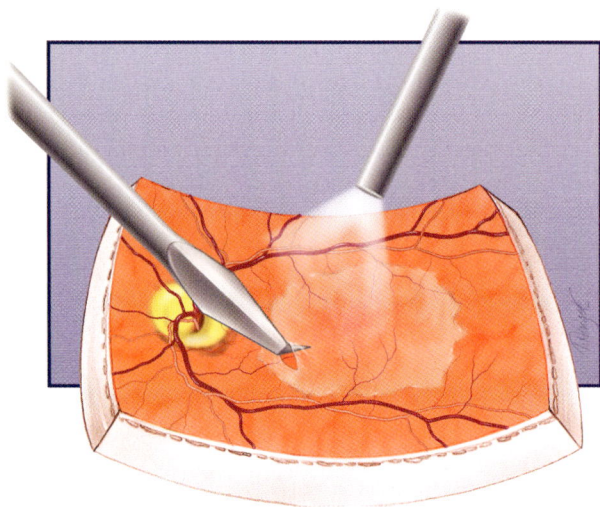

FIGURE 51.7 The technique of removal is similar to the fibrotic membrane, but a sharp blade is more commonly necessary to create an edge to peel. Frequently, a finer forceps is necessary and may need to be used earlier in the course of the peeling maneuver to extricate the membrane. It is common that both the ILM and the ERM are removed together in this type of membrane.

Vitreomacular Traction

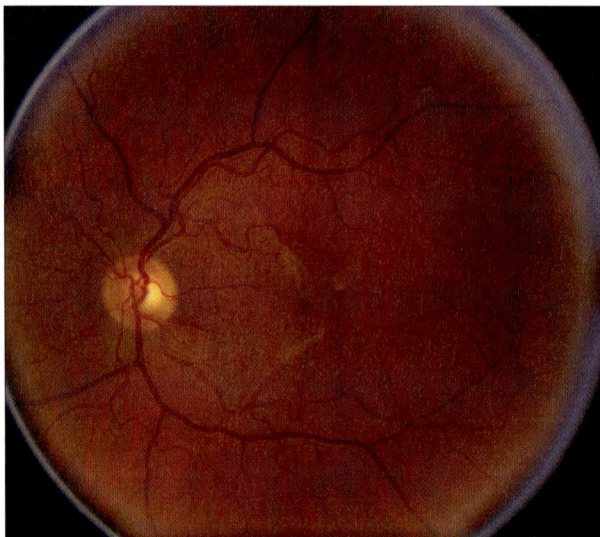

FIGURE 51.8 The vitreomacular traction syndrome is a variant of the epiretinal membrane, in which the posterior vitreous separation is incomplete and commonly attaches prominently at the edges of the preretinal tissue. Commonly, the preretinal tissue extends over a broad zone including the macula and the disc, and even more peripherally.

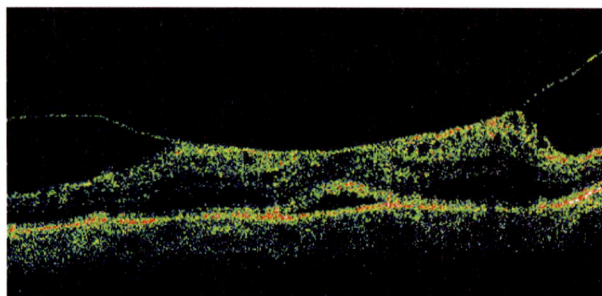

FIGURE 51.9 The vitreoretinal attachment and preretinal tissue is visible with the OCT. The fovea is commonly flattened or even elevated. Intraretinal edema is common, and the traction may give rise to a focal retinal separation.

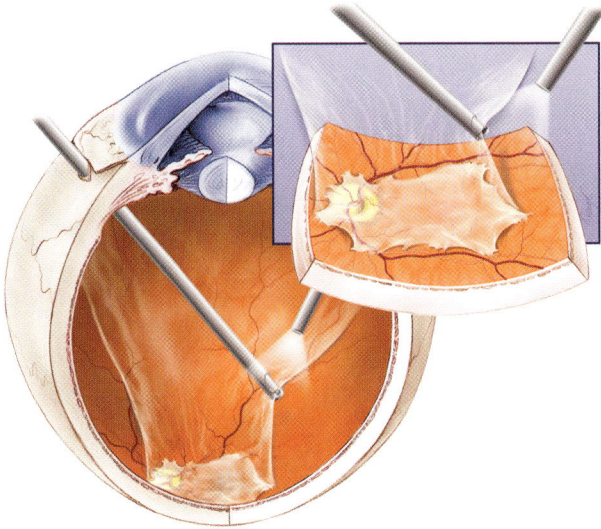

FIGURE 51.10 The surgical anatomy of vitreomacular traction syndrome involves recognizing the anterior to posterior alignment of the partial, peripheral vitreous detachment. A strategy is to remove this traction first, by excising the vitreous, rendering the remaining preretinal tissue amenable to techniques such as those described with epiretinal membrane peeling.

Macular Hole

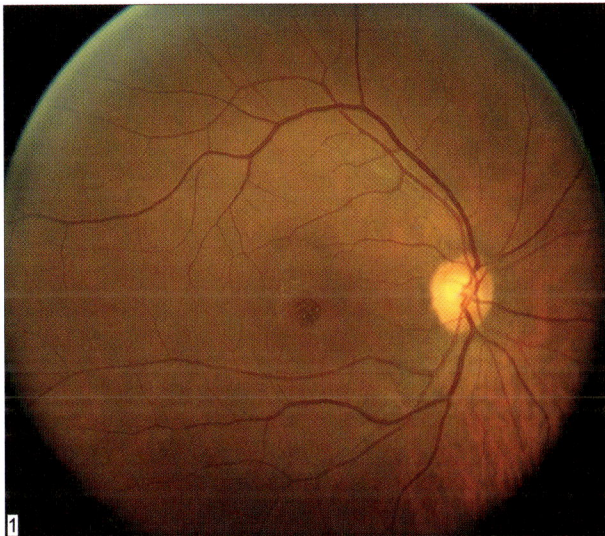

FIGURE 51.11 A full-thickness macular hole classically appears as a circular, fovea-centered defect. The edges of the retina are commonly elevated or thickened, blurring the underlying choroidal appearance. White spots in the level of the RPE and the base of the hole have been correlated with macrophages histologically, and are pathognomonic. The hole might be small, making it difficult to distinguish from other preretinal entities.

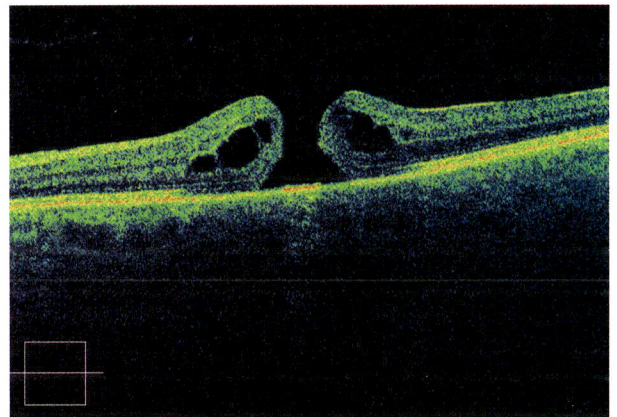

FIGURE 51.12 The OCT is diagnostic, as it shows the discontinuity in the retina. The edges of the hole are commonly rounded and the margins are variably elevated. There is also commonly a variable degree of intraretinal edema. An overlying operculum or posterior hyaloid may also be present.

(a)

(b)

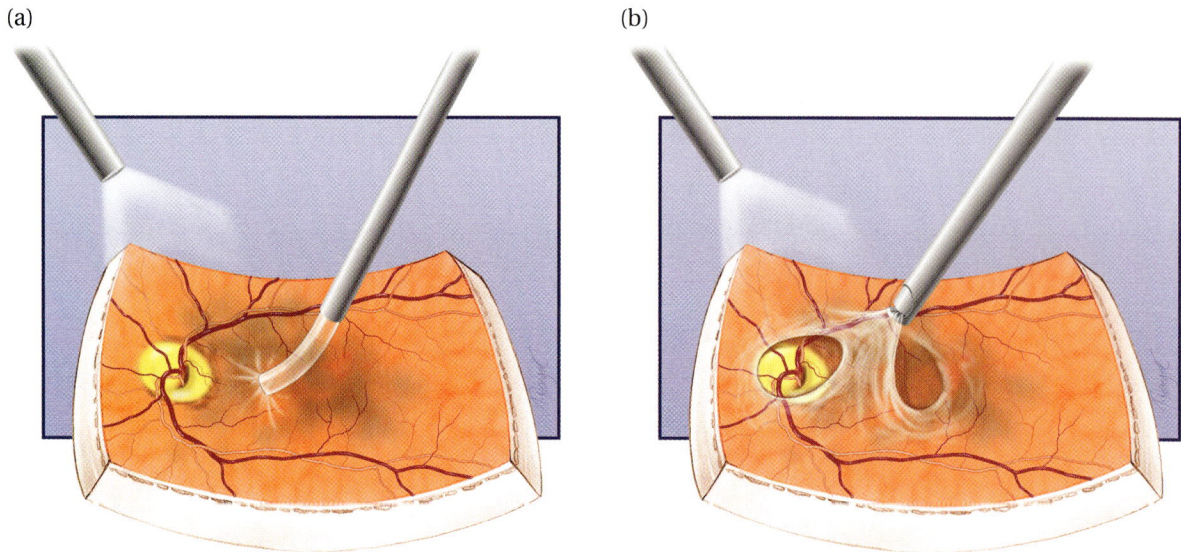

FIGURE 51.13 (a) After performing a core vitrectomy, the surgeon should remove the posterior hyaloid, or demonstrate that it has fully separated by using a flexible silicone-tipped extrusion needle. As the residual vitreous layer is engaged, the silicone tip deviates in what has been called the "fish strike sign." (b) Sequentially making posterior- to anterior-elevation motions, in a variety of locations throughout the macula, elevates the posterior hyaloid so the vitreous cutter, on suction mode only, engages the vitreous more firmly than the needle, so the Weiss ring can be dehisced from the optic nervehead. The remaining vitreous is then removed in the standard fashion.

(a)

(b)

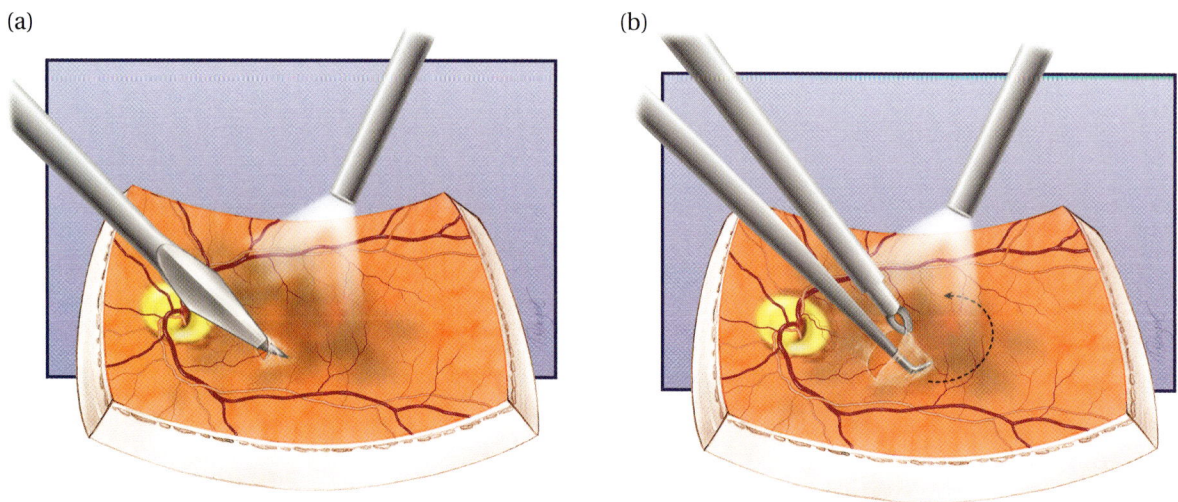

FIGURE 51.14 Internal limiting membrane peeling might be the reason for the increased success rates seen in recent years for macular hole, and has been applied to numerous other conditions including epiretinal membranes, vitreofoveal traction, myopic traction maculopathy, and diabetic macular edema. (a) The basic technique involves puncturing the internal limiting membrane with a sharp blade to expose a leading edge that may be developed more broadly using a vitreoretinal pick or forceps across the macula. (b) The dissection is executed by using gentle elevation and side-to-side motions to elevate the internal limiting membrane from the retinal surface. At some point, it is convenient to switch to a fine forceps to peel the elevated ILM (pictured together with the pick, but never used simultaneously). Usually, the ILM is more firmly attached around the margins of the macular hole, and a doughnut-shaped elevation is accomplished yielding a funnel-shaped configuration of the internal limiting membrane. Adjunctive dyes can facilitate ILM peeling, but may not be necessary in a majority of cases.

Subretinal Surgery

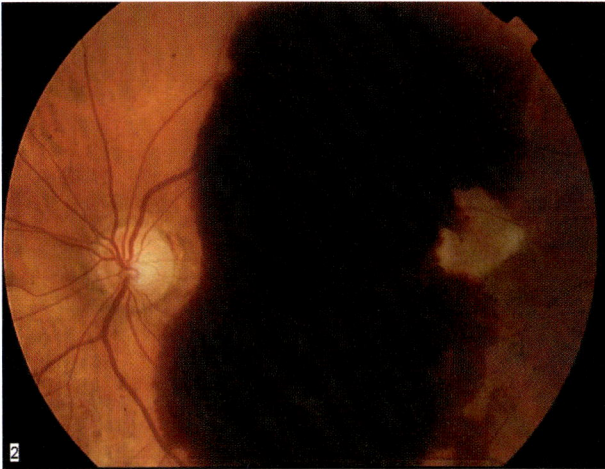

FIGURE 51.15 A massive subretinal hemorrhage is a dreaded complication of choroidal neovascularization. A variety of therapeutic approaches have been recommended for this occurrence, but the prognosis, especially when due to age-related macular degeneration, is usually poor. Exceptional cases might be considered for surgery, however. This patient had a vision of 2/200 due to a massive disciform scar in the right eye, and presented within 24 hours of having lost vision from 20/25.

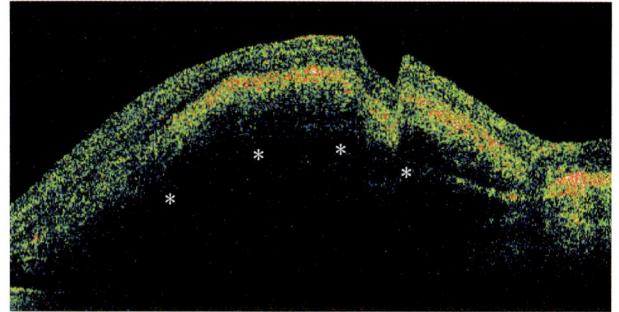

FIGURE 51.16 The OCT demonstrates the subretinal hemorrhage, which appears to include subretinal pigment epithelial (*) hemorrhage.

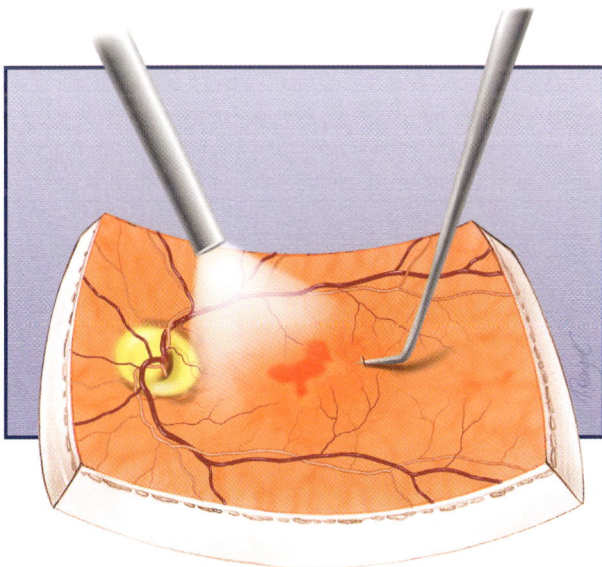

FIGURE 51.17 When subretinal surgery is performed, retinal penetrator consisting of a fine, 36 or smaller, gauge instrument is used to access the subretinal space.

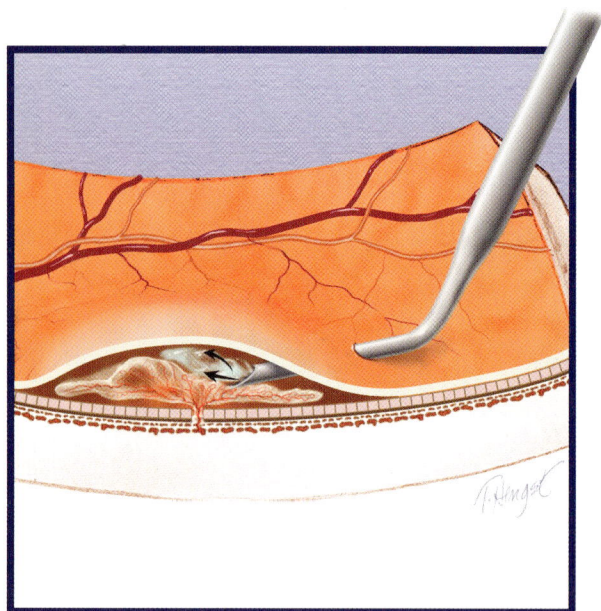

FIGURE 51.18 Using a fine cannula, balanced salt that might include tissue plasminogen activator is infused into the subretinal space to raise a focal retinal detachment. This allows room to facilitate removal of clot components or neovascular tissue, which is depicted in this figure using a fine forceps. When possible, a membrane is ideally dissected from the retina and underlying retinal pigment epithelium before being extracted. Postoperatively, a gas-bubble may be used to re-approximate the retina at the tiny retinotomy (which may not require retinopexy) and to push residual subretinal hemorrhage elements inferiorly, away from the foveal center.

TABLE 51.2 *Potential Complications of Surgery*

Retinal detachment

Induced cataract (through direct lens touch, or more commonly months after vitrectomy)

Endophthalmitis

Choroidal hemorrhage

SELECTED REFERENCES

Brooks HL Jr. Macular hole surgery with and without internal limiting membrane peeling. *Ophthalmology.* 2000;107:1939–1948.

Kelly NE, Wendel RT. Vitreous surgery for idiopathic macular holes. Results of a pilot study. *Arch Ophthalmol.* 1991;109:654–659.

Michels RG. Vitrectomy for macular pucker. *Ophthalmology.* 1984;91:1384–1287.

Peyman GA, Nelson NC, Alturki W, et al. Tissue plasminogen activator factor assisted removal of subretinal hemorrhage. *Ophthalmic Surg.* 1991;22:575.

Smiddy WE Michels RG, Glaser BM, deBustros S. Vitrecotmy for macular traction caused by incomplete vitreous separation. *Arch Ophthalmol.* 1988;106:624–628.

Thomas MA, Kaplan HJ. Surgical removal of subfoveal neovascularization in the presumed ocular histoplasmosis syndrome. *Am J Ophthalmol.* 1991;111:1.

52 Vitreoretinal Complications of Cataract Surgery

Saad El-Naggar, MD, Frank L. Myers, MD, and Jay S. Duker, MD

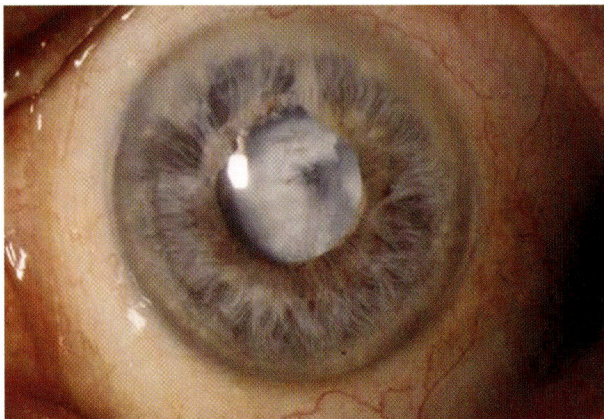

FIGURE 52.1 Anterior segment photograph of an eye with retained cortical material following cataract surgery. A pars plana approach ensures that the retained lens material behind the intraocular lens is removed as well.

Posterior Capsular Rupture during Cataract Surgery

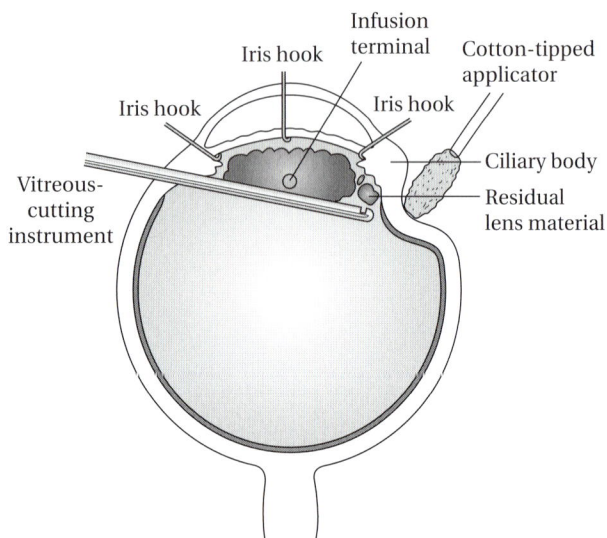

FIGURE 52.2 Following inadvertent posterior capsule rupture during extracapsular cataract extraction, vitreous may enter the anterior chamber and residual lens material may be difficult to remove via the corneoscleral wound. A pars plana approach to the removal of residual lens material and vitreous may be required. Iris retraction with hooks improves visualization. Scleral depression is used to bring lens fragments into view.

Loss of Lens Material into the Vitreous during Cataract Surgery

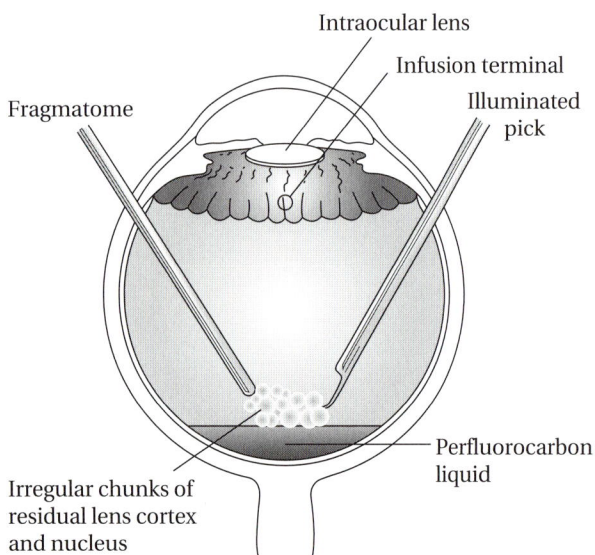

FIGURE 52.3 Dislocation of fragments of the crystalline lens into the vitreous cavity may occur after rupture of the posterior capsule during extracapsular cataract procedure. Dislocated lens fragments may produce uveitis, increased intraocular pressure, corneal edema, vitreous opacification, and cystoid macular edema. A 3-port pars plana vitrectomy with phacofragmentor is used for removal of retained nucleus and cortical material. An illuminated pick is helpful to "hold" lens fragments. Liquid perfluorocarbon may be used to elevate lens fragments from the retinal surface and protect the macula from dropped nuclear material.

Intraocular Lens Dislocation into the Vitreous

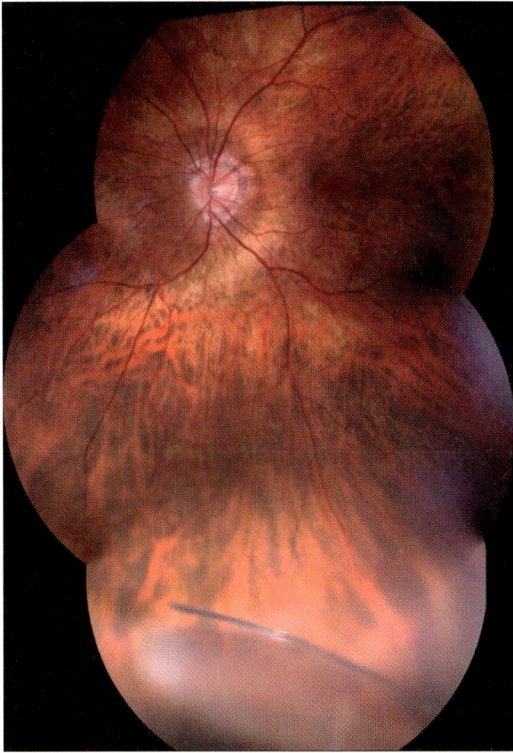

FIGURE 52.4 A montage photograph of a dislocated intraocular lens in the inferior vitreous cavity. Suturing of the lens to the ciliary body or iris is possible. Alternatively, a pars plana vitrectomy can be used to remove the intraocular lens and replace it with an anterior chamber IOL.

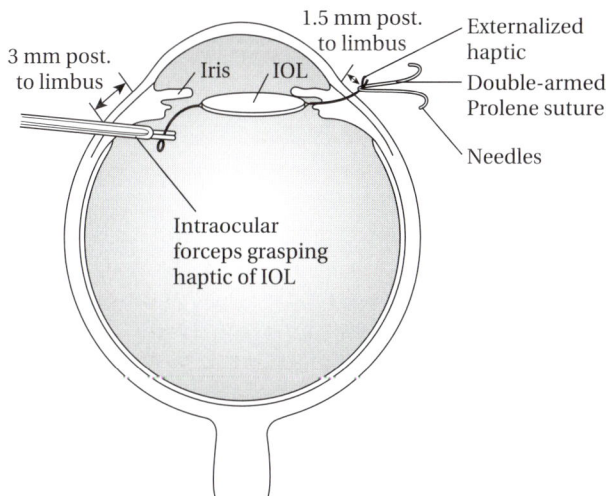

FIGURE 52.5 Dislocation of an intraocular lens (IOL) may occur in eyes with pseudoexfoliation, improper sulcus fixation, improper implant size, or trauma. The IOL may be retrieved after pars plana vitrectomy to remove vitreous attachments to the IOL, anterior chamber, and limbal wounds. The lens may be removed via the anterior chamber, replaced in the sulcus, or scleral fixated. Scleral fixation may be achieved by externalizing the haptics through sclerotomies 1.5 mm posterior to limbus. Double-armed polypropylene (Prolene) sutures are tied to the haptics. The sutures are secured to the sclera after the haptics are reposited in the eye.

Hemorrhage Associated with Cataract Surgery

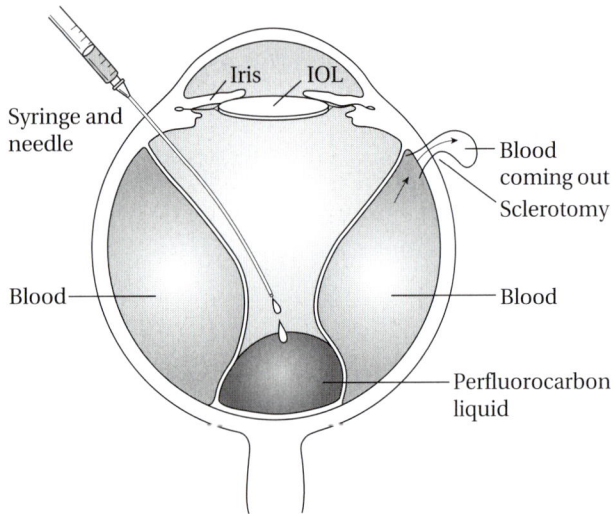

FIGURE 52.6 Suprachoroidal hemorrhage may occur during or after cataract extraction. Associated retinal detachment, appositional choroidals, elevated intraocular pressure, retained lens material, and intractable pain are indications for vitreoretinal surgery. The surgical objective is drainage of hemorrhage through posterior sclerotomies while maintaining intraocular pressure with vitreous substitutes, such as balanced salt solution or perfluorocarbon liquid injected via the pars plana or anterior chamber. After drainage of the suprachoroidal hemorrhage, a standard pars plana vitrectomy may be performed.

Aminoglycoside Retinal Toxicity

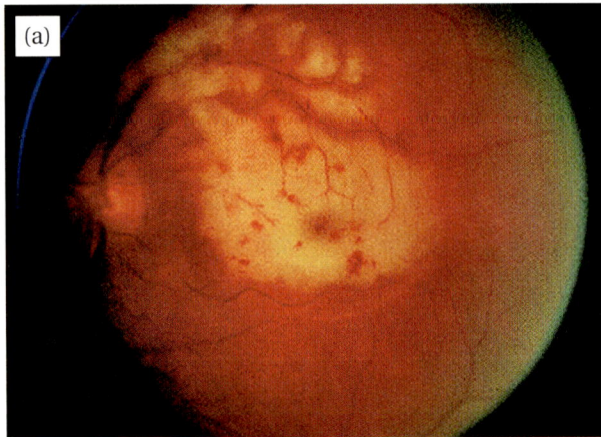

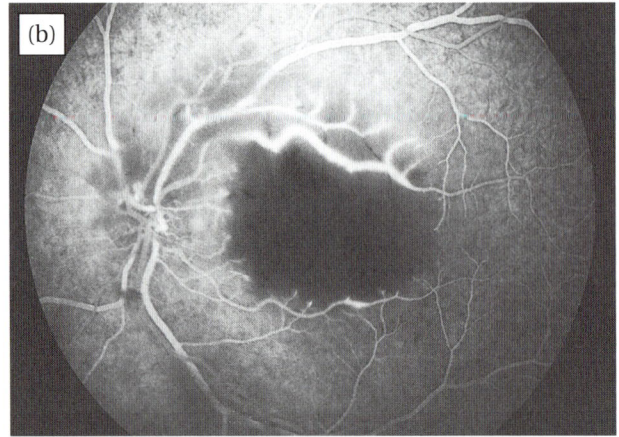

FIGURE 52.7 Accidental injection of intracameral gentamicin sulfate has been reported as a complication of cataract surgery, resulting in acute retinal toxicity. Immediate findings include macular vascular nonperfusion, intraretinal hemorrhage, and retinal edema. (a) Fundus photograph of gentamicin-induced retinal toxicity. (b) Fluorescein angiogram of same eye showing nonperfusion of posterior pole.

Cystoid Macular Edema

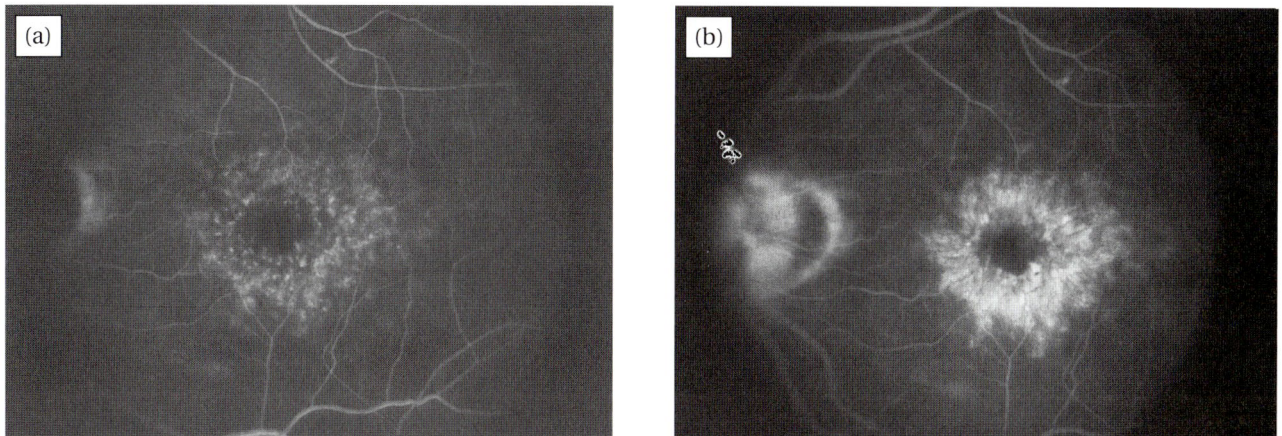

FIGURE 52.8 Cystoid macular edema may occur following cataract extraction. It occurs more commonly in the presence of vitreous loss, disruption of anterior hyaloids membrane, adherence of vitreous to IOL or operative wound, or chronic inflammation. (a) Early-phase fluorescein angiogram of aphakic cystoid macular edema showing perimacular capillary dilation. (b) Late-phase fluorescein angiogram of aphakic cystoid macular edema showing leakage of dye from capillaries into cystoid spaces surrounding the macula.

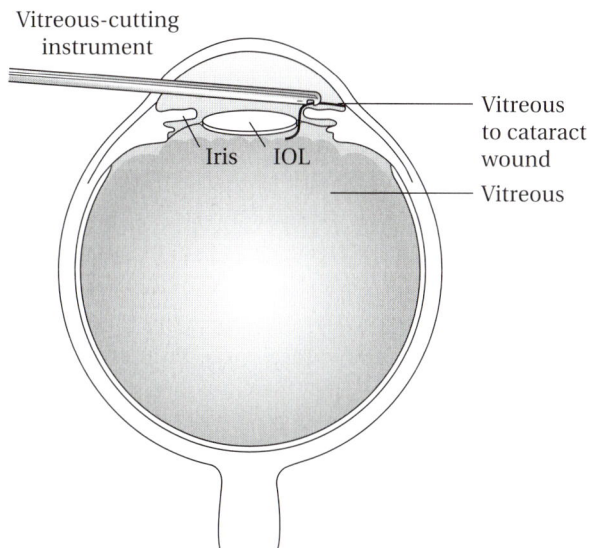

FIGURE 52.9 Most cases of cystoid macular edema resolve spontaneously, or with pharmacologic therapy with cyclooxygenase inhibitors. Vitreous incarceration in the surgical wound, or deformation of the iris by vitreous in the anterior chamber, may cause chronic inflammation and cystoid macular edema. Vitrectomy via a limbal or pars plana approach may be useful to remove vitreous bands.

Retinal Detachment After Cataract Extraction

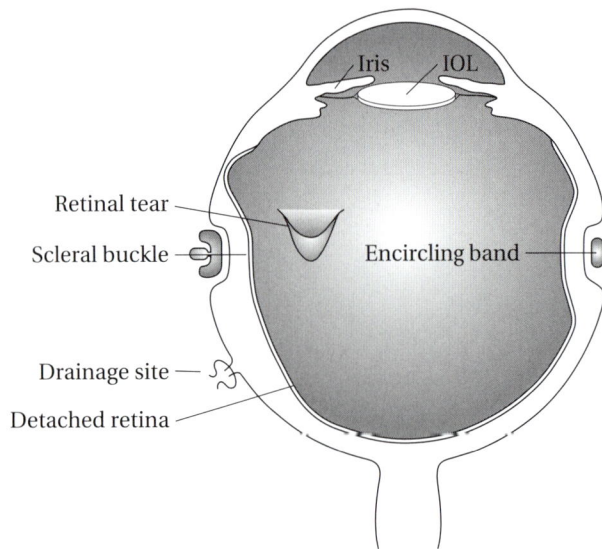

FIGURE 52.10 Scleral buckling of pseudophakic retinal detachment, with drainage of subretinal fluid posterior to the bed of the buckle via sclerotomy. An increased incidence of retinal detachment is associated with cataract extraction. Retinal breaks in aphakic and pseudophakic eyes tend to be small, peripheral, and at or anterior to the vitreous base.

Light-induced Retinopathy from the Operating Microscope

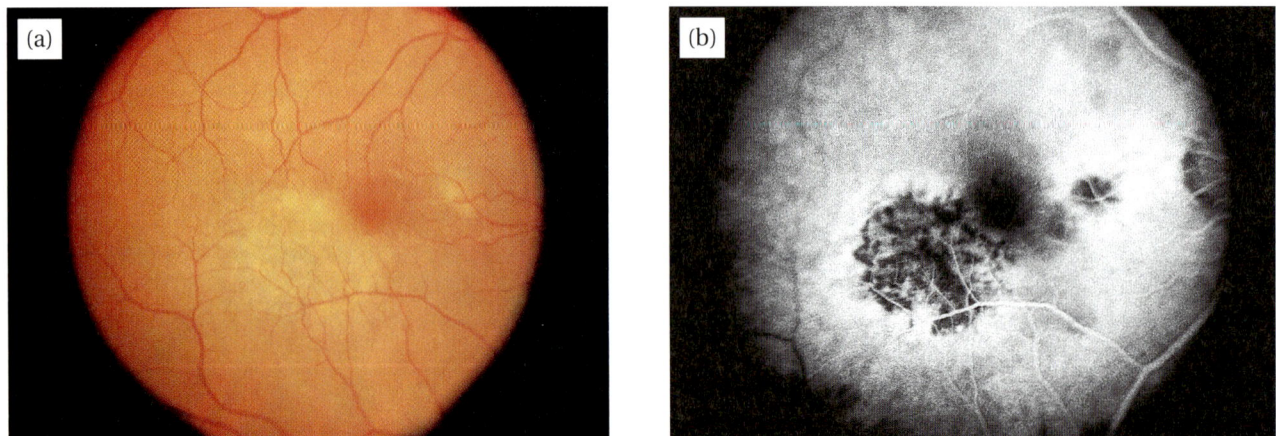

FIGURE 52.11 Photic retinopathy resulting from use of the operating microscope is believed to be caused by photochemical damage from the focusing of high-intensity coaxial light on the retina. The most significant risk factor in the development of photic retinopathy from the operating microscope is a prolonged operating time. (a) Fundus photograph of light-induced chorioretinal lesions nasal and inferotemporal to the macula following vitrectomy. (b) Fluorescein angiogram of the same lesion showing retinal pigment epithelial changes.

SELECTED REFERENCES

Ling R, Cole M, James C, Kamalarajah S, Foot B, Shaw S. Suprachoroidal haemorrhage complicating cataract surgery in the UK: epidemiology, clinical features, management, and outcomes. *Br J Ophthalmol.* 2004;88(4):478–480.

Lois N, Wong D. Pseudophakic retinal detachment. *Surv Ophthalmol.* 2003;48(5):467–487.

Merani R, Hunyor AP, Playfair TJ, Chang A, Gregory-Roberts J, Hunyor AB, Azar D, Cumming RG. Pars plana vitrectomy for the management of retained lens material after cataract surgery. *Am J Ophthalmol.* 2007;144(3):364–370.

53

Pediatric Retinal Disorders

Tushar M. Ranchod, MD and Antonio Capone, Jr, MD

TABLE 53.1 *Indications for Surgery*

Retinopathy of Prematurity (ROP)

Stage 4: Partial retinal detachment with (4B) or without (4A) macular involvement

Lens-sparing vitrectomy through the pars plicata is indicated if adequate space exists between the lens and detached retina to safely enter the vitreous cavity. This type of surgery consists primarily of releasing transvitreal traction.

Stage 4B/5: Retinal detachment (total retinal detachment with prior laser ablation)

Lensectomy may be necessary in cases with prior peripheral laser ablation and detachment of all non-lasered retina (this is technically stage 4B, since the lasered retina is attached). This type of surgery consists primarily of removing proliferative tissue on the retinal surface.

Stage 5: Total retinal detachment (no prior laser ablation)

Lensectomy and vitrectomy are performed using limbal incisions rather than pars plicata, since adequate surgical space usually does not exist between the lens and detached retina in these eyes. Drainage of subretinal blood is sometimes appropriate when both tractional and exudative retinal detachment components are significant (TERD).

Familial Exudative Vitreoretinopathy (FEVR)

Stage 4: Partial retinal detachment with macular involvement

Pars plicata lens-sparing vitrectomy is indicated if a safe surgical space exists between the lens and detached retina, whereas a combined lensectomy and vitrectomy is indicated via limbal approach when the detached retina or proliferative tissue extend to the lens centrally.

Stage 5: Total retinal detachment

The surgical approach and technique are similar to Stage 5 ROP (see above).

Persistent Fetal Vasculature Syndrome (PFVS)

Pars plicata vitrectomy is indicated when stalk tissue exerts traction on the posterior segment. When lens opacity is minimal or eccentric, lens-sparing vitrectomy often suffices, whereas lensectomy may be necessary in cases of central lens opacity in order to prevent amblyopia.

TABLE 53.2 *Complications of Surgery*

In all pediatric cases, the creation of an iatrogenic retinal break is a dreaded complication. The proliferative response to rhegmatogenous retinal trauma is so great that progression to complete tractional retinal detachment, and ultimately phthisis, is difficult to prevent.

If a retinal break is created in a tractional pediatric detachment, residual proliferative tissue may prevent apposition of a break to retinal pigment epithelium, thereby preventing effective retinopexy unless extensive surgical relaxation is performed.

Anatomic and visual outcomes tend to be poor after a rhegmatogenous component is introduced. A conservative approach to pediatric vitrectomy is appropriate, particularly since the relief of pathologic vitreoretinal traction rarely requires vitreous shaving near the retinal surface.

Retinopathy of Prematurity (ROP) and Familial Exudative Vitreoretinopathy (FEVR)

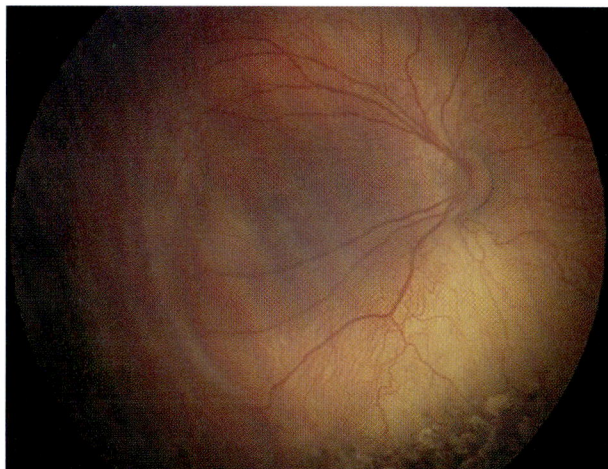

FIGURE 53.1 Preoperative photograph of Stage 4A retinal detachments in retinopathy of prematurity (ROP). Stage 4A is a macula-sparing partial retinal detachment. The etiology of the detachment is primarily transvitreal traction, without significant proliferative tissue on the retinal surface.

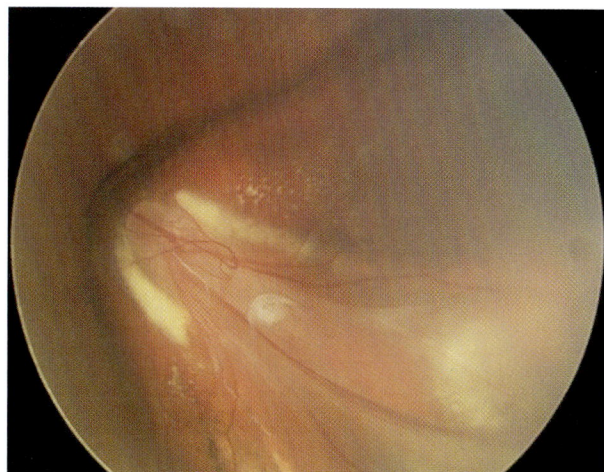

FIGURE 53.2 Preoperative photograph of Stage 4B retinal detachment in familial exudative vitreoretinopathy (FEVR). *Stage 4* denotes a partial retinal detachment with macular involvement, while the "B" denotes the presence of exudation. The retinal detachment is both tractional and exudative in nature (TERD), without significant proliferative tissue on the retinal surface.

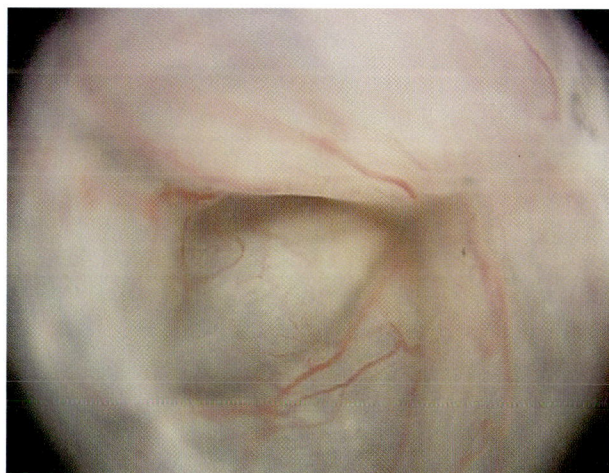

FIGURE 53.3 Preoperative photograph of Stage 5 ROP. A total retinal detachment is present. While subretinal exudate and blood is inevitably present, the closed funnel shape of the detachment is due to retinal surface proliferation. A similar anatomic configuration, consisting of surface proliferation greater than subretinal exudation, characterizes Stage 5 FEVR as well.

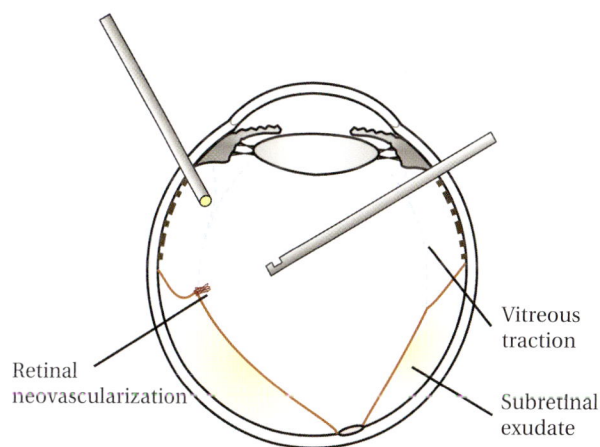

FIGURE 53.4 Cross-sectional diagram of Stage 4B ROP before surgery. The blue lines represent the vectors of transvitreal traction extending from the ridge between vascular and avascular retina to the lens and ciliary bodies. The goal of surgery is the release of this transvitreal traction. Because no significant surface proliferative component is present, shaving of the vitreous cortex near the retinal surface introduces the risk of iatrogenic retinal breaks, without contributing to the surgical goal.

Lasered
retina

Resorbing
subretinal
exudate

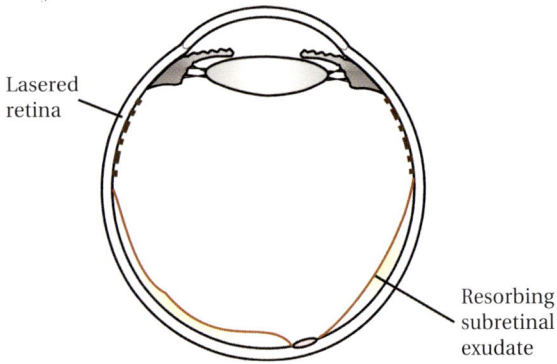

FIGURE 53.5 Cross-sectional diagram of Stage 4B ROP following surgery. Once transvitreal traction has been released with vitrectomy, an immediate relaxation of the retina is often observed. In some cases, retinal redundancy (due to prolonged traction) or subretinal exudation may delay complete retinal reattachment.

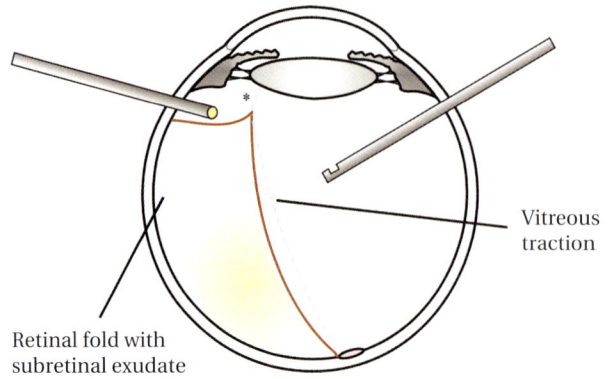

Vitreous
traction

Retinal fold with
subretinal exudate

FIGURE 53.6 Cross-sectional diagram of Stage 4B FEVR. Similar to Stage 4 ROP, Stage 4 FEVR is defined by transvitreal traction vectors from the retina to the lens/ciliary body diaphragm. A large temporal fold, extending temporally from the optic disc and anteriorly towards the lens, is characteristic of FEVR. Depending on the surgical space (indicated in the figure by the asterisk) between the fold and the posterior aspect of the lens, a lens-sparing approach may or may not be feasible. Postoperative relaxation of the retinal fold may take months, as subretinal exudate gradually resorbs, similar to Stage 4 ROP.

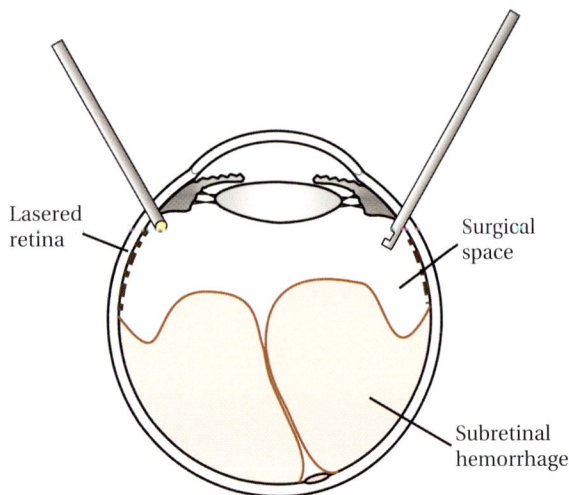

Lasered
retina

Surgical
space

Subretinal
hemorrhage

FIGURE 53.7 Cross-sectional diagram of Stage 4B/5 ROP surgery. Stage 4B/5 is characterized by the complete detachment of the retina posterior to the areas of prior peripheral photocoagulation. The retinal detachment may take on a funnel configuration, with significant surface proliferation. A surgical working space is present between the lens–ciliary body diaphragm, the attached peripheral retina, and the detached retina. The lens can usually be spared if the surgeon is able to safely enter this space. The goals of surgery are both the relief of transvitreal traction (similar to Figure 53.4), as well as the removal of surface proliferative tissue. Since the retina is often atrophic, great care must be taken to peel proliferative tissue without creating an iatrogenic retinal break. The complete removal of all surface proliferation is often not necessary to allow retinal reattachment.

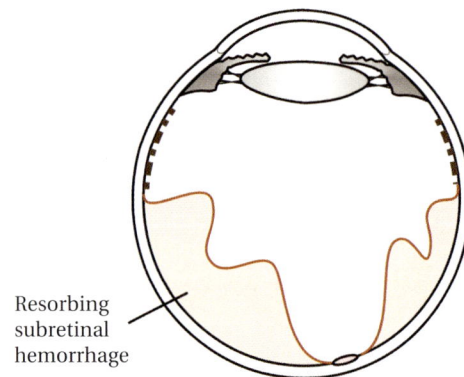

Resorbing
subretinal
hemorrhage

FIGURE 53.8 Cross-sectional diagram of Stage 4B/5 ROP following surgery. Subretinal blood and exudate may take many months to reabsorb following surgery. Retinal redundancy is often present due to prolonged traction, and peripheral retinal folds may form subsequently.

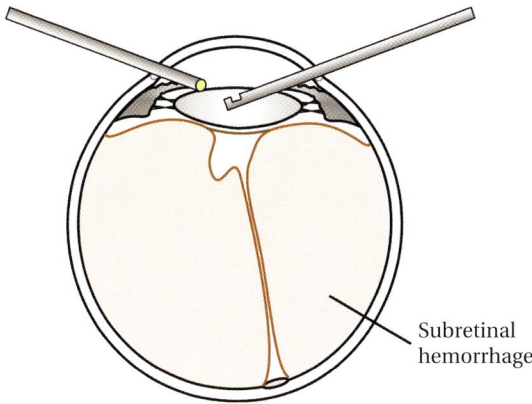

FIGURE 53.9 Cross-sectional diagram of Stage 5 ROP/FEVR surgery. In previously untreated total retinal detachments from ROP or FEVR, a surgical working space posterior to the lens–ciliary body diaphragm is generally absent. In order to safely address retinal surface proliferation, a limbal approach is used and the lens is removed. The lens capsule should be removed entirely, in contrast to surgery for congenital cataract, in which a rim of capsule is left in place for future intraocular lens implantation. In Stage 5 disease, capsular remnants serve as a scaffold for anterior proliferation and retinal redetachment, making complete capsulectomy critical.

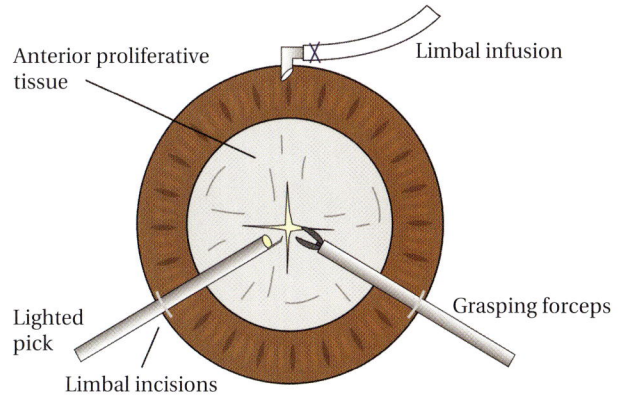

FIGURE 53.10 Surgical approach to Stage 5 ROP/FEVR. Once the lens has been removed through limbal incisions, a superficial cruciate incision is created in the proliferative tissue on the retinal surface. A lighted pick and grasping forceps are useful instruments for this purpose, as the sharp pick can incise the fine proliferative tissue with minimal traction on the atrophic underlying retina.

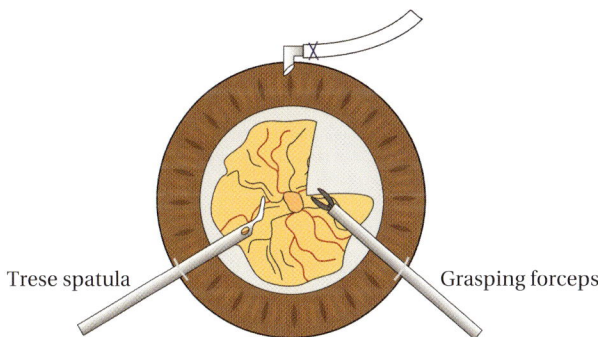

FIGURE 53.11 Surgical removal of proliferative tissue in Stage 5 disease. Once the cruciate incision has been successfully created (Figure 53.9), proliferative tissue is gently peeled from the retinal surface. Once a surgical plane has been created between the proliferative tissue and underlying retina, the sharp lighted pick is exchanged for the Trese irrigating spatula. The spatula edges are useful in continuing the surgical plane without traumatizing the underlying retina.

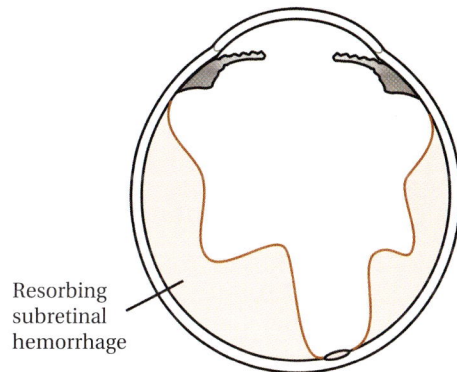

FIGURE 53.12 Cross-sectional diagram of Stage 5 ROP/FEVR following surgery. As with Stage 4B/5 ROP, retinal redundancy and subretinal exudate or blood are frequently present, and may result in retinal folds or delayed retinal reattachment over a period of months. An air–fluid or air–sodium hyaluronate exchange at the end of surgery, with postoperative face-down or upright positioning, may assist in opening a funnel detachment once the anterior proliferation has been removed. Some residual surface proliferative tissue usually remains at the end of surgery, given the increased marginal risk of creating a retinal break with continued membrane peeling. Partial retinal reattachment is often a realistic best-case outcome, given the constrictive effect of residual proliferation.

Persistent Fetal Vascular Syndrome (PFVS)

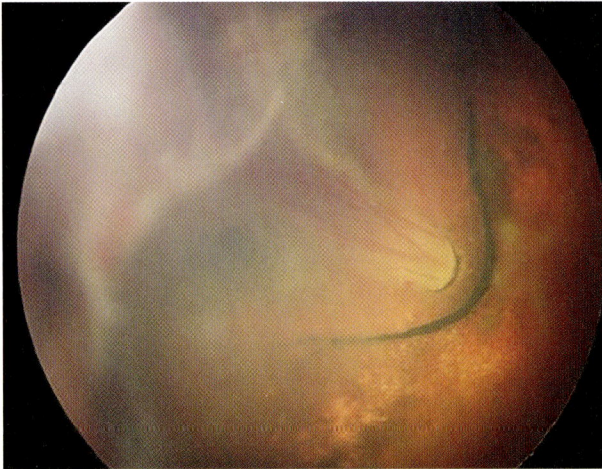

FIGURE 53.13 Preoperative photograph of persistent fetal vasculature syndrome (PFVS). The stalk is highly vascularized near the optic disc, and the retina is pulled into folds around the disc, demarcated by a dense pigment line.

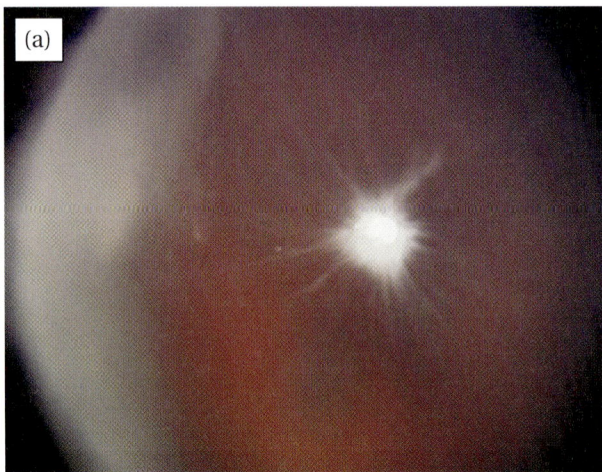

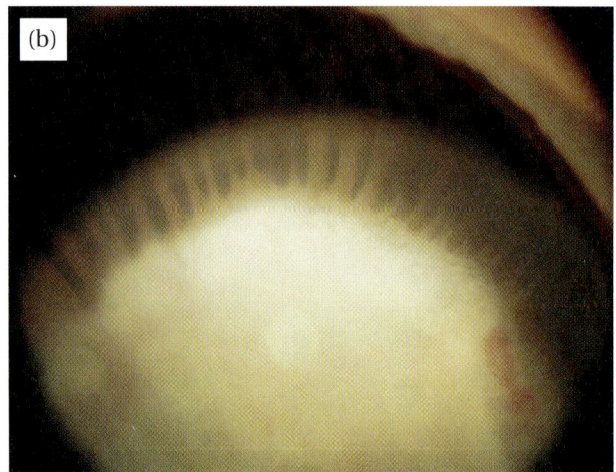

FIGURE 53.14 Preoperative photographs of PFVS. A wide variety of stalk configurations may be seen anteriorly, ranging from a small central or eccentric lens opacity (a) to a large posterior plaque extending to (and sometimes pulling on) the ciliary processes (b).

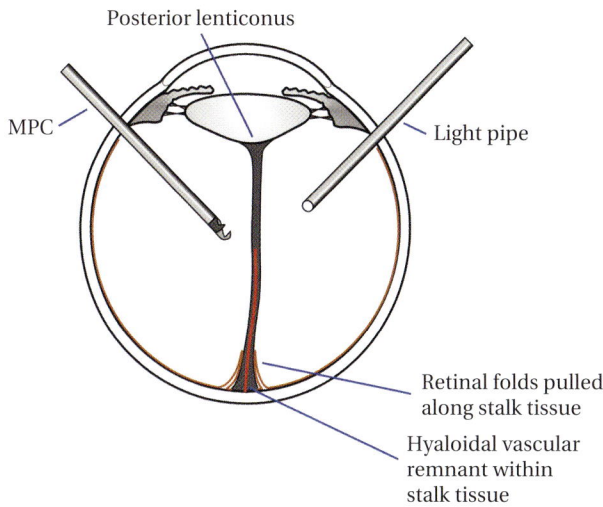

FIGURE 53.15 Cross-section diagram of PFVS surgery. If the anterior aspect of the stalk is associated with a small non-central lens plaque, the lens may be spared using a pars plicata approach. A mild tractional posterior lenticonus may be present prior to stalk segmentation. The primary goal of surgery is segmentation of the stalk to prevent constriction of globe growth. The retina is frequently pulled into folds along the base of the stalk. These folds may be difficult to identify even intraoperatively, and caution must be taken to segment the stalk anterior to any folds. Similarly, active vasculature is often present within the posterior aspect of the stalk, and the stalk should be segmented relatively anteriorly to prevent significant intraoperative bleeding. A membrane-peeler-cutter (MPC) scissor is useful for segmenting the stalk.

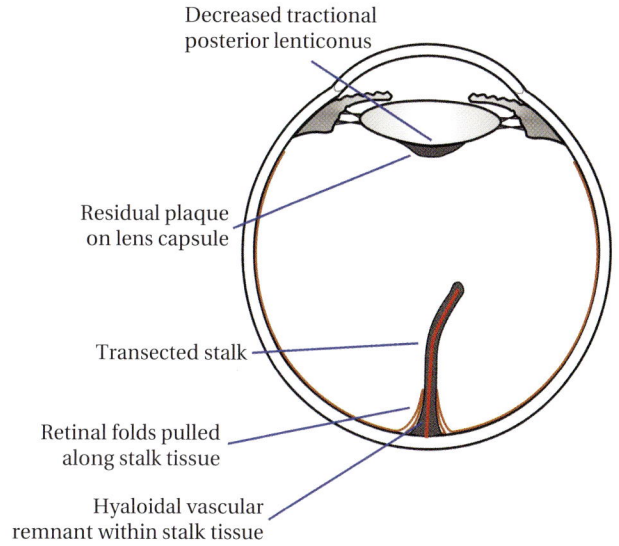

FIGURE 53.16 Cross-sectional postoperative diagram of lens-sparing vitrectomy for PFVS. Following stalk segmentation and removal of vitreous around the stalk, and between the stalk and lens, the stalk tissue should fall away from the lens, demonstrating a lack of anterior tractional vectors.

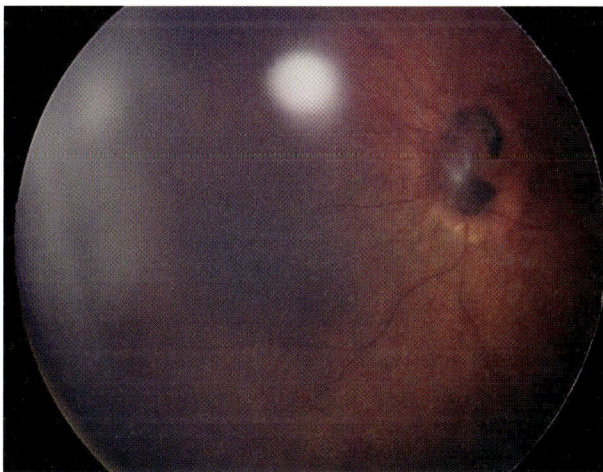

FIGURE 53.17 Postoperative photograph of lens-sparing vitrectomy for PFVS, with a residual small eccentric posterior lens capsular opacity. The contracted and fibrotic stalk remnant is visible over the optic disc.

Complications

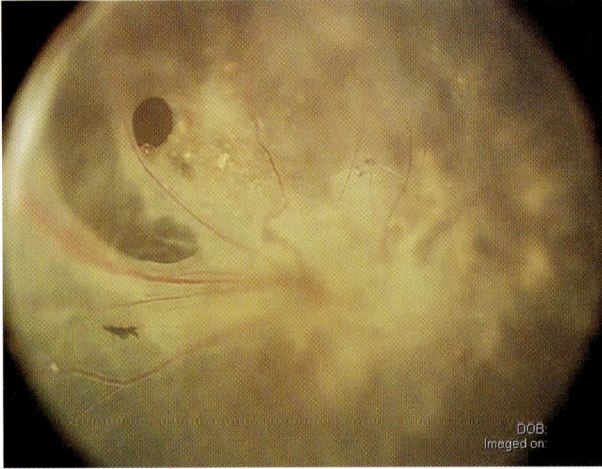

FIGURE 53.18 Proliferative vitreoretinopathy (PVR) following iatrogenic retinal break during ROP surgery. Infants and small children tend to mount a rapid and severe proliferative response to full-thickness retinal breaks. In addition, residual proliferative tissue often prevents complete retinal reattachment in the absence of a retinal break. If a retinal break occurs, apposition of the break to retinal pigment epithelium may not be possible, thereby preventing effective retinopexy unless extensive surgical relaxation is performed. Anatomic and visual outcomes tend to be poor after such a complication. For this reason, a conservative, relatively minimalist surgical approach is warranted in pediatric retinal surgical cases.

SELECTED REFERENCES

Capone A, Jr., Trese MT. Lens-sparing vitreous surgery for tractional stage 4A retinopathy of prematurity retinal detachments. *Ophthalmology*. 2001;108(11):2068–2070.

Capone A, Jr., Trese MT. Pediatric rhegmatogenous retinal detachment. In: Hartnett ME, ed. *Pediatric Retina*. Philadelphia: Lippincott Williams & Wilkins, 2005: 365–376.

Fivgas GD, Capone A, Jr. Pediatric rhegmatogenous retinal detachment. *Retina*. 2001;21(2):101–106.

Joshi MM, Ciaccia S, Trese MT, Capone A, Jr. Posterior hyaloid contracture in pediatric vitreoretinopathies. *Retina*. 2006;26(7 Suppl):S38–S41.

Maguire AM, Trese MT. Visual results of lens-sparing vitreoretinal surgery in infants. *J Pediatr Ophthalmol Strabismus*. 1993;30(1):28–32.

Pendergast SD, Trese MT. Familial exudative vitreoretinopathy. Results of surgical management. *Ophthalmology*. 1998;105(6):1015–1023.

Prenner JL, Capone A, Jr., Trese MT. Visual outcomes after lens-sparing vitrectomy for stage 4A retinopathy of prematurity. *Ophthalmology*. 2004;111(12):2271–2273.

Shaikh S, Trese MT. Lens-sparing vitrectomy in predominantly posterior persistent fetal vasculature syndrome in eyes with nonaxial lens opacification. *Retina*. 2003;23(3):330–334.

Trese MT, Capone A, Jr. Surgical approaches to infant and childhood retinal diseases: Invasive methods. In: Hartnett ME, ed. *Pediatric Retina*. Philadelphia: Lippincott Williams & Wilkins, 2005, pp. 359–364.

Amol D. Kulkarni, MD and Daniel M. Albert, MD, MS, FACS

Amyloidosis

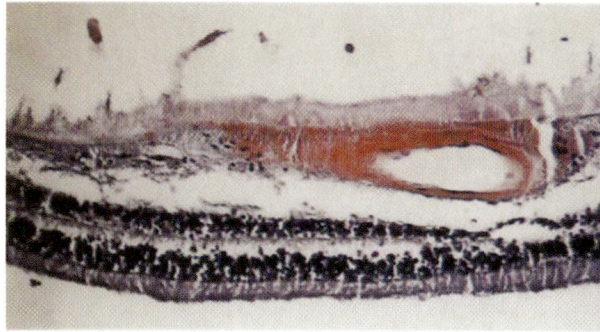

FIGURE 54.1 Amyloids are proteins with beta-pleated sheet configuration, and can be derived from large serum or tissue proteins. Ocular involvement occurs in primary, secondary, and heredofamilial amyloidosis. Vitreous amyloid deposits may be the first manifestation of systemic amyloidosis. The amyloid passes through the retinal vessels and ciliary body, and subsequently accumulates in the vitreous and other ocular structures. Note the deposits of eosinophilic, congophilic material within the wall of a retinal blood vessel in a case of familial amyloidotic polyneuropathy. (Reprinted with permission from Ciulla TA, Tolentino F, Morrow JF, Dryja TP. Vitreous amyloidosis in familial amyloidotic polyneuropathy. Report of a case with the Val30Met transthyretin mutation. *Surv Ophthalmol.* 1995 Nov–Dec;40(3):197–206.)

Epiretinal Membrane

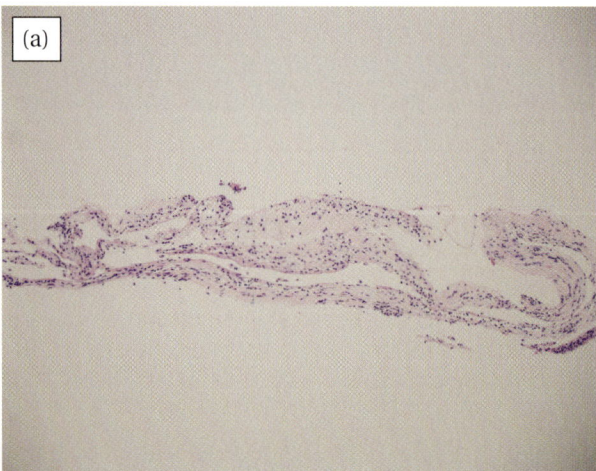

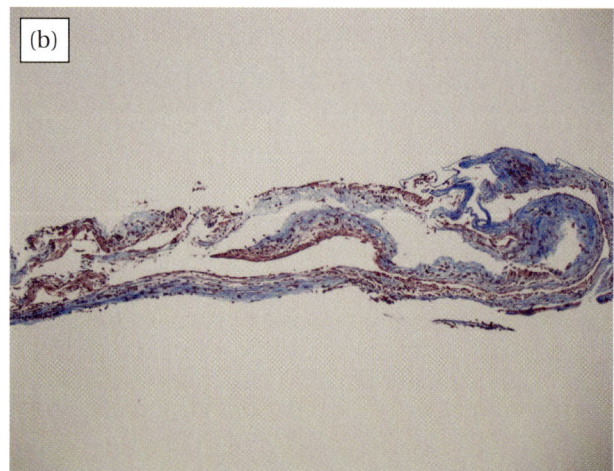

FIGURE 54.2 At least two subtypes of epiretinal membranes can occur: hypocellular with intracortical vitreoschisis, and thick, proliferative, contractile cells with cortical remnants after posterior vitreous detachment. (a) Epiretinal membrane with predominance of retinal pigment epithelium-derived fibroblast-like cells (hematoxylin-eosin, original magnification × 100). (b) Epiretinal membrane with blue staining of the collagen (Masson's trichrome, original magnification × 100).

Diabetic Retinopathy

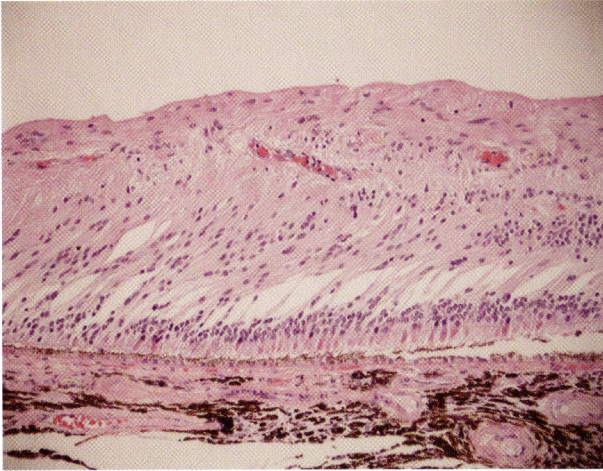

FIGURE 54.3 The pathologic process in diabetic retinopathy is a microangiopathy characterized by capillary microaneurysm formation, dilation, and hyperpermeability, with exudates, hemorrhages, edema, and capillary occlusion. This figure shows cystoid retinal edema, an important complication of diabetic retinopathy (hematoxylin-eosin, original magnification × 200).

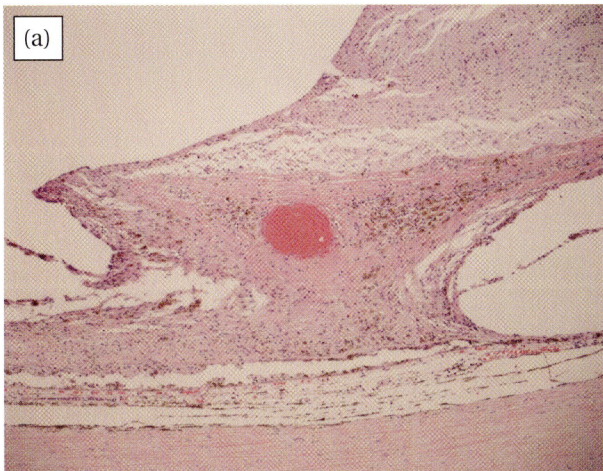

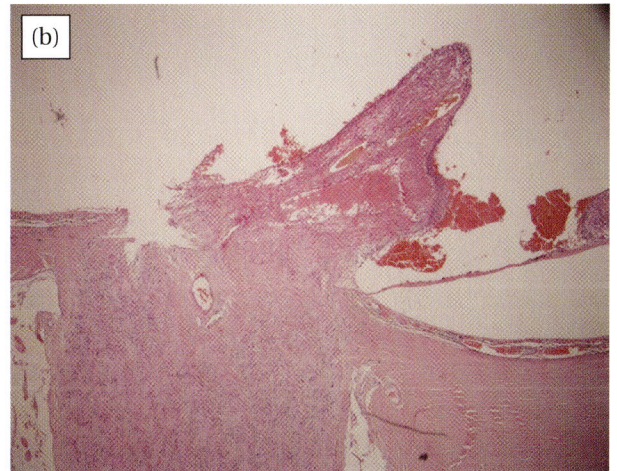

FIGURE 54.4 Proliferative diabetic retinopathy is characterized by breakdown of the blood–retinal barrier, vitreoretinal adherence provoked by gliovascular proliferation, partial posterior vitreous detachment, and preretinal neovascular formation. (a) Thickening of the inner retina secondary to gliosis with preretinal fibrovascular proliferation (hematoxylin-eosin, original magnification × 100). (b) Neovascularization of the disk with vitreous hemorrhage (hematoxylin-eosin, original magnification × 40).

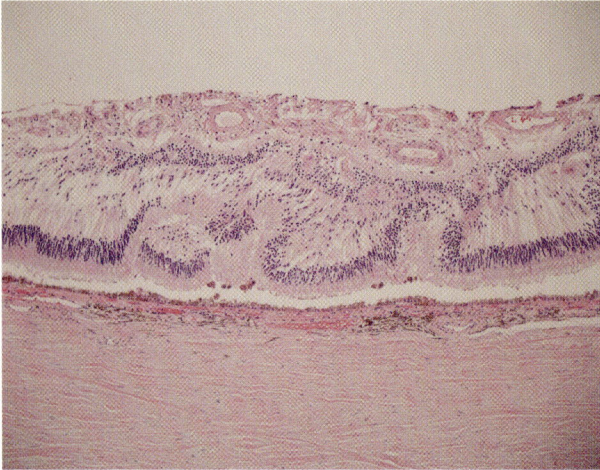

FIGURE 54.5 Proliferative diabetic retinopathy with preretinal fibrovascular proliferation leading to tangential traction and retinal folds. (hematoxylin-eosin, original magnification × 60).

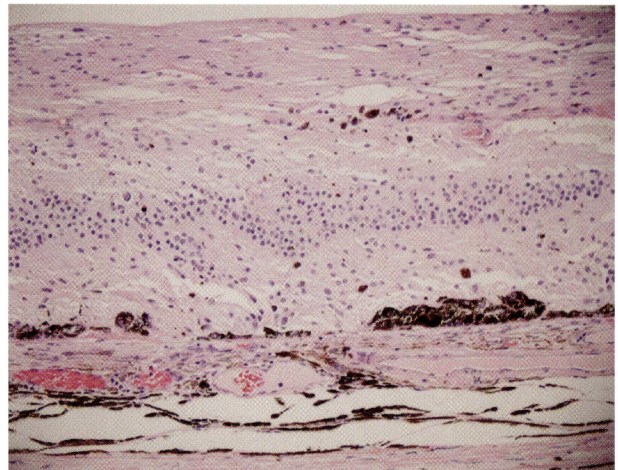

FIGURE 54.6 Photocoagulation scars in proliferative diabetic retinopathy. These are characterized by clumping and inner retinal migration of the retinal pigment epithelium (pseudoretinitis pigmentosa) with gliosis, and epiretinal membrane formation (hematoxylin-eosin, original magnification × 200).

Retinal Detachment and Proliferative Vitreoretinopathy

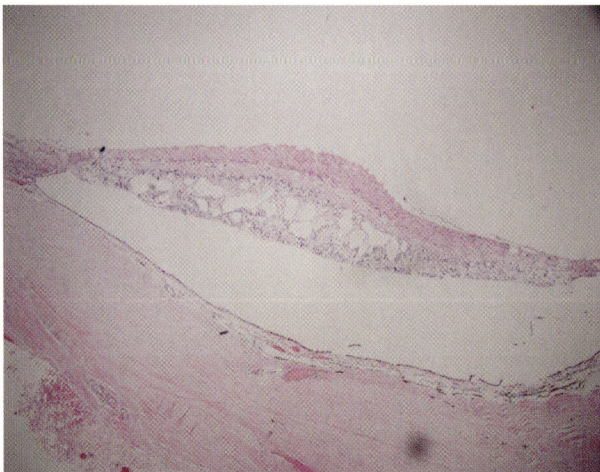

FIGURE 54.7 This eye had a total retinal detachment. Note the absence of photoreceptors and atrophy of outer plexiform and outer nuclear layers. There is epiretinal membrane formation, macular pucker, and cystoid macular edema. (hematoxylin-eosin, original magnification × 40).

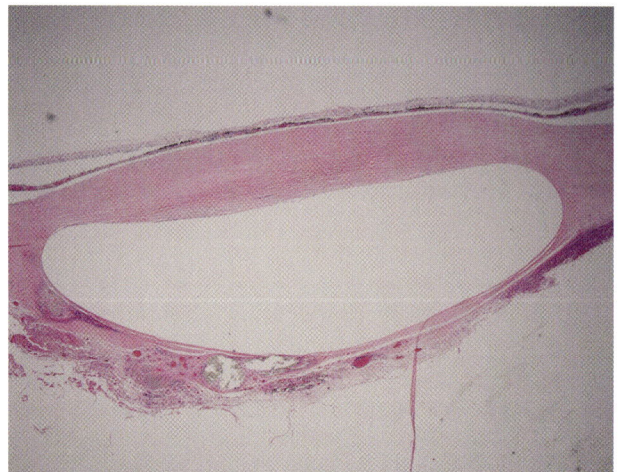

FIGURE 54.8 Postmortem removed eye after successful repair of retinal detachment with sclera buckle. The retina overlying the site of buckle is attached. The sclera shows a fibrous tunnel around the site of the buckle, with suture remnants on the episcleral side. (hematoxylin-eosin, original magnification × 20).

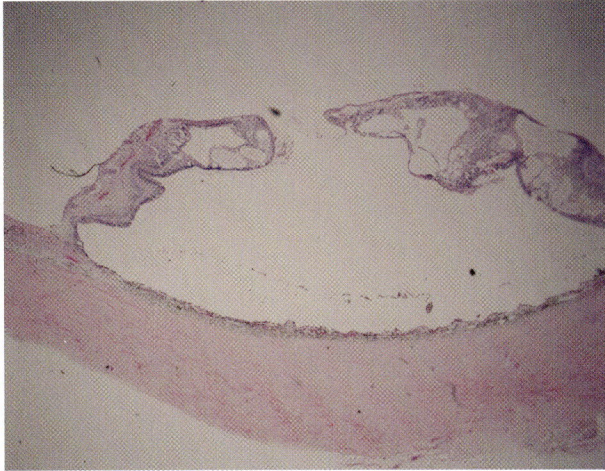

FIGURE 54.9 Rhegmatogenous retinal detachment caused by a retinal hole. Note the rounded edges of the retinal tissue on the either side of the true hole. There is atrophy and cystoid changes in the outer plexiform and outer nuclear layers. (hematoxylin-eosin, original magnification × 20).

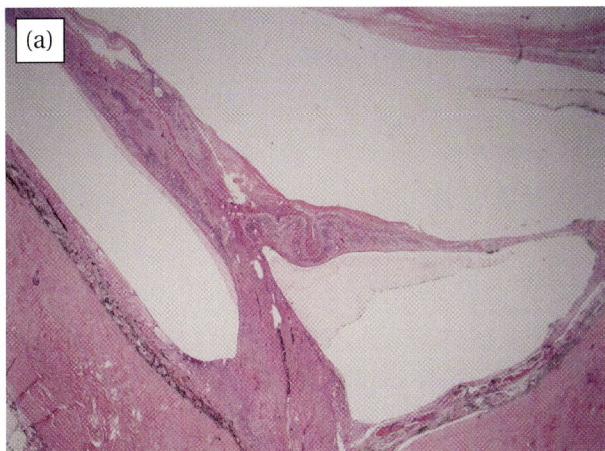

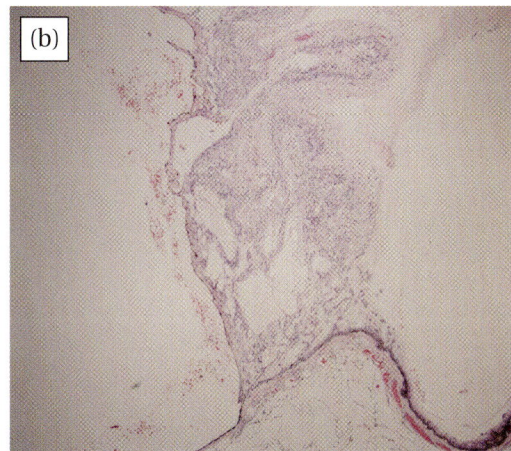

FIGURE 54.10 Proliferative vitreoretinopathy (PVR) is a major cause of failure of primary retinal detachment surgery. (a) A complex PVR membrane is seen, composed of densely organized vitreous and glial tissue, causing a closed funnel detachment that overlies the optic disk. The retina is folded, with an absence of photoreceptors and the presence of underlying subretinal fluid. The PVR membrane contains proliferated metaplastic pigment epithelial cells, embedded in fibrous extracellular matrix (hematoxylin-eosin, original magnification × 40). (b) In anterior PVR, there is glial proliferation at the vitreous base with tight adherence to the retinal surface, causing tractional separation of nonpigmented and pigmented neuroepithelial layers at the pars plana and pars plicata (hematoxylin-eosin, original magnification × 40).

SELECTED REFERENCES

Ciulla TA, Tolentino F, Morrow JF, Dryja TP. Vitreous amyloidosis in familial amyloidotic polyneuropathy. Report of a case with the Val30Met transthyretin mutation. *Surv Ophthalmol.* 1995 Nov–Dec;40(3):197–206.

Elner SG, Elner VM, Diaz-Rohena R, et al. Anterior PVR, Part II: Clinicopathologic, light microscopic, and ultrastructural findings. In: Freeman HM, Tolentino FI, eds. *Proliferative Vitreoretinopathy (PVR).* New York, NY: Springer-Verlag; 1989, pp. 34–45.

Sahel JA, Brini A, Albert DM. Pathology of the retina and vitreous. In: Albert DM, Jakobiec FA, eds. *Principles and Practice of Ophthalmology*, Philadelphia, PA: WB Saunders; 1994, p. 2247.

Pediatric Ophthalmology and Strabismus Surgery

Edited by **Edward G. Buckley**

Anatomy

Edward G. Buckley, MD

SELECTED REFERENCES

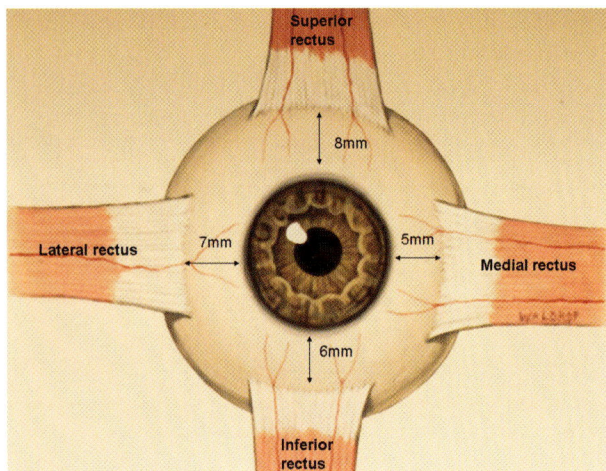

FIGURE 55.1 Right eye anterior view: The rectus muscles attach to the globe anterior to the equator. The relative distances of the insertions from the limbus form a spiral (spiral of Tilaux) with the medial rectus the closest, increasing clockwise to the superior rectus. This distance needs to be taken into account when isolating the rectus muscles during surgery.

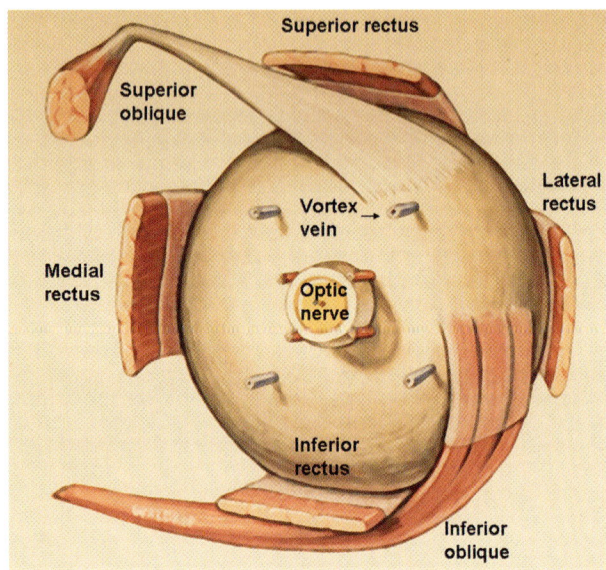

FIGURE 55.2 Right eye posterior view: The oblique muscles attach posterior to the equator, and thus rotate the eye in the opposite direction when compared to the rectus muscles. The superior rectus muscle depresses and the inferior oblique muscle elevates the eye. The insertions of these muscles are in close proximity to the vortex veins, and care must be taken during surgery on these muscles not to hook or injure them.

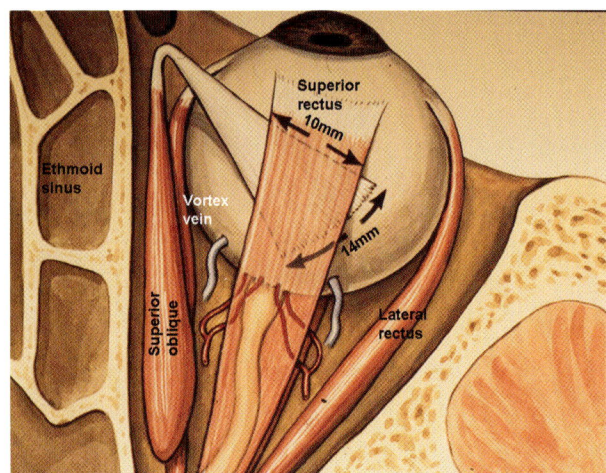

FIGURE 55.3 Right eye superior view: The superior oblique tendon lies underneath the superior rectus and extends for about 14 mm. Because of the close proximity of the medial border of the superior rectus muscle to the insertion of the superior oblique muscle, it is possible to inadvertently hook the superior oblique tendon when isolating the superior rectus muscle. The vortex vein is located near the medial border of the insertion, and must be avoided during surgery on the superior oblique.

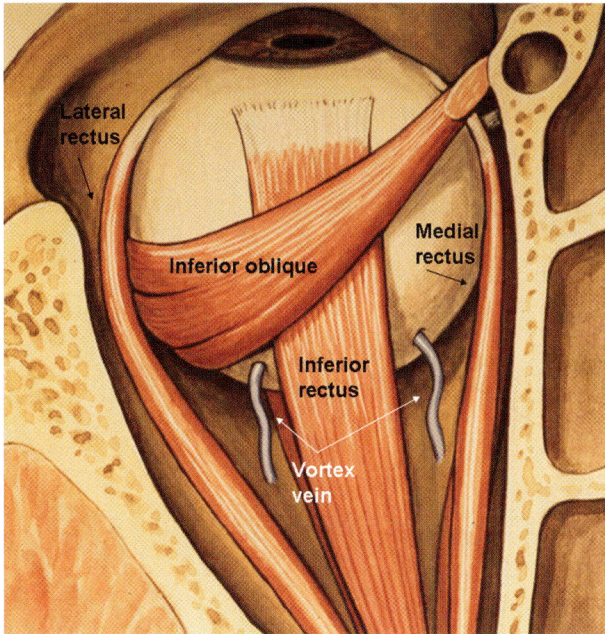

FIGURE 55.4 Right eye inferior view: The inferior oblique muscle passes under the inferior rectus, and attaches to the lateral aspect of the lacrimal bone. The posterior border is in close proximity to the vortex vein, and care must be exercised when hooking this muscle to avoid injuring the vein.

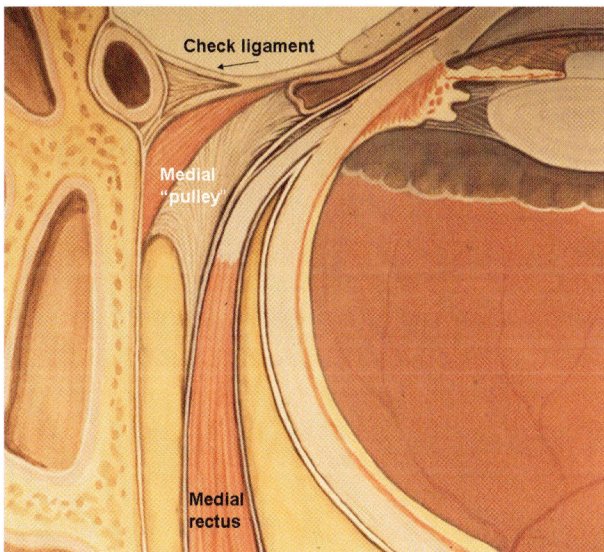

FIGURE 55.5 Right eye view from above: The rectus muscles pass through connective tissue structures, which act like "pulleys" guiding the movement. These pulleys wrap around the muscle and attach to the adjacent bone. These structures limit the excursion of the muscle and effect the rotational movement of the eye. Similar structures (check ligaments) also provide resistance to rotation.

TABLE 55.1 *Length, Origin, Insertion, and Innervation of the Extraocular Muscles*

Muscle	Origin	Insertion, Distance from Limbus (mm)	Muscle Length (mm)	Tendon Length (mm)	Insertion Width (mm)	Innervation	Action
Medial rectus	Annulus of Zinn	4.7–6.2	37.7–40.8	2.4–3.0	10.4–11.3	Superior division, oculomotor	Adduction
Lateral rectus	Annulus of Zinn	6.3–7.7	36.3–40.6	7.0–7.2	9.6–10.7	Abducens	Abduction
Superior rectus	Annulus of Zinn	6.6–8.5	37.3–41.8	4.0–4.3	10.4–11.5	Superior division, oculomotor	Elevation, adduction, incyclotorsion
Inferior rectus	Annulus of Zinn	5.3–7.0	37.0–40.0	2.7–4.7	8.6–9.8	Inferior division, oculomotor	Depression, adduction, excyclotorsion
Superior oblique	Annulus of Zinn	10.8	40.0	20.0	7–18	Trochlear	Incyclotorsion, depression, abduction
Inferior oblique	Maxilla antero-medially	—	37.9	0.0	4–15	Inferior division, oculomotor	Excyclotorsion, elevation, abduction

TABLE 55.2 *Muscle Actions Primary, Secondary, and Tertiary Actions of the Extraocular Muscles*

Muscle	Primary	Secondary	Tertiary
Medial rectus	Adduction	—	—
Lateral rectus	Abduction	—	—
Superior rectus	Elevation	Incycloduction	Adduction
Inferior rectus	Depression	Excycloduction	Adduction
Superior oblique	Incycloduction	Depression	Abduction
Inferior oblique	Excycloduction	Elevation	Abduction

SELECTED REFERENCES

Apt L. An anatomical reevaluation of rectus muscle insertions. *Trans Am Ophthalmol Soc.* 1980;78:365–375.

Buckley EG, Shields MB. *Strabismus and Glaucoma Surgery, Vol III.* St. Louis, MO: Mosby, 1995.

Souza-Dias C, Prieto-Diaz J, Uesugui CF. Topographical aspects of the insertions of the extraocular muscles. *J Pediatr Ophthalmol Strabismus.* 1986;23:183–189.

von Noorden GK. *Binocular Vision and Ocular Motility, Theory, and Management of Strabismus.* 5th ed. St. Louis, MO: Mosby-Year Book; 1996:41–52.

Equipment and Suture Technique

Edward G. Buckley, MD

SELECTED REFERENCES

0.5- and 0.3-mm Castroviejo forceps

(1)

Bishop Harmon toothed forceps

(2)

Moody locking forceps, curved

(3)

Small straight hemostat

(4)

Tying forceps

(5)

Jameson muscle clemp, left and right

(6)

Fine needle holder, curved, locking

(7)

Solid-blade Barraquer or lancater
speculum, adult and infant size

(8)

Desmarres lid speculum, small and medium

(9)

Malleable retractor, 10-15 mm wide

(10)

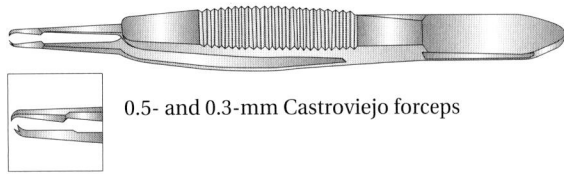

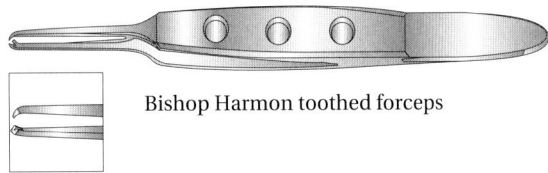

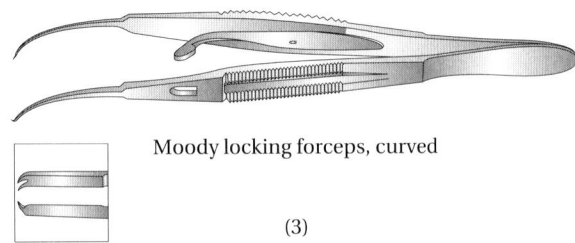

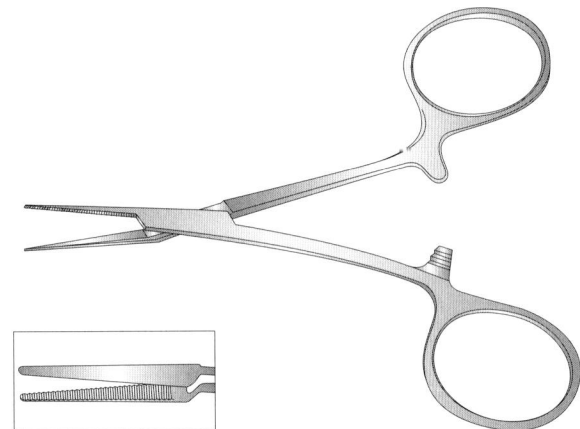

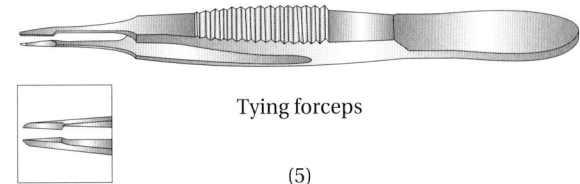

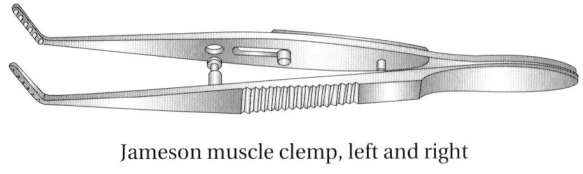

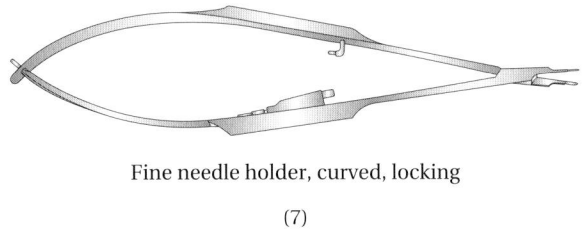

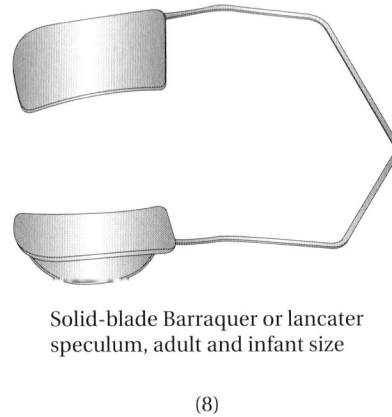

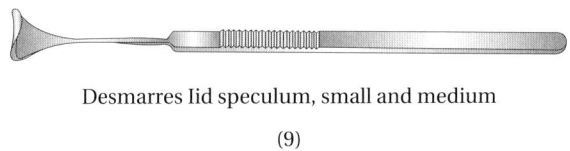

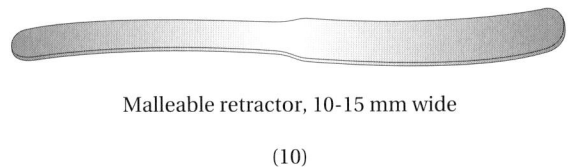

FIGURE 56.1 Instruments used in strabismus surgery will vary somewhat among procedures, and surgeons can perform the same procedure using different instruments. However, certain basic instruments should be available for all strabismus procedures, and should compose a minimal surgical set.

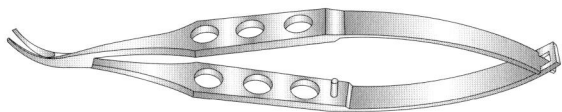

Westcott curved scissors

(11)

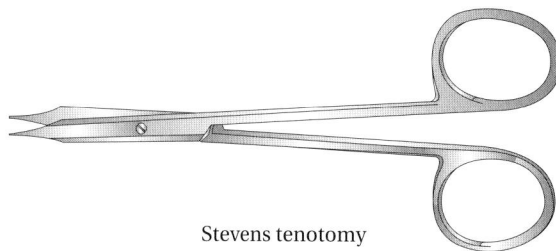

Stevens tenotomy

(12)

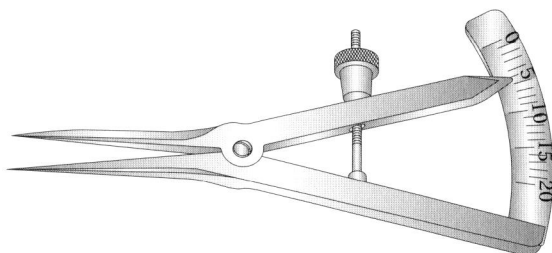

Castroviejo calipers

(13)

FIGURE 56.1 (a) (*continued*).

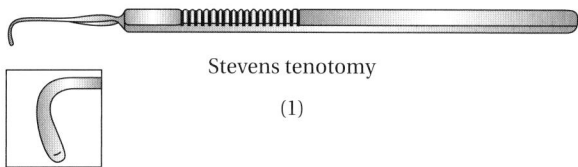

Stevens tenotomy

(1)

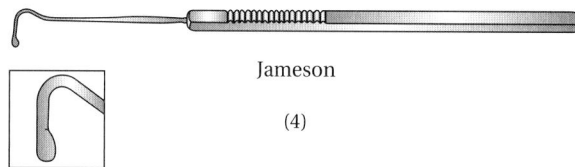

Jameson

(4)

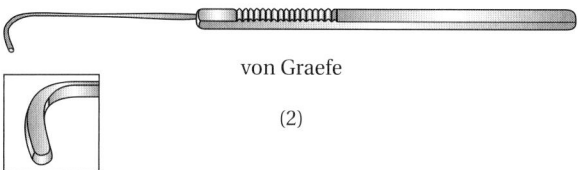

von Graefe

(2)

Bishop tendon tucker

(5)

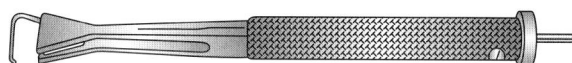

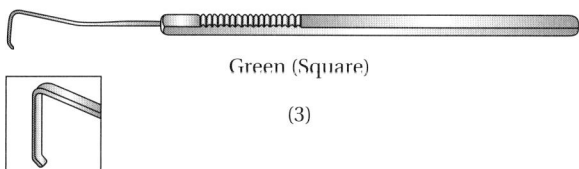

Green (Square)

(3)

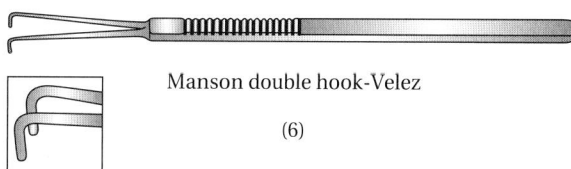

Manson double hook-Velez

(6)

FIGURE 56.1 (b) (*continued*).

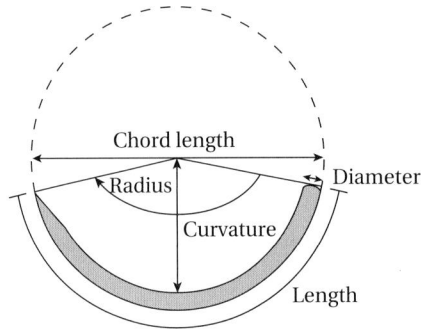

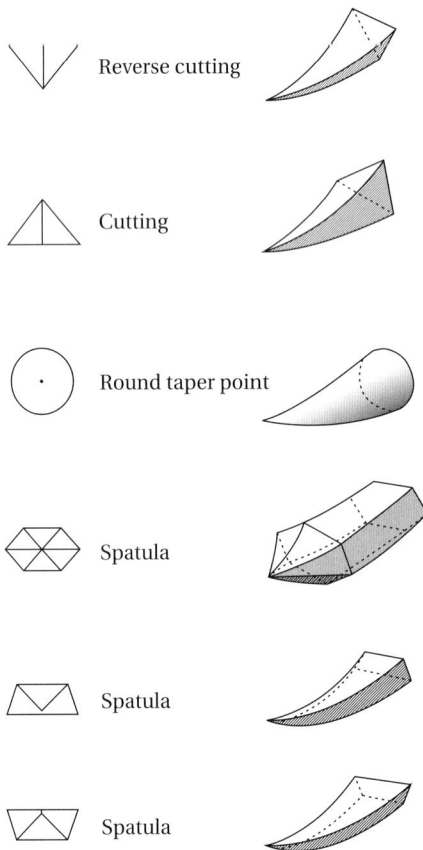

FIGURE 56.2 Safe, accurate placement of the needle prevents perforation of the sclera and allows secure anchoring of the reattached muscle. Spatulated needles cut on the lateral surfaces and, when held properly in the tangential angle to the sclera, have less potential for scleral perforation or erosion. Polyglactin and polyglycolic acid braided material is available in a variety of calibers, ranging from 2-0 to 8-0. The most popular caliber for muscle surgery has been 6-0. The tensile strength of the suture is sufficient to allow strabismus surgery with a caliber of 6-0 or smaller. Nearly full tensile strength is maintained for 14–21 days.

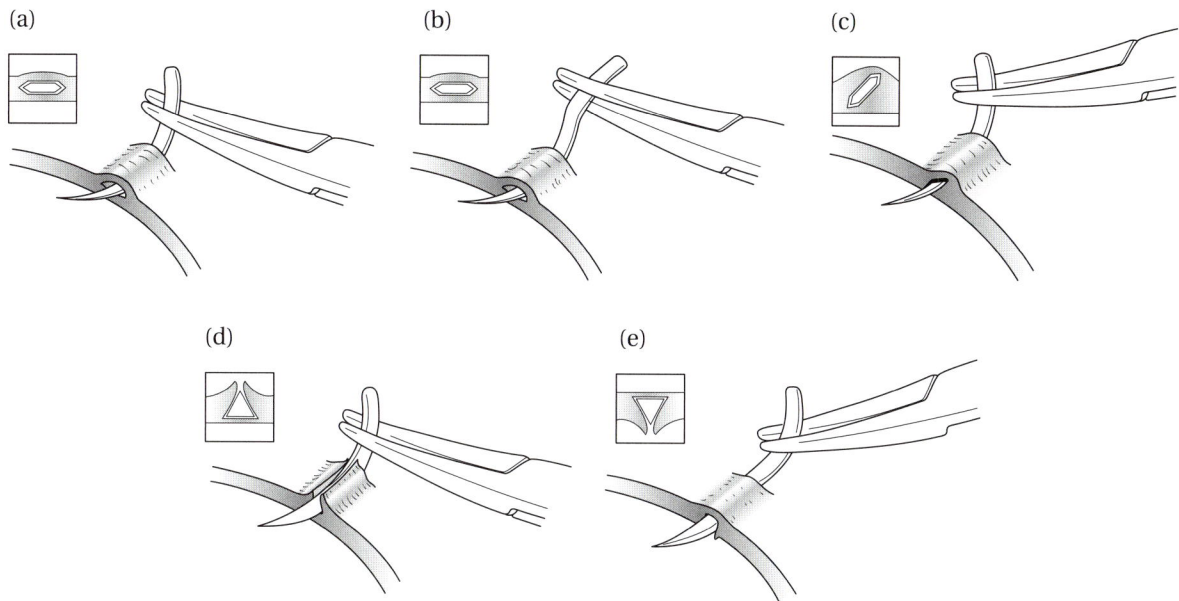

FIGURE 56.3 Scleral suture technique. Understanding the needle design is important to understand proper surgical technique. (a) The suture should be passed with its curvature perpendicular to the scleral surface. The depth of the pass should allow firm attachment, but the needle should be visible within the translucent sclera, approximately 0.2 mm. (b) Excessive torque or rotational force applied against the curvature of the needle can easily bend the small needles, making passage difficult. (c) Tilting the needle so that the curvature is not perpendicular to the scleral surface will turn the cutting edges across the sclera, risking perforation or weakening the suture pass. (d) Cutting needles, with a cutting edge inside the curve of the needle, risk weakening the scleral pass or cutting out of the sclera completely. (e) Reverse cutting needles risk perforation into the eye on scleral passage, and should not be used for strabismus surgery.

SELECTED REFERENCES

Apt L. An anatomical reevaluation of rectus muscle insertions. *Trans Am Ophthalmol Soc.* 1980;78:365–375.

de Gottrau P, Gajisin S, Roth A. Ocular rectus muscle insertions revisited: an unusual anatomic approach. *Acta Anat* (*Basel*).1994;151:268–272.

de Gottrau P, Gajisin S. Anatomic, histologic, and morphometric studies of the ocular rectus muscles and their relation to the eye globe and Tenon's capsule. *Klin Monatsbl Augenheilkd.* 1992;200:515–516.

Helveston EM. Sutures and needles for strabismus surgery. *Int Ophthalmol Clin.* 1976;16:39–45.

Schwartz RL, Koller HP. Survey of sutures used in strabismus surgery—1980. *J Pediatr Ophthalmol Strabismus.* 1981;18:39–41.

Souza-Dias C, Prieto-Diaz J, Uesugui CF. Topographical aspects of the insertions of the extraocular muscles. *J Pediatr Ophthalmol Strabismus.* 1986;23:183–189.

von Noorden GK. *Binocular Vision and Ocular Motility, Theory, and Management of Strabismus.* 5th ed. St. Louis, MO: Mosby-Year Book; 1996:41–52.

Zide BM, Jelks GW. Surgical anatomy of the orbit. *Plast Reconstr Surg.* 1984;74:301–305.

Edward G. Buckley, MD

TABLE 57.1 *Surgical Amounts—Esodeviations*

Amount of Deviation (Prism Diopters)	Medial Rectus Recession OU	Lateral Resection OU	Medial Rectus Recession/Lateral Rectus Resection OD or OS	Medial Rectus Recession OU 5.5 mm + Lateral Rectus Resection(s)
15	3.0	4.0	3.5/4.0	—
20	3.5	5.0	4.0.5/5.0	—
25	4.0	5.5	4.5/5.5	—
30	4.5	6.0	5.0/6.0	—
35	5.0	6.5	5.5/6.5	—
40	5.5	7.0	5.5/7.0	—
50	6.0	—	—	4.0
60	(7.0)	—	—	6.0
70	(7.0)	—	—	4.0 OU
80	(7.0)	—	—	6.0 OU
90	(7.0)	—	—	7.0 OU

TABLE 57.2 *Surgical Amounts—Exodeviations*

Amount of Deviation (Prism Diopters)	Lateral Recession OU	Medial Resection OU	Lateral Recession/ Medial Resection, 1 Eye	Lateral Recession OU 8.0 mm + ½ Medial Resection(s)
15	4.0	3.0	4.0/3.0	—
20	5.0	4.0	5.4/4.0	—
25	6.0	5.0	6.0/5.0	—
30	7.0	5.5	7.0/5.5	—
35	7.5	6.0	7.5/6.0	—
40	8.0	6.5	8.0/6.5	—
50	9.0	—	(9.0/7.0)	5.0
60	—	—	(10.0/8.0)	7.0
70	—	—	(10.0/9.0)	5.0 OU
80	—	—	(10.0/10.0)	6.0 OU
90	—	—	—	76.0 OU

TABLE 57.3 *Surgical Amounts—Vertical Deviations*

Amount of Deviation (Prism Diopters)	Superior or Inferior Recession, 1 Eye	Superior or Inferior Resection, 1 Eye	Vertical Rectus Recession/ Resection, 1 Eye
10	3.5	3.5	—
15	5.0	5.0	4/3
20	—	—	5/4
25	—	—	6/5
30	—	—	7/5
35	—	—	7/6

Forced Duction Testing

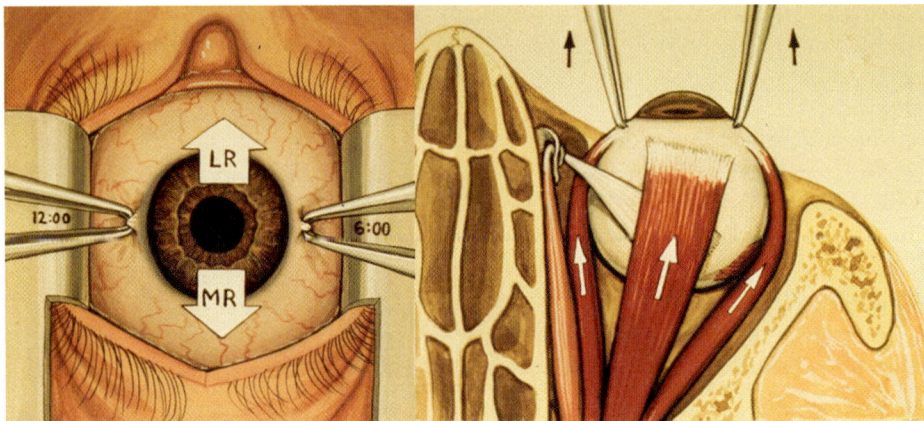

FIGURE 57.1 To test the horizontal rectus muscles, grasp the limbus at the 12 and 6 o'clock positions, and gently lift the eye. Rotate the eye nasally to test the lateral rectus and laterally to test the medial rectus. The eye should freely move in either direction. If a restriction is encountered (a positive forced duction), retropulse the eye to see if the restriction improves. If it does not improve with this maneuver, the restriction may be caused by a nonrectus muscle abnormality, such as periocular scarring or other orbital causes.

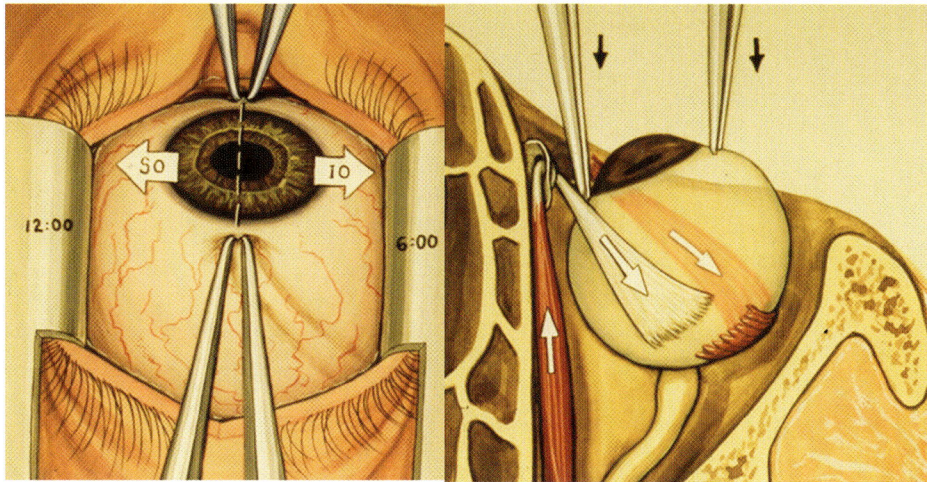

FIGURE 57.2 To evaluate the oblique muscles, grasp the limbus with toothed forceps at the 3 and 9 o'clock positions. The eye should be rotated nasally and retropulsed, placing the oblique muscles on maximum stretch. The superior oblique muscle is tested by moving the eye upward, and the inferior oblique is tested by moving the eye downward. While performing this test, the most important forceps is the one located nasally over the medial rectus muscle insertion. It is in the nasal forceps that the examiner will first "feel" the restriction. As the eye is elevated or depressed, the nasal forceps will become limited and the eye will begin to twist or tort. This feeling is different than when testing rectus muscles, in which the restriction is felt "equally" in both forceps. It is important to keep the "imaginary" line between the forceps parallel to the floor of the orbit while moving the eye superiorly and inferiorly in adduction.

Muscle Exposure Techniques/Issues

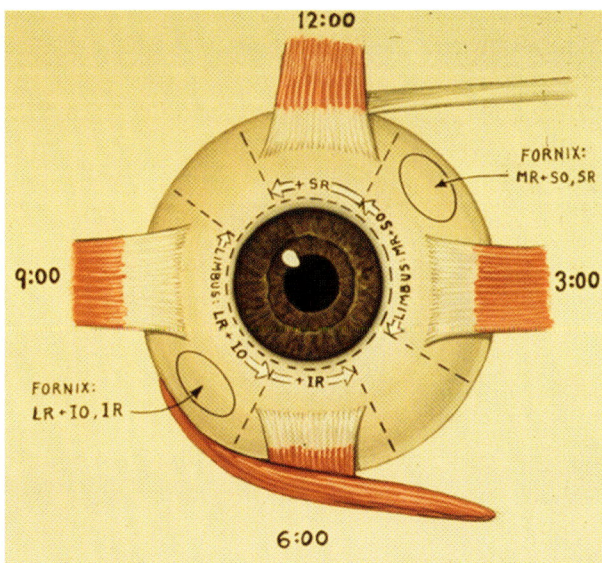

FIGURE 57.3 When operating on more than one muscle per eye is necessary, surgeons often find it advantageous to modify the conjunctival incision to allow exposure of the additional muscle through a single incision. This figure illustrates the various openings that can be used to accomplish this task. For example, if both the medial and superior rectus muscles are to be modified, a limbus-based incision can be extended from 11 o'clock to 4 o'clock to allow adequate exposure of both muscles. Likewise, a fornix-based incision can be placed in the superior nasal fornix to allow exposure of both muscles. For combination lateral rectus and inferior oblique surgery, the limbus-based incision can be extended just slightly more inferiorly to allow exposure of the inferior oblique muscle. No modification is necessary for a fornix-based incision for this combination of muscles. Additional variations are shown in the diagram.

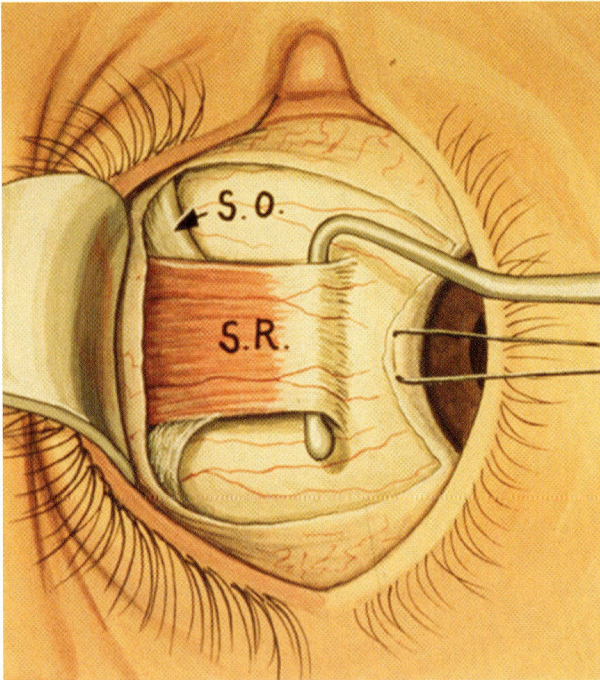

FIGURE 57.4 Exposure of the superior rectus and superior oblique can be facilitated by removing the lid speculum and using a Desmarres lid retractor in its place. By inserting a Desmarres lid retractor underneath the upper lid, both the superior rectus and the superior oblique tendon are easily exposed. The same maneuver can be used on the inferior rectus muscle.

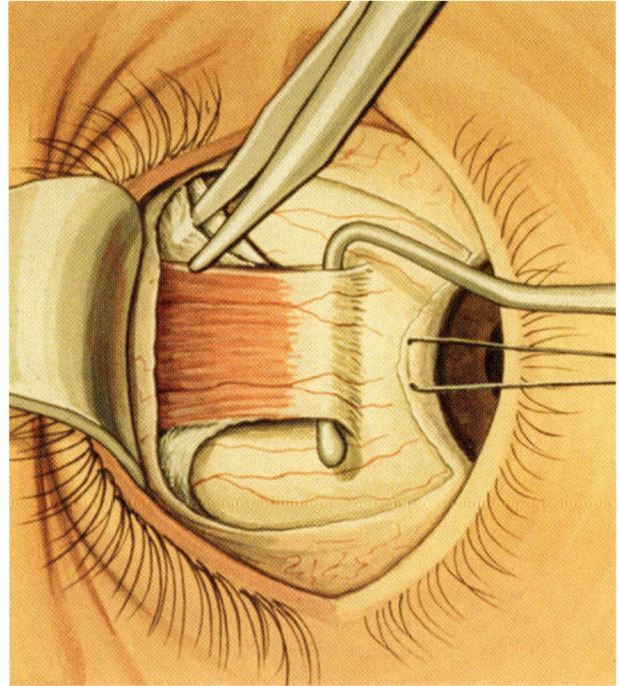

FIGURE 57.5 Caution must be used in severing attachments in intermuscular septum along the nasal border of the superior rectus, because the *superior oblique tendon* is often pulled forward toward the superior rectus insertion and could accidently be cut.

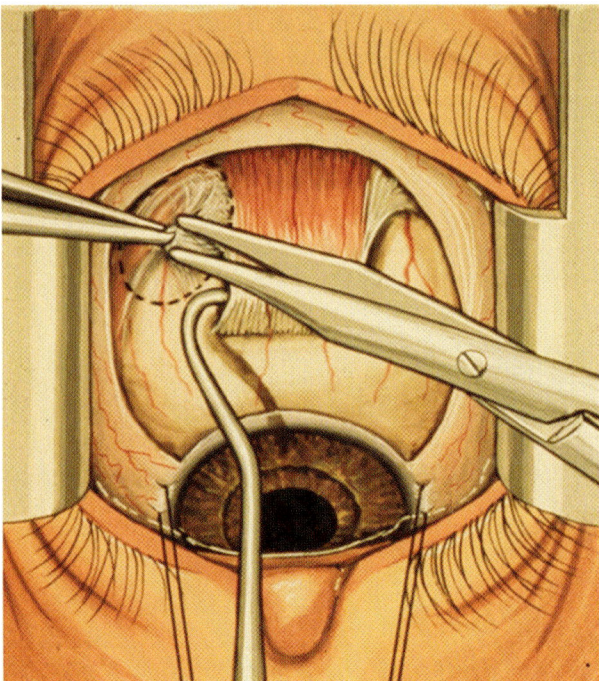

FIGURE 57.6 When exposing the lateral rectus muscle, the *inferior oblique* can sometimes be caught up in the connective tissue attachments, and end up displaced anteriorly toward the lateral rectus insertion. One should be careful not to cut into it. One must be especially careful in reoperations, since the inferior oblique muscle is often displaced anteriorly and can be located very near the lateral rectus muscle insertion.

Conjunctival Incisions—Limbal Approach

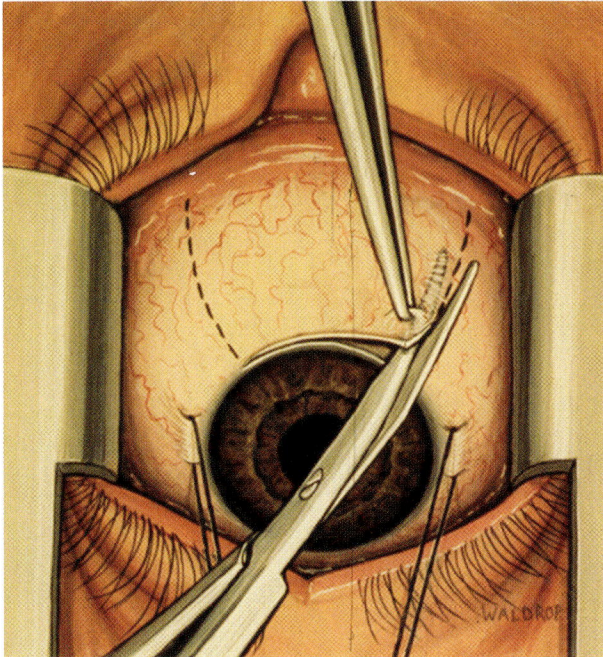

FIGURE 57.7 Using a toothed forceps, elevate the conjunctiva and Tenon's tissue at a distance approximately 2–3 mm from the limbus on one side of the insertion of the muscle to be exposed. Using Westcott scissors, create a small opening through this tissue, exposing bare sclera. Insert both blades of the Westcott scissors into the opening and use a spreading technique to create a tunnel near the limbus. Insert the bottom blade into the opening while the top blade of the scissors remains external. Gently press the internal scissor blade against the limbus while cutting the tissue. This will ensure a smooth-edged incision. While still grasping the original edge of the conjunctival opening with forceps, approximate the cut edge (corner) to its original location. The beginnings of a small radial incision will be seen. Using the opening as a guideline, extend the incision posteriorly for approximately 7–8 mm (or to the semilunar fold for the medial rectus) in a slightly oblique fashion from the limbus. This radial incision should be perpendicular to the limbus. A similar radial incision is made at the other end of the limbal opening.

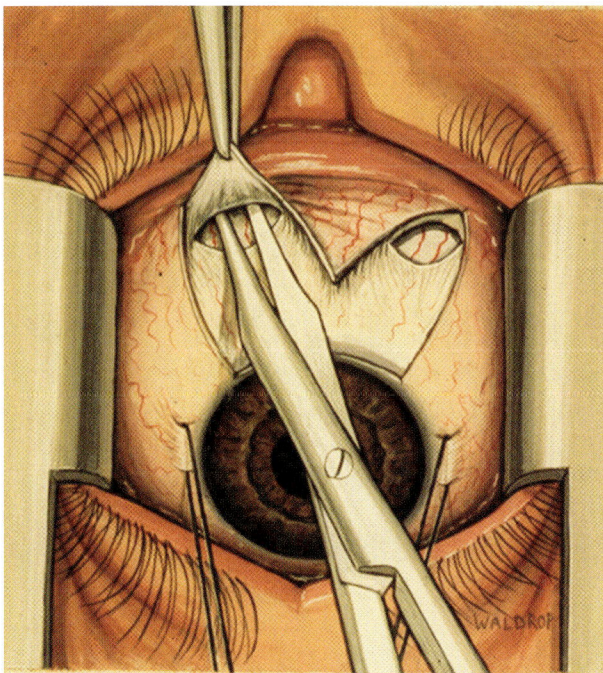

FIGURE 57.8 With forceps, grasp the edge of the conjunctival incision near its base on one side of the muscle insertion. Gently elevating the forceps will put the underlying Tenon's tissue on stretch. Push the closed blades of the Westcott scissors into this tissue until resistance is met. Then allow the points to spread (blunt dissection). Continue to push and spread until an opening is created through Tenon's capsule. This has been accomplished when *bare sclera* is seen through this opening. Try to direct the tips of the scissors away from the presumed location of the muscle, to avoid injuring the muscle capsule and causing an unwanted hemorrhage. After an opening has been created that is large enough to insert a small Stevens tenotomy hook, perform the same maneuver on the other side of the muscle.

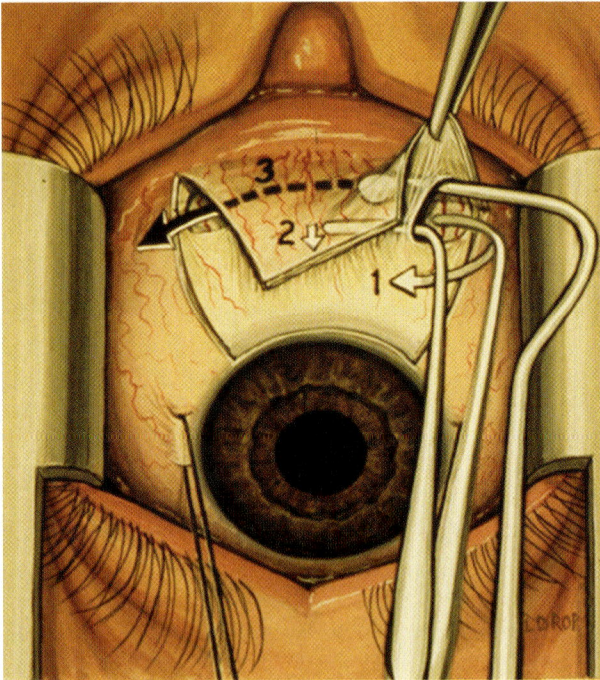

FIGURE 57.9 With toothed forceps, grasp the previously created opening through Tenon's capsule on one side of the muscle. Insert a small Stevens tenotomy hook through the opening, keeping the point of the hook against the sclera. Slide the hook in the direction of the muscle insertion *(Step 1)* and then slowly withdraw the hook toward the limbus to firmly engage the muscle *(Step 2)*. Marked resistance should be felt with continued retraction of the hook. The edge of the rectus muscle can usually be seen at this time. Once certain that the tip of the Stevens muscle hook is underneath the edge of the muscle insertion, pass a Jameson muscle hook just posterior to the Stevens tenotomy hook to isolate the entire rectus muscle insertion *(Step 3)*. The tip of the Jameson muscle hook should pass easily underneath the rectus muscle and out the opposite opening in Tenon's capsule. Sometimes it is necessary to grasp the opposite opening and maneuver the Jameson hook tip through it. The tip of the Jameson muscle hook should appear shiny, indicating that no tissue is overlying it.

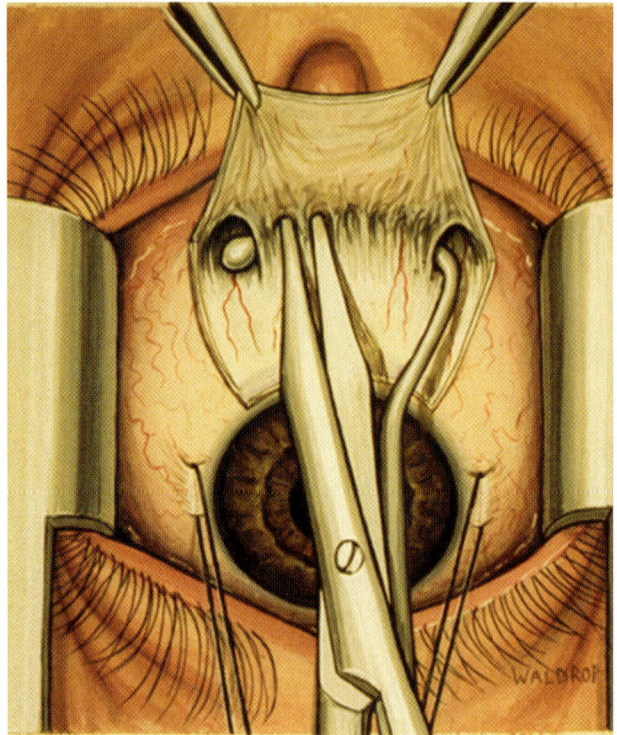

FIGURE 57.10 With two toothed forceps, have the assistant tent up the conjunctiva by grasping the cut ends that were previously attached to the limbus. This will stretch the anterior Tenon's capsule and remaining fascial attachments, facilitating sharp dissection from the rectus muscle. Westcott scissors can be used to sever these attachments from the sclera and muscle by a blunt dissection. The tips of the Westcott scissors are inserted into the tissue and spread gently, only cutting tissue that is clearly identified as being Tenon's or fascial attachments. This separation of tissues can also be accomplished with a cotton-tipped applicator, which is moved over the anterior surface and down the sides of the rectus muscle. This often strips off muscle capsule in addition to other attachments. With either technique, bleeding may occur and light cautery may be necessary to maintain adequate visualization. Care must be taken to avoid opening posterior Tenon's capsule, thereby allowing orbital fat to prolapse forward. This can be avoided by staying close to the muscle while dissecting tissue free.

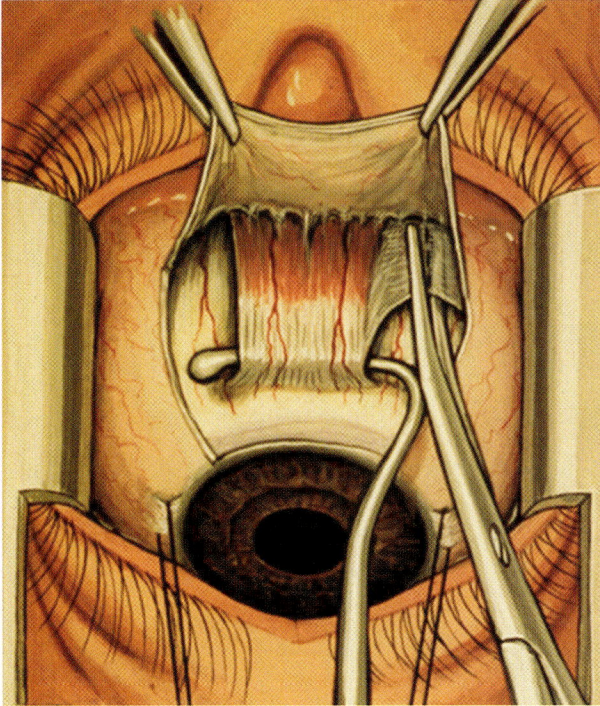

FIGURE 57.11 To cut the remaining intermuscular septal attachments, grasp the septum with forceps and stretch the tissue by pulling away from the muscle edge. After clearly identifying the edge of the rectus muscle, sever the attachments posteriorly for approximately 5–6 mm. Care must be exercised to avoid opening the subTenon's tissue, thereby exposing the fat pad. Additional light cautery can be applied to the muscle capsule vessels to prevent bleeding.

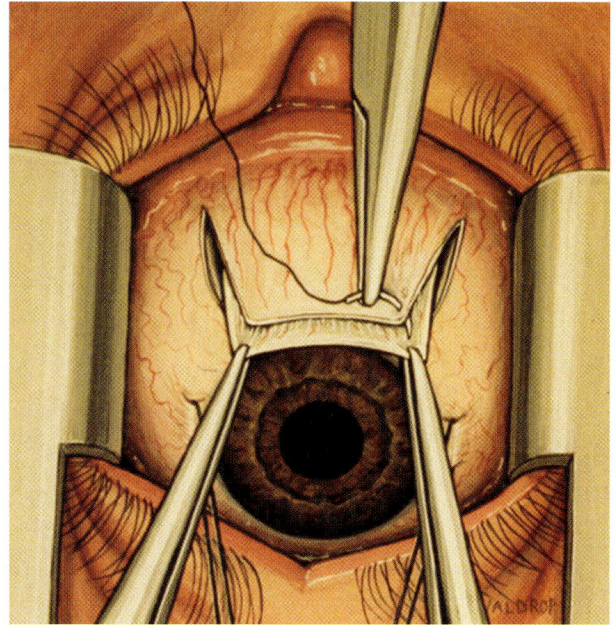

FIGURE 57.12 When closing the limbal incision, it is important to identify the conjunctival edge so it can be accurately re-approximated. To aid in its identification, grasp *Tenon's capsule* with two forceps and place it on stretch by pulling it toward the limbus. The edge of conjunctiva will become visible. After locating one corner of the conjunctiva, place the needle through it, 1 mm posterior to the edge, taking care not to include the underlying Tenon's capsule. The edge of Tenon's capsule is then released and allowed to retract posteriorly. Use an absorbable suture such as 8-0 Vicryl.

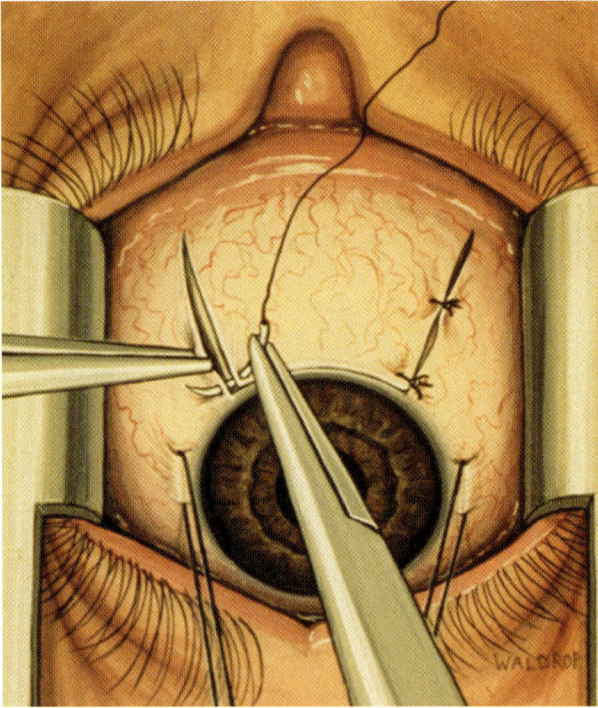

FIGURE 57.13 The conjunctival edge is then sutured to the limbal conjunctiva; this is performed at both ends of the limbal incision. An additional suture can be placed posteriorly midway along the incision, if Tenon's capsule prolapses through the opening. Any excess conjunctiva that is draped over the cornea should be excised at this time.

Conjunctival Incision—Fornix Approach

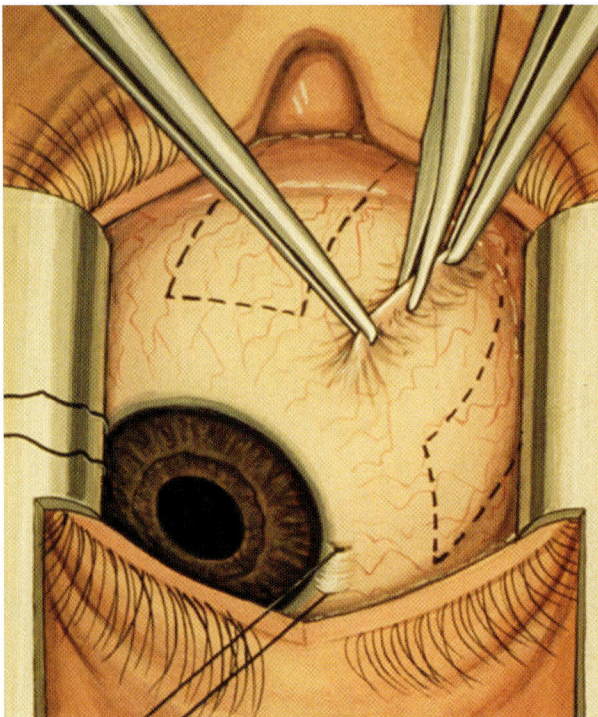

FIGURE 57.14 Rotate the eye up and out, exposing the inferior fornix area between the medial and inferior rectus. Using two toothed forceps, tent up the conjunctiva approximately 8–10 mm from the limbus. This should be done on a radial line perpendicular to the limbus extending backward. With the Westcott scissor blades parallel to the limbus, make an opening in the conjunctival tissue by cutting along the apex of the tented conjunctiva. Enlarge the opening if necessary.

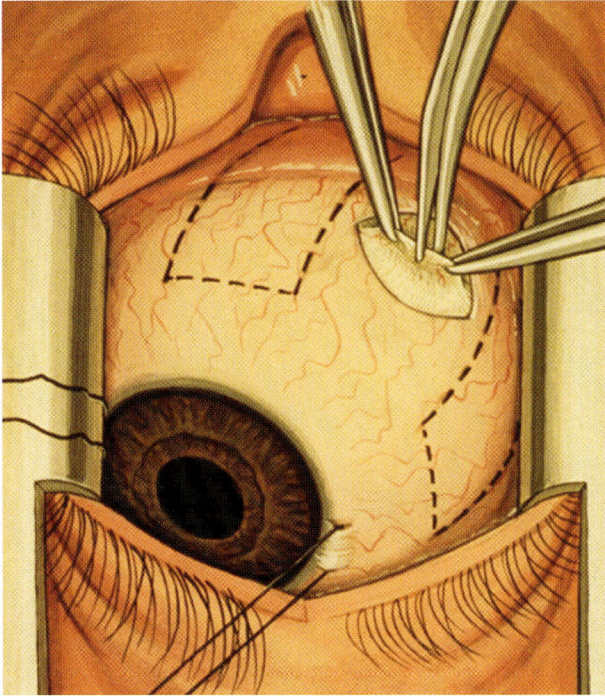

FIGURE 57.15 Through the conjunctival opening, grasp and elevate the intermuscular septum and Tenon's tissue with forceps. Tent up this tissue in a similar manner as the conjunctiva, but rotated 90 degrees from the previous incision. Using Westcott scissors, turn the blades perpendicular to the limbus; with pressure against the sclera, make an incision through the elevated tissue to expose bare sclera. Moderate downward pressure on the Westcott scissors is necessary to accomplish this task. Using this technique, two elliptical openings are created. One is through conjunctiva, with the long end of the opening parallel to the limbus, and the other is through Tenon's capsule and intermuscular septum, with the long opening perpendicular to the limbus. The edge of the conjunctival opening should be approximately 6–8 mm from the limbus, and extend to within 1–2 mm of the fornix or, in the case of the medial rectus, the semilunar fold.

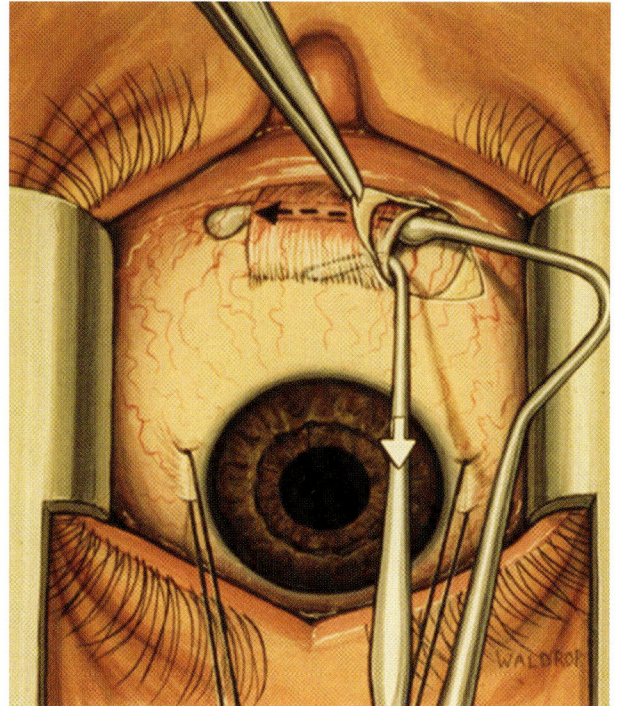

FIGURE 57.16 Grasp the edge of the Tenon's capsule/intermuscular septum opening near the inferior border of the rectus muscle. Insert a Stevens tenotomy hook into the opening, rotating the point against bare sclera; with a sweeping motion, pass the hook underneath the inferior edge of the muscle. Gently elevate the Stevens muscle hook, thereby creating a small tunnel underneath the muscle insertion. Pass a Jameson muscle hook just posterior to the Stevens hook and slide it underneath the rectus muscle. The Jameson muscle hook should meet little resistance. This is best accomplished by slightly rotating the tip of the Jameson muscle hook downward so it maintains contact with sclera.

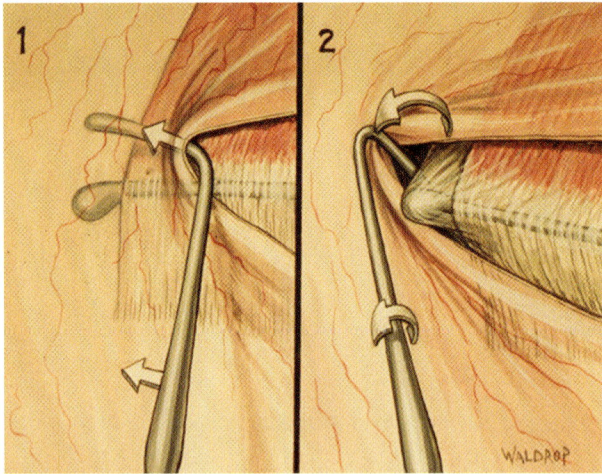

FIGURE 57.17 Remove the Steven's tenotomy hook from underneath the muscle insertion and use it to stretch the conjunctival tissue over the end of the Jameson muscle hook. Rotate the Jameson muscle hook approximately 10–15 degrees upward so that it will remain free of the conjunctival tissue once it is passed over its end.

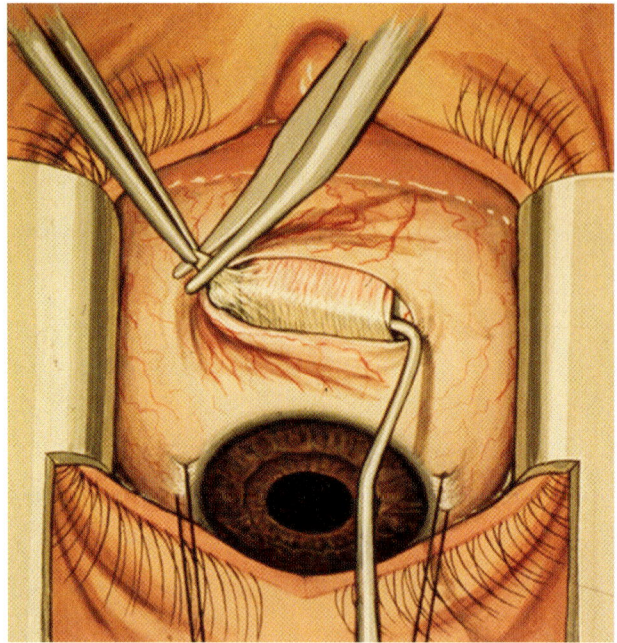

FIGURE 57.18 While continuing to rotate the Jameson muscle hook slightly upward, have the assistant elevate the intermuscular septum and Tenon's tissue, which is covering the end of the Jameson muscle hook. Using Westcott scissors, make a small opening in this tissue and pass the muscle hook through this opening. The end of the Jameson muscle hook should now appear shiny, indicating no tissue over its surface. Excise the remaining anterior Tenon's capsule from the surface of the muscle by gently lifting the edge of this tissue near the muscle insertion with a forceps. Any remaining intermuscular septum attachments can be severed in a similar matter.

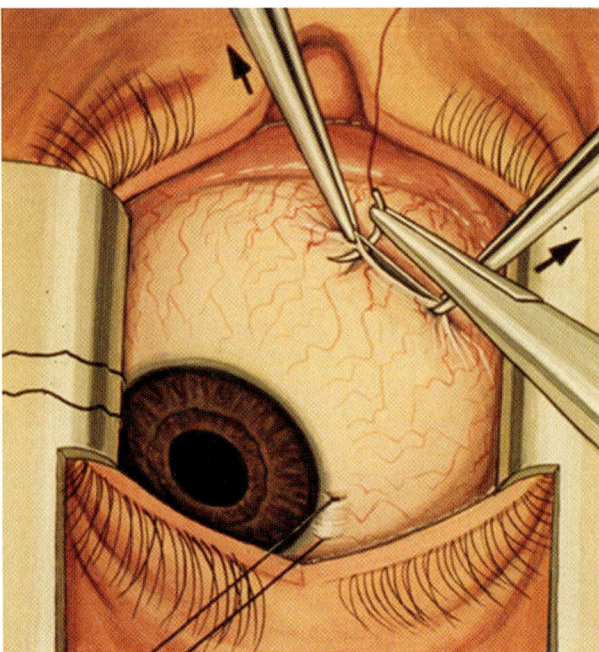

FIGURE 57.19 Fornix conjunctival incision closure is facilitated by grasping the ends of the conjunctival incision with a toothed forceps and elevating. This allows the cut ends of the conjunctiva to re-approximate. Care should be taken not to include Tenon's capsule. Interrupted 8-0 Vicryl suture can be used. The number of sutures placed depends on the size of the opening. Occasionally, no sutures are necessary because the incision is self-sealing.

TABLE 57.4 *Potential Complications of Limbal Incisions*

Dellen

Conjunctival cyst

Prolapse of Tenon's capsule

Advancement of the semilunar fold

Allergic reaction-Persistent hyperemia

Fat adherence syndrome

Lid fissure abnormalities

SELECTED REFERENCES

Buckley EG, and Shields MB. Strabismus and Glaucoma. In *Atlas of Ophthalmic Surgery, Vol. III*. St. Louis: Mosby, 1995.

Guyton DL. Exaggerated traction test for the oblique muscles. *Ophthalmology*. 1981;88:1035.

Helveston EM, Allorn DM, Ellis ED. Inferior oblique inclusion after lateral rectos surgery. *Graefe's Arch Exp Ophthalmol*. 1998;226:102–105.

Parks MM. Fornix incision for horizontal rectus muscle surgery. *Am J Ophthalmol*. 1998;65(6):907–915.

Plager DA. Traction testing in superior oblique palsy. *J Pediatr Ophthalmol Strabismus*. 1990;27(3):136–140.

von Noorden A. The limbal approach to surgery of the rectus muscles. *Arch Ophthalmol*. 1968;80:94–97.

von Noorden OK. Modification of the limbal approach to the rectus muscles. *Arch Ophthalmol*. 1969;82:349–350.

58 Rectus Muscle Surgery

Monte D. Mills, MD

TABLE 58.1 *Indications for Rectus Muscle Surgery*

Strabismus that interferes with binocular visual function, including binocular fusion, stereopsis, or binocular visual fields

Strabismus associated with symptoms including diplopia, visual confusion, or asthenopia

Strabismus associated with disfiguring facial appearance

Strabismus associated with compensatory abnormal head posture

Manifest nystagmus, either with compensatory abnormal head posture, or with a component of visual impairment related to reduced foveation time

TABLE 58.2 *Preoperative Considerations*

Direction and angle of deviation, best measured with functional testing with prisms (prism cover tests) or corneal light reflex testing (Hirschberg or Krimsky test), in primary position (looking straight ahead with head held straight)

Relative eye alignment in eccentric positions, especially reading position (downward). If the angle of deviation is similar in eccentric positions, it is considered comitant. Strabismus with angle of deviation that varies depending on the direction of gaze is incomitant. Strabismus may also vary depending on the distance of the visual target (e.g., near-distance incomitance, side-gaze incomitance)

Relative motor function of the relevant rectus and oblique muscles

Restrictions of ocular rotation

Sensory adaptations or abnormalities, including amblyopia, diplopia, and suppression, and the sensory response to optical correction (prism adaptation)

Refractive error

Patient expectations

Rectus Muscle Surgery

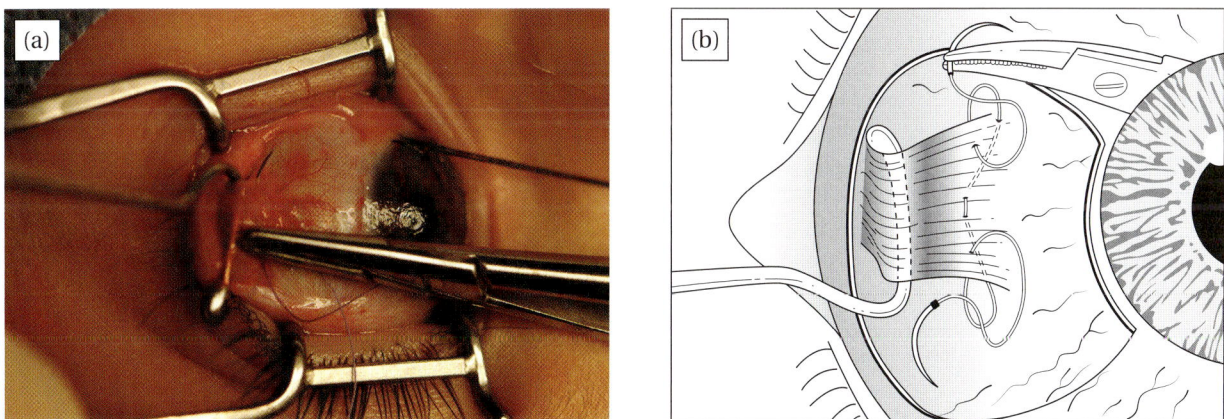

FIGURE 58.1 (a) The rectus muscles are exposed with a variety of incision techniques, including limbal incision and fornix incision (Chapter 57, Surgical Basics). In this and the following photographs and drawings, limbal incisions are used for improved anatomical visualization. Surrounding Tenon's capsule and check ligaments are separated from the muscle insertion, exposing the insertion. The suture is passed through the rectus muscle tendon within 1 mm of the scleral insertion, taking care to leave sufficient space between sclera and suture to cut the tendon. The muscle hook is used to elevate the tendon from the sclera, to prevent inadvertent passage of needle into sclera. (b) A locking knot is created at each margin of the rectus muscle tendon by a second pass of the suture through the tendon, to retain the width of the original tendon.

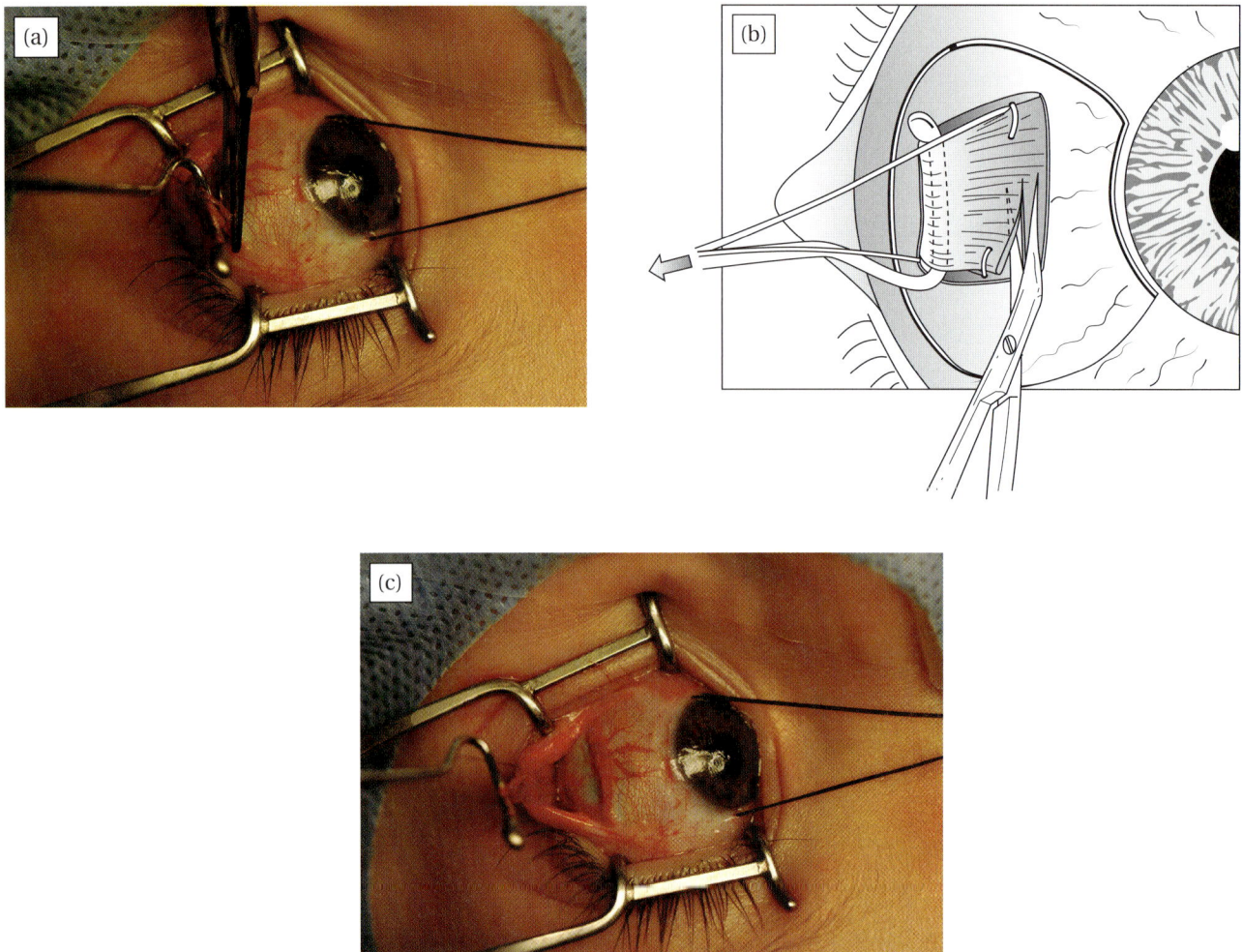

FIGURE 58.2 (a) The muscle tendon is cut from the sclera with scissors. Care is taken that the suture is not cut. (b) Placement of the suture and locking knot at the appropriate distance from the scleral insertion allows the tendon to be cut without cutting the suture, and minimizes the advancement effects of residual tendon anterior to the suture. (c) After the tendon is completely transected, the suture and tendon are inspected to insure the suture is intact, and that the muscle is entirely separated. The stump of the scleral insertion is visible.

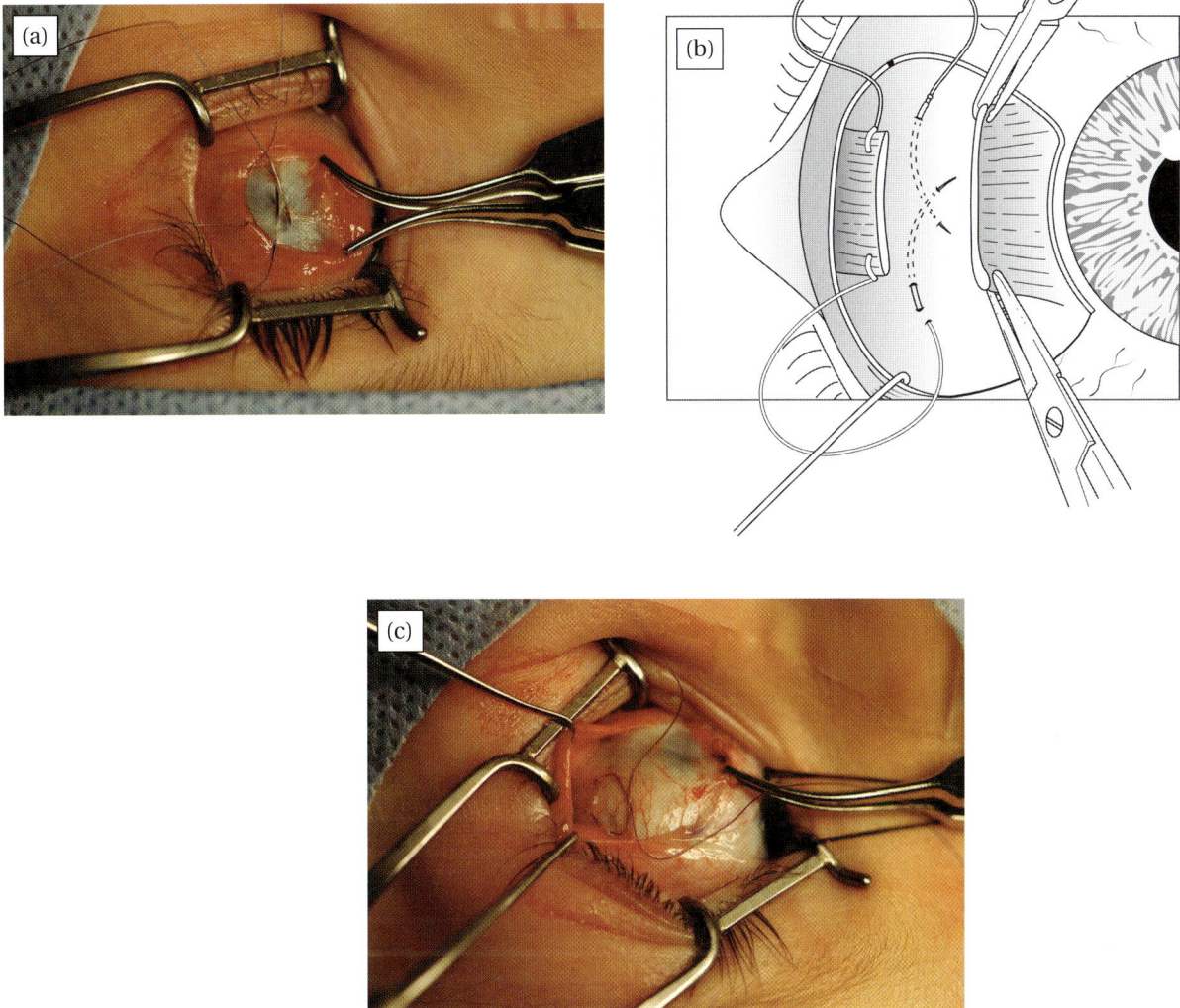

FIGURE 58.3 (a) The rectus muscle is reattached to the sclera at the planned site of recession, passing the suture needles through the sclera. The appropriate scleral depth of the needle passage allows the needle to be seen through the translucent sclera. The globe is fixated with forceps placed at the cut scleral insertion. (b) Perpendicular scleral suture passage (crossed-swords technique) may be used as shown, or sutures may be passed parallel to the rectus muscle. The point of entry of the suture needle will become the new point of insertion of the rectus muscle. (c) The suture needles are pulled through the sclera, and the sutures drawn through until the muscle is tightly attached to the sclera at the planned site of recession. The sutures are then tied and cut, before closing the conjunctiva over the recessed muscle.

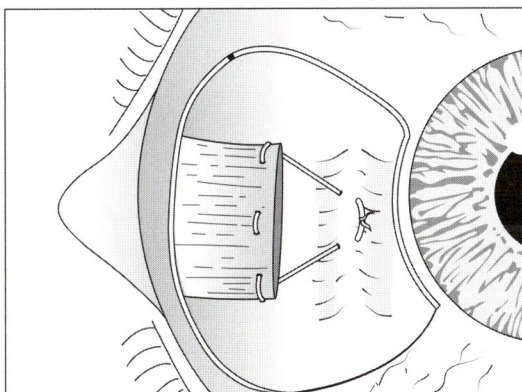

FIGURE 58.4 As an alternative technique to standard rectus muscle recession with direct reattachment of the tendon to the sclera, the muscle may be reattached to the original insertion and allowed to "hang back" on a suture loop. The recession distance may be measured by pulling the muscle all the way forward to the original insertion, and measuring the sutures past the scleral attachment to the knot. This technique can also be used for postoperative suture adjustment, if a sliding noose or slip knot is used to attach the sutures (Chapter 60, Adjustable Sutures).

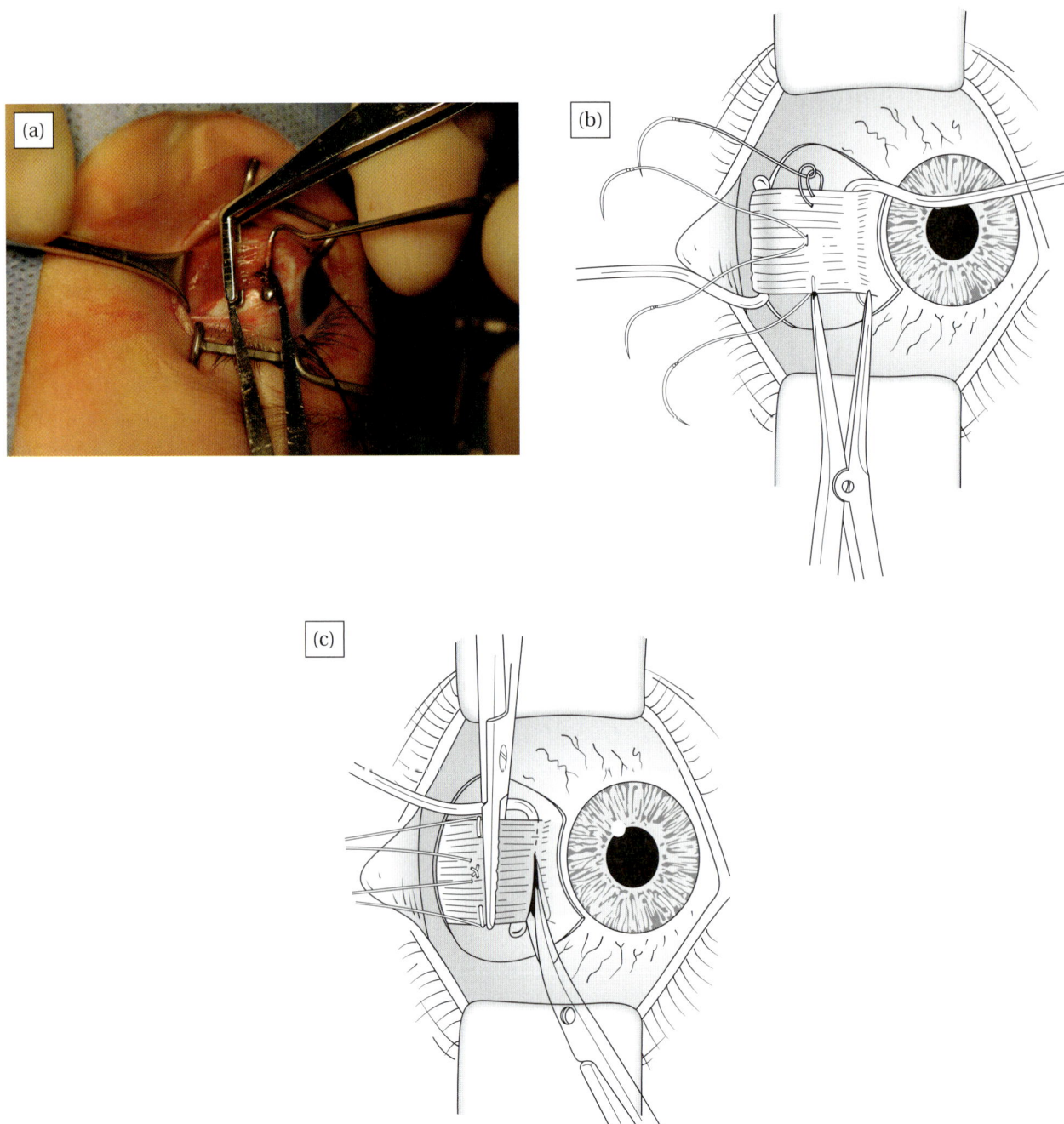

FIGURE 58.5 (a) Rectus muscle resections are measured from the scleral insertion to the point of suture placement in the muscle. A Jameson muscle resection clamp and calipers are used to measure from the insertion to the posterior edge of the clamp (where the sutures will be placed). It is important to provide tension between the clamp and muscle hook, in order to measure the resection consistently. (b) It is also possible to place sutures prior to placing the muscle clamp, measuring the resection between the muscle insertion and sutures. Using two double-armed sutures allows secure, precise reattachment of the resected muscle. Because the resection may involve suture placement in muscle tissue rather than tendon, special care must be taken to secure the locking knots and avoid tearing the muscle with the suture needle. (c) After placement of the sutures, the rectus muscle is separated from the sclera at the insertion. Excess muscle anterior to the sutures (anterior to the clamp) is removed, and the muscle stump is cauterized, before reattaching and releasing the clamp at the original insertion.

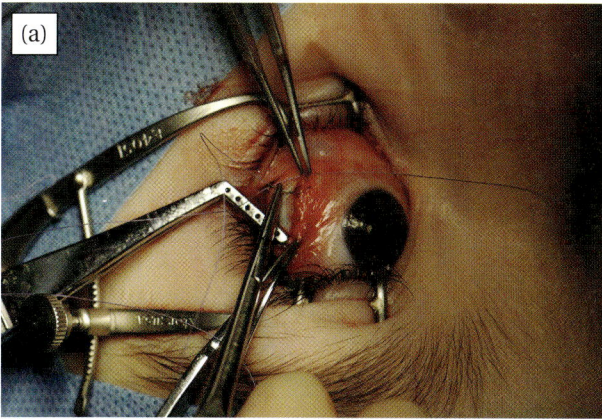

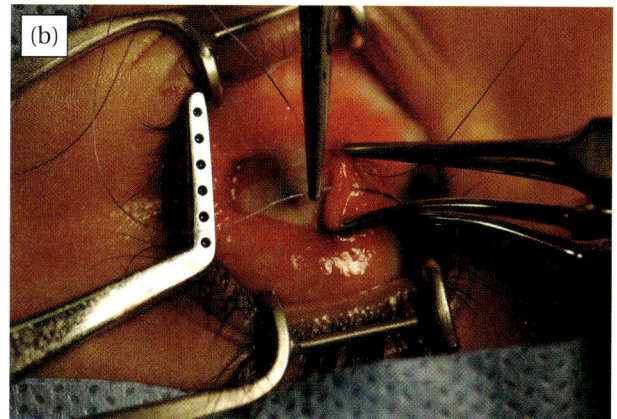

FIGURE 58.6 (a) While the clamp is still in place, the sutures are passed through the cut rectus muscle insertion stump to reattach the resected muscle. (b) After passing the sutures through the cut insertion stump, the sutures are tied securely before removing the clamp.

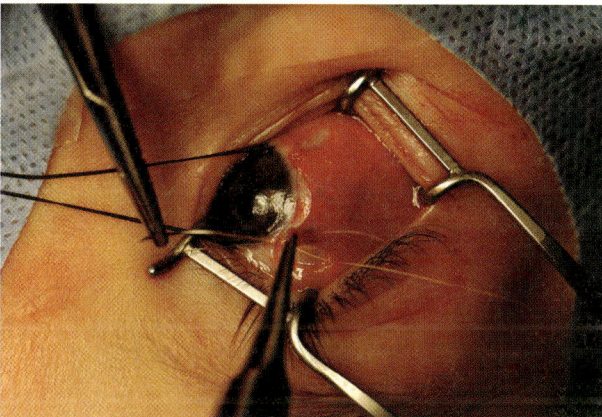

FIGURE 58.7 The conjunctiva is closed over the resected or recessed muscle. With the limbal incision, sutures are placed at the margins of the incision. When large recessions are performed, conjunctival recession may be necessary if passive rotation of the eye is limited by tethering of the conjunctiva. The conjunctival flap may be reattached to the sclera posterior to the original limbus, and the gap between the limbus and the flap allowed to heal by secondary intention.

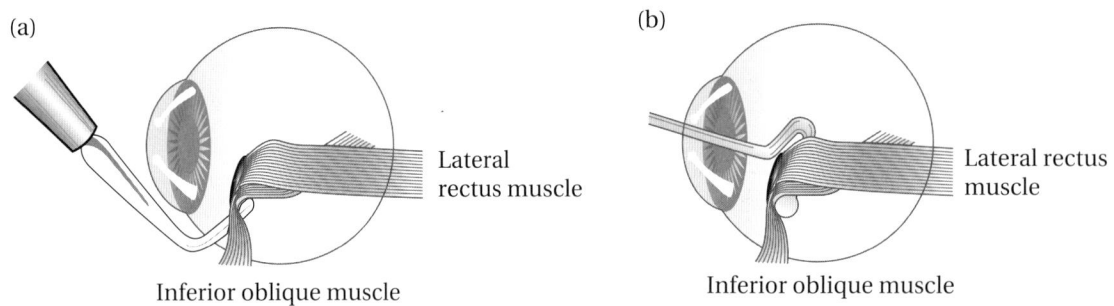

FIGURE 58.8 (a) Inadvertent inclusion of inferior oblique muscle in muscle hook, inferior approach. The inferior oblique muscle passes adjacent to the inferior margin of the lateral rectus muscle, and is attached to the lateral rectus by check ligaments and connective tissues. Because of this relationship, the inferior oblique muscle is frequently inadvertently included in the muscle hook when attempting to hook the lateral rectus muscle, especially when hooking the muscle from inferiorly. Careful inspection of the muscle, avoiding passing the muscle hooks deeply into the orbit, and cautious dissection will reduce this hazard. (b) Inadvertent inclusion of inferior oblique muscle in muscle hook, superior approach. It is possible to hook the inferior oblique with the lateral from superiorly, also. Careful inspection of the muscle, avoiding deep passage of the muscle hooks, and cautious dissection will reduce this hazard. The superior oblique tendon must also be avoided when approaching the superior rectus muscle; the superior oblique tendon is underneath the superior rectus and should be carefully separated from the superior rectus, particularly for large superior rectus recessions.

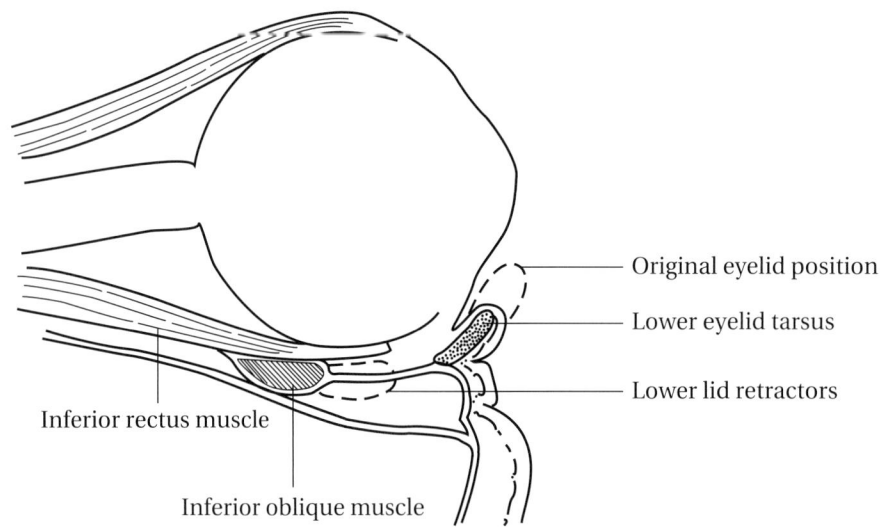

FIGURE 58.9 The retractors of the lower eyelid are closely attached to the capsule of the inferior rectus muscle and the inferior oblique muscle. Changes in the position of the inferior rectus muscle (resection or recession) will change the lower eyelid position. In general, recessions of the inferior rectus of 5 mm or more will cause retraction of the lower lid, unless these attachments are severed and advanced relative to the inferior rectus.

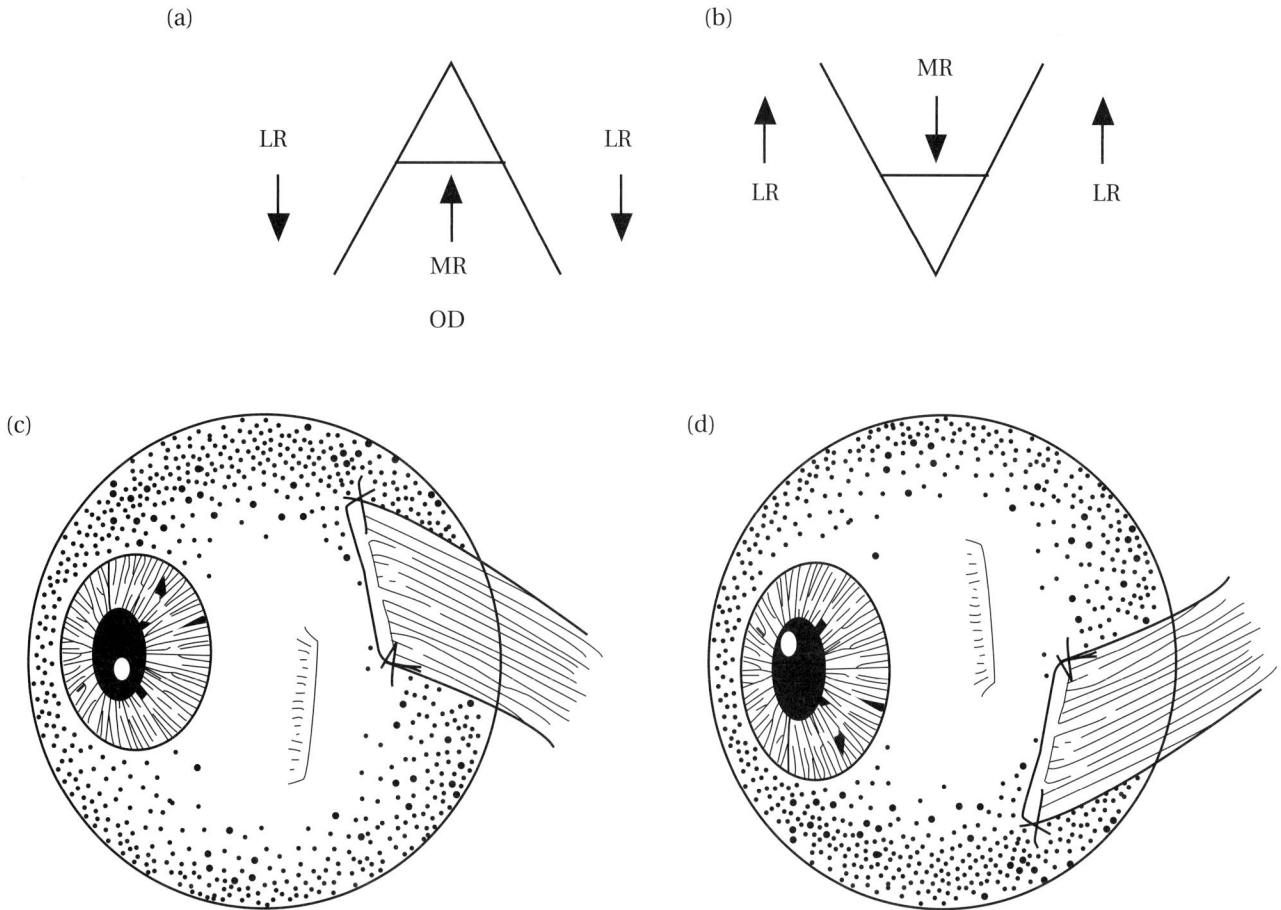

FIGURE 58.10 (a) Incomitant horizontal strabismus with an A or V pattern (larger esotropia or exotropia in upgaze or downgaze, relative to primary position) can be corrected by shifting the position of the insertion of the horizontal rectus muscles, usually one-half to one tendon width (5–10 mm) vertically. For A-pattern incomitance, the medial rectus insertion is shifted up and/or the lateral shifted down. (b) For V-pattern incomitance, the medial rectus insertion is shifted down and/or the lateral shifted up. (c) Recession of the horizontal rectus, with upward vertical transposition one tendon width. (d) Recession of the horizontal rectus, with downward vertical transposition one tendon width.

TABLE 58.3 *Complications of Rectus Muscle Surgery*

Complication	Relative Risk	Associated Factors	Causes	Prevention/Treatment
Overcorrection, undercorrection	High	• Amblyopia or other causes of poor vision • Abnormal muscle elasticity • Abnormal muscle contractility • Restrictive strabismus	• Excessive recession or resection • Migration of site of muscle reattachment • Unpredictable restrictive or paretic muscle factors • Deviation measurement artifacts	• Accurate preoperative measurements and careful surgical planning • Accurate, secure reattachment of muscle to sclera • Recognition and consideration of abnormal muscle contractile or elastic factors and ocular restrictions in surgical plan • Adjustable suture techniques • Reoperation
Scleral perforation	Low	• Faden suture • Large recession • Inexperienced surgeon	• Deep scleral pass	• Spatulated needle • Surgical magnification • Hang-back suture technique
Infection	Very low	• Concurrent dacryocystitis or blepharitis • Inadequate operative antisepsis	• Preoperative or postoperative surgical site contamination	• Preoperative treatment of blepharitis, dacryocystitis • Adequate perioperative antisepsis • Avoid postoperative contamination • Postoperative topical antibiotic
Anterior segment ischemia syndrome	Very low	• Simultaneous or sequential surgery on adjacent rectus muscles • Systemic microvascular disease (hypertension, smoking, etc.)	• Occlusion of blood supply to the anterior ocular segment at muscle insertion	• Avoiding simultaneous surgery on adjacent rectus muscles • Ciliary vessel-sparing surgical techniques • Treatment with topical steroid
Pyogenic granuloma	Low	• Unknown	• Unknown	• Treatment with topical steroid or excision
Diplopia	Low	• Overcorrection • Disruption of sensory adaptations (suppression)	• Residual or recurrent ocular misalignment	• Careful surgical planning • Adjustable suture techniques (Chapter 60, Adjustable Sutures) • Reoperation

TABLE 58.3 (*continued*)

Complication	Relative Risk	Associated Factors	Causes	Prevention/Treatment
Corneal dellen	Low	• Elevated limbal conjunctival incision	• Abnormal tear film with corneal dehydration	• Fornix incision technique • Topical rewetting and lubrication • Temporary eyelid closure
Conjunctival scarring and distortion	Low	• Limbal conjunctival incision	• Improper conjunctival closure • Conjunctival incision crossing plica similunaris	• Fornix incision (Chapter 57, Surgical Basics) • Careful conjunctival closure
Orbital fat adherence syndrome	Low	• Reoperation • Rectus muscle or orbital scarring • Deep orbital penetration when hooking rectus muscles	• Penetration of Tenon's fascial sleeve surrounding rectus muscle • Postoperative adhesion of orbital fat to muscle and sclera	• Avoid sweeping deeply into orbit with muscle hooks • Avoid deep dissection through Tenon's muscle sheath • Intraoperative steroid infiltration
Eyelid position changes	Low	• Thyroid eye disease • Restrictive strabismus • Large recession or resection of inferior rectus muscle	• Fascial attachments between eyelid and vertical rectus muscles	• Avoid large recession or resection of inferior rectus (>5 mm) • Careful dissection of fascial attachments of inferior rectus (Lockwood ligament)

SELECTED REFERENCES

Keech RV. Rectus muscle surgery. In Albert DA, ed. *Ophthalmic surgery: Principles and technique,* 857–873. Malden, MA: Blackwell Science; 1999.

Mills, MD. Fundamentals principles of strabismus surgery. In Albert DA, ed. *Ophthalmic surgery: Principles and technique,* 810–856. Malden, MA: Blackwell Science; 1999.

59 Oblique Muscle Surgery

David A. Plager, MD

Inferior Oblique Procedures

Inferior Oblique Procedures

TABLE 59.1 *Indications for Inferior Oblique (IO) Procedures*

IO Recession

Inferior oblique overaction—Recession may be preferred when primary position deviation is small and degree of inferior oblique overaction is mild; e.g., 1–2+ on 4-point scale.

IO Anterior Transposition

Main indication is for treatment of inferior oblique overaction in association with dissociated vertical deviation. A V-pattern would normally be present. Not typically done unilaterally unless an asymmetric relative restriction to upgaze is a desired outcome.

IO Myectomy

Inferior oblique overaction—particularly when IO overaction is moderate to marked. Can be done unilaterally or bilaterally.

General Exposure for Inferior Oblique

General—The approach through conjunctiva and Tenon's capsule in the inferior temporal quadrant can be identical for all inferior oblique procedures including myectomy, recessions, and anterior transpositions.

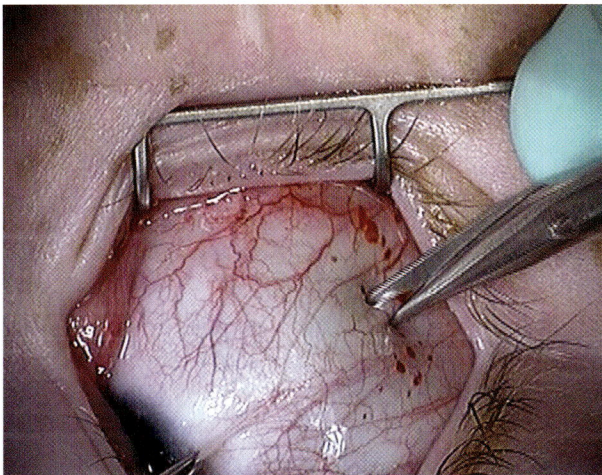

FIGURE 59.1 The eye (right eye shown in this series) is brought up into an elevated adducted position by grasping the inferior temporal limbus with a locking curved forceps. Incision is made through conjunctiva just inferior to the inferior border of the lateral rectus muscle. The scissors cut is made in line with the proposed conjunctival incision. After gentle spreading between the conjunctiva and Tenon's capsule, Tenon's is grasped with forceps and incision is made straight down to the sclera, perpendicular to the direction of the conjunctival incision.

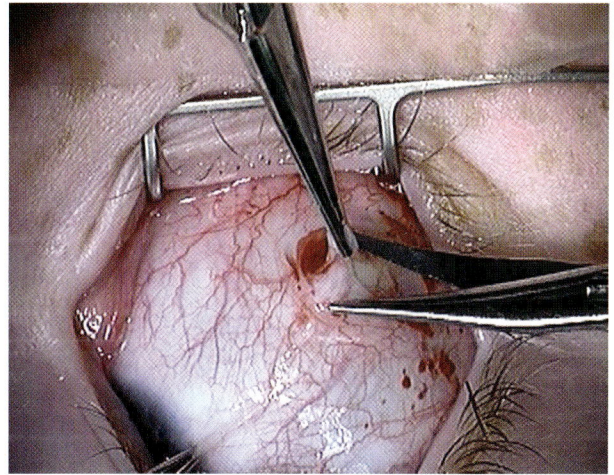

FIGURE 59.2 Excess Tenon's capsule can be excised. This is particularly advantageous in children with excess Tenon. This maneuver helps with exposure and also helps prevent prolapse of Tenon's capsule through the conjunctival incision postoperatively.

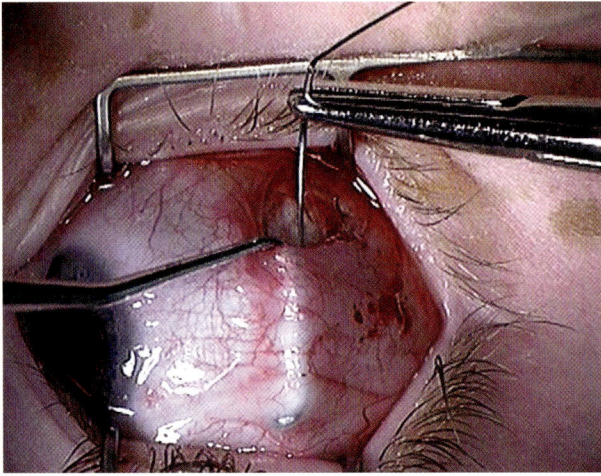

FIGURE 59.3 The lateral rectus muscle is hooked on a muscle hook, and a silk traction suture is placed beneath the lateral rectus muscle. The traction suture is used to bring the eye into an elevated adducted position, and the suture is clamped to the drape. It is imperative that the cornea be above the suture, in order to get appropriate exposure of the inferior oblique muscle. Do not let the lateral rectus muscle slip across the globe superiorly, which will cause the cornea to orient lower than the suture.

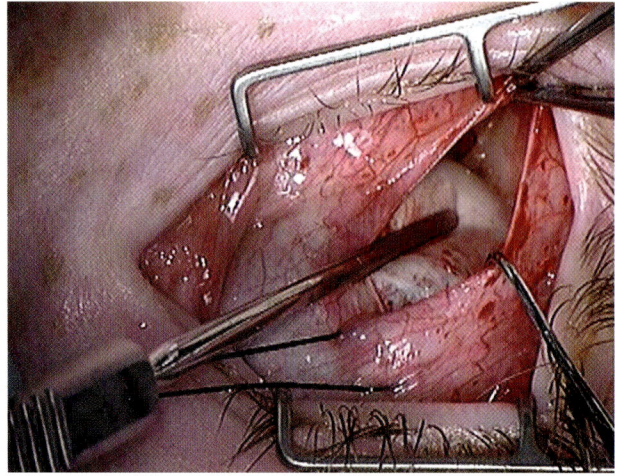

FIGURE 59.4 A long muscle hook, such as a Jameson hook, is placed in the inferior temporal quadrant and firmly retracts the inferior oblique away from the globe. An iris repositor can be used to help retract the globe, and a second muscle hook is used underneath the lateral rectus muscle in order to aid exposure. This view of what Parks termed the "triangle of white," where the triangle bound by the superior oblique muscle on one side, the globe on the bottom side, and the vortex vein on the opposite side, can always be obtained if the traction hooks are in the right position. This frequently requires a repositioning of the initial long hook in the inferior temporal quadrant.

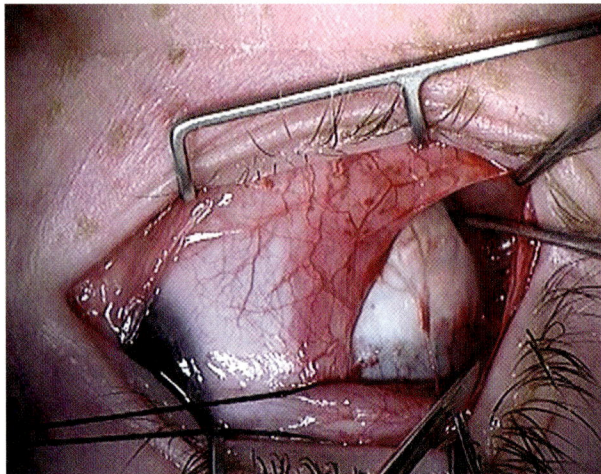

FIGURE 59.5 Another muscle hook is used to hook the inferior oblique under direct observation, with the hook pointed toward the lateral orbital wall. The hook is brought up into the operative field. Included on the hook will be the inferior oblique, as well as surrounding extraconal fat.

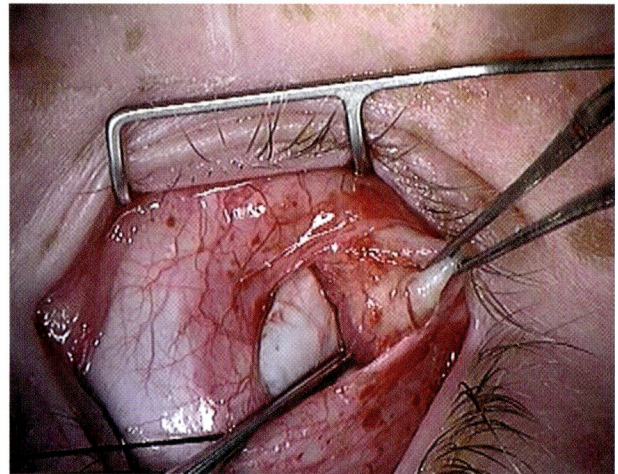

FIGURE 59.6 It is crucial to carefully maneuver the hook such that only the inferior oblique muscle remains on the hook. The extraconal fat is carefully lifted off the hook with a forceps.

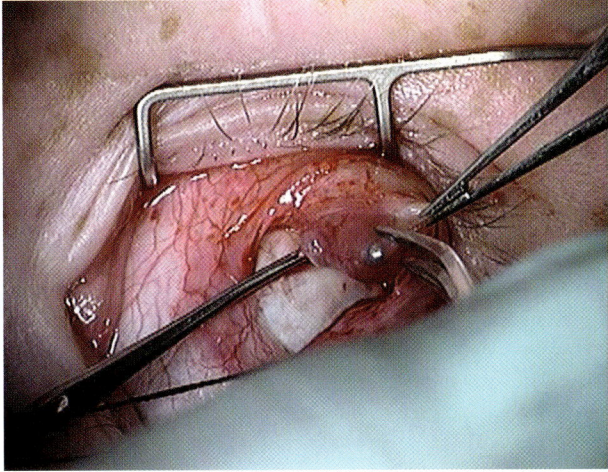

FIGURE 59.7 A cut is then made in the intramuscular septum on the posterior surface of the small muscle hook. Once the tip of the hook is completely exposed, a second hook is placed.

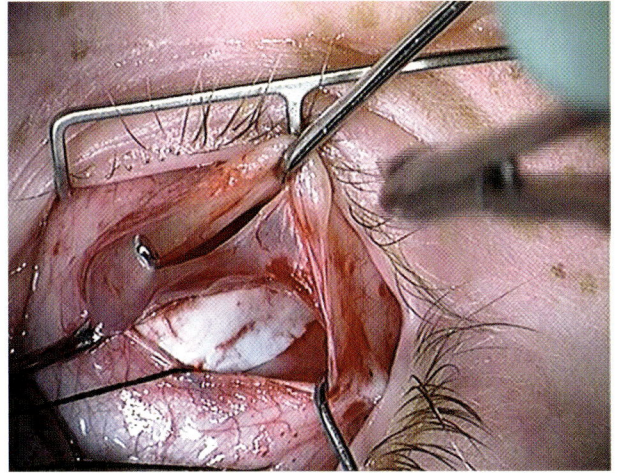

FIGURE 59.8 A second Green hook is placed in the incision, oriented 180° away from the hook holding the inferior oblique. This places the intramuscular septum on stretch, allowing dissection back to the inferior oblique insertion.

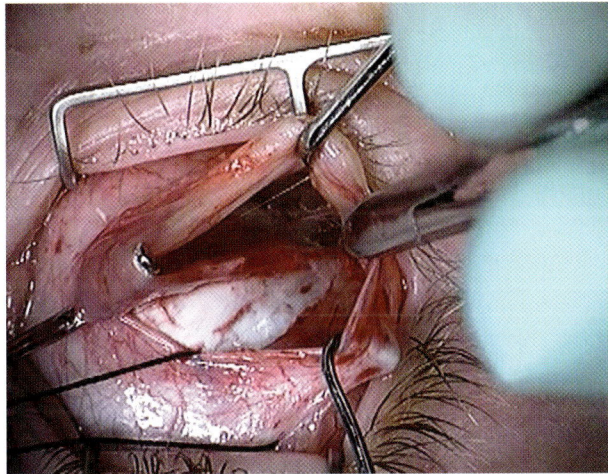

FIGURE 59.9 Careful dissection is carried out to expose the inferior oblique insertion. Care is taken to be sure the dissection is along the surface of the inferior oblique and does not violate the extraconal fat pad.

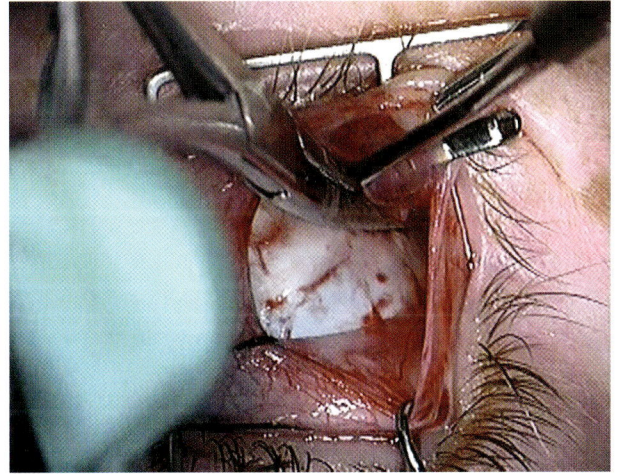

FIGURE 59.10 A curved hemostat is then placed across the inferior oblique insertion, leaving just enough room behind the hemostat to allow scissors to cut the muscle from the globe.

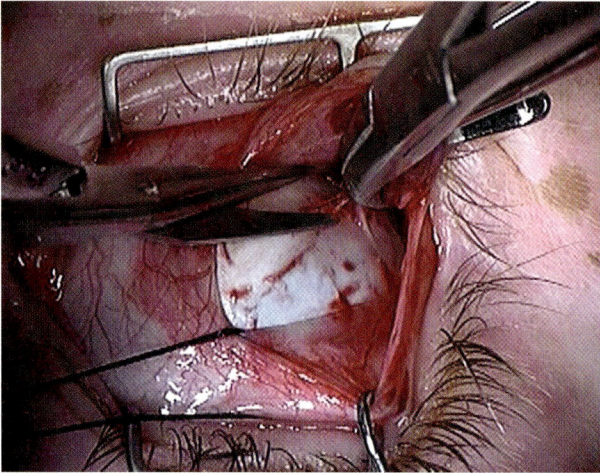

FIGURE 59.11 The hemostat is tilted forward to allow the scissors behind the hemostat. The transection of the muscle off the globe is done under direct observation, being sure not to cut into the globe.

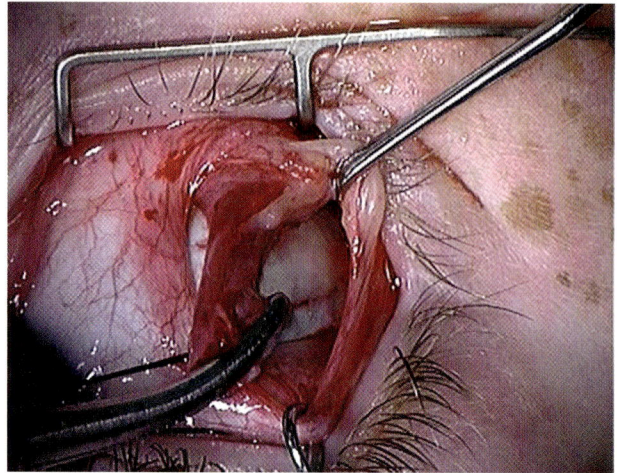

FIGURE 59.12 Once disinserted, the inferior oblique muscle is brought up into the operative field, still maintained on the hemostat. At this point, the muscle can be secured with a double-armed 6-0 polyglactin suture if a recession or anterior position is to be performed. If, instead, a myectomy is to be performed, the clamp is maintained in place.

Myectomy

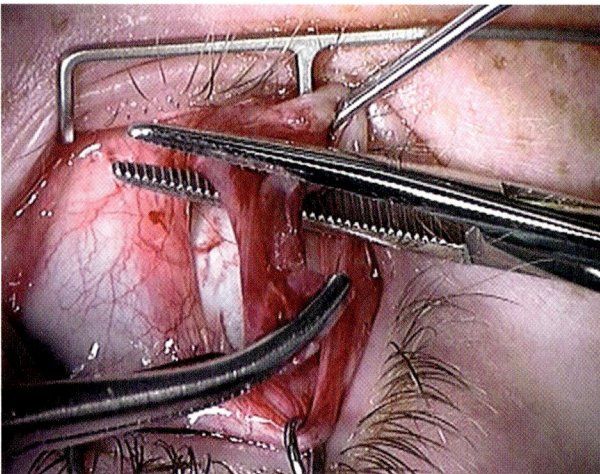

FIGURE 59.13 For a myectomy, a second hemostat is used to cross-clamp the inferior oblique just as it penetrates through Tenon's capsule.

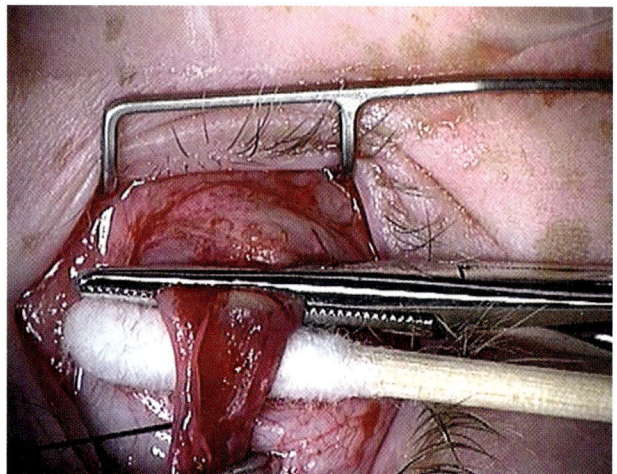

FIGURE 59.14 A cotton swab is placed underneath the inferior oblique muscle in order to protect the globe.

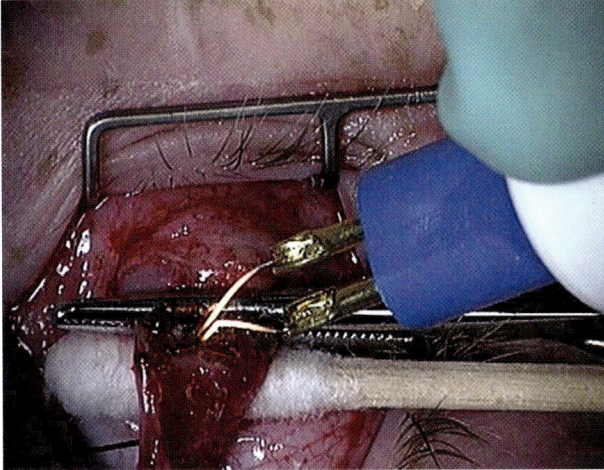

FIGURE 59.15 A hot handheld cautery can be used to transect the inferior oblique muscle, being sure the cautery does not touch any other surrounding tissues. Alternatively, the muscle can be transected with scissors and then the cut end cauterized.

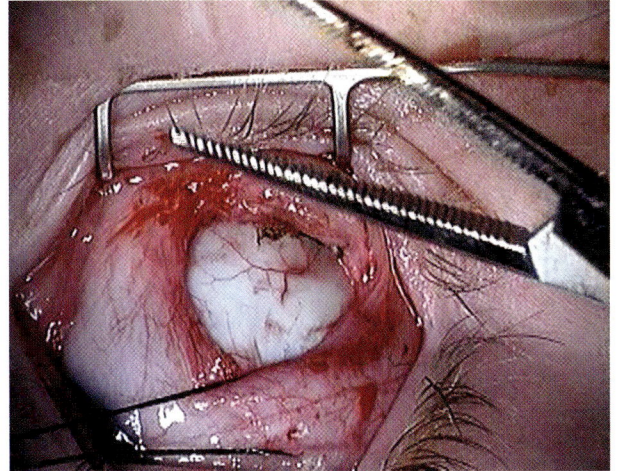

FIGURE 59.16 The muscle is released from the hemostat, and the muscle will be seen to retract back into Tenon's capsule.

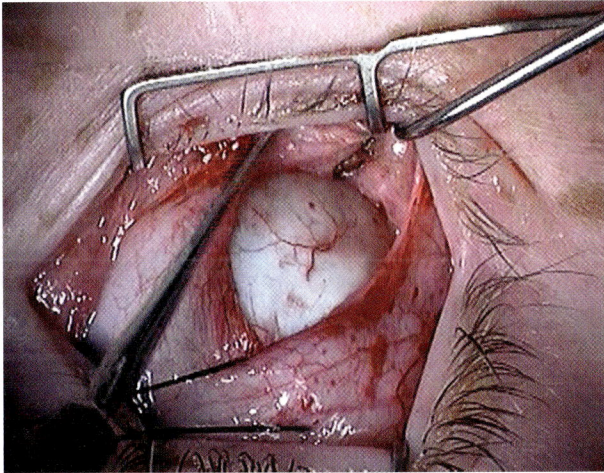

FIGURE 59.17 The muscle end can be pushed back through the opening or, alternatively, one can suture closed the rent in Tenon's capsule over the surface of the muscle, although this is not usually necessary.

Inferior Oblique Recession

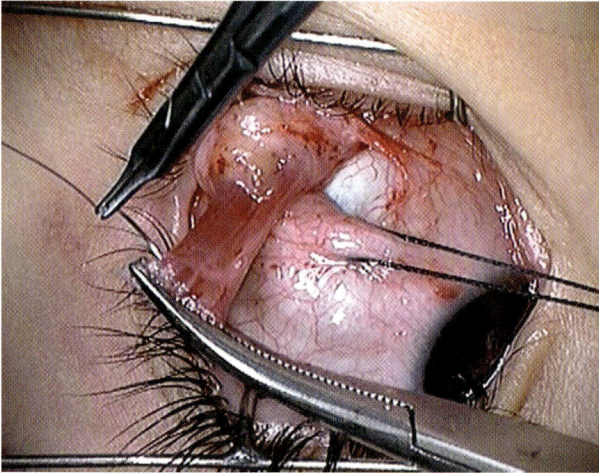

FIGURE 59.18 Exposure and isolation of the inferior oblique muscle is done as described in Figures 59.1–59.12 above. In this left eye shown, the inferior oblique is secured on a double-armed 6.0 polyglactin suture with locking bites on each side of the muscle. Once both locking bites are in position in the muscle, the clamp is removed.

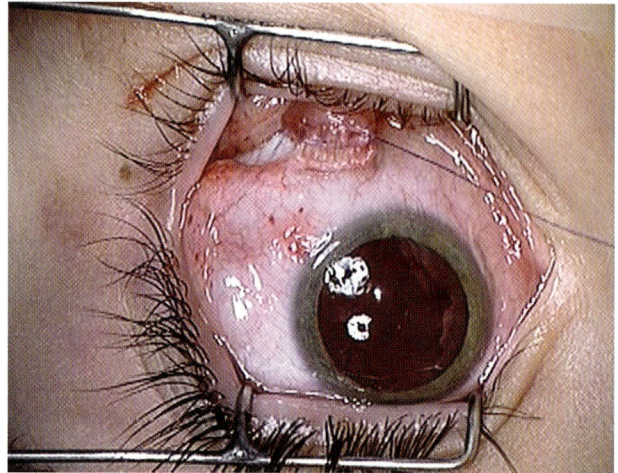

FIGURE 59.19 Care is taken to be sure the muscle is well secured on the double-armed suture.

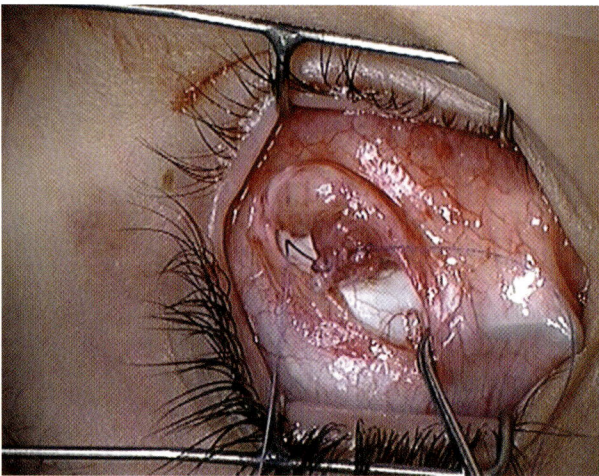

FIGURE 59.20 The inferior rectus muscle is hooked on a muscle hook, and the eye retracted superiorly. The cornea is underneath the upper lid.

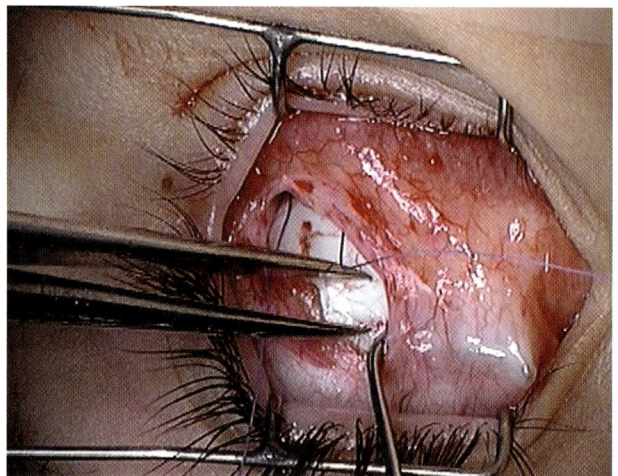

FIGURE 59.21 Calipers can be used to measure 3 mm posterior to the temporal edge of the inferior rectus insertion.

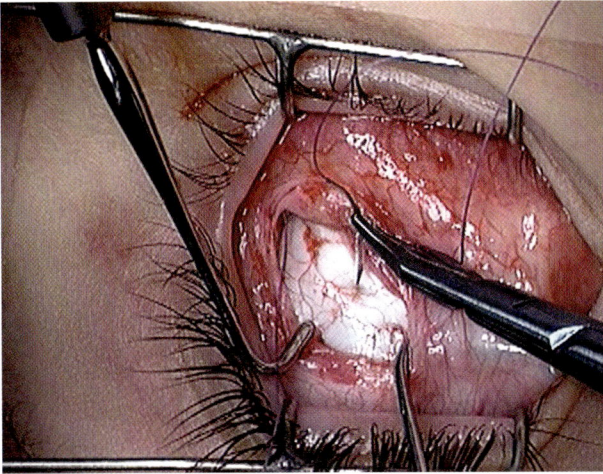

FIGURE 59.22 Then, 2 mm temporal to that mark, is the so-called "10 mm recession" mark. The inferior oblique muscle is then reattached to the globe at that point.

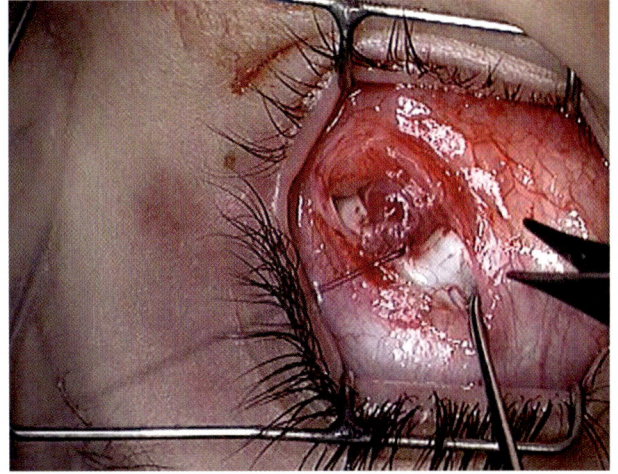

FIGURE 59.23 The two ends of the suture are placed relatively close together, to bunch up the inferior oblique insertion.

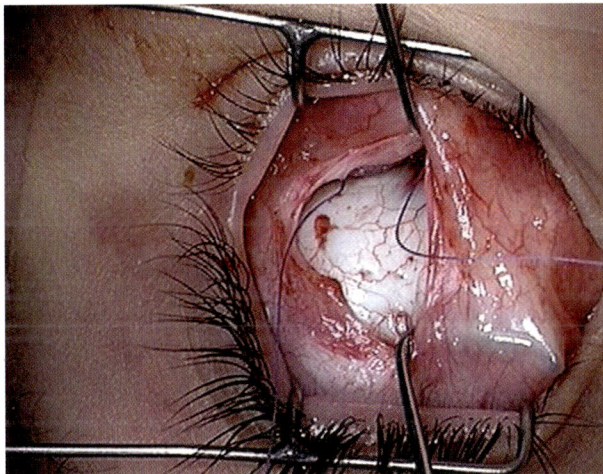

FIGURE 59.24 A 14 mm recession is performed by resuturing the inferior oblique such that each of the two arms of the suture are passed on either side of the inferior temporal vortex vein.

Anterior Transposition

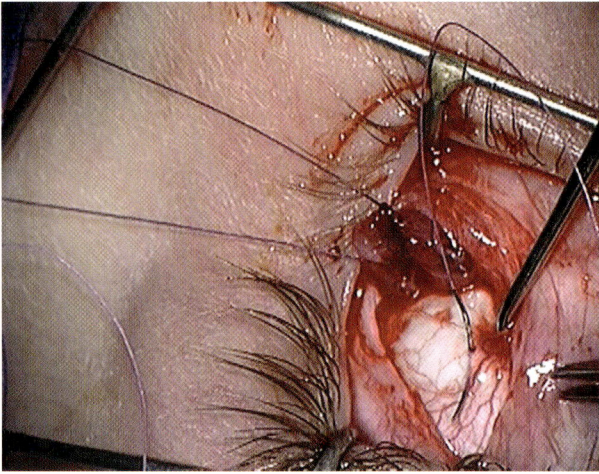

FIGURE 59.25 One suture arm is passed 1 mm anterior to the lateral border of the inferior rectus.

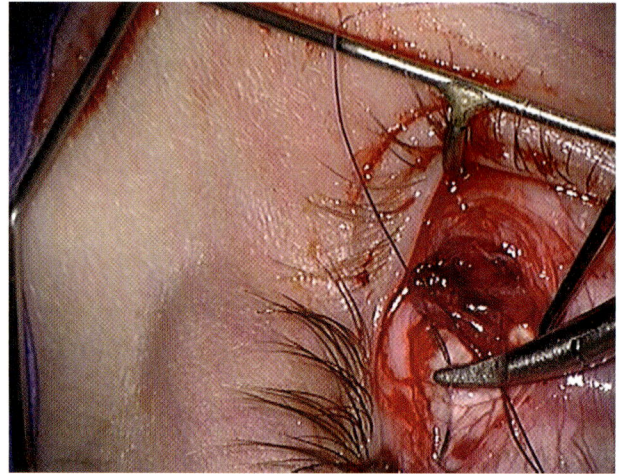

FIGURE 59.26 The second arm is passed nearby, taking care not to stretch out the insertion too widely.

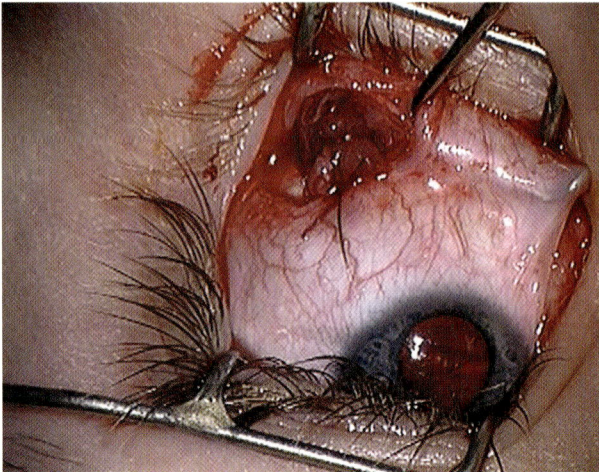

FIGURE 59.27 Appearance of muscle tied in place.

TABLE 59.2 *Complications of Inferior Oblique Surgery*

- Incomplete isolation of the muscle, particularly for myectomy, where not including the entire muscle will result in failure to weaken the overacting muscle.
- Violation of the extraconal fat pad, which will result in an adherence syndrome.
- Excessive traction on the neurovascular bundle to the IO, which may result in transient or permanent pupil dilation.
- Excessive spreading or temporal placement of IO insertion with anterior transposition can cause anti-elevation syndrome.

Superior Oblique Procedures

TABLE 59.3 *Indications for Superior Oblique (SO) Procedures*

SO Tenotomy

• Marked superior oblique overaction, usually in presence of large A pattern when bilateral.

SO Spacer

• Used for SO weakening when there is heightened concern regarding overcorrection, particularly in unilateral cases. Brown syndrome is the most common indication.

SO Tuck

• Strengthening of a superior oblique tendon, as in some cases of SO palsy. Particularly indicated when the involved tendon is considered lax in relation to the opposite SO tendon.

Harada-Ito

• Used for reduction of large degrees of excyclotorsion, particularly in cases of acquired SO palsy where more than 10 degrees of excyclotorsion is present.

General Exposure for Superior Oblique

The same exposure to the temporal side of the SO tendon can be used for SO tenotomy, SO spacer, and SO tuck as described below in Figures 59.28–59.31.

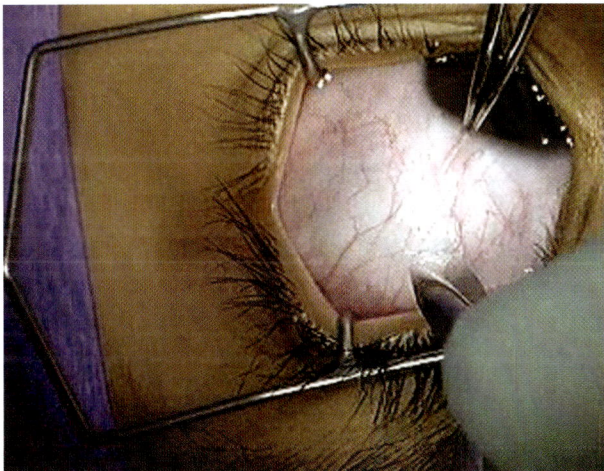

FIGURE 59.28 The eye is brought into an infraducted adducted position by grasping the superior temporal limbus with a locking curved forceps.

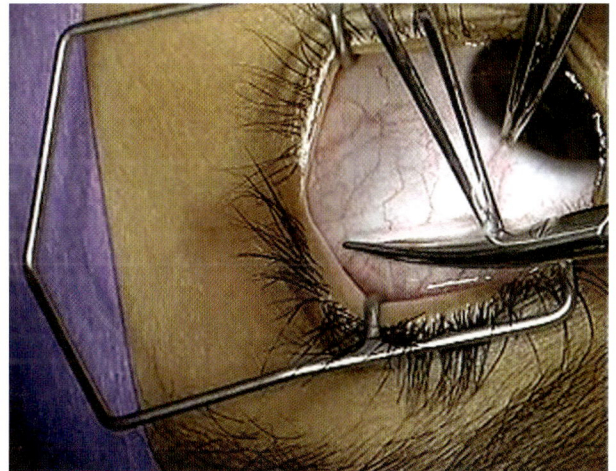

FIGURE 59.29 A superotemporal fornix incision is made through conjunctiva, starting the incision just temporal to the temporal edge of the superior rectus muscle.

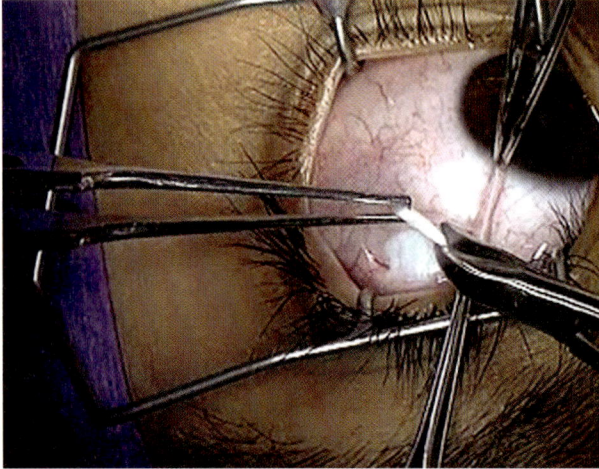

FIGURE 59.30 The conjunctiva is retracted inferiorly as the Tenon's capsule is grasped. A cut through Tenon's capsule is made straight down to sclera in the opposite orientation as the conjunctival incision. Excess Tenon's capsule can be excised.

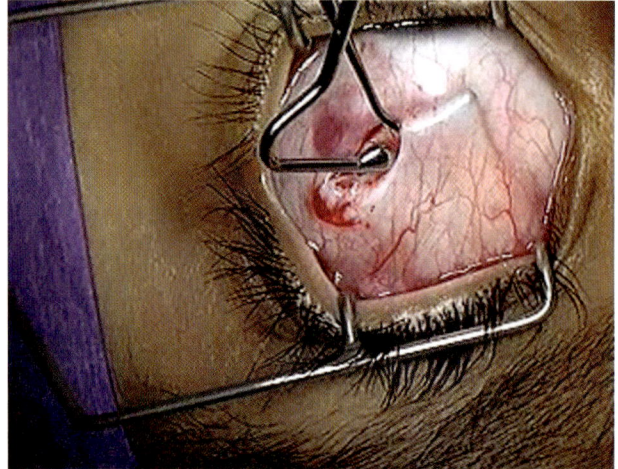

FIGURE 59.31 The superior rectus muscle is hooked with a small (Stevens) muscle hook. A second, larger hook, such as a Jameson or Green hook, is used to hook the superior rectus insertion.

Superior Oblique Tenotomy

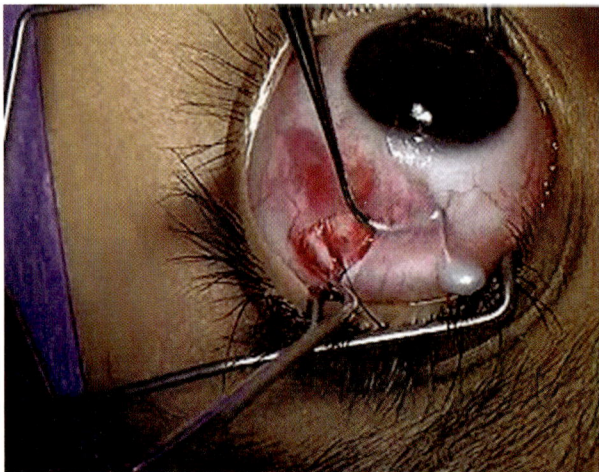

FIGURE 59.32 A second small muscle hook is used to retract conjunctiva over the muscle hook.

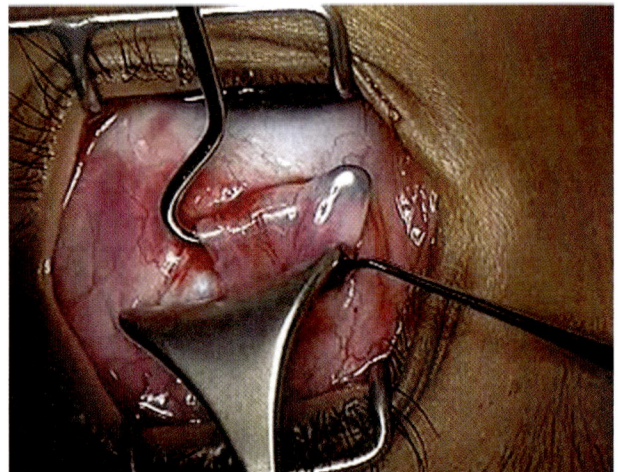

FIGURE 59.33 A Desmarres retractor is placed beneath the conjunctiva.

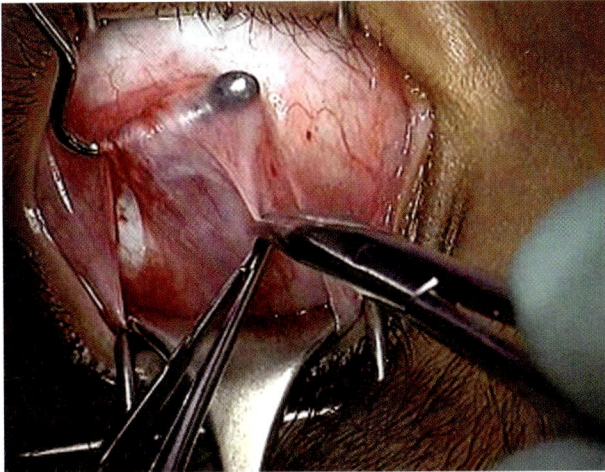

FIGURE 59.34 The diagonal check ligament across the surface of the superior rectus is grasped with forceps, and a small buttonhole is made with Westcott scissors.

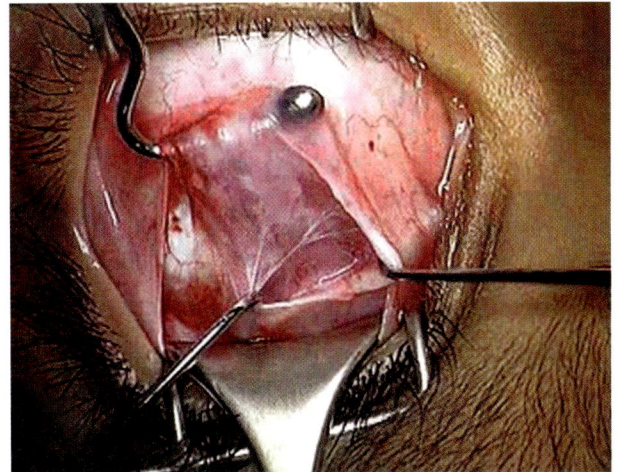

FIGURE 59.35 Two small muscle hooks are placed in the opening and spread large enough for the Desmarres retractor to go into the next layer.

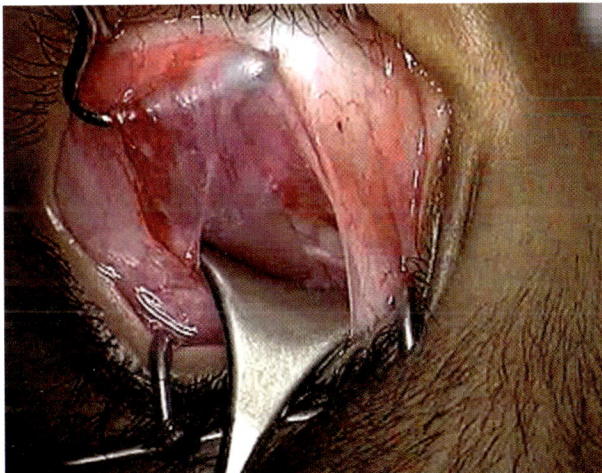

FIGURE 59.36 Inspection of the nasal side of the superior rectus will typically reveal the fibers of the superior oblique tendon stretching from the trochlea toward the insertion underneath the superior rectus muscle.

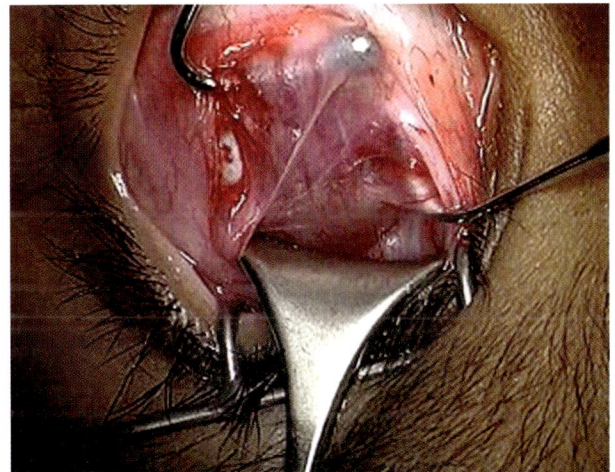

FIGURE 59.37 A small Stevens muscle hook is used to hook the superior oblique tendon.

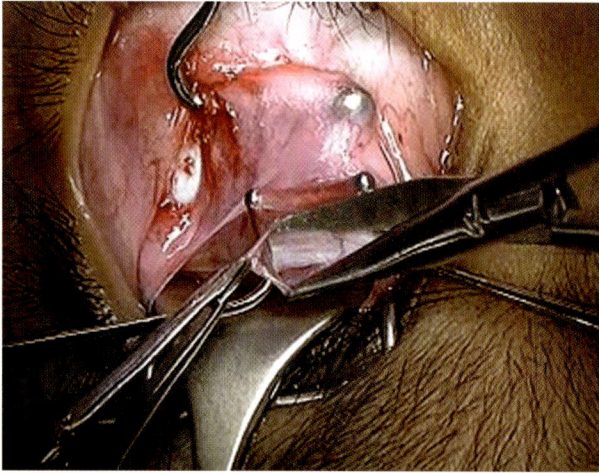

FIGURE 59.38 The capsule of the superior oblique can be opened further with Westcott scissors.

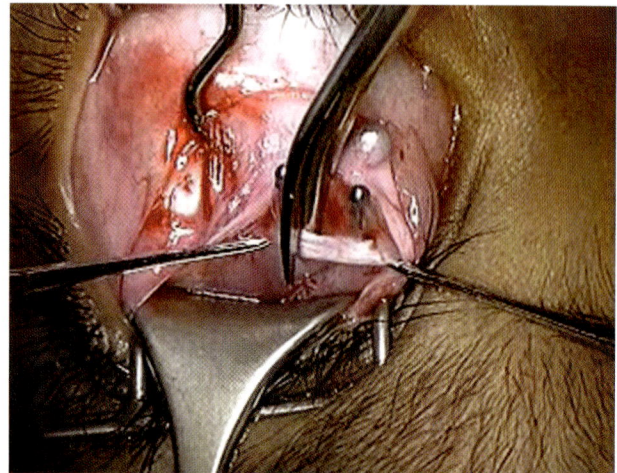

FIGURE 59.39 The superior oblique tendon is then cut on the nasal side of the superior rectus muscle and the two ends allowed to retract.

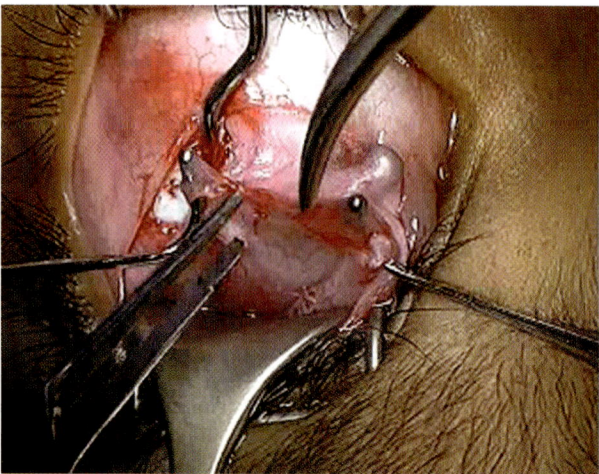

FIGURE 59.40 Careful inspection of the area should be carried out to be sure there are no residual tendon fibers left. Repeat traction testing is the best way to be sure the tendon has been transected completely.

Superior Oblique Spacer

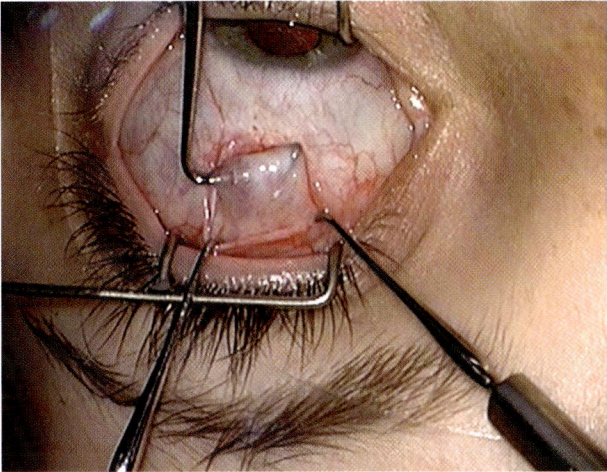

FIGURE 59.41 The SO is exposed as described in Figures 59.28–59.31 above. Two muscle hooks are placed underneath the conjunctiva to make room for placement of a Desmarres retractor.

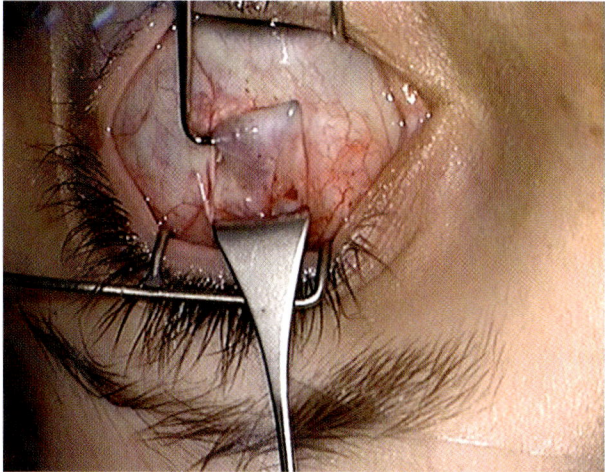

FIGURE 59.42 A Desmarres retractor is placed to provide further exposure.

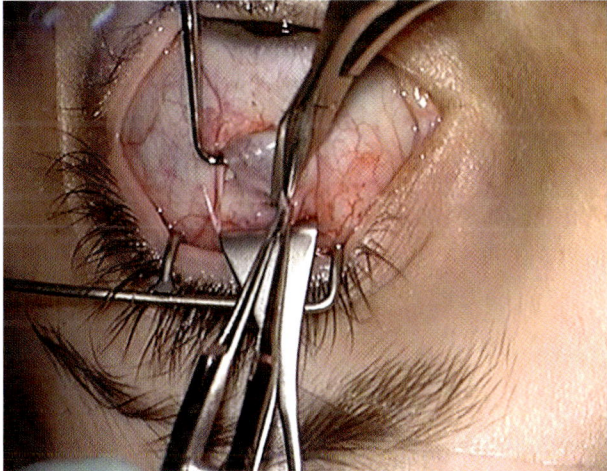

FIGURE 59.43 The diagonal check ligament across the surface of the superior rectus is grasped with a forceps, and a small rent made with scissors.

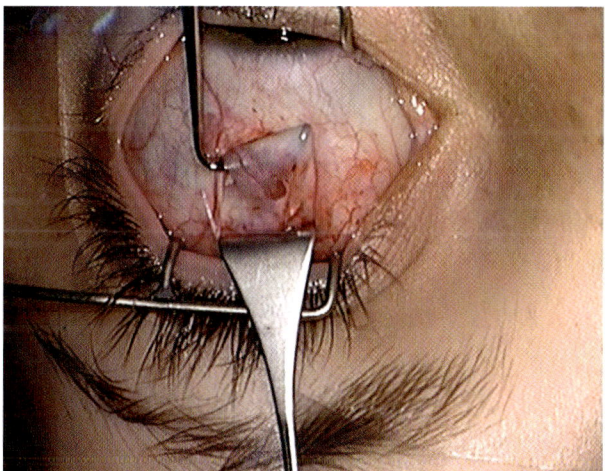

FIGURE 59.44 The small rent is apparent on the surface of the superior rectus muscle.

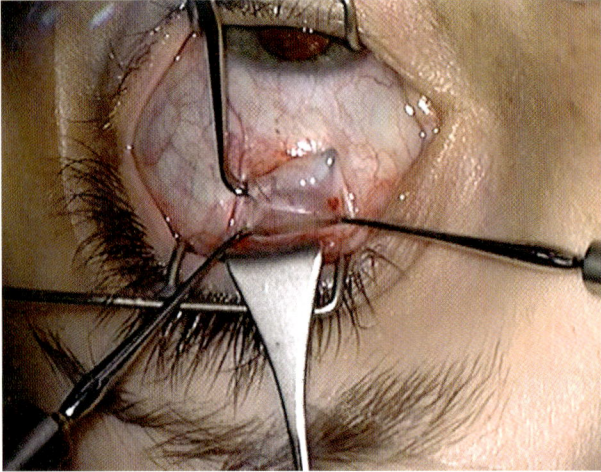

FIGURE 59.45 The two Stevens hooks are placed through the rent, and the rent stretched enough for the Desmarres retractor to be placed through the opening.

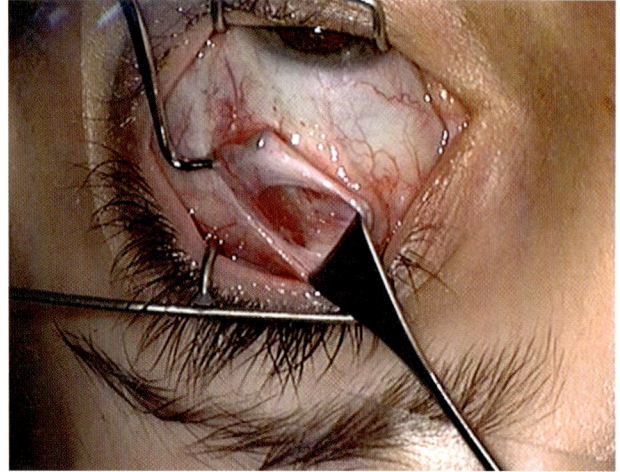

FIGURE 59.46 The Desmarres is in position, and inspection along the nasal border of the superior rectus will usually reveal the fibers of the superior oblique tendon coursing from the trochlea underneath the superior rectus muscle.

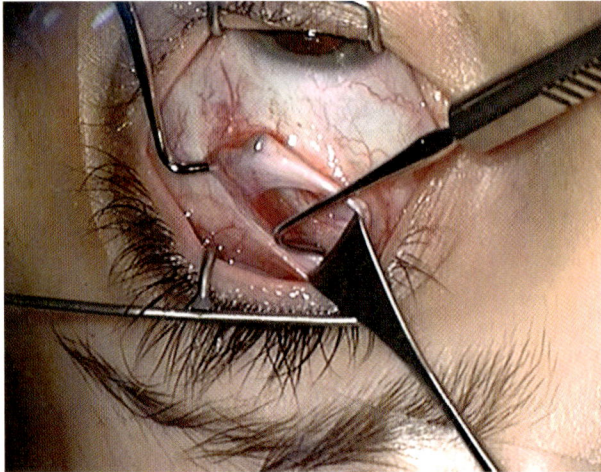

FIGURE 59.47 The superior oblique tendon is hooked with a small muscle hook and brought up into the operative field.

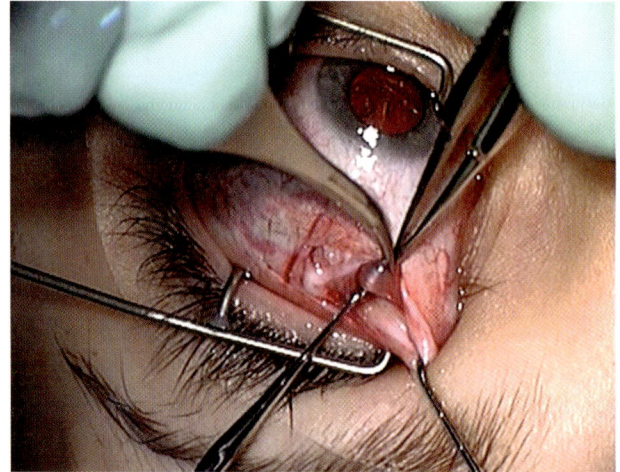

FIGURE 59.48 A small rent is made to the sheath of the superior oblique tendon with Westcott scissors.

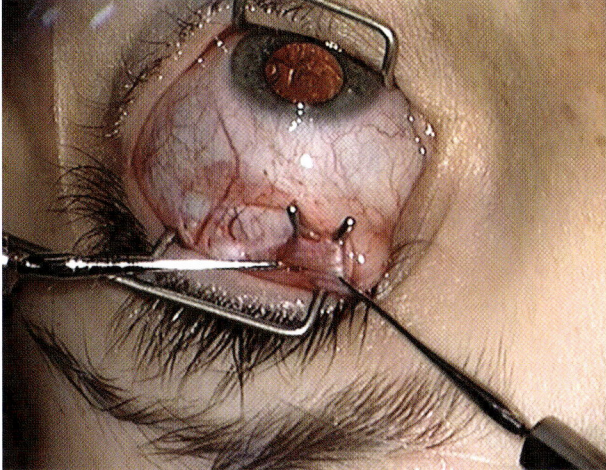

FIGURE 59.49 A second muscle hook is placed beneath the superior oblique tendon.

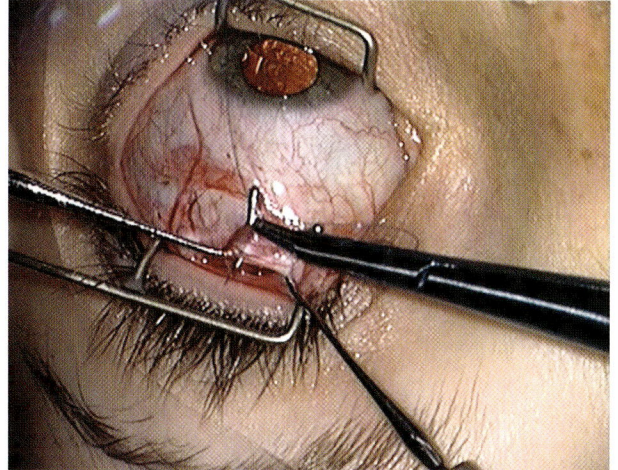

FIGURE 59.50 7-0 nonabsorbable monofilament suture, such as polypropylene, is used to secure the superior oblique tendon.

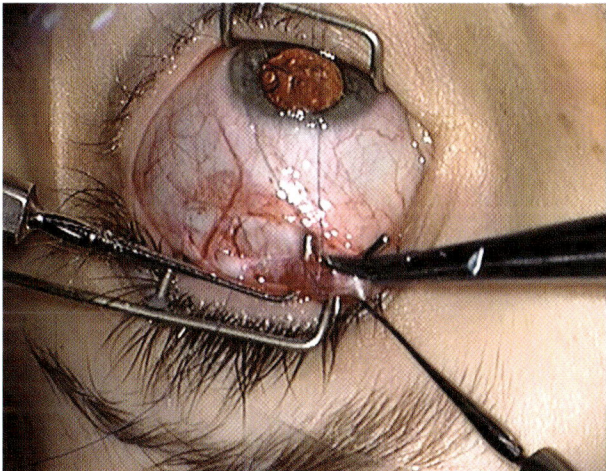

FIGURE 59.51 A second double-armed 7-0 suture is then placed adjacent to the first one, leaving several millimeters in between the two sutures.

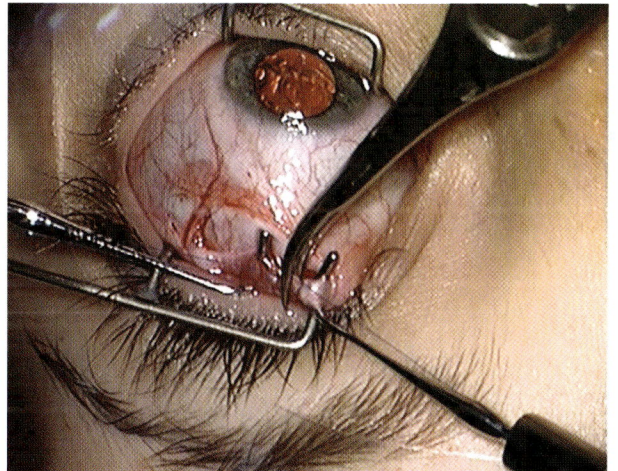

FIGURE 59.52 Westcott scissors are used to perform a complete tenotomy between the two sutures.

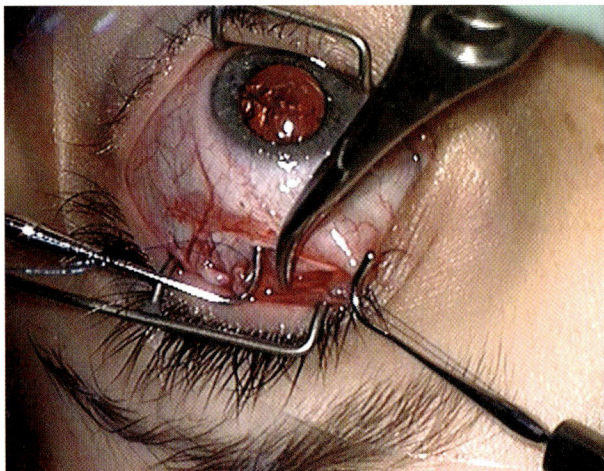

FIGURE 59.53 Inspection is carried out to be sure the entire superior oblique has been included. It is imperative that traction testing of the superior oblique be carried out at this point, in order to be sure the entire superior oblique tendon has been included. The globe should be able to be retropulsed in an elevated adducted position without feeling any resistance from a superior oblique tendon. This should be in stark contrast to the traction test findings at the beginning of the procedure.

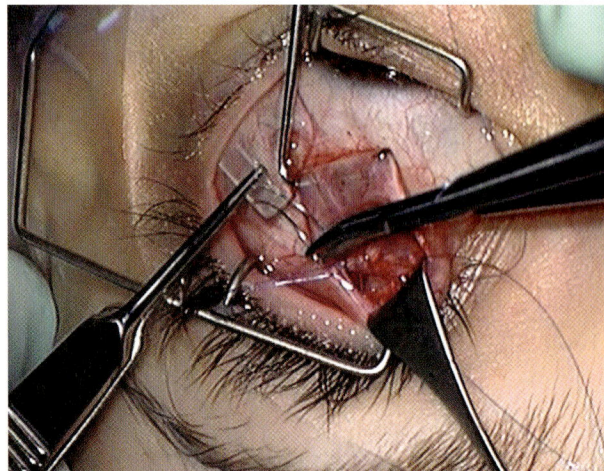

FIGURE 59.54 A 240 silicone retinal band can be used as the spacer material. Each of the two double-armed sutures are brought out through the butt end of one end of the silicone spacer.

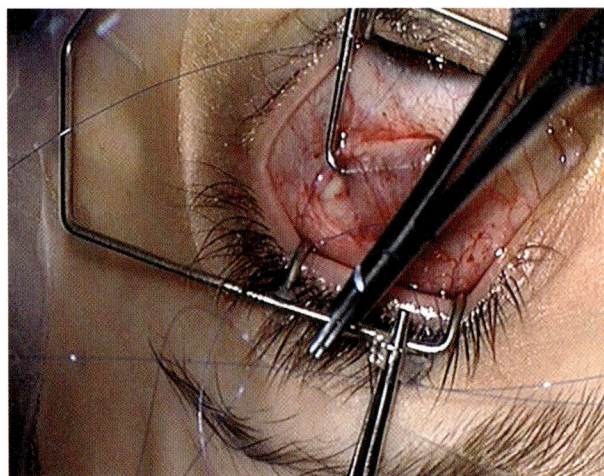

FIGURE 59.55 The two needles from the suture of the opposite side of the superior oblique are then passed through the butt end of the opposite side of the silicone spacer.

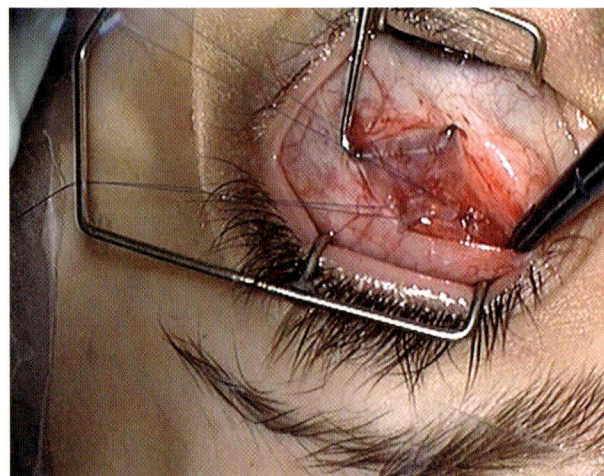

FIGURE 59.56 The ends of the superior oblique are pulled up flush against the silicone spacer and the sutures tied down.

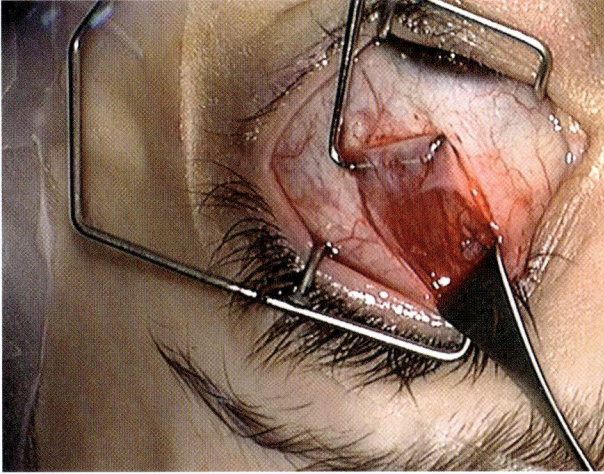

FIGURE 59.57 The silicone spacer is allowed to fall back into its position along the course of the superior oblique tendon. Ideally, the underside of the superior oblique tendon sheath has remained intact throughout this procedure. Traction testing can be repeated to be sure the tendon feels to be of the appropriate length. This maneuver should not be terribly vigorous, in order to not pull out the delicate sutures, but the maneuver should be enough to be convincing that the superior oblique–spacer complex is intact and is not causing an abnormal restriction to elevation in adduction. The superior temporal conjunctival incision is closed with one interrupted polyglactin suture

Superior Oblique Tuck

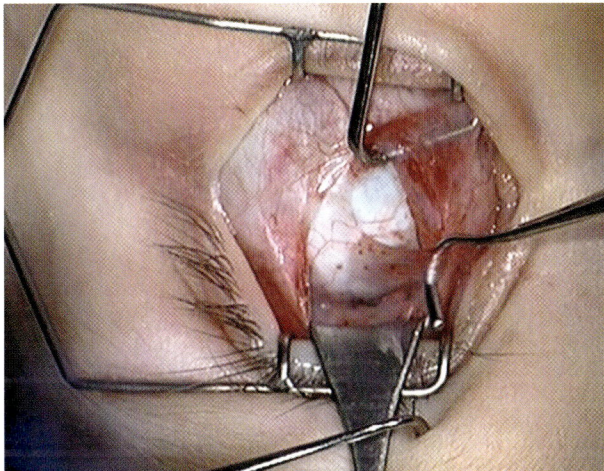

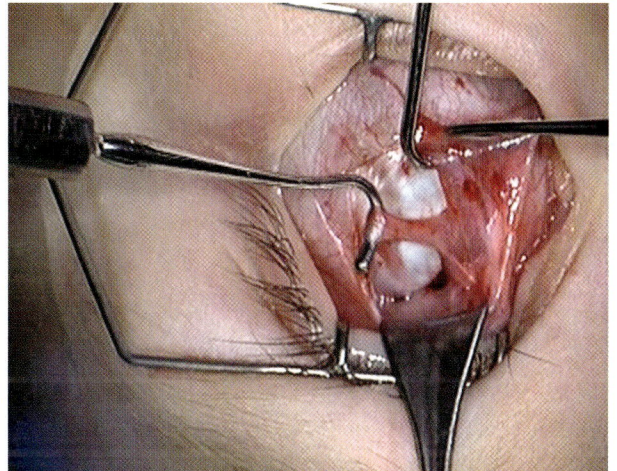

FIGURE 59.58 The exposure of the superior oblique tendon for superior oblique tuck is identical to that described in Figures 59.28–59.31 for superior oblique weakening procedures. Once the superior rectus muscle has been hooked on a muscle hook, the superior oblique tendon fibers can be seen attaching to the globe underneath the temporal border of the superior rectus muscle. Here, the superior oblique tendon is hooked with a small muscle hook on the temporal side of the superior rectus muscle.

FIGURE 59.59 Care is taken to be sure the entire superior oblique tendon has been identified and hooked.

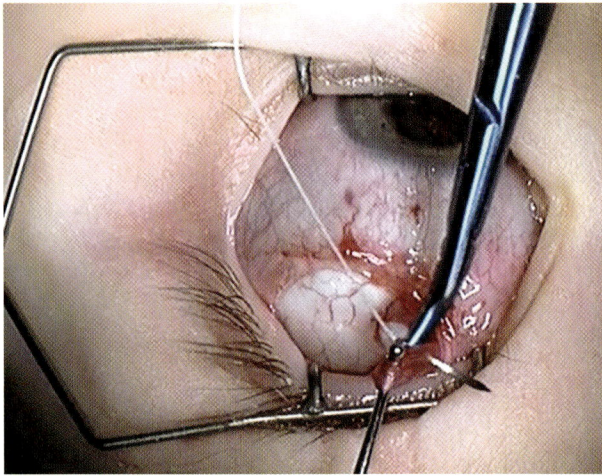

FIGURE 59.60   A 5-0 nonabsorbable suture is placed through each arm of the superior oblique tendon as it hangs beneath the muscle hook. The amount of tendon to be tucked cannot be known from the preoperative clinic exam—the proper amount is based on the excess laxity found in the superior oblique tendon at the time of surgery.

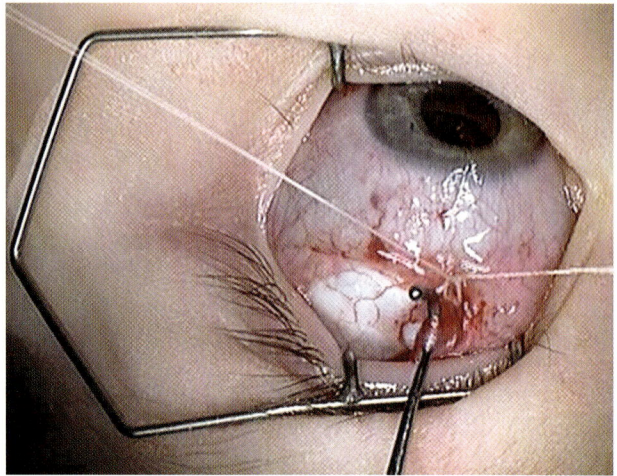

FIGURE 59.61   The suture is tied down, incorporating approximately one-third of the width of the superior oblique tendon.

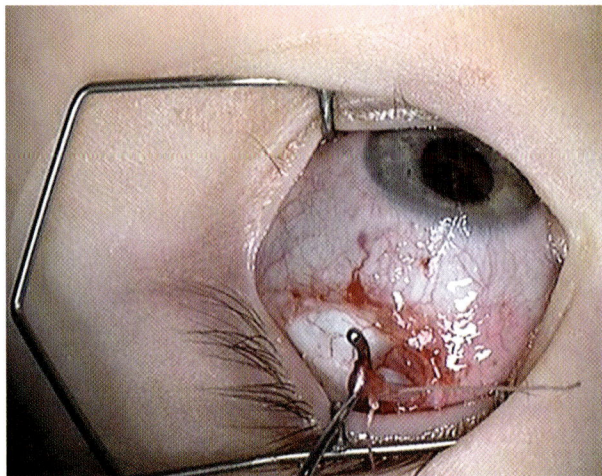

FIGURE 59.62   A second double-arm suture is passed through the opposite borders of the superior oblique tendon at the same level as that of the initial suture.

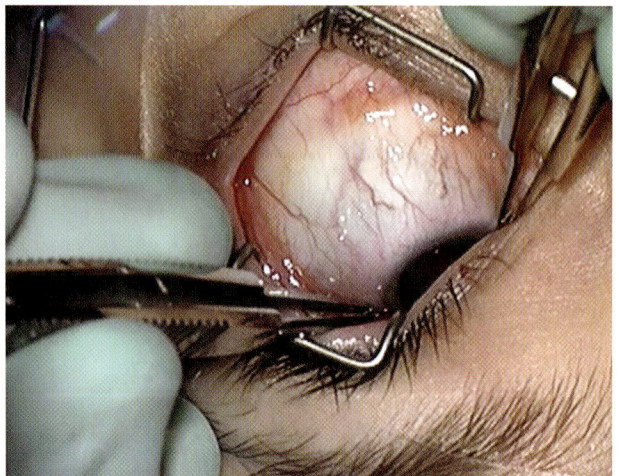

FIGURE 59.63   The superior oblique tendon is not sutured to the globe—it is allowed to find its own place in the superior temporal quadrant. It is imperative to repeat the traction testing of the superior oblique muscle to be sure a proper amount of tautness is present. In the case of a unilateral tendon tuck, the proper end point for tuck tightness is to make the superior oblique on the tuck side feel approximately equal to the tautness of the superior oblique on the opposite eye. The tucked side can be slightly more taut, since the tuck typically loosens somewhat over time. If a significant Brown syndrome is present on the traction testing, the tuck should be taken down and made smaller. Conversely, if there is still excess tendon laxity based on the traction test finding, a large tuck should be done.

Harada-Ito Procedure

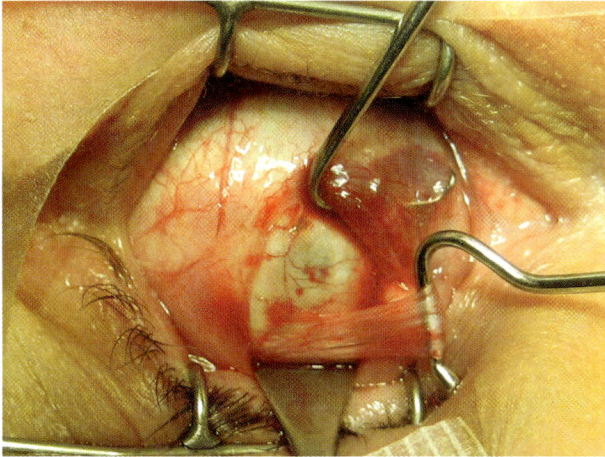

FIGURE 59.64 The exposure is done in the superior temporal quadrant in a fashion identical to that used for other superior oblique procedures, including SO tenotomy, spacer, or tuck. The superior rectus is hooked with a large square (Green) hook through the superior temporal fornix incision. The tenuous fibers of the fanned-out superior oblique insertion are hooked as it lies under the superior rectus muscle.

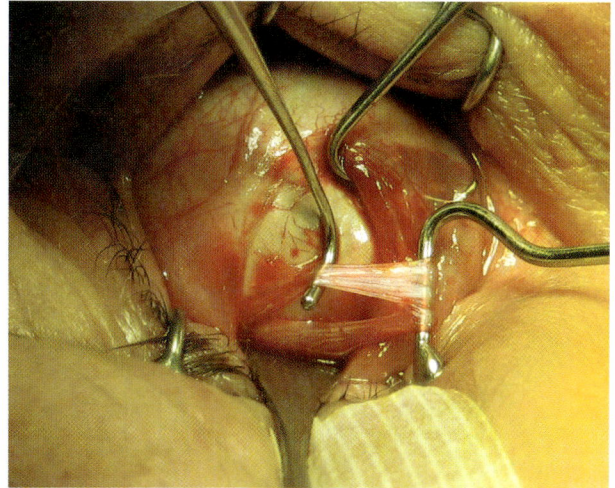

FIGURE 59.65 The superior oblique tendon is split in half horizontally.

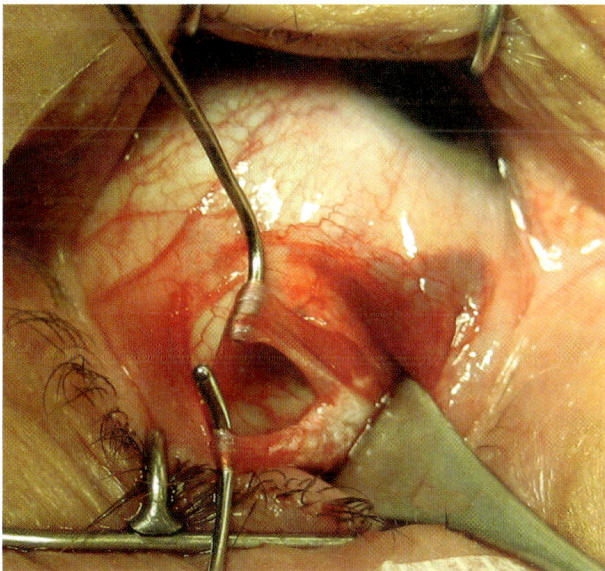

FIGURE 59.66 The split is extended by cutting with scissors in line with the tendon fibers. Here, the tendon is fully split enough to perform the procedure by advancing the anterior half of the tendon without disturbing the posterior half.

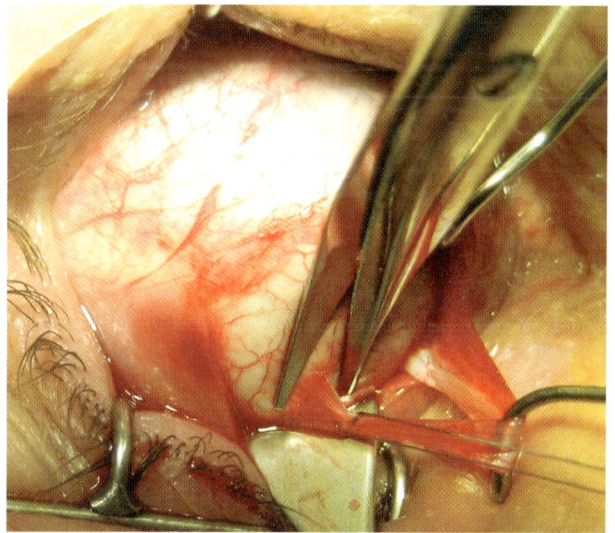

FIGURE 59.67 After securing the anterior half of the tendon on a double-armed 6-0 absorbable suture, the tendon is disinserted.

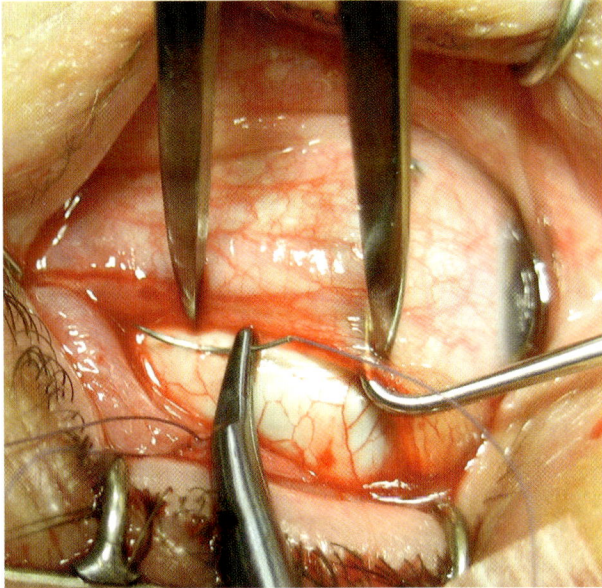

FIGURE 59.68 The spot for reattachment of the SO tendon is 8 mm posterior to the insertion of the lateral rectus, at the superior border of the lateral rectus.

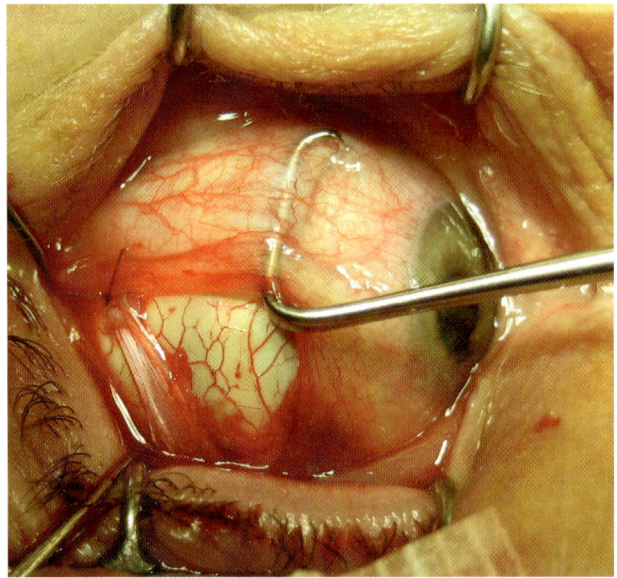

FIGURE 59.69 The SO tendon has been advanced and attached securely to the sclera at the point described.

TABLE 59.4 *Complications of Superior Oblique Surgery*

Tenotomy
- Incomplete tenotomy will result in failure of weakening.

Spacer
- Excessive dissection around SO tendon sheath can lead to adherence of spacer to globe or surrounding tissues.
- Extrusion of the silicone spacer. Extrusion more likely if a large spacer is used; e.g., greater than 7 mm.

Tuck
- Iatrogenic Brown syndrome from too aggressive tuck. Can be prevented by careful traction testing after the tuck is completed to be sure passive elevation in adduction is not restricted.

Harada-Ito
- Inadequate separation of the anterior and posterior tendon fibers can lead to Brown syndrome.

SELECTED REFERENCES

Plager DA, ed. *Strabismus Surgery: Basic and Advanced Strategies.* Chapter 3. New York: Oxford University Press; 2004, pp. 35–68.

Rosenbaum AL, Santiago AP, eds. *Clinical Strabismus Management: Principles and Surgical Techniques.* Philadelphia: WB Saunders; 1999.

60   Adjustable Sutures

David L. Guyton, MD

TABLE 60.1 *Strong Indications for the Use of Adjustable Sutures*

Reoperations in general

Thyroid myopathy

Restrictive strabismus in general

Operating around scleral buckles

Extraocular muscle tightening secondary to anesthetic myotoxicity

TABLE 60.2 *Optional Indications for the Use of Adjustable Sutures*

Diplopia requiring a precise surgical result

Adult strabismus in general

Pediatric strabismus in general, with propofol anesthesia, if needed, for adjustment

All strabismus surgery except inferior oblique muscle procedures

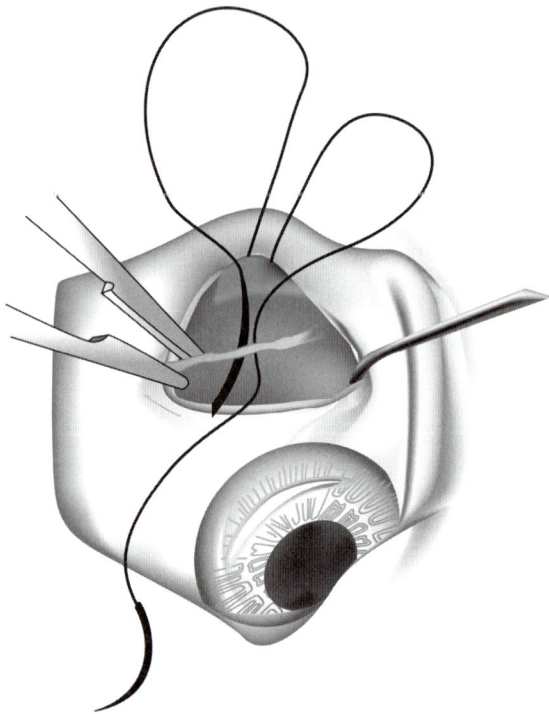

FIGURE 60.1 Reattachment of muscle to sclera. After the muscle is secured with a double-armed, 6-0 absorbable suture, the muscle is disinserted and is reattached at the original insertion site, passing the sutures approximately 2 mm apart. A preferred, small cul-de-sac conjunctival incision is used here, as well as being illustrated in subsequent figures.

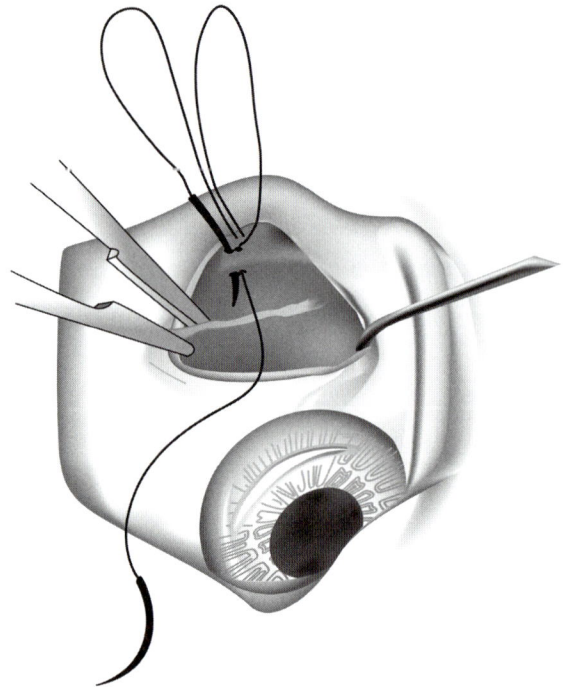

FIGURE 60.2 Reattachment of muscle using non-absorbable sutures. When non-absorbable sutures are used—for example, almost always on the inferior rectus muscle and with large recessions of the medial rectus muscle—the sutures are passed through the sclera approximately 4 mm posterior to the original insertion, so that the permanent suture ends can be fully buried to minimize the chance of erosion through the conjunctiva months to years later.

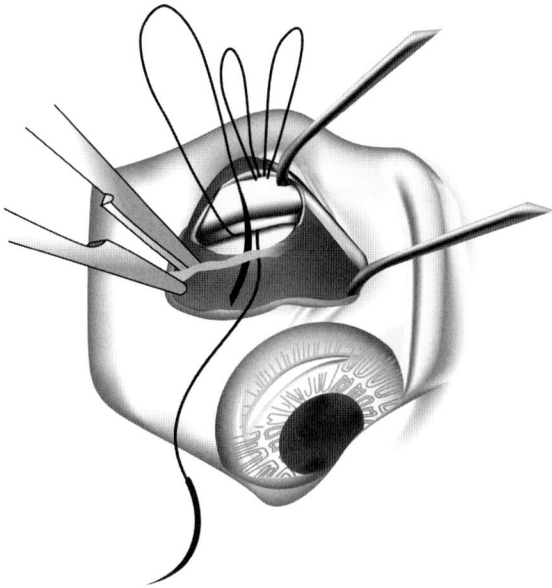

FIGURE 60.3 Threading sutures/muscle under scleral buckle. When a scleral buckle is present, a muscle can be effectively recessed by burrowing beneath the scleral buckle anteriorly to posteriorly, passing a small curved hemostat beneath the scleral buckle, and pulling the sutures and muscle beneath the scleral buckle from behind, to ensure proper adherence to the sclera during healing.

(a)

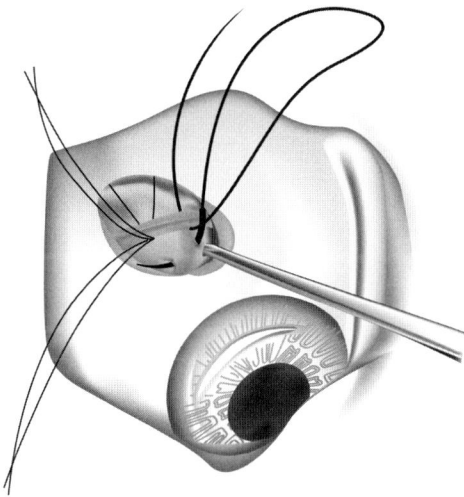

(b)

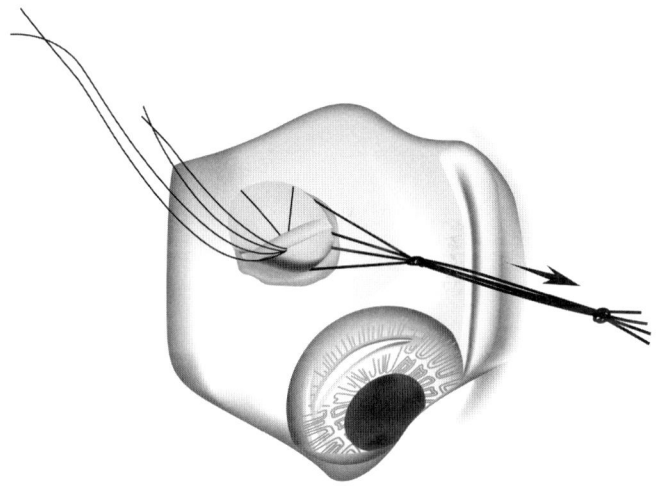

FIGURE 60.4 (a, b) Placing traction suture for exposure during adjustment. A 6-0 polyester suture on a spatula needle is passed through the insertion on the side of the muscle sutures where the conjunctiva has been retracted, and again in front of the muscle sutures, to provide four-suture retraction of the conjunctiva for access to the sliding noose at the time of adjustment.

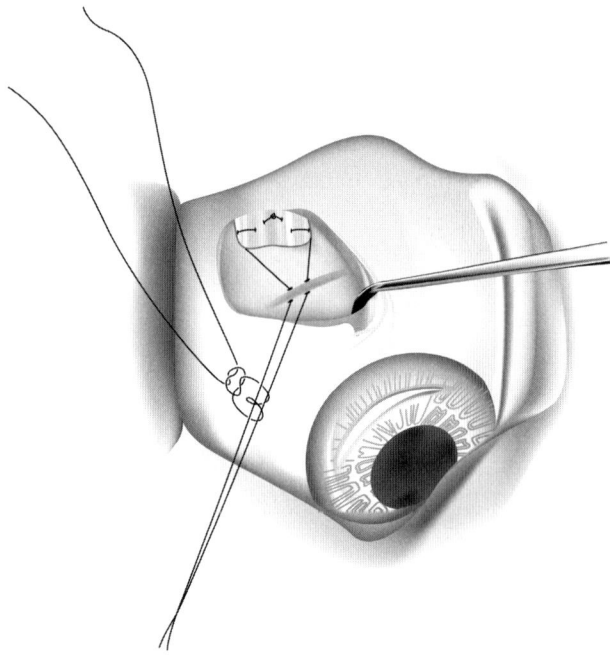

FIGURE 60.5 Tying sliding noose. A piece of absorbable suture cut from one end of the muscle sutures is passed twice around the muscle sutures and then tied in a tight square knot. This provides a stable knot, with good friction during adjustment.

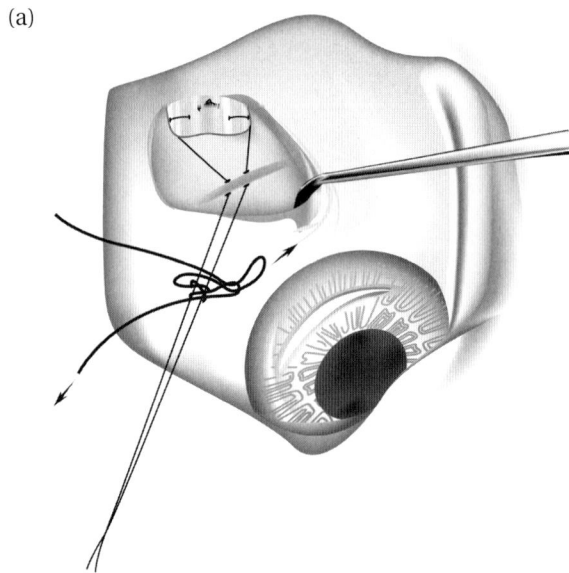

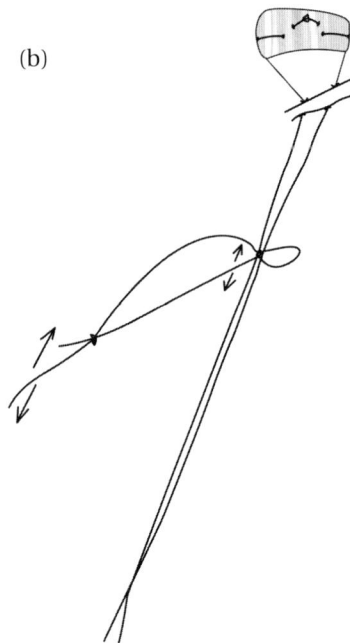

(a)

(b)

FIGURE 60.6 (a, b) Tying removable sliding noose. In order to leave less suture material behind for resorption, the noose knot can later be removed, still with good friction during adjustment, if the noose is fashioned in the form of a clove hitch with two successive slipknots, as shown. After the two successive slipknots are tied tightly, the two ends of the noose suture are tied together with an overhand knot, and part of the loop of the second slipknot is pulled through the noose knot. This reduces the size of the loop to minimize tissue capture, and also identifies the short suture arm by which the noose is moved back and forth. Alternatively, the noose may be moved back and forth by grasping the noose suture distal to the overhand knot.

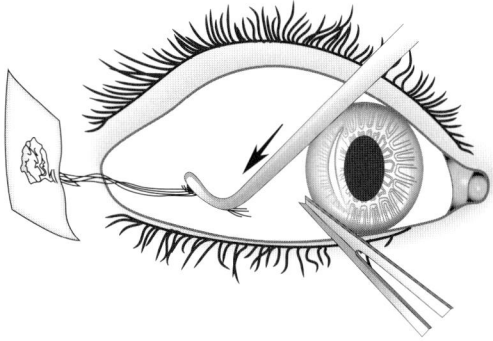

FIGURE 60.7 Closing conjunctiva and taping of adjustable suture ends. With small-incision cul-de-sac surgery, the conjunctival incision can simply be milked closed, and the adjustable suture ends are taped to the side of the cheek or to the bridge of the nose.

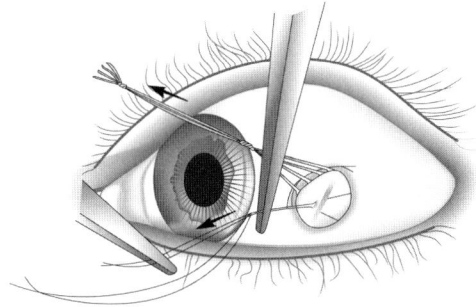

FIGURE 60.8 Suture adjustment: Loosening. The muscle sutures are pulled forward enough to allow a needle holder to grasp the muscle sutures posterior and close to the sliding noose. The noose is then pulled forward with another needle holder, sliding it along the muscle sutures for the desired number of millimeters of loosening.

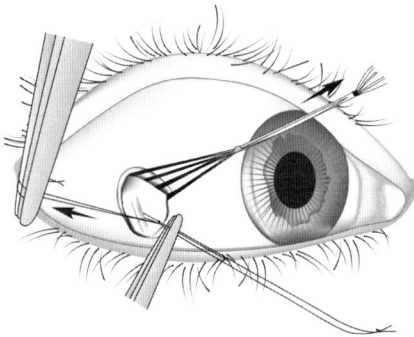

FIGURE 60.9 Suture adjustment: Tightening. The muscle sutures are grasped with a needle holder near the sliding noose, they are pulled forward, and another needle holder is used to slide the noose backward along the muscle sutures.

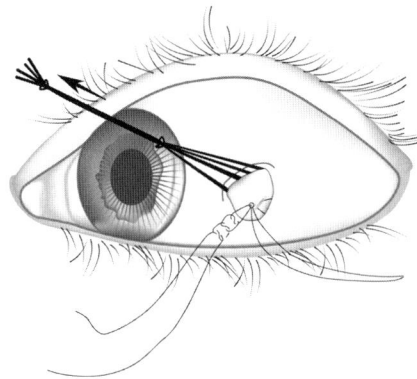

FIGURE 60.10 Tying off sutures. Once the muscle is adjusted to the desired position, as confirmed by cover testing or visual inspection, the muscle sutures are tied in a 3-throw square knot, being careful not to tie the first throw so tightly that the sliding noose is pushed backward. The suture ends are then trimmed to about 4 mm, the traction suture is removed, and the conjunctiva is milked closed over the remaining suture ends and noose knot.

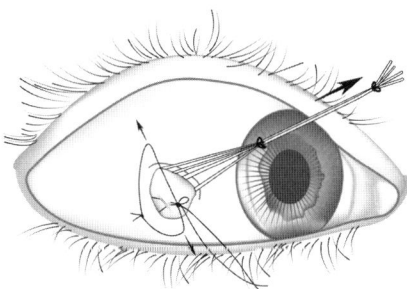

FIGURE 60.11 Removing removable sliding noose. If a removable sliding noose has been used, most commonly on recessions, it is removed entirely by separating the two noose sutures and pulling sideways with two needle holders.

(a)

(b)

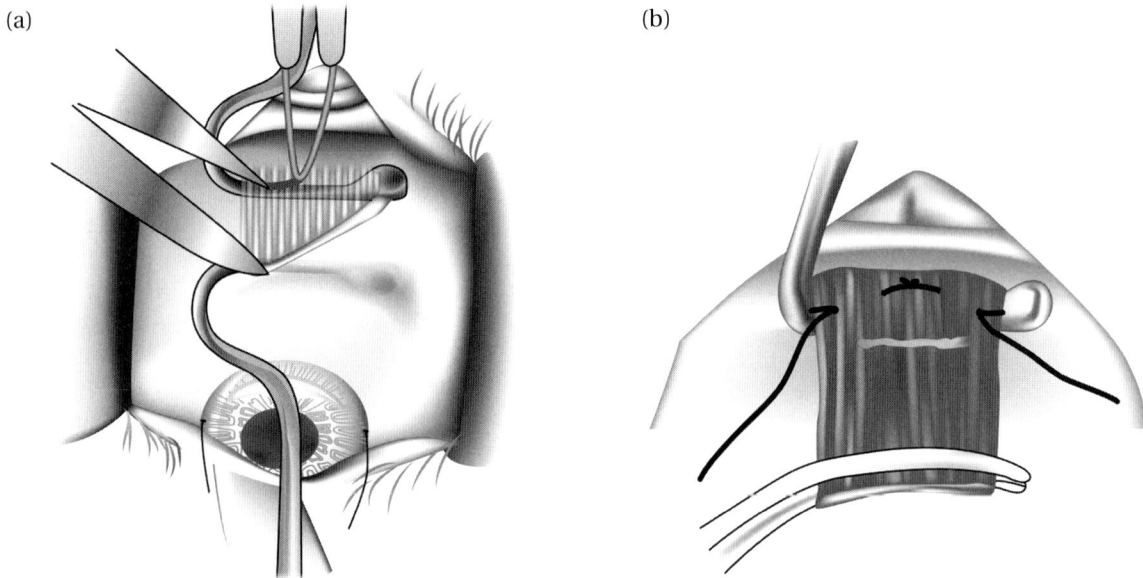

FIGURE 60.12 (a, b) Adjustable resections: Disinsertion and suture placement. The amount of resection is first marked with cautery. The muscle is then clamped with a small curved hemostat, and disinserted. Disinserting the muscle before suture placement enables large resections, while keeping the conjunctival incision small. The muscle on the clamp is pulled forward, and a large hook is placed behind the muscle by the assistant to provide exposure. The surgeon secures the muscle with a double-armed suture with a central knot and locking passes to both sides, such that the suture ends emerge from the front surface of the muscle approximately 2 mm from the edges and 2 mm posterior to the mark on the muscle.

FIGURE 60.13 Adjustable resections: Reattachment to sclera. The resected muscle is attached to the original insertion site in the same manner as a recessed muscle, but it is allowed to hang backward 2 mm to enable subsequent adjustment forward as well as backward.

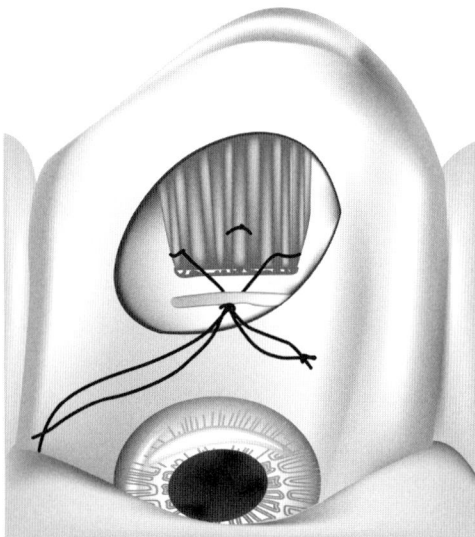

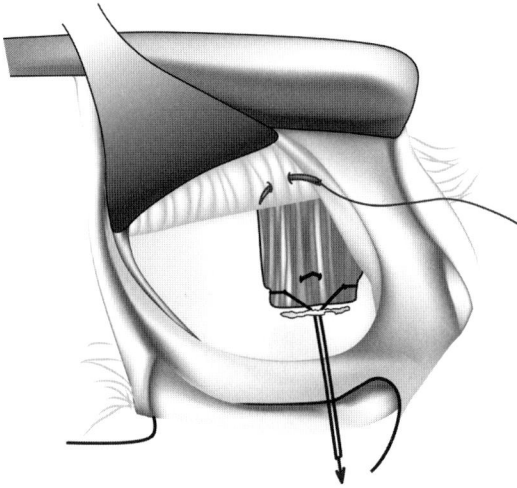

FIGURE 60.14 Adjustment of lower lid level with inferior rectus muscle recessions. The lower lid is often pulled down by inferior rectus muscle recessions, especially in elderly individuals. This retraction can be minimized by full dissection of the "capsulopalpebral head" of the inferior rectus muscle away from the front surface of the muscle, marking the capsulopalpebral tissue with cautery at the site of the primary attachment. After the muscle is disinserted and reattached, it is pulled forward to the insertion, and an adjustable absorbable suture is passed with a mattress bite through the capsulopalpebral lid tissue at the marked position. This tissue is suspended backward to its original position with the adjustable suture, with the adjustable suture attached to the original muscle insertion on the sclera. If there is retraction of the lower lid at the time of adjustment, the adjustable suture holding the lid tissues can be pulled forward to minimize or correct the retraction of the lid.

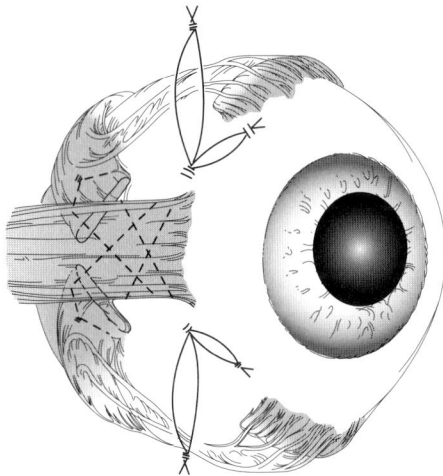

FIGURE 60.15 Adjustable Knapp-type transposition procedure. In this case, the superior and inferior rectus muscles of the right eye are transposed temporally to help compensate for a right sixth nerve palsy. A vessel-sparing technique is used by passing a taper-point needle beneath the large vessels on the surface of the inferior and superior rectus muscles. Each vessel group is dissected from the front surface of the respective muscle, along with a few muscle fibers, for a distance of 7–10 mm from the insertion, and the vessel group is reflected nasally. The underlying muscles are secured with absorbable sutures and are disinserted approximately 2 mm from their insertions. The muscle sutures are passed beneath the lateral rectus muscle and are secured to the sclera at the respective opposite corners of the lateral rectus muscle. Postoperatively, both muscle sutures may be tightened or loosened to adjust the horizontal position of the eye, or may be differentially adjusted to eliminate an induced vertical misalignment.

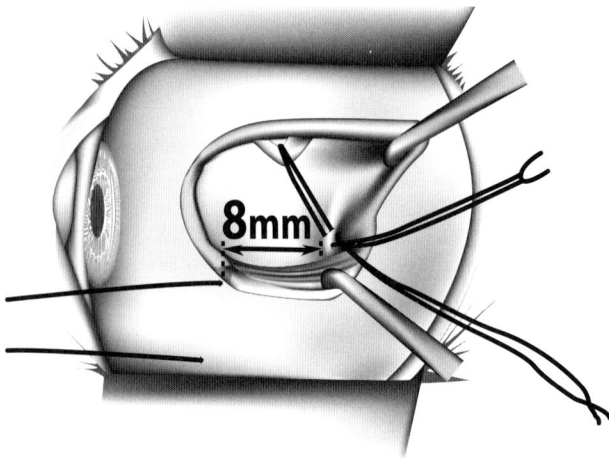

FIGURE 60.16 Adjustable Harada-Ito procedure. The superior rectus muscle is first hooked through a superotemporal conjunctival incision. The anterior third of the superior oblique tendon is identified, is hooked with a small muscle hook, and is separated from the remainder of the tendon for a distance of about 10–12 mm from its insertion. This portion of the tendon is secured with a double-armed 6-0 absorbable suture at the 10 mm point. The suture is brought temporally, as shown, to reinsert into the sclera just superior to the upper border of the lateral rectus muscle, approximately 8 mm posterior to the insertion of the lateral rectus muscle. An adjustable noose is placed at this point, as well as a subsequent traction suture.

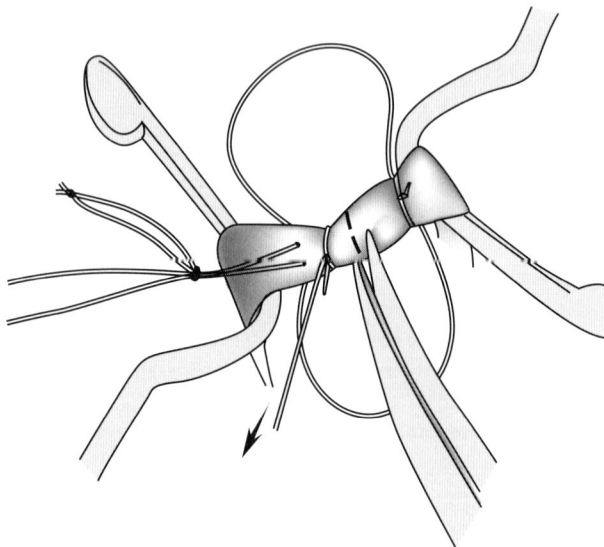

FIGURE 60.17 Adjustable superior oblique tendon surgery. The superior oblique tendon is first isolated through a superonasal conjunctival incision and displayed between two large muscle hooks. A double-armed 6-0 polyester suture is used to secure the tendon just nasal to the superior rectus muscle, to the right in the figure. The two suture ends are then passed through the nasal end of the exposed tendon, and an absorbable sliding noose is placed on these ends for subsequent adjustment. A fragment of the polyester suture is used to secure the tendon at a second position, with one end of this suture left long for traction purposes. The tendon is divided between the two securing sutures and the adjustable suture is adjusted for the desired initial separation. (The superior oblique tendon may be shortened in a similar manner by placing the securing sutures farther apart and performing a tenectomy in between them.) During adjustment, an upper lid retractor is used, and the patient is advised to look upward rather than downward, in order to loosen the superior oblique tendon so that the nasal end can be pulled forward, out of the wound, for adjustment.

TABLE 60.3 *Complications and Remedies*

Complications	Remedies
Broken suture during adjustment	Repair under topical anesthesia or return to operating room.
Frozen noose	Avoid tissue in knot. Separate muscle sutures and pull sideways to move noose. If removable noose, pull on loop to loosen.
Increased effect upon removal of removable noose	Pull knot forward and tie new noose behind knot.
Poor patient cooperation for exam	Face adults downward until able to open eyes. Hold young children up, looking down, to encourage opening eyes.

SELECTED REFERENCES

Awadein A, Sharma M, Bazemore MG, Saeed HA, Guyton DL. Adjustable suture strabismus surgery in infants and children. *J AAPOS.* 2008;12:585–590.

Goldenberg-Cohen N, Tarczy-Hornoch K, Klink DF, Guyton DL. Post-operative adjustable surgery of the superior oblique tendon. *Strabismus.* 2005;13:5–10.

Guyton DL. Strabismus: fornix approach with adjustable sutures. In Gottsch JD et al. (eds). *Ophthalmic surgery (Rob & Smith's operative surgery).* London: Arnold; 1999, pp. 85–91.

Mallette RA, Kwon JY, Guyton DL. A technique for repairing strabismus after scleral buckling surgery. *Am J Ophthalmol.* 1988;106:364–365.

Pacheco EM, Guyton DL, Repka MX. Changes in eyelid position accompanying vertical rectus muscle surgery and prevention of lower lid retraction with adjustable surgery. *J Ped Ophthalmol Strabismus.* 1992; 29:265–272.

Parsa CF, Sanjari MS, Guyton DL. Non-absorbable sutures should be used for inferior rectus muscle recessions. In de Faber JT (ed.). *Transactions of the 29th European Strabismological Association Meeting.* 2005, pp. 81–84.

Wisnicki HJ, Repka MX, Guyton DL. Reoperation rate in adjustable strabismus surgery. *J Ped Ophthalmol Strabismus.* 1988;25:112–114.

61 Transposition Procedures

Federico G. Velez, MD and Arthur L. Rosenbaum, MD[†]

[†] Deceased.

TABLE 61.1 *Indications for Transpositions*

Limitation to ocular rotations due to rectus muscle paralysis
Limitation to ocular rotation due to extraocular muscle absence
Limitation to ocular rotation due to muscle trauma
Monocular or bilateral elevation or depression deficiency
Cranial misinnervation syndromes

TABLE 61.2 *Preoperative Considerations*

	Positive	Negative
Rotation past midline	Resection	Transposition
Saccadic movement	Resection	Transposition
Force generation test	Resection	Transposition

TABLE 61.3 *Force Duction Test*

Positive	Negative
Full tendon or partial tendon transposition	Full tendon transposition
Weakening procedure antagonist muscle	
• Ciliary sparing procedure	
• Recession	
• Chemical denervation	

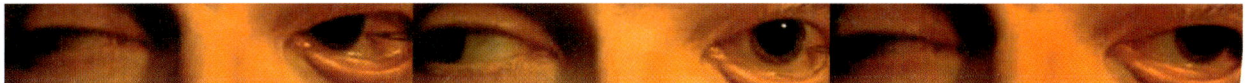

FIGURE 61.1 Force duction and force generation test. The conjunctiva is grasped with a forceps from the limbus opposite to the paralyzed muscle while the patient directs fixation in the field of action of the paralyzed muscle (middle). In the absence of restriction, the eye can be rotated in the field of action of the paralyzed muscle (left). Forced generation test confirms muscle weakness if the eye can be rotated in the opposite direction while the patient is still fixing in the direction of the field of action of the paralyzed muscle (right).

Full Tendon Transposition

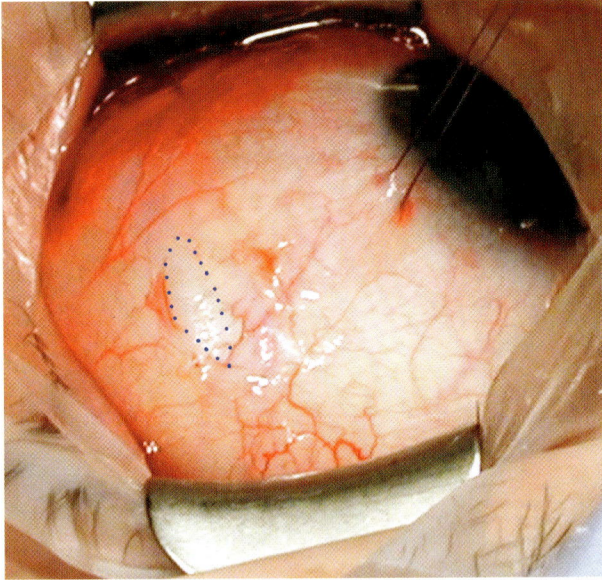

FIGURE 61.2 Conjunctival fornix incision between the paralyzed muscle and the muscle to be transposed at approximately 8.0 mm from the limbus. A circumferential incision parallel to the limbus creates a wider field for better visualization.

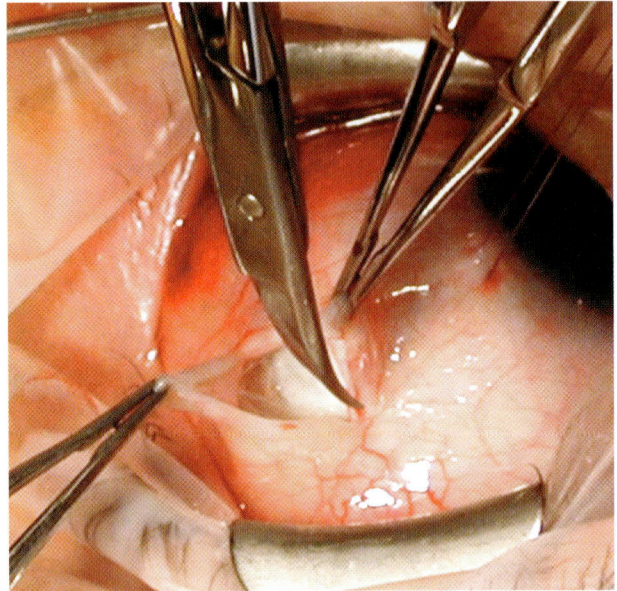

FIGURE 61.3 Dissection through Tenon's capsule to expose the sclera.

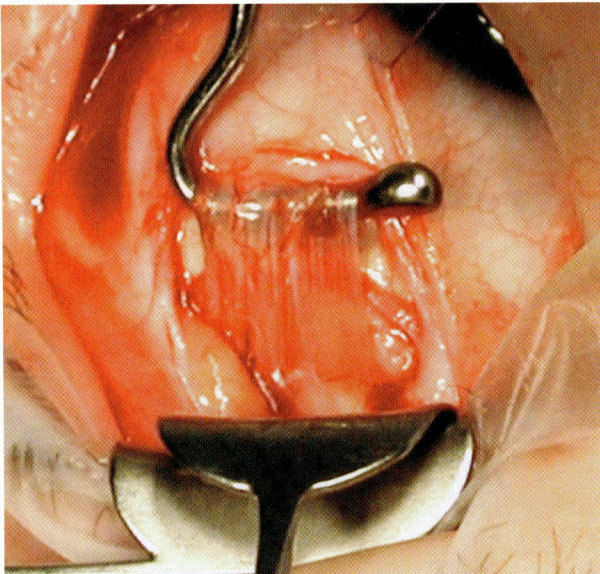

FIGURE 61.4 Superior rectus muscle dissection.

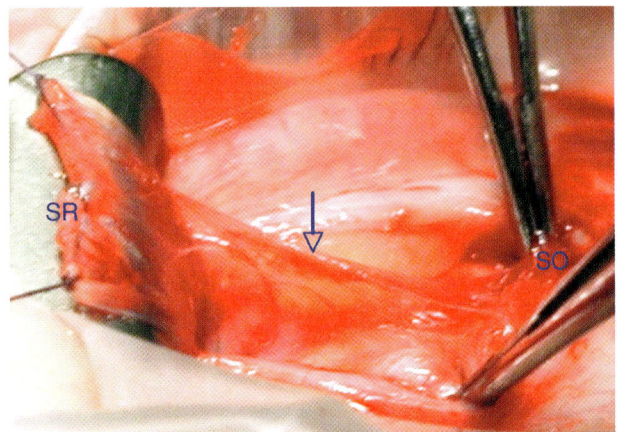

FIGURE 61.5 The frenulum (arrow) between the superior oblique tendon (SO) and the superior rectus muscle (SR) is identified.

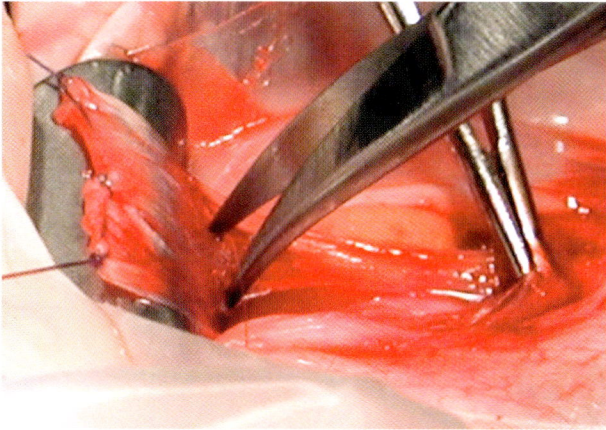

FIGURE 61.6 The frenulum is carefully dissected from the superior rectus muscle. This is essential to avoid dragging the superior oblique tendon during the superior rectus muscle transposition.

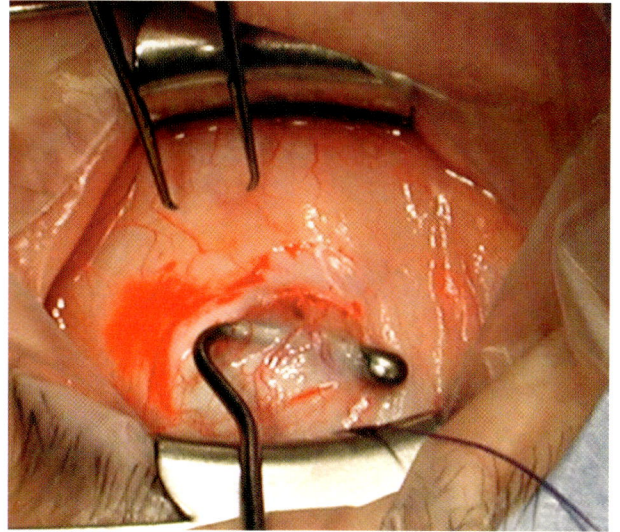

FIGURE 61.7 Inferior rectus muscle dissection.

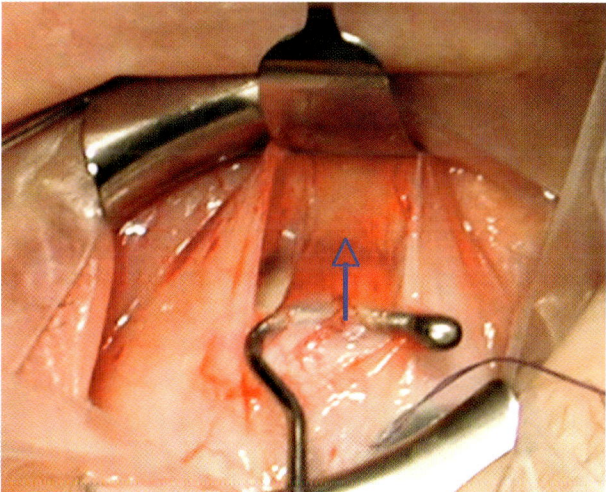

FIGURE 61.8 The attachments between the inferior rectus muscle and the eyelid retractors and Lockwood ligaments (arrow) are identified.

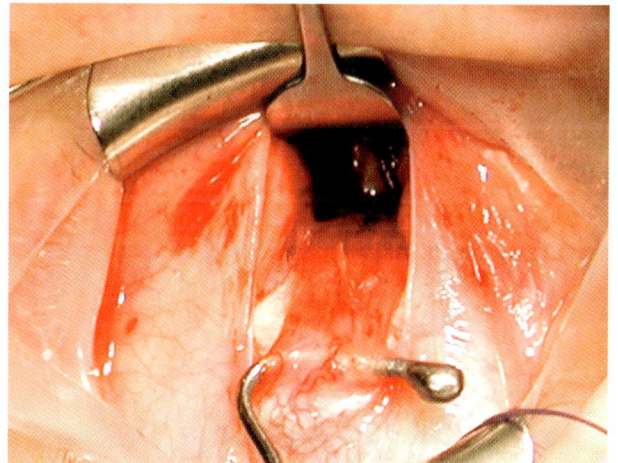

FIGURE 61.9 Careful dissection of the attachments between the eyelid retractors, Lockwood ligaments, and the inferior rectus is essential. Avoid orbital fat prolapse.

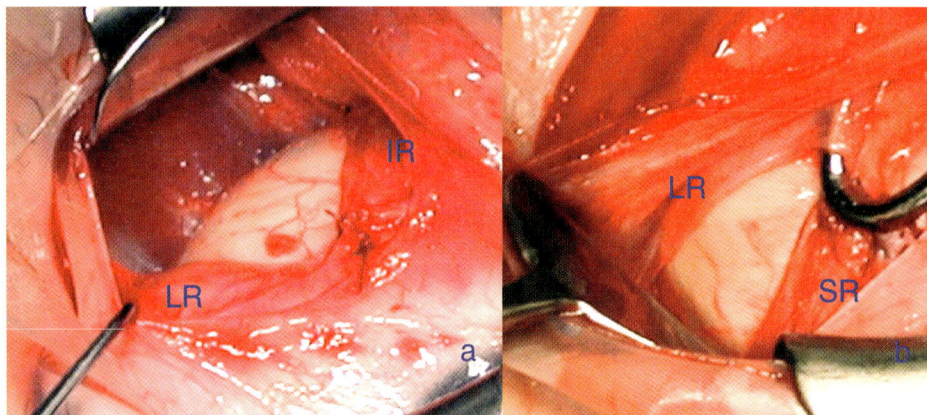

FIGURE 61.10 The transposed muscle is reinserted in the sclera using a 6-0 absorbable suture on a spatulated needle. One corner of the new insertion is adjacent to insertion of the paralyzed rectus muscle, and the opposite corner is inserted parallel to the spiral of Tillaux. (a) Inferior rectus muscle (IR) and (b) superior rectus muscle (SR) after a full tendon transposition toward the lateral rectus muscle (LR).

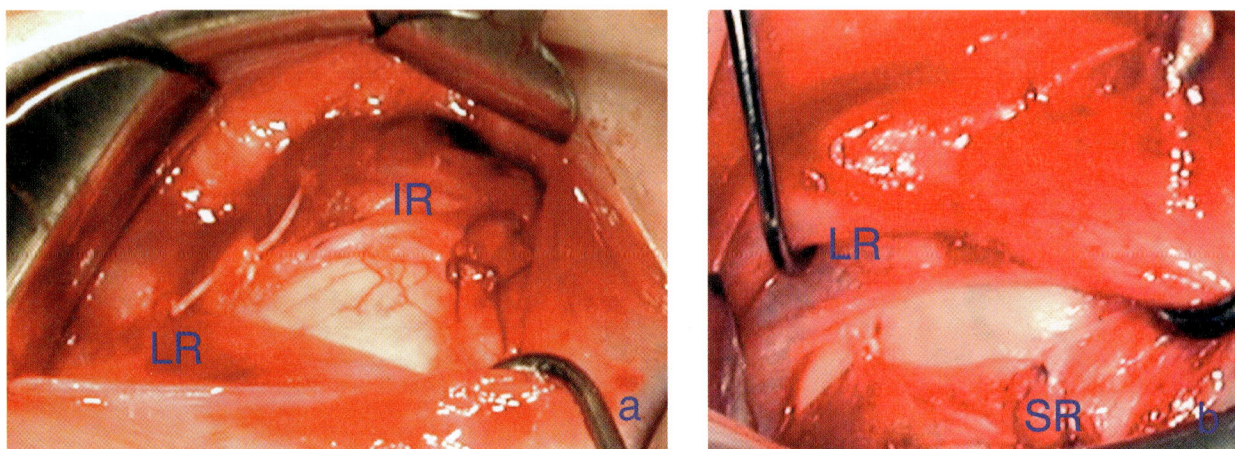

FIGURE 61.11 Posterior fixation suture. A 6-0 non-absorbable suture on a flat spatulated needle is passed between one-third of the belly of the transposed muscle and the sclera adjacent to the paralyzed muscle belly at 8–10 mm posterior to the paralyzed muscle insertion. The belly of the transposed (a) inferior rectus (IR) muscles and (b) superior rectus muscle (SR) is dragged closer to the adjacent paralyzed lateral rectus muscle (LR) to enhance the effect of the transposition.

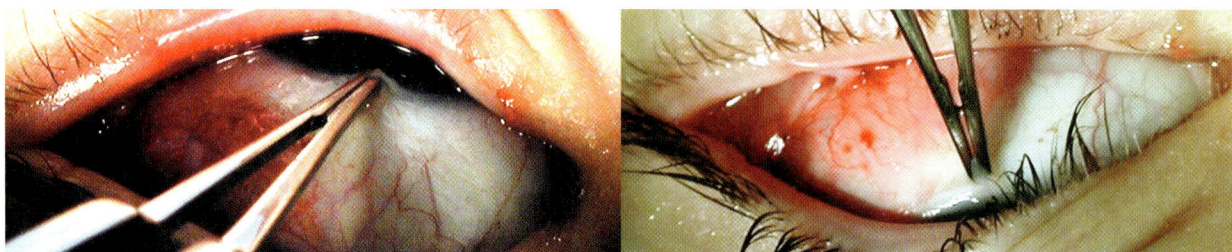

FIGURE 61.12 Intraoperative force duction test after both muscles are transposed to confirm symmetry. Explore the transposed muscles and the posterior fixation suture if the force duction test is restrictive or asymmetric.

Partial Rectus Muscle Transposition

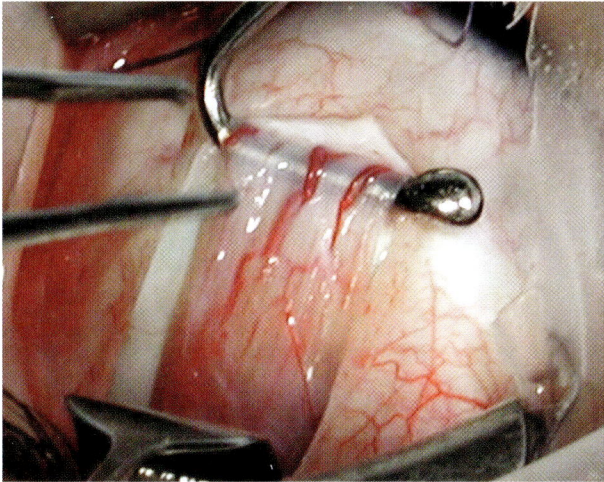

FIGURE 61.13 Identify the anterior ciliary vessels.

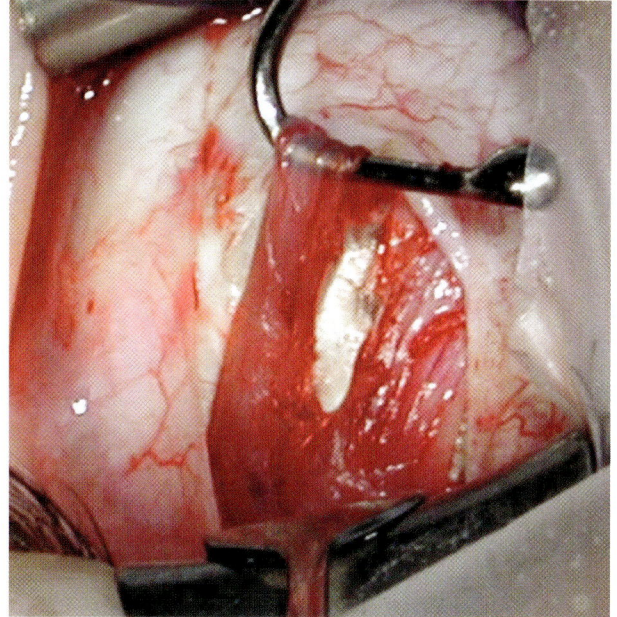

FIGURE 61.14 The muscle is split, leaving at least one anterior ciliary vessel intact.

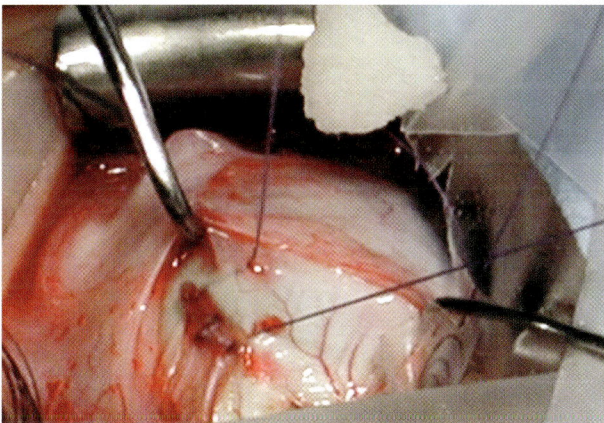

FIGURE 61.15 The partial-width tendon is transposed toward the paralyzed muscle insertion. The transposed muscle is reinserted in the sclera using a 6-0 absorbable suture on a spatulated needle. One corner of the new insertion is adjacent to insertion of the paralyzed rectus muscle, and the opposite corner is inserted parallel to the spiral of Tillaux.

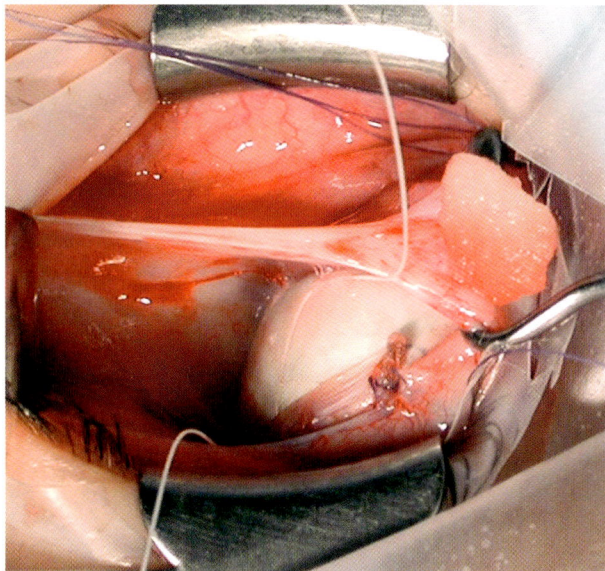

FIGURE 61.16 Posterior fixation suture placement of the partial width. A 6-0 non-absorbable suture on a flat spatulated needle is passed between one-third of the belly of the transposed muscle and the sclera adjacent to the paralyzed muscle belly at 8–10 mm posterior to the paralyzed muscle insertion.

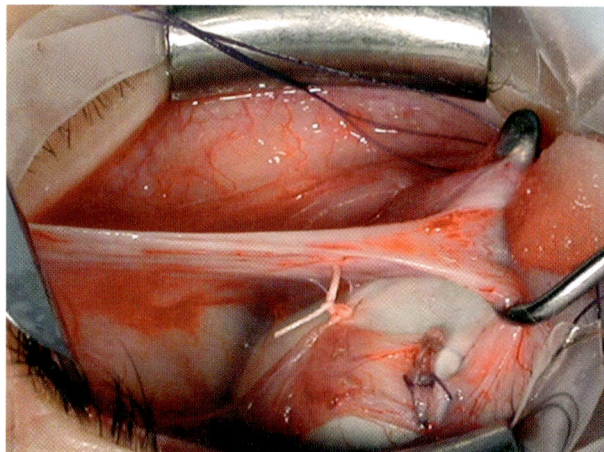

FIGURE 61.17 The transposed muscle belly is dragged closer to the belly of the paralyzed muscle by the posterior fixation suture.

TABLE 61.4 *Selected Entities*

Abduction deficiency	• Superior rectus and inferior rectus muscles transposition to lateral rectus muscle
	• Posterior fixation sutures
Adduction deficiency	• Superior rectus and inferior rectus transposition to medial rectus muscle
	• Resection of both transposed muscles 5 mm
	• Posterior fixation sutures
Elevation or depression deficiency	• Vertical transposition of the medial rectus and lateral rectus muscles
	• Posterior fixation sutures
Combined vertical and horizontal deficiency	• Resection and recession of the transposed muscles to correct the associated deviation
	• Posterior fixation sutures

TABLE 61.5 *Potential Complications*

Undercorrection
Overcorrection
Induced vertical deviation
Scleral perforation
Anterior segment ischemia
Selecting the wrong patient

SELECTED REFERENCES

Britt MT, Velez FG, Thacker N, Alcorn D, Foster RS, Rosenbaum AL. Partial rectus muscle-augmented transpositions in abduction deficiency. *J AAPOS.* 2003 Oct;7(5):325–332.

Buckley EG, Townshend LM. A simple transposition procedure for complicated strabismus. *Am J Ophthalmol.* 1991 Mar 15;111(3):302–306.

Clark RA, Rosenbaum AL, Demer JL. Magnetic resonance imaging after surgical transposition defines the anteroposterior location of the rectus muscle pulleys. *J AAPOS.* 1999 Feb;3(1):9–14.

Coats DK, Brady-McCreery KM, Paysse EA. Split rectus muscle modified Foster procedure for paralytic strabismus: A report of 5 cases. *Binocul Vis Strabismus Q.* 2001;16(4):281–284.

Dawson EL, Boyle NJ, Lee JP. Full-tendon nasal transposition of the vertical rectus muscles: A retrospective review. *Strabismus.* 2007 Jul–Sep;15(3):133–6.

Foster RS. Vertical muscle transposition augmented with lateral fixation. *J AAPOS.* 1997 Mar;1(1):20–30.

Hong S, Chang YH, Han SH, Lee JB. Effect of full tendon transposition augmented with posterior intermuscular suture for paralytic strabismus. *Am J Ophthalmol.* 2005 Sep;140(3):477–483.

Metz HS. Rectus muscle transposition surgery. *J Pediatr Ophthalmol Strabismus.* 1981 Nov–Dec;18(6):51–54.

Mohamed SR, Ainsworth JR. Vertical augmented transposition surgery. *Eye* (Lond). 2004 Jan;18(1):81–84.

Paysse EA, Brady McCreery KM, Ross A, Coats DK. Use of augmented rectus muscle transposition surgery for complex strabismus. *Ophthalmology.* 2002 Jul;109(7):1309–1314.

Paysse EA, Saunders RA, Coats DK. Surgical management of strabismus after rupture of the inferior rectus muscle. *J AAPOS.* 2000 Jun;4(3):164–167.

Rosenbaum AL, Kushner BJ, Kirschen D. Vertical rectus muscle transposition and botulinum toxin (Oculinum) to medial rectus for abducens palsy. *Arch Ophthalmol.* 1989 Jun;107(6):820–823.

Rosenbaum AL. Costenbader Lecture. The efficacy of rectus muscle transposition surgery in esotropic Duane syndrome and VI nerve palsy. *J AAPOS.* 2004 Oct;8(5):409–419.

Ruth AL, Velez FG, Rosenbaum AL. Management of vertical deviations after vertical rectus transposition surgery. *J AAPOS.* 2009 Feb;13(1):16–19.

Struck MC. Augmented vertical rectus transposition surgery with single posterior fixation suture: Modification of Foster technique. *J AAPOS.* 2009 Aug;13(4):343–349.

Velez FG, Foster RS, Rosenbaum AL. Vertical rectus muscle augmented transposition in Duane syndrome. *J AAPOS.* 2001 Apr;5(2):105–113.

62 Fadenoperation

Edward G. Buckley, MD

SELECTED REFERENCES

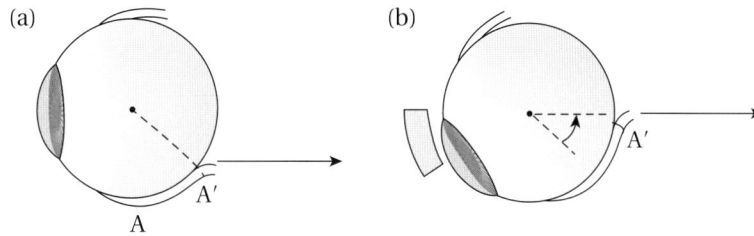

FIGURE 62.1 The fadenoperation is used to create a limitation in the primary field of action of a muscle without affecting the straight-ahead gaze position of the eye. A suture is used to fix the muscle to the globe at a point posterior (point A′) to the muscle's original insertion (point A) as illustrated on the inferior rectus in figure (a). The location of the suture becomes the new functional insertion, and as the muscle pulls to rotate the eye, the point of maximum rotation occurs earlier than before, limiting the full rotation of the eye only in that direction (b). The primary use for this procedure is to match a weakness in rotation that is present in the fellow eye.

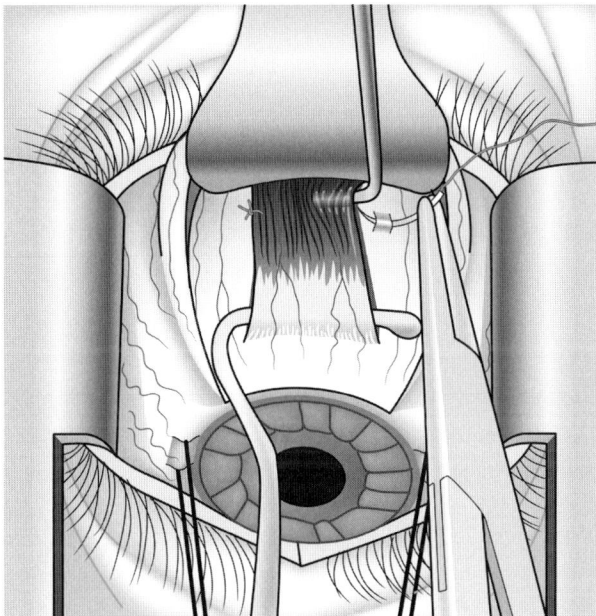

FIGURE 62.2 The technique requires placement of a non-absorbable suture into the sclera and then the muscle, incorporating approximately 1/4 of the muscle at each border, posterior to the muscle's original insertion. The distance from the insertion should be at least 10 mm, but ideally 13–15 mm. The procedure requires good exposure and is best accomplished with a small flat (1/8 circle) spatulated needle and a narrow blade retractor, such as a Fison or Helveston Barbee. The location of the vortex veins often limit the posterior extent of the suture placement, and must be tied firmly in order to insure a tight adherence of the muscle to the sclera.

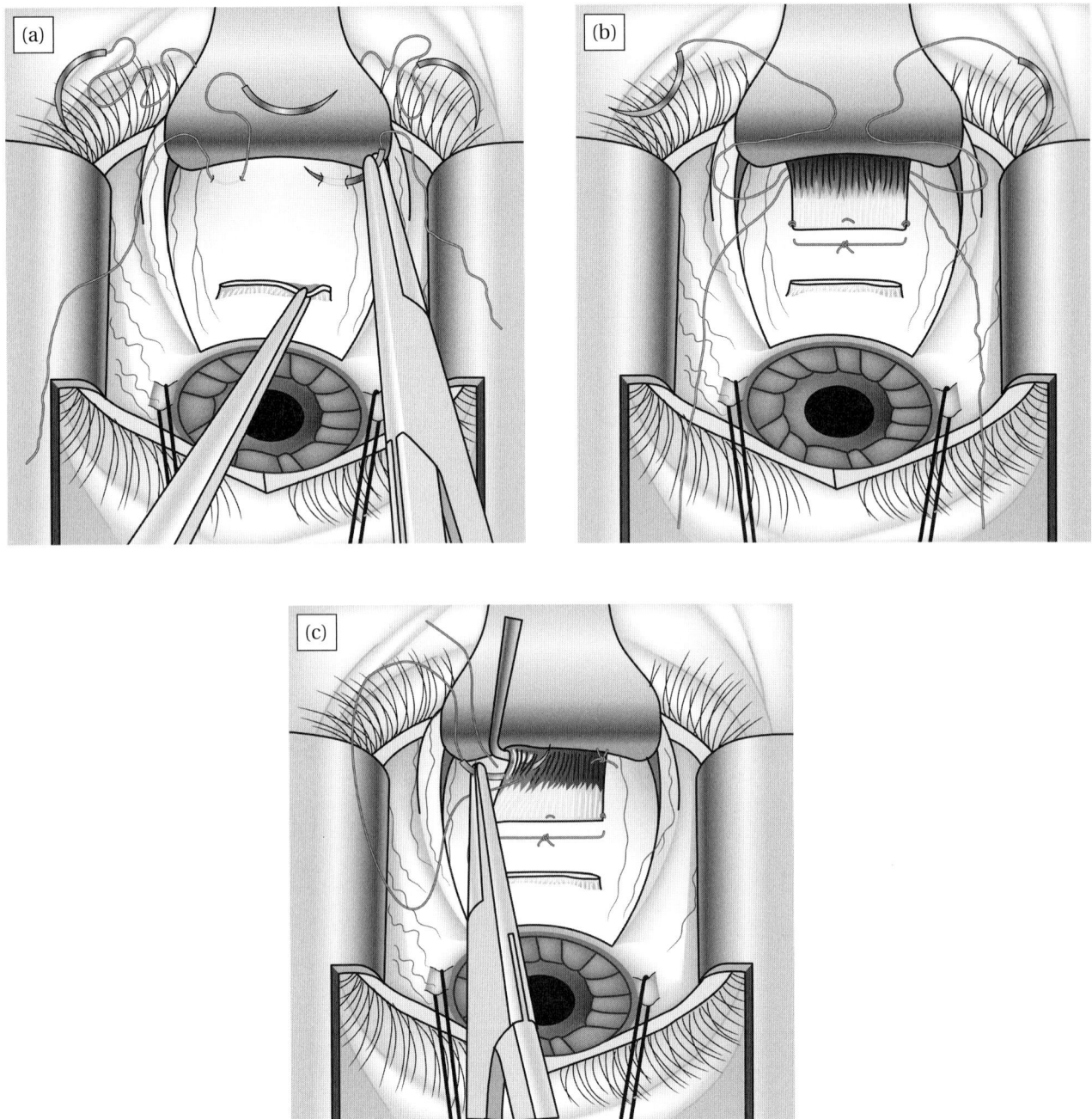

FIGURE 62.3 (a) The fadenoperation can be combined with a recession or resection of the muscle if a change in primary position is required along with a reduction in ocular rotation in the muscle's field of action. This is accomplished by performing the recession or resection in the standard manner as illustrated in Chapter 58. Before reattaching the muscle, the fixation suture is preplaced in the sclera at the desired location, usually 13–15 mm behind the original insertion. (b) The muscle is then reattached at the desired recessed or resected position. (c) The previously preplaced suture is now attached to the muscle making sure to incorporate about 1/4 of the muscle on each side.

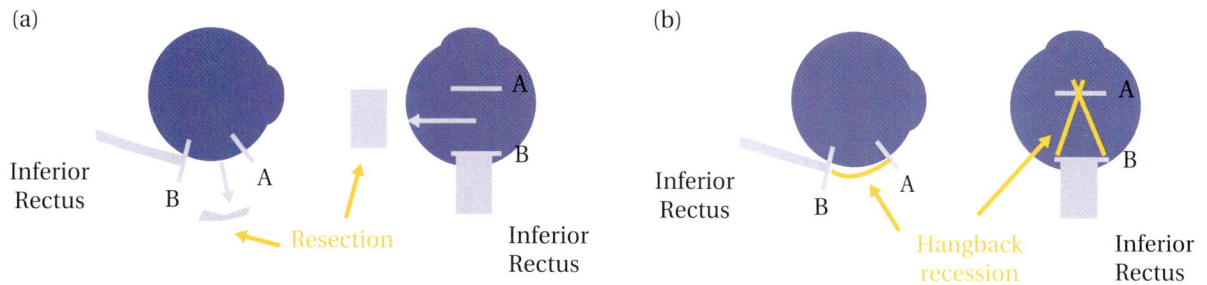

FIGURE 62.4 (a) An operation which produces the same outcome as a fadenoperation but can be adjusted postoperatively can be created by performing a combined resection and then recession of the same muscle. After the standard fadenoperation the muscle between the insertion and the suture is functionally no longer active. One can achieve the same effect by removing the muscle (resection) and then reattaching the cut end of the muscle (b) to the sclera at the distance of the resection from the insertion (recession). A resection of 10 mm (A to B), combined with a recession of the cut end of 10 mm yields the same result as a suture attaching the muscle to the sclera 10 mm behind the insertion. (b) After resecting a portion of the muscle (A to B) it is then recessed using the hangback technique an equal or greater amount depending on the amount of correction desired in the primary gaze position. This location can then be adjusted postoperatively using the same technique as a standard "adjustable" operation. While adjustment is often desired, this technique can be used to get a "fadenoperation-like effect" without having to suture the muscle to the sclera. This is especially useful when trying to limit the rotation of the lateral rectus, which is often difficult to do using the standard approach, due to the long arc of contact of the muscle requiring placement of the suture 15 or more millimeters behind the insertion, which is very difficult.

TABLE 62.1 *Fadenoperation Complications*

Complicated reoperations

Scleral perforation

Duction limitation

SELECTED REFERENCES

Bock CJ, Buckley EG, Freedman SF. Combined resection and recession of a single rectus muscle in the treatment of incomitant strabismus. *J AAPOS.* 1999;3:263–268.

Buckley EG, Shields MB. *Strabismus and Glaucoma Surgery.* Vol. III. St Louis: Mosby, 1995.

Buckley EG. Fadenoperation. In AP Santiago and AL Rosenbaum (eds.). *Clinical Strabismus Management —Principles and Surgical Technique* (Chapter 37). Philadelphia: W. B. Saunders Co., 1999.

63 Pediatric Cataracts

Fatema Esmail, MD and Scott R. Lambert, MD

TABLE 63.1 *Indications for Cataract Surgery*

Size	Blockage of visual axis, usually diameter >3 mm
Vision	Best corrected visual acuity <20/40
Signs of Sensory Deprivation	Development of nystagmus, fixation preference, or strabismus
Diagnostic	To facilitate examination of posterior segment

TABLE 63.2 *Perioperative Considerations*

Medications	Preparation	Equipment	Position
Cyclopentolate 1%	5% povidone-iodine to ocular surface	Venturi pump	Surgeon at head of bed
Phenylephrine 2.5%	Eyelashes taped down with adhesive drape	Consider keeping capsular stain available for cases with poor red reflex	
Consider topical antibiotic	Wick into inferior fornix to direct fluid away from surgical site		
	4-0 silk superior rectus bridle suture to rotate the eye inferiorly		

TABLE 63.3 *Difference in Approach when Considering IOL Implantation*

	Lensectomy	Lensectomy with PCIOL implant
Incisions	2 paracenteses	1 paracentesis
		3 mm limbal or scleral tunnel incision
Anterior Chamber Maintenance	Maintained with irrigation only	Need OVD at time of IOL insertion, and also may use it while creating tunnel incision to maintain globe tension
Need for Anterior Vitrectomy	Always	In patients 5 years old or younger, to reduce incidence of visual axis opacification

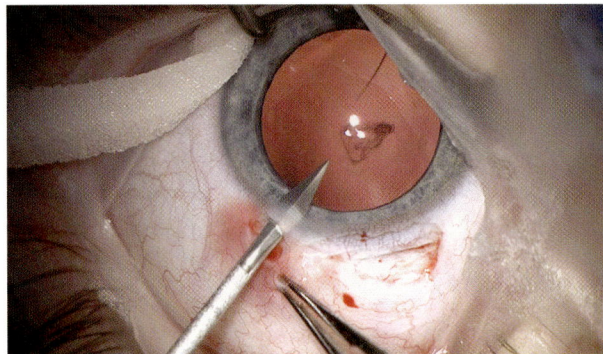

FIGURE 63.1 Peritomies are created in the superonasal and superotemporal quadrants. A larger peritomy, on the surgeon's dominant side, is needed if an IOL will be inserted. **Scleral Groove**: The crescent blade is used to make a 3 mm partial thickness groove in the sclera. It should be located in the superior quadrant of the surgeon's dominant side. **Scleral Tunnel:** The crescent blade is then used to create a planar incision, at a depth of half thickness of the sclera, spanning the 3 mm width. Care is taken to stop after reaching clear cornea; the surgeon must not penetrate the anterior chamber at this time. The MVR blade is used to make a paracentesis at the limbus in the superior quadrant on the surgeon's non-dominant side. The paracentesis should be at least 90 degrees away from the main incision, to optimize control of instruments in both hands.

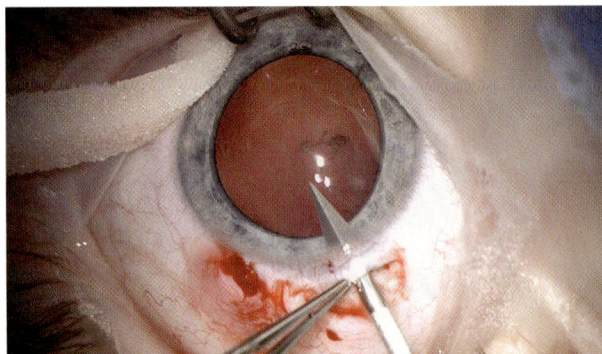

FIGURE 63.2 After the anterior chamber is filled with an ophthalmic viscosurgical device (OVD) through the paracentesis, a MVR blade is used to enter the anterior chamber through the center of the scleral tunnel. The small incisions allow a snug fit for the 20 gauge instruments; this ensures maintaining anterior chamber integrity.

Anterior Capsulorhexis Options

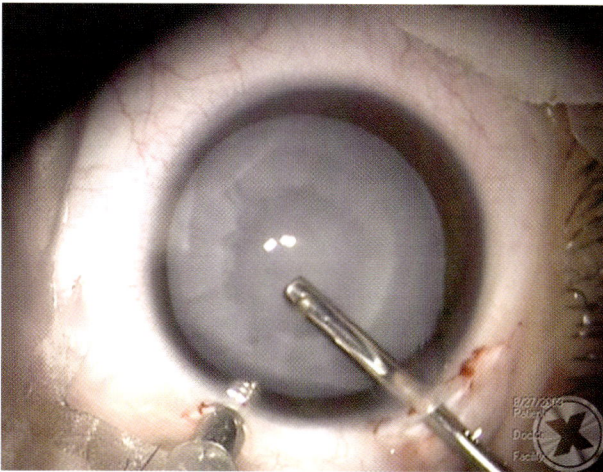

FIGURE 63.3 Vitrectorrhexis. After the insertion of the irrigation cannula through the paracentesis, the vitrector is inserted into the anterior chamber through the main incision. The OVD in the anterior chamber is aspirated. The port of the vitrector is then directed posteriorly in order to engage the anterior capsule and create a central opening. Recommended settings are Cut Rate: 100 cuts per minute; Aspiration: 150. The vitrectorrhexis is especially useful in cases when a red reflex is not visible.

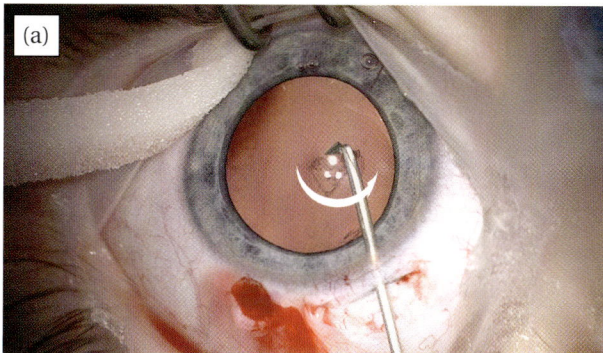

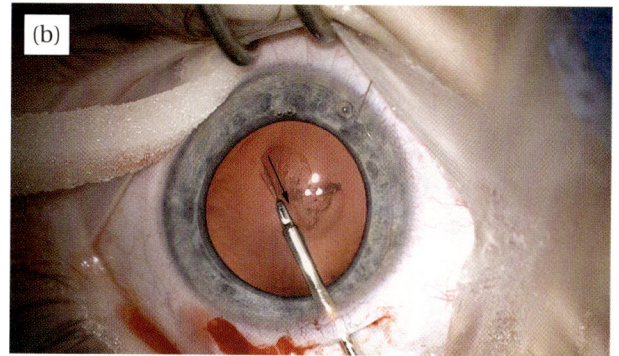

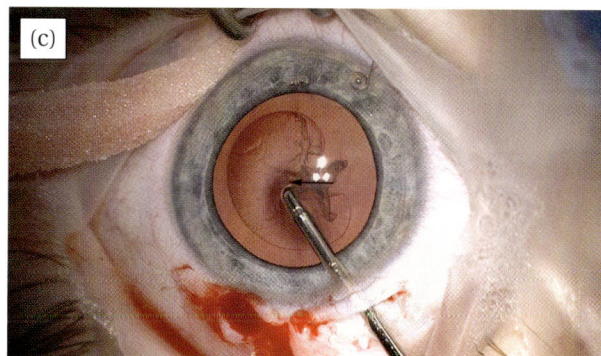

FIGURE 63.4 Continuous Curvilinear Capsulorhexis. (a, b, c) After filling the anterior chamber with an OVD, the cystotome is introduced and rotated to orient the tip to be perpendicular to the capsular surface. A small radial tear is created just beyond the center of the anterior capsule, and the edge is folded over to create a flap (white arrow; Figure a). The edge of the flap is then grasped by Katena forceps, and the anterior capsular opening is extended to complete the continuous curvilinear capsulorhexis. The edge of the flap is frequently regrasped as needed to direct the movement of the capsule. Of note, the vector of force in pediatric capsulorhexis should be directed toward the center of the opening, as noted by the arrows in Figures (b) and (c). This is necessary because the anterior capsule in children is quite elastic, and the leading edge will often extend too far peripherally otherwise.

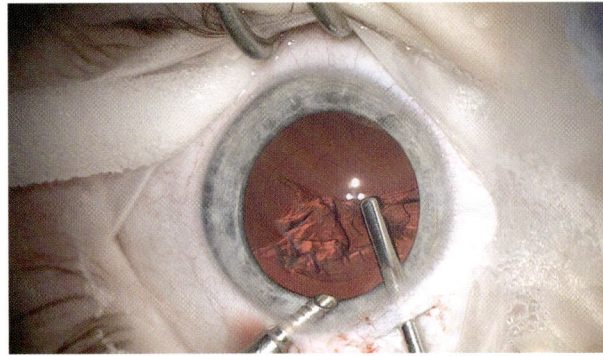

FIGURE 63.5 After completion of the anterior capsulorhexis, an irrigation cannula is inserted through the paracentesis. A 20 gauge Lewicky chamber maintainer is shown in the figure—it is a stationary cannula that is affixed to the drapes with steri-strips. A bimanual irrigating cannula may also be used if the surgeon prefers. Pediatric cataracts are usually very soft, and the lens material can simply be aspirated with a vitrector; however bursts of cutting may be helpful when removing denser material, or if the port becomes plugged. The vitrector is directed into the equatorial cortex, with the port turned toward the bulk of the lens material to achieve maximal occlusion of the port. The foot pedal is used to linearly increase the aspiration rate, as the lens material is stripped toward the center of the eye. The instruments can be interchanged between openings in order to reach all the lens material. This is very useful for removing subincisional cortex. The recommended starting settings are Cut Rate of 100 cuts per minute, and Aspiration of 150. The aspiration can be increased if needed.

TABLE 63.4 *Anterior Vitrectomy Options*

	Through Anterior Chamber prior to IOL	**Through Pars Plana after IOL**	**Through Anterior Chamber after IOL**
Key Points	Illustrated in this chapter	• Scleral tunnel incision is closed after IOL insertion • Stab incision made 2 mm posterior to limbus in the pars plana with MVR blade • The vitrector is first directed with the port facing up until it engages the center of the posterior capsule. A posterior capsulotomy is then performed. Afterwards, an anterior vitrectomy is carried out in a standard fashion • Irrigation is maintained through the original paracentesis using the anterior chamber maintainer • 8-0 polyglactin used to close the pars plana incision site	• After IOL insertion, the vitreous cutting instrument is directed posteriorly, around the edge of the IOL, to reach the center of the posterior capsule • The posterior capsulotomy and anterior vitrectomy are performed in the same manner illustrated in the chapter
Benefits	2 incisions only	• Easier IOL insertion • Lower risk of IOL displacement	2 incisions only
Risks	Risk IOL dislocating posteriorly during insertion	• Risk of damage to retina • An extra incision in the pars plana is needed	• Technically most difficult • Risk dislocating IOL posteriorly or into the anterior chamber during procedure

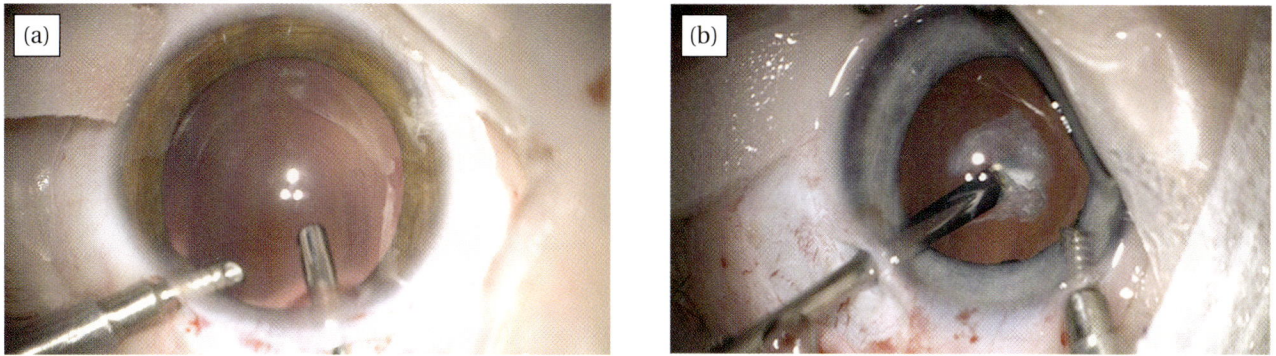

FIGURE 63.6 Primary Posterior Capsulotomy. (a) With settings of cut rate 600 cuts per minute and aspiration rate of 100, the vitrector is turned port down to engage the posterior capsule and create a central opening. This opening is also extended circumferentially, to achieve a diameter of about 4.5 mm. It should be slightly smaller than the anterior capsulorrhexis in order to optimize visualization of the anterior and posterior capsular leaflets during IOL insertion. When performing a lensectomy without IOL implantation, sufficient capsular support should be left behind to allow for secondary IOL implantation when the child is older. If the capsulotomies are made about the same size (ideally 5 mm) they will fuse together and form a Soemmerring ring. The Soemmerring ring can then be opened at the time of secondary IOL implantation and after aspirating regenerated lens cortex, the IOL can often be positioned in the capsular bag. (b) If there is a plaque on the posterior capsule, as is often the case with pediatric cataracts, the vitrector is directed through an opening in the posterior capsule and the plaque is removed using a posterior approach. This approach allows for better visualization and purchase of the plaque by the vitreous cutting instrument.

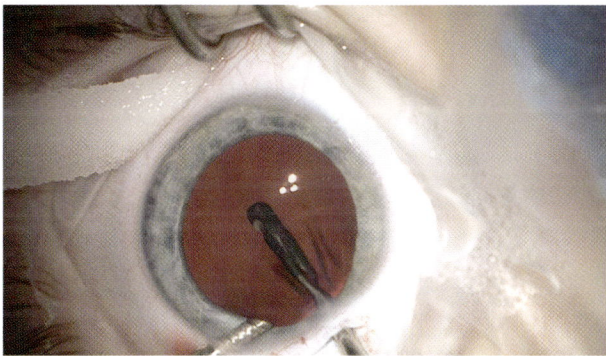

FIGURE 63.7 The vitrector is then directed posteriorly through the posterior capsulotomy to perform the anterior vitrectomy. The settings are maintained at 600 cuts per minute and aspiration of 100. About one-third of the anterior vitreous should be removed. Of note, in order to prevent vitreous being drawn into the anterior chamber, the irrigation should be turned off before withdrawing the instruments from the eye.

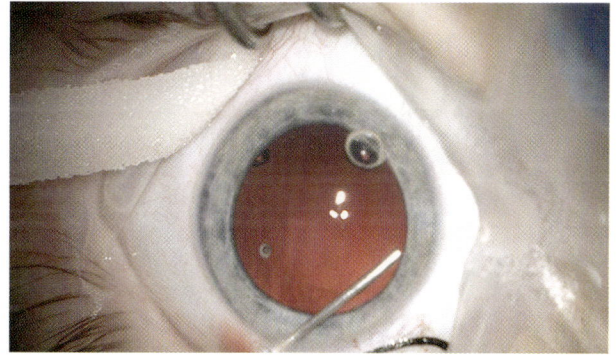

FIGURE 63.8 A high density OVD is injected into the capsular bag in order to separate the anterior and posterior leaflets of the capsule in preparation for insertion of the IOL.

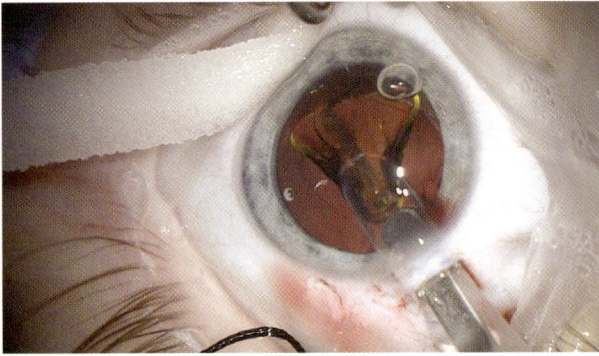

FIGURE 63.9 IOL insertion: A 3 mm keratome is then introduced through the scleral tunnel to enlarge the incision to accommodate the IOL. When implanting the foldable posterior chamber intraocular lens, the surgeon should keep the IOL in the horizontal plane to avoid the risk of the IOL dislocating through the posterior capsulotomy. The leading haptic should be guided into the capsular bag, followed by the optic.

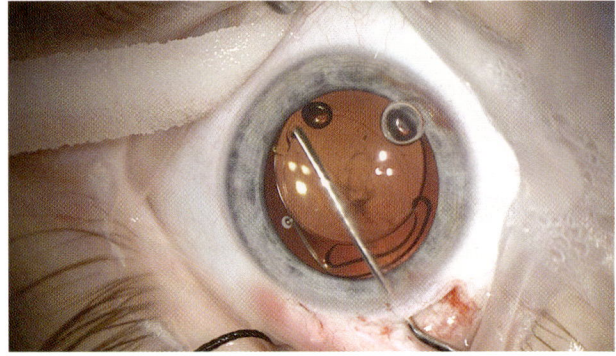

FIGURE 63.10 A variety of instruments are available to rotate the IOL into good position; an angled Lester IOL pusher is shown here. Care must be taken to ensure that the IOL is positioned entirely within the capsular bag and not in the sulcus. This is particularly important when implanting a one-piece IOL.

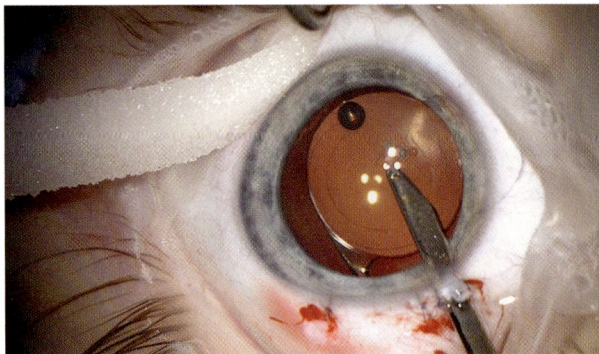

FIGURE 63.11 The incisions have been closed with interrupted 9-0 polyglactin sutures. Before tying down the final suture, a Simcoe cannula is used to manually remove the OVD from the anterior chamber. The knots on the sutures should also be rotated away from the cornea.

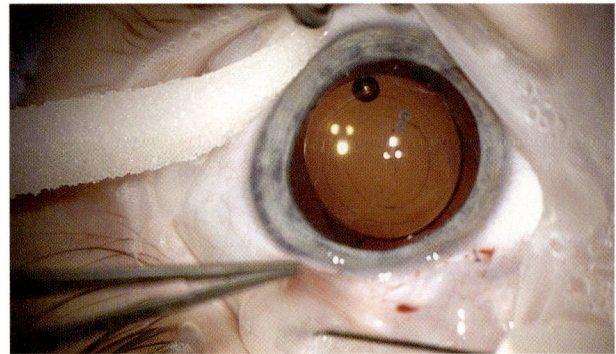

FIGURE 63.12 After ensuring adequate anterior chamber integrity, antibiotics and steroids are injected subconjunctivally to balloon the conjunctiva over the incision sites. Suturing the conjunctival peritomies closed is optional.

TABLE 63.5 *Intraoperative Complications*

Iris prolapse
Retained cortex
Peripheral tears in anterior capsule
Tears in posterior capsule
Suprachoroidal hemorrhage
Lens material dropped into vitreous
IOL dislocated into vitreous

TABLE 63.6 *Postoperative Complications*

Hyphema	Capsulophimosis
Corectopia	Glaucoma
Pupillary capture of IOL	Endophthalmitis
Visual axis opacification	Retinal detachment
Posterior synechiae	Pthisis bulbi
Precipitates on IOL optic	Corneal decompensation
Iris atrophy	

SELECTED REFERENCES

BenEzra D. Cataract surgery and intraocular lens implantation in children, and intraocular lens implantation in children. *Am J Ophthalmol.* 1996;121:224–226.

Dahan E, Salmenson BD. Pseudophakia in children: precautions, technique, and feasibility. *J Cataract Refract Surg.* 1990;16:75–82.

Fallaha N, Lambert SR. Pediatric cataracts. *Ophthalmol Clin North Am.* Sep 2001;14:479–492.

Hutcheson KA, Drack AV, Ellish NJ, Lambert SR. Anterior hyaloid face opacification after pediatric Nd:YAG laser capsulotomy. *J AAPOS.* 1999;3:303 307.

Lambert SR, Amaya L, Taylor D. Detection and treatment of infantile cataracts. *Int Ophthalmol Clin.* Spring 1989;29:51–56.

Lambert SR, Buckley EG, Drews-Botsch D et al. for the Infant Aphakia Treatment Study Group. The infant aphakia treatment study: design and clinical measures at enrollment. *Arch Ophthalmol.* 2010;128:21–27.

Lambert SR, Buckley EG, Drews-Botsch D et al for the Infant Aphakia Treatment Study Group. A randomized clinical trial comparing contact lens with intraocular lens correction of monocular aphakia during infancy: grating acuity and adverse events at 1 year. Arch Ophthalmol 2010;128:810–818.

Wilson ME, Englert JA, Greenwald MJ. In-the-bag secondary intraocular lens implantation in children. J AAPOS 1999;3:350–355.

Wilson ME, Jr., Trivedi RH, Buckley EG, et al. ASCRS white paper. Hydrophobic acrylic intraocular lenses in children. *J Cataract Refract Surg.* 2007;33:1966–1973.

Wilson ME, Saunders RA, Roberts EL, Apple DJ. Mechanized anterior capsulectomy as an alternative to manual capsulorhexis in children undergoing intraocular lens implantation. *J Pediatr Ophthalmol Strabismus.* 1996;33:237–240.

64 Pediatric Glaucoma Surgery

Tammy L. Yanovitch, MD MHSc and Sharon F. Freedman, MD

TABLE 64.1 *Indications for Pediatric Glaucoma Surgery*

Procedure	Description	Indication(s)
Angle Surgery		
Goniotomy	Incision of the uveal trabecular meshwork under direct visualization	• Primary Congenital Glaucoma • Other Primary Glaucomas • Aniridia (with progressive angle closure)*
Trabeculotomy ab Externo	Cannulation of Schlemm canal and tearing through the trabecular meshwork	• Primary Congenital Glaucoma • Other Primary Glaucomas • Aniridia (with progressive angle closure)*
Filtration Surgery (covered in Chapter 34: Trabeculectomy)		
Trabeculectomy	Removal of a segment of the angle tissue under a partial thickness scleral flap, creating a filtering "bleb"	Glaucoma in an eye that has reasonable visual potential and unscarred conjunctiva, with IOP uncontrolled on medications after angle surgery failure (or unlikely success with angle surgery)
Combined Trabeculectomy/ Trabeculotomy	Creation of filtering "bleb" and canalization of Schlemm canal with tearing through the trabecular meshwork	Glaucoma in an eye in which: • Trabeculotomy cannot be completed (failure to cannulate Schlemm's) • Angle surgery alone has failed or unlikely to succeed
Aqueous Drainage Device Surgery	Placement of a flexible tube into the eye to conduct aqueous humor posteriorly to a reservoir (plate) sewn against the sclera	Primary congenital and aphakic glaucoma that has failed angle surgery Glaucoma in an eye with: • Failed trabeculectomy with intraoperative mitomycin C and reasonable visual potential • High risk for complications with trabeculectomy (i.e., Sturge-Weber Syndrome, aphakia) • High risk for failure with trabeculectomy from scarring (i.e., after multiple conjunctival surgeries)
Cycloablation (covered in Chapter 32: Cyclophotocoagulation and Cryotherapy)		
Cyclocryotherapy	Freezing of the ciliary processes from an external approach	Reserved for extremely severe cases of glaucoma in which altered anatomy makes laser cycloablation unlikely to succeed
Transscleral Laser Cyclophotocoagulation	Laser ablation of the ciliary processes from an external approach	Glaucoma that is refractory to medical or other surgical interventions

TABLE 64.1 *(continued)*

Procedure	Description	Indication(s)
Endoscopic Laser Cyclophotocoagulation	Application of laser energy to the ciliary processes under direct visualization	Glaucoma that is refractory to medical or other surgical interventions and amenable to endoscopy
Enucleation (covered in Chapter 83)	Removal of the eye	Glaucoma resulting in a blind, painful eye

*Angle surgery for aniridia should be undertaken only by those experienced in these techniques, due to unprotected lens. The use of angle surgery for prophylactic treatment of glaucoma in aniridia is controversial.

Goniotomy

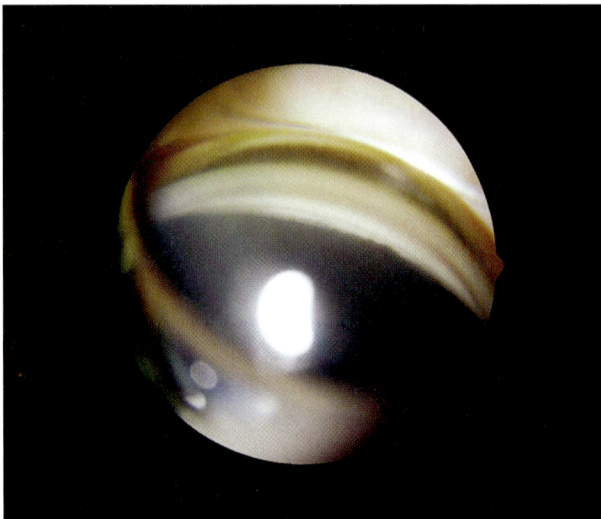

FIGURE 64.1 This photograph shows the gonioscopic view of an eye with congenital glaucoma following a successful goniotomy procedure. The whitish line (goniotomy cleft) appears in the central portion of the photograph, where the angle is notably widened, revealing the ciliary body band.

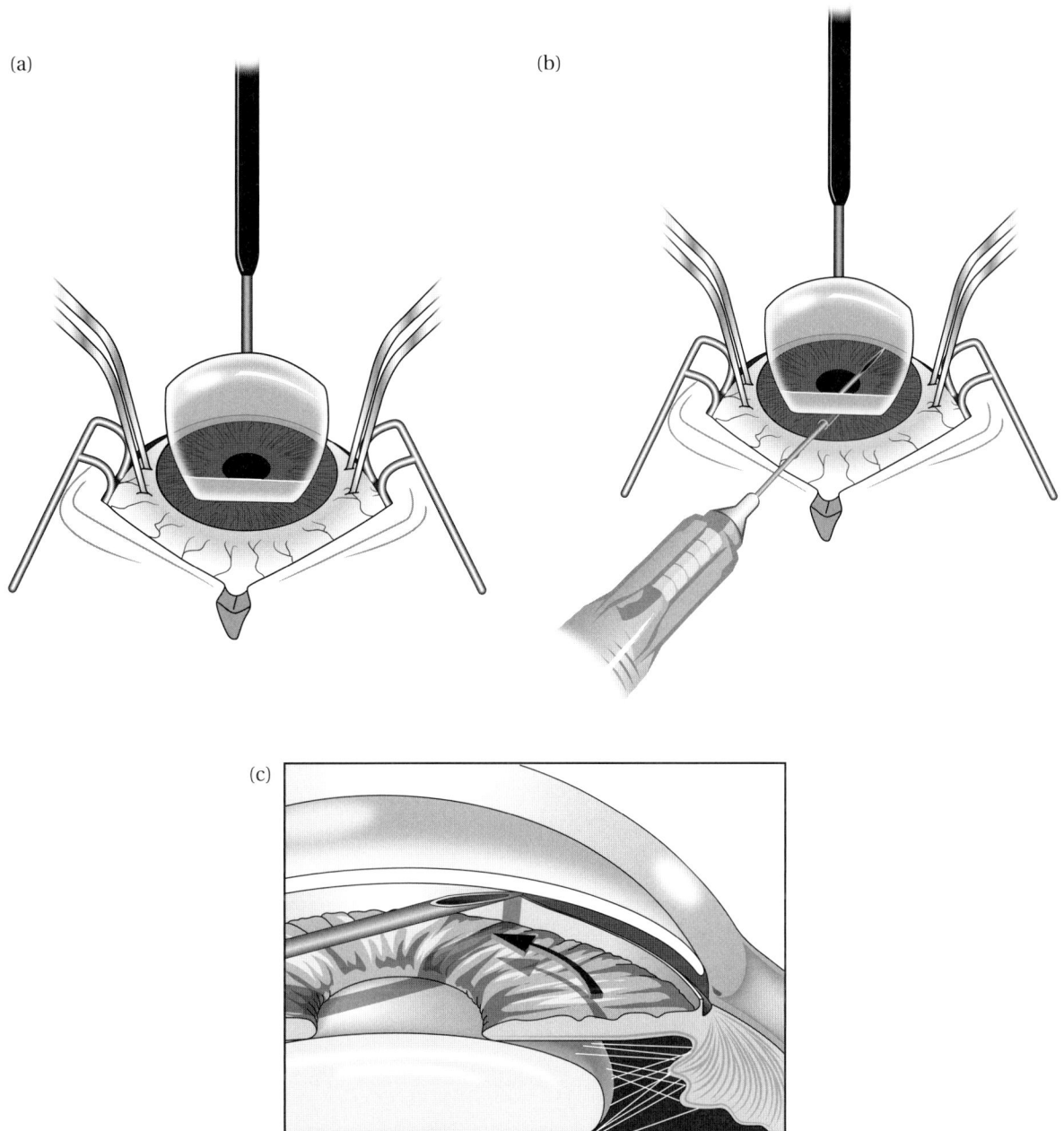

FIGURE 64.2 (a) One of the most difficult aspects of performing a goniotomy is correctly positioning the eye to allow an adequate view of the angle structures. The operating microscope is tilted at 45 degrees. The eye is then stabilized by an assistant with Moody locking forceps, which are placed near the limbus at 12 and 6 o'clock (for nasal or temporal goniotomy). A Barkan goniotomy lens (or similar lens of the surgeon's choice) is held on the cornea by the surgeon. For a nasal goniotomy, the assistant gently holds the eye in adduction to facilitate the surgeon's view of the angle. Prior to surgery, the eye has is treated with pilocarpine 2% and apraclonidine 0.5%. (b) A 25 gauge needle (1 ¼ in) on a syringe filled with viscoelastic is used to enter the peripheral cornea on the side opposite to the intended angle incision. Therefore, for a nasal goniotomy, the needle would enter the eye temporally. The needle is guided over the iris and lens to engage the anterior portion of the trabecular meshwork. (c) Once the trabecular meshwork is engaged, the assistant cautiously rotates the eye in either direction. The incision creates a cleft with the peripheral iris moving posteriorly as the angle widens. The needle is then carefully withdrawn from the eye. A small amount of viscoelastic may be injected just as the needle is removed from the eye. The chamber is then refilled with balanced salt solution (if it shallows) and the entry site is closed with a single 10-0 polyglactin suture. A bubble of filtered air may be placed to help confirm a formed chamber in an infant on the first postoperative day. Subconjunctival antibiotic and short-acting steroid are injected, and a shield is placed over the eye. Postoperative medications typically include a topical antibiotic, steroid and miotic.

Trabeculotomy

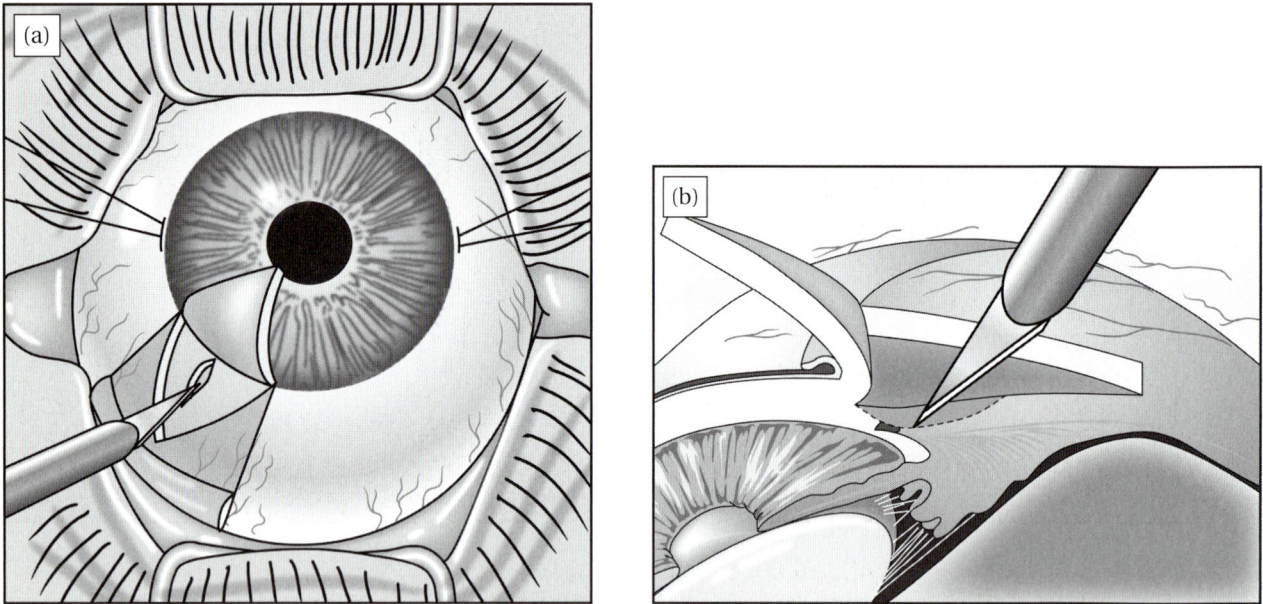

FIGURE 64.3 (a) Unlike goniotomy, trabeculotomy ab externo does not require a view of the angle structures. A limbal conjunctival incision is made with Westcott scissors. A supersharp 15-degree blade is followed by Beaver 64 and 66 blades to create a triangular, partial-thickness scleral flap (~3–4 mm wide). The supersharp blade is then used to make a radial "scratch" incision under the flap. (b) Each layer of sclera is "scratched" away until Schlemm canal is identified. A small egress of fluid (which may be admixed with blood) is often seen, once Schlemm's canal has been entered. At this point, a 6-0 polypropylene suture (blunted on one end using a disposable cautery to create a small "mushroom cap") is introduced into one cut end of Schlemm canal to confirm that the canal has been correctly identified. The suture should feed smoothly into the canal with little resistance, and may sometimes be viewed on 4-mirror gonioscopy intraoperatively. A small amount of viscoelastic may be used at the cut ends of Schlemm canal to facilitate the suture's introduction. A paracentesis is made, and a small amount of viscoelastic injected into the anterior chamber at this point, to help prevent its collapse once Schlemm's canal has been entered and the trabecular meshwork disrupted (see Figures 64.3c and 64.3d).

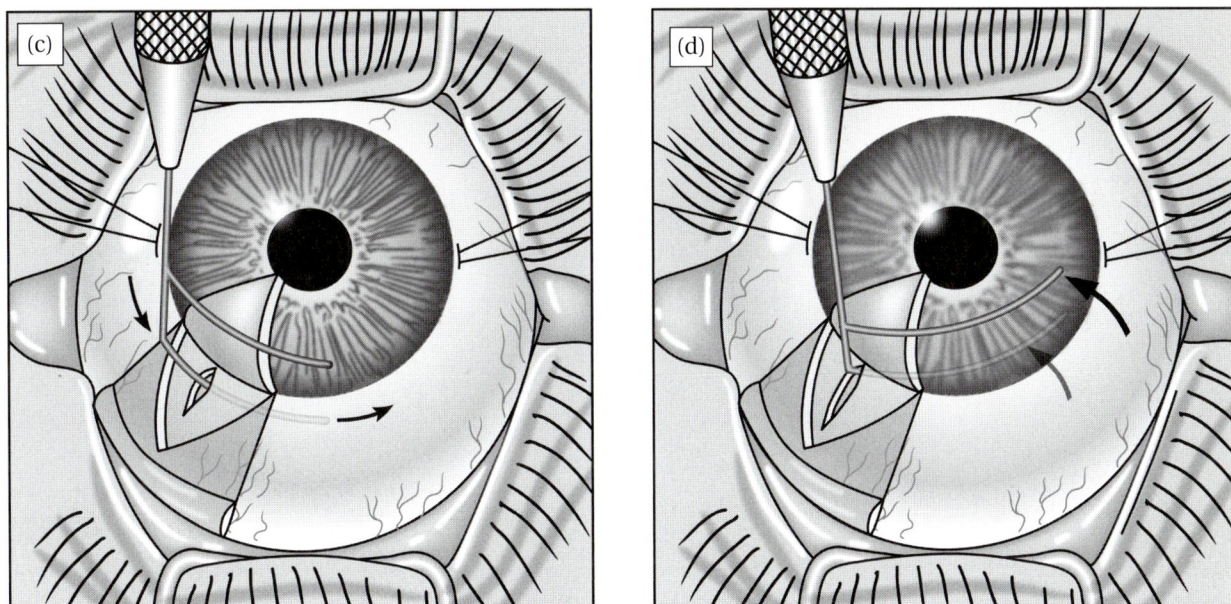

FIGURE 64.3 (*continued*) (c, d)A curved metal trabeculotome is then carefully advanced into one cut end of Schlemm canal maximally until resistance is encountered, and is then gently rotated inward to tear the trabecular meshwork, taking care to avoid entering the peripheral cornea or the iris root, and watching the "outer arm" of the trabeculotome as a guide to the position of the probe within the canal. The trabeculotome is then carefully withdrawn from the anterior chamber. The trabeculotome (pointing the opposite direction) is then entered into the other cut end of Schlemm canal, and the same procedure is performed to open an additional several clock hours of the trabecular meshwork). The anterior chamber may be refilled with isotonic fluid or additional viscoelastic prior to, and again after, the second trabeculotome advancement. The scleral flap is then closed with interrupted 10-0 polyglactin sutures. The scleral flap closure should be watertight. The conjunctiva is then closed with one or two interrupted polyglactin sutures at the limbus. As with the goniotomy, a bubble of filtered air may be placed to help confirm a formed chamber in an infant on the first postoperative day. Subconjunctival antibiotic and short-acting steroid may be injected, and a shield is placed over the eye. Postoperative medications typically include a topical antibiotic, steroid, and miotic.

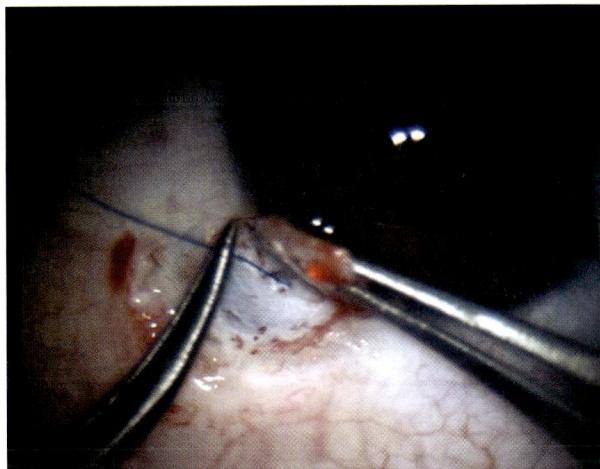

FIGURE 64.4 This photograph shows an eye with primary congenital glaucoma undergoing a 360-degree suture trabeculotomy. The 6-0 polypropylene suture is being advanced with a forceps through one cut end of Schlemm canal. When it appears from the other cut end, it will have traversed the canal 360 degrees. The next step will be to gently pull both free ends of the suture to tear open the trabecular meshwork.

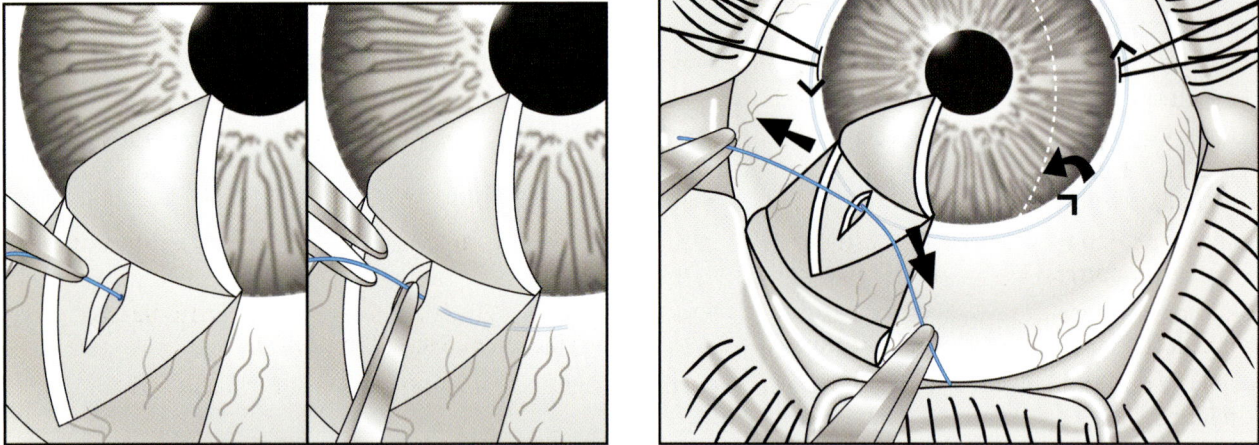

FIGURE 64.5 The procedure for a *trabeculectomy* ab externo with suture is similar to a trabeculotomy ab externo with a trabeculotome, except that a 6-0 prolene suture is used instead of a trabeculotome. The suture is advanced through either cut end of Schlemm canal (a, b). In order to facilitate threading into the canal, the tip of the suture is melted with cautery into a small mushroom-shaped cap. This procedure is facilitated by deepening the anterior chamber with viscoelastic, and monitoring the progress of the suture using intraoperative gonioscopy when corneal clarity permits. The same procedure may also be performed using the iScience endoscopic probe, which is illuminated to identify its position as it traverses the canal circumferentially. Once the canal has been cannulated 360 degrees, with either a suture or the iScience (iScience Interventional™, Menlo, CA) endoscopic probe, the ends of the suture (or probe) can be pulled in opposite directions, "cheese-wiring" into the anterior chamber and thereby disrupting trabecular meshwork circumferentially for the entire angle (c). Significant bleeding will occur unless the anterior chamber is well-filled with viscoelastic.

TABLE 64.2 *Pediatric-Specific Modifications for Non-Angle Surgery*

Trabeculectomy (usually with mitomycin C)

- Place a traction suture (7-0 vicryl) in the peripheral cornea at two places opposite the intended operative site to optimize exposure and stabilization.
- Use a fornix-based incision to optimize future bleb morphology (consider limbus-based in selected cases).
- Use mitomycin C (0.2–0.4 mg/ml for 2–5 minutes). Apply to a broad area of uncut sclera and Tenon's capsule. Keep away from conjunctival edges and cornea.
- Cut a fairly thick, rectangular (4 × 4 mm) flap with a hinge at the limbus. After making a paracentesis elsewhere, enter under the flap into the cornea with a supersharp. Punch a large (1 × 2 mm), anteriorly placed opening. Then make an iridectomy, taking care to avoid ciliary processes.
- Close the flap with 10-0 nylon sutures at the back corners and two anterior (+/– releasable) sutures buried into clear cornea. Titrate flap closure to adequate flow.
- Use a running suture (8-0 polyglactin) on a vascular needle to close each "wing" of the fornix-based incision. Place two horizontal mattress sutures (10-0 polyglactin) between the "wings."
- Fill the anterior chamber and "bleb" with balanced salt solution (add a small amount viscoelastic if needed).

Aqueous Drainage Device Surgery

- Use a fornix incision unless scarring prevents this approach.
- Determine the type and size of implant based on the need for immediate pressure reduction and the size of the eye.
  - An S-2 or FP-7 Ahmed requires an axial length of at least 21 mm (would trim posterior portion of plate if the axial length is <22 mm and adjust distance from limbus for shorter eyes)
  - The Ahmed and other valved implants provide immediate pressure reduction compared with the Baerveldt, which requires time for the capsule to form (and therefore requires ligated tubing or two-stage surgery)
- Place the implant in the superotemporal quadrant if possible. Secure with 8-0 nylon suture through positioning holes.
- Ligate non-valved devices with suture (6-0 polyglactin) before placing against sclera.
- Position the tube into the anterior chamber, parallel to the iris (as far back as practical to prevent exposure and corneal-tube touch) and almost parallel to the superior limbus. Use a 30 gauge finder needle on viscoelastic before 23 gauge entry, for tube placement in the anterior chamber. Consider posterior chamber/pars plana positioning in cases with shallow anterior chamber (in conjunction with pars plana vitrectomy by retinal surgeon).
- Secure tube to sclera with suture (9-0 nylon), then use that needle to make venting slits proximal to polyglactin ligature for Baerveldt implants (not recommended for eyes with choroidal hemangioma). Close the conjunctiva with a double running suture (8-0 polyglactin on vascular needle, Tenon's, and conjunctiva separately, for fornix incision).
- Fill anterior chamber with viscoelastic in cases of valved implant placement (Ahmed).
- Maintain anti-inflammatory treatment for several months (topical steroid then a nonsteroidal) and use aqueous suppression liberally to decrease risk of bleb capsule thickening/encapsulation. Watch for low-grade anterior chamber inflammation.

TABLE 64.2 *(continued)*

Cycloablation

- Determine the optimal type of ablation.
  - Transscleral and endoscopic (diode laser)—most commonly used.
  - Cryotherapy—limited to cases with altered anatomy where other types of cycloablation are unlikely to succeed.
- Limit treatment to three quadrants with transscleral and endoscopic laser, and two quadrants with cryotherapy, to avoid hypotony and phthisis.
- Document location of treatments and rarely allow 360 degrees of cumulative treatment.
- Use adequate anti-inflammatory treatment to prevent inflammation. Usually, topical steroid for four weeks, titrated to inflammation level, with oral steroids for cases of hypotony.
- Discuss limitations of treatment fully with parents to achieve mutual understanding of risks and alternatives.

TABLE 64.3 *Common Complications of Glaucoma Surgery in Pediatric Patients*

Procedure	Early Complications	Late Complications
Angle Surgery		
Goniotomy	• Intraoperative or postoperative bleeding/hyphema • Anterior chamber collapse • Lens or capsule injury • Endophthalmitis*	Failure to adequately control IOP Cataract
Trabeculotomy ab Externo	• Intraoperative or postoperative bleeding/hyphema • Wound leak • False passage • Tearing or stripping of Descemet's membrane • Endophthalmitis*	Failure to adequately control IOP Corneal scar Cataract
Filtration Surgery (covered in Chapter: 34: Trabeculectomy)		
Trabeculectomy	• Intraoperative or postoperative bleeding/hyphema • Wound leak • Shallow anterior chamber • Hypotony-maculopathy or choroidal detachment • Aqueous misdirection • Cataract • Endophthalmitis	• Encapsulated bleb/elevated pressure • Bleb thinning/leaking • Infection (blebitis, endophthalmitis)

TABLE 64.3 *(continued)*

Procedure	Early Complications	Late Complications
Combined Trabeculectomy/ Trabeculotomy	See trabeculectomy and trabeculotomy	
Aqueous Drainage Device Surgery	• Tube malposition or blockage • Shallow anterior chamber • Cataract • Hypotony • Choroidal detachment • Retinal detachment • Endophthalmitis	• Tube malposition or blockage • Tube/plate exposure • Pupil abnormalities • Motility disturbance • Corneal scarring/decompensation • Hypotony • Encapsulated bleb/elevated pressure • Retinal detachment • Endophthalmitis

Cycloablation (covered in Chapter 32: Cyclophotocoagulation and Cryotherapy)

Cyclocryotherapy	• Visual loss • Uveitis • Hyphema • Retinal detachment • Chronic hypotony	• Phthisis • Scleral thinning
Transcleral Laser Cyclophotocoagulation	• Visual loss • Retinal detachment • Chronic hypotony	

*Endophthalmitis has rarely been reported with goniotomy and trabeculotomy procedures.

SELECTED REFERENCES

Barkan O. Goniotomy for the relief of congenital glaucoma. *Br J Ophthalmol.* 1948;32(9):701–728.

Beck AD, Lynch MG. 360 degrees trabeculotomy for primary congenital glaucoma. *Arch Ophthalmol.* 1995;113(9):1200–1202.

Coleman AL, et al. Initial clinical experience with the Ahmed Glaucoma Valve implant in pediatric patients. *Arch Ophthalmol.* 1997;115(2):186–191.

Mandal AK, et al. Safety and efficacy of simultaneous bilateral primary combined trabeculotomy-trabeculectomy for developmental glaucoma. *Indian J Ophthalmol.* 2002;50(1):13–19.

Molteno AC, Ancker E, Van Biljon G. Surgical technique for advanced juvenile glaucoma. *Arch Ophthalmol.* 1984;102(1):51–57.

Neely DE, Plager DA. Endocyclophotocoagulation for management of difficult pediatric glaucomas. *J AAPOS.* 2001;5(4):221–229.

O'Malley Schotthoefer E, Yanovitch TL, Freedman SF. Aqueous drainage device surgery in refractory pediatric glaucomas: I. Long-term outcomes. *J AAPOS.* 2008:12(1):33–39.

O'Malley Schotthoefer E, Yanovitch TL, Freedman SF. Aqueous drainage device surgery in refractory pediatric glaucoma: II. Ocular motility consequences. *J AAPOS.* 2008;12(1):40–45.

Susanna R Jr., et al. Mitomycin as adjunct chemotherapy with trabeculectomy in congenital and developmental glaucomas. *J Glaucoma.* 1995;4(3):151–157.

65 Pediatric Ptosis

William R. Katowitz, MD

Preoperative Evaluation

TABLE 65.1 *Oculoplastic Evaluation of a Child with Ptosis*

Vision testing: Screening for amblyopia

Eyelid exam

Margin reflex distance

The 2.5% phenylephrine test (Figure 65.1a and 65.1b)

Levator function (without brow use)

Presence of Bell's phenomenon

Corneal sensation

Frontalis function

Chin position

Cycloplegic refraction

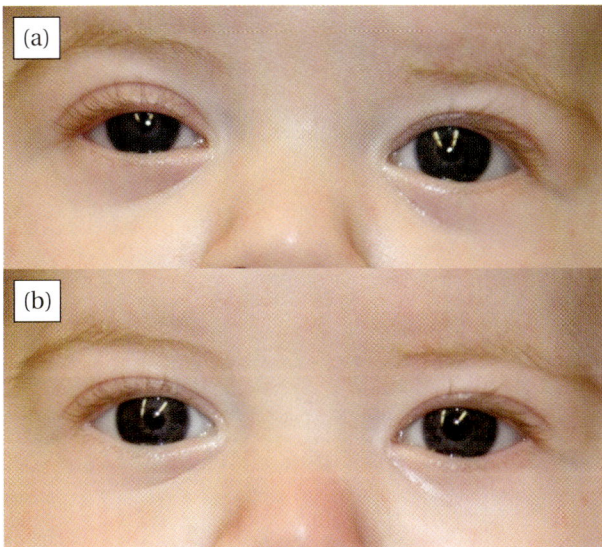

FIGURE 65.1 The 2.5% Phenylephrine Test. (a) Right upper eyelid ptosis in a patient with a right Horner's syndrome. (b) Right upper eyelid response 5 minutes after one drop of 2.5% phenylephrine to the right eye.

TABLE 65.2 *Indications for Surgery*

Deprivation amblyopia

Induced astigmatism (including refractive amblyopia)

Excessive chin up position

Family wishes, including psychosocial concerns

Trauma

TABLE 65.3 *Choice of Procedure*

Modified Fasanella-Servat procedure (tarsal-conjunctival Müllerectomy)

    Good response to 2.5% phenylephrine (Figure 65.1b)

    Poor or missing Bell's phenomenon

Anterior levator resection

    Good to fair levator function (at least 5 mm or better)

Frontalis sling with silicone sling material

    Poor levator function (≤4 mm)

    Age below 4 years (insufficient leg length autogenous fascia lata harvesting)

    Potential need for removal (e.g., mechanical ptosis due to infantile capillary hemangioma)

Frontalis sling with autogenous fascia lata

    Poor levator function (≤4 mm)

    Age above 4 years (adequate leg length for autogenous fascia lata harvesting)

Modified Fasanella-Servat Procedure (Tarsal-Conjunctival-Müllerectomy)

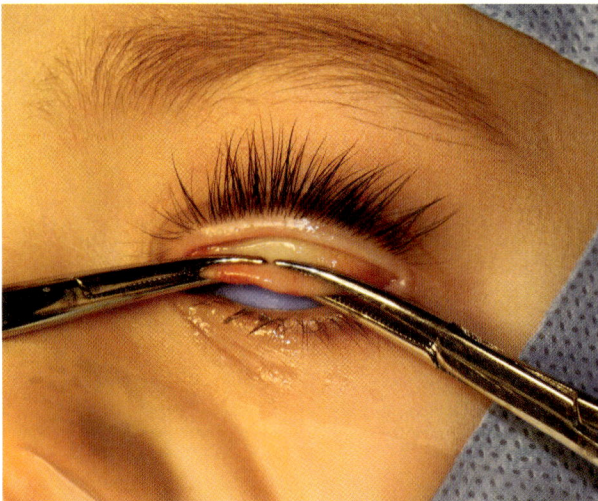

FIGURE 65.2 The tarsus is grasped with two matching curved hemostats, approximately 3–4 mm from the superior tarsal border.

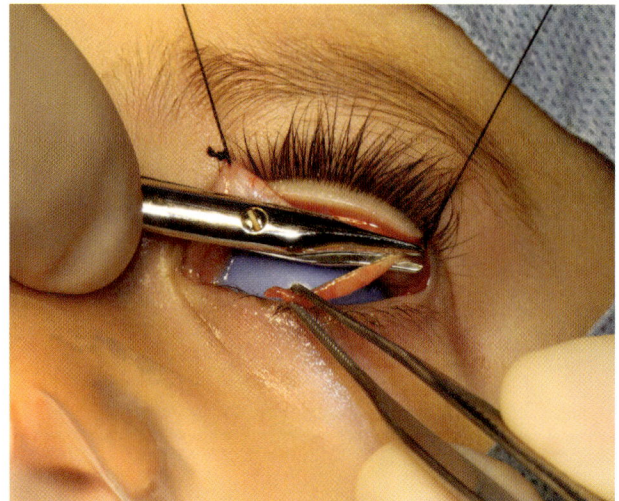

FIGURE 65.3 Two 4-0 silk traction sutures are tied to the conjunctiva laterally and medially, and the clamped tarsus, conjunctiva, and Müller's muscle are excised.

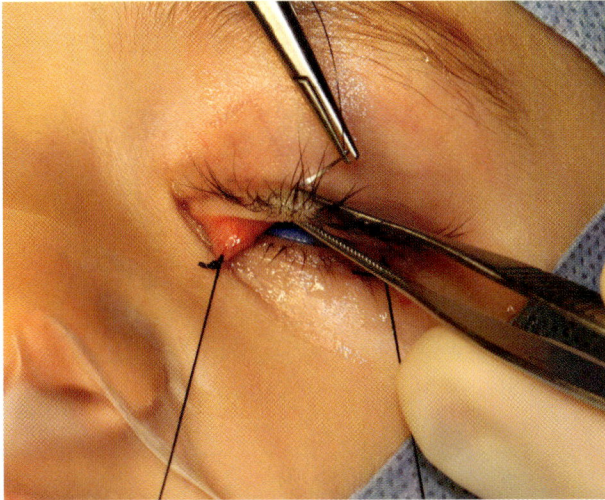

FIGURE 65.4 A 5-0 nylon suture on a P-3 needle (Ethicon) is passed from the medial eyelid skin crease to the medial edge if the trimmed Müller's muscle.

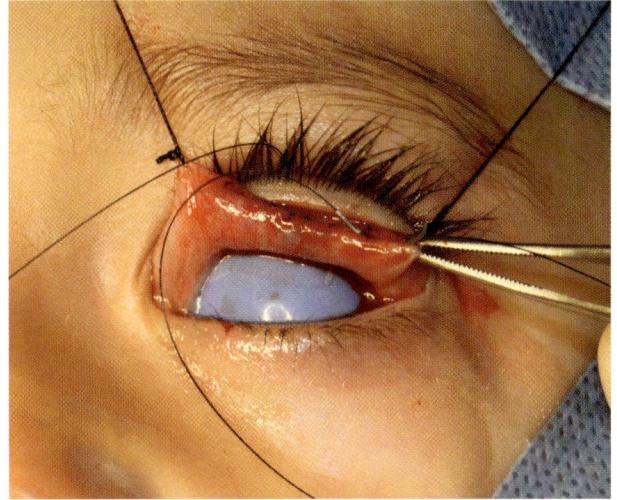

FIGURE 65.5 The nylon suture is passed through Müller's muscle and vertically through the tarsus. The suture is buried below the conjunctiva.

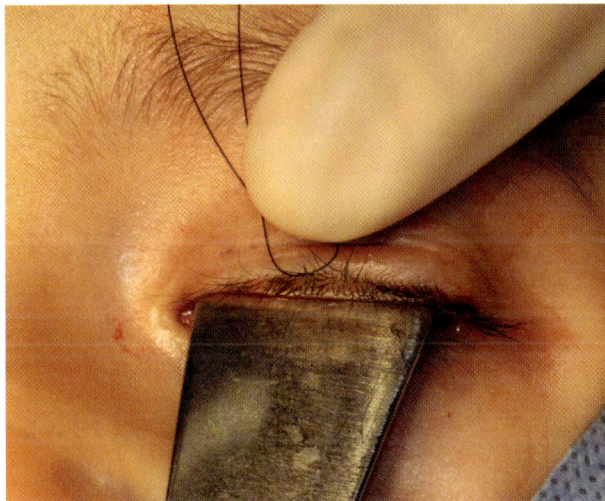

FIGURE 65.6 After passing the nylon suture through tarsus back to the lateral eyelid skin crease, the silk sutures are removed and the tissue is flattened over a shoehorn retractor.

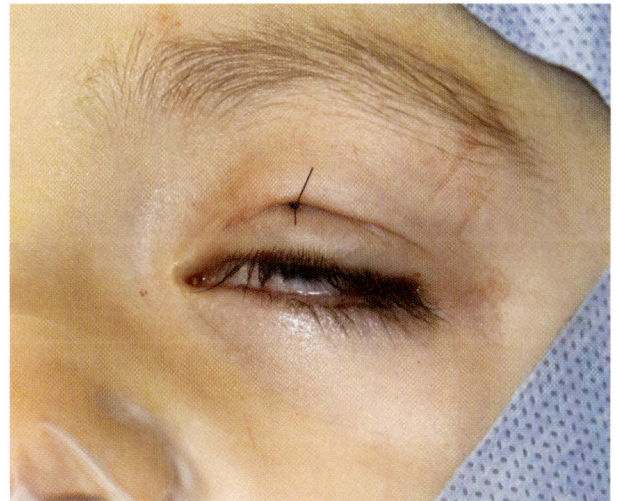

FIGURE 65.7 The suture is tied anteriorly and should be removed after 5–7 days.

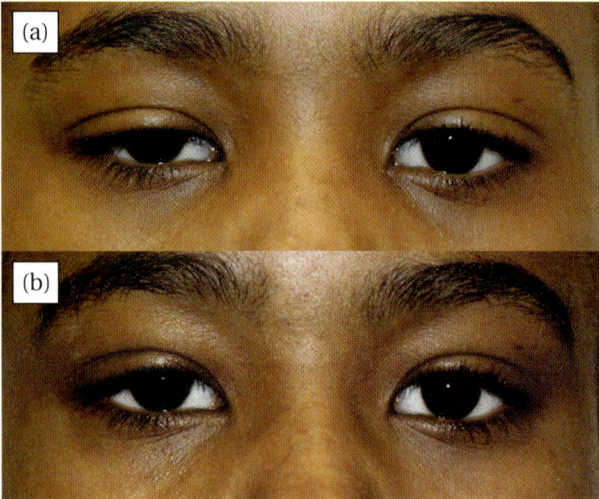

FIGURE 65.8 (a) 12-year-old patient with right upper eyelid ptosis. (b) Postoperative photo one year after a right eyelid modified Fasanella-Servat surgery.

Anterior Levator Resection

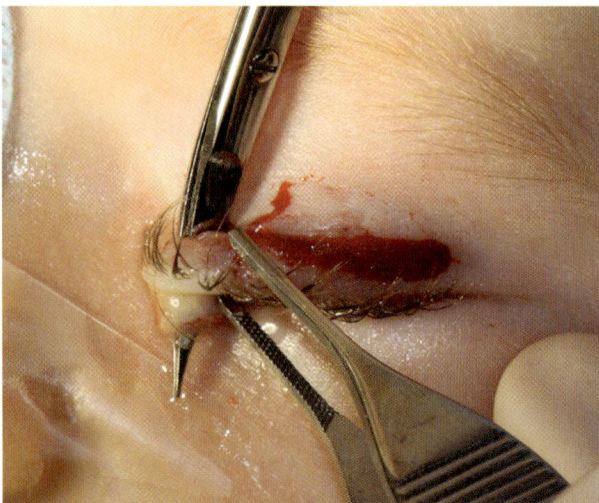

FIGURE 65.9 The skin crease is marked and the skin is incised with a #15 blade (not pictured). This incision is continued through the orbicularis with electrocautery (not pictured). The medial levator/Müller's and conjunctiva complex are punctured medially above the tarsus with curved iris scissors.

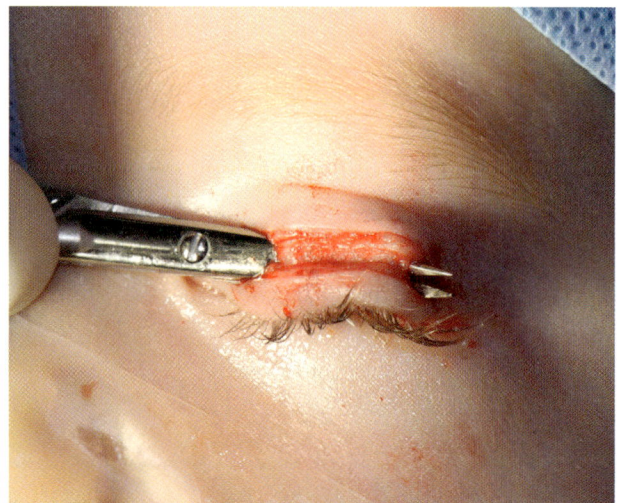

FIGURE 65.10 The scissors are extended laterally and the posterior eyelid tissue is punctured again above the tarsus.

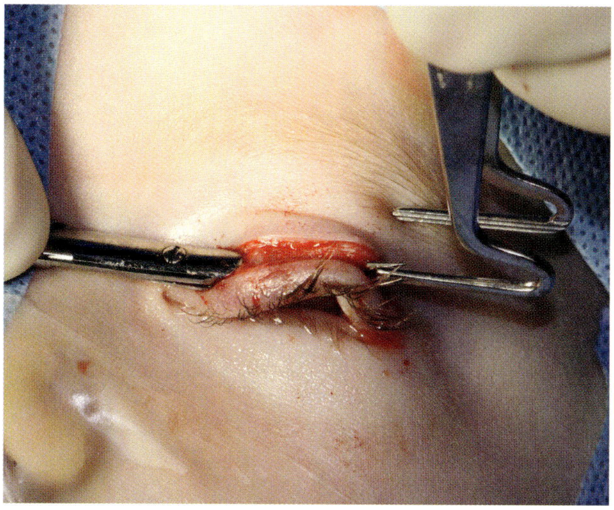

FIGURE 65.11 The posterior arm of a levator muscle clamp is grasped with the iris scissors. While holding the levator clamp, the scissors are retracted medially allowing the clamp to grasp the eyelid tissue above the tarsus.

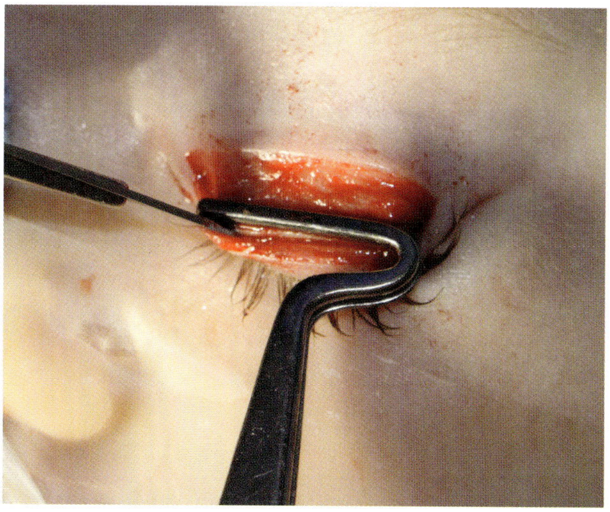

FIGURE 65.12 With the levator clamp clasped and locked, the levator-Müller's-conjunctiva complex is severed from the superior border of the tarsus using a #15 blade.

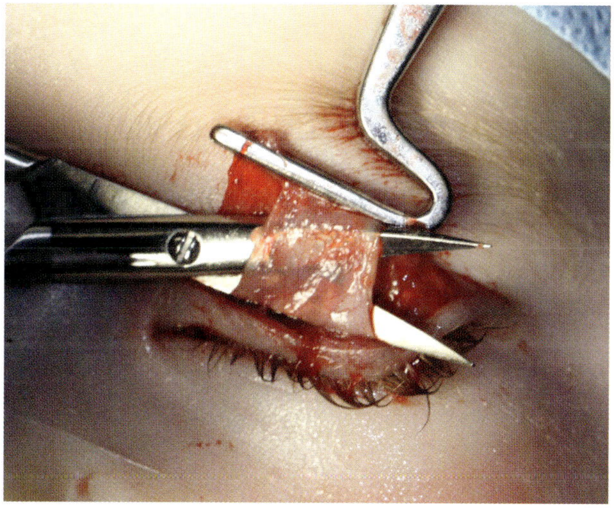

FIGURE 65.13 The conjunctiva is dissected from Müller's muscle with iris scissors. This excess conjunctiva is excised (not pictured) and the conjunctiva is advanced onto the superior tarsal border with three to four 6-0 plain gut sutures (not pictured).

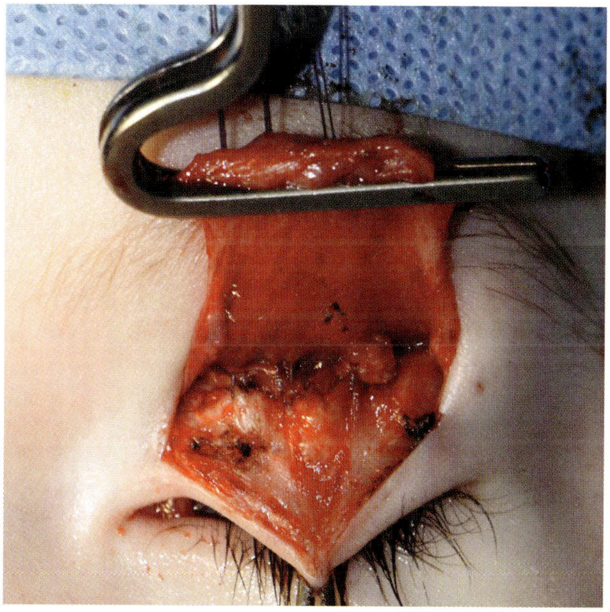

FIGURE 65.14 The levator clamp is reflected downward and the orbital septum is dissected off the superior surface of the levator aponeurosis (not pictured). The levator is advanced onto the tarsus with three 5-0 double-armed polyglactin sutures on an S-29 needle (Ethicon). The polyglactin sutures may be tied on a slipknot to set the eyelid height (usually an MRD1 of 4–5 mm).

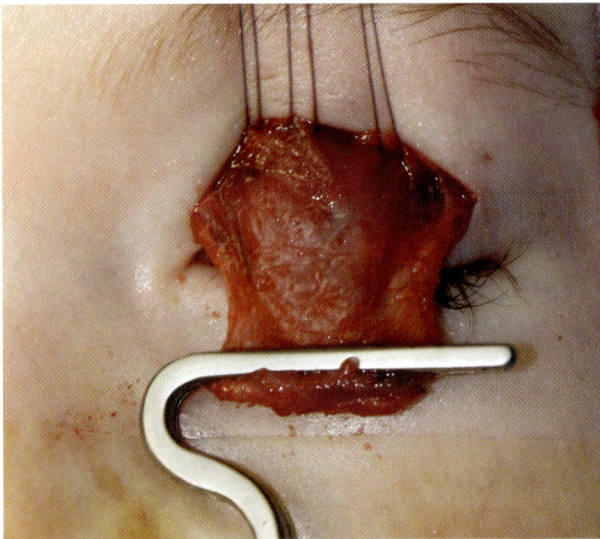

FIGURE 65.15 The levator is pulled downward to allow better apposition of the underlying tarsus when tying the polyglactin sutures. Excess levator is excised, leaving a 2 mm stump (not pictured). To determine the amount of levator aponeurosis and muscle to resect, one may prefer to use the tables modified from Berke or Beard (see References). The lid crease is reformed with three interrupted 7-0 polyglactin sutures passed from the skin and orbicularis from the upper incision to the levator aponeurosis stump, and to the orbicularis and skin of the lower incision (not pictured). The incision is further closed with a running 6-0 fast absorbing gut suture (not pictured).

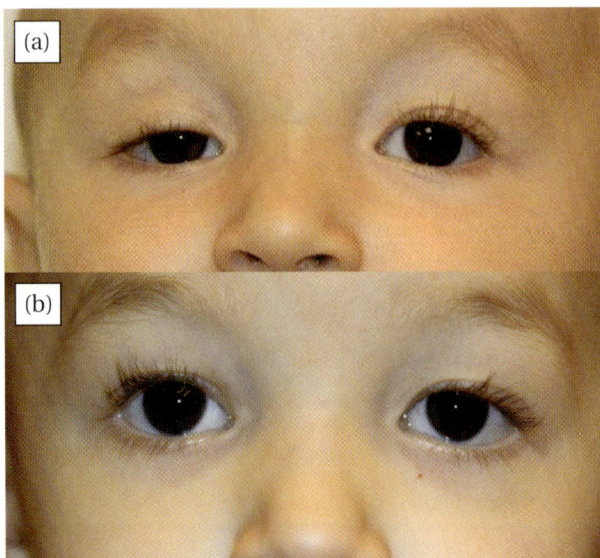

FIGURE 65.16 (a) Preoperative photo of a 10-month-old boy with right upper eyelid ptosis and 8 mm of levator function. (b) Postoperative photo 8 months after a right anterior levator resection.

Frontalis Sling Using a Silicone Rod (with a Lateral Suture Tarsorrhaphy)

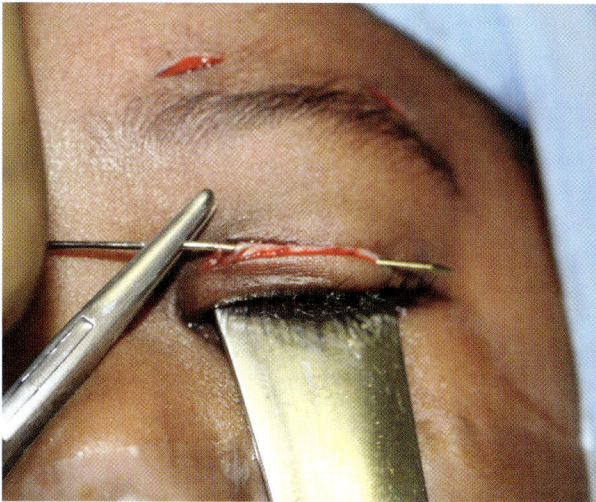

FIGURE 65.17 An upper eyelid crease incision is made with a #15 blade along with two supra-brow stab incisions laterally and medially. A shoehorn retractor can be placed under the eyelid to protect the eye, and a silicone rod sling suaged to a steel needle (BD Visitec 585192) is held with a Webster needle holder and passed from medial to lateral. Care is taken to pass the needle in the pretarsal, sub-orbicularis plane. Care must be taken to confirm there is no silicone exposed on the undersurface of the tarsus.

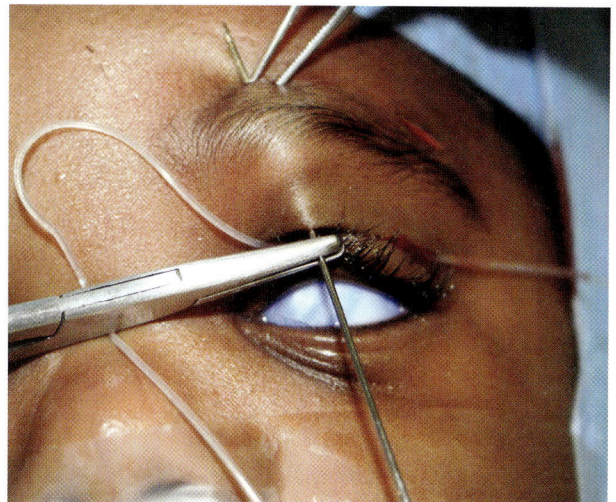

FIGURE 65.18 The steel needle is advanced under the skin and orbicularis over the superior orbital rim to the medial supra-brow stab incision. Care is taken to not puncture the dermis of the stab incision as this would lead skin dimpling at the incision site.

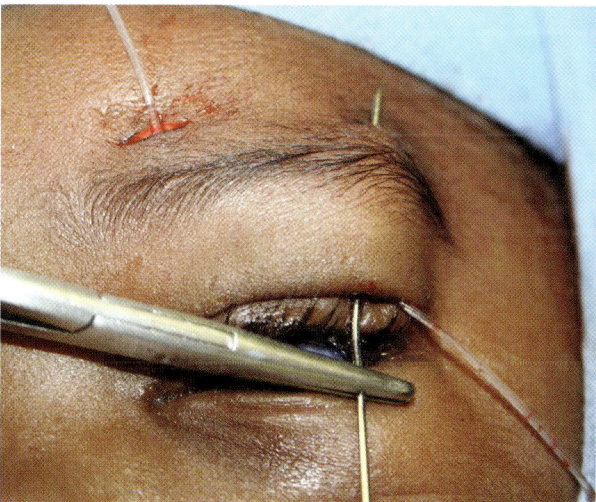

FIGURE 65.19 The same maneuver is accomplished with the lateral silicone rod.

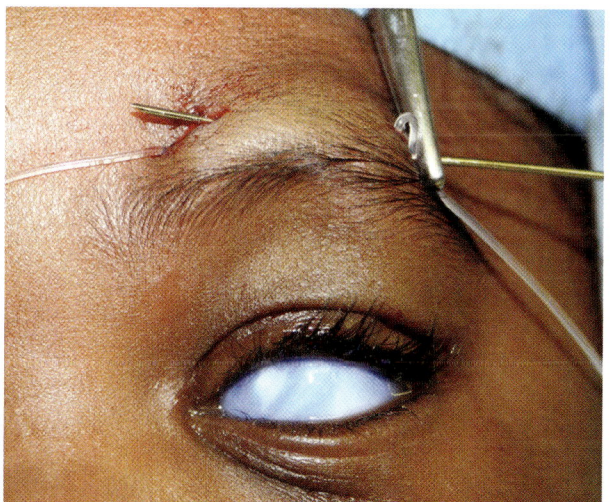

FIGURE 65.20 The steel needle is advanced from the lateral incision to the medial incision. Care must be taken to not nick the silicone rod with the needle, as this may lead to silicone rod breakage when tightening the sling.

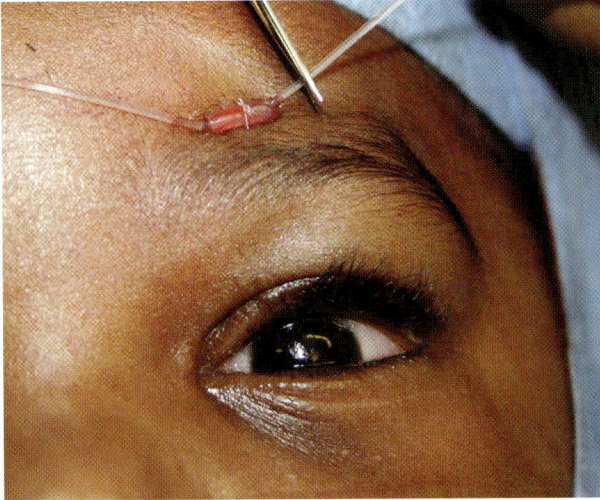

FIGURE 65.21 Before tightening the sling material, the skin crease is closed with a running 6-0 fast absorbing gut suture (not pictured). Each end of the silicone is passed through a silicone sleeve (BD Visitec 585192). After removal of a scleral shell, the eyelid height is set to an MRD1 of 4.5 mm. A 5-0 clear nylon suture is tied over the silicone sleeve, and excess silicone is trimmed at the sleeve ends.

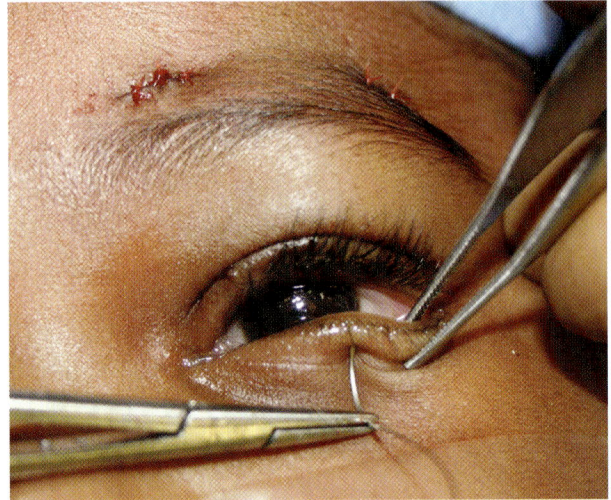

FIGURE 65.22 The sleeve is buried in the medial supra-brow incision, and the brow wounds are closed with a 6-0 polyglactin suture. A lateral suture tarsorrhaphy is made with a 5-0 black nylon suture at the level of the lateral limbus. This suture enters the lower eyelid near or above the crease and exits the eyelid margin at the gray line.

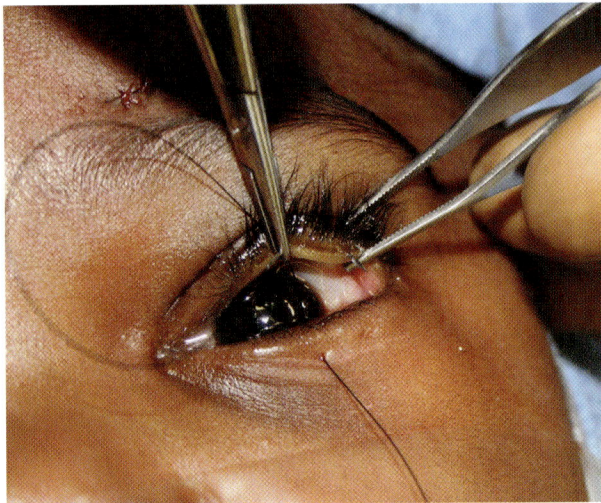

FIGURE 65.23 The nylon suture is passed through the upper eyelid at the gray line.

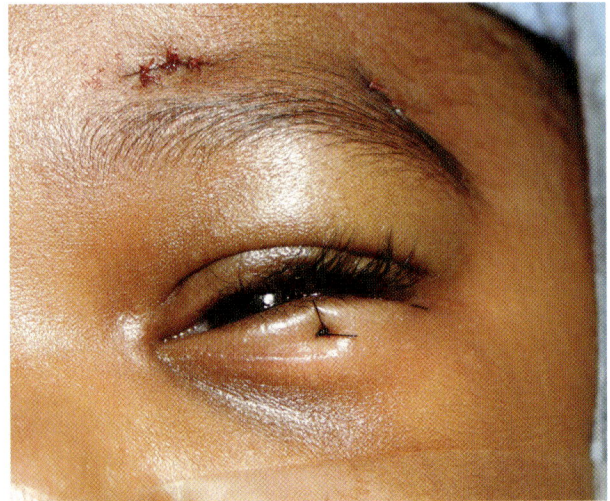

FIGURE 65.24 The lateral end of the suture is passed back into the eyelid margin at the gray line (not pictured) a knot is tied in the lower eyelid. This suture should allow visibility medially, and should be removed 3–5 days after the procedure, to provide adequate postoperative corneal protection.

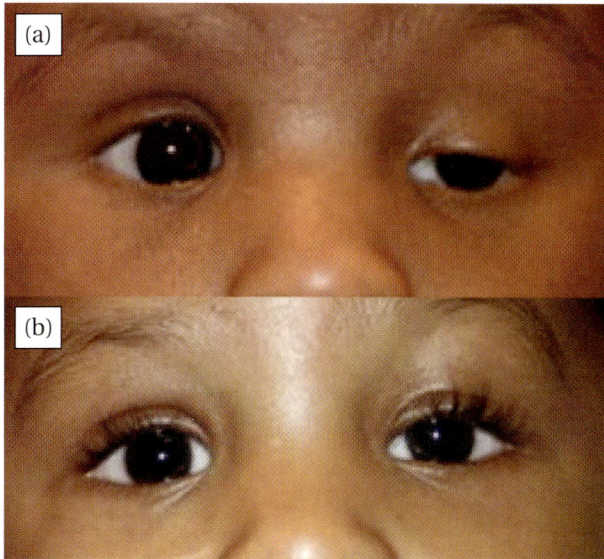

FIGURE 65.25 (a) Preoperative photo of a 12-month-old boy with congenital left upper eyelid ptosis and poor levator function. (b) Postoperative photo 18 months after a left frontalis sling with a silicone rod.

Frontalis Sling with Autogenous Fascia Lata

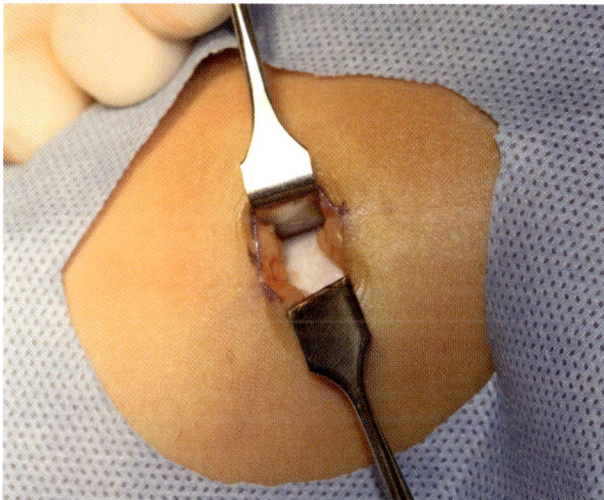

FIGURE 65.26 After the patient is positioned intraoperatively with the donor leg flexed, a 15 mm linear incision is made in the lateral leg (not pictured). The incision should be approximately 2–3 cm above the lateral condyle of the femur. Dissection is carried down to the fascia lata.

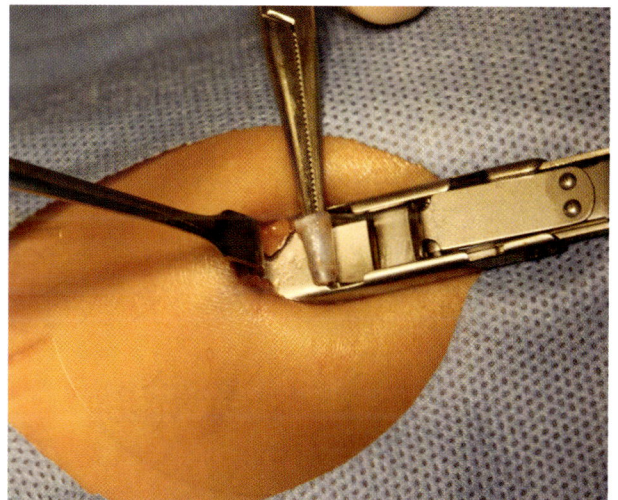

FIGURE 65.27 A flap of fascia lata is raised with a #15 blade. This flap is extended through the tip of a fascia stripper and grasped with a straight hemostat. While holding tension on the fascia lata, the stripper is advanced superiorly toward the iliac crest. Care should be taken to push the stripper in one motion. The stripper should be advanced up to the 15–20 cm marking.

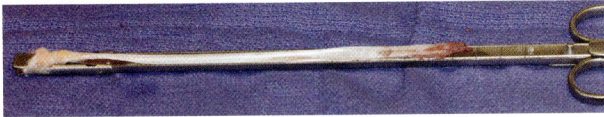

FIGURE 65.28 The fascia stripper with autogenous fascia lata tissue (note 17 cm of tissue stripped). The graft is then placed on a cutting board, and the adherent fat is removed from the graft. The graft is then split lengthwise into 4 strips (enough to use for a bilateral case). The leg wound is closed with 3–4 vertical mattress 4-0 polyglactin sutures and a running subcuticular 5-0 poliglecaprone 25 (Monocryl) suture. The wound is sealed with cyanoacrylate tissue adhesive (not pictured).

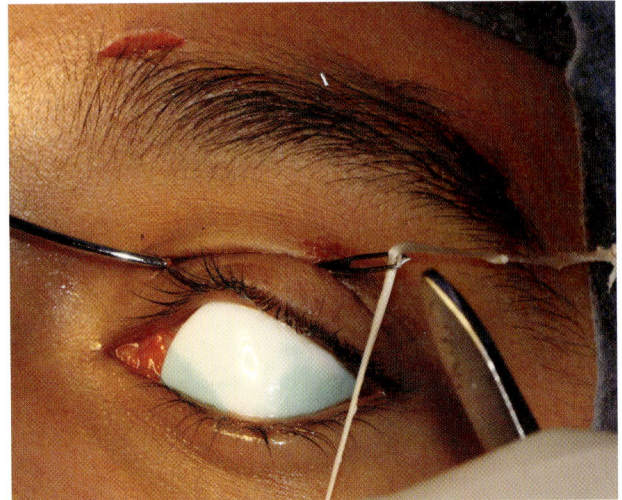

FIGURE 65.29 (Similar to Figure 65.17) The lid crease is incised with a #15 blade. Two stab wounds are made above the brow medially and laterally. A Wright fascia needle (FCI Ophthalmics) is passed from the medial wound in the sub-orbicularis and pretarsal plane to just beyond the middle of the eyelid. One strip of fascia lata graft is threaded through the needle, and the needle is retracted though the wound.

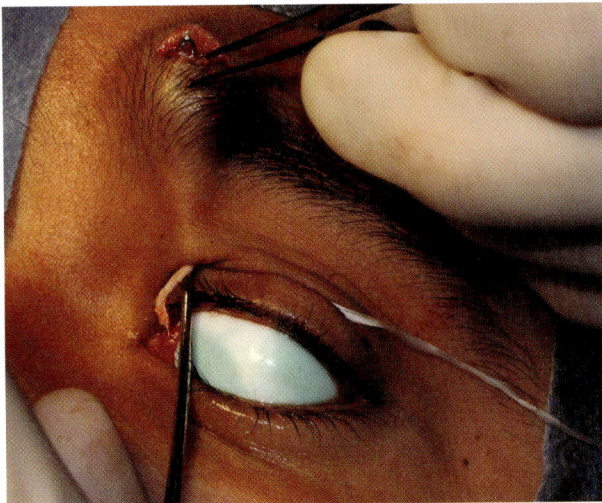

FIGURE 65.30 With the medial end of the fascia strip still threaded on the Wright needle, the graft is passed under the skin and orbicularis to the medial brow incision. Care is taken to be above the superior orbital rim and to avoid periosteum. The same procedure is performed with the lateral end of the fascia strip.

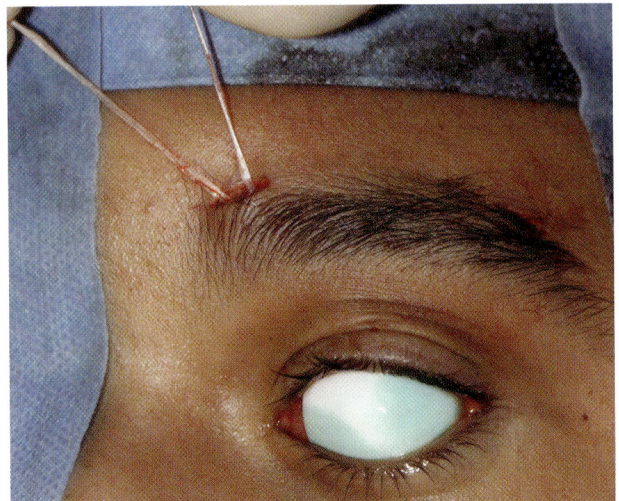

FIGURE 65.31 Good medial lid elevation is demonstrated with the medial strip in place alone.

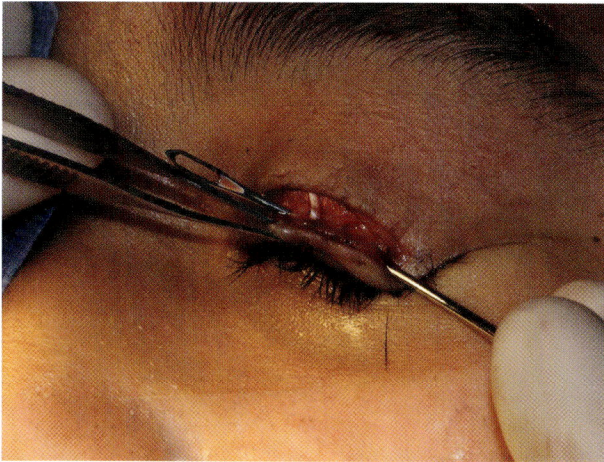

FIGURE 65.32 The Wright needle is passed in the same approximate sub-orbicularis and pretarsal plane from the lateral incision to overlap the medial tarsal strip.

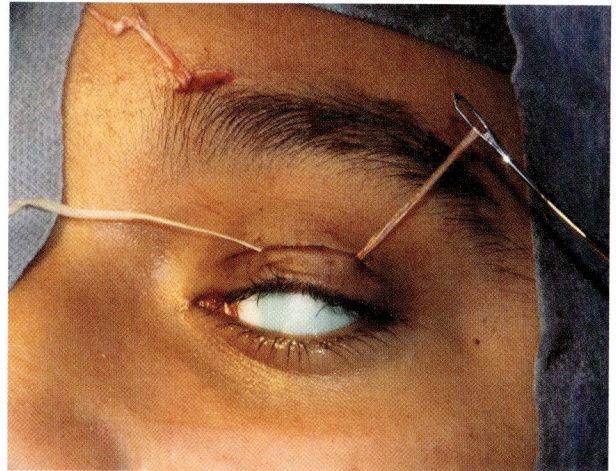

FIGURE 65.33 A second autogenous fascia lata strip is threaded into the Wright needle eyelet and the needle is retracted. This strip is passed to the lateral supra-brow incision.

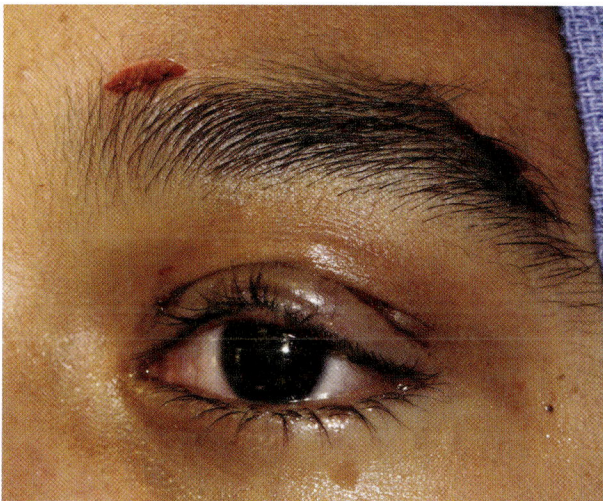

FIGURE 65.34 Excess upper eyelid tissue (skin, orbicularis and septum) may be removed before closing the eyelid crease incision. The skin is then closed with a running 6-0 fast absorbing gut suture (not pictured). The fascial strips are tied above the brow forming two triangles. The eyelid is lifted to an MRD1 of approximately 4 mm. A 5-0 clear nylon suture is tied through each of the fascial strip knots (not pictured), excess fascia lata is cut, and the knots are buried in the supra-brow incisions. These incisions are closed with interrupted 6-0 polyglactin sutures.

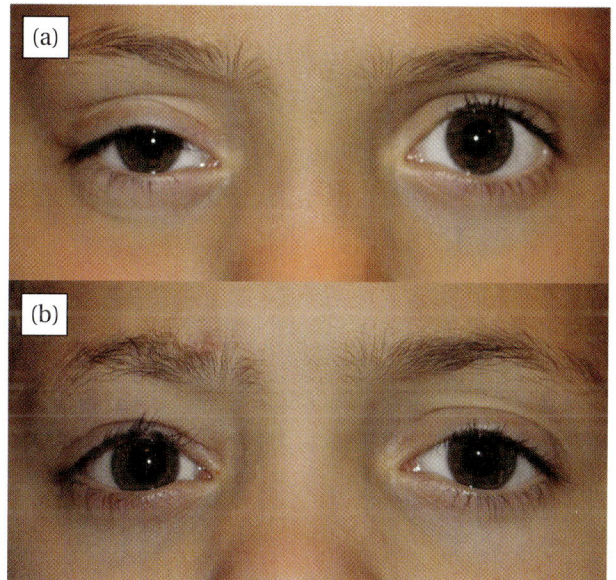

FIGURE 65.35 (a) Preoperative photo of a 5-year-old boy with right congenital ptosis and poor levator function. (b) Postoperative photo 6 months after a right autogenous fascia sling.

Complications from Ptosis Surgery

TABLE 65.4   *Complications from Ptosis Surgery*

Under correction
Over correction
Eyelid retraction (see Figure 65.36)
Chronic lagophthalmos (see Figure 65.37)
Corneal abrasion or ulceration
Suture or sling granuloma (see Figure 65.38)
Eyelid and eyelash ectropion
Eyelid asymmetry (lateral or medial droop) infection

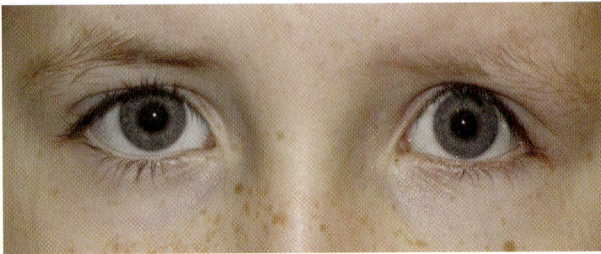

FIGURE 65.36   Left upper eyelid retraction after a left anterior levator resection.

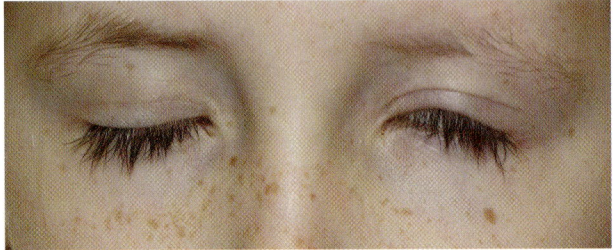

FIGURE 65.37   Chronic lagophthalmos 6 months after a left anterior levator resection.

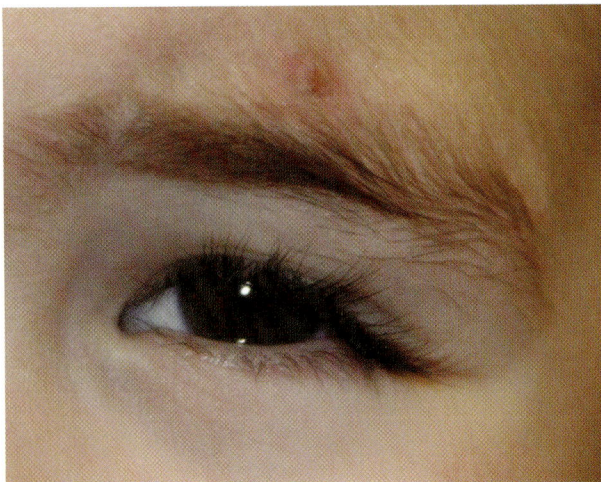

FIGURE 65.38   Left brow wound granuloma that persisted 7 months after a silicone rod frontalis sling.

SELECTED REFERENCES

Berke RN. Resection of the levator muscle through the external approach for congenital ptosis. *Trans Pac Coast Otoophthalmol Soc Annual Meet.* 1964;45:207–214

Callahan M. Levator maldevelopment ptosis. In Callahan M, Beard C, eds. *Beard's ptosis*, 4th edition. (p. 116). Birmingham, Alabama; 1990.

Carter SR, Meecham WJ, Seiff SR. Silicone frontalis slings for the correction of blepharoptosis: indications and efficacy. *Ophthalmology.* 1996;103:623–630.

Heher LH, Katowitz JA. Pediatric Ptosis. In: Katowitz JA, ed. *Pediatric oculoplastic surgery* (pp. 253–288). New York: Springer-Verlag; 2002.

Rathbun JE. Anterior approach to correction of levator maldevelopment ptosis. In: Levin M, ed. *Manual of oculoplastic surgery* (p. 79). Boston: Butterworth-Heinemann;1996.

Wiggs EO. The Fasanella-Servat operation. *Ophthalmic Surg.* 1978;9:48–57.

Oculofacial Plastic, Orbital, and Lacrimal Surgery

Edited by **Don O. Kikkawa**

Subsection Editors **Cat Nguyen Burkat and Bobby S. Korn**

66

Surgical Anatomy of the Orbit, Eyelids, and Lacrimal System

Gregory J. Griepentrog, MD and Mark J. Lucarelli, MD, FACS

Orbital Anatomy

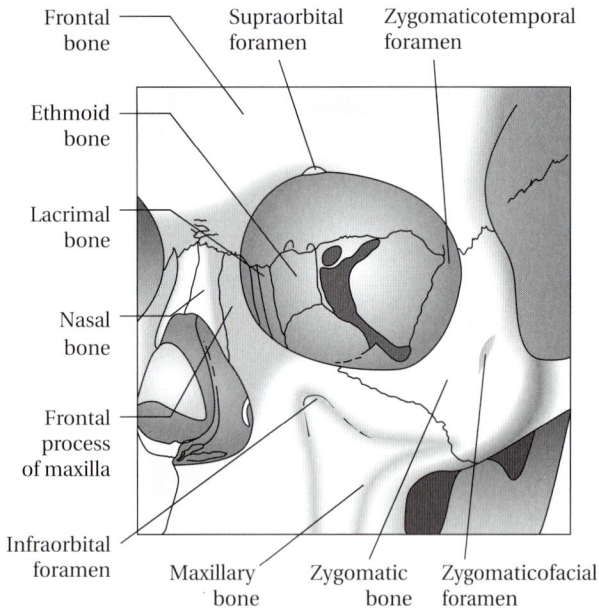

FIGURE 66.1 Frontal view of the orbital osteologic structure.

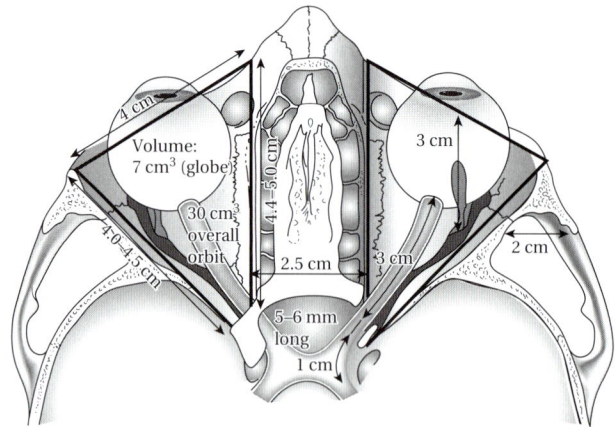

FIGURE 66.2 Axial view of the orbits shows gross dimensions and relationships.

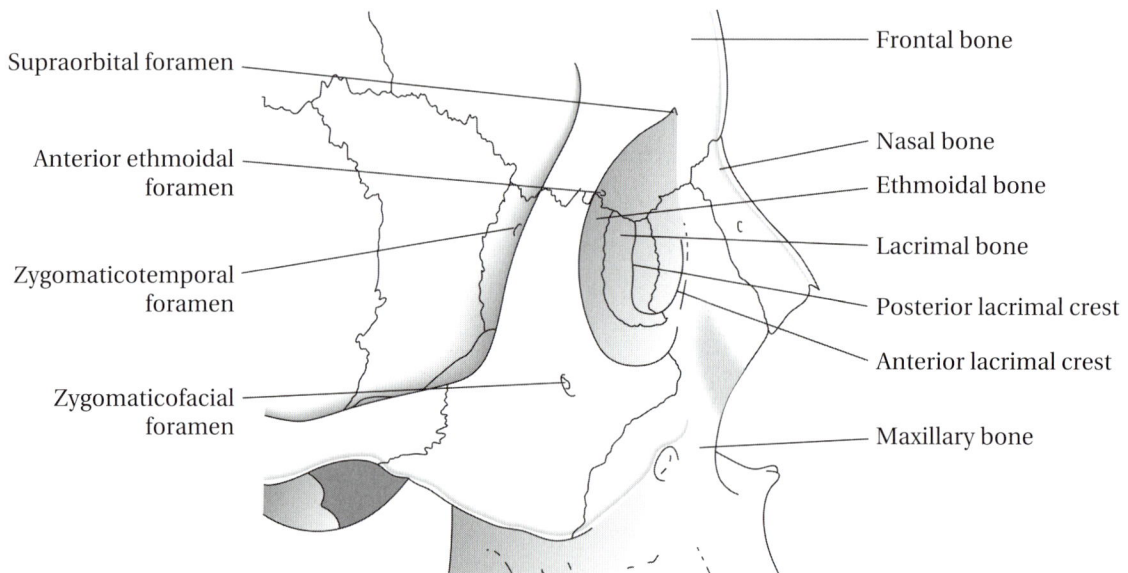

FIGURE 66.3 Lateral view of the orbital bones.

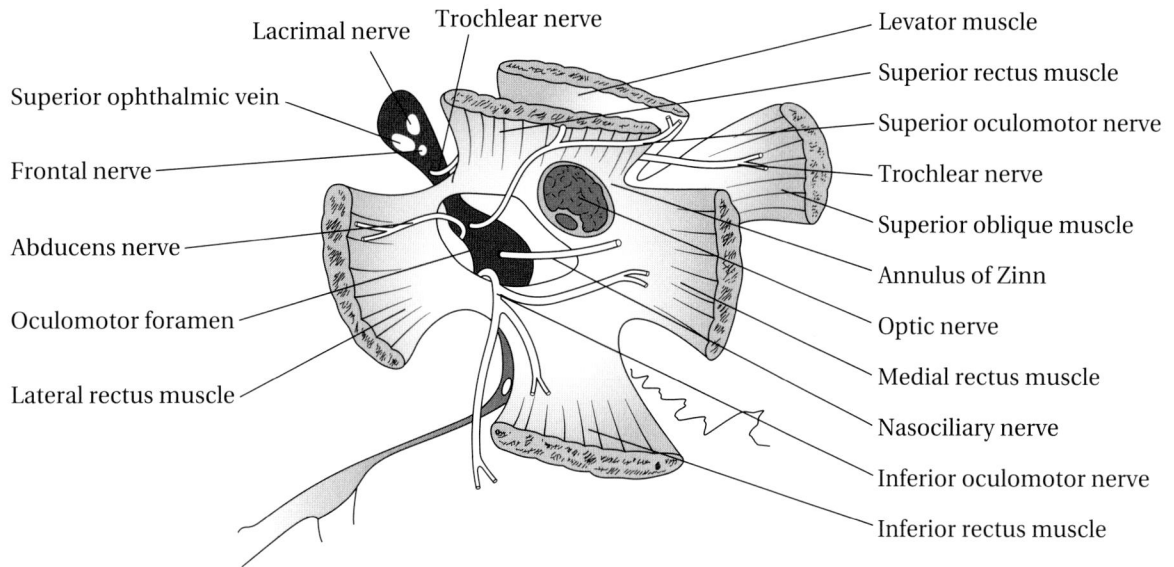

FIGURE 66.4 Anterior view of the right orbital apex.

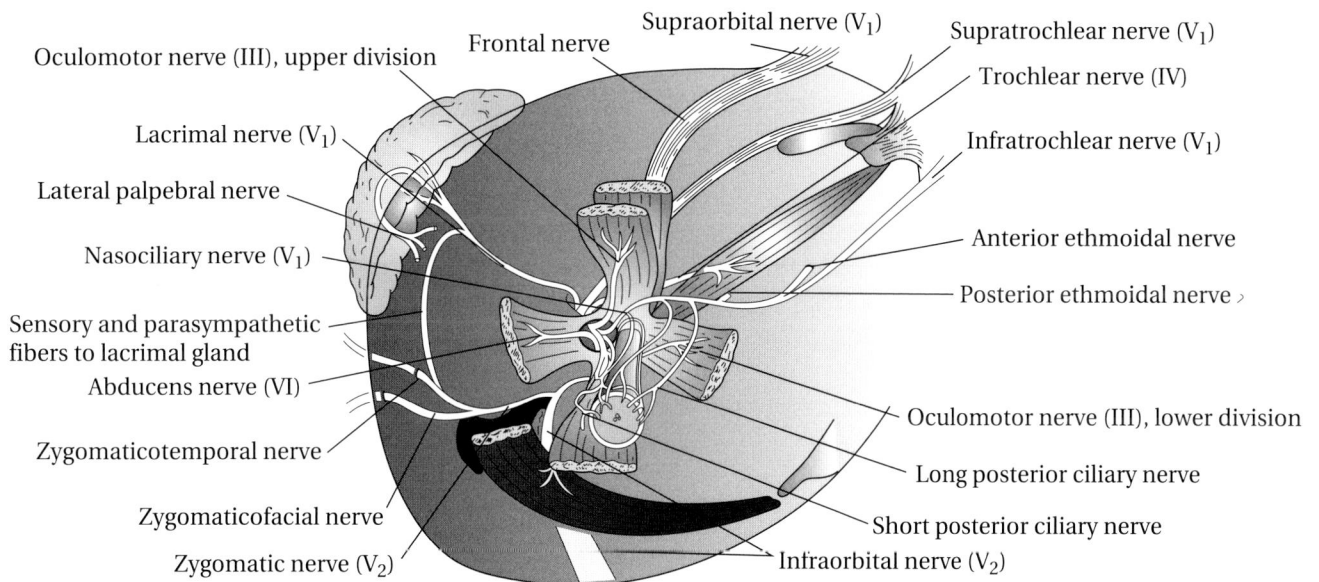

FIGURE 66.5 Foreshortened view emphasizes the major relationships of the neural structures within the orbit and the superior orbital fissure.

Lateral muscular artery Zygomaticotemporal artery Anterior ethmoidal artery

Lacrimal artery Posterior ethmoidal artery Supraorbital artery

Recurrent meningeal artery Supratrochlear artery

Nasofrontal artery

Dorsal nasal artery

Medial palpebral artery

Muscular artery

Posterior ciliary artery

Middle meningeal artery Central artery of retina

Medial muscular artery

Maxillary meningeal artery Zygomaticofacial artery Infraorbital artery Angular artery

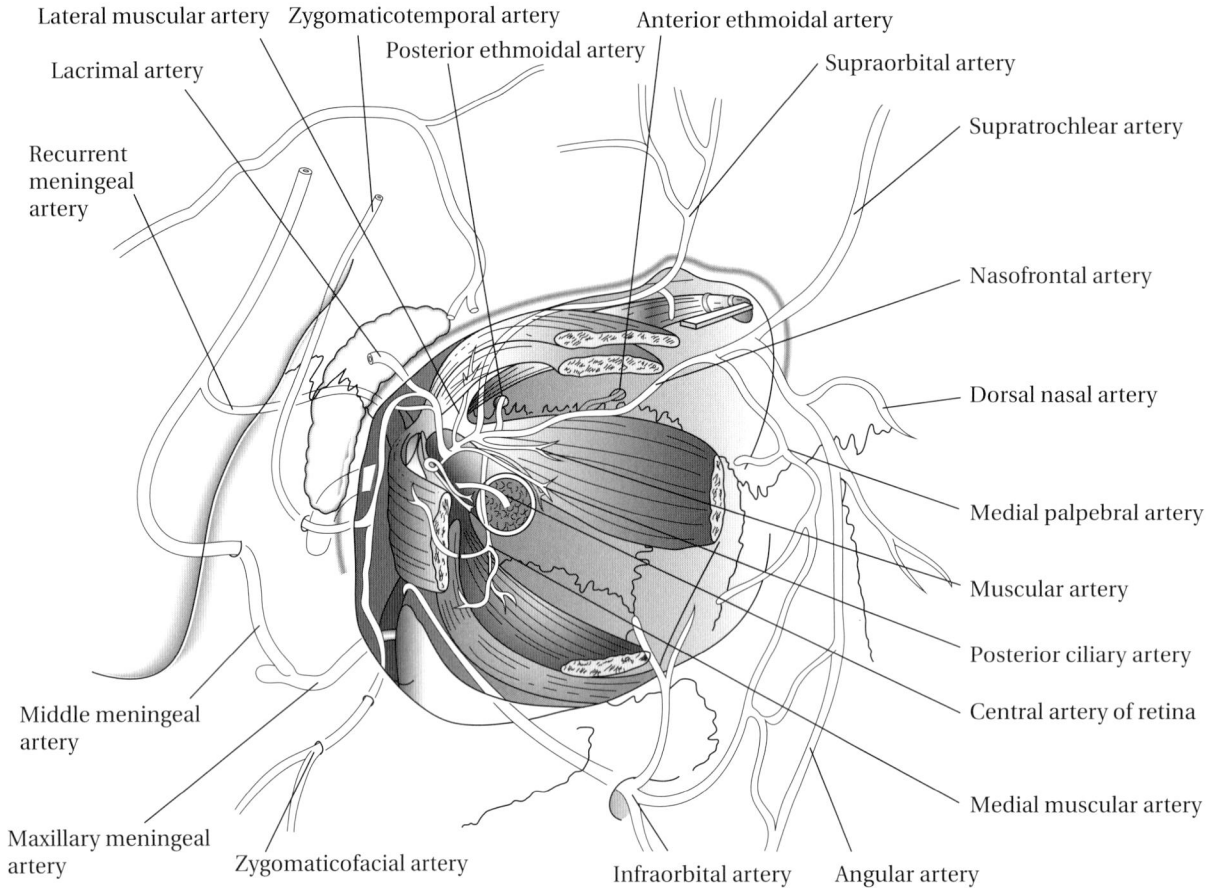

FIGURE 66.6 Direct anterolateral view of the arteries of the orbit.

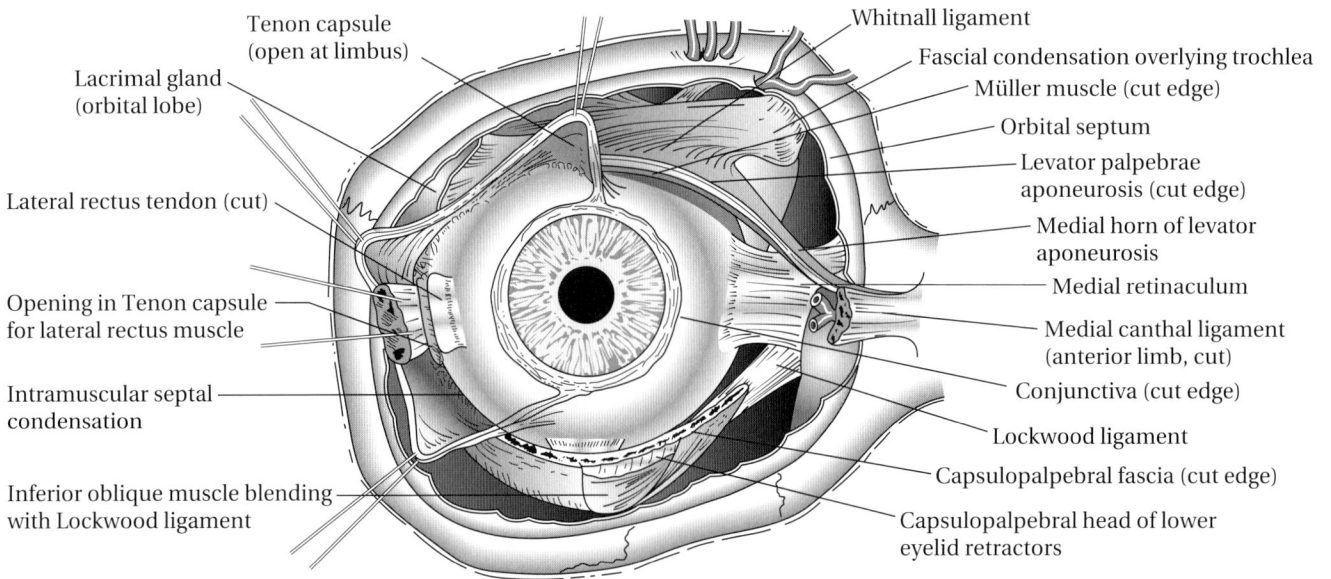

Tenon capsule (open at limbus) Whitnall ligament

Lacrimal gland (orbital lobe) Fascial condensation overlying trochlea

Müller muscle (cut edge)

Orbital septum

Levator palpebrae aponeurosis (cut edge)

Lateral rectus tendon (cut) Medial horn of levator aponeurosis

Medial retinaculum

Opening in Tenon capsule for lateral rectus muscle Medial canthal ligament (anterior limb, cut)

Conjunctiva (cut edge)

Intramuscular septal condensation Lockwood ligament

Capsulopalpebral fascia (cut edge)

Inferior oblique muscle blending with Lockwood ligament Capsulopalpebral head of lower eyelid retractors

FIGURE 66.7 Tenon's capsule and anterior orbital structures and septa.

Superior ophthalmic vein

Frontal nerve

Levator palpebrae
superioris muscle

Superior rectus muscle

Ophthalmic artery

Abducens nerve

Lateral rectus muscle

Oculomotor nerve,
branch to medial
rectus muscle

Oculomotor nerve,
branch to inferior
oblique muscle

Inferior rectus muscle   Periorbita

Whitnall ligament

Levator aponeurosis

Orbital septum

Lockwood ligament

Inferior oblique muscle

Inferior ophthalmic vein

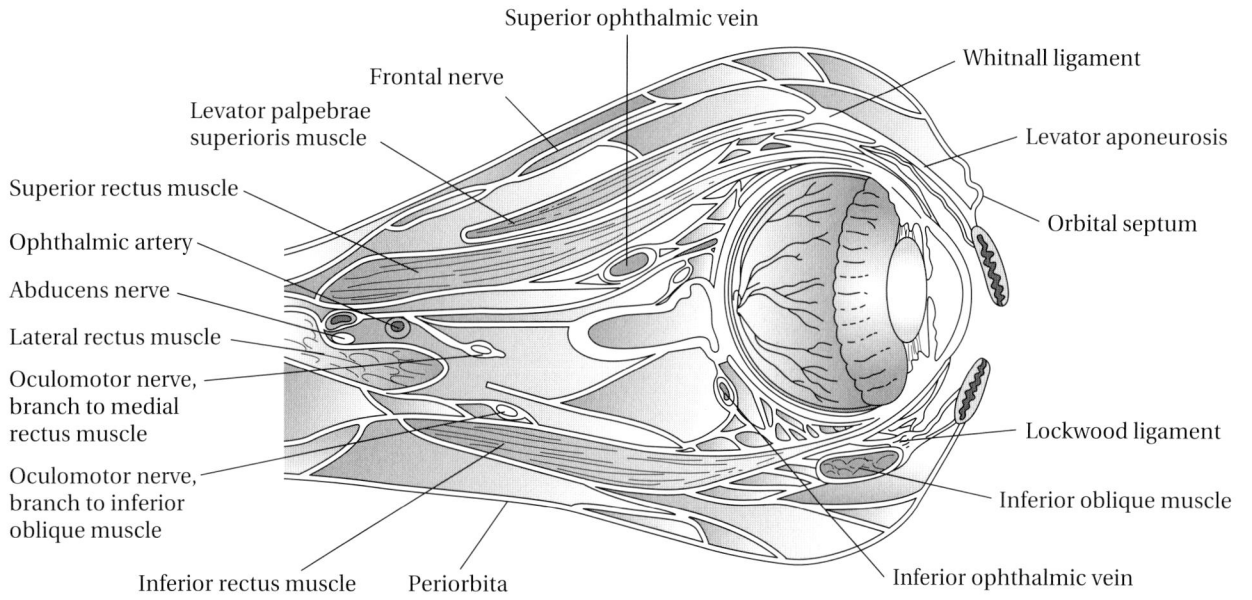

FIGURE 66.8 Lateral view of the central orbital fascial system.

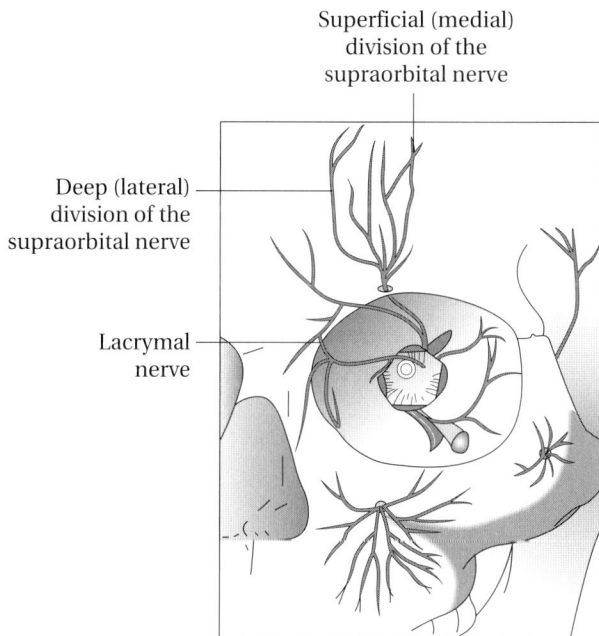

Superficial (medial)
division of the
supraorbital nerve

FIGURE 66.9 Sensory nerve distribution of the eyelids.

Deep (lateral)
division of the
supraorbital nerve

Lacrymal
nerve

Eyelid, Brow, and Midface Anatomy

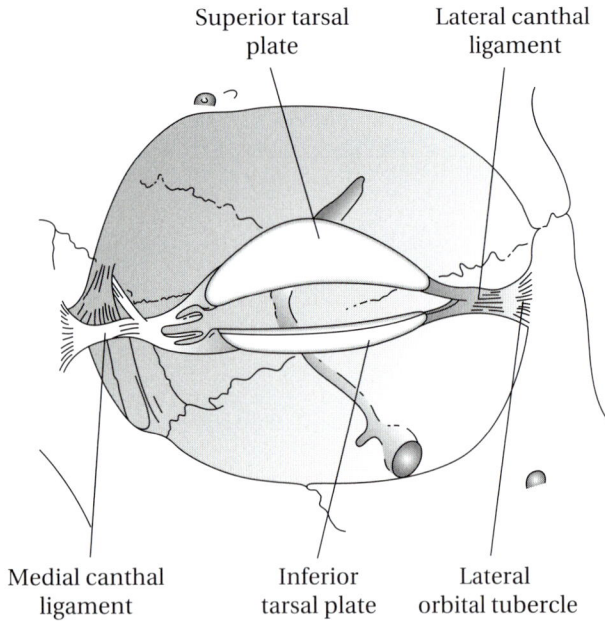

FIGURE 66.10 Deep structural elements of the eyelids.

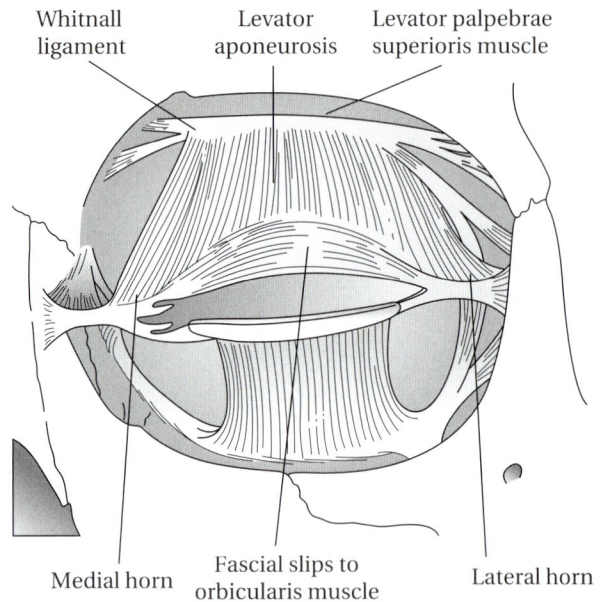

FIGURE 66.11 Eyelids, levator aponeurosis, and ligamentous support.

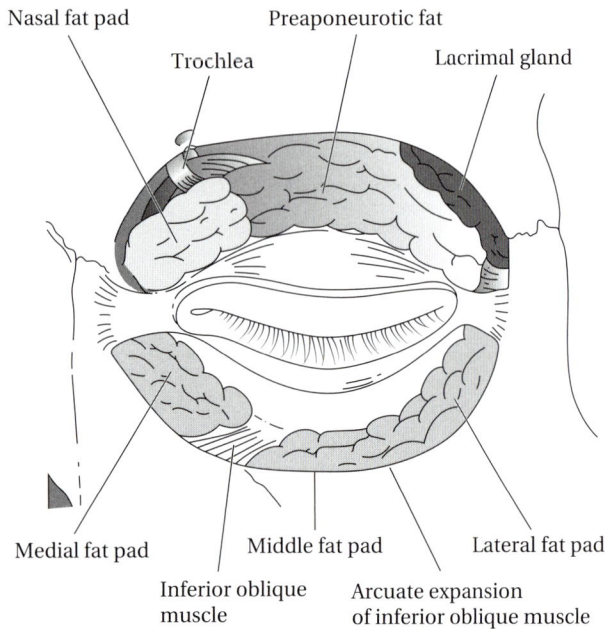

FIGURE 66.12 Anterior orbital fat pads after removal of the orbital septum. Deeper dissection of orbital fat pads shows fascial extensions of the trochlea dividing fat pads in the upper eyelid. The inferior oblique muscle and the anterior expansion of Lockwood ligament (arcuate expansion of the inferior oblique) divide the fat pads of the lower eyelid into medial, middle (central), and lateral portions.

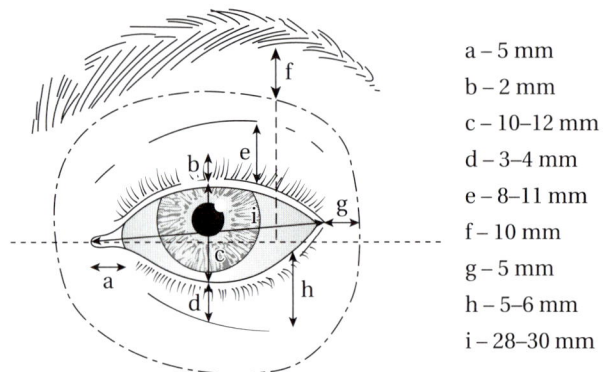

a – 5 mm
b – 2 mm
c – 10–12 mm
d – 3–4 mm
e – 8–11 mm
f – 10 mm
g – 5 mm
h – 5–6 mm
i – 28–30 mm

FIGURE 66.13 Average measurements of the superficial anatomy of the eyelids in occidental, or non-Asian, population. The female brow is arched, with the highest point at the lateral limbus. The male brow is horizontal and somewhat lower. The eyelid crease and lateral canthus also tend to be lower in men than in women.

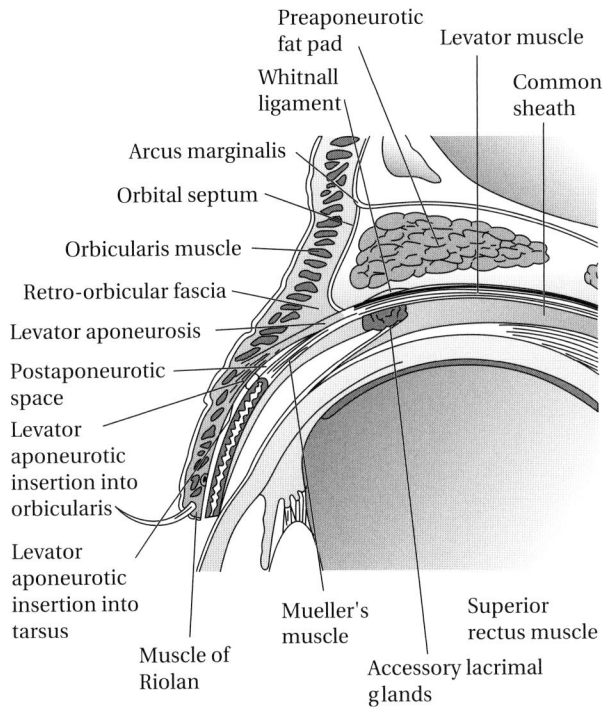

FIGURE 66.14 Anatomy of the upper eyelid retractors.

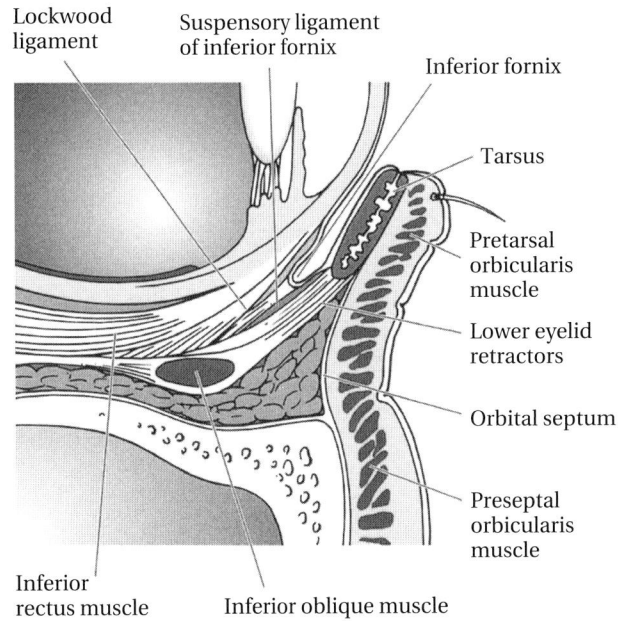

FIGURE 66.15 Anatomy of the lower eyelid retractors. Note the orbital septum joins the capsulopalpebral fascia before jointly inserting around the inferior border of the tarsus. Also note the fine connective tissue strands that pass through the orbital fat to insert on the periorbita of the orbital floor.

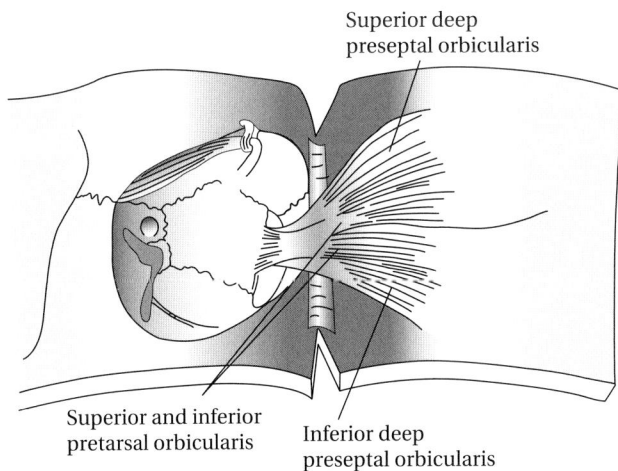

FIGURE 66.16 The eyelid skin and muscle are reflected medially. Note the superior and inferior deep, pretarsal orbicularis joining to form Horner or Duverney muscle, and inserting on the posterior lacrimal crest. The inferior and superior sections of the deep preseptal orbicularis join and insert on the lacrimal fascia.

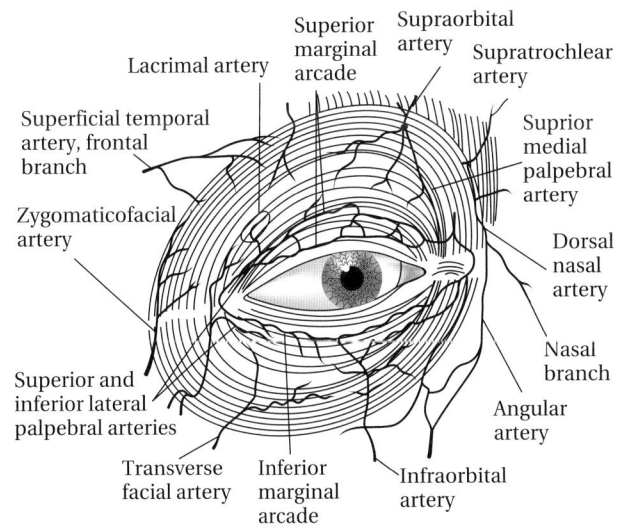

FIGURE 66.17 Superficial arteries of the eyelids.

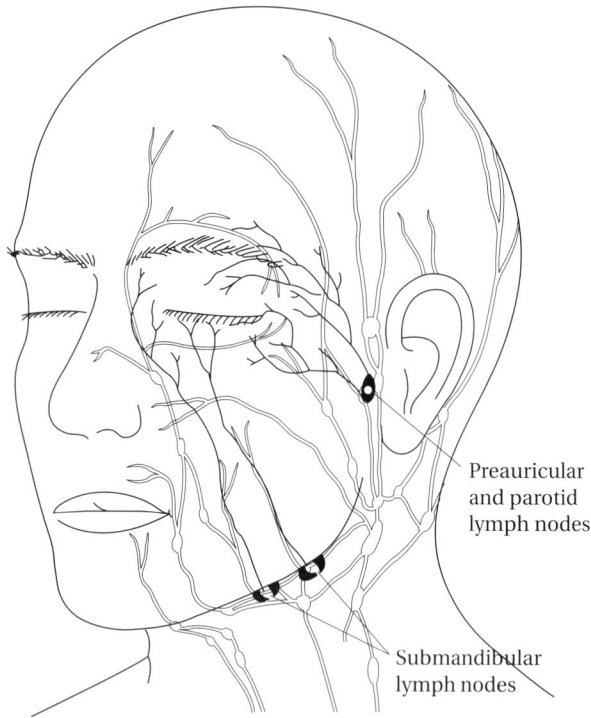

FIGURE 66.18 Lymphatic drainage pattern of the eyelids.

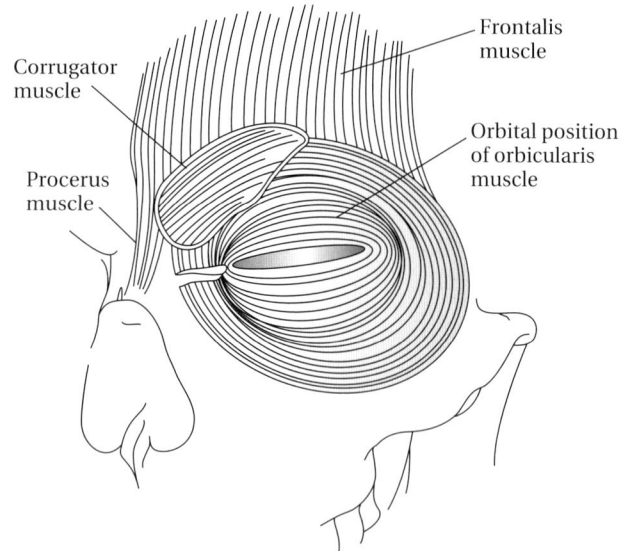

FIGURE 66.19 Muscles of the eyelids and eyebrows.

(a)

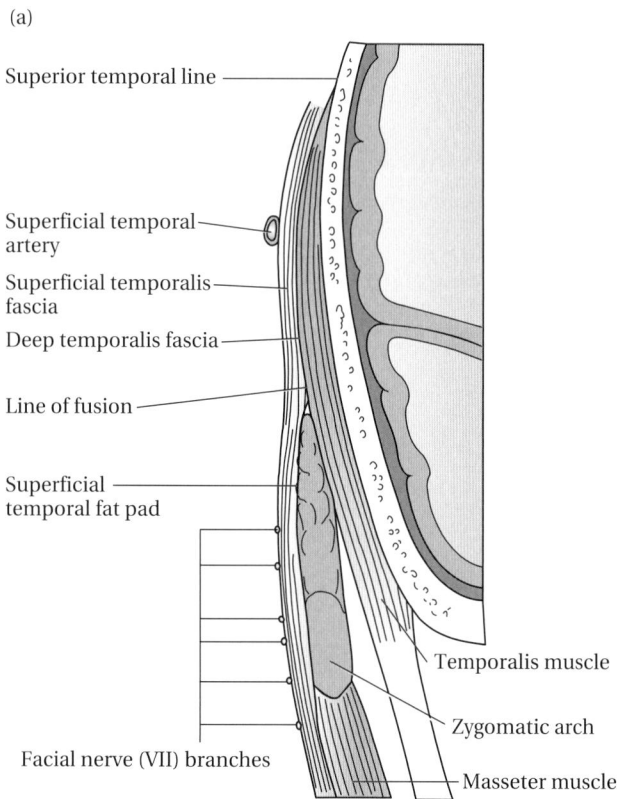

(b)

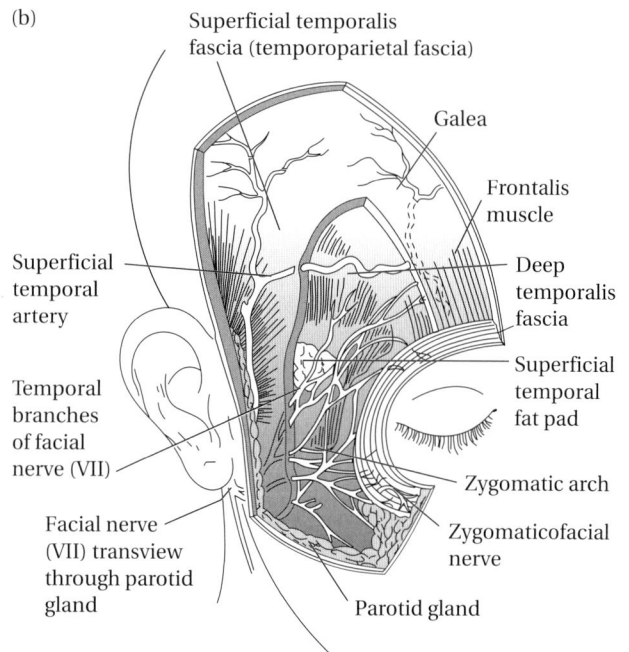

FIGURE 66.20 (a) Sagittal cross section of temporalis fascia and zygomatic arch. (b) Seventh cranial nerve and temporal artery branches show relationships in the region of the temporalis fascia.

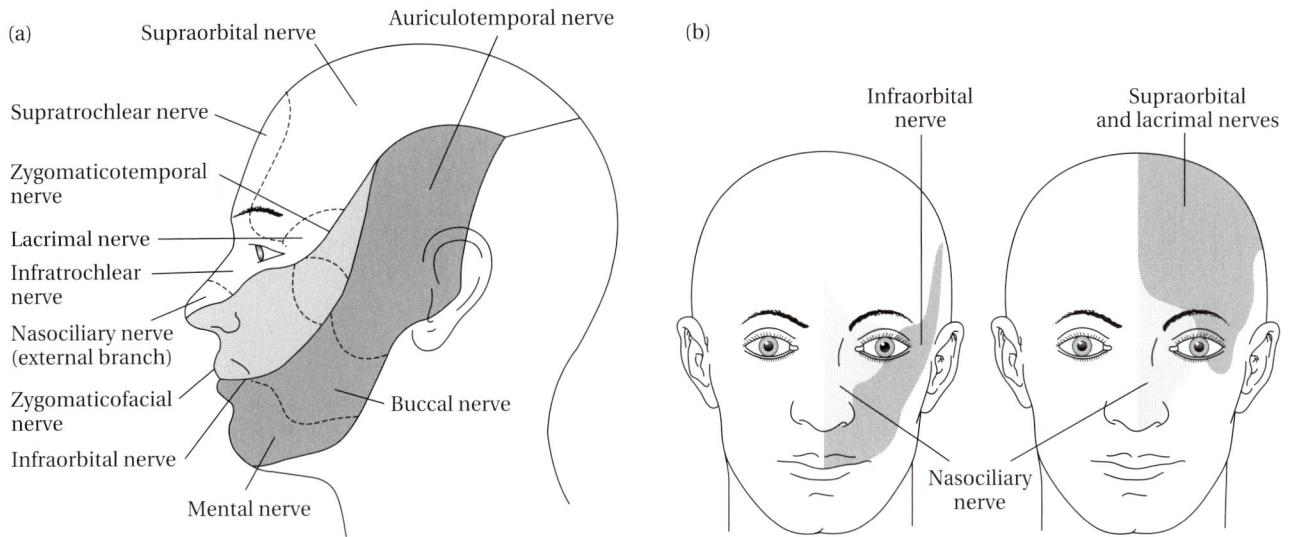

FIGURE 66.21 (a) Sensory dermatomes of the fifth nerve: V_1, ophthalmic division (white); V_2, maxillary division (gray); and V_3, mandibular division (black). (b) Cutaneous distribution of select branches of cranial nerve V.

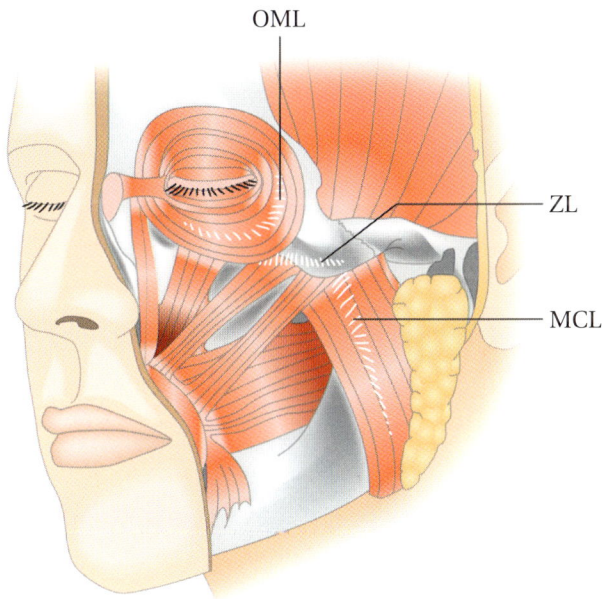

FIGURE 66.22 Midface anatomy and ligamentous support. OML, Orbitomalar ligament; ZL, Zygomatic ligaments; MCL, Masseteric cutaneous ligaments.

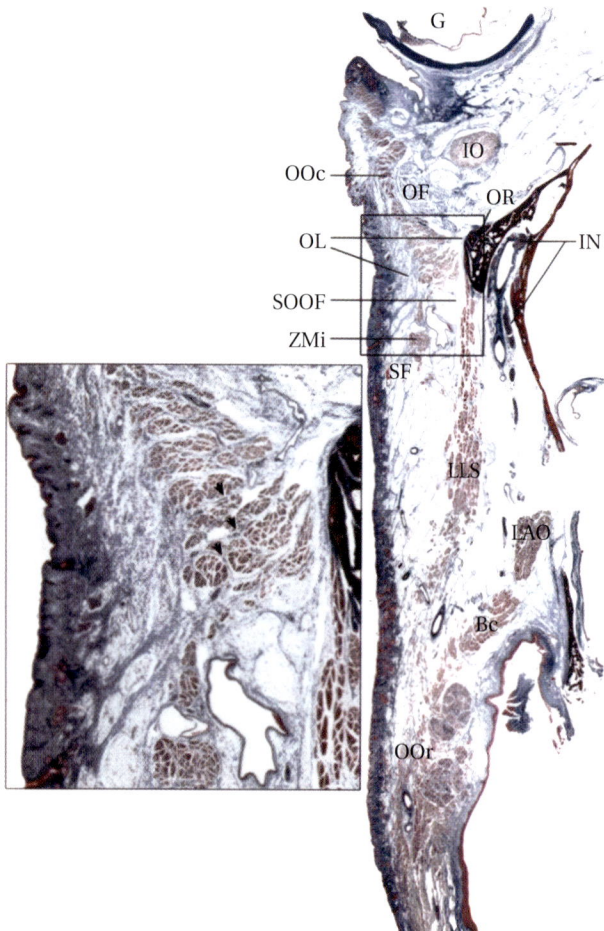

FIGURE 66.23   Merged sections through central lower eyelid extending to the oral commissure from specimen with midfacial ptosis (Masson trichrome staining). The globe (G), inferior oblique (IO), and orbital fat (OF) are visible superiorly. The orbitomalar ligament (OL) extends off the orbital rim (OR) and passes through the orbicularis oculi muscle (OOc) to the dermis. The nasolabial fold (NLF) is seen inferiorly. The subcutaneous fat (SF) can be seen anterior to the orbicularis oculi and zygomatic minor (ZMi) muscles. The suborbicularis oculi fat (SOOF) rests posterior to the orbicularis oculi muscle and surrounds the proximal portion of the levator labii superioris muscle (LLS). Note the continuity of the inferior SOOF and the subcutaneous fat. The infraorbital nerve (IN) and accompanying vessel can be seen traversing the SOOF deep to the levator labi superloris muscle. The levator anguli oris (LAO) arises from the maxilla inferior to the infraorbital foramen. The orbicularis oris (OOr) and buccinator (Bc) are visible in the inferior portion of the specimen. The inset details the orbitomalar ligament (arrowheads) traversing the orbicularis oculi muscle. (From Lucarelli MJ et al: Ophthal Plast Recontr Surg 16(1):7-22, 2000.)

Lacrimal Anatomy

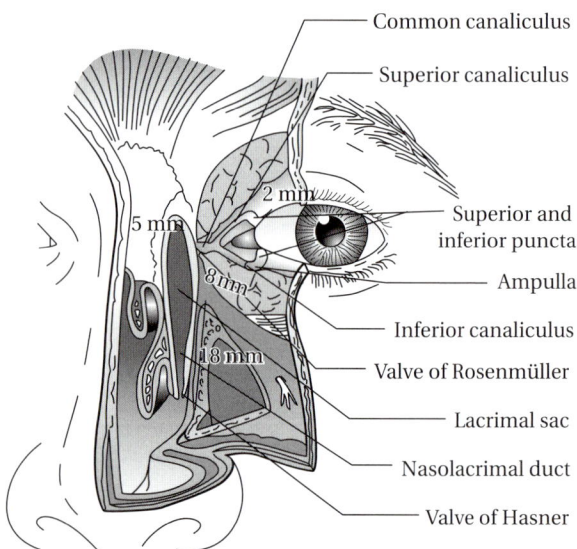

FIGURE 66.24   Nasolacrimal excretory system.

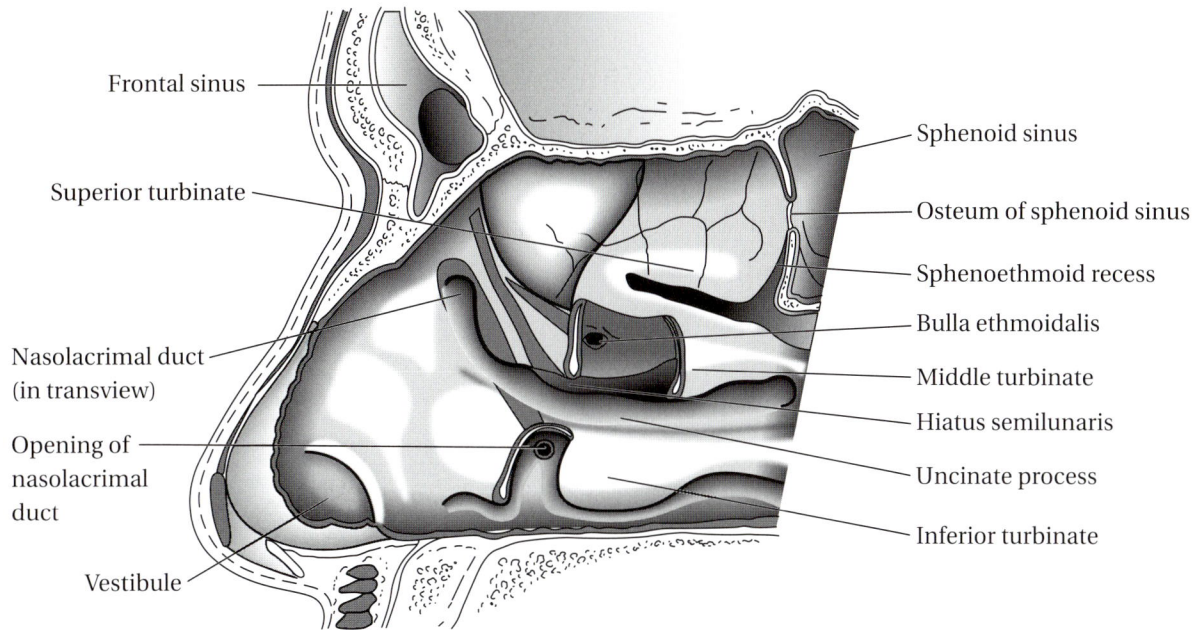

FIGURE 66.25 Lateral wall of the nose, with sinuses, ostia, and lacrimal system.

SELECTED REFERENCES

Dutton JJ. *Atlas of clinical and surgical orbital orbital anatomy*. Philadelphia: WB Saunders; 1994.

Kikkawa DO, Lemke BN, Dortzbach RK. Relations of the superficial musculoaponeurotic system to the orbit and characterization of the orbitomalar ligament. *Ophthal Plast Reconstr Surg*. 1996;12(2):77–88.

Knize DM. *The forehead and temporal fossa*. Philadelphia: Lippincott Williams & Wilkins; 2001.

Lemke BN, Lucarelli MJ. Anatomy of the ocular adnexa, orbit, and related facial structures. In Nesi FA, Lisman RD, Levine MR, eds. Smith's ophthalmic plastic and reconstructive surgery, St. Louis: Mosby-Year Book, 1998; pp. 3–78.

Zide BM. *Surgical anatomy around the orbit: The system of zones*. Philadelphia: Lippincott Williams & Wilkins; 2006.

Zide BM, Jelks GW. *Surgical anatomy of the orbit*. New York: Raven Press; 1985.

67 Energy-Based Skin Therapy

E. Victor Ross, MD and Sang-Rog Oh, MD

TABLE 67.1 *Various Energy-Based Modalities and their Common Indications and Considerations*

Modality	Common Indications	Special Considerations
Green/yellow visible light laser and Intense pulsed light (IPL)	Vascular lesions: telangiectasia, rosacea, vascular malformations, and hemangiomas; pigmented lesions, skin rejuvenation	May require multiple sessions, use caution in darker skin
Red and near red light laser and Nd:YAG laser	Pigmented lesions, vascular lesions, hair removal, fine wrinkles,	May require multiple sessions
Nonfractional "full coverage" ablative laser	Fine and deep wrinkles, pigmented lesions, scars, xanthelasma, syringomas	Extensive downtime (1–3 weeks), risk of hypopigmentation with deeper injury
Fractional ablative laser	Wrinkles, scars, pigmented lesions	Occasionally longer downtime when compared to fractional non-ablative laser
Fractional non-ablative laser	Wrinkles, scars, pigmented lesions	May require multiple sessions

TABLE 67.2 *Relative Contraindications to Energy-Based Skin Treatments*

Infections secondary to bacteria, viral, or fungal origin in the treatment areas

Use of oral isotretinoin within 6 months (which may impede re-epithelialization when performing ablative laser therapy)

Family or personal history of keloids in the treatment areas when performing ablative laser therapy

Active acne vulgaris

History of gold ingestion when performing Q-switch (e.g. Nd:YAG) laser therapy, as it may induce pigmentation in treated areas

Patients with Fitzpatrick classes V–VI skin types who are at high risk of postinflammatory hyperpigmentation(PIH)

TABLE 67.3 *Preoperative Considerations for Ablative Therapy*

Oral antibiotics may be started at least one day prior to surgery and continued for 10 days. Commonly used antibiotics are ciprofloxacin and dicloxacillin. The use of oral antibiotics should be at the discretion of the physician. With close follow-up in low-risk patients, their use is optional.

Oral antiviral medication is started 1 to 2 days before surgery and continued for one week. Either acyclovir or valacyclovir is used.

Diagrams Depicting the Targets of Various Laser Therapies

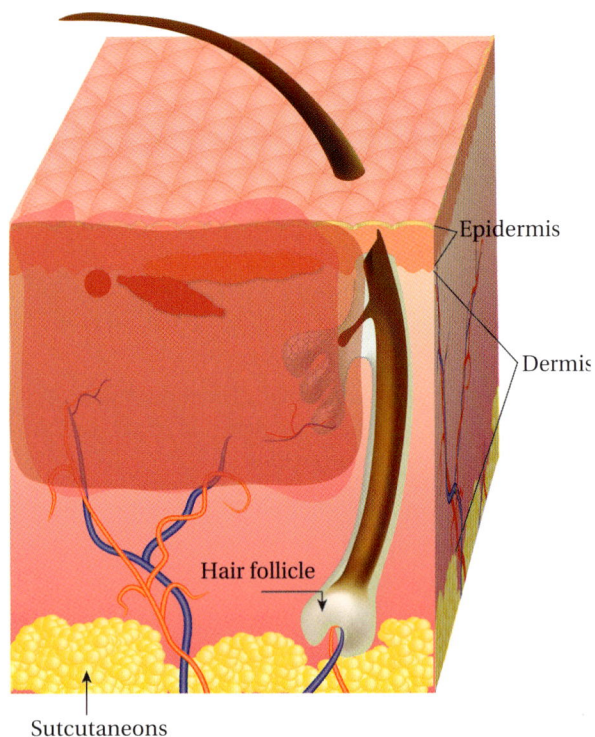

FIGURE 67.1 Ablative laser treatment. The epidermis and dermis are ablated together (Dark red). Thermal injury to the dermis promotes collagen remodeling and tightening of photoaged skin. Despite removal of the basal cell layer of the epidermis, new epidermis is regenerated from the pluripotent epithelial cells of the outer root sheath of hair follicles.

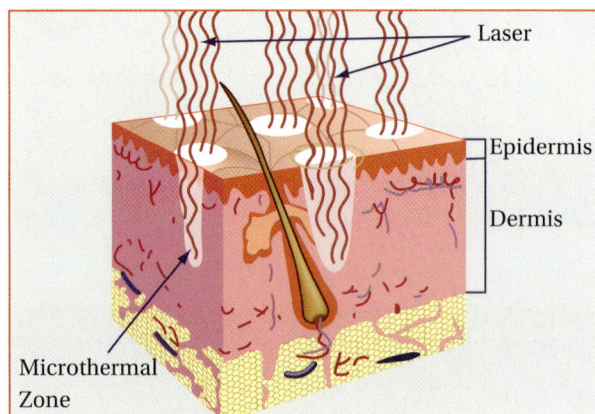

FIGURE 67.2 Fractional laser with array of microthermal zones of ablation. The intervening areas of intact epidermis allow for rapid re-epithelialization of ablated areas.

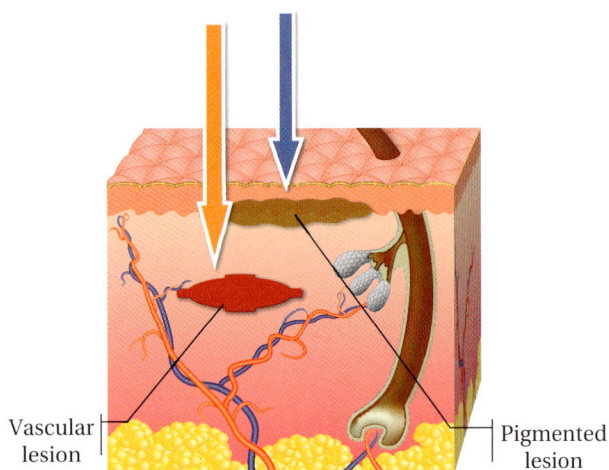

FIGURE 67.3 Selective photothermolysis. Using various wavelengths of light, specific structures or tissues are targeted with the intention of absorbing light into that target area alone. The energy directed into the target area produces sufficient heat to damage the target while allowing the surrounding area to remain relatively undisturbed. For example, hemoglobin in vascular lesions is targeted with pulsed dye laser (orange arrow) whereas pigmented lesions is treated with pulsed Q-switched alexandrite laser (blue arrow).

Ablative Fractional CO_2 Laser Therapy

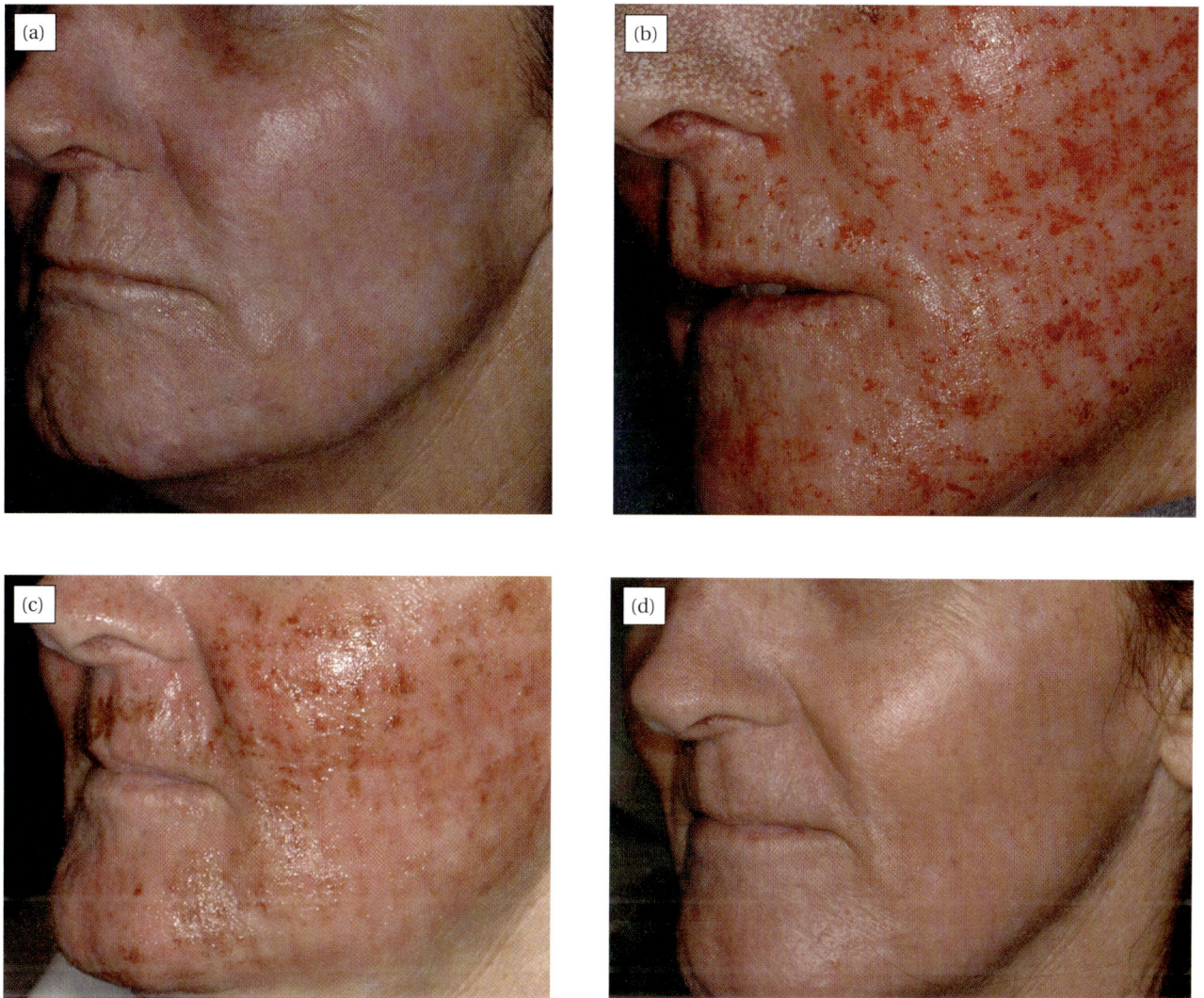

FIGURE 67.4 (a) Preoperative photograph of a patient with diffuse cutaneous scarring. (b) Immediate post-treatment photograph. (c) Post-treatment photograph at 5 days. (d) Post-treatment photograph at 6 weeks.

Nd:YAG Laser Therapy

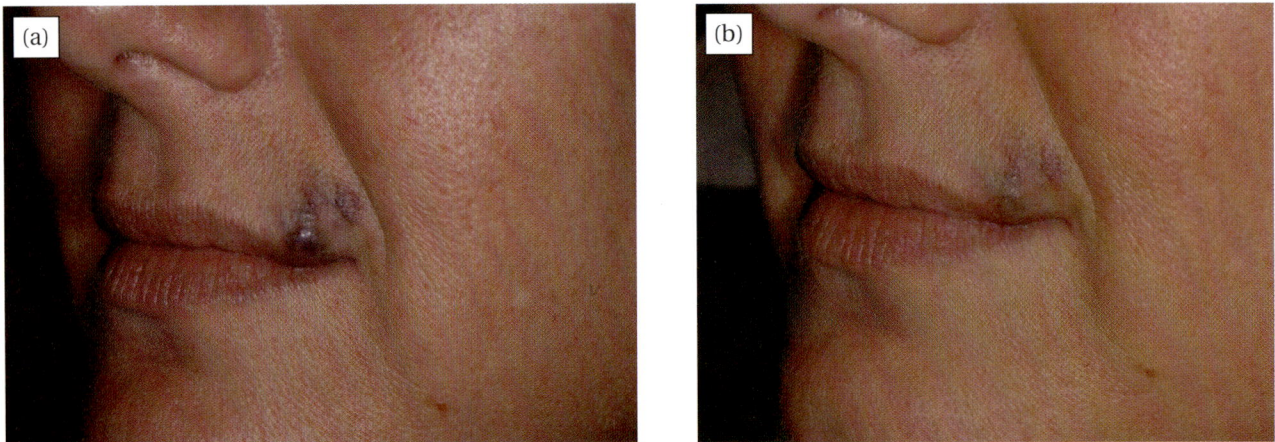

FIGURE 67.5   (a) Pretreatment photograph of a patient with arteriovenous malformation (AVM). (b) Post-treatment photograph after one treatment with Nd:YAG laser.

Ablative CO$_2$ Laser Therapy

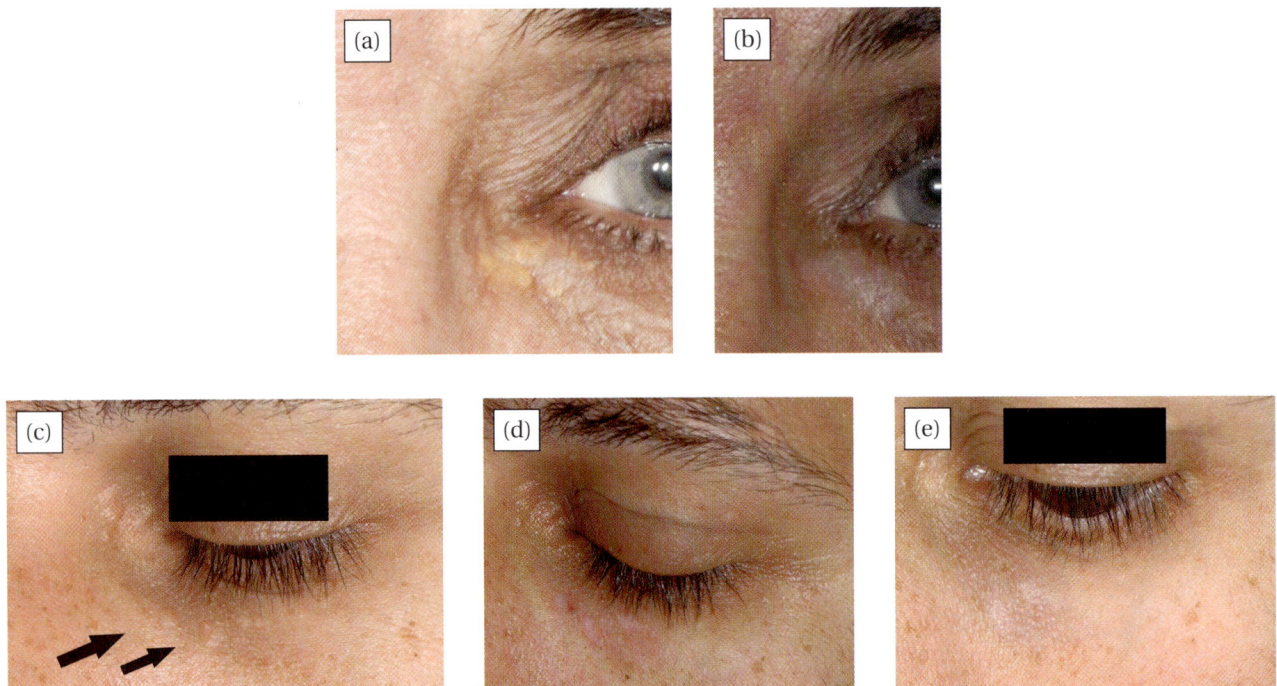

FIGURE 67.6   (a) Pretreatment photographs of patient with xanthelasma of left lower lid. (b) Post-treatment photograph at 6 weeks. (c) Pretreatment photograph of a patient with lower eyelid syringomas (arrows). (d) Immediate post-treatment photograph. (e) Post-treatment photograph at 6 weeks. Note the mild hypopigmentation at the treatment sites.

Potassium Titanyl Phosphate (KTP) YAG Laser Therapy

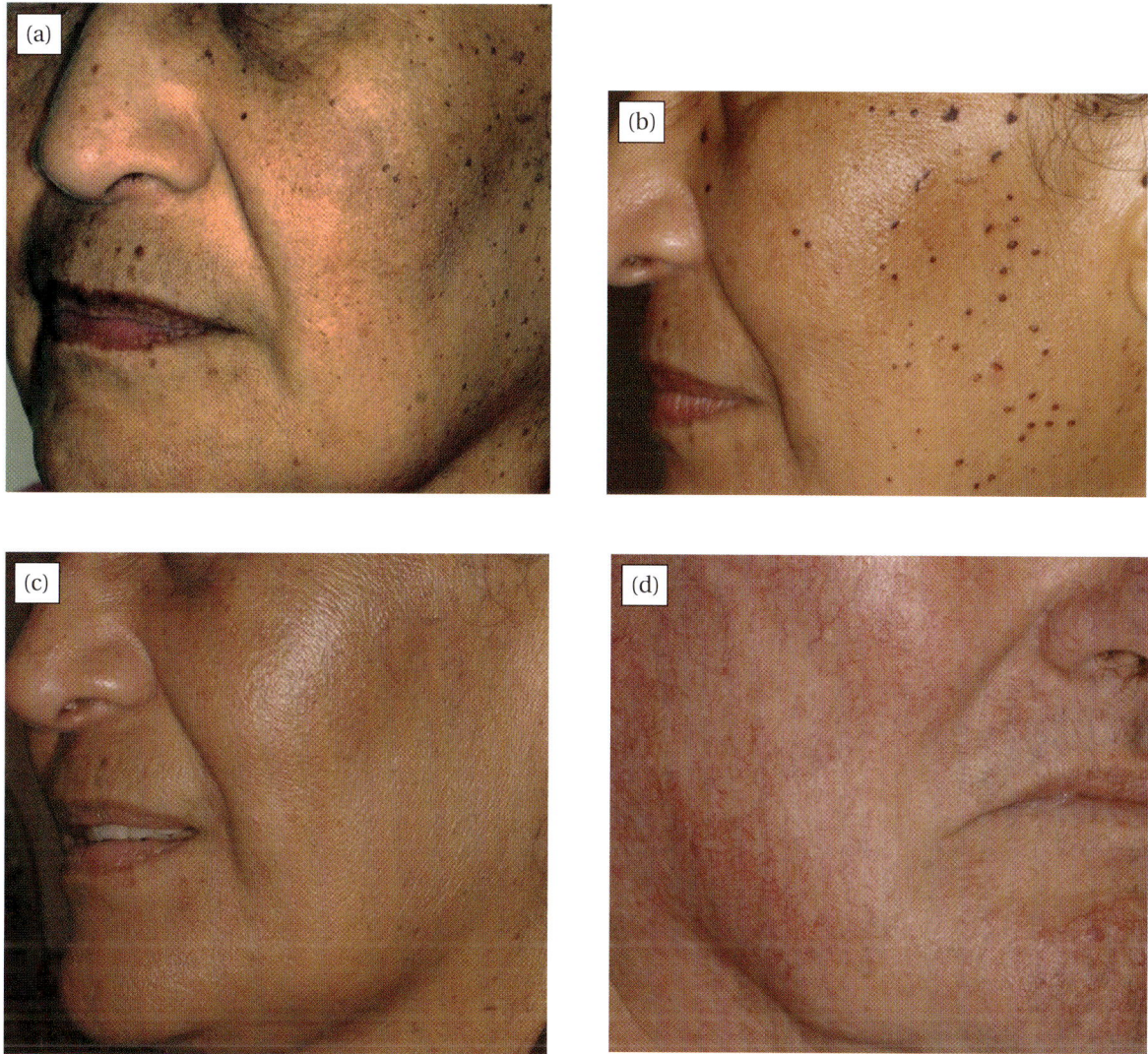

FIGURE 67.7 (a) Pretreatment photograph of a patient with dermatosis papulosa nigra. (b) Post-treatment photograph at 10 days. The KTP YAG laser has the advantage of being able to deposit energy over a longer period of time due to longer pulse widths. This allows for adequate thermal damage to the target, while minimizing damage to surrounding tissues. Note the crusting at the areas of treatment. (c) Post-treatment photograph at 6 weeks. (d) Pretreatment photograph of a patient with facial telangiectasias.

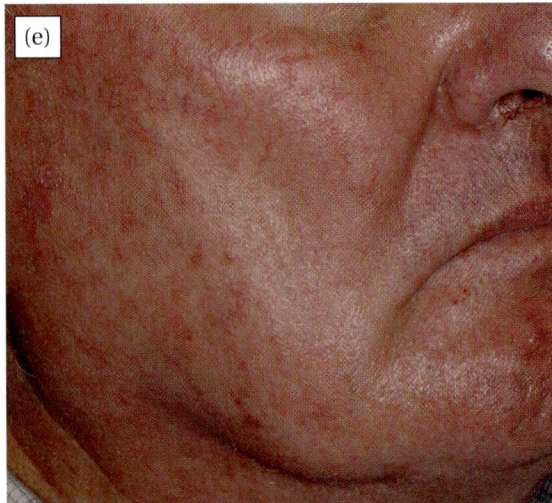

FIGURE 67.7 (*continued*) (e) Post-treatment photograph at 6 weeks.

Pulse Dye Laser (PDL) and Pulsed Q-switched YAG Laser

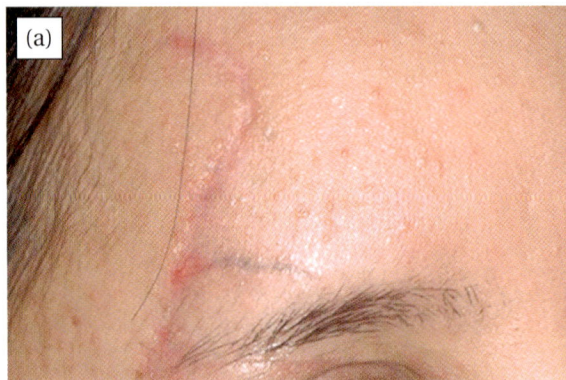

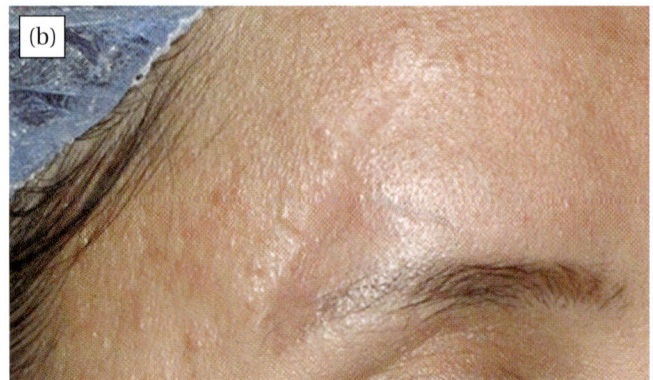

FIGURE 67.8 (a) Pretreatment photograph of a patient with scarring of the brow after a motor vehicle accident. Note that the majority of the scar is erythematous along with an inferior pigmented area. (b) Immediate post-treatment photograph. The PDL targets the erythematous scar, whereas the YAG laser targets the pigmented area.

TABLE 67.4 *Possible Complications*

Prolonged erythema

Hyperpigmentation

Hypopigmentation

Activation of herpes simplex virus

Skin fragility, peeling, and redness

Milia and acneiform eruptions

Scarring

SELECTED REFERENCES

Bogdan Allemann I, Kaufman J. Fractional photothermolysis—an update. *Lasers Med Sci.* 2010 Jan;25(1):137–144.

Brightman LA, et al. Ablative and fractional ablative lasers. *Dermatol Clin.* 2009 Oct;27(4):479–489, vi–vii.

Hantash BM, Mahmood MB. Fractional photothermolysis: a novel aesthetic laser surgery modality. *Dermatol Surg.* 2007 May;33(5):525–534.

Hunzeker CM, Weiss ET, Geronemus RG. Fractionated CO2 laser resurfacing: our experience with more than 2000 treatments. *Aesthet Surg J.* 2009 Jul–Aug;29(4):317–322.

Ross EV, et al. Full-face treatments with the 2790-nm erbium: YSGG laser system. *J Drugs Dermatol.* 2009 Mar;8(3):248–252.

Ross EV, Smirnov M, Pankratov M, Altshuler G. Intense pulsed light and laser treatment of facial telangiectasias and dyspigmentation: some theoretical and practical comparisons. *Dermatol Surg.* 2005 Sep;31(9 Pt 2):1188–1198.

SELECTED REFERENCES

Neurotoxins

TABLE 68.1 *Indications for Botulinum Toxin Treatment*

Cosmetic	Medical
Forehead furrows	Dystonias
Glabellar folds	Hemifacial spasm
Eyebrow contouring	Abberent seventh nerve regeneration
Crow's feet	Eyelid retraction
Nasal wrinkles	Ptosis
Lipstick lines	Neurogenic pain
Melomental/Labiomental folds	Hyperhidrosis
Chin dimpling	
Platysmal bands	
Hypertrophic orbicularis	

TABLE 68.2 *Contraindications for Botulinum Toxin Treatment*

- Prior allergic reaction
- Injection into areas of infection or inflammation
- Pregnancy Category C
- Breastfeeding (unknown if excreted in human milk)
- Diseases of the neuromuscular junction (e.g., myasthenia gravis or Lambert-Eaton neuropathy) or peripheral motor neuropathic diseases (e.g., amyotrophic lateral sclerosis)
- Aminoglycosides or agents that interfere with neuromuscular transmission
- Sensitivity or concern for human blood products (albumin)

TABLE 68.3 *Pre-treatment Considerations*

- Per FDA regulations, a copy of the Medication Guide must be distributed directly to each patient every time he/she receives a botulinum injection
- A detailed patient chart/procedure note outlining injection pattern, units injected per site, type of botulinum injected, lot number of botulinum vial(s) used, and response/reactions to previous treatments should be kept for each treatment
- Rhytids that are not dynamic in nature do not respond to treatment (e.g., caused by alteration in collagen, fat, or skin texture, such as in age-related changes, gravitational descent, or photodamage)
- Treatment effects will not be visible for 2–5 days
- Duration of treatment is variable, with 3–4 months being average
- Set appropriate expectations for the outcome of treatment (i.e., deep, longstanding rhytids may not completely resolve with one treatment)

TABLE 68.4 *Botulinum Toxin Preparations*

	Units per vial	Standard Dilution (mL)	Concentration per 0.1mL (units)
Botox® onabotulinumtoxinA	100	2	5
Dysport® abobotulinumtoxinA	300	2	30
Xeomin® incobotulinumtoxinA	50 or 100	1 (50 units)	5
		2 (100 units)	
Myobloc® rimabotulinumtoxinB	17,500	3.5*	500

Either preserved or unpreserved sterile, injectable saline (0.9% sodium chloride) is used for reconstitution. Final dilution is a matter of preference, however higher concentration solutions allow for more accurate delivery to a specific area by decreased diffusion due to volume effect.

*Myobloc is already in a 0.9% saline solution at a concentration of 5000 U per 1.0 cc, but may be further diluted if desired.

TABLE 68.5 *OnabotulinumtoxinA (Botox®) or IncobutulinumtoxinA Reconstitution (Xeomin®)*

Diluent Added	Resulting Units per 0.1 mL
1.0 mL	10.0 U
2.0 mL	5.0 U
2.5 mL	4.0 U
4.0 mL	2.5 U

Either preserved or unpreserved sterile, injectable saline (0.9% sodium chloride) is used for dilution.

TABLE 68.6 *AbobotulinumtoxinA (Dysport®) Reconstitution*

Diluent Added	Resulting Units per 0.1 mL
1.0 mL	30.0 U
1.5 mL	20.0 U
3.0 mL	10.0 U
4.0 mL	7.5 U

Either preserved or unpreserved sterile, injectable saline (0.9% sodium chloride) is used for dilution.

TABLE 68.7 *Botulinum Storage and Handling*

- Prior to reconstitution, store at 2–8°C for up to 36 months (note Xeomin can be refrigerated, but it is not required).
- Once reconstituted, refrigerate at 2–8°C.
- There is no consensus as to the amount of time reconstituted botulinum can be stored without losing efficacy. Generally up to one week is acceptable (Note this differs from package insert).
- In theory, Botulinum may be denatured by agitation.
- When reconstituting or diluting there is no need to "shake" the vial.

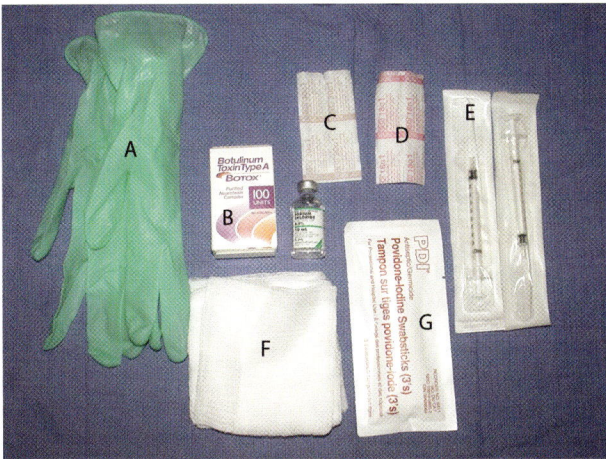

FIGURE 68.1 Recommended Supplies. A: Gloves—sterile or nonsterile. B: Appropriate dilution of botulinum toxin. C: 1″ 30 gauge needle for injecting patient. D: 1″ 18 gauge needle for drawing up botulinum toxin. E: 1cc syringe. F: Gauze—sterile or nonsterile. G: Betadine swab to prep injection sites.

TABLE 68.8 *Anesthesia*

- Based on patient's pain tolerance
- Majority of patients do not require anesthetic
- If anesthetic is required, ice or topical EMLA (lidocine 2.5% and prilocain 2.5%, APP Pharmaceuticals, Schaumburg, IL) or the equivalent and be used
- Vibratory stimulus may also be of use in decreasing perceived injection discomfort

TABLE 68.9 *Injection Technique*

- Mark injection sites with patient in seated, upright position activating the desired muscle(s)
- Needle depth—tip should be located in or on top of muscle being treated
- Typically inject at a 45-degree angle
- Skin "pinch" may decrease discomfort and aid localization of injection point
- Apply pressure if ecchymosis develops

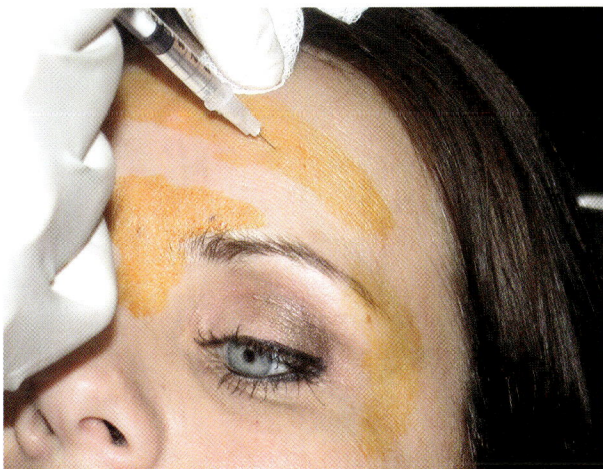

FIGURE 68.2 Injection Technique—Frontalis Injection. Areas of injection have been prepped with 10% povidone-iodine solution (Betadine; Solution Swabsticks, Purdue Products, L.P., Stamford, CT). Alternatively, an isopropyl alcohol prep can be used; however, there is no consensus as to the benefit of antisepsis prep prior to injection. As the injector becomes knowledgeable and comfortable with treatment, marking the injection areas prior to treatment may become unnecessary. If not employing the "skin" pinch injection method, the non-injecting hand should be used to stabilize the patient's head. Note the injection angle of approximately 45 degrees, and the injected solution beginning to form a skin elevation at the site of injection.

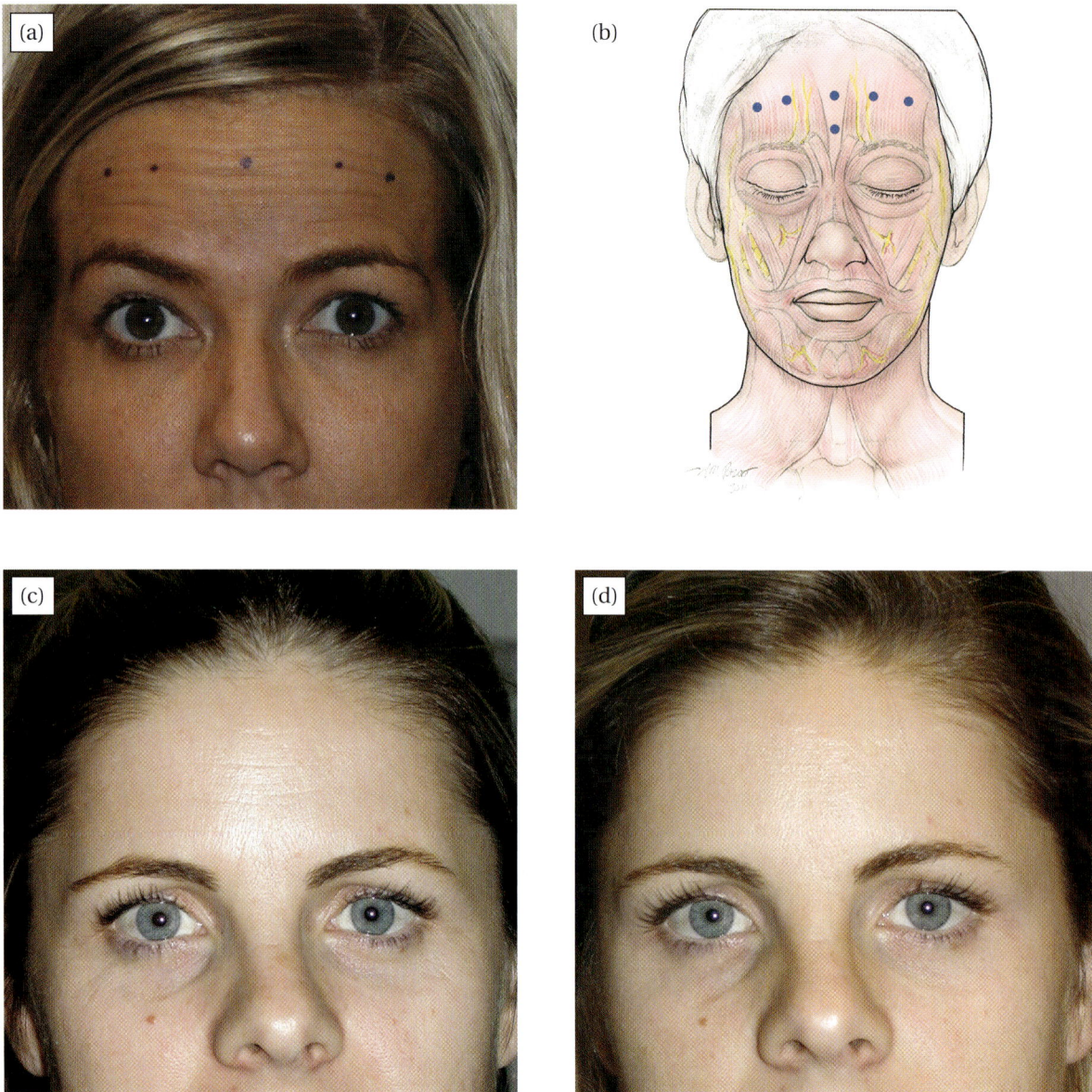

FIGURE 68.3 Forehead Furrows. (a) Injection sites are marked for the specific patient. (b) Anatomical diagram illustrating possible injection sites and the underlying musculature. *Muscle*: frontalis. *Injection Sites*: 2–7; location varies with individual anatomy. *Botox* 7.5–15 total units. *Dysport* 25 total units. *Pearl*: Avoid overtreating the frontalis, as it will result in brow ptosis. (c) Pre-treatment. (d) Post-treatment.

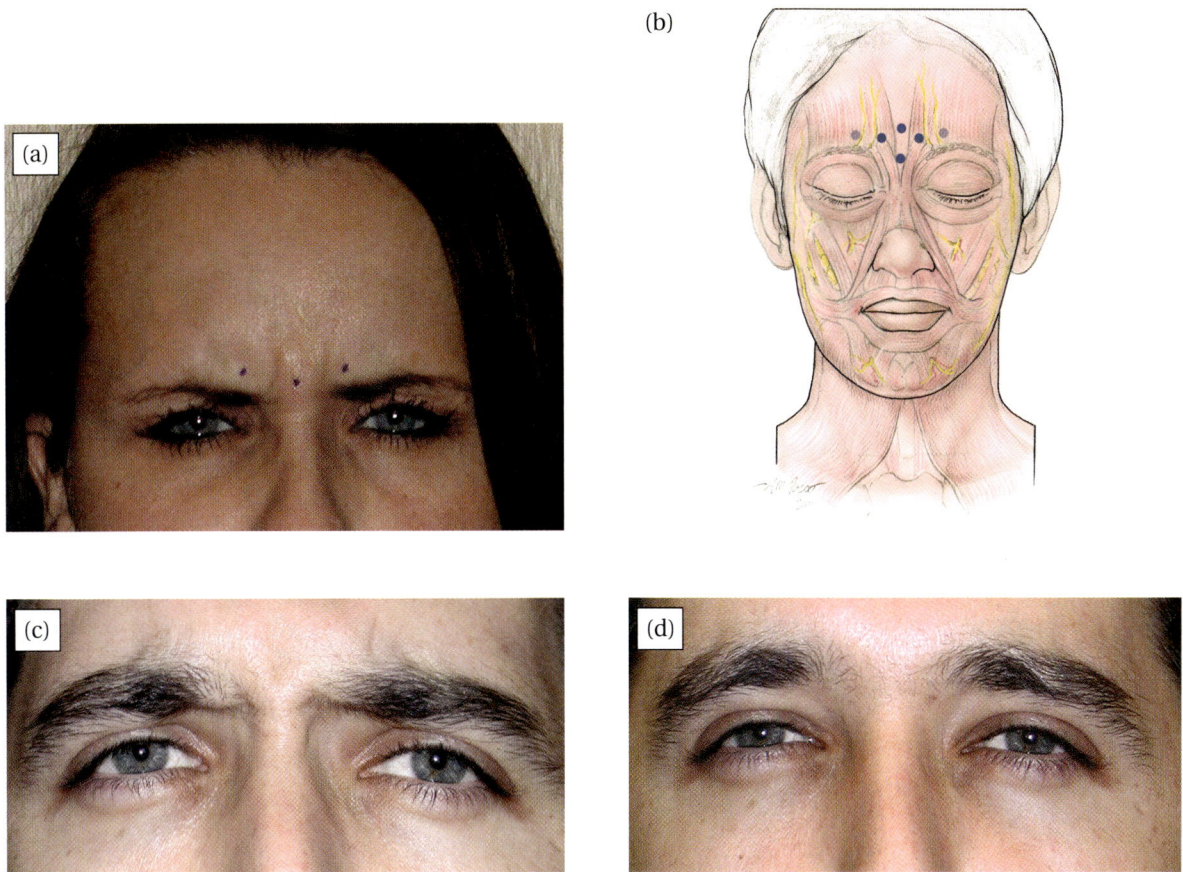

FIGURE 68.4 Glabellar Folds. (a) Injection sites are marked for the specific patient. (b) Anatomical diagram illustrating possible injection sites and the underlying musculature. Lighter blue marks correspond to optional injection sites. *Muscles*: corrugator supercillii, depressor supercillii & procerus. *Injection sites*: 2–6. *Botox* 15–40 units total. *Dysport* 45–90 units total. *Pearl*: Follow the muscle bulges for injection sites. (c) Pre-treatment. (d) Post-treatment.

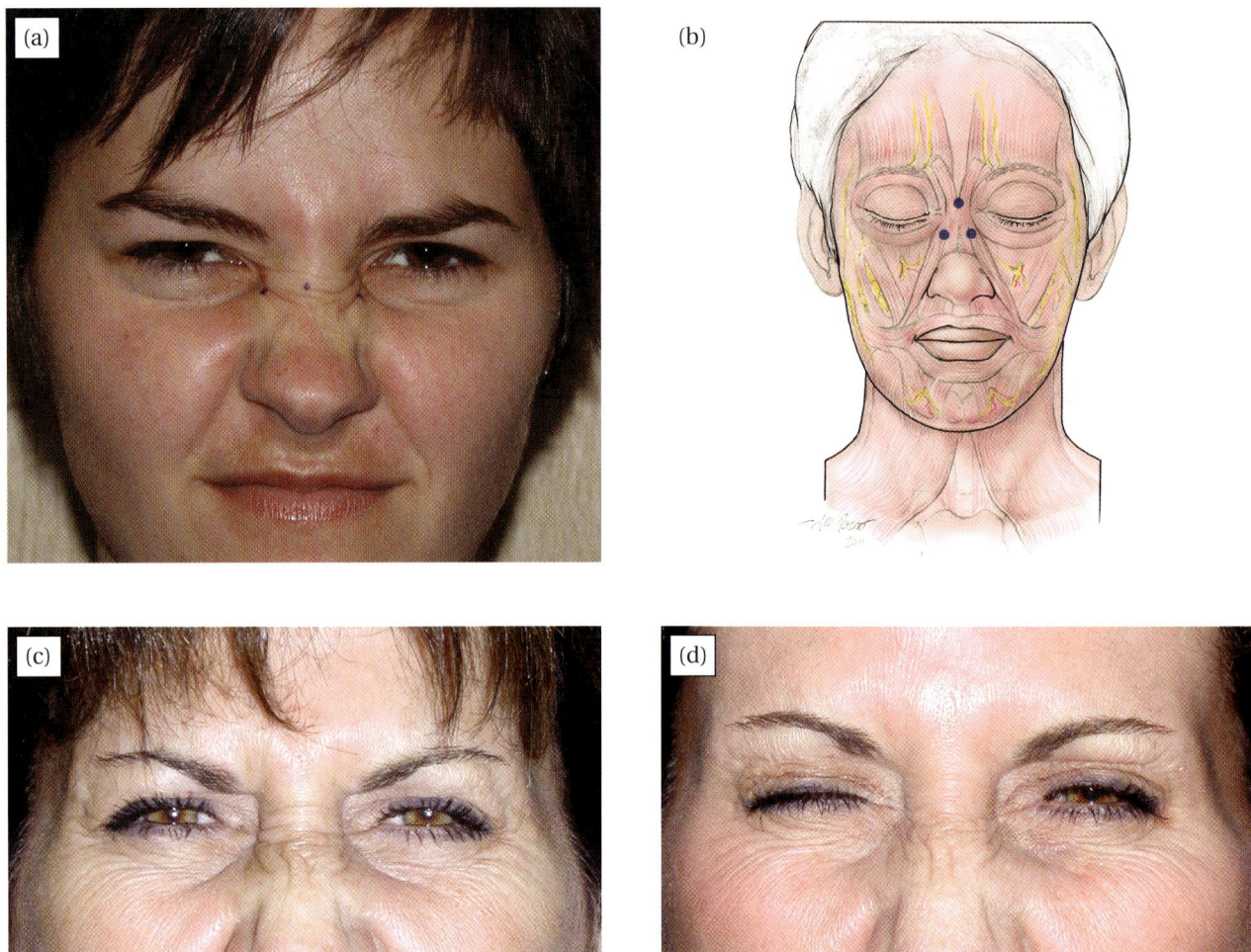

FIGURE 68.5 Nasal Wrinkles (Bunny Lines). (a) Injection sites are marked for the specific patient. (b) Anatomical diagram illustrating possible injection sites and the underlying musculature. *Muscles*: nasalis and procerus. *Injection sites:* 1–3. *Botox* 2–2.5 units per site. *Dysport* 7.5 units per site. *Pearl*: When simultaneously treating the glabella, the central area is often already treated, but one may wish to treat a little lower on the central injection if the horizontal nasal lines warrant it. (c) Pre-treatment. (d) Post-treatment.

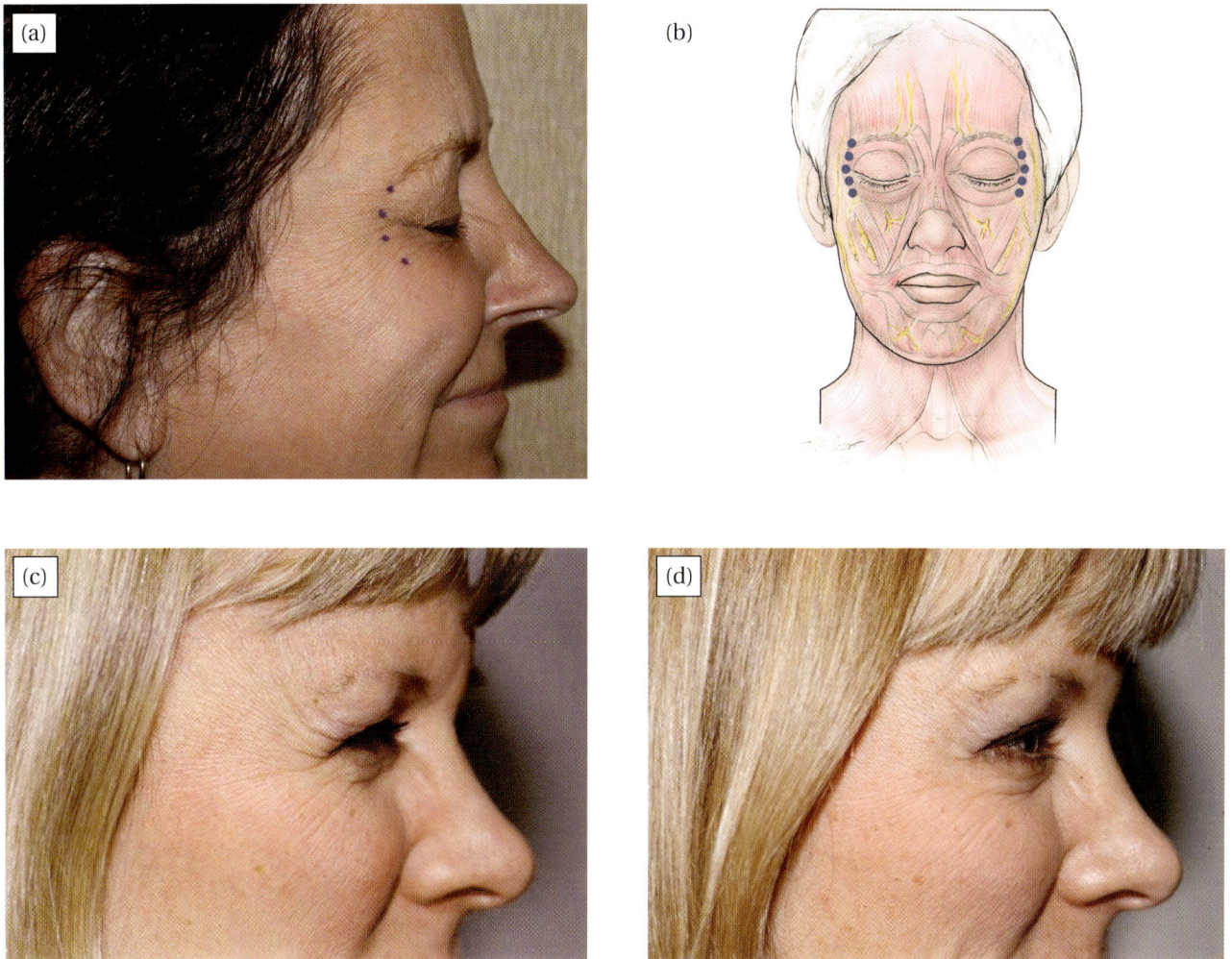

FIGURE 68.6 Lateral Periocular Wrinkles (Crow's Feet). (a) Injection sites are marked for the specific patient. (b) Anatomical diagram illustrating possible injection sites and the underlying musculature. *Muscle*: orbicularis oculi. *Injection sites*: 2–5 per side. *Botox* 15–25 units total. *Dysport* 45–80 units total. *Pearl*: Injection depth should be superficial as this region is prone to ecchymosis. (c) Pre-treatment. (d) Post-treatment.

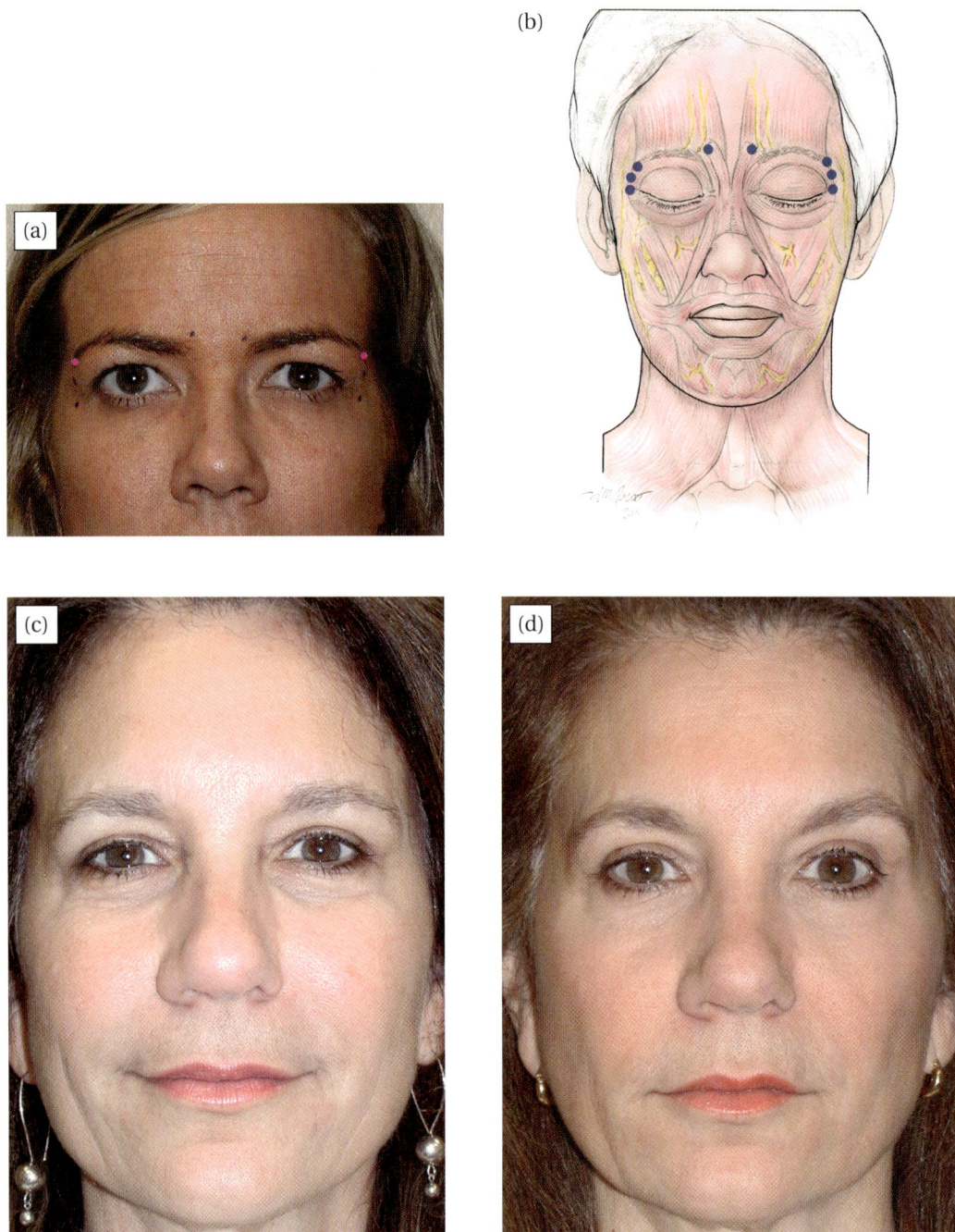

FIGURE 68.7 Brow Contouring. (a) Injection sites are marked for the specific patient (Note lateral brow injection site marking has been digitally enhanced for improved visibility). (b) Anatomical diagram illustrating possible injection sites and the underlying musculature. *Muscles*: orbicularis oculi and corrugator supercillii/procerus. *Injection sites*: 3–4 per side, including one paracentral nasal injection. *Botox* 2.5 units per site lateral, 5–10 units per site nasal. *Dysport* 7.5 units per site lateral, 10–20 units per site nasal. *Pearl*: Keep nasal injection low, to avoid frontalis. (c) Pre-treatment. (d) Post-treatment.

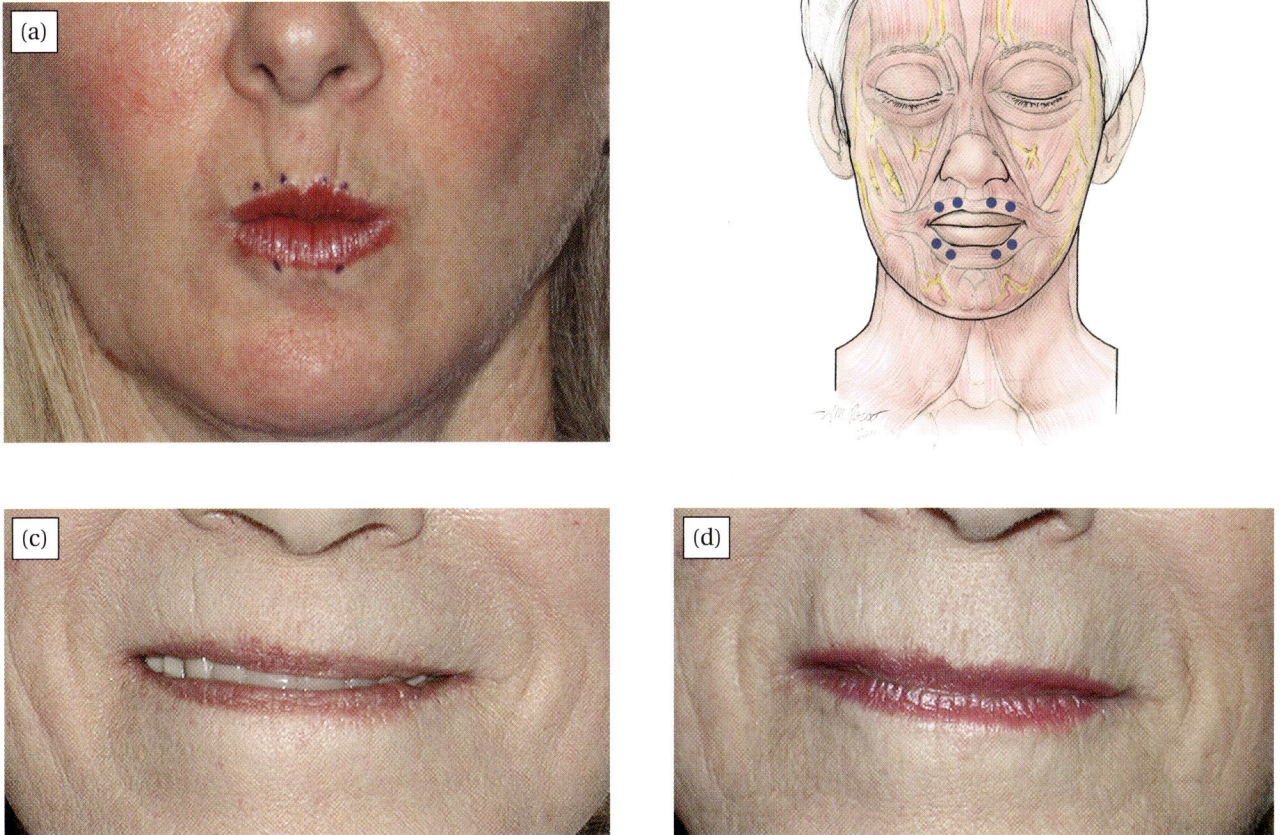

FIGURE 68.8 Perioral Wrinkles (Lipstick Lines). (a) Injection sites are marked for the specific patient. (b) Anatomical diagram illustrating possible injection sites and the underlying musculature. *Muscles*: orbicularis oris. *Injection sites*: 2–8. *Botox* 1–6 units total. *Dysport* 3–18 units total. *Pearl*: Treat symmetrically (even if the wrinkles aren't) to keep mouth movement natural. (c) Pre-treatment. (d) Post-treatment.

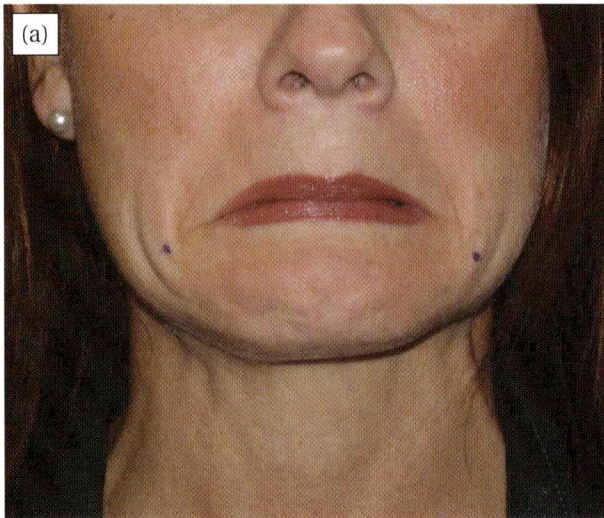

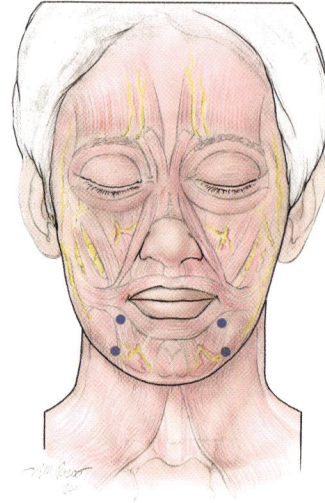

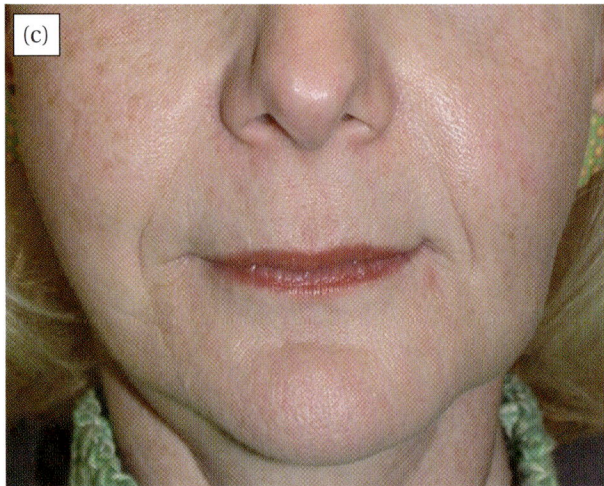

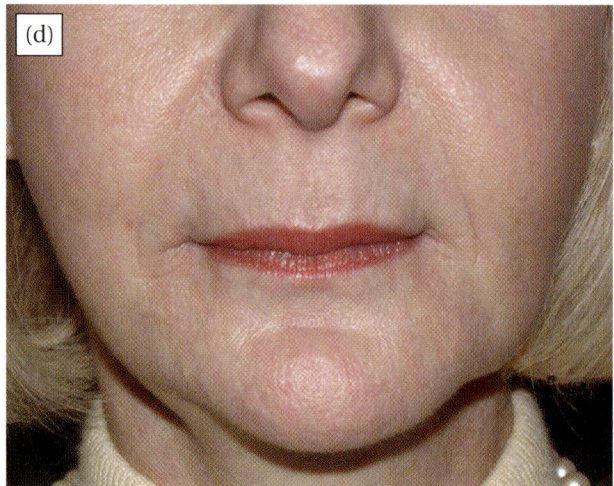

FIGURE 68.9 Labiomental (Melolabial) Folds. (a) Injection sites are marked for the specific patient. (b) Anatomical diagram illustrating possible injection sites and the underlying musculature. *Muscle*: Depressor anguli oris. *Injection sites*: 2–4. *Botox* 2–2.5 units per site. *Dysport* 5–7.5 units per site. *Pearl*: Stay lateral to avoid the depressor labii. (c) Pre-treatment. (d) Post-treatment.

(b)

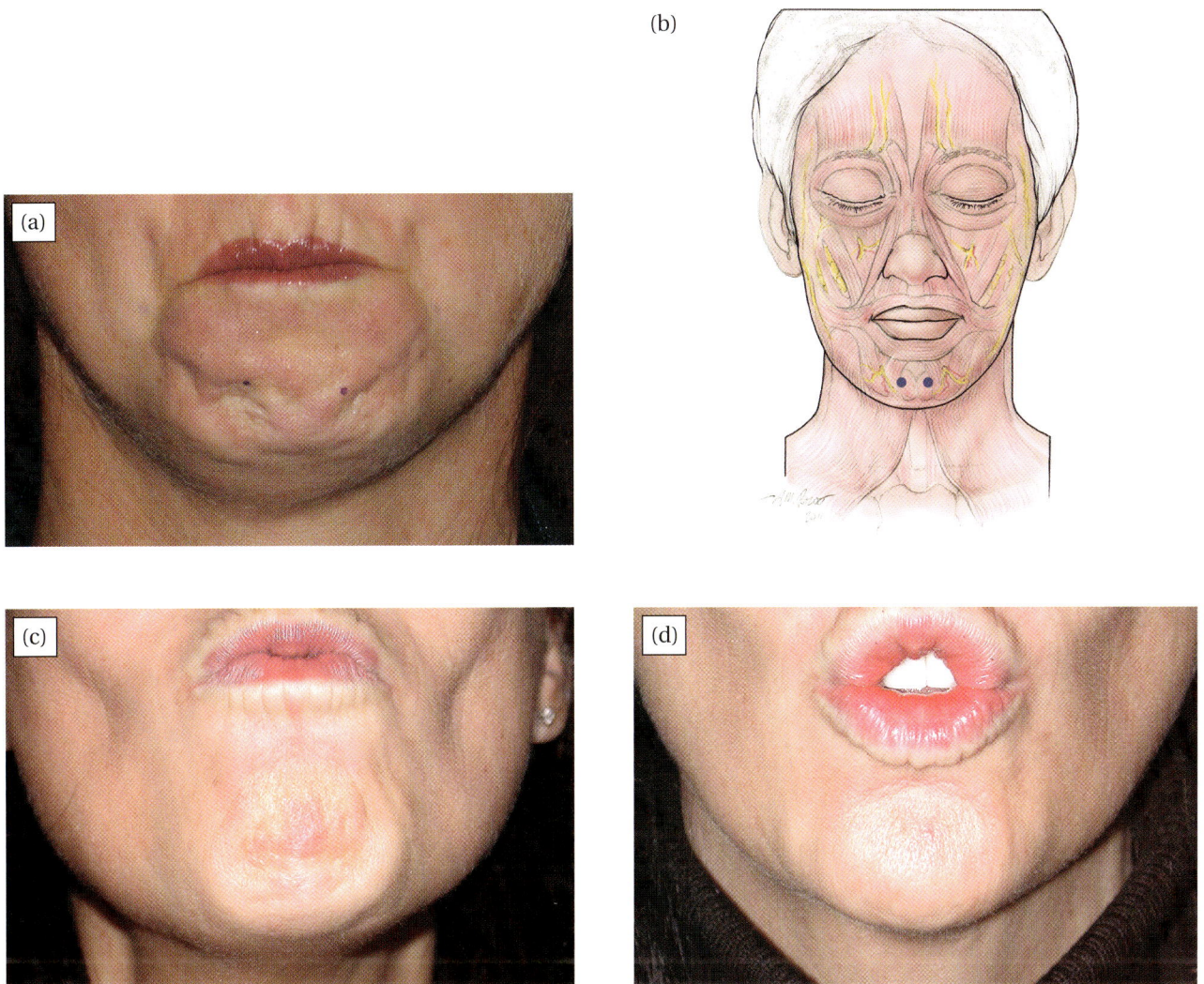

FIGURE 68.10 Chin Dimpling. (a) Injection sites are marked for the specific patient. (b) Anatomical diagram illustrating possible injection sites and the underlying musculature. *Muscle*: Mentalis. *Injection sites*: 2. *Botox* 2.5 units per site. *Dysport* 5–7.5 units per site. *Pearl*: Inject deeply to avoid depressor labii. (c) Pre-treatment. (d) Post-treatment.

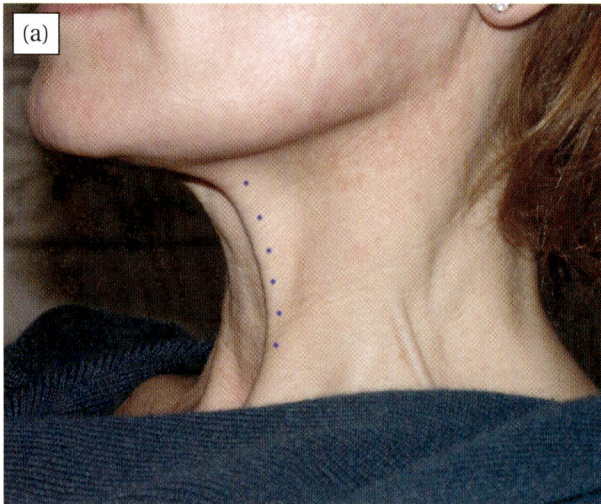

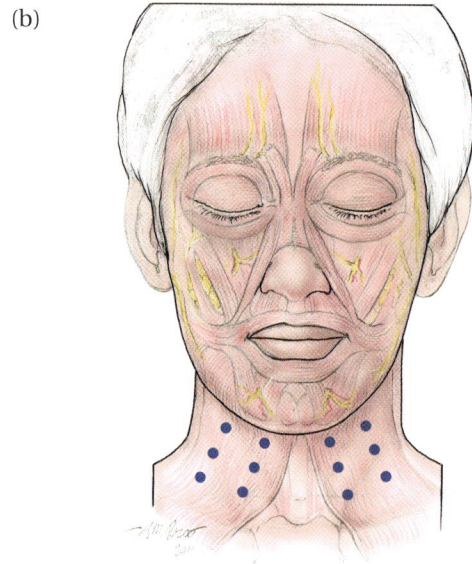

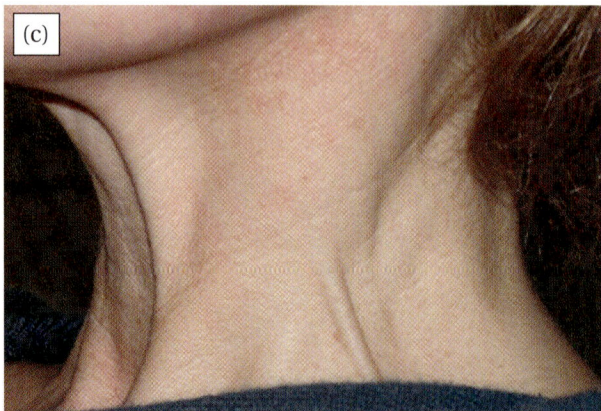

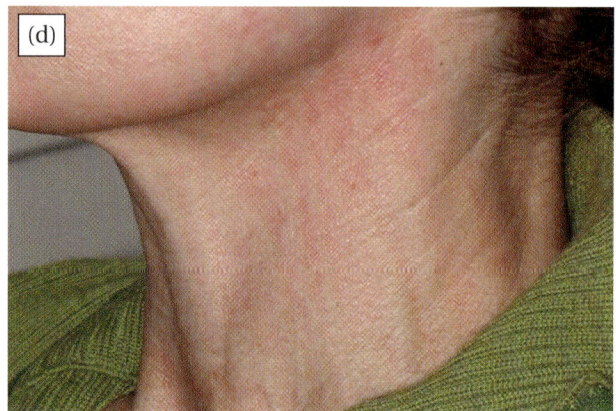

FIGURE 68.11 Platysmal Bands. (a) Injection sites are marked for the specific patient (note neck injection site markings have been digitally enhanced for improved visibility). (b) Anatomical diagram illustrating possible injection sites and the underlying musculature. *Muscle*: Platysma. *Injection sites*: 2–6 per band. Some patients have multiple bands. *Botox* 30–60 units; 2–2.5 units per site. *Dysport* 60–180 units total. *Pearl*: Use superficial injections to avoid surrounding structures. (c) Pre-treatment. (d) Post-treatment.

TABLE 68.10 *Complications and Management of Neurotoxins*

Injection Area	Complication	Management
Forehead	Brow ptosis	Obs/Treat brow depressors
	Uneven weakening/treatment	Treat non-weakened areas to achieve symmetry
Glabellar	Upper eyelid ptosis	Obs/brimonidine gtts
Brow	"Spocked" brow	Treat ipsilateral frontalis
	Upper eyelid retraction	Obs/Treat frontalis
	Sulcus reveal	Obs/Address underlying sulcus volume issues
Crow's Feet	Lagophthalmos	Obs/lubrication
	Inferior scleral show	Obs/lubrication
Nasal	Lip drop	Obs/treat contralateral levator labii for symmetry
Lipstick Lines	Drooling, inability to use straw	Obs
Labiomental	Rolling in of vermillion border on lower lip	Obs/treat contralateral depressor labii if asymmetric
	"Chipmunk" food storage in lower lip when eating	Obs
Chin	Accidental depressor labii block, and labiomental complications	Obs, treat asymmetry with contralateral injection
Platysma	Swallowing difficulty or voice changes	Obs
	Difficulty lifting head off pillow in AM	Obs

Just as treatment is individualized to each patient, management of complications varies based on multiple factors, including the potential further complications any intervention may cause. This table should be used as a generalized guideline for management of complications. The universal complications of ecchymosis and bleeding can be encountered at all injection areas. Primary treatment should be localized pressure to the area. Ice is a useful adjunct to pressure; however, it has been postulated the decreased tissue temperature caused by the ice might interfere with the botulinum mechanism of action.

Obs = Observation, gtts = drops.

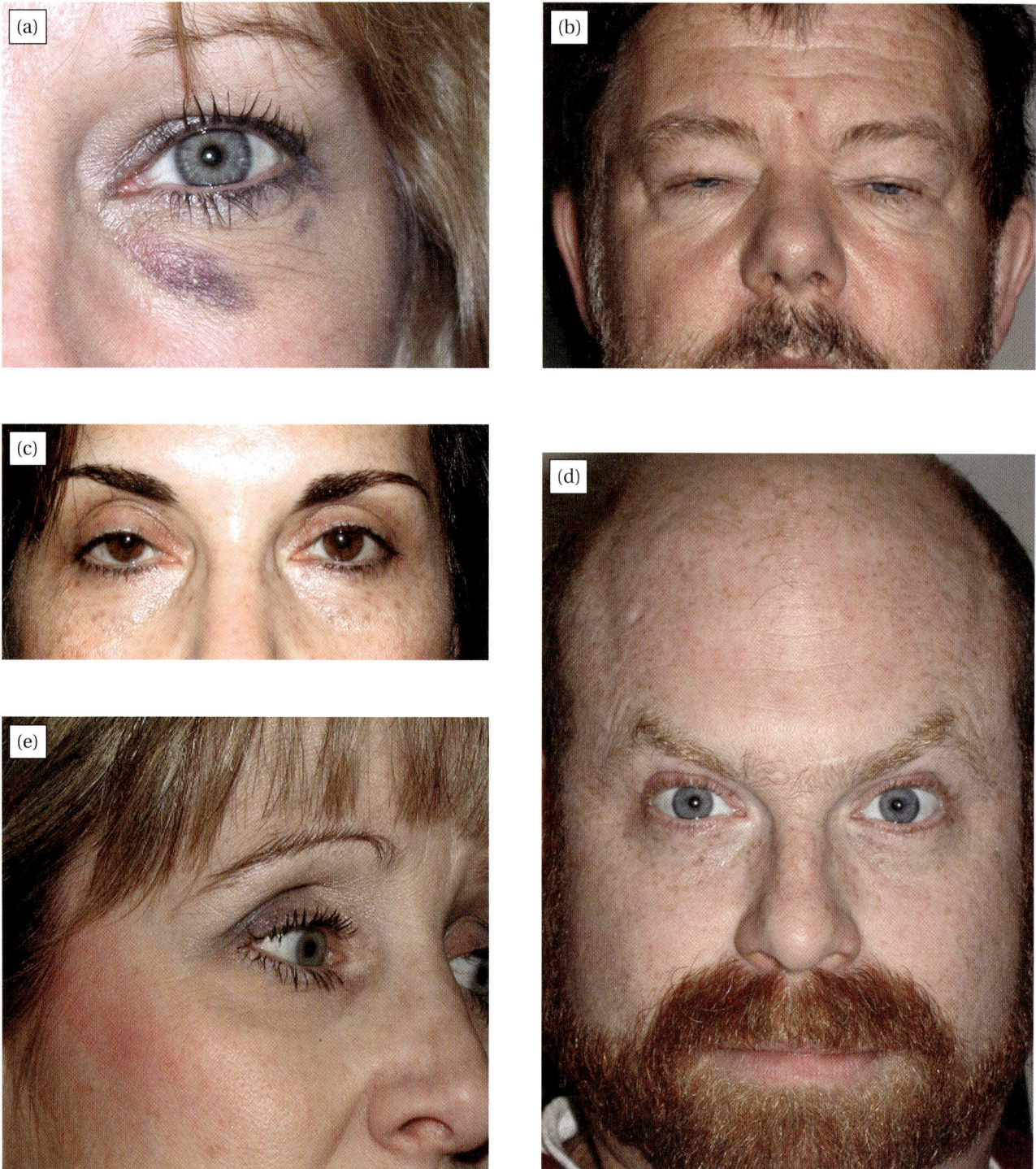

FIGURE 68.12   Common complications of botulinum treatment. (a) Ecchymosis from venopuncture during orbicularis (crow's feet) injection. (b) Brow ptosis resulting from unopposed action of the brow depressors. (c) Right upper eyelid ptosis resulting from diffusion of botulinum to the levator muscle. (d) Bilateral "Spocked" brow resulting from unopposed action of the frontalis laterally with medial weakening. (e) Prominent deep superior sulcus resulting from treatment of the brow depressors and an underlying sulcus volume deficiency.

Soft Tissue Fillers

TABLE 68.11 *FDA Approved Soft Tissue Fillers*

- **Autologous**
  Fat
  Dermis
- **Hyaluronic Acids**
  Synthetic/Bacteria
  Restylane®
  Perlane®
  Juvedérm™ and Juvéderm Ultra Plus™
  Prevelle Silk™
  Elevess™
  Captique™*
  Hydrelle™
  Animal derived
  Hylaform®* and Hylaform Plus®*
- **Silicone**
  Silikon® 1000#
  AdatoSil 5000
- **Poly-L-Lactic Acid**
  Sculptra®

- **Calcium Hydroxylapatite Microspheres**
  Radiesse®
- **Polymethylmethacrylate (PMMA) Microspheres and Bovine Collagen**
  Artefill©*
  ArteColl®*
- **Collagen**
  Bovine
  Zyderm®
  Zyplast®
  Human
  Cosmoderm™
  Cosmoplast™
  Porcine
  Evolence®*

* No longer commercially available in the United States, included as background for previously treated patients.

Reformulated as Prevelle Silk.

TABLE 68.12 *Comparison of Hyaluronic Acids*

	Restylane Perlane	Juvéderm Ultra Juvéderm UltraPlus	Prevelle Silk	Hylaform Plus
Source	Bacteria	Bacteria	Bacteria	Animal
Cross-linking agent/ degree of cross-linking	BDDE <2%	BDDE 6–11%	DVS >20%	DVS 20%
Total HA concentration	20 mg/mL	24 mg/mL	5.5 mg/mL	4.5–6.0 mg/mL
Average particle size	250 um 1000 um	Various sizes	300 um	750 um

BDDE = 1,4-Butanediol diglycidyl ether, DVS = divinyl sulphone.

TABLE 68.13   *Indications for Soft Tissue Fillers*

• **Cosmetic**	• **Medical**
Glabellar folds	Craniofacial asymmetry
Eyebrow contouring	Tissue loss/Wasting
Superior sulcus shaping	Correction of surgical complications
Crow's feet	Scar revision
Nasal contouring	
Tear trough	
Cheek augmentation	
Nasolabial folds	
Melomental folds/Oral commisure	
Lip shaping	
Labiomental fold	
Pre-jowl sulcus	
Temporal hollowing	
Pre-parotid hollowing	

TABLE 68.14   *Contraindications for Soft Tissue Fillers*

- Prior allergic reactions
- Hypersensitivity to any of the components of the product including allergy to Gram-positive bacterial proteins, porcine products, avian proteins, or collagen
- Injection into areas of infection or inflammation
- Pregnancy/breastfeeding safety unknown

These contraindications are generalized and may vary between filler products. See package insert for details specific to product.

TABLE 68.15   *Treatment Precautions for Soft Tissue Fillers*

- Possible risk of inflammatory reaction at site of implantation, with procedures causing a dermal response (laser, chemical peels)
- Immunosuppressive therapy
- Bleeding disorders or anticoagulant therapy
- History of keloid formation or hypertrophic scarring
- History of recurrent herpetic eruptions

The table describes generalized precautions for treatment as stated by the product inserts. Use caution and clinical discretion when treating individuals, and refer to package insert for specific product for details, as precautions may vary between filler products.

TABLE 68.16 *Pre-treatment Considerations*

Universal Pre-treatment Considerations for all Soft Tissue Filler Types

- Set appropriate expectations for the outcome of treatment
- Differentiate dynamic from static shape changes
- Use a patient chart/procedure note detailing injection pattern, volume injected per site, type of filler injected, lot number of syringes used, and response/reactions to previous treatments
- Photograph full face, not just areas undergoing treatment. Pre-treatment photographs should be available for review at time of treatment
- Assess the patient's needs for anesthesia
- Prep injection areas with antiseptic solution

TABLE 68.17 *Post-treatment Considerations*

- New patient follow-up visit in 2–4 weeks to assess results
- Patient should avoid excessive sun (UV lamp) and extreme heat or cold until initial swelling and redness have resolved
- Patients should avoid strenuous exercise and alcoholic beverages for 24 hours
- Consider ice for swelling and comfort within 24 hours (avoid direct contact of ice with the skin)
- Calcium hydroxylapatite fillers are radiopaque on CT scans and possibly plain radiography

Generalized post-treatment considerations, which may vary between products. See specific product insert for details.

TABLE 68.18 *Filler Handling and Storage*

- Store at room temperature*
- Do not freeze
- Avoid exposure to sunlight
- All soft tissue fillers are indicated for single use. Literature has suggested storage and reuse is possible.
- There is no literature available describing the efficacy of filler materials after storage
- Literature suggests no increased risk of infection with reuse

* "Room Temperature" range varies between products. See product insert for specific ranges. Generally 15°C to 30°C is an acceptable storage range.

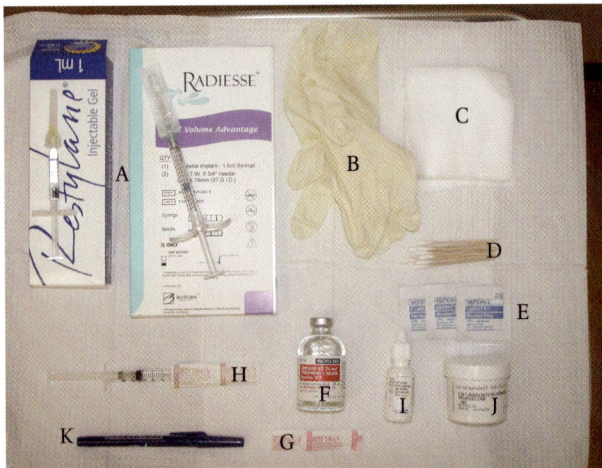

FIGURE 68.13 Recommended Supplies for Hyaluronic Acid Injection. A: Injectable filler compound of choice. B: Gloves—sterile or nonsterile. C: Gauze—sterile or nonsterile. D: Cotton swabs. E: Alcohol or betadine swab to prep injection sites. F: Local anesthetic. G: 1″ 18 gauge needle for drawing up local anesthetic. H: 1″ 30 gauge needle for injecting local anesthetic (area dependent— 1.5″, 1″, 0.5″ 30 or 27 gauge can be used). I: Tetracaine for oral topical. J: Topical anesthetic. K: Surgical marking pen.

TABLE 68.19 *Topical Anesthesia*

- 20% benzocaine, 8% lidocaine. 4% Tetracaine, with a Lipoderm cream base
- "BLT" Formulation—not FDA approved
- Must be prescribed by a physician and compounded by a pharmacy

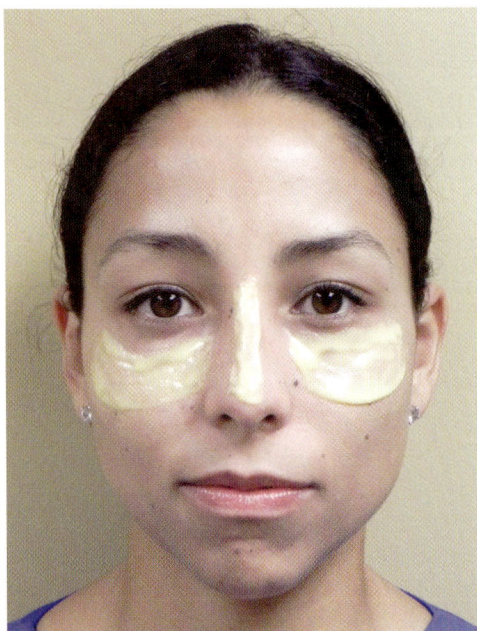

FIGURE 68.14 Topical Anesthesia Application. Although the comfort of injection has been improved by the addition of anesthetic to the products, some patients will still have a more pleasant experience if efforts are made to further diminish the pain of injection. Topical, local or regional anesthesia techniques may be employed. If it is determined the patient requires topical anesthesia for comfort, the BLT compound is placed on the treatment areas 20 minutes prior to treatment. Other FDA approved topical compounds such as a mixture of lidocaine 2.5% and prilocaine 2.5% (EMLA˙, APP Pharmaceuticals, Schaumburg, IL) or Ela-Max˙ (Ferndale Laboratories Inc., Ferndale, MI) [Ela-Max – LMX 4˙ (4% lidocaine) and LMX 5˙ (5% lidocaine)]can also be used. Efficacy with time of placement prior to treatment is unique for each compound.

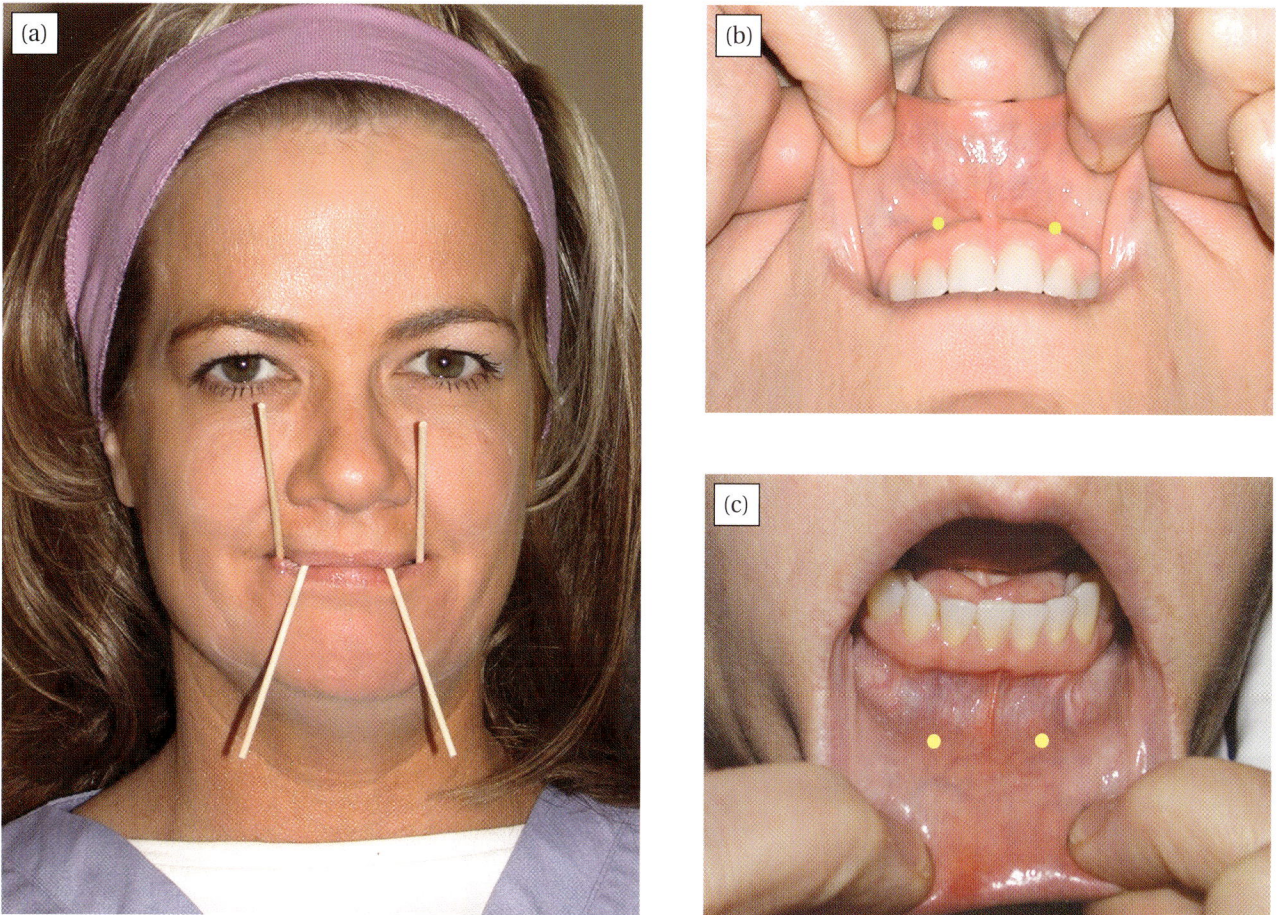

FIGURE 68.15 Topical and Local Anesthesia. The lip area is a location with tremendous sensitivity. Some patients will tolerate the filler/anesthetic mix without additional numbing, but for others, topical, local or regional anesthesia techniques may be employed to diminish injection pain. When augmenting the lips alone, a local block may be all that is necessary, rather than a regional nerve block. (a) The oral mucosa of the buccal gingival cul-de-sacs is pretreated with tetracaine topical anesthetic on cotton applicators. (b, c) Small amounts of local anesthetic (0.2 cc to 0.3 cc per site) can be placed at two to four locations in the buccal gingival cul-de-sacs as indicated by the yellow dots.

(a)

(b)

Area of anesthetic effect   Infraorbital nerve

(c)

Infraorbital
nerve

Mental nerve

Area of   Mental
anesthetic effect   nerve

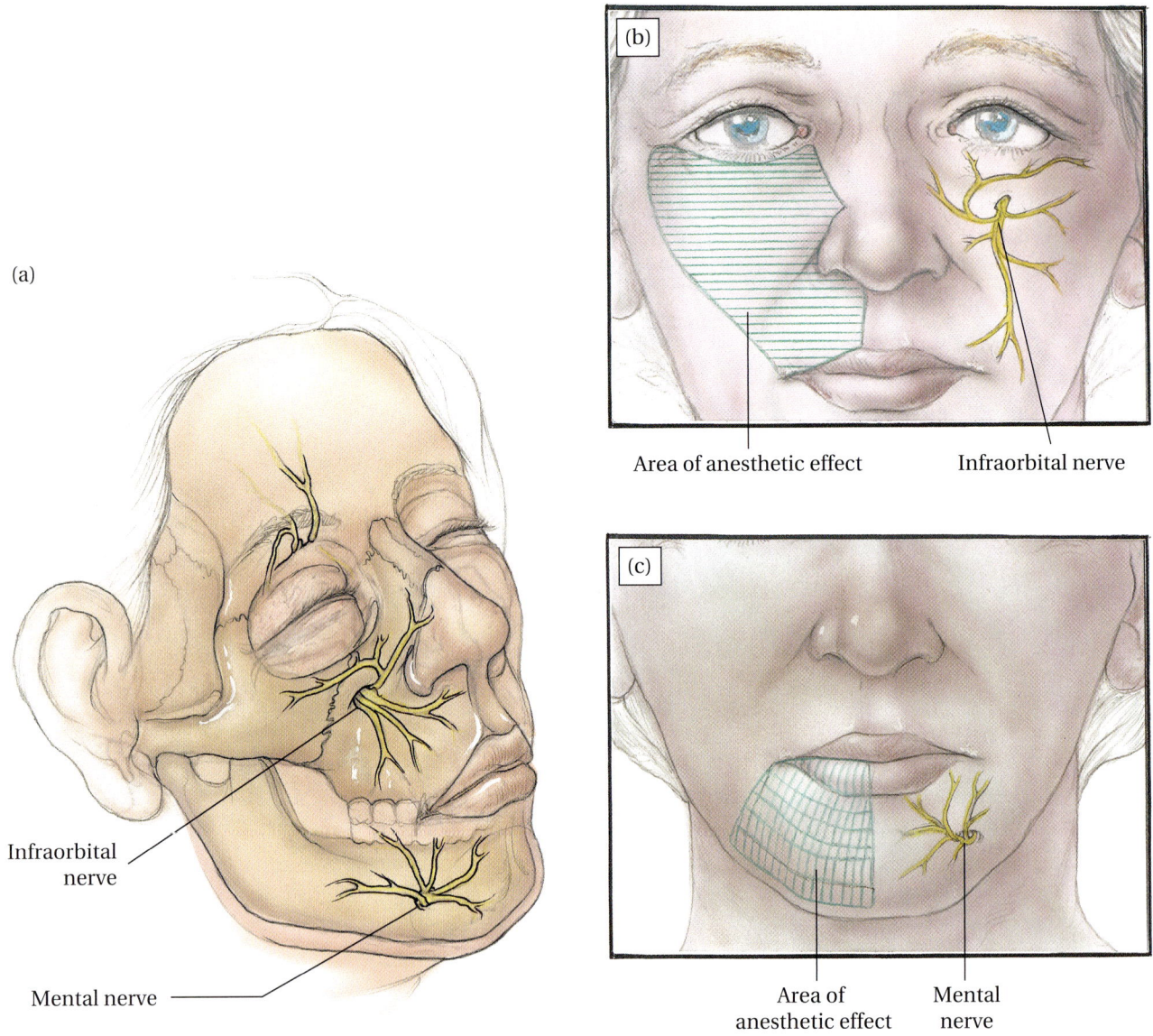

FIGURE 68.16 Regional Anesthesia. (a) Pertinent nerve anatomy. (b, c) Corresponding dermatomes of effect.

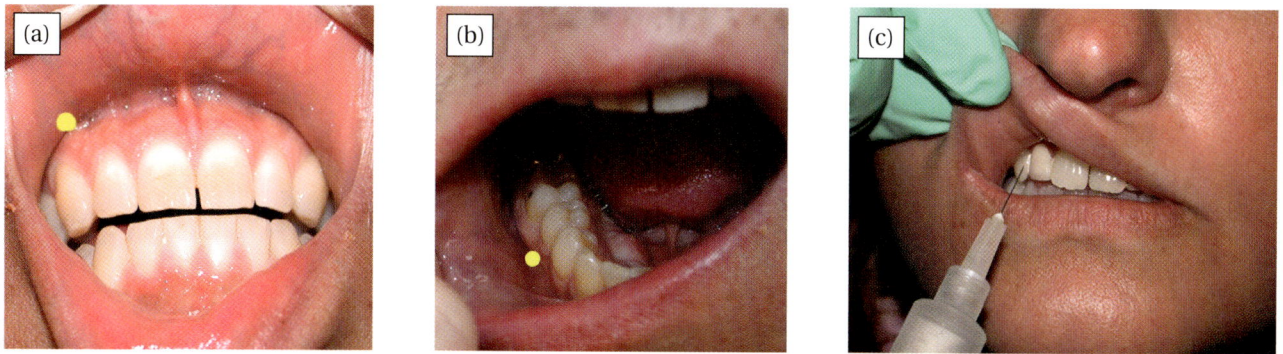

FIGURE 68.17 Regional Anesthesia Application. (a) Infraorbital nerve block in placed above the canine tooth as indicated by yellow dot. (b) Mental nerve block is placed below the second bicuspid tooth as indicated by yellow dot. (c) The lip is distracted and inverted. providing exposure of the injection site. A 1″ or 1.5″ 30 or 27 gauge can be used for injection.

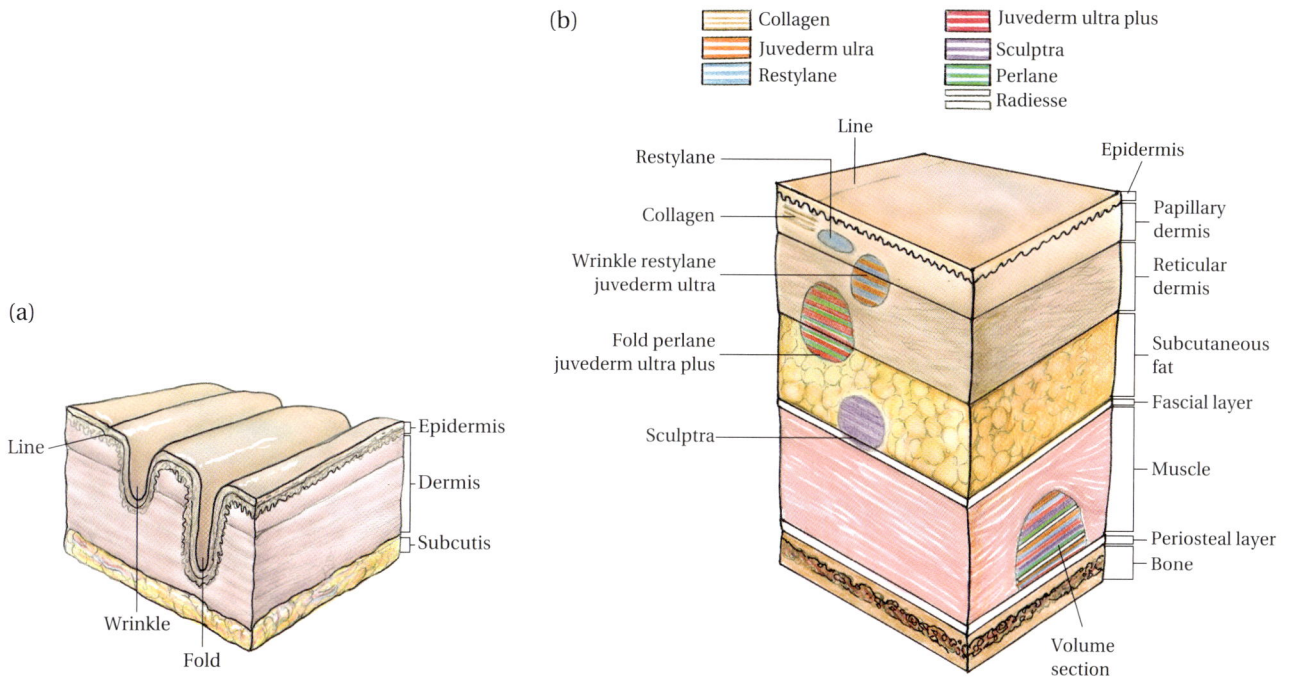

FIGURE 68.18 Tissue Anatomy and Level of Filler Placement. (a) Tissue level of cosmetic defects: lines, wrinkles and folds. (b) Skin and soft tissue anatomy. The tissue level of filler placement is shown for the corresponding defects from (a). In general, the less pliable the filler, the deeper the dermal placement. Sculptra is placed subcutaneously or just above the periosteum.

(a)

(b)

(c)

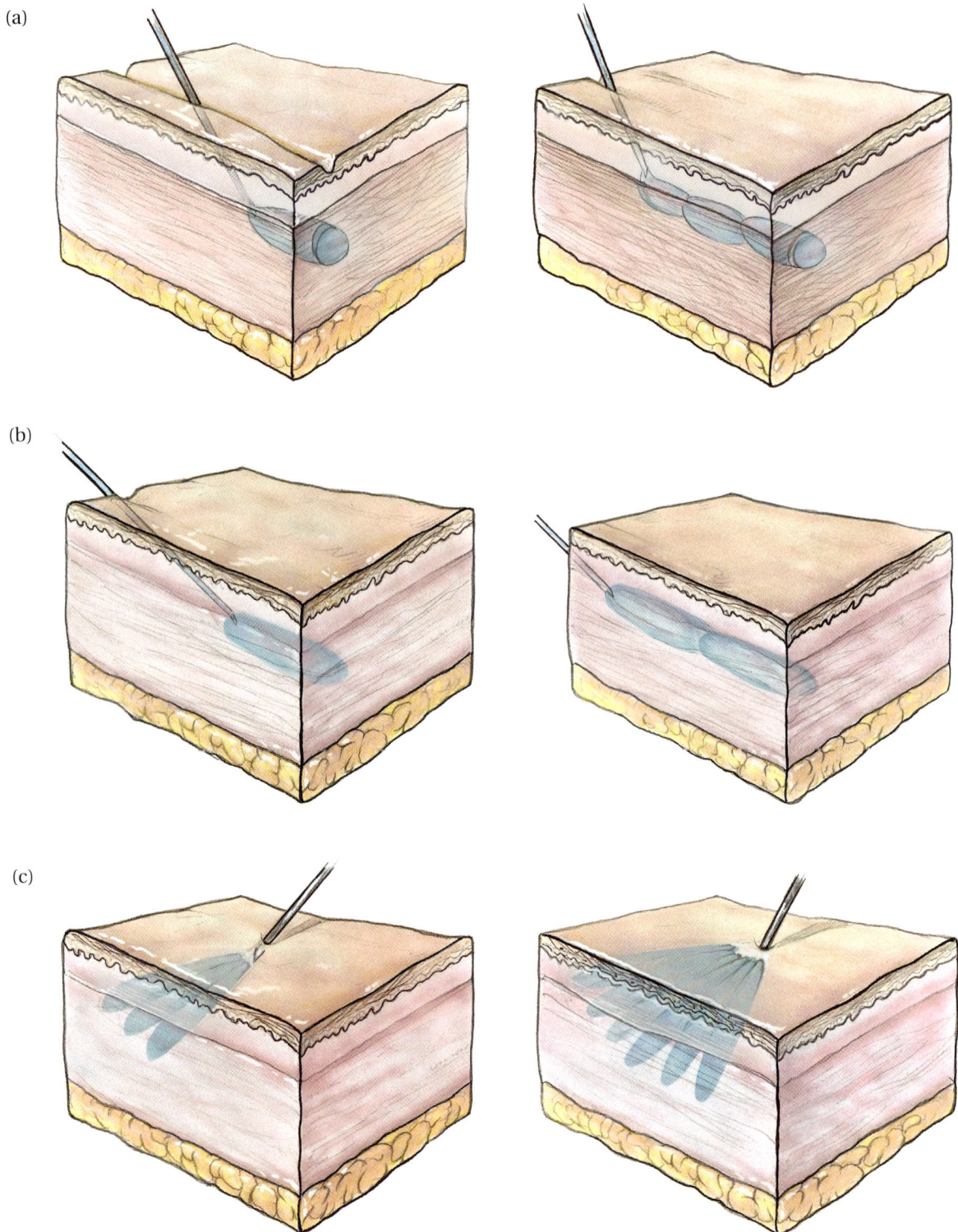

FIGURE 68.19 Injection Techniques. (a) *Serial Puncture/Depot*. A small "bead" or a series of little "beads" of filler are placed at the injection site. Massage is used to flatten the filler. (b) *Linear Threading*. Insert the needle through the middle of the defect. Inject the material while pulling the needle slowly backward and repeat as needed forming a continuous line. Linear threading may also be accomplished in an anterograde fashion with a "push ahead" technique, where a small amount of injected filler clears the way to advance the needle. (c) *Fanning*. Injection technique mirrors linear threading. After injecting each line, without withdrawing the needle, change the direction of injection, repeating to form a fan-shaped pattern.

(d)

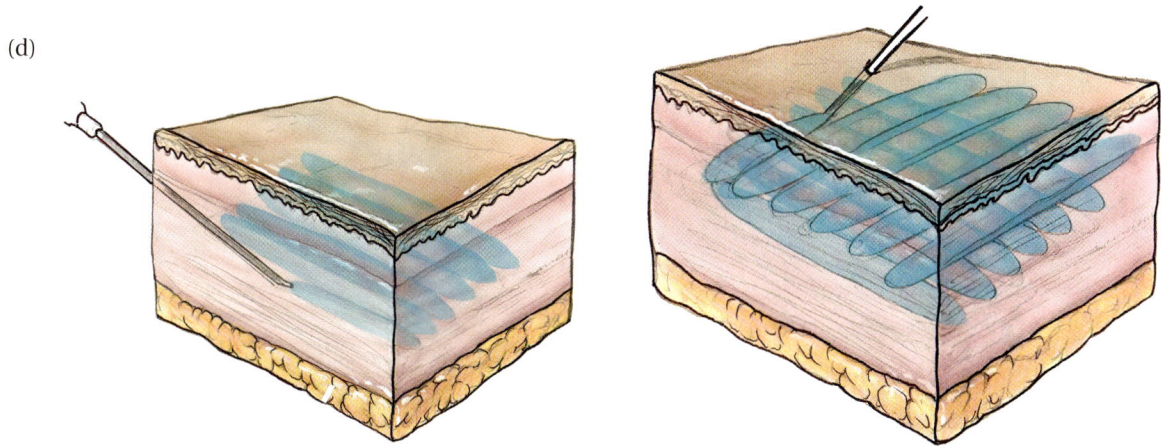

FIGURE 68.19 (*continued*) (d) *Crosshatching*. Injection technique mirrors linear threading. After injecting each line, withdraw the needle and reinsert to form a series of linear threads. Change the angle of injection to form a new series of threads at a slightly different tissue level.

TABLE 68.20 *Hyaluronic Acid Injection Pearls*

- To improve symmetry, mark treatment areas with patient in upright position. Markings are most helpful for volume replacement locations. Consider injecting with the patient in upright position as well.
- Provide anesthesia to assist patient comfort.
- 30 or 27 gauge needle, 1", 1.5", or 0.5" depending on area and type of material.
- Inject small amounts (0.05 cc) **slowly** in multiple passes. Larger, deeply placed aliquots may be used for volumizing injections.
- Plan and minimize puncture sites. Stop injecting prior to needle withdrawal to avoid superficial injections.
- Massage and mold area for desired contour.
- Avoid overcorrection. If indicated, plan sequential injections to provide full correction. This is particularly important in the lips, where shape is as important as volume, and volume is sometimes the enemy of shape.
- Try to avoid intravascular injection.

TABLE 68.21 *Glabellar Furrows*

- This is an area with some danger for occlusion of terminal arteries. Watch for blanching and treat promptly.
- Filler type: "Softer" filler such as Juvéderm or Restylane should be used.
- Injection technique: Linear threading. The material is placed below the furrows with retrograde threading. This technique is easier with the patient in a slightly reclined position.
- Typical volume: 0.2 cc to 0.4 cc
- Pearl: Pretreating or concomitantly treating the furrows with botulinum toxin is recommended.

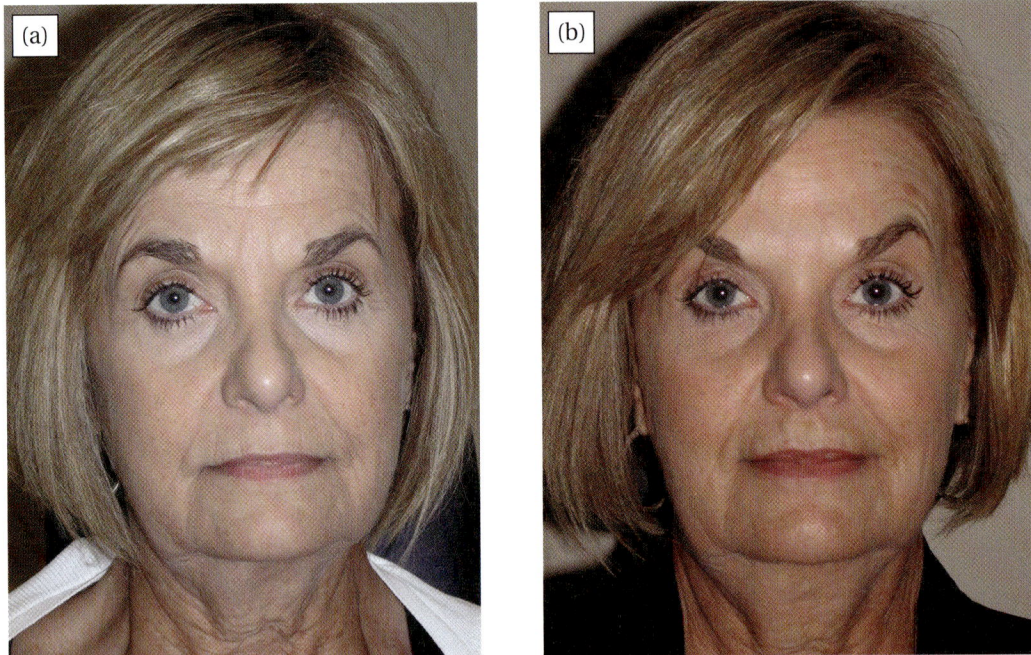

FIGURE 68.20 Glabellar furrows. (a) Pre-treatment. The patient has deep glabellar furrows. (b) Post-treatment. The glabellar area is softened following filling of the furrows with Juvéderm and neurotoxin treatment of the corrugators. Note the high arched brow contour is the patient's preference, not a complication of treatment.

TABLE 68.22 *Brow Contouring*

- The eyebrow has a three-dimensional shape, and fat/volume loss in the AP dimension increases lateral brow ptosis. Replacement of the lateral brow fat with filler improves projection and appearance.
- Filler type: "Thicker" filler such as Juvéderm UP or Perlane
- Injection technique: Crosshatching. Material is placed beneath the brow cilia at the lateral and more inferior aspect of the brow hair to restore shape.
- Typical volume: 0.1 cc to 0.3 cc per side
- *Pearl*: Brow filler injections cause minimal discomfort. Topical anesthetic alone is almost always adequate.

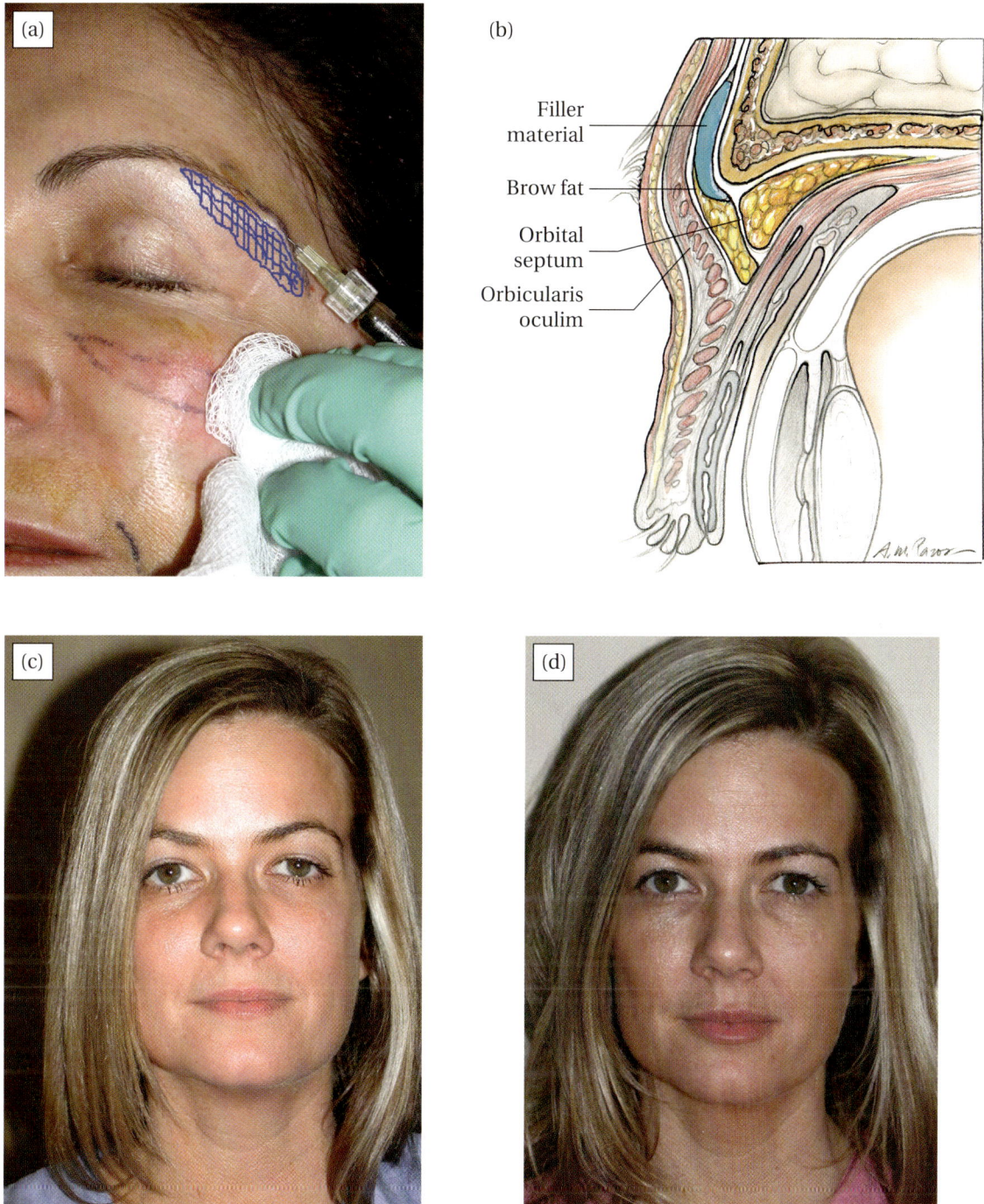

FIGURE 68.21 Brow contouring. Injection proceeds in a crosshatching manner as indicated by blue lines. (b) Cross section indicating anatomical location and tissue level of filler placement. (c) Pre-treatment. (d) Post-treatment. Patient also had Restylane placed in tear trough and lips.

TABLE 68.23 *Superior Sulcus Shaping*

- Hollowing of the superior sulcus may occur from orbital volume changes, or iatrogenically as a result of blepharoplasty. Fillers offer a minimally invasive technique for augmentation.
- Filler type: Restylane
- Injection technique: Serial puncture/depot. Serial depot injections are placed below the orbicularis and anterior to the orbital fat below the orbital rim.
- Typical volume: 0.2 cc to 0.5 cc per side
- Pearl: Highly vascular area (especially medially); avoid intravascular injection

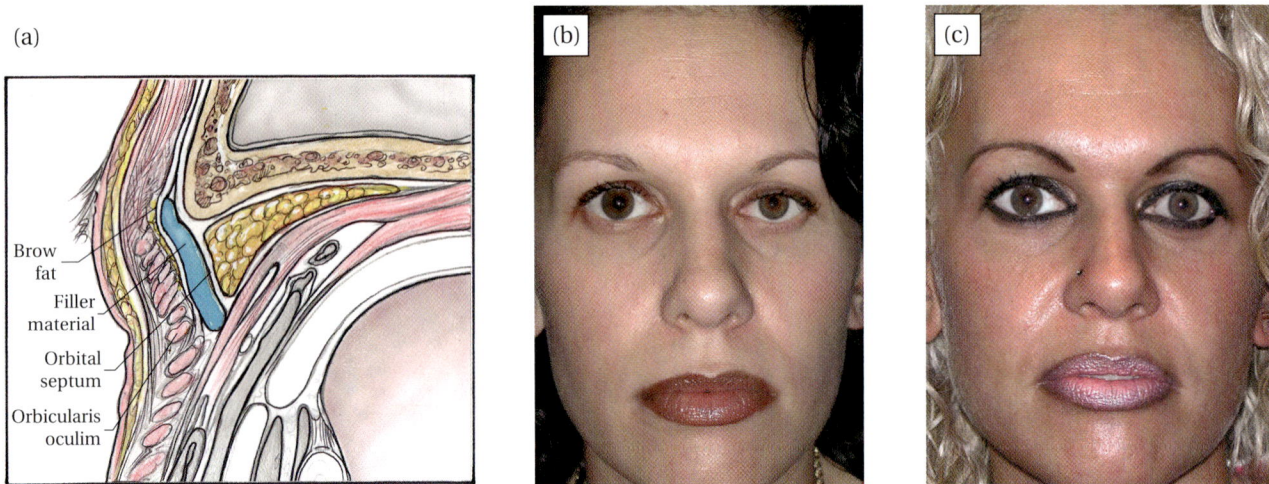

FIGURE 68.22 Superior sulcus shaping. (a) Cross section indicating anatomical location and tissue level of filler placement. (b) Pre-treatment. Note the hollowing of the left sulcus. (c) Post-treatment. The left sulcus has been reshaped with Restylane to better match the right side.

TABLE 68.24 *Crow's Feet*

- Botulinum toxin is favored over fillers in this area, as the majority of wrinkles in this area are dynamic, not static. Filler tends to lump and look irregular.
- Filler type: Collagen, Juvéderm, or Restylane
- Injection technique: Linear threading
- Typical volume: 0.1 cc to 0.2 cc per side
- Pearl: If you choose to treat with fillers, use a fine gauge needle 30 or 32

TABLE 68.25 *Nasal Contouring*

- Smooth irregular nasal bridge and/or improve contour irregularities
- Filler type: Juvéderm Ultra or Restylane
- Injection technique: Linear threading/depot
- Typical volume: 0.1 cc to 0.25 cc
- Pearl: Inject between the index finger and thumb to direct the injection location

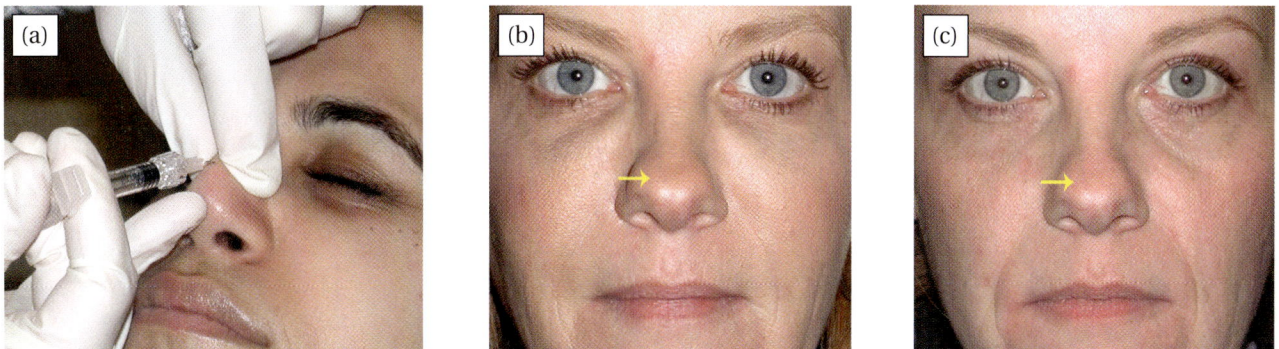

FIGURE 68.23 Nasal contouring. (a) Injection to nasal bridge. Note placement of index finger and thumb to control injection dispersion. (b) Pre-treatment. Note the contour irregularity of the nasal tip with shadowing (yellow arrow). (c) Post-treatment. The nasal tip irregularity is reduced with filler placement.

TABLE 68.26 *Tear Trough*

- Prior to tear trough treatment, cheek augmentation is often performed to improve cheek contour.
- In the tear trough, almost all patients experience post injection bruising and edema. This may not be the first location that one will choose to inject in a new filler patient.
- Filler type: "Softer" filler such as Restylane. Anecdotally, Restylane may incite less post-treatment edema than other HA fillers.
- Injection technique: Retrograde threading and depot. Inject horizontally across the lower eyelid/tear trough using retrograde threading and small depot injections on top of the periosteum. The depot injections are immediately "pancaked" to flatness with massage.
- Typical volume: 0.1 cc to 0.4 cc per side.
- Pearl: Although some physicians prefer more superficial placement, layering the filler material below the orbicularis or on top of the periosteum is less likely to create superficial irregularities or Tyndall effect.

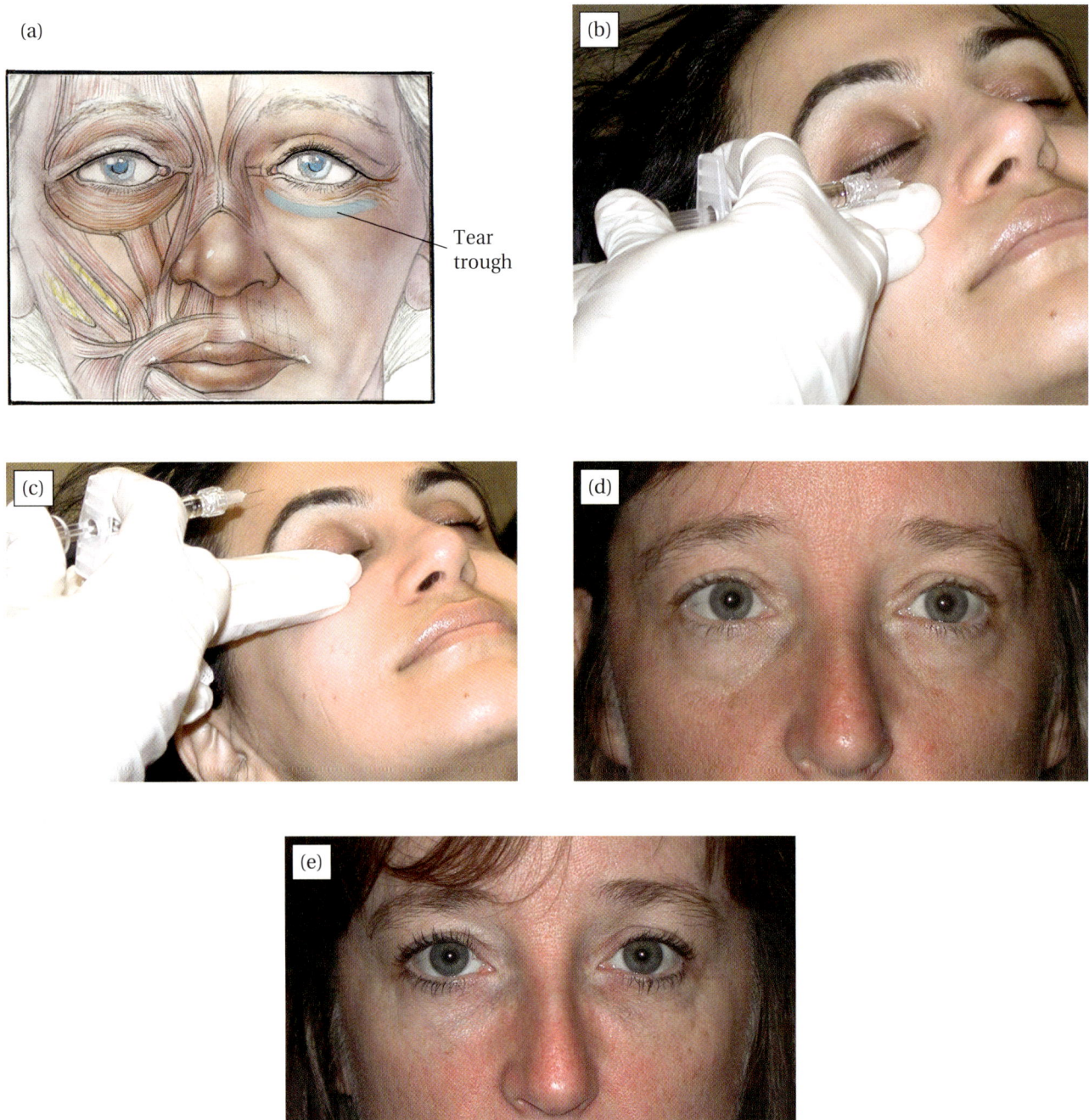

FIGURE 68.24 Tear trough injection. (a) Injection pattern for tear trough contouring. (b) Injection above the periosteum in a retrograde threading manner. (c) The non-injecting hand is used to flatten the filler material. (d) Pre-treatment. (e) Post-treatment.

TABLE 68.27 *Cheek Augmentation*

- Midfacial descent, loss of fat, and bone loss all contribute to diminished anterior projection of the cheek. Augmenting with filler adds volume and the opportunity to improve contour.
- Filler type: "Thicker" filler such as Radiesse, Perlane, or Juvéderm UP deep, and "softer" fillers such as Restylane layered anterior to the deep material.
- Injection technique: Fanning. Entering above the nasolabial fold, a fanning technique is used in three locations across the cheek from medial to lateral, elevating the entry site and shortening the length of the fan with each lateral move. The superior extent of the fan stops at the inferior orbital rim.
- Typical volume: 0.5 cc to 1.5 cc per side.
- Pearl: Intraoral filler injection techniques are also described. These may diminish swelling and bruising, but introduce the filler through a nonsterile plane.

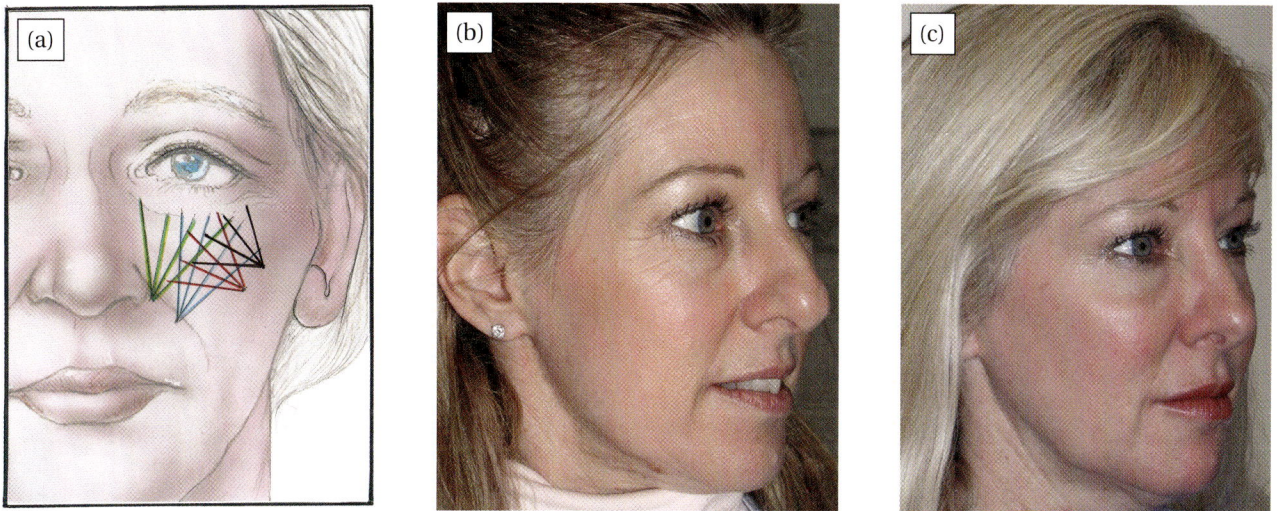

FIGURE 68.25 Cheek augmentation. (a) Injection pattern for cheek augmentation. The pattern is the same for both deep and superficial filler levels. (b) Pre-treatment. (c) Post-treatment. One syringe of Juvéderm UP each cheek and neurotoxin to the Crow's feet lines. One vial of Sculptra was also injected in the temple and cheek regions for generalized volume augmentation. The tear trough was not treated. In practice, both the tear trough and cheek are usually treated simultaneously. These examples were selected to show individual treatment results.

TABLE 68.28 *Nasolabial Folds (NLF)*

- Prior to isolated treatment of the NLF, determine if some of the gravitational descent and volume loss is amenable to cheek volume augmentation.
- Some contour modification between the cheek and upper lip is desirable, so complete obliteration of the NLF looks abnormal.
- Filler type: "Thicker" filler such as Radiesse , Juvederm Ultra Plus, or Perlane deep, and "softer" fillers such as Restylane or Juvederm Ultra layered anterior to the deep material.
- Injection technique: Fanning, linear/retrograde threading, crosshatching. The NLF is an area where layering of thicker and thinner materials is beneficial. Filler material is placed below the groove of the nasolabial fold. At the top of the fold near the nostril, fanning is used. Linear threading or retrograde threading is used in the thinner layers of the fold more inferiorly.
- Typical volume: 0.5 cc to 1.5 cc per side.
- Pearl: Lightly crosshatching horizontally below the fold helps a deep wrinkle line.

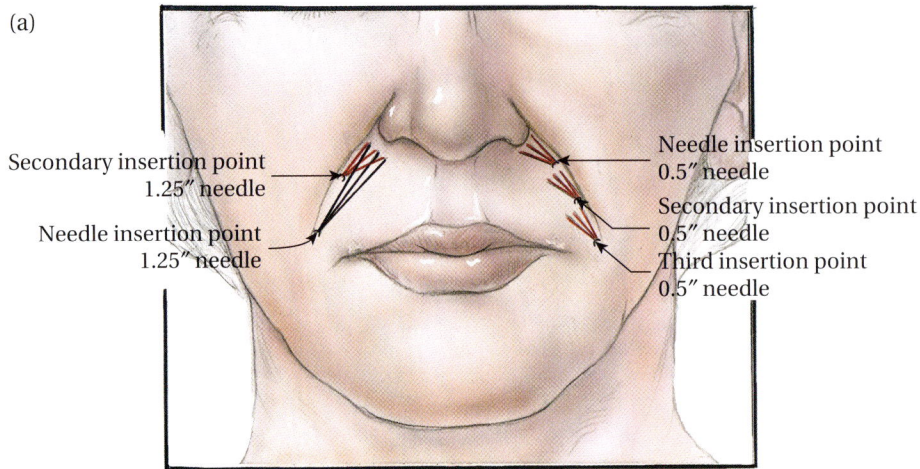

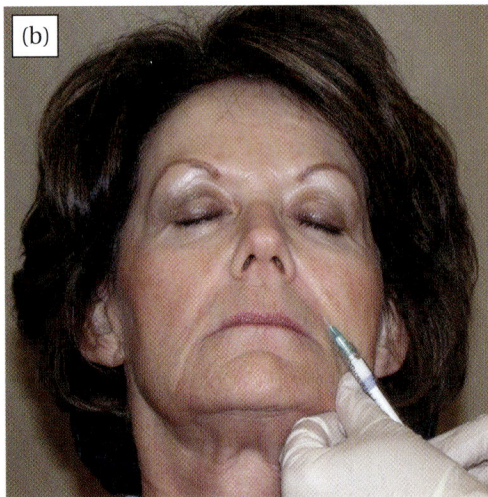

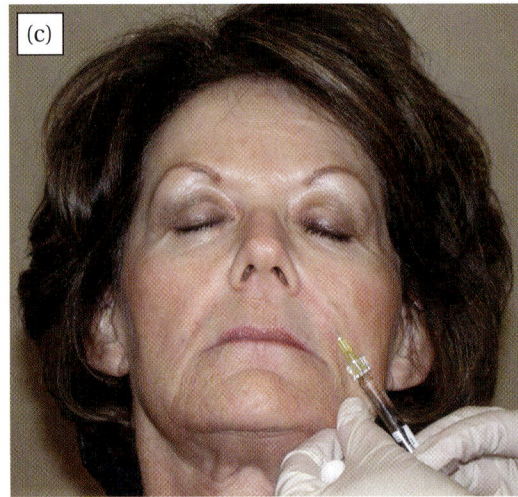

FIGURE 68.26 Nasolabial fold injection. (a) Injection pattern for nasolabial fold. A fanning pattern is used deep, and linear threading is used for superficial filler levels. (b) Radiesse is injected into the deep dermis of the nasolabial fold. Note how the thumb of the non-injecting hand provides traction of skin in injection area. (c) Restylane is layered superficially to the Radiesse. Layering "heavier" fillers with "lighter" fillers allows for filling of deep folds by forming a deep base for volume, and lighter fillers are placed superficially for shaping.

TABLE 68.29 *Melomental folds (Marionette Lines) and Oral Commissure*

- Filler type: For marionette lines, start with thicker filler such as Radiesse, Perlane, or Juvéderm UP. Closer to lip and for commissure—use thinner filler such as Juvéderm or Restylane. For milder lines or if one product must be chosen, use the "lighter" HA fillers.

- Injection technique: Linear threading and fanning. Fanning technique with retrograde threading to lift and fill the upper marionette line. Massage with thumb and forefinger to contour. Progressively bring to full correction with multiple passes.

- Typical volume: 0.3 cc to 0 .5 cc per side.

- Pearl: Support the lateral oral commissure with a vertical column of filler to elevate the corner Also assess the lateral corner of the upper lip. For rejuvenation of the lateral oral commisure, this sometimes needs volume added.

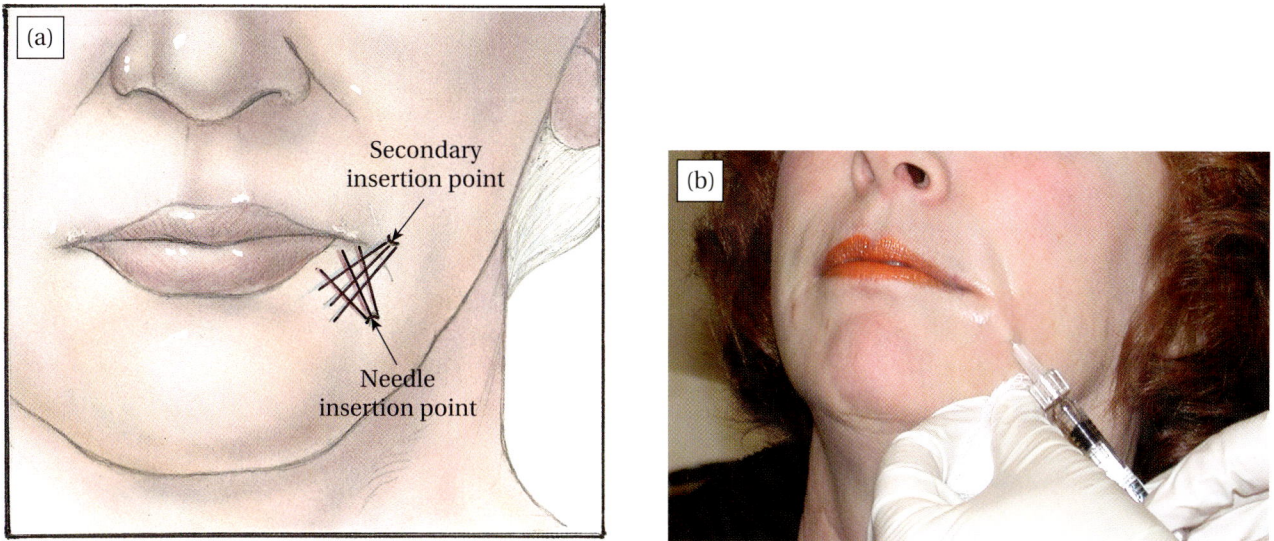

FIGURE 68.27 Melomental folds (marionette lines) and oral commissure injection. (a) Injection pattern for melomental folds. (b) Fanning with retrograde threading.

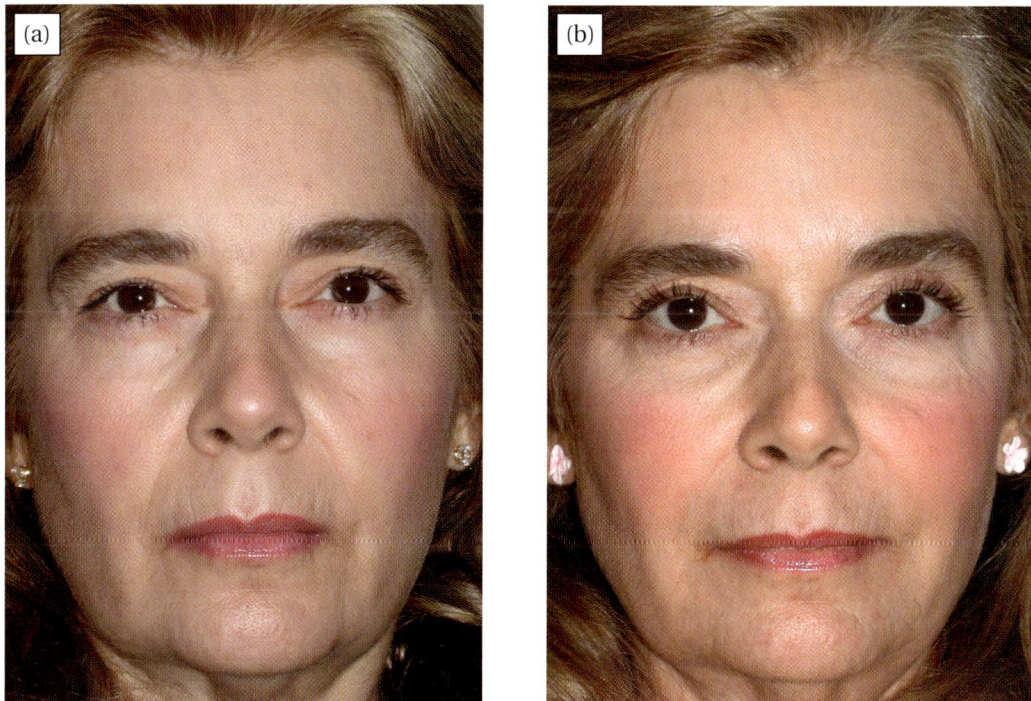

FIGURE 68.28 Before and after nasolabial and melomental fold injections. (a) Pre-treatment of nasolabial folds and melomental folds. (b) Post-treatment Radiesse (0.75 cc/side) deep for each nasolabial fold, and Restylane (0.2 cc/side) superficially in the NL folds. Restylane (0.6 cc/side) was placed in the marionette lines, and 0.2 cc/side in the lateral oral commissure.

TABLE 68.30 *Lip Shaping*

- Filler type: "Soft" fillers such as Restylane and Juvederm, or if available, collagen for outlining. Hyaluronic acid filler for volume.
- Injection technique:
  - Vermillion border—outline with linear threading or retrograde threading.
  - Philtrum—outline with retrograde threading while holding the tissue between the index finger and thumb to limit spread.
  - Pink lip—volumize with depot injections focusing on 4 central quadrants; horizontal linear threading is also sometimes helpful for balance.
- Check lateral upper lip commissure area for a dimple that may need to be filled.
- Lightly crosshatch between nose and vermillion border lateral to philtrum for bone volume loss (particularly in denture wearers this helps to prevent "duck lip").
- Typical Volume: 0.4 cc to 1.0 cc per lip.
- Pearl: Don't try to create big lips from small lips in one treatment.

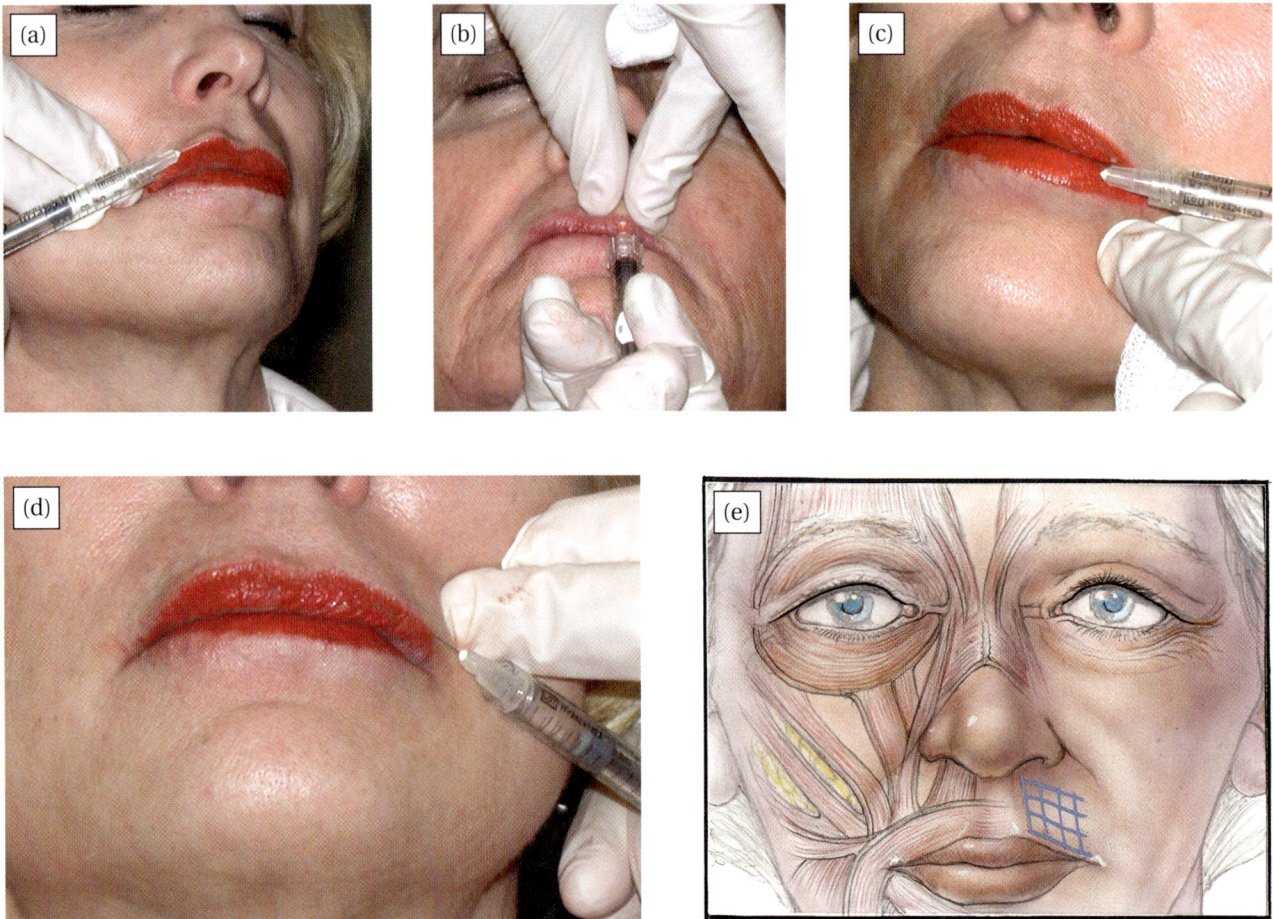

FIGURE 68.29 Lip shaping. (a) Outlining vermillion border. (b) Philtral shaping. (c) Pink lip volume augmentation. (d) Adjusting upper lateral oral commissure. Note the indentation just above the upper lip on the right. This area has been filled on the left side. (e) Crosshatching injection pattern for overall upper lip volume. Crosshatching is only required in more severe cases of volume loss, where augmentation of pink volume causes "duck lip."

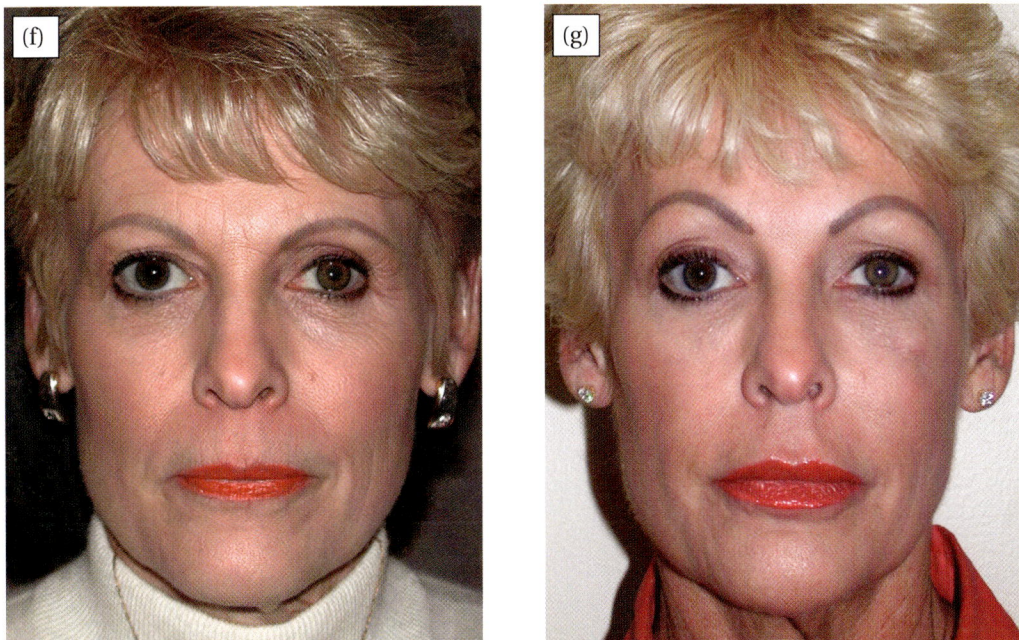

FIGURE 68.29 (*continued*) (f) Pre-treatment. (g) Post-treatment. Vermillion border, philtrum, and pink lip have been treated with Restylane. This patient has also had a surgical brow lift and volume augmentation to the left superior sulcus.

TABLE 68.31 *Labiomental Fold and Chin*

- Filler type: "Soft" fillers such as Restylane or Juvéderm Ultra.
- Injection technique: Fanning and/or linear threading.
- Linear threading can be used to soften a deep mental crease. Fanning is used to improve overall anterior projection of the chin.
- Typical volume: 0.1 cc to 0.3 cc.
- Pearl: Complete eradication of mental groove is not desirable, especially in males.

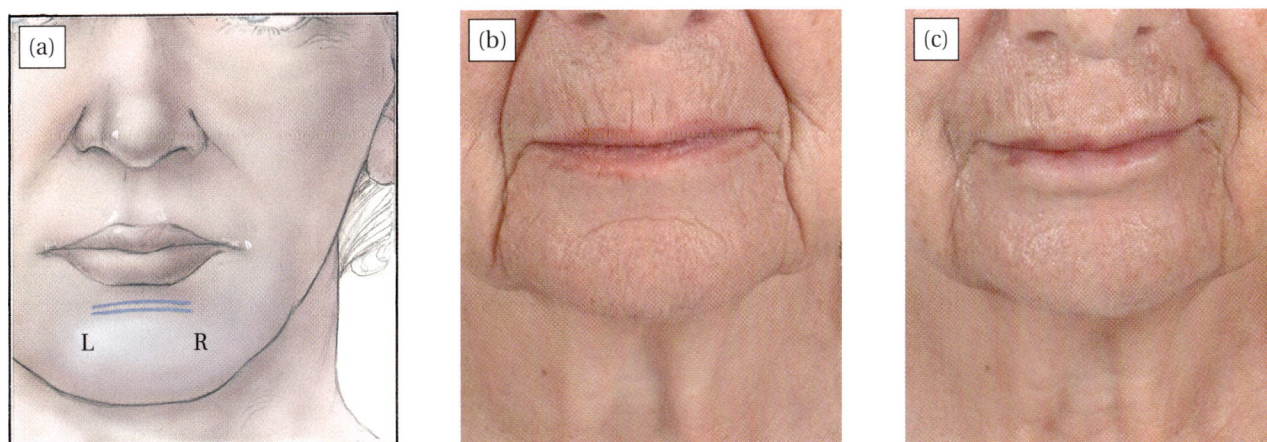

FIGURE 68.30 Labiomental fold injection. (a) Injection pattern. (b) Pre-treatment. (c) Immediate post-treatment. (Photographs courtesy of Allan E. Wulc, MD, FACS.)

TABLE 68.32 *Pre-jowl Sulcus*

- Filler type: "Thicker" filler, such as Radiesse, Perlane, or Juvéderm UP deep, and "softer" fillers such as Restylane or Juvederm Ultra layered anterior to the deep material.
- Injection technique: Fanning, linear threading (border of mandible).
- Typical volume: 0.2 cc to 0.4 cc per side.
- Pearl: Inject inferior to the jowl and be sure to include area immediately inferior to mandible.

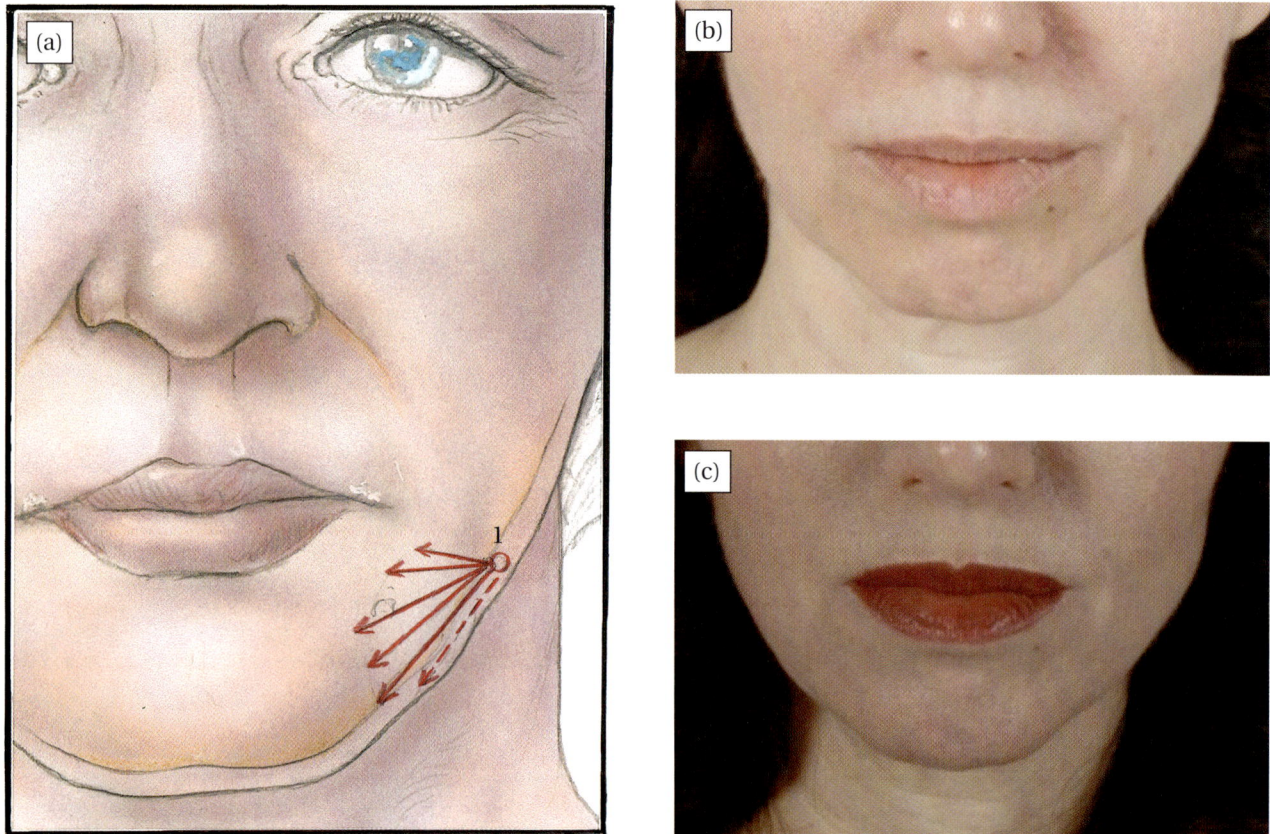

FIGURE 68.31 Pre-jowl sulcus. (a) Injection pattern. (b) Pre-treatment. (c) Post-treatment. (Photographs courtesy of Allan E. Wulc, MD, FACS.)

TABLE 68.33 *Radiesse Applications and Contraindications*

- Good for cheek volume augmentation and nasolabial folds
- Radiesse can be mixed with lidocaine to enhance anesthesia
- Not typically used for lips
- Contraindications
  - Identical to those listed for HAs
  - Generalized treatment precautions are similar to those listed for HAs

TABLE 68.34 *Sculptra Applications and Contraindications*

- Unique mechanism of action
- Generalized volume replacement rather than focal contouring
- Delayed response based on individual reaction to the component particles of the material
- Useful for temporal and preparotid hollowing
- Contraindications
  - Hypersensitivity to any of the components of the product (poly-L-lactic acid, sodium carboxymethylcellulose, non-pyrogenic mannitol)
  - Pregnancy/breastfeeding safety unknown
  - Generalized treatment precautions are similar to those listed for HAs

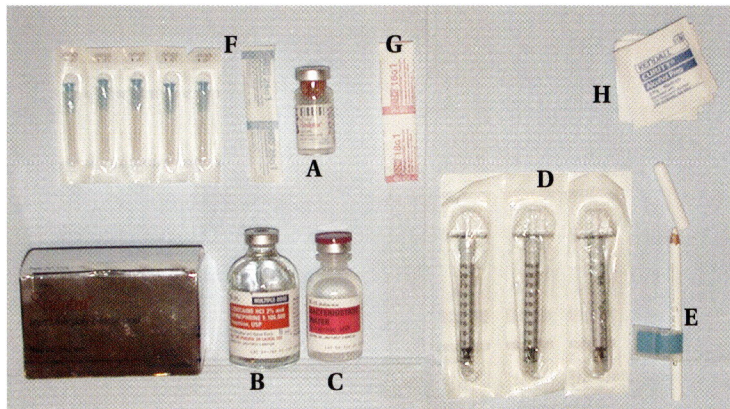

FIGURE 68.32 Recommended Supplies for Sculptra Injection. A: Sculptra vial. B: Local anesthetic. C: Sterile water. D: Minimum two single-use 1–3 mL sterile syringes. E: Skin marking pencil. F: Several 1" or ½" 25 gauge needles for injecting product. G: Two 1" 18 gauge needles. H: Alcohol or Betadine swab to prep injection sites. Single-use 5 mL sterile syringe for dilution (not pictured). Gloves—sterile or nonsterile (not pictured).

TABLE 68.35   *Sculptra Storage, Preparation, Considerations, and Injection Techniques*

Storage

- Store at room temperature, up to 30°C.
- Do NOT freeze.
- Refrigeration is not required following reconstitution.

Preparation

- Must be prepared 48 hours prior to use.
- Lidocaine is added at time of treatment, sterile water 48 hours prior.
- Room temperature storage following reconstitution.
- The vial should not be agitated 24 hours following hydration.
- Vial should be agitated immediately prior to usage, forming a uniform translucent suspension.
- Should be used within 72 hours of reconstitution.
- Reconstitute with a combination of lidocaine and sterile water. The variable dilution ratio is still evolving. Changes in the reconstitution process and the dilution ratio have been recommended to try to prevent clustering of the particles and post treatment nodules.
  - For facial injection— 6 cc sterile water and 2 cc lidocaine for a total of 8 cc
  - For hand injection—8–10 cc sterile water and 2 cc lidocaine for a total of 10–12 cc

Injection Techniques

- Pre-mark the areas of desired volume enhancement.
- In the temporal region, 1 cc per side of material may be placed in a depot injection below the temporalis muscle
- In the upper zygoma region, 1 cc per side of material may be placed in a depot injection deep to the orbicularis oculi muscle, inferior to the infraorbital rim and anterior to the maxilla. (i.e. not anterior to the orbital septum)
- Everywhere else, the solution is injected in the deep dermis or subcutaneous layer in small aliquots, using a combination fanning, linear threading, and crosshatching technique with a 1-inch needle (25 or 27 gauge).
- About 1 cc total of solution is injected in 2 inch square treatment area, with individual injections limited to 0.1–0.2 cc.
- Following each injection, especially depot, the area is massaged.

Post-treatment Considerations

- Patient should massage treatment areas at home (five minutes, five times per day for 5 days).
- Patient should avoid excessive sun and UV lamp exposure until initial swelling and redness have resolved.
- Consider ice for swelling and comfort within 24 hours (avoid direct contact of ice with the skin).
- Small papules may form in the treatment area but are typically asymptomatic and not visible unless skin is elevated by underlying nodule.
- Wait 6 weeks to see the degree of effect.
- Most patients require two to three treatments to obtain desired result.
- Retreat when indicated.

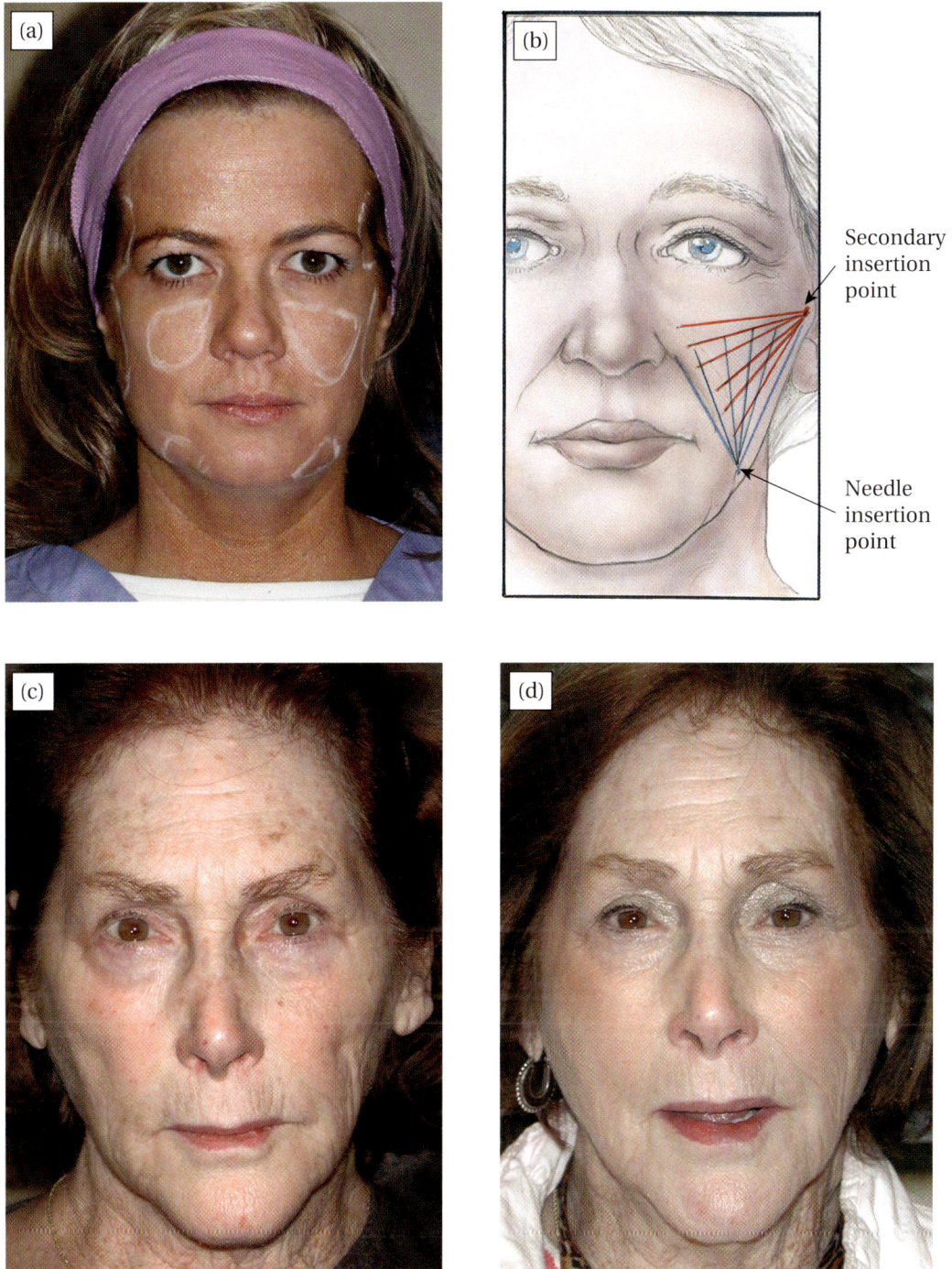

FIGURE 68.33 Sculptra injection. (a) Patient marking for Sculptra treatment. (b) Typical injection pattern linear threading, fanning, and crosshatching. (c) Pre-treatment. (d) Post-treatment with three vials of Sculptra. Patient also had 532nm wavelength laser for pigmentary irregularities and perioral HA filler.

TABLE 68.36 *Generalized Filler Complications*

Technique Based
- Asymmetry
- Over/undercorrection
- Erythema/Edema
- Ecchymosis
- Inflammatory hyperpigmentation/hemosiderin
- Infection
- Hematoma
- Vascular occlusion/infiltration
- Venous compression
- Vascular blanching
- Nodules
- Tyndall effect

Product Based
- Allergic reactions
- Granulomas

TABLE 68.37 *Managing Hyaluronic Acid Complications*

Edema, Bruising and Erythema
- Normal for first-time patients and lip injections
  - Edema will resolve over several hours to days
- Rule out causes other than injection technique or materials
  - Skin care products
  - Allergies to latex, topical anesthetic

Post-Inflammatory Hyperpigmentation or Hemosiderin Deposition
- Topical hydroquinones have minimal effect
- Topical or intralesional steroids
- Retinoic acid to increase turnover of skin

Hematoma
- Rare complication
- Can be seen most commonly in lips from compromise of labial artery
- Treat with ice compress for 48 hours, followed by warm compress until resolution

Granuloma
- Rare complication, less than 1%
- Onset is delayed and the result of the stimulation of memory macrophages
  - Treatment consists of oral antibiotic therapy if infection is included within the differential diagnosis
  - Intralesional steroid injections may also aid in resolution

(continued)

TABLE 68.37 *Managing Hyaluronic Acid Complications (continued)*

Vascular Occulusion/Infiltration/Blanching

- Results from proximity to terminal arterial vessal with occlusion or compression
- Patient will experience pain
- Can result in tissue hypoxia to necrosis
- Recognizing signs and acting quickly is key
  - Stop injecting
  - Do not use ice or steroids to area
  - Use warm compress to area, aspirin, and nitropaste
  - For HAs, hyaluronicdase
  - Consider hyperbaric oxygen chamber

Venous Compression

- Blue/purple hue of area NOT injected
- Patient experiences NO pain
- Treat with warm compress and aspirin

Nodules

- Results from clumping of the HA product
  - Treat with massage—if recalcitrant, hyaluronidase or extrusion

Tyndall Effect (blue discoloration)

- Results from visible HA due to superficial injection near the skin surface or in area of thin skin
- Treatment consists of hyaluronidase or extrusion

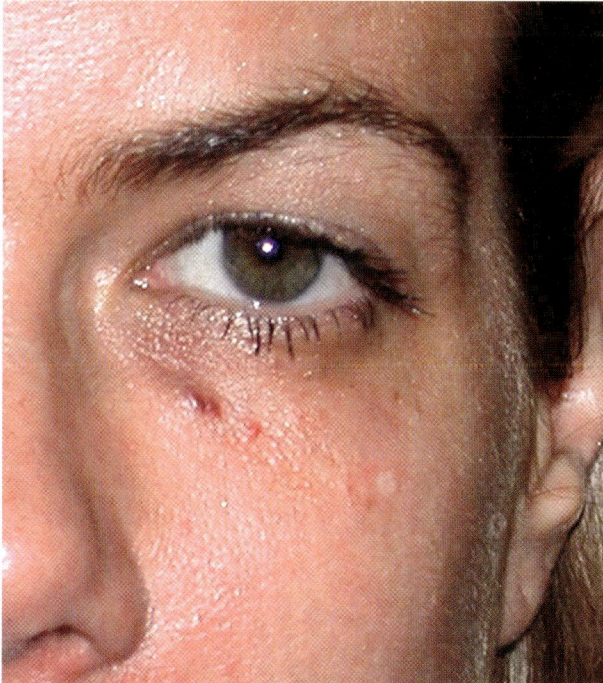

FIGURE 68.34 Tear trough ecchymosis following HA injection to the tear trough. This amount of ecchymosis is considered "normal" for injections in this region. If the ecchymosis causes distortion of the tissue architecture, injection should be delayed as proceeding may lead to injection into the improper tissue plane with less satisfactory results.

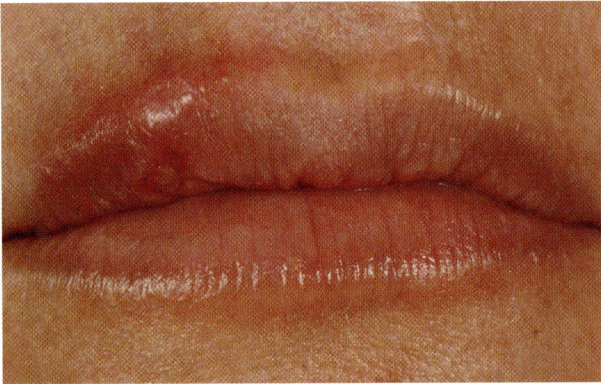

FIGURE 68.35 Herpes simplex infection following HA injection to the lips. Although the patient denied any previous herpetic episodes, lesions appeared three days post-injection. (Photography courtesy of Allan E. Wulc, MD, FACS.)

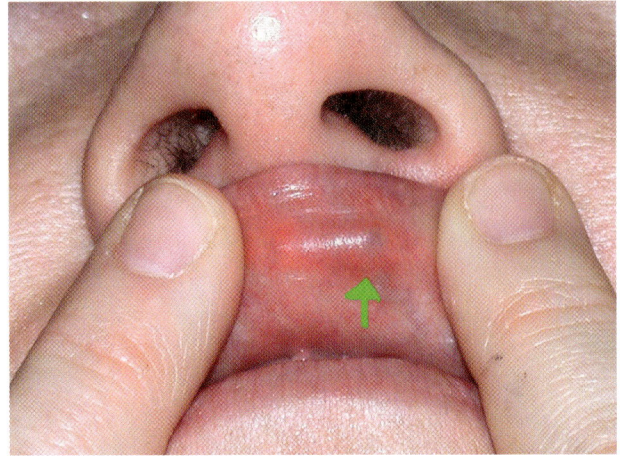

FIGURE 68.36 Tyndall effect and nodule following Restylane treatment to upper lip. Green arrow points to the HA nodule and area of blue discoloration.

TABLE 68.38 *Hyaluronidase*

Breaks down hyaluronic acid and temporarily makes tissues permeable to fluids
- Category C for pregnant patients
- Skin testing recommended 10–15 minutes prior to injection if question of allergy
- controversial in areas of infection
- FDA approved brands
  - Vitrase®
  - Wydase® (no longer manufactured)
  - Amphadase®
  - Hydase™
  - Hylenex™

TABLE 68.39 *Managing Radiesse Complications*

Semipermanent nodules, especially from lip injection
- Treatment requires surgical excision

Vascular Occlusion
- Dependent upon severity of occlusion
- No consensus as to "standard of care"
- Nitropaste (can combine with Aquaphor) q12hr to affected area
- Warm compress/heat to area as tolerated
- ASA 200–800 mg QID. Alternative: some have recommended enoxaparin sodium injection (Lovenox, Sanofi-Aventis, Bridgewater, NJ)
- Prophylaxis with topical antibiotic ointment and oral antibiotics if skin breakdown has or will occur
- Oral steroids has also been suggested, though no dosage range is available
- Local injection with hyaluronidase has also been proposed in doses ranging from 75 to 150u. One should be aware of the risks of anaphylaxis from hyaluronidase with certain preservatives

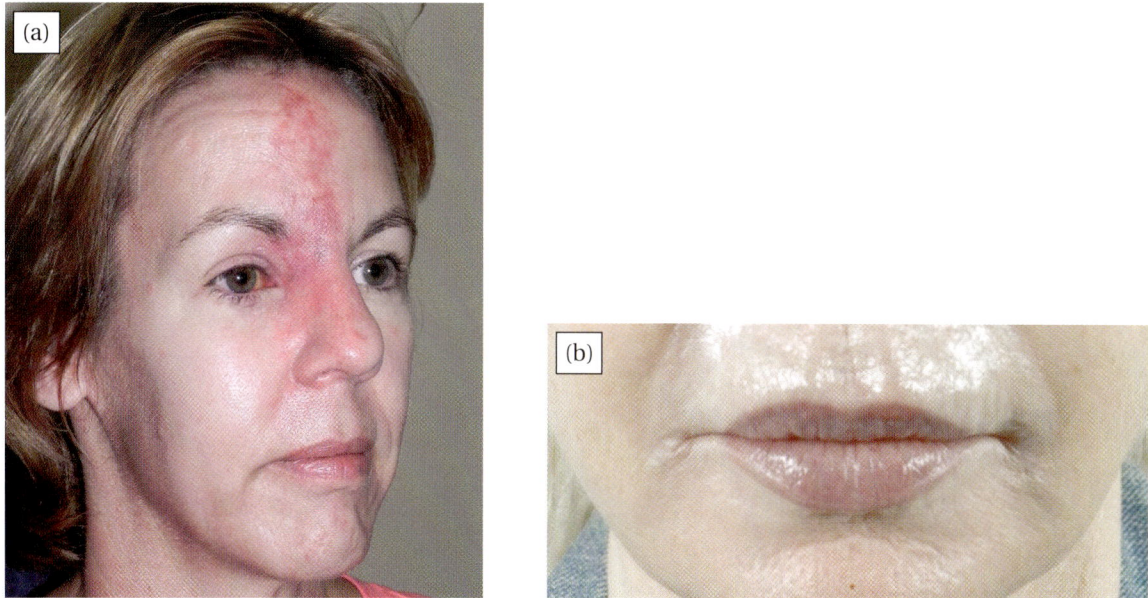

FIGURE 68.37 Radiesse Complications. (a) Vascular occlusion following Radiesse injection to the glabella. Note the area of distant necrosis under the right lower eyelid and the medial conjunctival hyperemia. These are both indicative of non-injection sites that can be affected from intravascular injection and material spread via anterograde and retrograde flow. (b) Perioral nodules following Radiesse injection to the lips and oral commissures. (Photograph courtesy of Allan E. Wulc, MD, FACS.)

TABLE 68.40 *Managing Sculptra Complications*

Reactive nodules and granulomas

• Thought to be related to (in part) higher concentration of solution used in initial treatments and clumping of PLLA
• Treat with massage and steroid injections

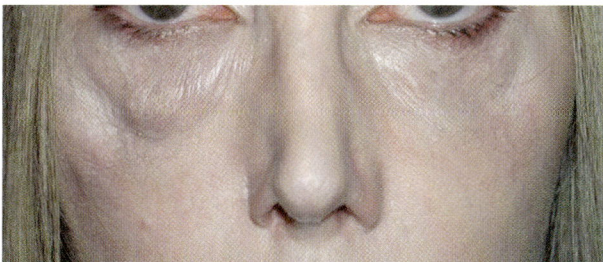

FIGURE 68.38 Midface granulomas and nodules following Sculptra injection. Nodules are bilateral and one large granuloma can be seen in the right lid–cheek junction. (Photograph courtesy of Michael E. Migliori, MD, FACS.)

SELECTED REFERENCES

Baumann L, Blyumia, M, and Saghari, S. Dermal fillers. In *Cosmetic dermatology: Principles and practice.* 2nd ed. New York: McGraw-Hill. 2009:191–211.

Bellew SG, Carroll KC, Weiss MA, Weiss RA. Sterility of stored nonanimal, stabilized hyaluronic acid gel syringes after patient injection. *J Am Acad Dermatol.* 2005 Jun;52(6):988–990.

Bhatia AC, Arndt KA, Dover JS, Kaminer M, Rohrer TE. Bacterial sterility of stored nonanimal stabilized hyaluronic acid-based cutaneous filler. *Arch Dermatol.* 2005 Oct;141(10):1317–1318.

Busso M, Applebaum D. Hand augmentation with Radiesse (Calcium hydroxylapatite). *Dermatol Ther.* 2007 Nov–Dec;20(6):385–387.

Carruthers J, Fagien S, Matarasso SL; Botox Consensus Group. Consensus recommendations on the use of botulinum toxin type a in facial aesthetics. *Plast Reconstr Surg.* 2004 Nov;114(6 Suppl):1S–22S.

Chasan PE. The history of injectable silicone fluids for soft-tissue considerations in soft-tissue contouring. *Plast Reconstr Surg.* 2006 Sep;118(3 Suppl):55S–63S.

Foster JA, Wulc AE, Holck DE. Cosmetic indications for botulinum A toxin. *Semin Ophthalmol.* 1998 Sep;13(3):142–148. Review.

Georgescu D, Jones Y, Mc Cann JD, Anderson RL. Skin necrosis after calcium hydroxylapatiet injection into the glabellar and nasolabial folds. *Ophthal Plast Reconstr Surg.* 2009 Nov–Dec;25(6):498–499.

Hexsel DM et al. Multicenter, double-blind study of the efficacy of injections with botulinum

toxin type A reconstituted up to six consecutive weeks before application. *Dermatol Surg.* 2003 May;29(5):523–529.

Huang W, Foster JA, Rogachefsky AS. Pharmacology of botulinum toxin. *J Am Acad Dermatol.* 2000 Aug;43(2 Pt 1):249–259.

Huang W, Rogachefsky AS, Foster JA. Browlift with botulinum toxin. *Dermatol Surg.* 2000 Jan;26(1):55–60.

Klein AW, Carruthers A, Fagien S, Lowe NJ. Comparisons among botulinum toxins: an evidence-based review. *Plast Reconstr Surg.* 2008 Jun;121(6):413e–422e.

Lam SM, Azizzadeh B, Graivier M. Injectable poly-L-lactic acid (Sculptra): technical augmentation. *Plast Reconstr Surg.* 2007 Dec;120(7):2034–2040; discussion 2041–2043.

Morley AS, Taban M, Malhotra R, Goldberg RA. Use of Hyaluronic Acid gel for upper eyelid filling and contouring. *Ophthal Plast Reconstr Surg.* 2009 Nov–Dec;25(6):440–444.

Narins RS. Minimizing adverse events associated with poly-L-lactic acid injection. *Dermatol Surg.* 2008 Jun;34 Suppl 1:S100–S104.

Pham T, Perry JD. Botulinum toxin type A injection without isopropyl alcohol antisepsis. *Ophthal Plast Reconstr Surg.* 2009 May–Jun;25(3):178–179.

Sami, MS, et al. Efficacy of botulinum toxin type A after topical anesthesia. *Ophthal Plast Reconstr Surg.* 2006 Nov–Dec,22(6).448–452.

Facial Fat Transfer

John B. Holds, MD, FACS

TABLE 69.1 *Indications for Fat Transfer*

Age-related facial volume loss
Malar volume loss and prominent tear trough
Traumatic facial defects

TABLE 69.2 *Preoperative Considerations*

Ensure the patient has an appropriate donor site.

May augment or replace traditional lifting techniques in the eyebrow and upper eyelid.

The midface is the key area. Volume loss is the most important cause of midface aging changes, such as prominent tear trough, malar triangle formation and midface ptosis.

Fat transfer may be used to augment results at the time of cosmetic blepharoplasty or facelift surgery.

Photo Series of Fat Grafting

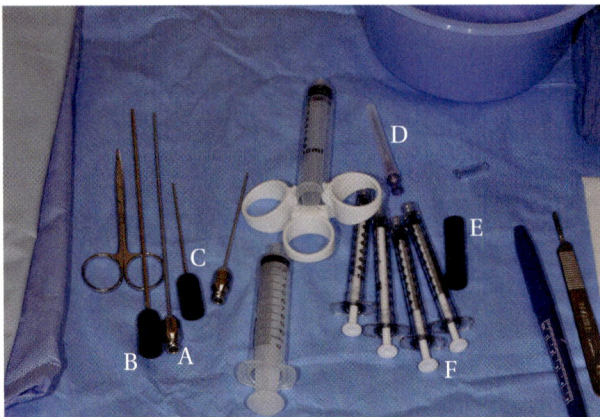

FIGURE 69.1 Equipment specific to fat transfer technique including: A. infiltrating cannula; B. fat harvest cannula; C. fat infiltrating cannulas; D. Nokor needle for entry stabs; E. female–female Luer-lock transfer adapter; F. polycarbonate 1mL syringes.

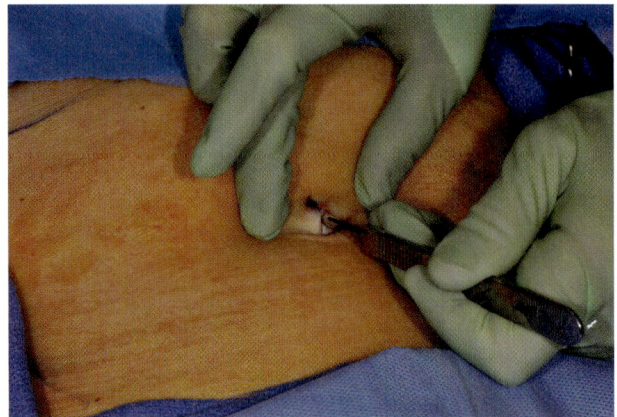

FIGURE 69.2 A suitable site for fat harvest is selected. Avoiding sites of prior liposuction, the lower abdomen, inner and outer thigh, hip, waist, and buttock can all be used. After achieving local anesthesia with dilute lidocaine with epinephrine (0.25% lidocaine, 1:800,000 epinephrine), an incision is made and additional dilute local anesthetic used to tumesce the harvest site.

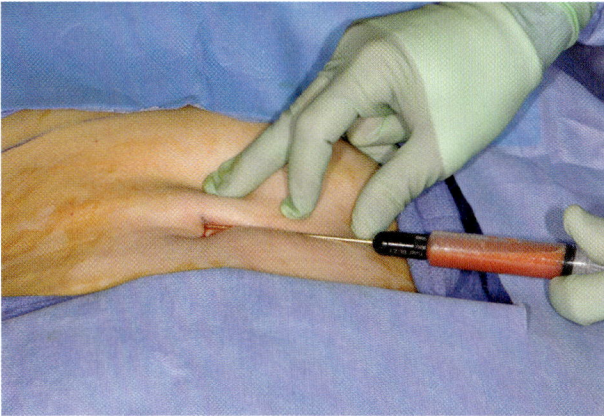

FIGURE 69.3 After 10–20 minutes for the anesthetic to infiltrate the tissues, a 10 mL syringe is used with a fat harvesting cannula (2.1 mm multiport fat harvest cannula, Tulip Medical Inc.). 1–2 mL of negative pressure is applied, as the nondominant hand stabilizes the harvest site. Be cognizant of the location of the cannula tip, and attempt to harvest from the mid-depth of the fat space, redirecting the cannula every 3–4 strokes in a fanning motion.

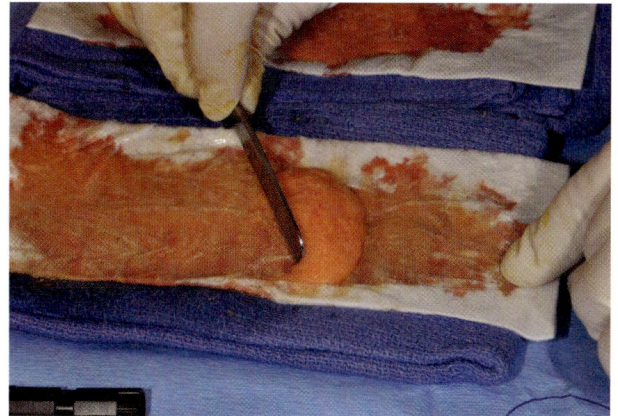

FIGURE 69.4 Fat is often processed in one of two ways: by draining onto Telfa and manually repacking into syringes, or by centrifuging the fat. This shows the fat after 5 minutes of drainage onto Telfa.

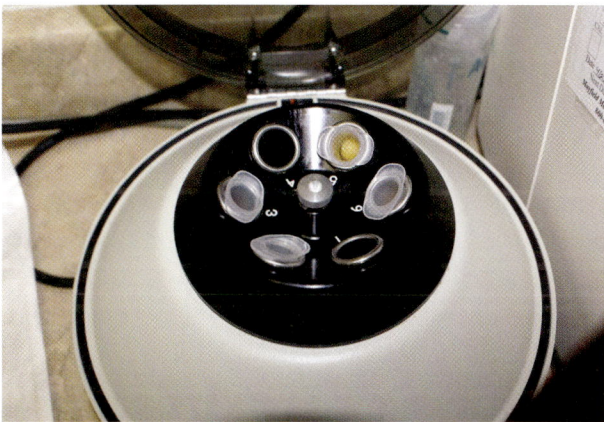

FIGURE 69.5 Alternatively, the fat harvest syringes are capped and centrifuged at 3000 rpm for 3 minutes. (Photograph courtesy of L. Mike Nayak, MD.)

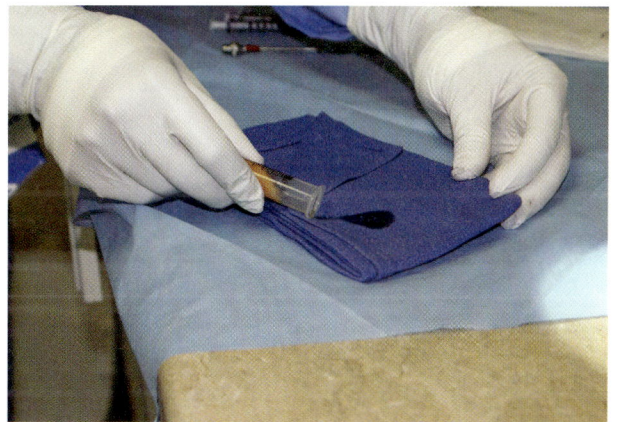

FIGURE 69.6 After centrifuging the syringes, the free lipid is poured off the top of the intact fat. (Photograph courtesy of L. Mike Nayak, MD.)

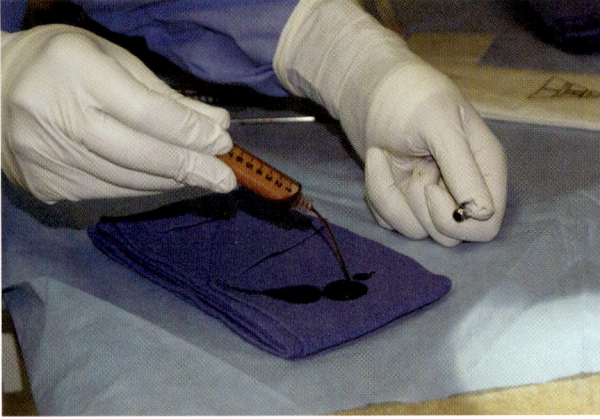

FIGURE 69.7 The Luer-lock cap is removed, and blood and serum below the fat poured off, leaving the processed fat. (Photograph courtesy of L. Mike Nayak, MD.)

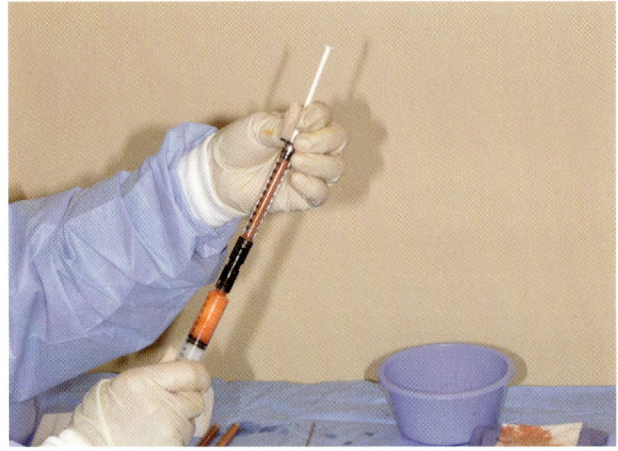

FIGURE 69.8 Heavy 1 mL syringes are filled using female–female adapter and avoiding air bubbles.

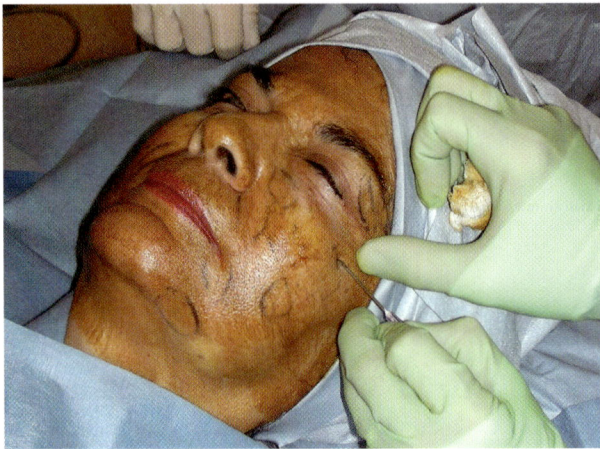

FIGURE 69.9 Preoperatively, the patient is marked at sites for fat transfer and entry sites. After local anesthesia, the entry sites are stabbed with the Nokor needle. The infiltrating cannulas are used to infiltrate dilute local anesthesia throughout the sites of proposed fat infiltration.

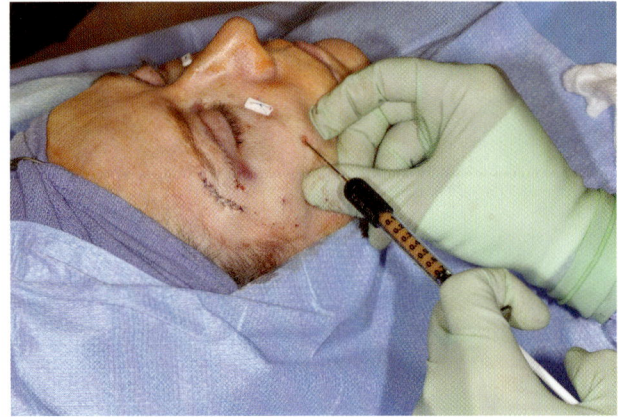

FIGURE 69.10 In a systematic fashion, fat is infiltrated following the preoperative surgical plan. Amounts deposited per pass vary from 0.03 mL under the thin tissues of the tear trough, to 0.1 mL/pass at deep sites in the medial canthus and pre-jowl area.

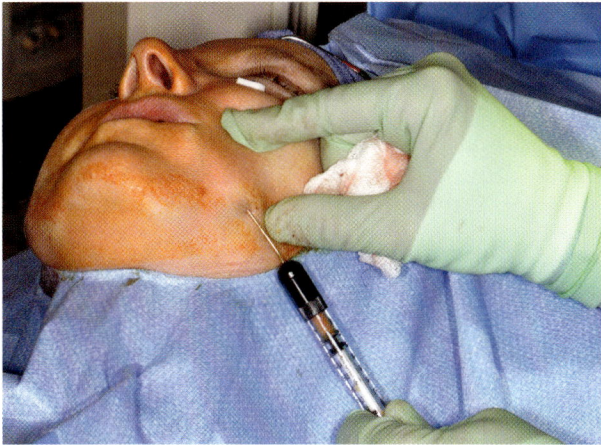

FIGURE 69.11 The jawline entry site may be used to inject the pre-jowl area, as well as the marionette lines and lateral lip.

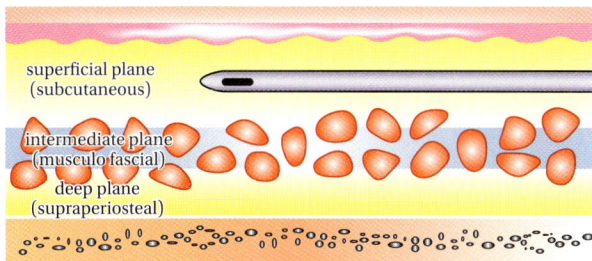

FIGURE 69.12 Under the thicker cheek tissues, fat is deposited in the deep, preperiosteal plane, the intermediate musculofascial plane, and the subcutaneous planes. The tear trough requires special attention, with very small aliquots of fat only in the deep plane. (From Lam SM, Glasgold MJ, Glasgold RA. *Complementary fat grafting.* Philadelphia: Lippincott, Williams and Wilkins, 2007; p. 61.)

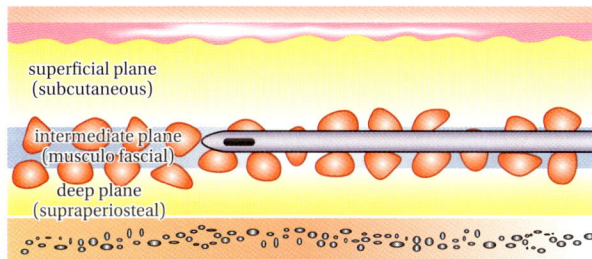

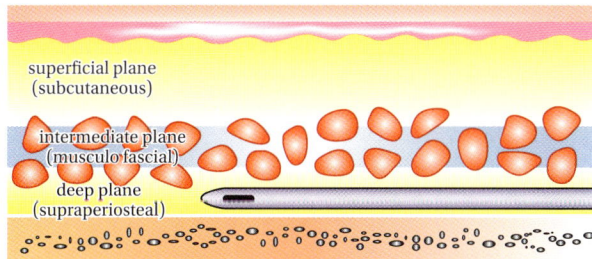

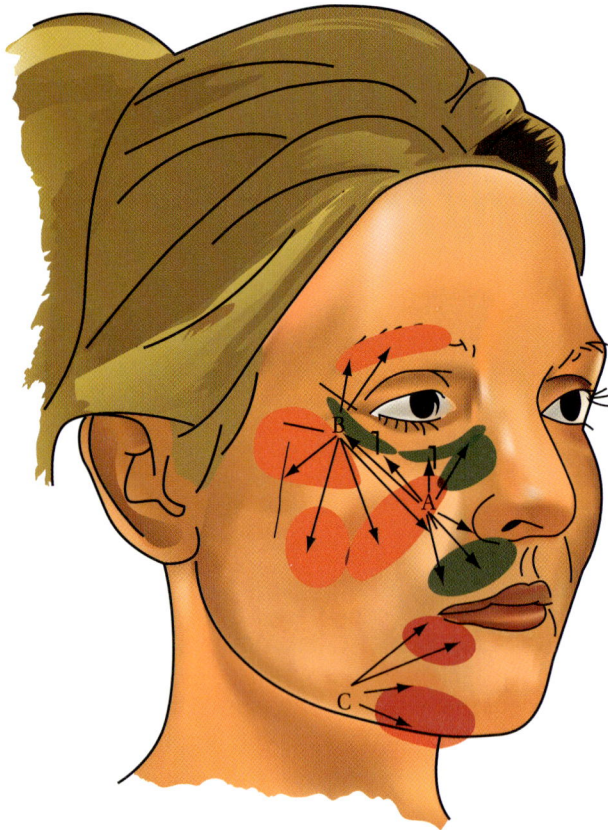

FIGURE 69.13   A basic foundation of transferred fat centering on the midface can be injected using three entry sites. Avoid injecting the tear trough through site B, instead using site A to approach the tear trough in a fanning fashion from below. Typical treatments will require 8–20 mL of fat per side. (From Lam, Glasgold, and Glasgold, p. 63 with minor modification.)

TABLE 69.3   *Table for Fat Infiltration*

Sequence	Site	Entry site	Volume (mL)	Fat/pass	Level*
1	Medial canthus	A	1–2	0.1	D
2	Medial orbital rim	A	0.5–1	0.03	D
3	Lateral orbital rim	A	0.5–1	0.03	D
4	Nasojugal groove	A	1–2	0.1	D,I,S
5	Nasolabial fold/lateral upper Lip	A	2–3	0.1	D,I,S
6	Lateral cheek	A	2	0.1	D,I,S
7	Buccal	A	2	0.1	I
8	Anterior cheek	A	2	0.1	D,I,S
9	Lateral brow	B	0.5–1	0.03	D
10	Lateral canthus	B	0.5–1	0.03	D
11	Lateral cheek	B	1–2	0.1	D,I,S
12	Malar septum	B	2	0.1	D,I,S
13	Buccal	B	1–2	0.1	I
14	Pre-jowl sulcus	C	2–3	0.1	D,I,S
15	Marionette line	C	1–2	0.1	I,S

* D=Deep; I=Intermediate; S=Superficial.
Modified from Lam, Glasgold, and Glasgold, p. 60.

Before and After Fat Grafting

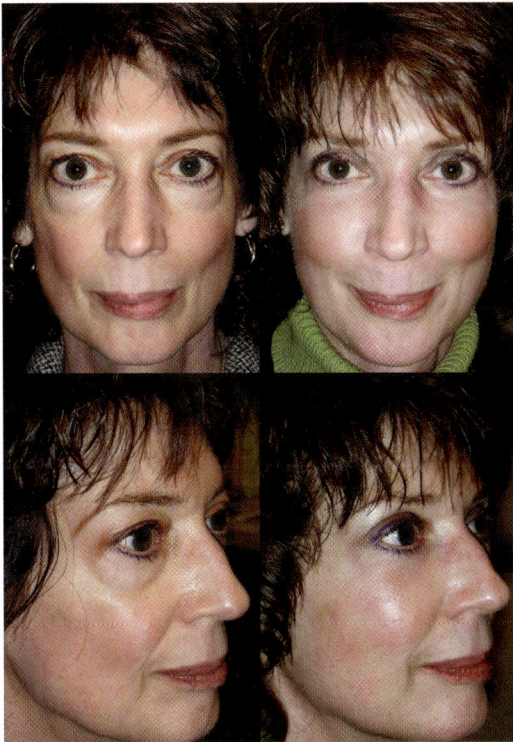

FIGURE 69.14 Patient before and six months after upper and lower blepharoplasty surgery and facial fat transfer (28 mL total; 14 mL per side). The periocular zone alone may have had similar benefit with the blepharoplasty alone, but the convexity of the brows, and cheek and facial fullness, could not have been achieved without fat transfer.

TABLE 69.4 *Potential Complications of Facial Fat Transfer*

Undercorrection

Overcorrection/bulges

Subcutaneous nodules/lumps

Persistent malar edema

Vascular embolization

SELECTED REFERENCES

Amar RE. *Microinfiltration Adipocytaire au nuveau de la fac ou restructuration tissulaire par greffe de tissue adipeux* [Microinfiltration of fat cells of the face or reconstruction of the tissue with grafts of fat tissue]. *Ann Chir Plast Esthet.* 1999;44:593–608.

Coleman SR. Facial recontouring with liposculpture. *Clin Plast Surg.* 1997;24(2):347–367.

Coleman SR. Structural fat grafts: the ideal filler? *Clin Plast Surg.* 2001;28(1):111–119.

Cook T, Nakra T, Shorr N, et. al. Facial recontouring with autologous fat. Facial Plast Surg. 2004;20(2):145–147.

Donofrio L. Structural autologous lipoaugmentation: a panfacial technique. *Dermatol Surg.* 2000;26:1129–1134.

Lam SM, Glasgold, MJ, Glasgold RA. *Complementary fat grafting.* Philadelphia, Lippincott Williams & Wilkins; 2007.

Pontius AT, Williams EF. The evolution of midface rejuvenation: combining the midface-lift and fat transfer. *Arch Facial Plast Surg.* 2006;8(5):300–305.

Spector JA, Draper L, Aston SJ. Lower lid deformity secondary to autogenous fat transfer: a cautionary tale. *Aesthetic Plast Surg.* 2008;32(3):411–414.

Teimourian B. Blindness following fat injections. *Plast Reconstr Surg.* 1988;80:361.

Williams EF, ed. *Facial Plastic Surgery Clinics of North America.* 16(4), Nov. 2008. Fat Grafting and Transfer Techniques.

70 Surgery of the Eyebrow and Forehead

Shubhra Goel, MD, John G. Rose Jr., MD, Mark J. Lucarelli, MD, FACS, and Bradley N. Lemke, MD

TABLE 70.1 *Causes of Eyebrow Ptosis*

Age-related degeneration of the supporting tissues
Gravitational forces and volume loss
Scarring
Facial nerve paralysis
Underlying bony and tissue asymmetry

TABLE 70.2 *Functions of the Muscles in the Brow and Forehead*

Frontalis muscle—elevates the brow medially and centrally
Orbital orbicularis oculi—closes the eyes and draws the brow towards the eyes
Corrugator supercilii—depresses the nasal eyebrow and pulls it medially
Procerus—depresses the eyebrow
Depressor supercilii—depresses the medial eyebrow

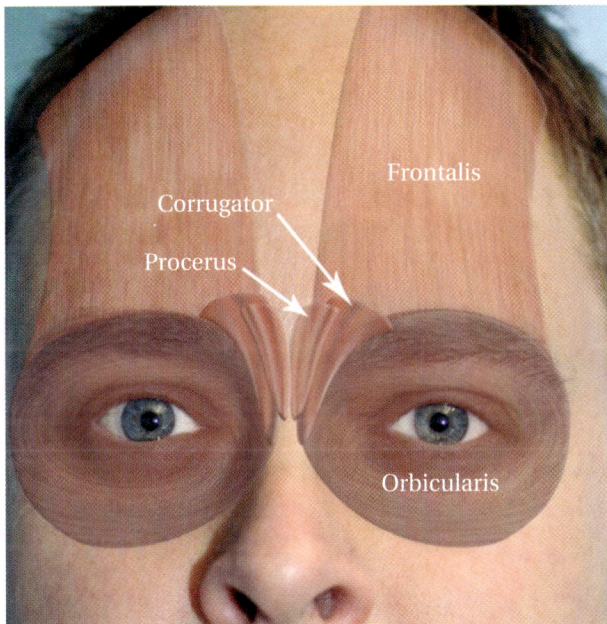

FIGURE 70.1 Anatomy of a Normal Eyebrow and Forehead. There are several muscles of facial expression that insert into the brow and forehead skin. These influence the position of the brow and upper facial expressions.

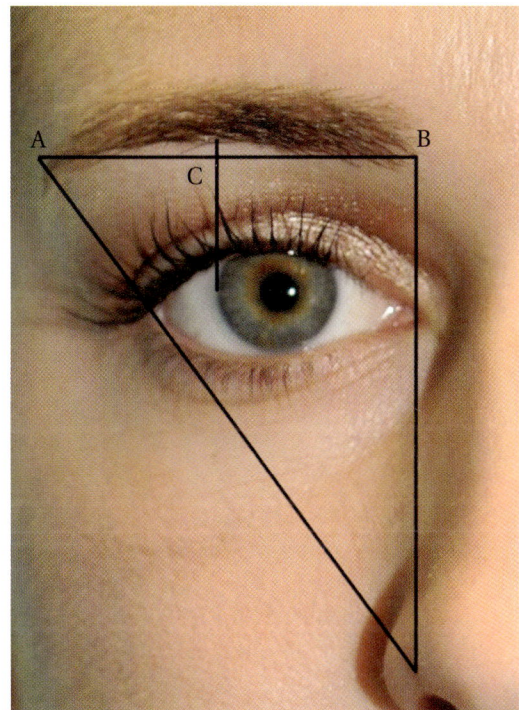

FIGURE 70.2 Eyebrow Dimensions and Relationships. The eyebrow forms a smooth arc in the region of supraorbital rim and is anchored along the supraorbital ridge by fascial attachment to the underlying brow fat. Medially the brow begins at point B along a line drawn through to the lateral ala of the nose and the inner canthus. It ends laterally at point A along an oblique line drawn from most lateral point of the ala to the lateral canthus. The medial and lateral ends of the brow lie almost at the same level. The apex of the brow lies on the vertical line directly above the lateral limbus (point C).

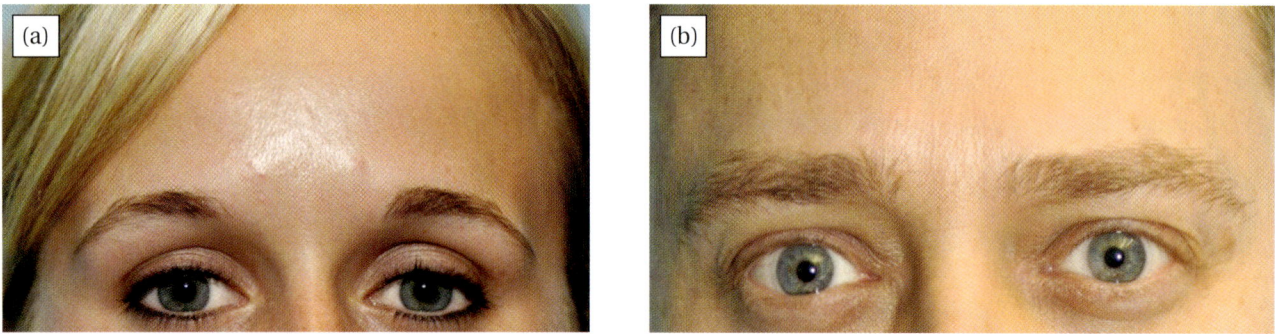

FIGURE 70.3 Topography of Female and Male Eyebrow. The typical youthful female brow is variable but generally rests 3–5 mm above the superior orbital rim and is gently arched (a). The typical male brow is more flat and lies at the level of the superior orbital rim (b).

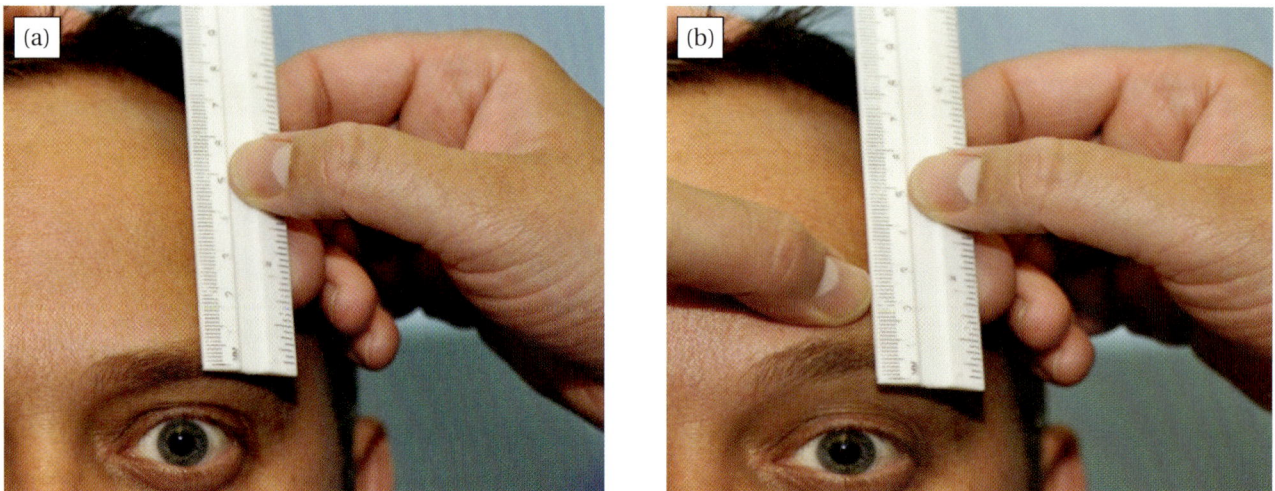

FIGURE 70.4 Measurement of Brow Ptosis. A ruler is placed with the zero mark at the upper border of the relaxed brow (a). The brow is manually lifted until the desired position is achieved and the measurement is taken (b). The degree of brow ptosis should be measured medially, centrally, and laterally.

TABLE 70.3 *Brow Assessment and Measurements*

The brow is an essential component of comprehensive facial rejuvenation.

Hairline

Forehead height

Forehead transverse rhytids

Eyebrow skin thickness, shape and symmetry

Eyebrow hair distribution: Plucking, loss, tattooing

Eyebrow mobility

Degree of dermatochalasis and eyelid ptosis

Periocular fat pads

Lacrimal gland proplapse

Goldman visual fields (if functional)

TABLE 70.4 *Indications for Brow and Forehead Lifting*

Brow ptosis leading to secondary dermatochalasis and visual field restriction.

Brow ptosis presenting together with significant upper dermatochalasis.

Temporal brow ptosis causing temporal hooding of the skin and visual field restriction.

Brow ptosis from facial palsy.

Brow ptosis resulting in a cosmetic concern.

TABLE 70.5 *Preoperative Considerations*

- Discontinuation anticoagulants and anti-inflammatory drugs preoperatively, unless medically contraindicated.
- Counseling of the patient, including discussion of realistic expectations.

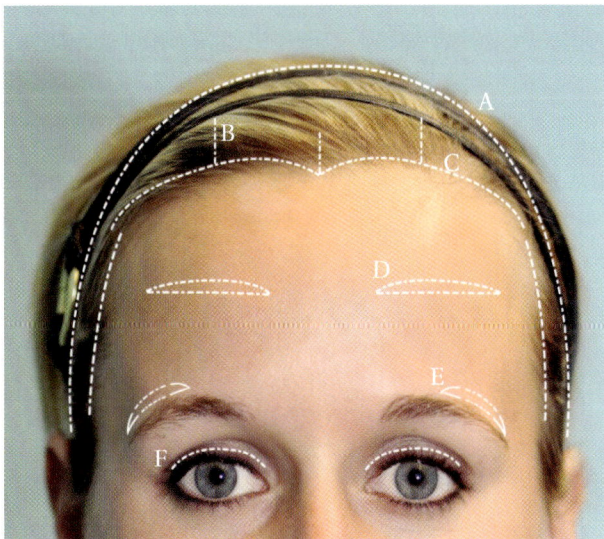

FIGURE 70.5 Incisions for Different Types of Brow Lifts. (A) Coronal. (B) Endoscopic. (C) Pretrichial. (D) Midforehead. (E) Supraciliary. (F) Transblepharoplasty. (G, not shown) Temporal. (Modified from Dailey RA, Saulny SM. Current treatment for brow ptosis. *Curr Opin Ophthalmol.* 2003;14:260–266.)

Surgical Procedures

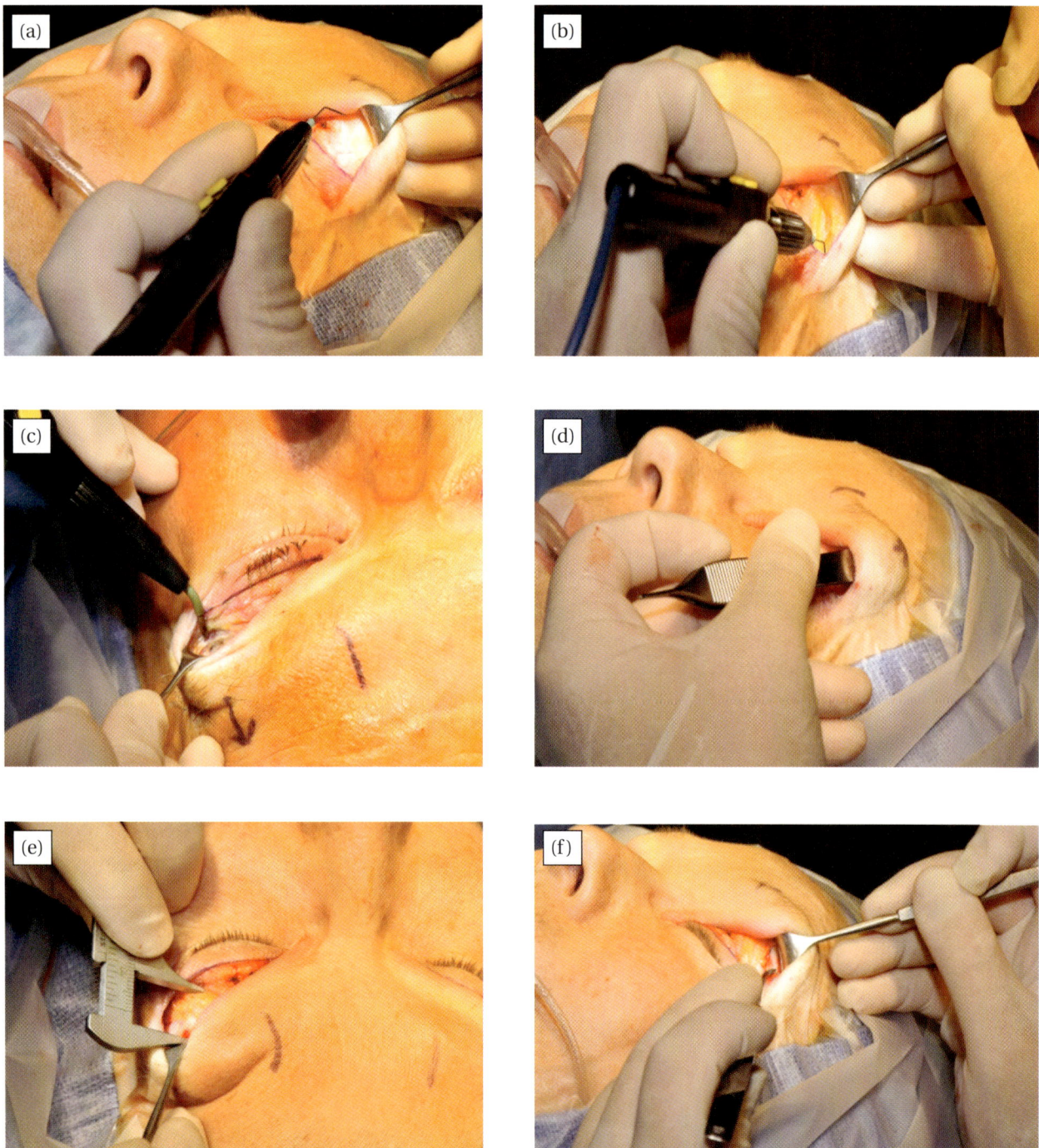

FIGURE 70.6 Internal Browlift with Suture Fixation. (a) Through the upper lid crease, the orbicularis oculi is opened and sharp dissection carried out to the superior orbital rim. (b) A preperiosteal dissection is the carried out under the central and lateral brow. (c) Lysis of the lateral attachments of the brow at the temporal fusion line. A vertical line also marks the course of the supraorbital nerve. (d) The brow is free centrally and laterally. (e) A measurement is then made from the inferior edge of the superior orbital rim to the point of suture fixation (typically 10–14 mm). (f) A 5-0 absorbable (Monocryl, Ethicon) suture is then passed through the periosteum of the frontal bone. A total of two sutures are placed.

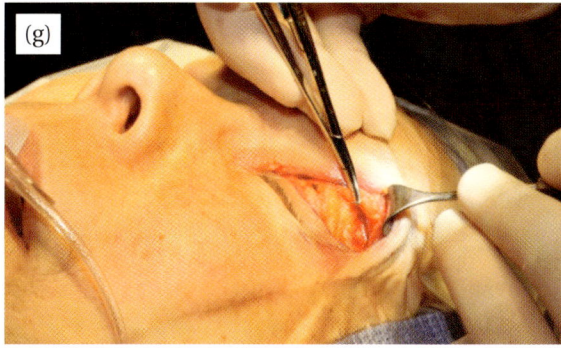

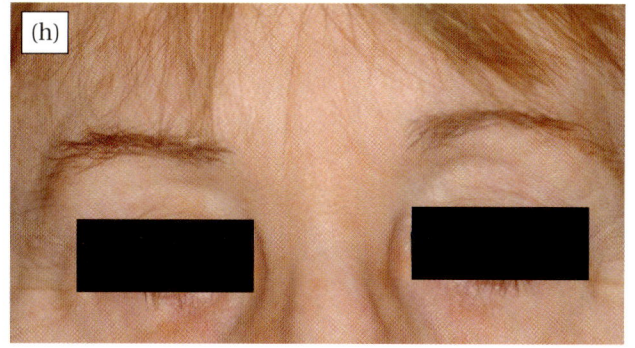

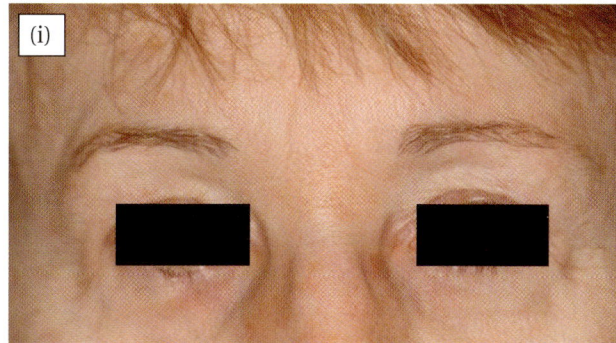

FIGURE 70.6 (*continued*) (g) These sutures are then passed through the inferior edge of the brow fat pad and tied. Skin closure is then performed. (h) Preoperative photo of a 55-year-old female with asymmetric lateral brow ptosis and dermatochalasis. (i) Postoperative of same patient following internal suture fixation brow ptosis surgery and upper lid blepharoplasty.

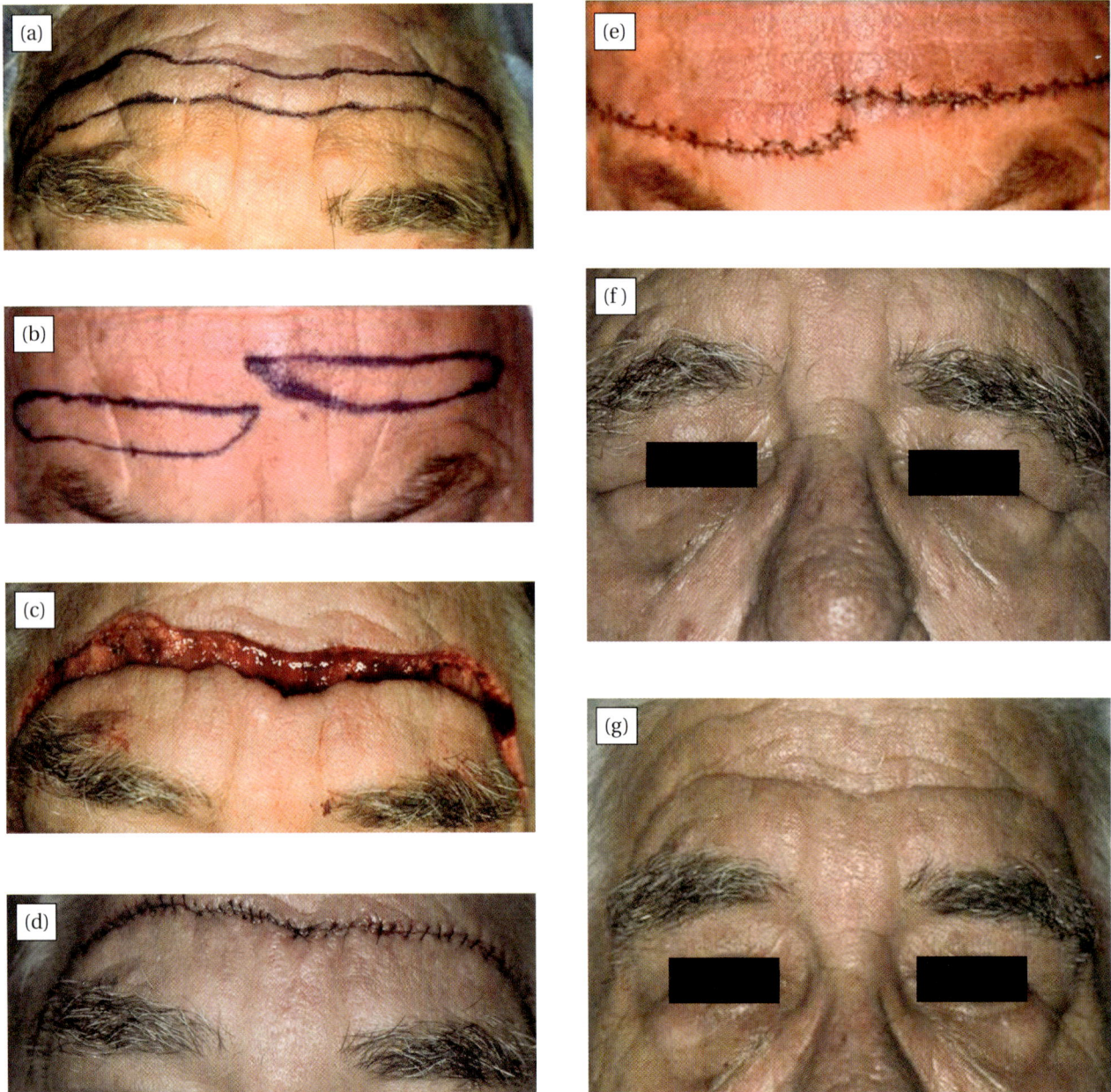

FIGURE 70.7 Midforehead Lift. (a) Markings are made along the natural forehead creases. This can be done as one incision, although many surgeons prefer excising midforehead crescents unilaterally at different levels. (b) Photo of a another patient showing midforehead crescents at different levels merging with the natural forehead creases. (c) The skin is incised and sharp dissection is carried out in the pre-frontalis plane to remove the skin and subdermal fibrofatty layer. (d) Skin closure with 5-0 nylon. Efforts are made to evert the skin edges. The patient (b) also underwent concurrent upper lid blepharoplasty. (e) Alternate technique on a different patient showing unilateral incisions after layered closure. Note the incisions fall within separate forehead creases. (f) Preoperative photo of a 70-year-old man with severe brow ptosis and dermatochalasis. (g) Postoperative photo of same patient, after single-incision midforehead lift and upper lid blepharoplasty.

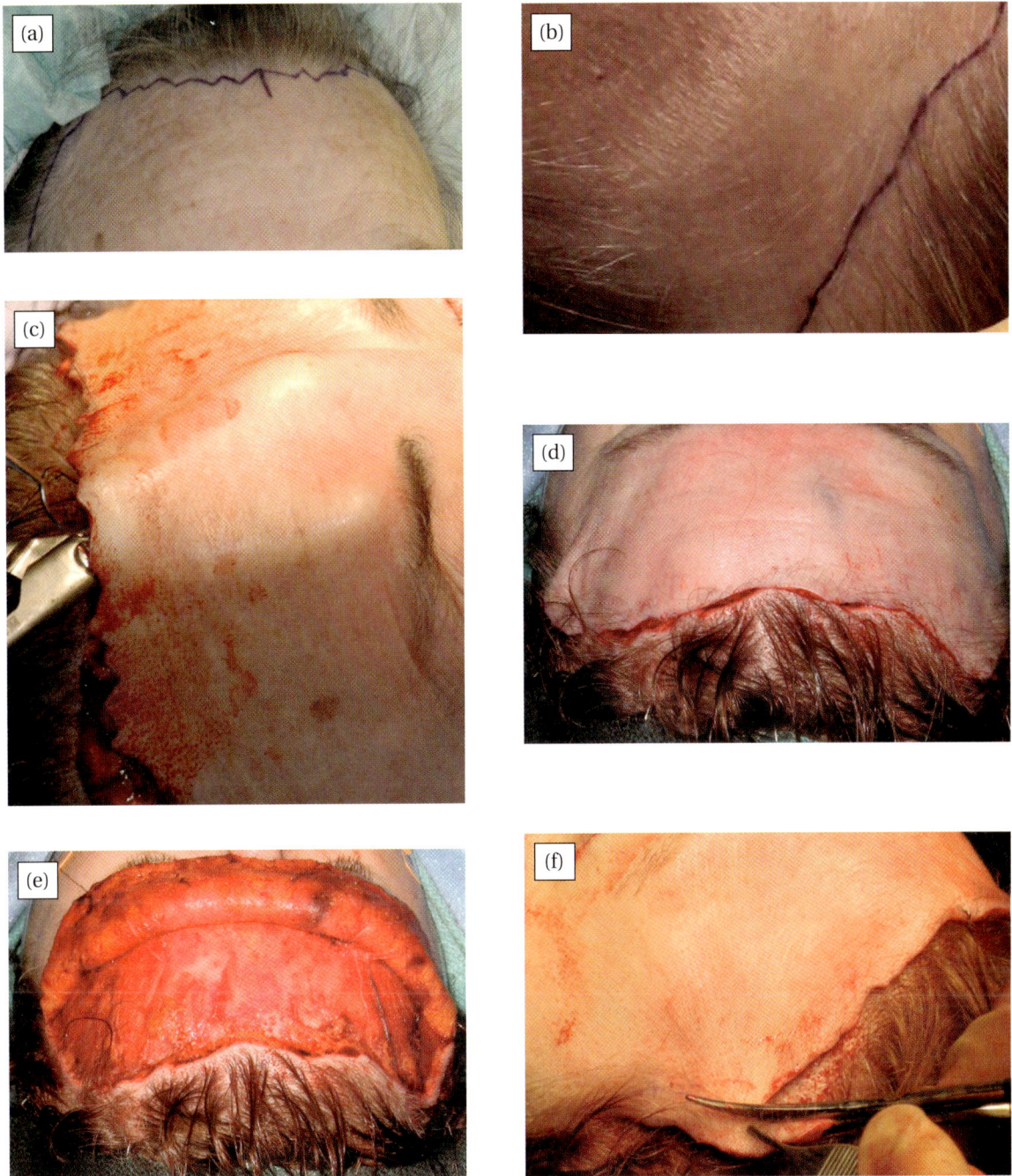

FIGURE 70.8 Pretrichial Browlift. (a) Skin markings are drawn along the anterior hairline where the incision will be made. Note the irregularly irregular marking, which helps to conceal the incision. (b) Magnified view of the pretrichial marking and location relative to the hair line. (c) After skin incisions are made, subcutaneous dissection is performed inferiorly to the level of the eyebrow. (d) After incision and subcutaneous undermining. (e) The forehead flap is turned inferiorly showing the plane of dissection. Note the beveled, irregularly-irregular incision line just anterior to the hairline. (f) The excess skin is then trimmed in a pattern matching the irregularities and bevel of the initial incision.

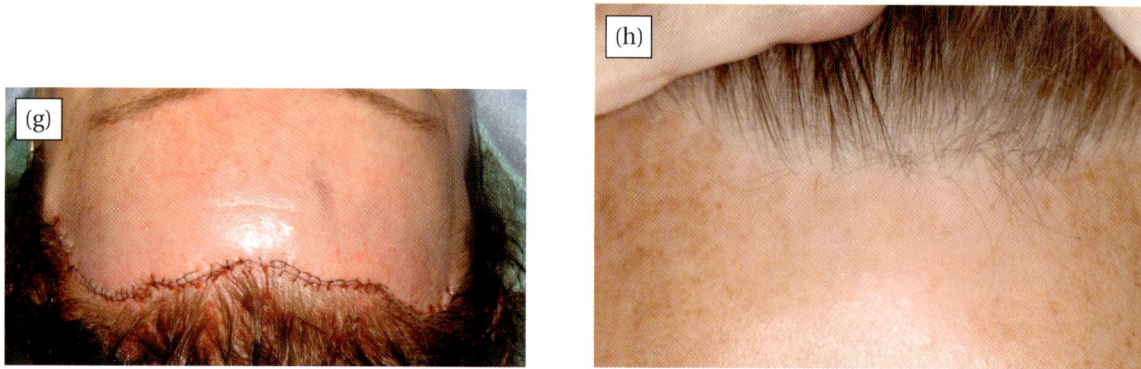

FIGURE 70.8 (*continued*) (g) Pretrichial lift with forehead flap resuspended with 2-layer closure. The subcutaneous layer is closed with interrupted 5-0 polyglactin sutures, and the skin is closed with a continuous running, locking 6-0 nylon suture. (h) Well-healed incision site 8 months postoperatively. Note the normal cilia growth along the beveled incision line.

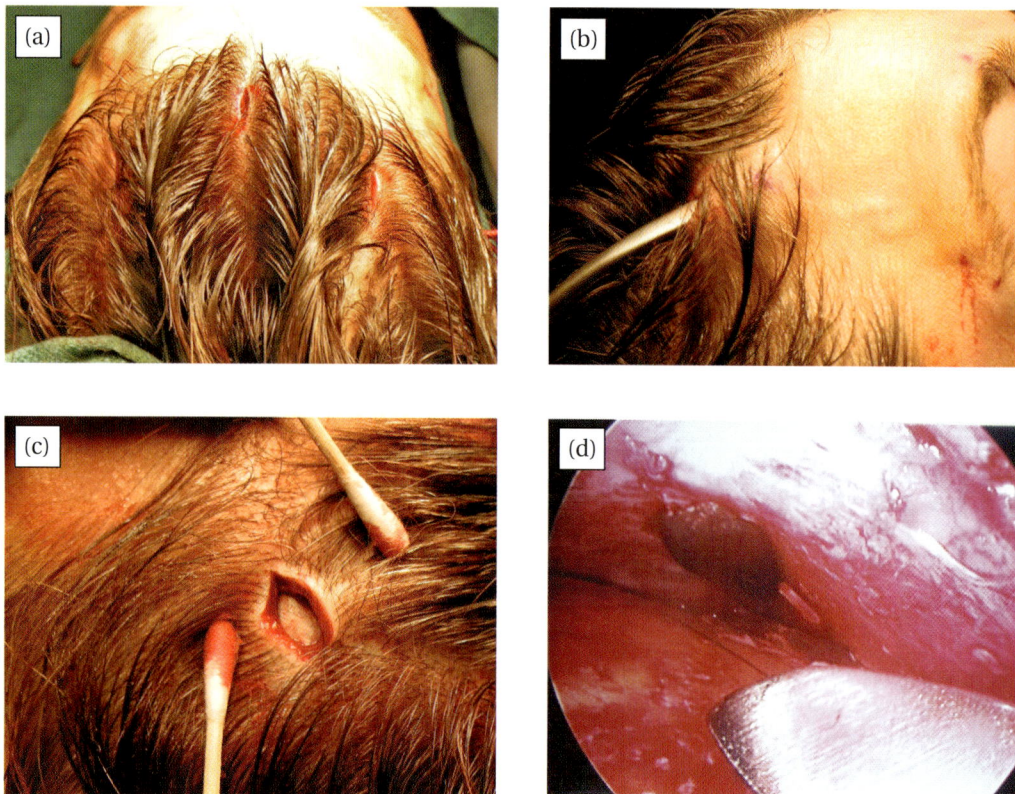

FIGURE 70.9 Endoscopic Browlift. (a) One midline and two parasagittal incision are made. (b) Through the parasagittal incisions, subperiosteal pocket is developed. (c) One temporal incision is made on each side. The deep temporalis fascia is visible through the temporal incision. The temporal dissection is performed between the superficial and deep layers of the temporalis fascia. (d) Endoscopic view of elevator and neurovascular bundle (arrow) inside subperiosteal dissection cavity.

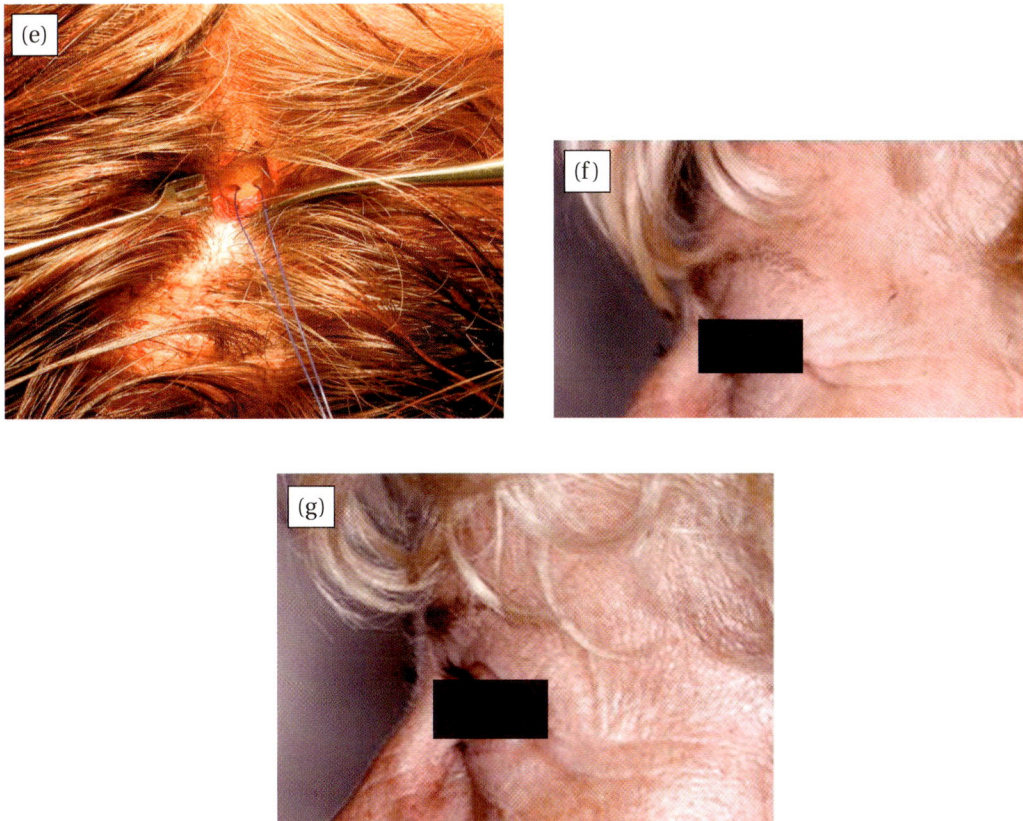

FIGURE 70.9 (*continued*) (e) After wide periosteal release along the temporal line of fusion and along the superior orbital rim to the lateral canthal area, the forehead flap is elevated and fixated through the parasagittal incision using bone tunnels and a 3-0 polydioxanone suture (PDS, Ethicon). (f) Preoperative, side view showing brow ptosis and dermatochalasis. (g) Postoperative, after endoscopic browlift and four-lid blepharoplasty.

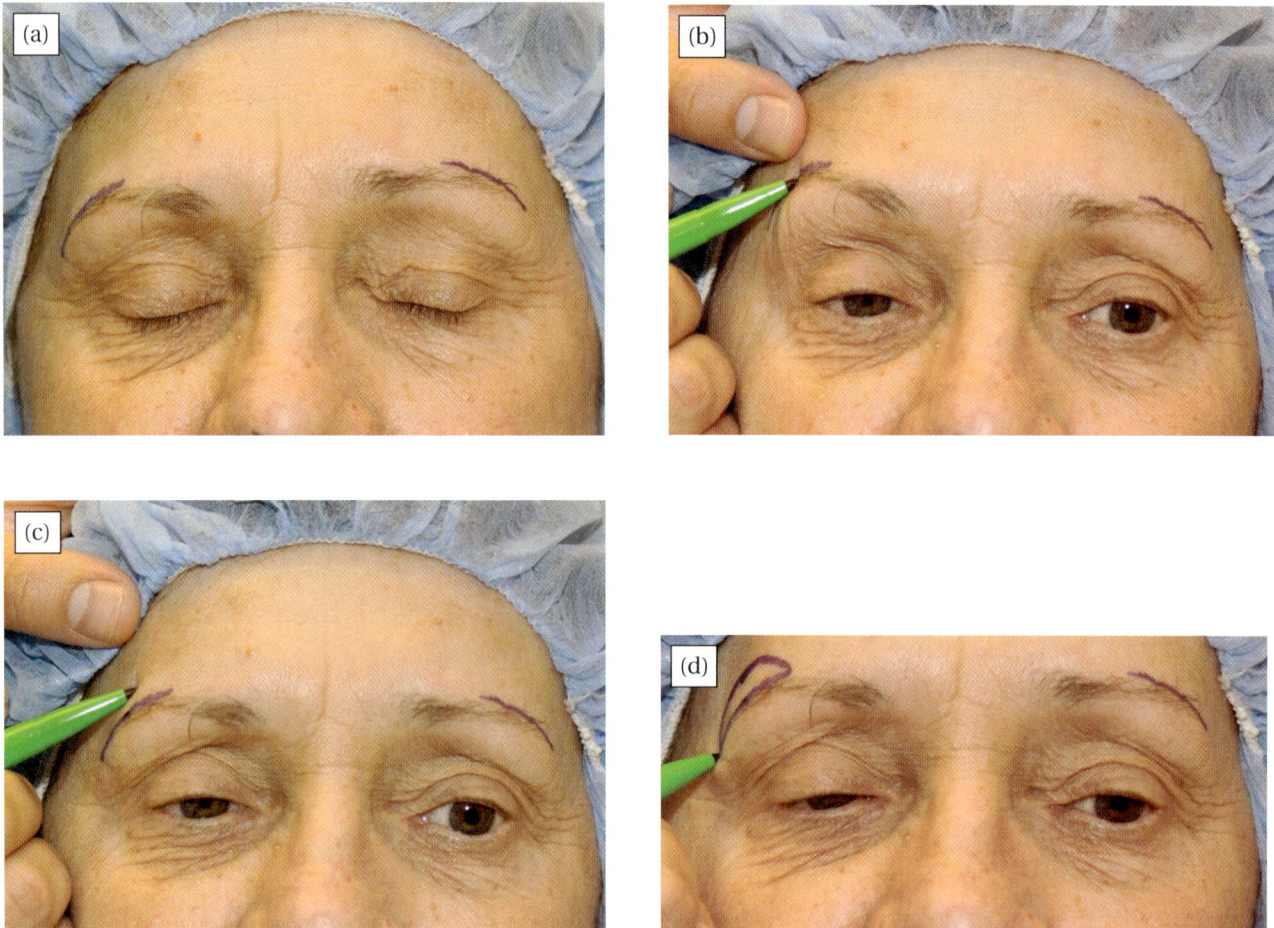

FIGURE 70.10 Supraciliary Browlift. (a) With patient in the sitting position, a line is drawn along the superior aspect of the brow (typically the lateral half to third) just above the first row of cilia. This patient has asymmetric brow ptosis from right facial palsy. (b) The eyebrow is raised to the desired level and a marking pen is placed as a reference point. (c) Keeping the pen suspended slightly away from the skin, the brow is released to fall with gravity. The skin is marked where the pen remains. The difference between the two marks represents the amount of skin to be excised. (d) Skin markings are completed.

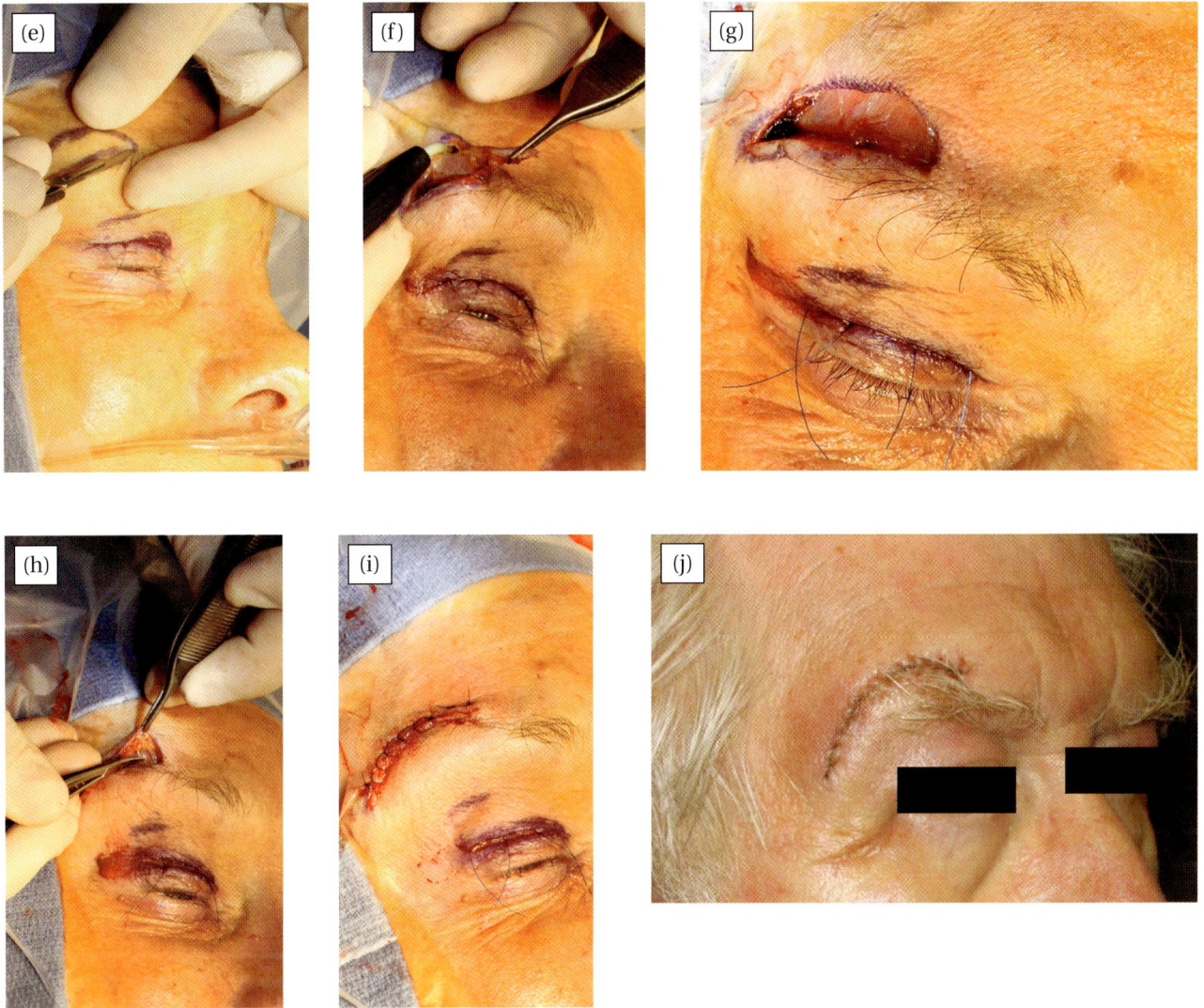

FIGURE 70.10 (*continued*) (e) The skin is incised with a # 15 blade. Note the blade is beveled parallel to the brow cilia to minimize hair follicle injury. (f) The crescent of skin and subcutaneous fibrofatty tissue is then excised. (g) Note the beveled skin edges and visible deep prefrontalis bed. (h) The subcutaneous layer is closed with interrupted buried 5-0 absorbable suture. (i) The skin is then closed with a running, locking 5-0 nylon. Note the everted skin edges. (j) Side view of a patient 7 days after direct supraciliary brow lift.

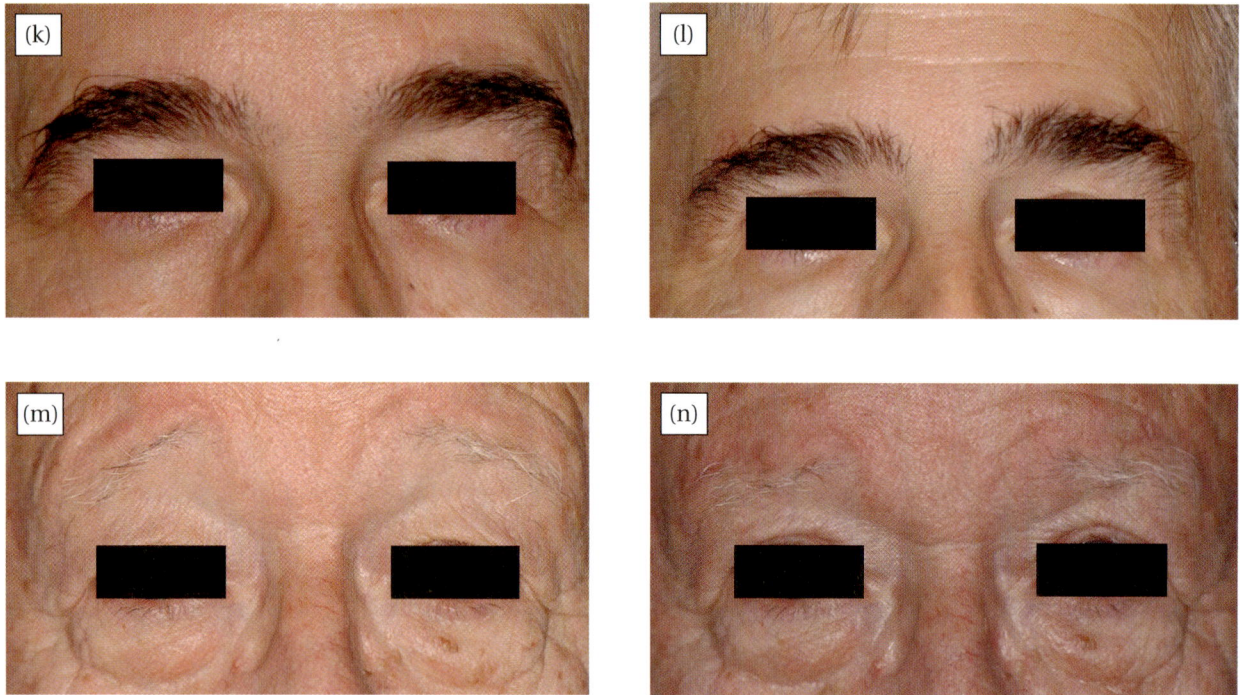

FIGURE 70.10 (*continued*) (k) Preoperative photo of a 50-year-old man with thick, bushy ptotic eyebrows and dermatochalasis. (l) Postoperative photo of same patient after supraciliary brow lift and upper lid blepharoplasty. Bushy eyebrows are ideal for hiding supraciliary scars. (m) Preoperative photo of an 80-year-old man with severe brow ptosis requiring frontalis muscle recruitment to clear the visual axis. (n) Postoperative, following supraciliary brow lift. Note the decreased use of frontalis muscle and the camouflaged scar along the brow.

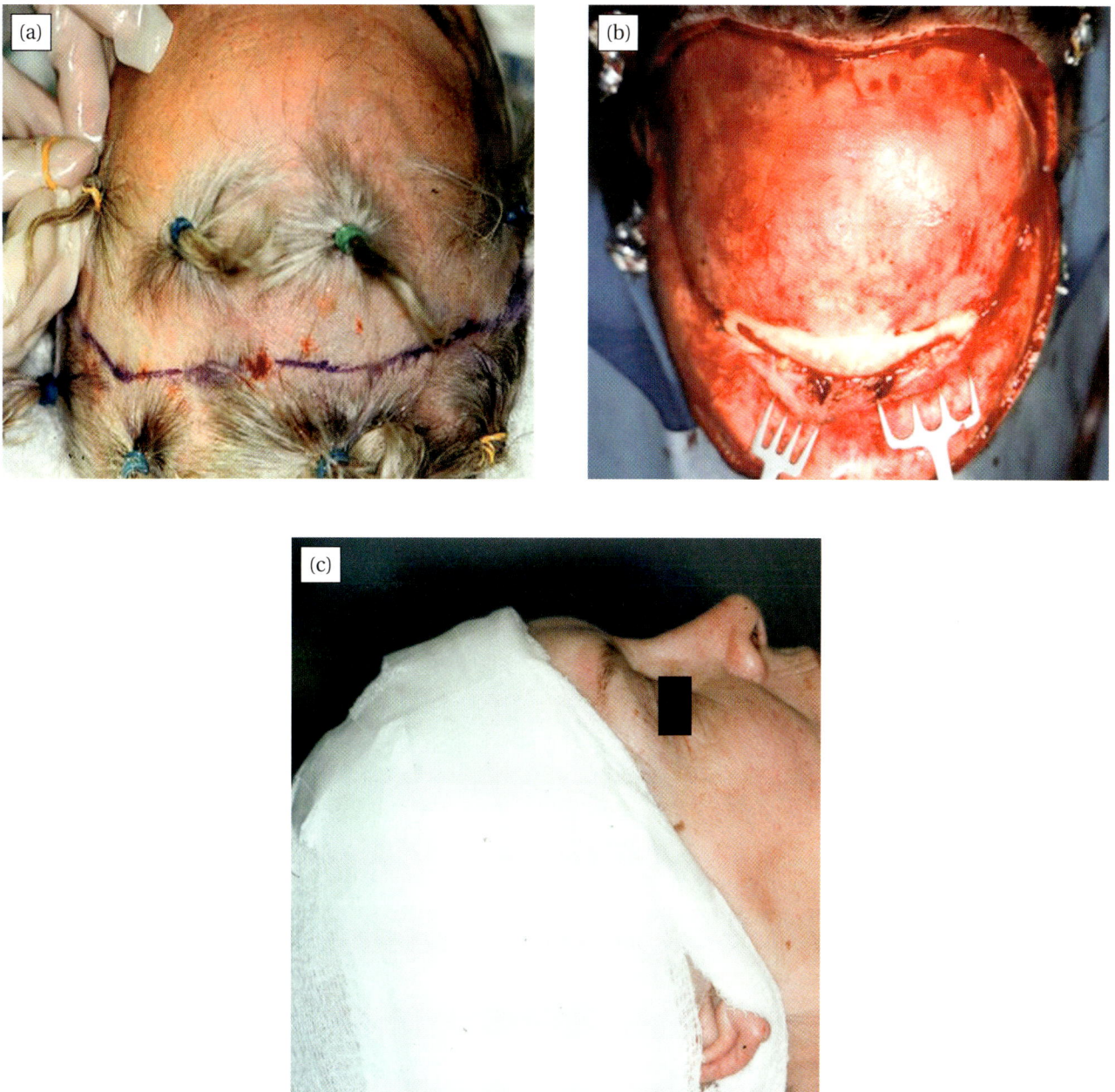

FIGURE 70.11 Coronal Browlift. (a) The hair is prepared using rubber bands and the scalp is marked. (b) The coronal flap is elevated in the subgaleal plane to a level 1.5 cm above the orbital rim. Here the dissection plane becomes subperiosteal. (c) The flap is then elevated, excess skin is excised and layered closure is performed. A pressure dressing is applied.

TABLE 70.6 *Postoperative Care*

Limited activities for at least a week.

Supine resting position with head elevated.

Cold compresses.

TABLE 70.7 *Common Complications in Brow Ptosis Surgeries*

Undercorrection/overcorrection

Asymmetry/contour issues

Neuralgia

Mild sensory dysfunction

Visible scar

TABLE 70.8 *Summary of Brow and Forehead Techniques*

Type of browlift	Specific indications	Advantages	Disadvantages	Complications
Coronal	Moderate to severe brow ptosis Forehead and glabellar rhytids Low or normal hairline Heavy forehead	Direct access Wide access for muscle transection Direct excision of redundant skin	Elevation of frontal hairline Long incision Sensory dysfunction	Alopecia Asymmetry Skin necrosis Permanent overcorrection Facial nerve dysfunction
Pretrichial	Heavy forehead ptosis Moderate to severe brow ptosis Forehead rhytids High hairline	Long lasting results Minimal damage to hairline Correction of medial and lateral brow ptosis and forehead rhytids Direct excision of the redundant skin	Scar along the frontal hairline Problematic with male pattern hair loss	Hematoma Alopecia Possible skin necrosis Damage to frontalis muscle and temporal branch of facial nerve
Midforehead	Mainly in men with prominent forehead furrows Patients with sparse frontal hairline	Simple Good camouflage of forehead rhytids if selected properly Good correction of asymmetry	Scar at the mid-forehead may remain visible	Hypesthesia Hematoma
Temporal	Predominantly lateral brow ptosis Patients who want to avoid full pretrichial incision Low temporal hairline Patients who do not want visible scar	Simpler and faster than coronal and pretrichial lifts Small scars, hidden in hairline Less dissection	Only addresses lateral lift	Hematoma Alopecia Receding temporal hairline may reveal scar Asymmetry

(continued)

TABLE 70.8 *Summary of Brow and Forehead Techniques (continued)*

Type of browlift	Specific indications	Advantages	Disadvantages	Complications
Supraciliary	Patients who do not want full forehead lift Male patients with thick, bushy eyebrows Paralytic brow ptosis	Simple Significant degree of lift Easy access to brow Minimally-invasive	Visible scar at the lateral end of brow	Hypesthesia if supraorbital neurovascular bundle is damaged Asymmetry
Internal (suture)	Patients undergoing blepharoplasty Patients wanting minimally-invasive surgical correction Mild lateral brow ptosis	No visible scar Simple and fast Minimally-invasive	Limited elevation No forehead rhytids correction Generally limited to lateral brow ptosis Prolonged discomfort at the fixation point (weeks-months)	Limited brow movement Possible brow dimpling
Internal (with absorbable implant)	Similar to internal suture brow surgery	Similar to internal suture brow surgery	Cost of the implant Bone drilling is required Palpable, tender implant in patients with thin skin	Infections Palpable mass Slow absorption may lead to lingering tenderness at implant site Displacement of implant Erosion of overlying skin Persistent neuralgia Inflammation adjacent to the implant
Endoscopic	Low to average hairline height Patients desiring invisible scars Mild to moderate brow ptosis in young patients	No scalp resection Minimal damage to motor and sensory nerve units Small incisions Limited scars Fast recovery	Expensive instrumentation Long learning curve Less direct exposure	Hematoma Sensory loss Asymmetry 7th nerve injury Elevation of hairline may create tall-appearing forehead and exaggerated upper-facial-third
Botox	Patients who want quick results and do not want surgery Very mild brow ptosis	Quick results Noninvasive Lower cost than surgery	Temporary results	Eyelid ptosis Diffusion to adjacent tissues

SELECTED REFERENCES

Booth AJ, Murray A, Tyres AG. The direct brow lift: Efficacy, complications and patient satisfaction. *Br J Ophthalmol.* 2004;88:688–691.

Burroughs JR, Bearden WH, Anderson RL, McCann J. Internal brow elevation at blepharoplasty. *Arch Facial Plast Surg.* 2006;8:36–41.

Dailey RA, Saulny SM. Current treatment for brow ptosis. *Curr Opin Ophthalmol.* 2003;14:260–266.

Fagien S. Eyebrow analysis after blepharoplasty in patients with brow ptosis. *Ophthal Plast Reconstr Surg.* 1992;3:210–214.

Fagien S. *Putterman's cosmetic oculoplastic surgery,* 4th ed. New York: Elsevier; 2008.

Frankel, Andrew S, Kamer, Frank M . Chemical brow lift. *Arch Otolaryngol Head Neck Surg.* 1998;124:321–323.

Goldstein SM, Katowitz JA. The male eyebrow: The topographic anatomic analysis. *Ophthal Plast Reconstr Surg.* 2005;21:285–291.

Guyuron, B, Davies B. Subcutaneous anterior hairline forehead rhytidectomy. *Aesth Plast Surg.* 1988; 12: 77–83.

Kahana A, Burkat CN, Lemke BN, Lucarelli MJ. Subcutaneous forehead lift: Technique and early results. *Am J Cosm Surg.* 2007;24(4):193–200.

Kikkawa DO, Miller SR, Batra MK, Lee AC. Small incision nonendoscopic brow lift. *Ophthal Plast Reconstr Surg.* 2000;16:28–33.

Knize DM. Limited-incision forehead lift for eyebrow elevation to enhance upper blepharoplasty. *Plast Reconstr Surg.* 1996;97:1334–1342.

Lemke BN, Stasior OG. Eyebrow incision making. *Adv Ophthal Plast Reconstr Surg.*1983;2:19–23.

Lemke BN, Stasior OG. The anatomy of eyebrows. *Arch Ophthalmol.* 1982;100:981–986.

Mccord C, Doxanas MT. Browplasty and browpexy: An adjuvant to blepharoplasty. *Plast Reconstr Surg.* 1990;86:248–254.

Paul MD. Evolution of the brow lift in the aesthetic plastic surgery. *Plast Reconstr Surg.* 2001;108:1409–1424.

Rohrich RJ, Beran SJ. Evolving fixation methods in endoscopically assisted forehead rejuvenation: controversies and rationale. *Plast Reconstr Surg.* 1997;100:1575–1582.

Steinsapir KD, Shorr N, Hoenig J, Goldberg RA, Baylis HI, Morrow D. The endoscopic forehead lift. *Ophthal Plast Reconstr Surg.* 1998;12:177–178.

Yeatts RP. Current concepts in brow lift surgery. *Curr Opin Ophthalmol.* 1997;8:46–50.

71 — Upper Eyelid Blepharoplasty

Cat Nguyen Burkat, MD, FACS and Nancy Kim, MD, PhD

TABLE 71.1 *Indications for Upper Eyelid Blepharoplasty*

Visually significant dermatochalasis

Cosmetically significant dermatochalasis or fullness

Absent or partial upper eyelid crease in a patient who desires aesthetic enhancement and creation of a distinct eyelid crease

Lash ptosis and upper lid entropion

TABLE 71.2 *Preoperative Considerations*

Assess amount of skin redundancy

Determine presence of fat prominence

Measure eyelid crease height and symmetry

Consider gender and racial differences

Look for concurrent eyelid ptosis, brow ptosis, forehead ptosis

Rule out lacrimal gland prolapse

Assess for eyelash ptosis, trichiasis, and entropion

Discuss with patient type of anesthesia: local or local with intravenous versus oral

Discuss with patient expectations regarding height and contour of the surgical lid crease

Be familiar with differences in eyelid anatomy of the Caucasian and Asian patients

Upper Eyelid Blepharoplasty

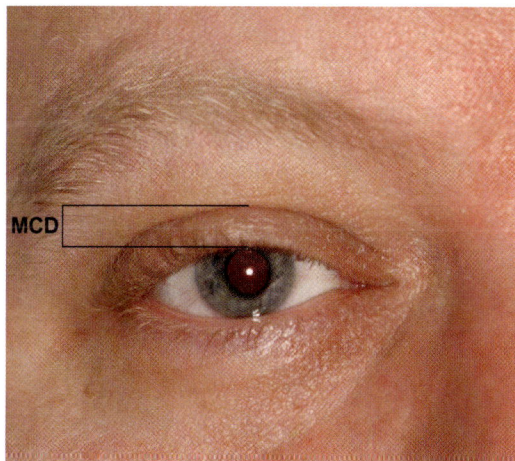

FIGURE 71.1 The margin-to-crease distance (MCD) should be measured bilaterally to make sure they are symmetric in height, and at the desired height for the patient's gender and race. An abnormally elevated MCD may suggest an underlying involutional ptosis that would require ptosis repair.

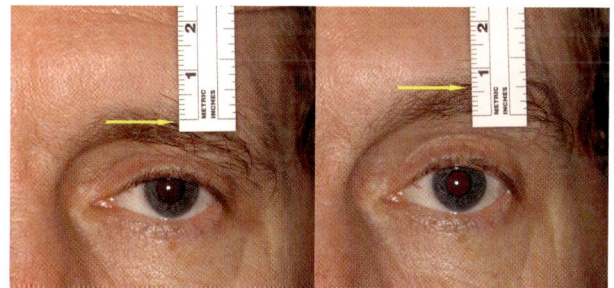

FIGURE 71.2 Prior to blepharoplasty, eyebrow ptosis can be measured with a ruler held to the ptotic brow (yellow arrow on the left shows alignment of upper brow cilia with "zero" mark on ruler). With manual elevation of the brow to the desired height, the amount of brow can be assessed (yellow arrow on the right now shows the same level of upper brow cilia at 7 mm; hence, 7 mm of brow ptosis exists). In general, a male brow typically rests at the level of the orbital rim, in contrast to a female brow that is located approximately 1 cm above the orbital rim.

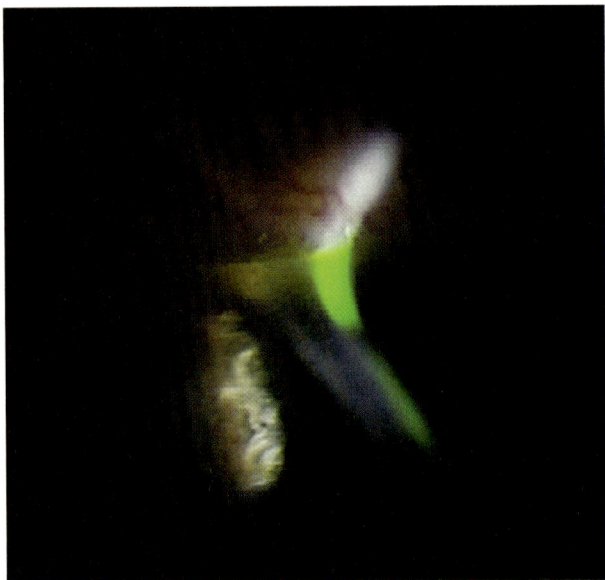

FIGURE 71.3   On preoperative examination, the tear meniscus and corneal surface should be evaluated for signs of dry eyes, as eyelid surgery may exacerbate dry eyes, and this should be discussed with the patient.

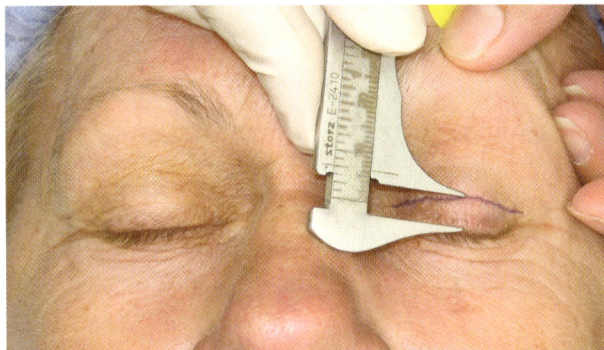

FIGURE 71.4   Placement of the skin marking for blepharoplasty is crucial. When possible, the inferior arc of the marking is placed in the lid crease. In females, the eyelid crease is typically 8–11 mm above the lid margin, and has a gentle curve or arc shape. In men, the crease is flatter and less-defined, and rests lower, at 6–8 mm above the lid margin. (In Asian patients the lid crease usually rests considerably lower.) The skin marking should not extend past the upper punctum to avoid medial canthal webbing.

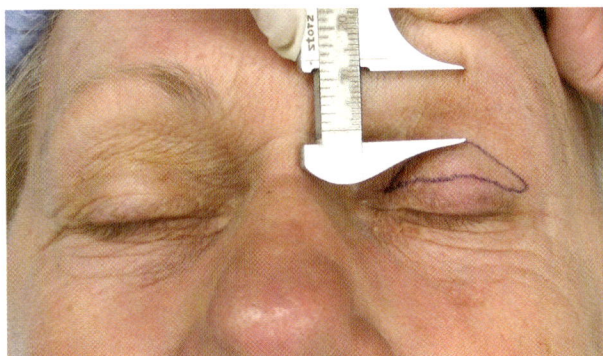

FIGURE 71.5   Approximately 20 mm of eyelid skin should be retained centrally in the upper lid in order to avoid postoperative retraction and lagophthalmos. Care is taken to measure from the junction of the thin eyelid skin to the thicker eyebrow skin, rather than from the eyebrow hairs.

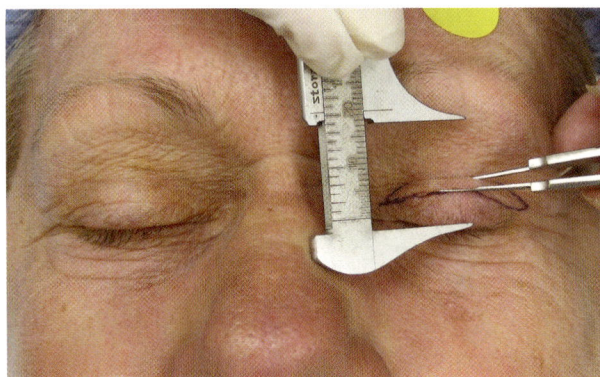

FIGURE 71.6   A skin pinch is performed to confirm that sufficient skin has been conserved without causing margin ectropion, retraction, or vertical tightening of the lid skin that would indicate anterior lamellar shortage.

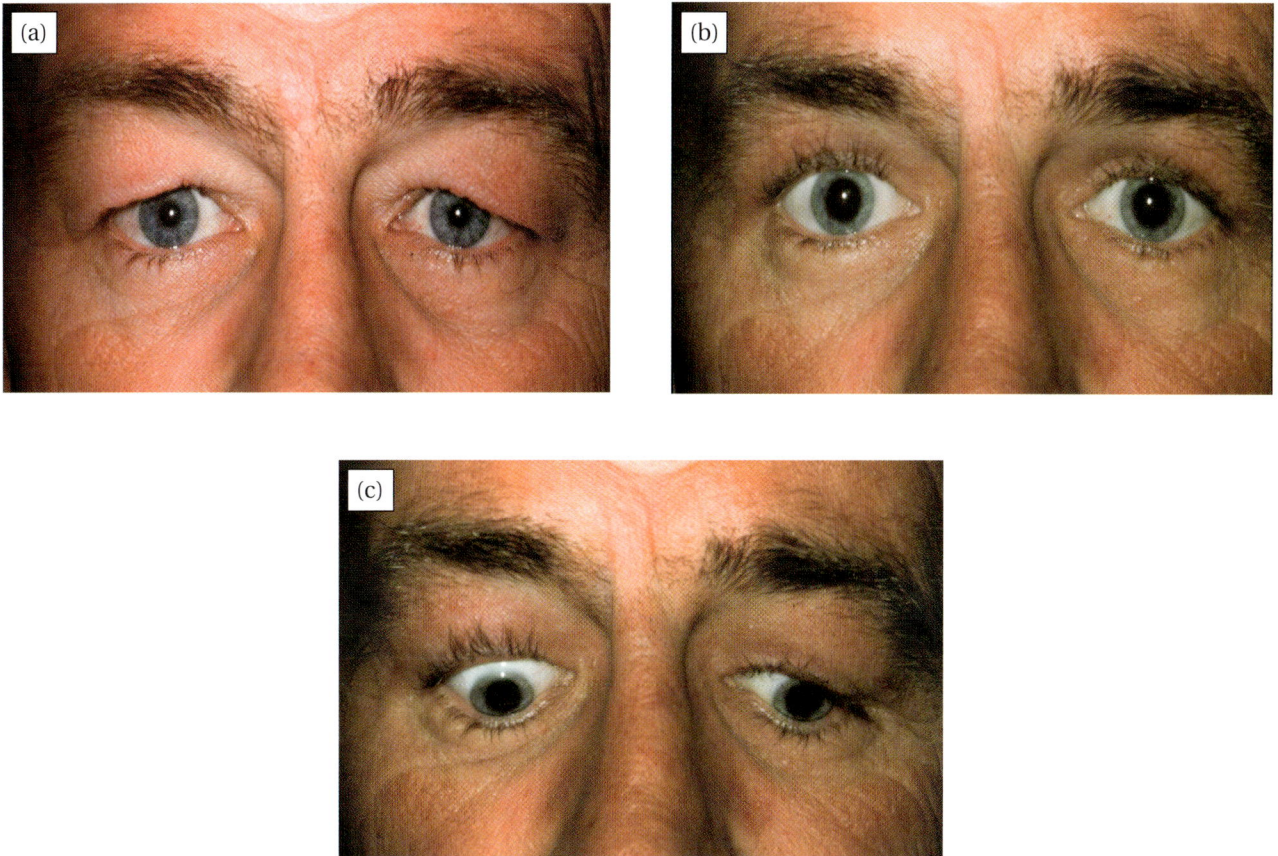

FIGURE 71.7 Excessive removal of upper lid skin may increase the risk of postoperative lagophthalmos and exposure keratopathy. (a) Preoperative dermatochalasis. (b) Following bilateral upper lid blepharoplasty. (c) Lid lag, lagophthalmos, and anterior lamellar shortage are present in right upper lid.

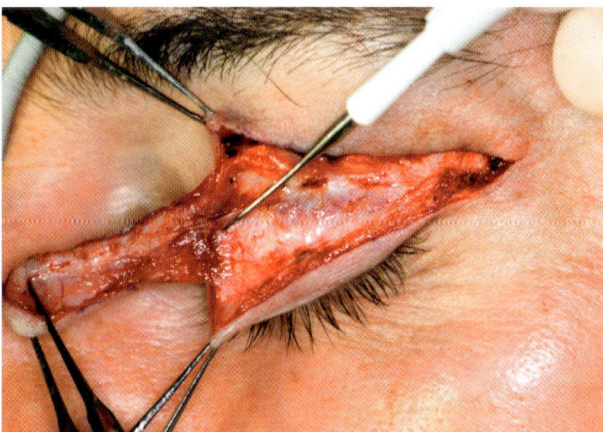

FIGURE 71.8 A CO_2 laser, radiofrequency unit, or a monopolar unit with a microdissection needle can be used to incise the skin and remove a skin-only or skin-muscle flap. (Courtesy of R.K. Dortzbach, MD.)

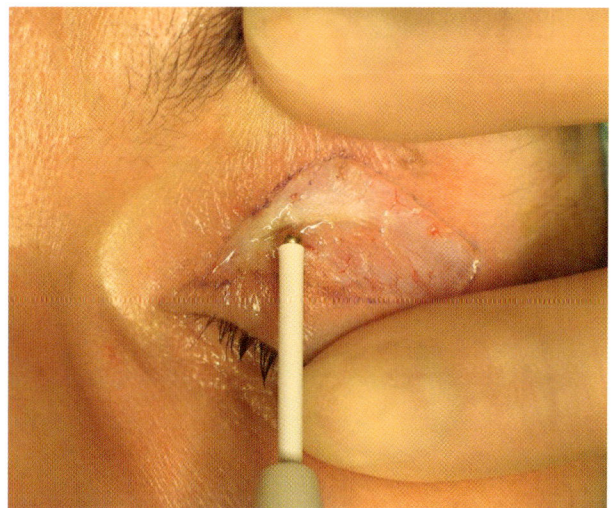

FIGURE 71.9 In upper lid blepharoplasty, volume preservation is associated with a youthful, rejuvenated appearance; therefore, conservative removal is important. Often, the orbital fat pads may be minimally sculpted with a cautery over an intact orbital septum.

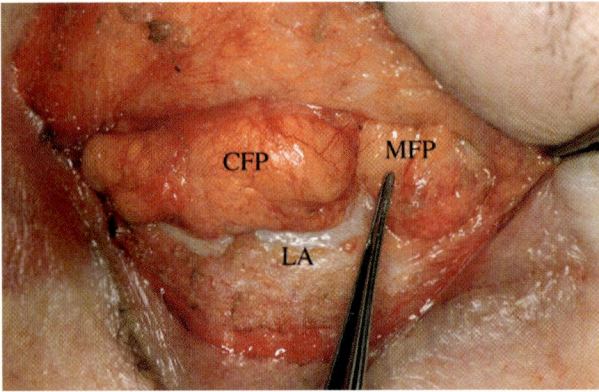

FIGURE 71.10 There are 2 upper lid fat pads posterior to the orbital septum, in contrast to the lower eyelid. Note medial fat pad (MFP), central preaponeurotic fat pad (CFP), and levator aponeurosis (LA). Avoid excessive fat removal, as this can result in a hollow superior sulcus. (Courtesy of R.K. Dortzbach, MD.)

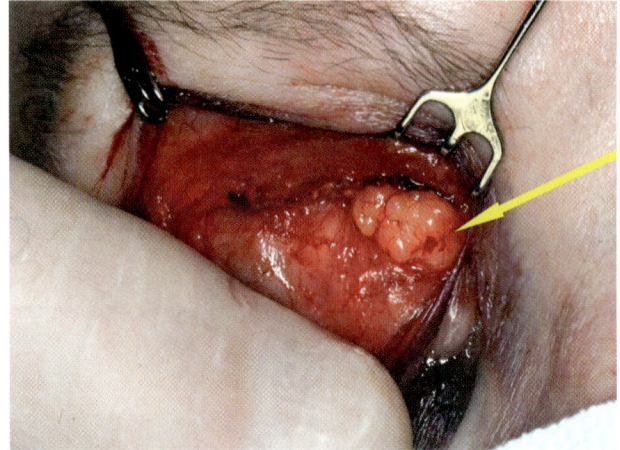

FIGURE 71.11 The medial fat pad (yellow arrow), which is whiter in color than the central preaponeurotic fat, can be exposed with gentle ballottement of the globe. (Courtesy R.K. Dortzbach, MD.)

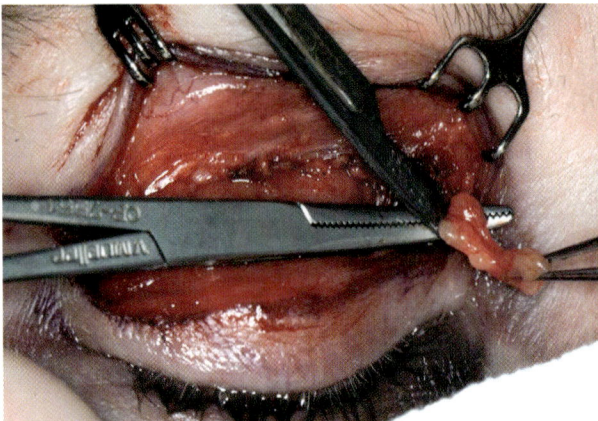

FIGURE 71.12 If conservative excision of the medial fat is indicated, care should be taken to avoid hemorrhage from the vessels traversing the medial fat pad. Injury to the superior oblique tendon or trochlea could result in diplopia. (Courtesy of R.K. Dortzbach, MD.)

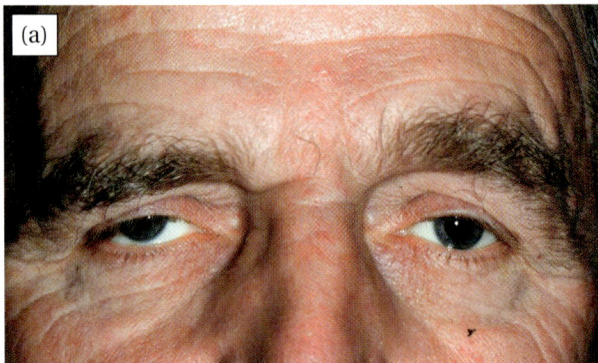

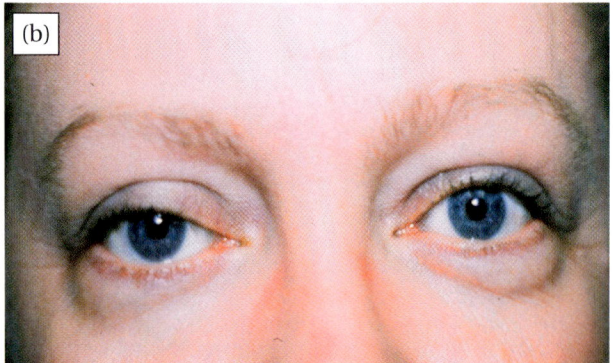

FIGURE 71.13 Concurrent conditions must be recognized prior to blepharoplasty surgery and addressed if indicated. (a) Severe eyebrow ptosis and eyelid ptosis are present, in addition to dermatochalasis. (b) Right involutional ptosis is also present.

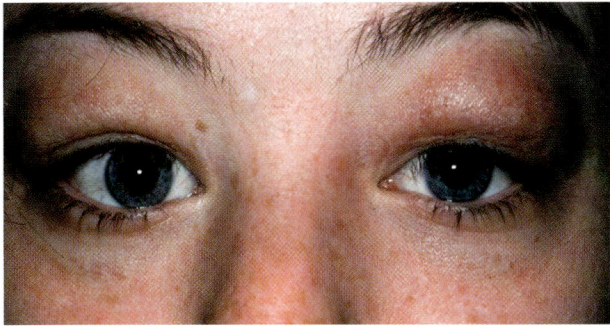

FIGURE 71.14 Blepharochalasis syndrome may be a form of localized angioedema that causes episodic exacerbations of eyelid inflammation and swelling. After the episodes have stabilized, skin redundancy may need to be treated with blepharoplasty.

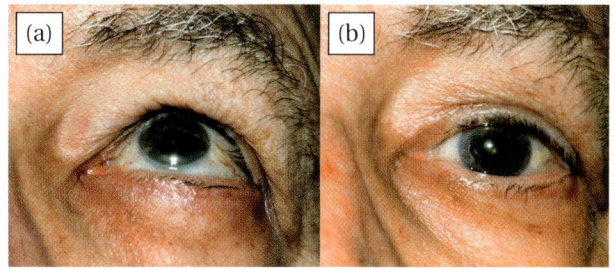

FIGURE 71.15 Secondary eyelash ptosis or trichiasis (a) may also occur from the mechanical weight of excess upper lid skin, which may be corrected with blepharoplasty surgery (b).

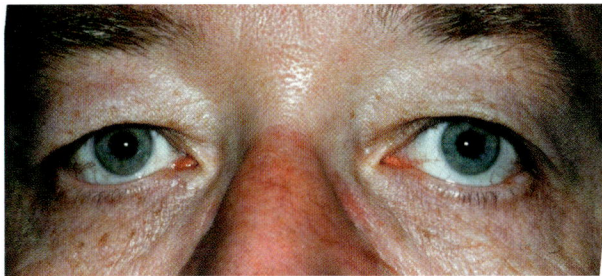

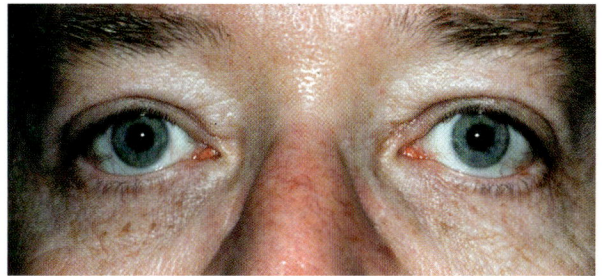

FIGURE 71.16 Clinical photos before and after upper eyelid blepharoplasty. Note the preserved eyelid fullness in this male patient.

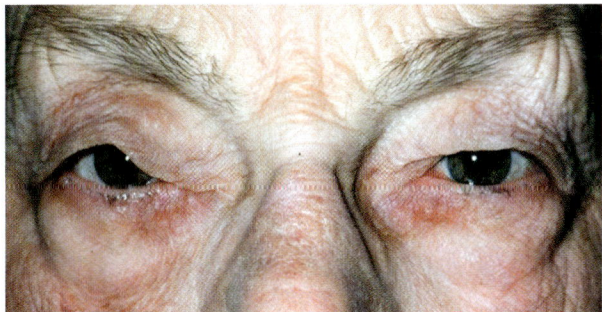

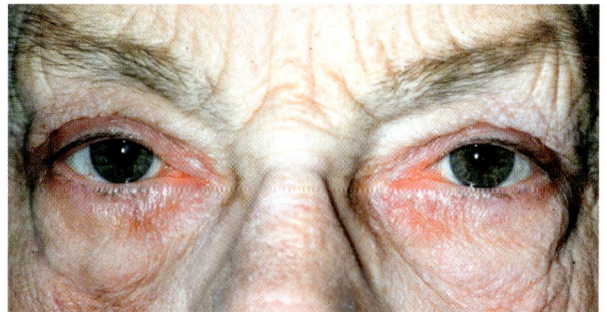

FIGURE 71.17 Clinical photos before upper eyelid blepharoplasty (left), and 2 weeks postoperatively (right).

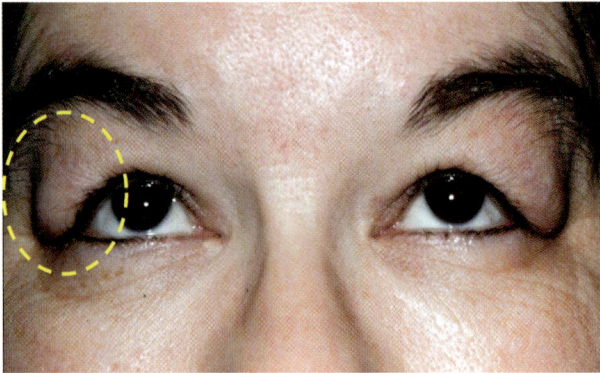

FIGURE 71.18   Bilateral lacrimal gland prolapse (encircled in right upper eyelid) should be considered if temporal eyelid fullness is present, as there is no lateral fat pad.

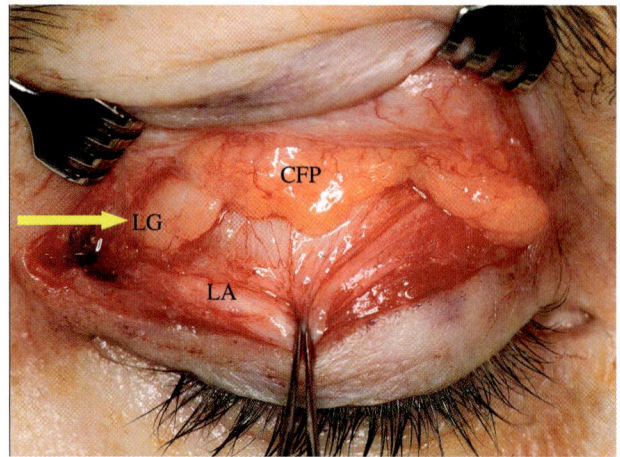

FIGURE 71.19   The lacrimal gland (LG, yellow arrow) has a characteristic temporal position, pink color, and lobulated shape. Failure to recognize a prolapsed gland during blepharoplasty may lead to partial lacrimal lobectomy and postoperative keratoconjunctivitis sicca. If uncorrected, persistent fullness could result in a poor cosmetic result. CFP = central preaponeurotic fat pad; LA = levator aponeurosis. (Courtesy of R.K. Dortzbach, MD.)

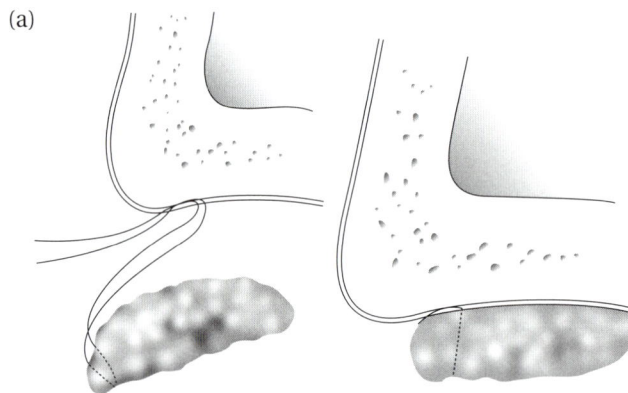

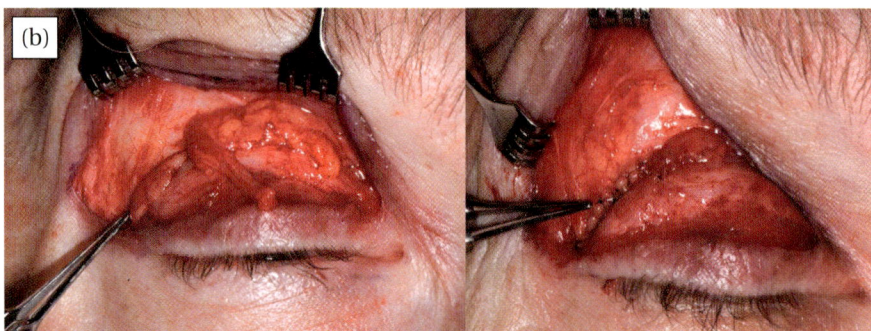

FIGURE 71.20   Surgical resuspension of the lacrimal gland back into the fossa of the superolateral frontal bone with 6-0 nonabsorbable suture may be indicated to improve the surgical outcome. (a) Schematic sagittal view. (b) Intraoperative views, right eye.

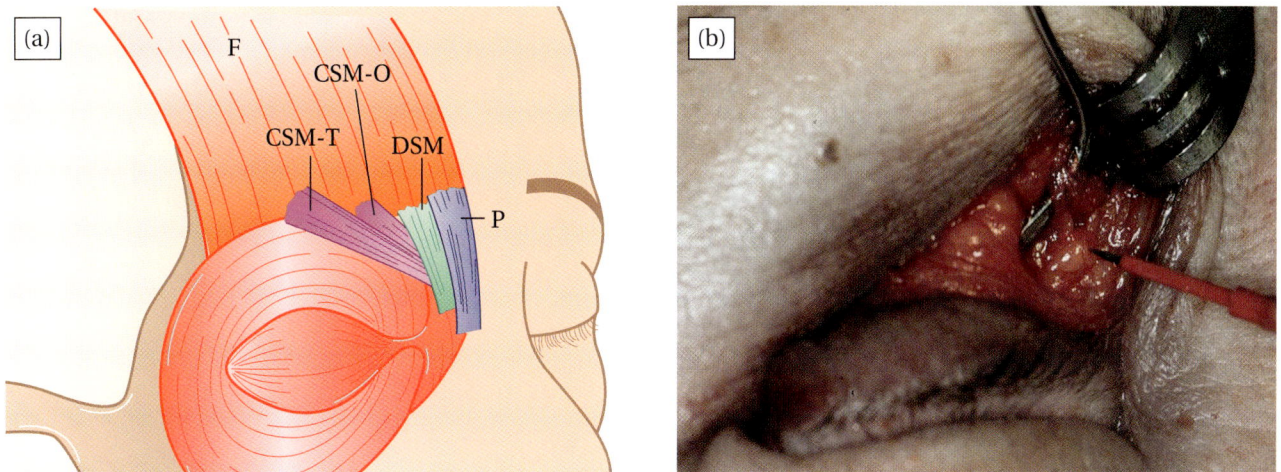

FIGURE 71.21 (a) Schematic of brow depressors. Adjunctive procedures may be performed during blepharoplasty, such as resection or weakening of the corrugator supercilii (CSM-O, CSM-T) and procerus (P) muscles through the medial incision to diminish the appearance of glabellar creases. DSM = depressor supercilii muscle; F = frontalis. (From: Burkat CN, Lucarelli MJ, Lemke BN. *Am J Cosm Surg.* 2005;22:7–24.) (b) Intraoperative view.

Complications of Upper Eyelid Blepharoplasty

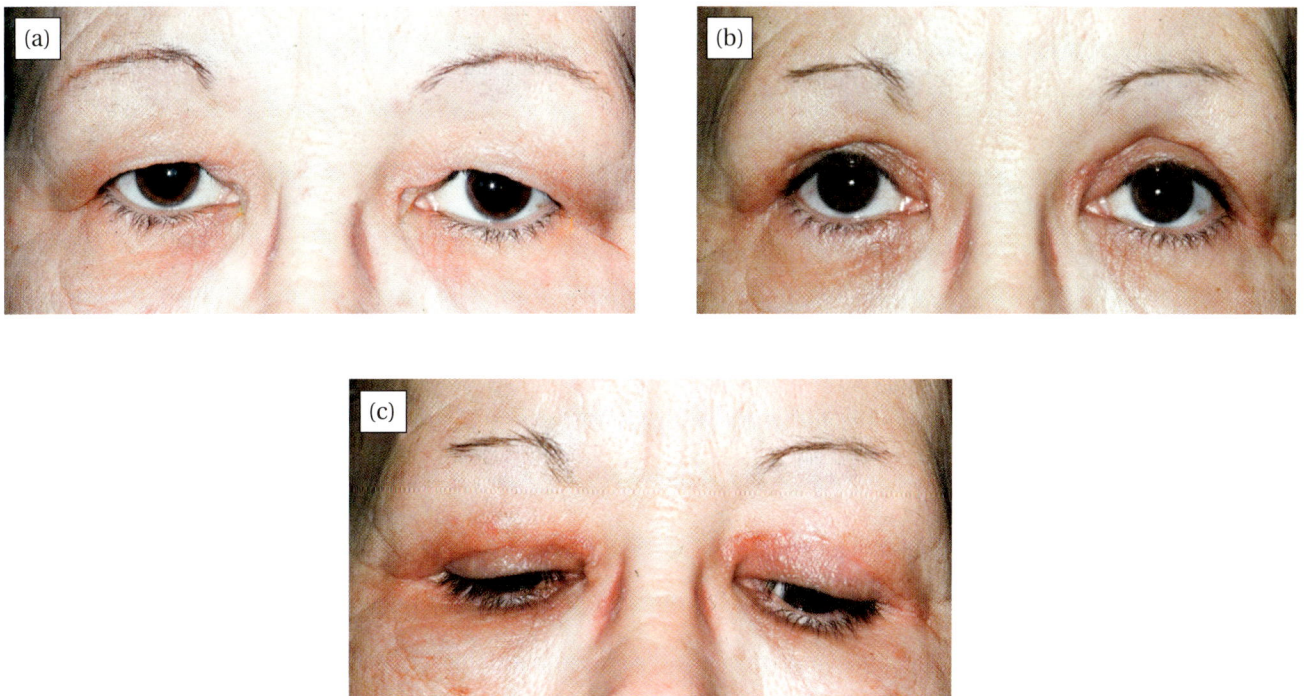

FIGURE 71.22 (a, b, c) 61-year-old female with postoperative asymmetric eyelid creases, as well as a hollow sulcus of left upper lid from aggressive fat removal.

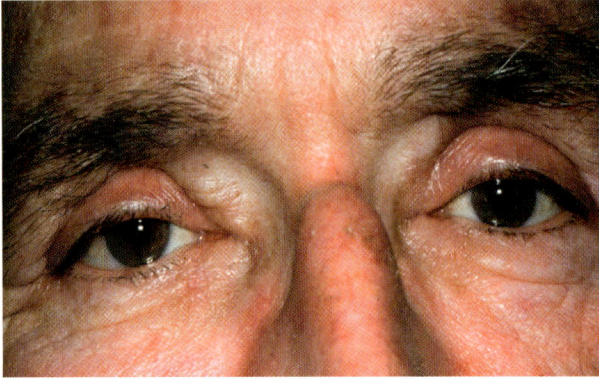

FIGURE 71.23 The eyelid creases were placed too high for a male, resulting in an unnatural, feminized appearance. (Courtesy R.K. Dortzbach, MD.)

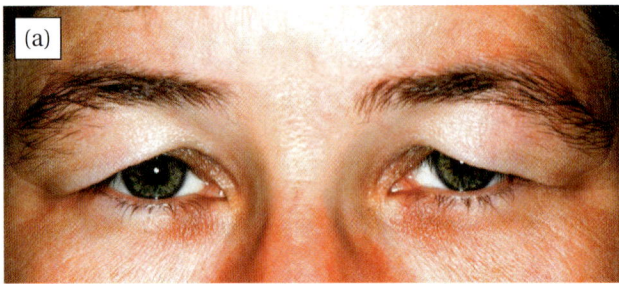

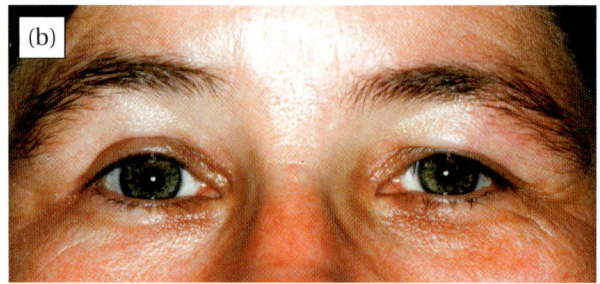

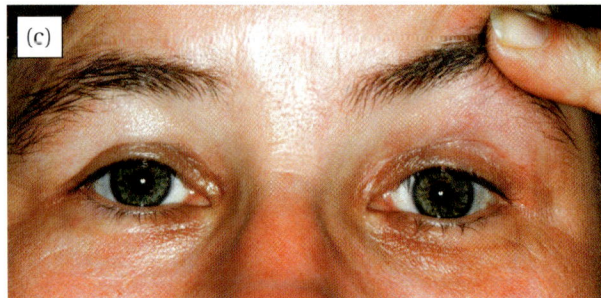

FIGURE 71.24 (a) Preoperative photograph of patient. Following blepharoplasty, the left eyelid still appeared droopy (b) secondary to pseudodermatochalasis from brow ptosis that was not addressed (c).

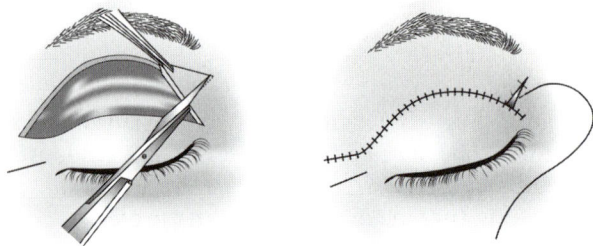

FIGURE 71.25 A Burow's triangle can be removed if excess medial eyelid tissue is present, rather than extending the incision past the level of the punctum.

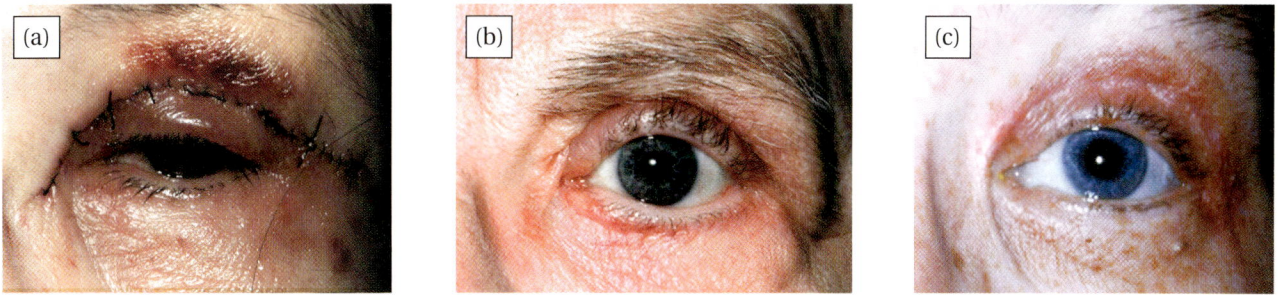

FIGURE 71.26 Medial canthal webbing. A medial incision that extends past the punctum into the medial canthus (a) may result in medial canthal webbing and unsightly scars (b, c) that are very difficult to correct. (Photos courtesy of R.K. Dortzbach, MD.)

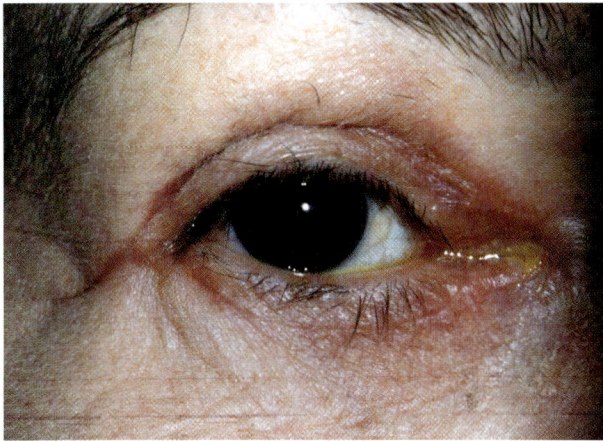

FIGURE 71.27 Suboptimal scarring can also occur laterally if the incision is carried inferiorly past the level of the lateral canthus, into the thicker temporal skin, or blended into the lateral canthoplasty incision.

Blepharoplasty in the Asian Patient

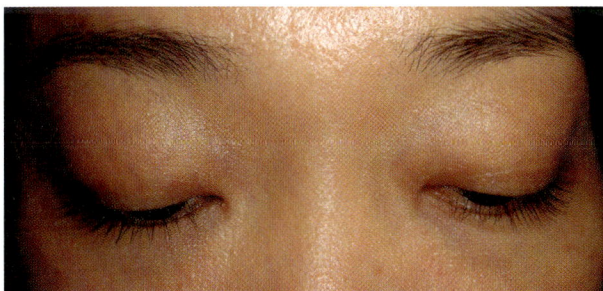

FIGURE 71.28 As a result of the lower point of fusion of the orbital septum, the orbital fat pad lies closer to the lid margin and gives the eyelids of Asians its characteristic fuller appearance. There is also a submuscular fat pad present superiorly in the Asians that is not typically seen in Caucasian lids.

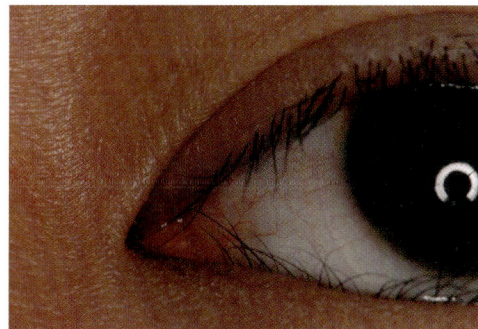

FIGURE 71.29 In blepharoplasty for the Asian patient, careful preoperative consideration should include discussion with the patient regarding the epicanthal fold, desired eyelid crease height, and the crease configuration. The incision should usually blend into the epicanthal fold medially.

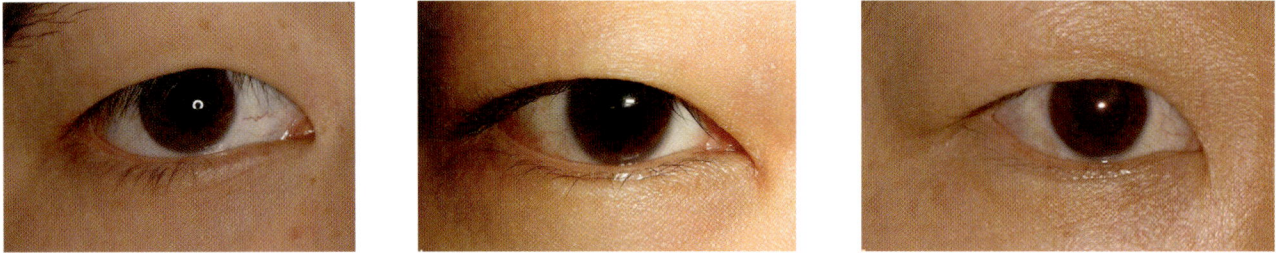

FIGURE 71.30 Clinical examples of the absent eyelid crease in both Asian males and females.

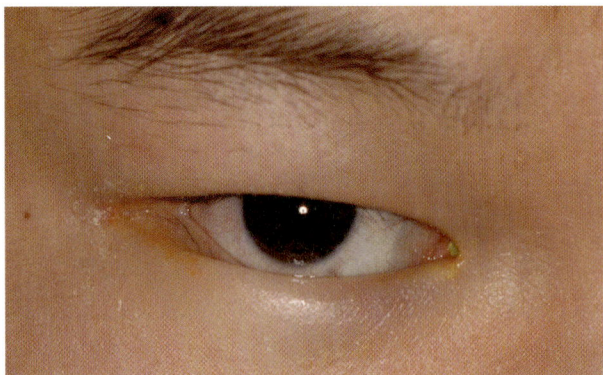

FIGURE 71.31 This 19-year-old Asian male demonstrates an absent upper eyelid crease, in addition to lower eyelid epiblepharon.

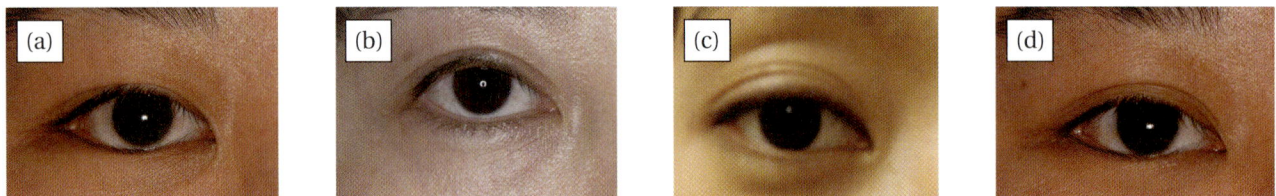

FIGURE 71.32 Eyelid crease configurations in Asian patients. (a) Inner fold with medial taper and gentle lateral flare, continuous. (b) Parallel continuous crease. (c, d) Multiple creases.

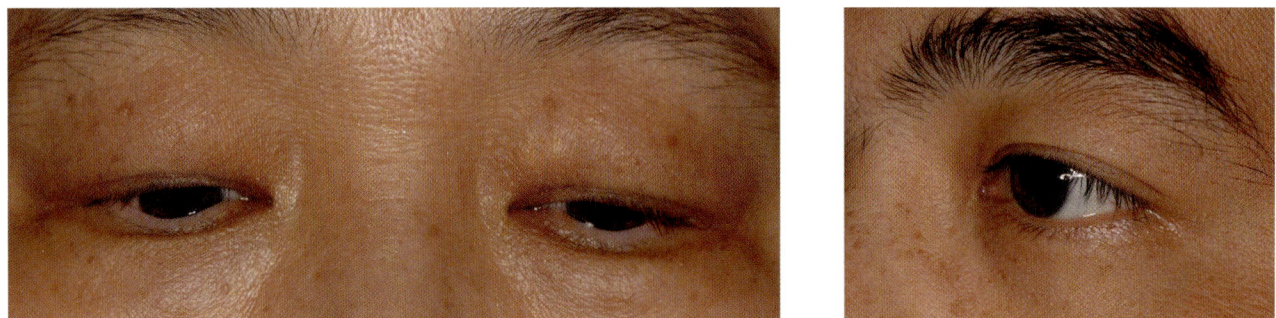

FIGURE 71.33 Note that the eyelid crease in Asian patients rests much closer to the lid margin than in the average Caucasian lid.

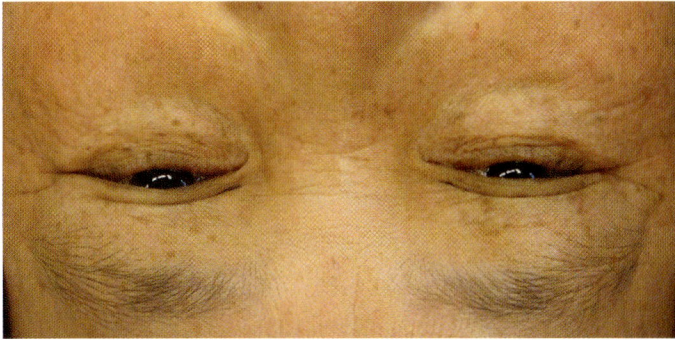

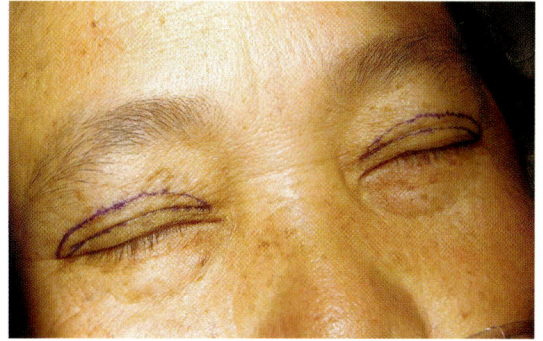

FIGURE 71.34 The placement of the surgical markings can be confirmed during surgery by having the patient open and close her eyes to ascertain that the skin excisions blend into the epicanthal fold medially. Note that the lid crease is drawn lower, to reflect the shorter height of the tarsus compared to Caucasian lids.

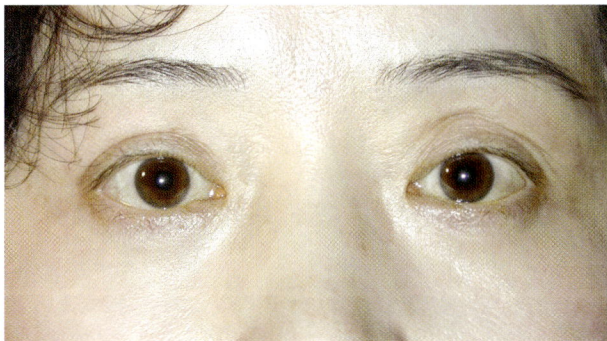

FIGURE 71.35 Following the flap excision, the preaponeurotic and submuscular fat pads should be minimally sculpted. As eyelids in Asians are typically fuller in appearance, a postoperative hollow sulcus deformity is an unnatural-looking complication after blepharoplasty, as seen in the left upper lid of this patient.

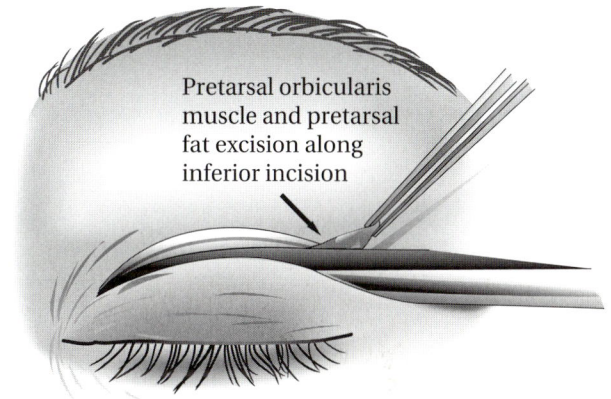

Pretarsal orbicularis muscle and pretarsal fat excision along inferior incision

FIGURE 71.36 The eyelids of Asians may contain more subcutaneous and suborbicularis fat, with a prominent pretarsal fat component; therefore, a small horizontal excision of pretarsal orbicularis muscle and fat may optimize the lid crease reformation and surgical outcome. (Adapted from Fagien S. *Putterman's cosmetic oculoplastic surgery*, 4th ed., Philadelphia PA: Saunders; 2007.)

Levator
aponeurosis

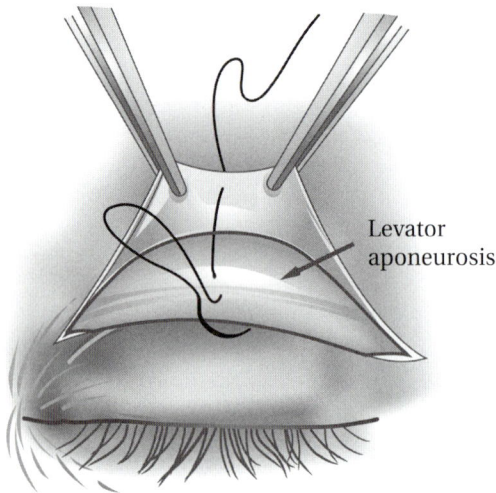

FIGURE 71.37   The crease is meticulously formed, using interrupted 6-0 nylon suture to secure the inferior skin edge to the levator aponeurosis at the superior tarsal edge, and then through the superior skin edge. After several of these sutures are placed along the length of the lid crease, the skin edges are closed with 6-0 fast absorbing plain gut or nylon suture in running fashion. (Adapted from Fagien S. *Putterman's Cosmetic Oculoplastic Surgery*, 4th ed., Philadelphia PA: Saunders; 2007.)

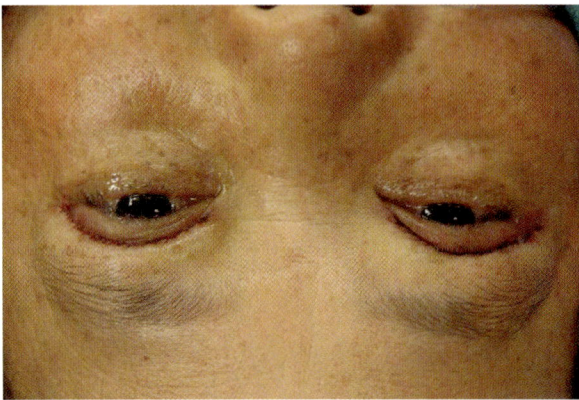

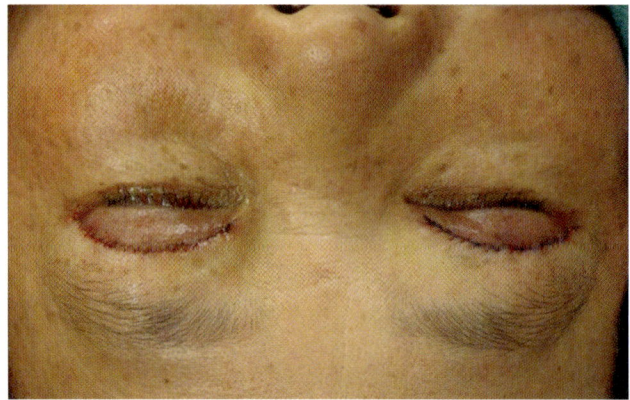

FIGURE 71.38   Immediately after an upper lid blepharoplasty in an Asian patient, with the medial incisions blended into the epicanthal fold to avoid webbing.

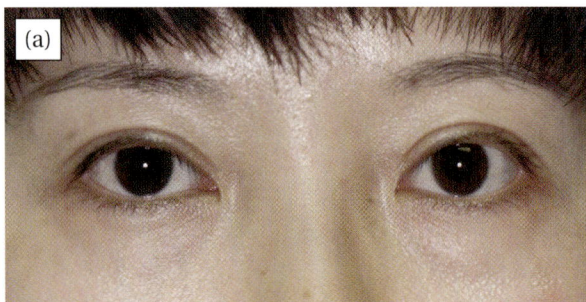

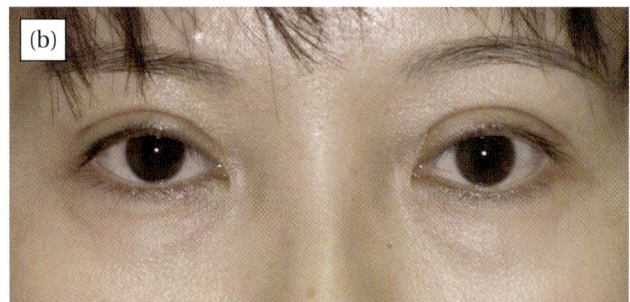

FIGURE 71.39   Preoperative (a) and 6-month postoperative (b) photo of an Asian female undergoing cosmetic blepharoplasty to create a subtle elevation of her eyelid creases. Note the left eyelid demonstrates a mild medial canthal web (b).

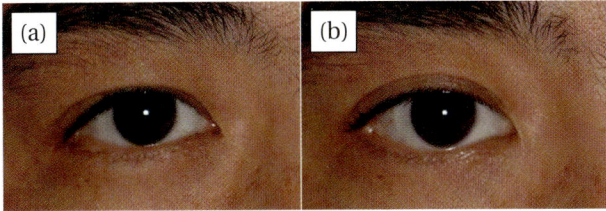

FIGURE 71.40 Preoperative (a) and 7-month postoperative (b) photo of a 31-year-old Asian male undergoing cosmetic upper lid blepharoplasty to enhance his eyelid crease, while still maintaining a low crease configuration.

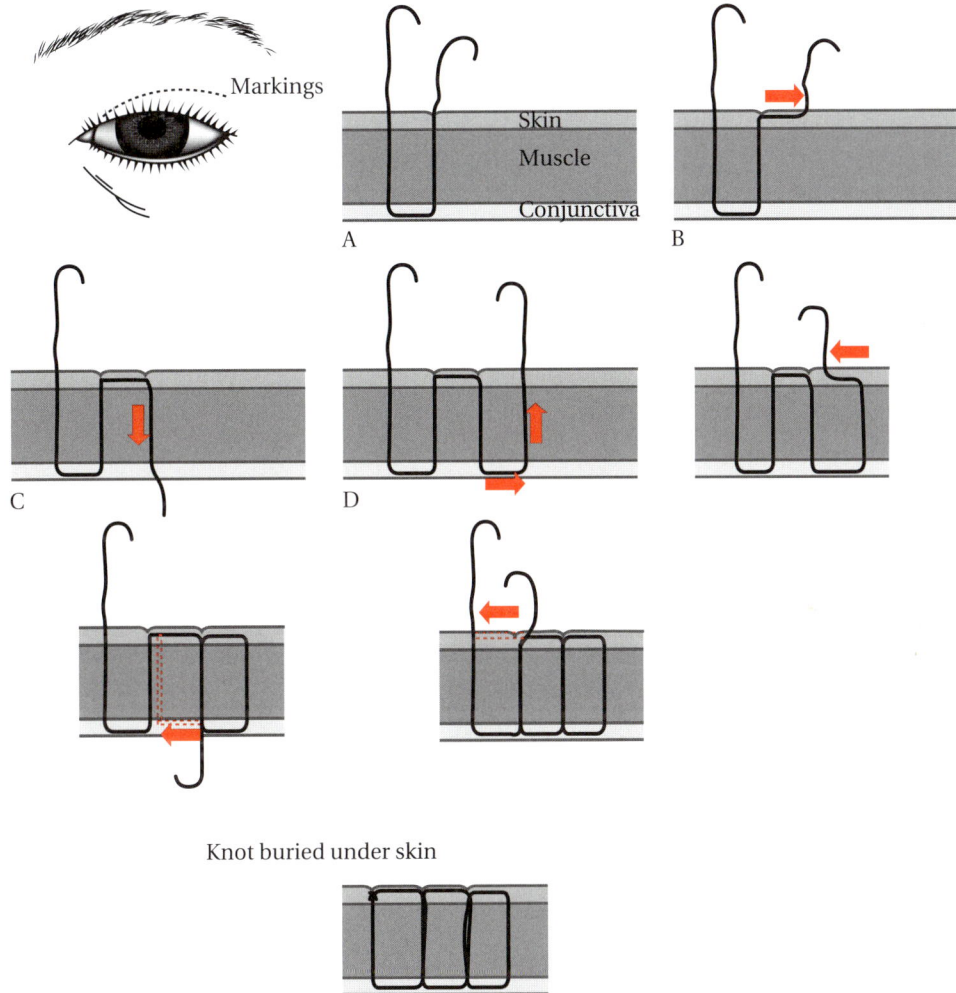

FIGURE 71.41 An example of a non-incisional simple continuous suture technique to create an eyelid crease, using 6-0 nylon suture along the desired eyelid crease. To avoid corneal irritation, the suture should not exit the conjunctival surface. There is a higher risk of failure and lack of permanence with non-incisional techniques. (Modified from Chen WP. Asian *Blepharoplasty and the Eyelid Crease*, 2nd ed. Philadelphia: Butterworth Heinemann, Elsevier; 2006.)

TABLE 71.3 *Potential Complications of Upper Eyelid Blepharoplasty*

Eyelid retraction, lagophthalmos

Exposure keratopathy, dry eyes

Retrobulbar or orbital hemorrhage with possible loss of sight

Asymmetry, multiple creases, or fading of the surgical creases over time

Excessive fat removal resulting in a hollow sulcus

Unnatural high crease placement and creation of a high sulcus

Infection, cellulitis

Hypertrophic scarring, canthal web formation

Undercorrection, need for additional surgery

SELECTED REFERENCES

Campbell JP, Lisman RD. Complications of blepharoplasty. *Facial Plast Surg.* 2000;8:303.

Chen WPD. Asian blepharoplasty. *Ophthal Plast Reconstr Surg.* 1987;3:135–140.

Collin JRO. Blepharochalasis: a review of 30 cases. *Ophthal Plast Reconstr Surg.* 1991;7(3):153–157.

Jeong S, Lemke BN, Dortzbach RK, Park YG, et al. The East Asian upper eyelid: an anatomical study with comparison to the Caucasian eyelids. *Arch Ophthalmol.* 1999;117(7):907–912.

McCord CD. Techniques in blepharoplasty. *Ophthalmic Surg.* 1979;10:40–55.

McKinney P, Byun M. The value of tear film breakup and Schirmer's test in preoperative blepharoplasty evaluation. *Plast Reconstr Surg.* 1999;104:566.

Millay DJ. Upper lid blepharoplasty. Skin versus pinch. *Laryngoscope.* 1991;101:1233.

Rubenzik R. Surgical revision of the Oriental eyelid. *Ann Ophthalmol.* 1977;9:1189.

Sheen JH. Supratarsal fixation in upper blepharoplasty. *Plast Reconstr Surg.* 1974;54:424.

72 Lower Eyelid Blepharoplasty

Bobby S. Korn, MD, PhD and Weerawan Chokthaweesak, MD

TABLE 72.1   *Indications for Lower Eyelid Blepharoplasty*

Cosmetically significant dermatochalasis with or
without fat prolapse

Lower eyelid double convex deformity

Visually significant lower eyelid fat prolapse
without infraorbital hollowing (infrequent)

TABLE 72.2   *Preoperative Considerations*

The transcutaneous approach with orbitomalar suspension is considered when excess
skin, orbital fat prolapse and midfacial ptosis are present.

The transconjunctival approach is performed when minimal lower eyelid
dermatochalasis is present in the setting of prolapsed orbital fat

Orbital fat redraping can be performed with both transcutaneous and
transconjunctival approaches. In the transconjunctival approach, a limited lateral
canthotomy provides improved surgical access.

Skin-pinch only lower eyelid blepharoplasty is ideally suited for lower eyelid
dermatochalasis and minimizes development of postoperative eyelid malposition.

Transcutaneous Lower Eyelid Blepharoplasty with Orbitomalar Suspension

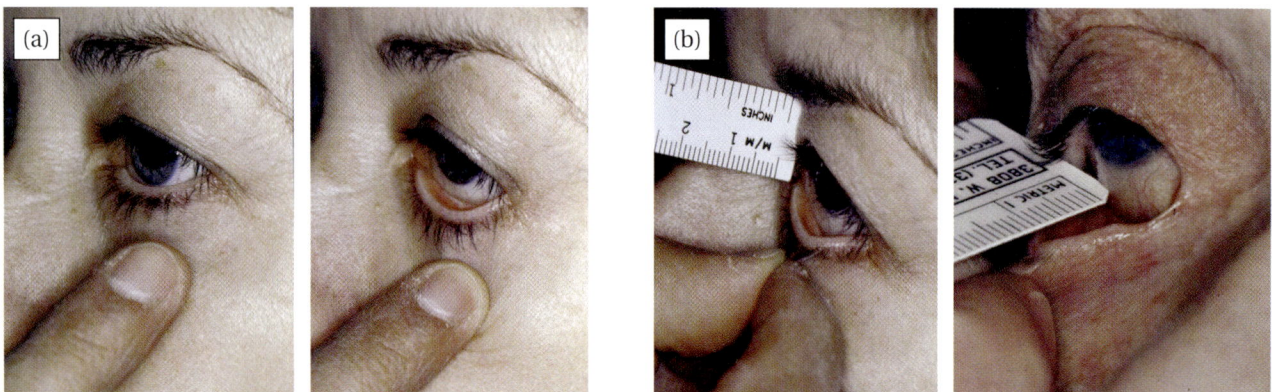

FIGURE 72.1   Assessment of Lower Eyelid Laxity. Lower eyelid laxity should be evaluated with the
snap back test (a) and the distraction test (b). Failure to address lower eyelid laxity at the time of
surgery can result in postoperative eyelid ectropion and lid retraction.

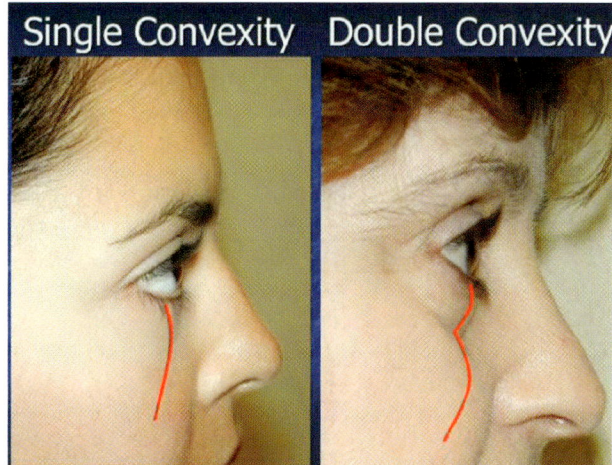

FIGURE 72.2 Assessment of Lower Eyelid Contour. In the youthful eyelid, there is a smooth junction between the lower eyelid and the midface as shown on the left panel. With age, there is unmasking of the inferior orbital rim, soft tissue deflation and midfacial descent, resulting in the double convexity as shown on the right panel. Fat repositioning during blepharoplasty or filler injections along the inferior orbital rim can address this contour change.

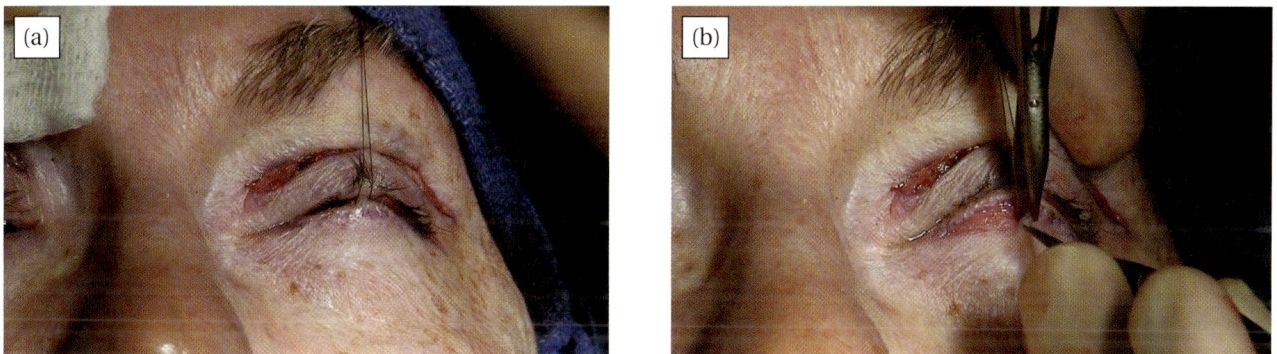

FIGURE 72.3 Infraciliary Incision. An infraciliary incision is marked close to the lower eyelid cilia to minimize visibility (a). Wescott scissors are used to create the infraciliary incision (b).

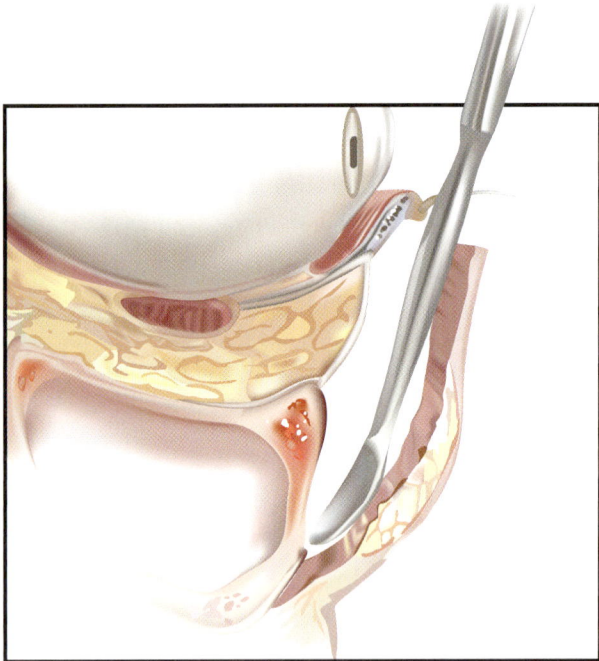

FIGURE 72.4 Preseptal Dissection and Exposure of Inferior Orbital Rim. Blunt dissection is then performed inferiorly in the avascular preseptal plane. (From Korn BS, Kikkawa DO, Cohen SR. Transcutaneous lower eyelid blepharoplasty with orbitomalar suspension: Retrospective review of 212 consecutive cases. *Plast Reconst Surg.* 2010;125(1):315–323.)

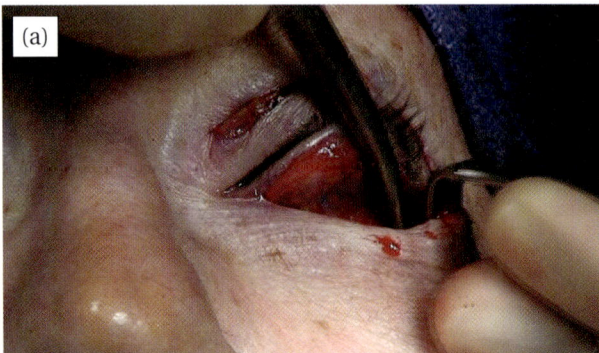

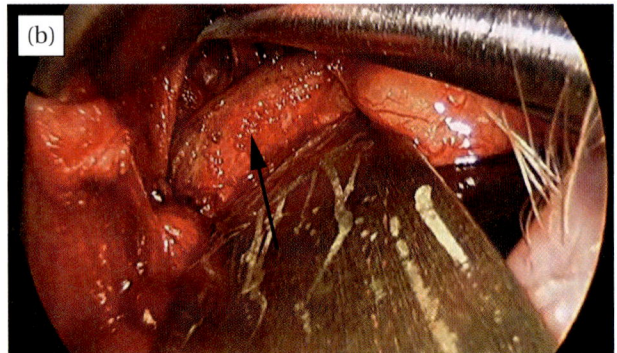

FIGURE 72.5 Release of Orbitomalar Ligament. After exposure of the inferior orbital rim, the orbitomalar ligament is released from its stout lateral attachments using a combination of blunt and sharp dissection (a). An endoscope is inserted for visualization, and the inferior orbital rim (arrow) is clearly seen (b). Excess orbital fat can be either excised or redraped.

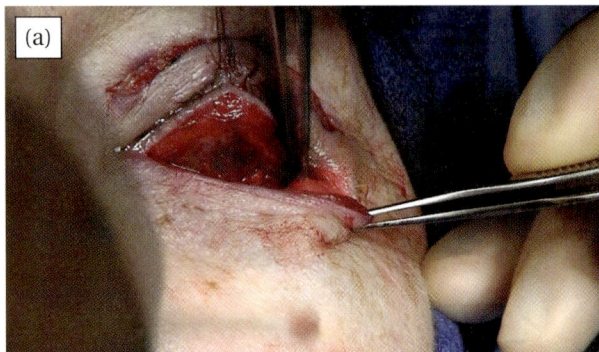

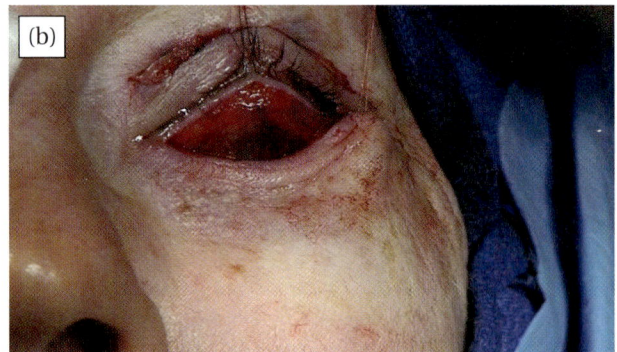

FIGURE 72.6 Grasping of Suborbicularis Oculi Fat (SOOF). The SOOF is grasped with Adson forceps (a) and secured with 5-0 polyglactin suture (b).

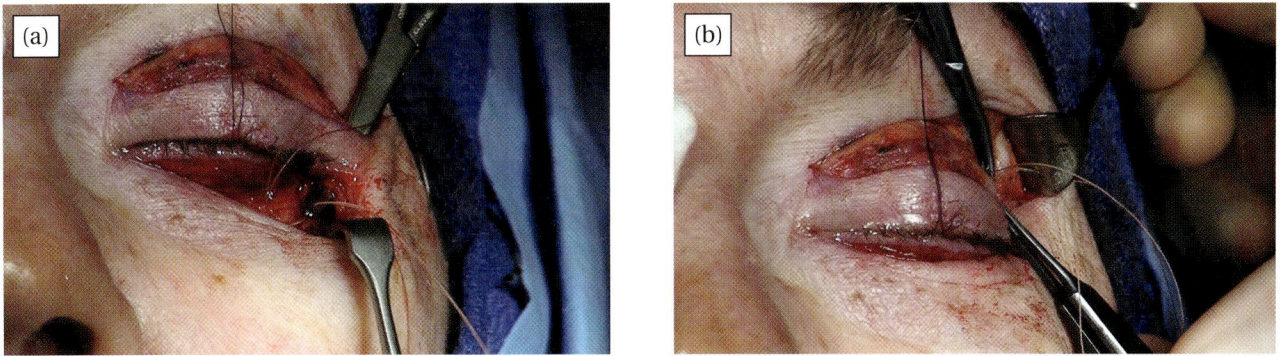

FIGURE 72.7 Orbitomalar Suspension. A tunnel from a lateral upper eyelid crease incision provides access to the lower eyelid, and the orbitomalar suspension suture is brought through this tunnel (a). The suture is then secured to the periosteum overlying the frontozygomatic suture (b).

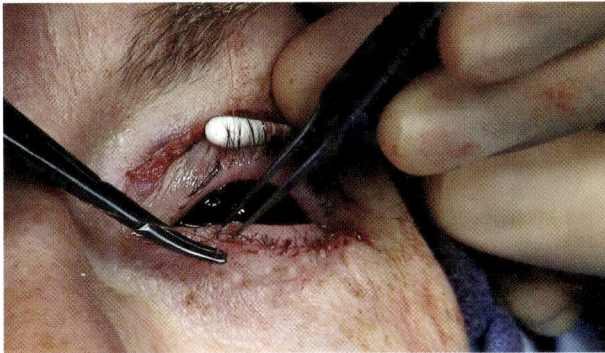

FIGURE 72.8 Closure of Skin. Conservative skin removal is performed, and the incision is closed from a temporal to nasal direction with 6-0 fast absorbing gut suture.

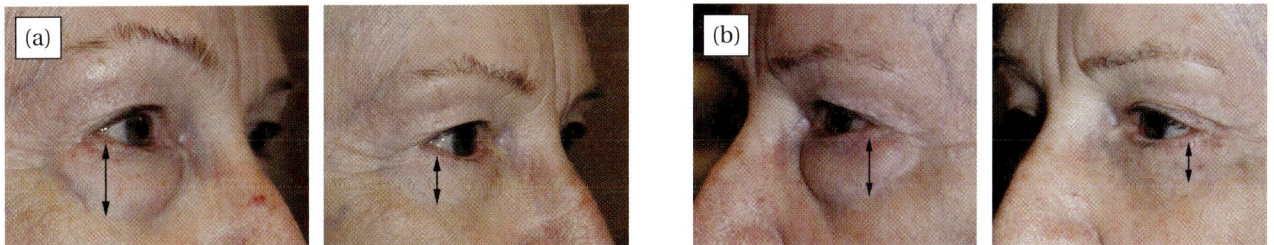

FIGURE 72.9 Preoperative and Postoperative Photographs. Profile views of same patient (a) and (b), showing before and after lower eyelid blepharoplasty with fat redraping and orbitomalar suspension. Note improvement in the lower eyelid contour as well as the volumetric enhancement of the midface and shortening of the lid-cheek junction as shown in the black arrows.

Transconjunctival Lower Eyelid Blepharoplasty with Orbital Fat Redraping

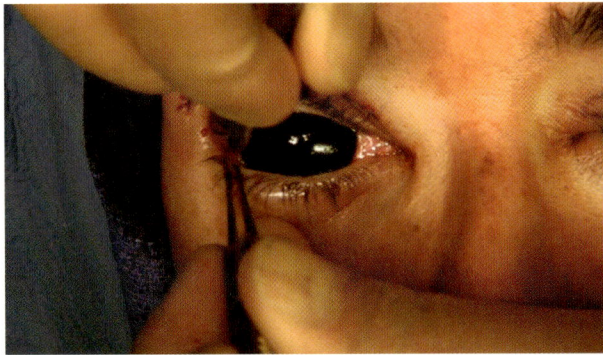

FIGURE 72.10 Lateral Canthotomy and Inferior Cantholysis. Using Westcott scissors, a small 1–2 mm lateral canthotomy and inferior cantholysis are performed to assist with lower eyelid access.

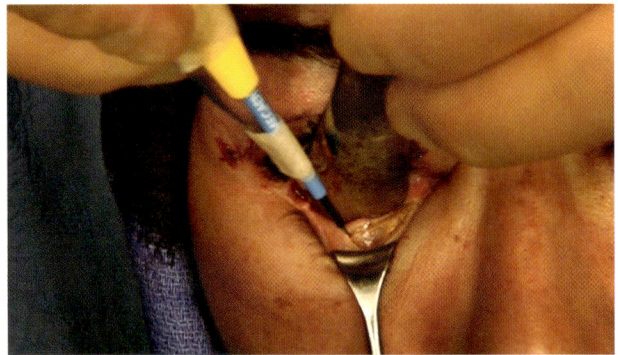

FIGURE 72.11 Transconjunctival Incision. A transconjunctival incision is made just below the interior tarsal border using the monopolar cautery with a needle point tip. A Desmarres retractor and Jaeger eyelid plate provide exposure and protect the cornea.

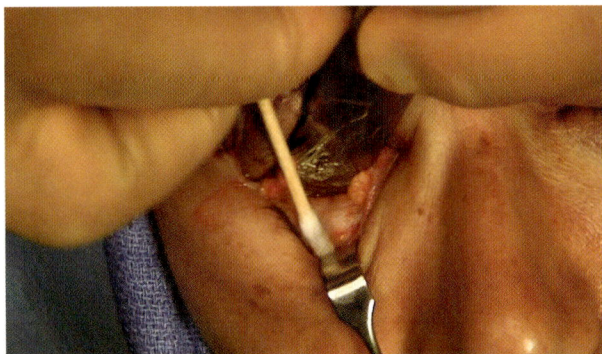

FIGURE 72.12 Preperiosteal Blunt Dissection. The dissection is carried inferiorly in the preperiosteal plane to expose the inferior orbital rim with cotton tipped applicators. Care is taken to preserve the periosteum, as this will be used for securing the redraped fat.

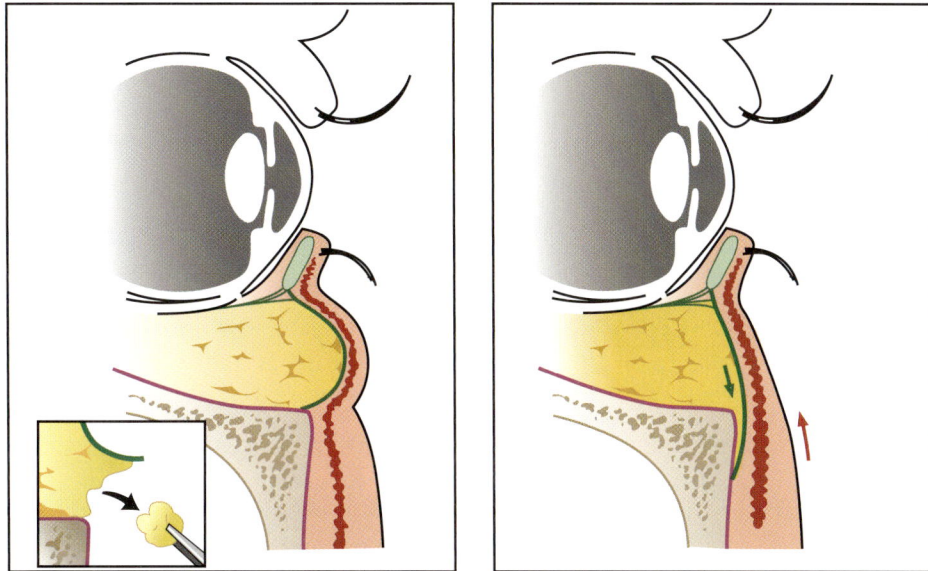

FIGURE 72.13 Schematic of Fat Redraping. The figure shows a schematic of orbital fat redraping along the inferior orbital rim. The orbital septum is then opened inferiorly above the arcus marginalis. Minimal fat excision is performed, and then fat pedicles are then dissected medially, centrally, and temporally. The fat pedicles are then secured to the anterior aspect of the inferior orbital rim. (© Elsevier 2010.)

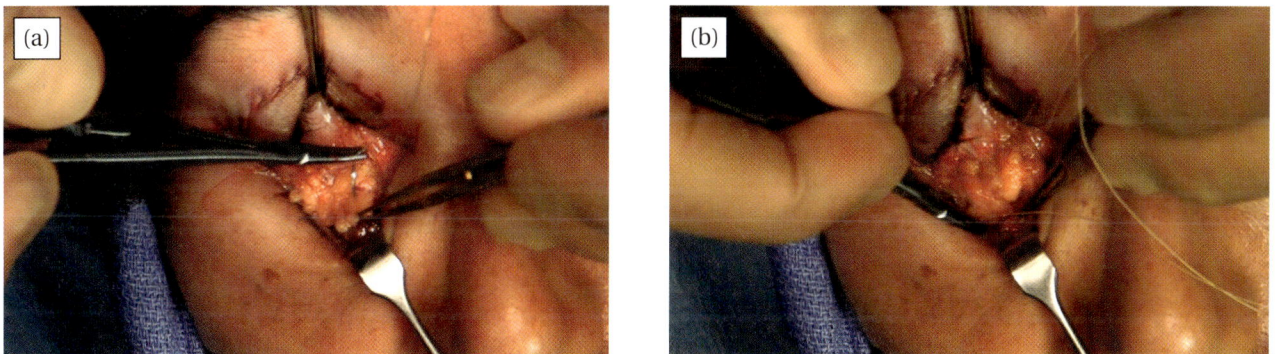

FIGURE 72.14 Redraping of Fat Pedicles. (a) The orbital septum is opened inferiorly and fat pedicles are exposed. The nasal, central, and temporal fat pedicles are then redraped onto the inferior orbital rim with a 5-0 polyglactin suture in a horizontal mattress fashion. Excess fat is judiciously removed or cauterized back. (b) The orbital septum is opened horizontally above the level of the fat pedicles to prevent lower eyelid retraction.

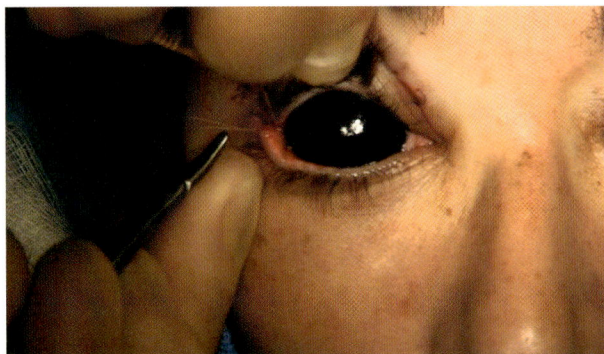

FIGURE 72.15 Closure of Incision. The conjunctiva is re-approximated with interrupted 6-0 fast absorbing gut suture. The canthus is reconstructed with 5-0 polyglactin suture by fixating the inferior eyelid to the superior crus of the lateral canthal tendon. Lateral canthal skin closure is performed with interrupted 6-0 fast absorbing gut suture.

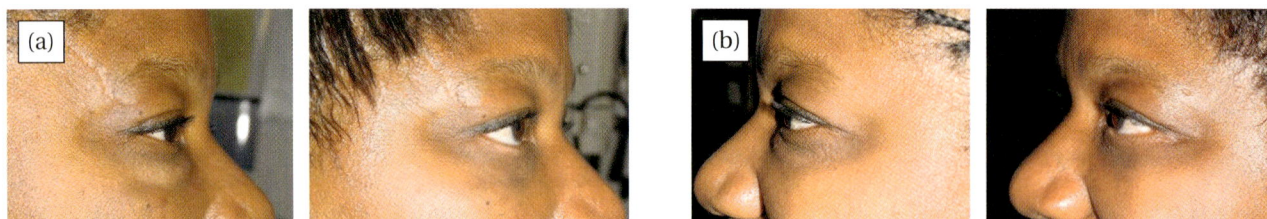

FIGURE 72.16 Preoperative and Postoperative Photographs. This patient underwent bilateral transconjunctival lower eyelid blepharoplasty. Before surgery (a) and after surgery (b).

TABLE 72.3 *Potential Complications of Lower Eyelid Blepharoplasty*

Lower eyelid ectropion and/or retraction

Lower eyelid hollowing

Asymmetry

Dry eye syndrome

Strabismus from damage to extraocular muscles

Lateral canthal angle rounding

Retrobulbar hemorrhage

Tissue bunching (typically resolves with time)

SELECTED REFERENCES

Kikkawa DO, Lemke BN, Dortzbach RK. Relations of the superficial musculoaponeurotic system to the orbit and characterization of the orbitomalar ligament. *Ophthal Plast Reconstr Surg.* 1996;12:77–88.

Korn BS, Kikkawa DO, Cohen SR. Transcutaneous lower eyelid blepharoplasty with orbitomalar suspension: Retrospective review of 212 consecutive cases. *Plast Reconst Surg.* 2010;125(1):315–323.

Morax S, Touitou V. Complication of blepharoplasty. *Orbit.* 2006 Dec;25:303–318.

73   Midfacial Surgery

Don O. Kikkawa, MD and Bobby S. Korn, MD, PhD

TABLE 73.1 *Indications for Midface Lifting*

Midfacial ptosis

Unmasking of the inferior orbital rim

Lower lid retraction with anterior lamellar shortage

TABLE 73.2 *Preoperative Considerations*

Consider the endoscopic approach for cases combined with endoscopic brow lifting

The transpalpebral approach is useful when posterior lamellar grafting is needed (in cases of post-blepharoplasty lid retraction and cicatricial ectropion)

The subperiosteal plane is more useful and safer in the endoscopic approach

Preperiosteal plane is more useful in cases of mild midfacial ptosis

Endoscopic Approach

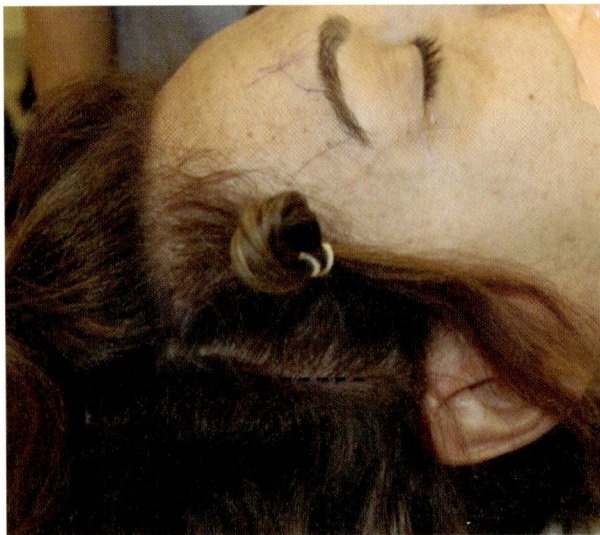

FIGURE 73.1 Temporal incision behind hairline.

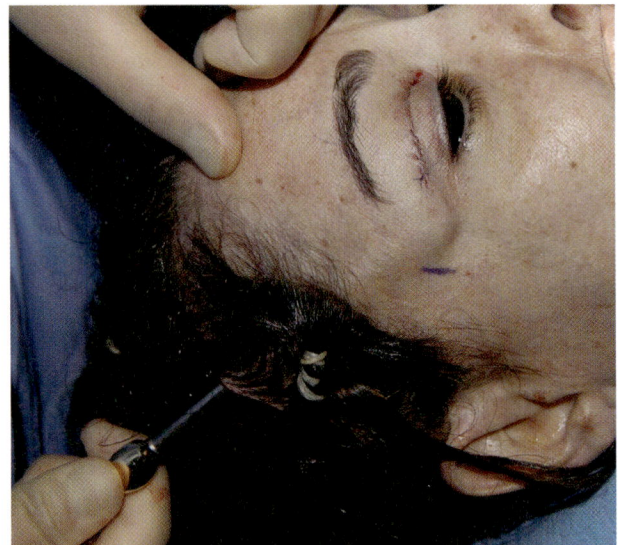

FIGURE 73.2 Dissection between superficial temporalis fascia and deep temporalis fascia with # 4 dissector (Snowden Pencer) to lateral canthus. Note 3 cm mark from lateral canthus indicating approximate position of temporal branch of facial nerve. Dissection should stay medial to this mark.

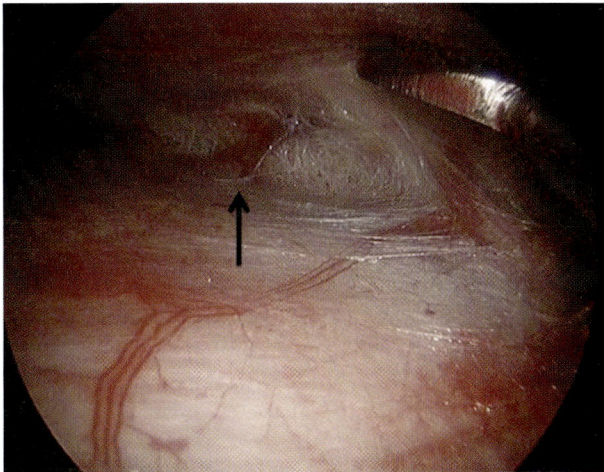

FIGURE 73.3 During temporal dissection, endoscopic view of dissection between deep temporalis fascia and superficial temporalis fascia. Note sentinel vein (arrow) is visible. The vein can preserved and dissected around, or cauterized.

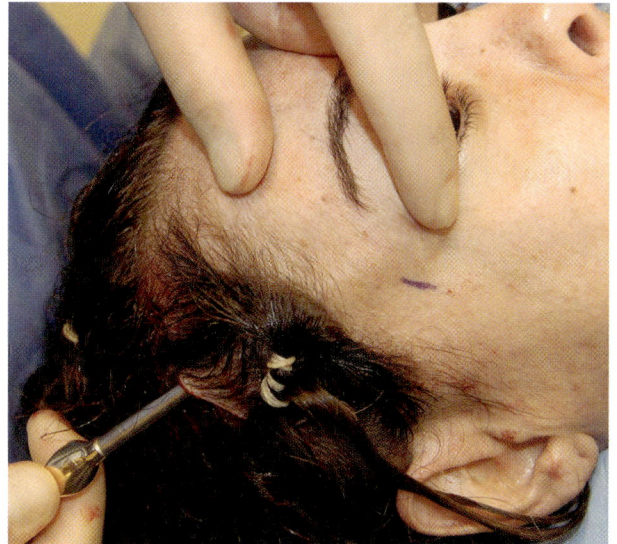

FIGURE 73.4 Conversion to subperiosteal plane at lateral orbital rim. This change in dissection plane is aided by digital palpation of the dissector tip.

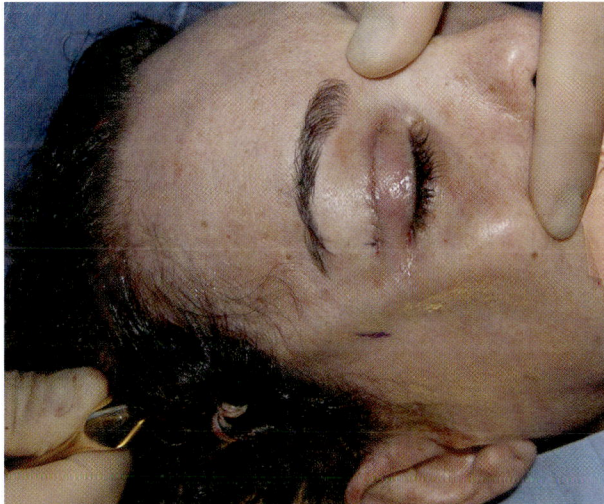

FIGURE 73.5 Subperiosteal plane dissection now mobilizes entire cheek. Inferior edge of periosteum must be completely released.

(a)   Subperiosted dissection-release (ZM)
Zygomaticus Major m. and Zygomaticus Minor m. (ZM)

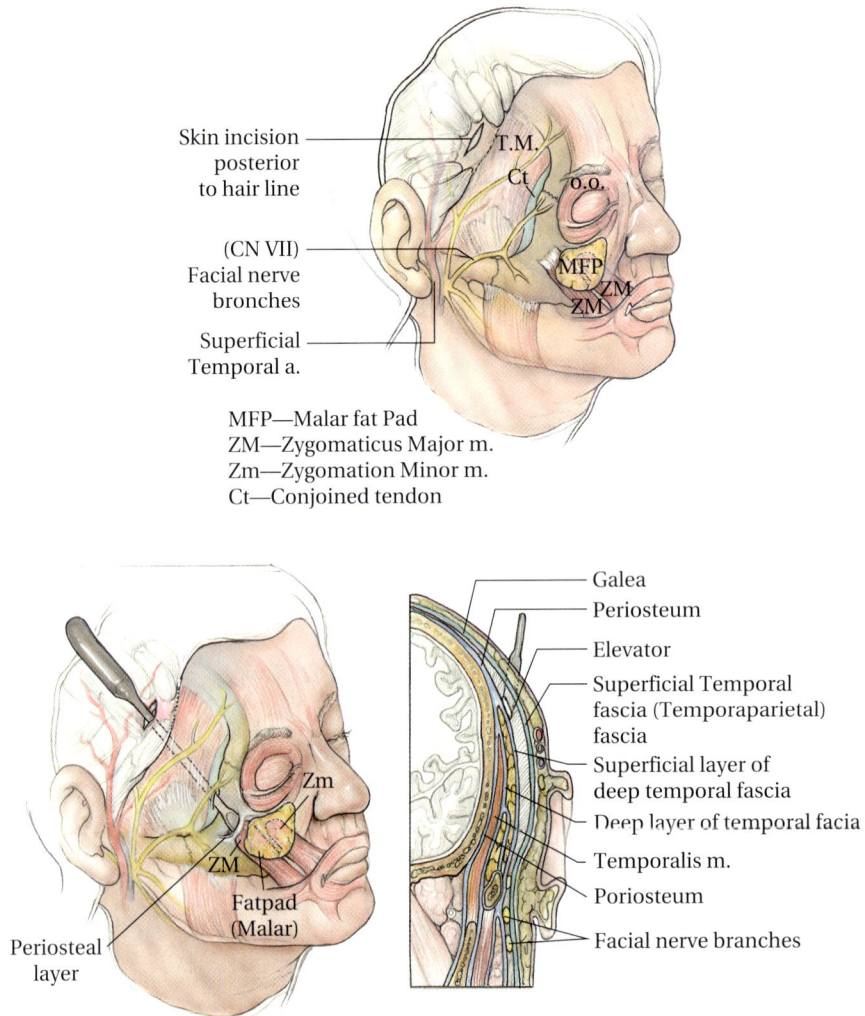

Skin incision
posterior
to hair line

T.M.

Ct

o.o.

(CN VII)
Facial nerve
bronches

MFP

ZM

ZM

Superficial
Temporal a.

MFP—Malar fat Pad
ZM—Zygomaticus Major m.
Zm—Zygomation Minor m.
Ct—Conjoined tendon

Zm

ZM

Fatpad
(Malar)

Periosteal
layer

Galea
Periosteum
Elevator
Superficial Temporal
fascia (Temporaparietal)
fascia
Superficial layer of
deep temporal fascia
Deep layer of temporal facia
Temporalis m.
Poriosteum
Facial nerve branches

(b)

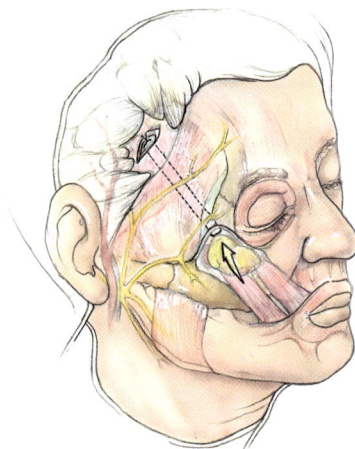

FIGURE 73.6   (a, b) Diagram showing dissection plane and suture placement.

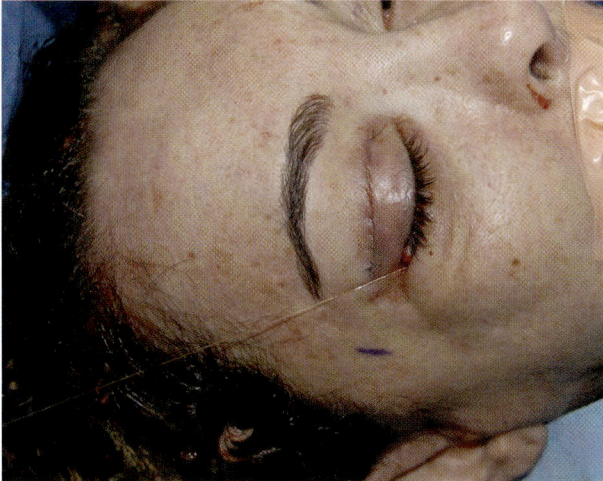

FIGURE 73.7   Monofilament polyglyconate (Maxon) 3-0 suture placed through transconjunctival and small canthotomy incision into SMAS of cheek.

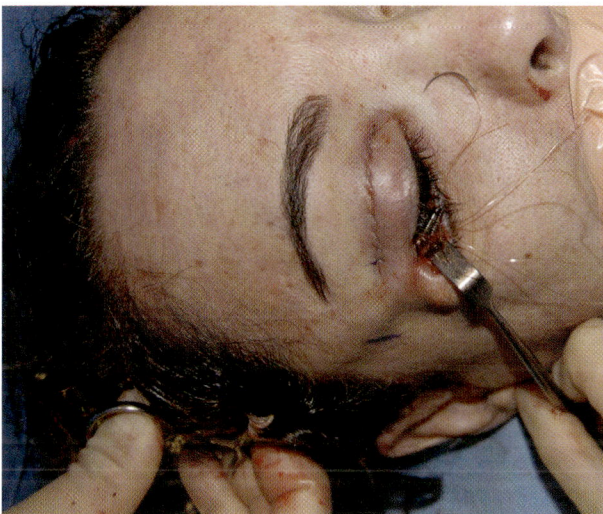

FIGURE 73.8   Retrieval of suture with long curved hemostat through temporal incision.

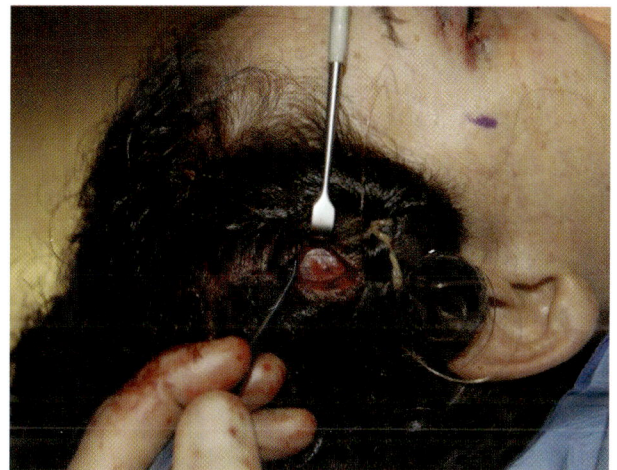

FIGURE 73.9   Fixation of suture to deep temporalis fascia. Wound is then closed with staples.

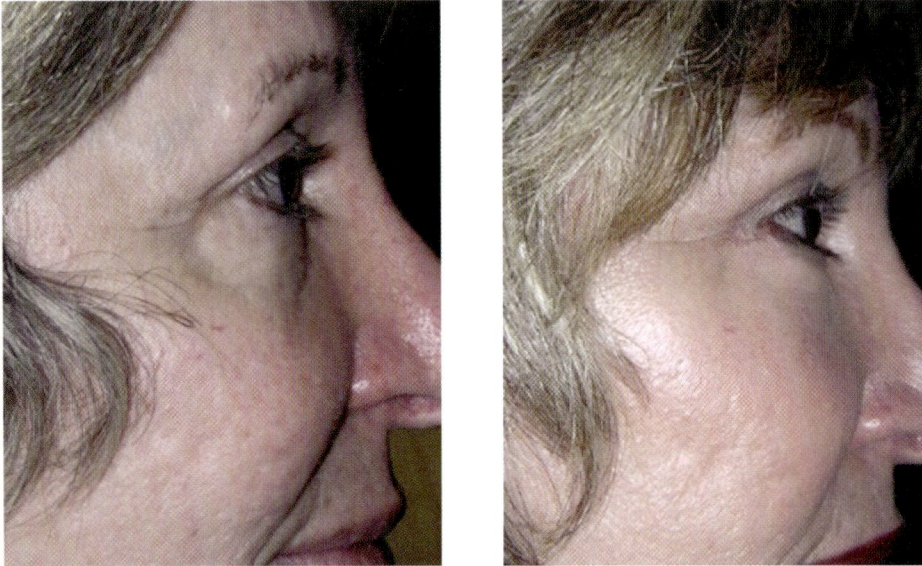

FIGURE 73.10 Profile view of patient before (left) and after (right) endoscopic midface lift. Note cheek elevation and restoration of volume along inferior orbital rim.

Transconjunctival Approach with Spacer Graft

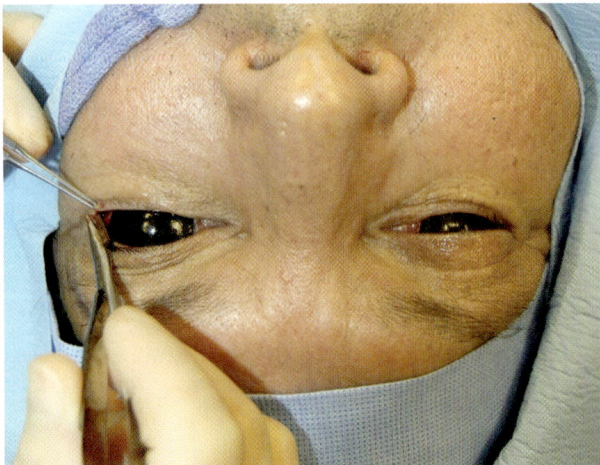

FIGURE 73.11 Lateral canthotomy and cantholysis.

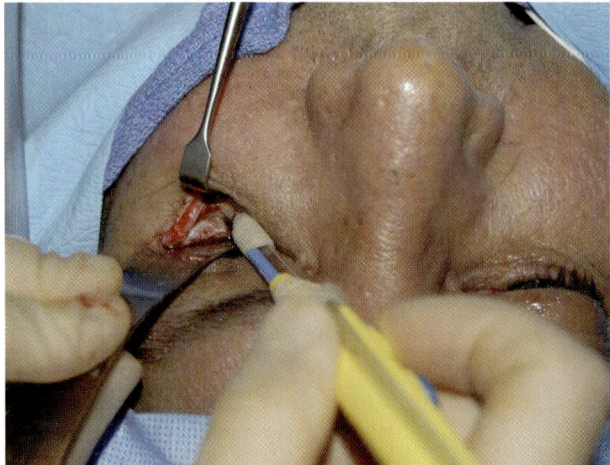

FIGURE 73.12 Transconjunctival incision below tarsal border.

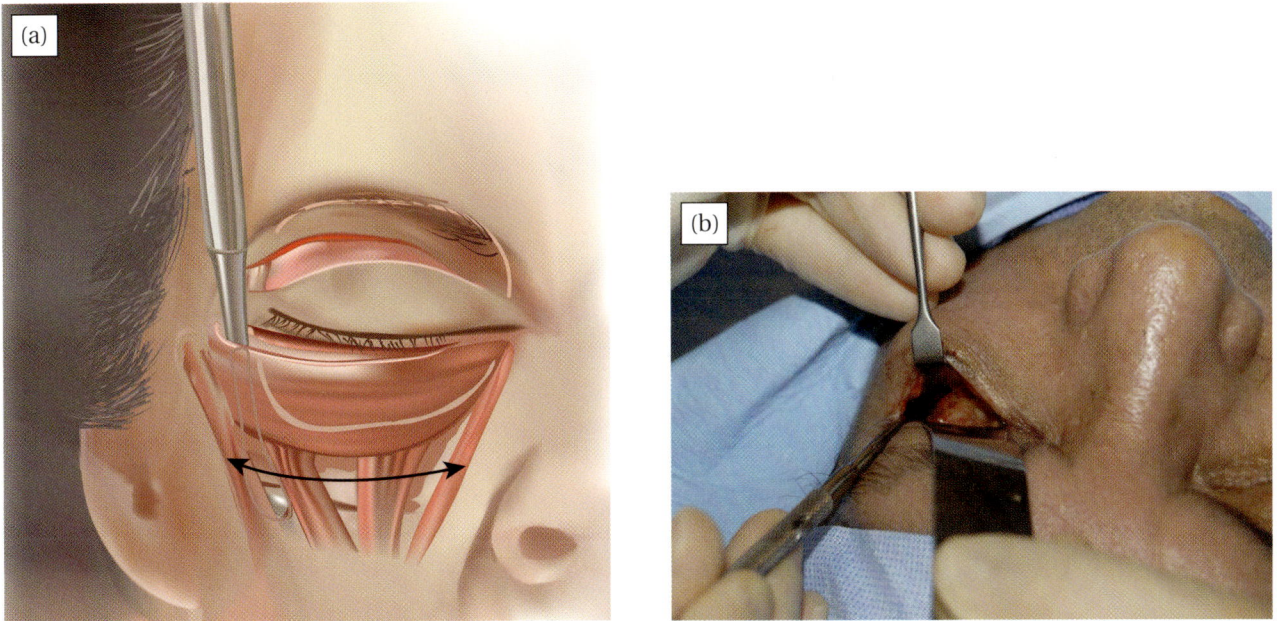

FIGURE 73.13 (a, b) Subperiosteal dissection with release of orbitomalar ligament. (Originally published in Korn BS, Kikkawa DO, Cohen SR. Transcutaneous lower eyelid blepharoplasty with orbitomalar suspension: Retrospective review of 212 consecutive cases. *Plast Reconst Surg.* 2010;125(1):315–323.)

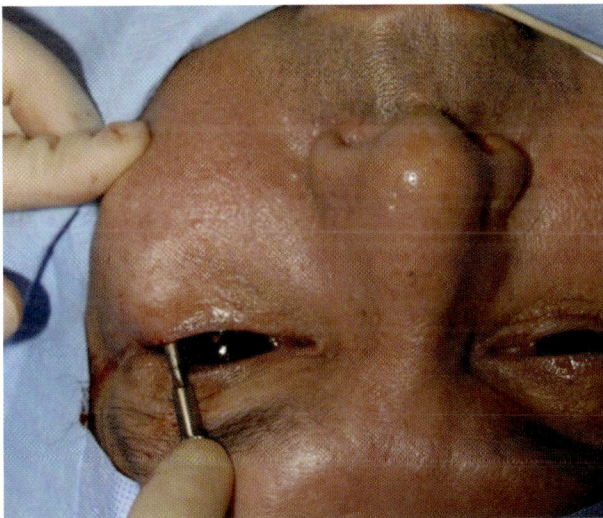

FIGURE 73.14 Inferior extent of subperiosteal dissection.

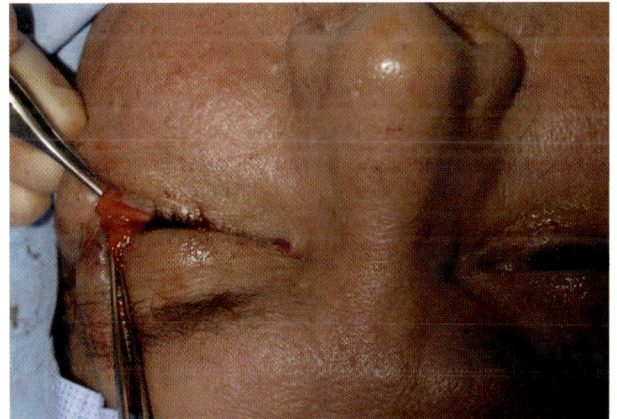

FIGURE 73.15 Fixation point where suture (4-0 polyglactin) is placed, along periosteal edge where orbitomalar ligament arises.

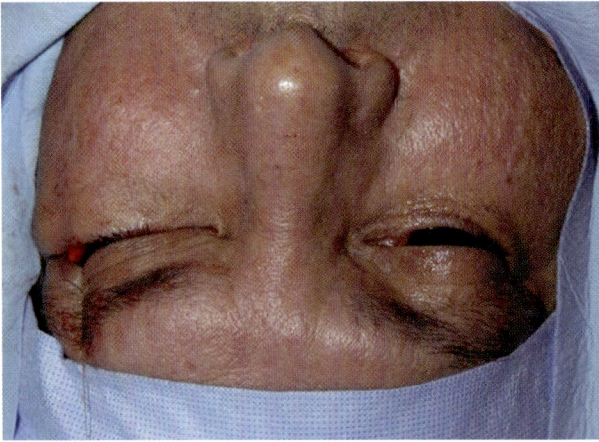

FIGURE 73.16 After suture placement, showing elevation of cheek with upward traction of suture. If completely dissected, cheek should elevate freely.

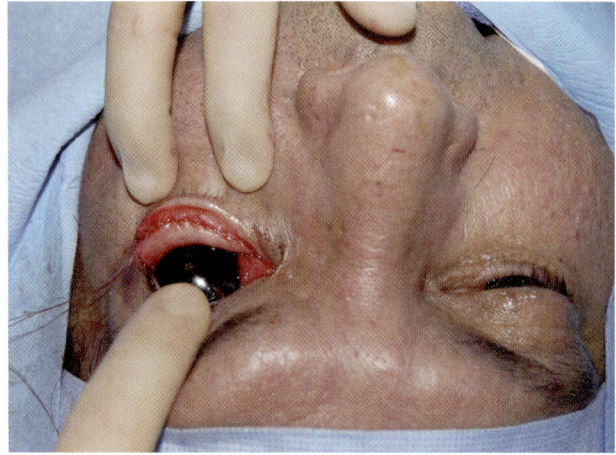

FIGURE 73.17 After placement of dermis fat graft between inferior tarsal border and lower eyelid retractors. Graft secured with 6-0 fast absorbing plain gut suture.

TABLE 73.3 *Posterior Lamellar Graft Options*

Hard palate mucosa

Dermis fat graft

Ear cartilage

Allografts (acellular dermis)

Xenografts (porcine decellularized collagen)

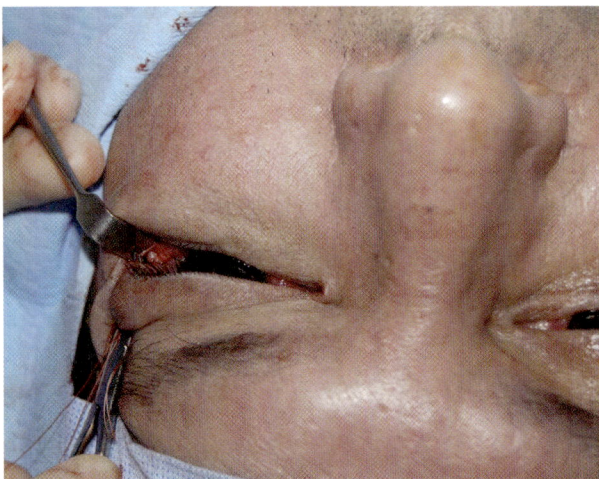

FIGURE 73.18 Retrieval of suture through lateral upper lid crease incision.

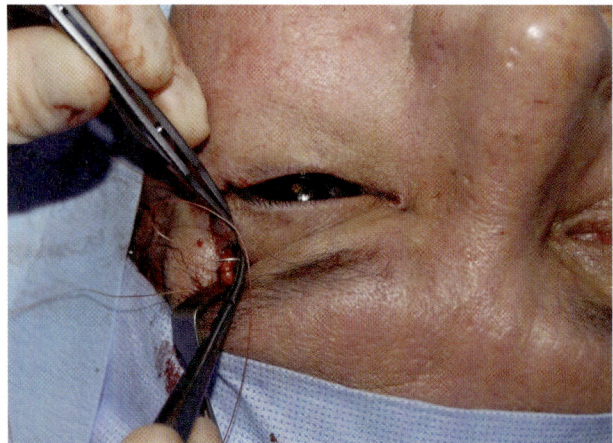

FIGURE 73.19 Fixation of suture to periosteum at the level of the frontozygomatic suture.

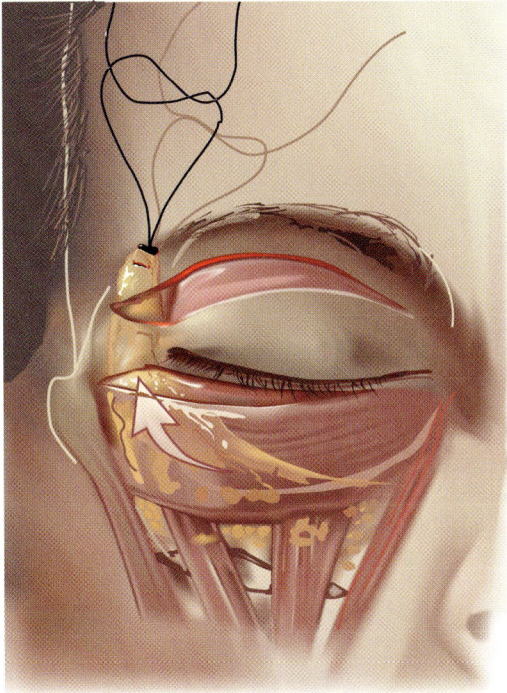

FIGURE 73.20 Diagram of suture placement
and suspension of midface to periosteum near
frontozygomatic suture. (Originally published in Korn
BS, Kikkawa DO, Cohen SR. Transcutaneous lower
eyelid blepharoplasty with orbitomalar suspension:
retrospective review of 212 consecutive cases. *Plast
Reconst Surg.* 2010;125(1):315–323.)

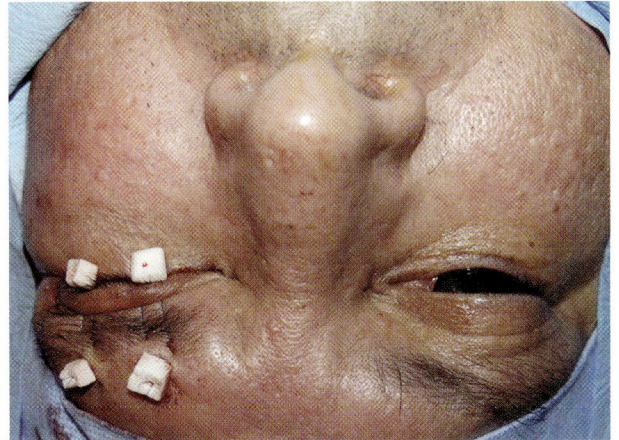

FIGURE 73.21 Placement of two Frost sutures
(5-0 double armed prolene) tied over foam bolsters.

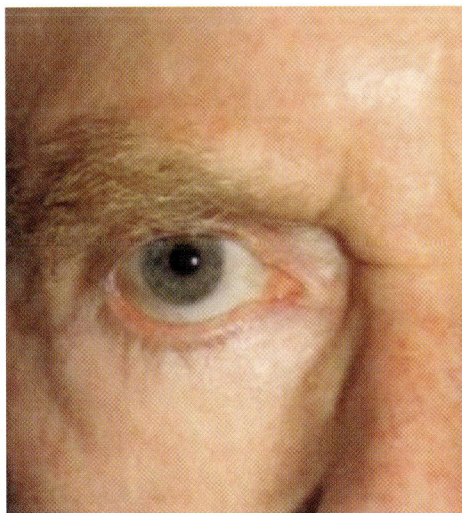

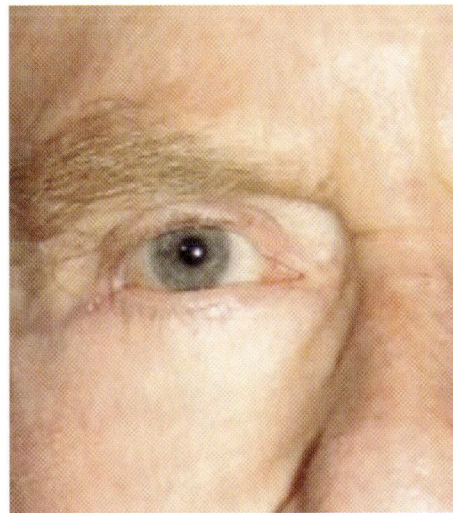

FIGURE 73.22 Before (left) and after (right) photo of patient after undergoing transconjunctival
midface lift and posterior lamellar spacer graft.

TABLE 73.4 *Potential Complications for Midface Lifting*

Inadequate lifting

Facial nerve damage

Sensory nerve damage (hypesthesia)

Recurrence of lower lid retraction

Tissue bunching (typically resolves with time)

SELECTED REFERENCES

Codner M. Modifying the subperiosteal cheek lift. *Aesthet Surg J.* 2003;23(3):203–204.

Goldstein SA, Goldstein SM. Anatomic and aesthetic considerations in midfacial rejuvenation. *Facial Plast Surg.* 200;22(2):105–111.

Lucarelli MJ, Khwarg SI, Lemke BN, Kozel JS, Dortzbach RK. Anatomy of midfacial ptosis. *Ophthal Plast Reconstr Surg.* 2000;16(1):7–22.

Patipa M.Transblepharoplasty lower eyelid and midface rejuvenation: part I. Avoiding complications by utilizing lessons learned from the treatment of complications. *Plast Reconstr Surg.* 2004;113(5):1459–1468; discussion 1475–1477.

Ramirez OM. Three-dimensional endoscopic midface enhancement: a personal quest for the ideal cheek rejuvenation. *Plast Reconstr Surg.* 2002;109(1): 329–340; discussion 341–349.

Sullivan SA, Dailey RA. Endoscopic subperiosteal midface lift: surgical technique with indications and outcomes. *Ophthal Plast Reconstr Surg.* 2002;18(5):319–330.

Williams III EF, Lam SM. Midfacial rejuvenation via an endoscopic browlift approach: a review of technique. *Facial Plast Surg.* 2003;19(2):147–156. Review.

Face-lifting

David E.E. Holck, MD, Manuel A. Lopez, MD, Bobby S. Korn, MD, PhD, and Don O. Kikkawa, MD

TABLE 74.1 *Indications for Face-lifting*

Jowl formation

Lower facial descent

Blunting of the cervicomental angle

Marionette lines

TABLE 74.2 *Preoperative Considerations*

Have the patient identify areas of concern using a handheld mirror.

Examine old photographs.

Elicit past medical history, including prior surgery and anticoagulant use.

Cessation of smoking is mandatory prior to surgery.

Patients with minimal jowling and excess skin may be candidates for the short incision technique; significant jowling is best addressed with a deep plane technique.

Neck liposuction and platysmaplasty may be necessary as additional procedures for subcutaneous neck lipomatosis and platysmal banding.

TABLE 74.3 *Operative Considerations*

Tumescent infiltration of the face with modified Klein solution (1000 cc normal saline, 500–1000 mg lidocaine, 0.65–1.0 mg epinephrine, 10 mEq sodium bicarbonate) facilitates dissection and helps with hemostasis.

Incision placement is preauricular, posttragal in women and preauricular, pretragal in men.

General anesthesia is typically preferred for the deep plane technique, while monitored anesthesia care can be used for the short incision technique.

Counter-traction is critical to maintain uniform skin and SMAS flaps. Transillumination through the flap further facilitates development of the skin flap.

Dissection of the SMAS flap below the inferior border of the mandible or above the zygomatic arch places the marginal mandibular and frontal branches of the facial nerves (respectively) at risk of trauma.

Leaving the skin at the inferior ear lobule slightly "bunched" helps to avoid lobule pull down in the postoperative period and "Pixie-ear" deformity.

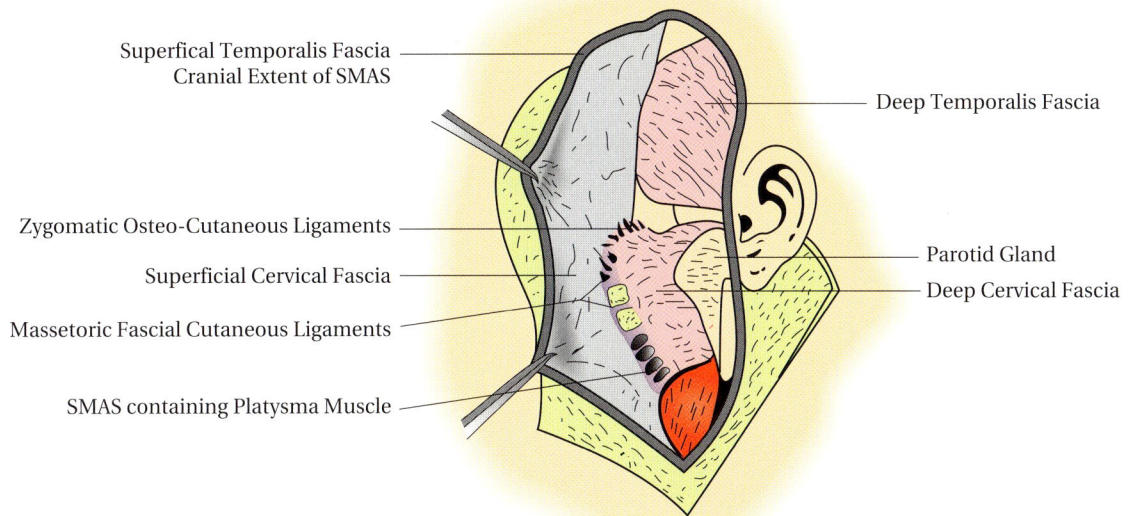

FIGURE 74.1 Relevant Facial Rhytidectomy Anatomy. The superficial musculoaponeurotic system (SMAS) lies in the superficial cervical fascia, and manipulation of this layer through plication, imbrication, or flap advancement allows optimal facial rejuvenation.

Deep Plane Technique

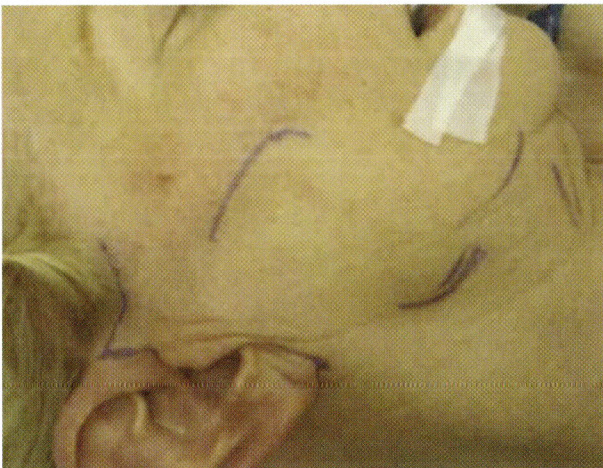

FIGURE 74.2 Surface anatomy markings. It is helpful to mark preoperatively the inferior border of the zygomatic arch, the angle of the mandible, inferior jowling, and platysmal bands.

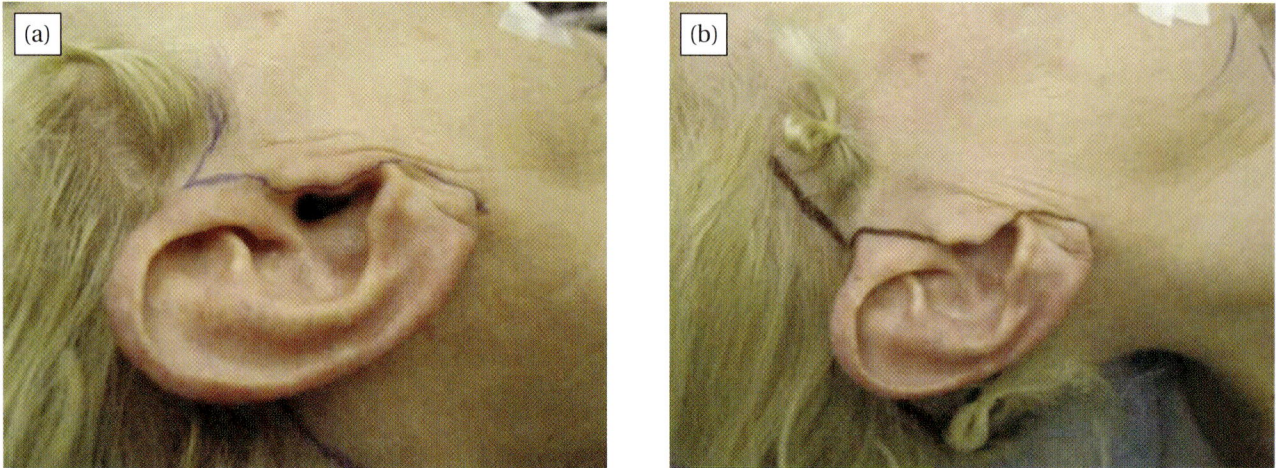

FIGURE 74.3 Anterior incision markings. With a high temporal hairline, a curvilinear incision along the anterior hairline of the temporal tuft is used to avoid posterior migration of the temporal tuft (a). With a normal or low temporal hairline, an incision may be continued into the temple (b).

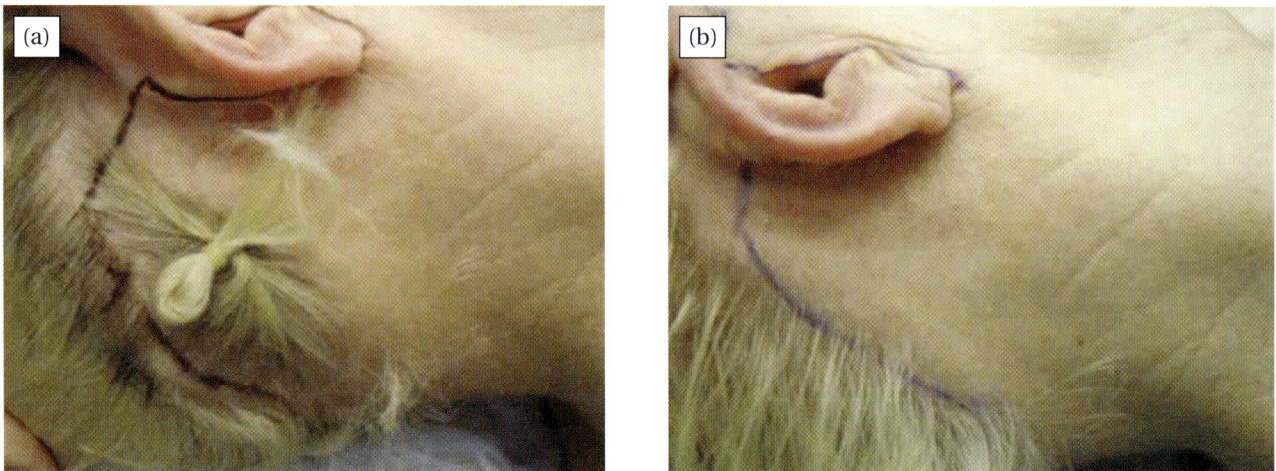

FIGURE 74.4 Posterior incision markings. In the retroauricular region, the incision is carried into the posterior hair approximately 5–6 cm. The incision is carried in a gentle curve, roughly bisecting the hairline and its tangent (a). Alternatively, if a large amount of neck skin is planned for excision, the incision may be carried along the hairline (b). In this case, the patient should be cautioned against wearing their hair pulled back, or the incision may be visible.

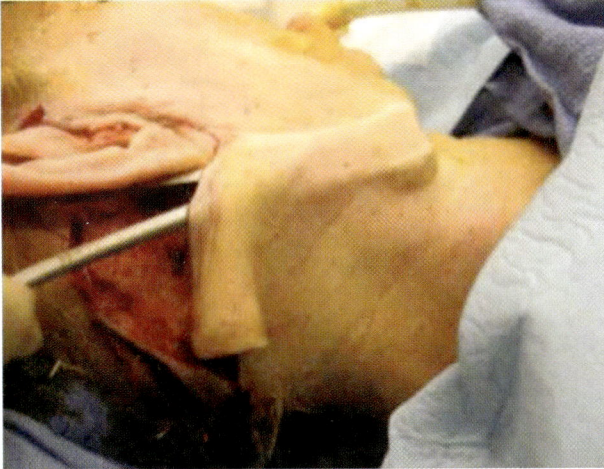

FIGURE 74.5 A skin flap is developed and the dissection in the neck is continued to the midline. The dissection is advanced to the prominence of the zygoma superiorly, and to the angle of the mandible inferiorly. Skin dissection is greatly enhanced by tumescence.

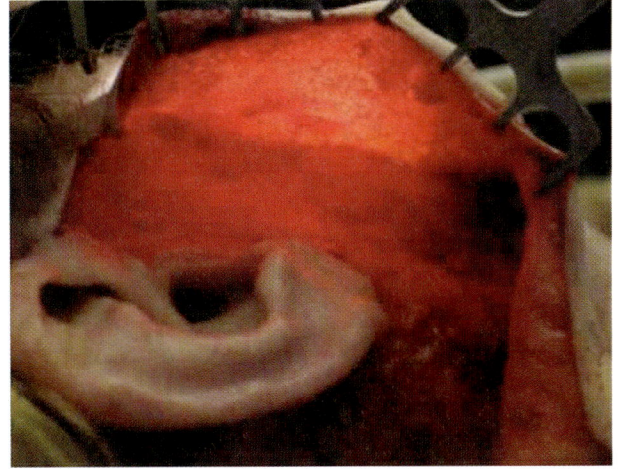

FIGURE 74.6 Transillumination of the skin flap allows evaluation of the uniformity of the subcutaneous fat layer. The fat should appear in a cobblestone pattern.

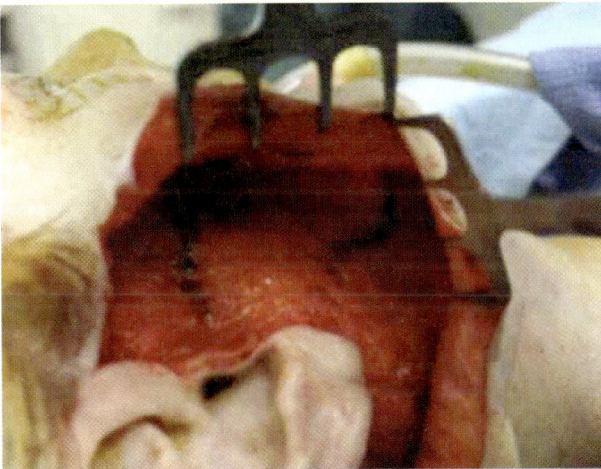

FIGURE 74.7 After completion of the skin flap, the inferior border of the zygomatic arch is marked, as well as the inferior border and the angle of the mandible. A SMAS flap is started from the junction of the zygomatic arch and body, and continued down to the inferior angle of the mandible.

(a)

(b)

FACE   NECK

SC

Platysma

Subcutaneous (SC)

SubSMAS

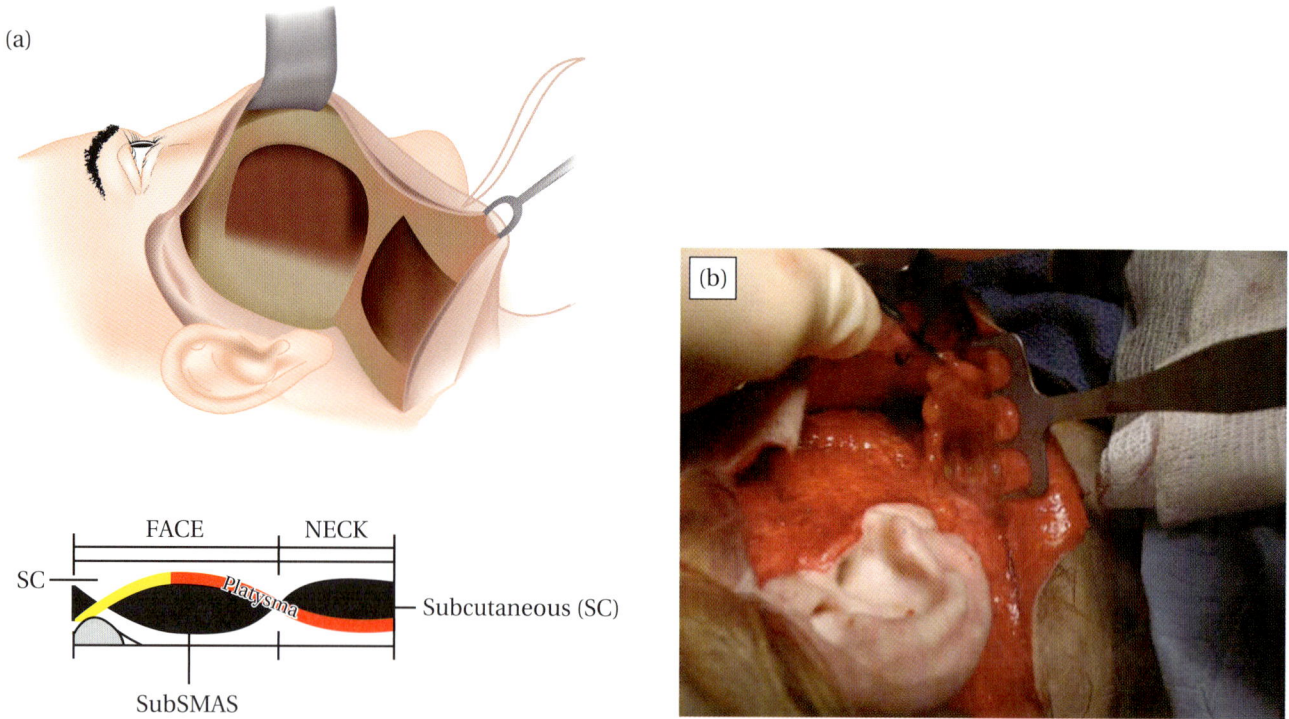

FIGURE 74.8 Schematic illustration (a) and intraoperative dissection (b) demonstrating the sub-SMAS dissection plane in the midface. The platysma muscle is superficial to the dissection plane in the midface region. The dissection below the inferior border of the mandible is subcutaneous (supraplatymsal).

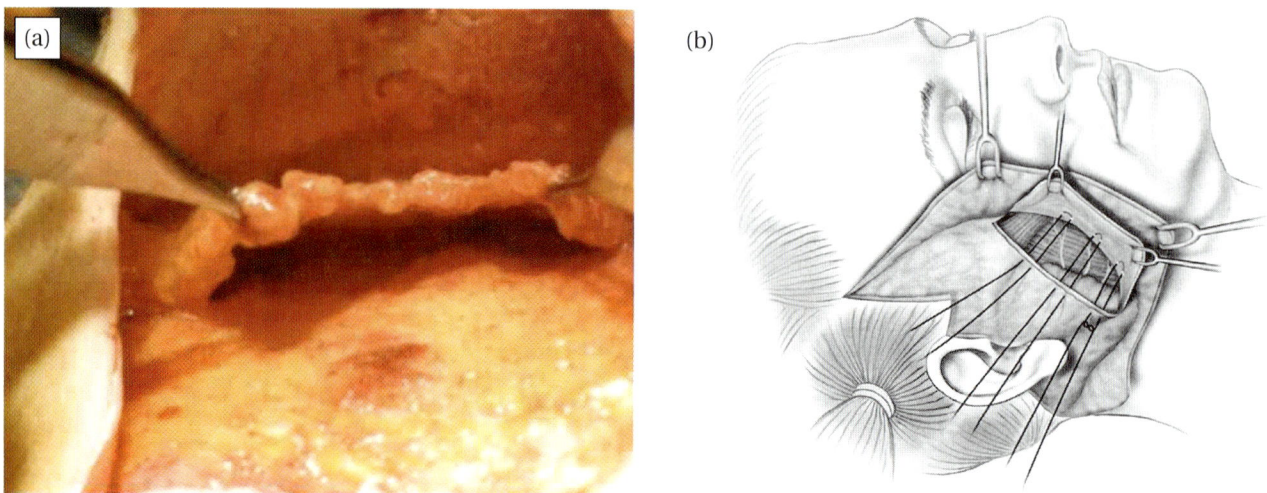

(a)

(b)

FIGURE 74.9 (a, b) A superficial musculoaponeurotic system (SMAS) flap is dissected and held with a forceps. Superior to the SMAS is the skin and subcutaneous tissue. Inferior to the SMAS flap lies the anterior portion of the parotid and the deep cervical fascia. It is in this layer that branches of the facial nerve maybe seen in the loose areolar tissue overlying the masseter muscle. The portion of the SMAS flap from the angle of the mandible is advanced to the inferior tragal border and sutured to the pretragal SMAS with a 3-0 polydioxanone (PDS) or polypropylene (Prolene) suture. The SMAS from the oral commissure is advanced to the superior tragal border and sutured in a similar fashion. (Credit for image (b): Baker SR, MD. Multiplane rhytidectomy. *Operative Techniques in Otolaryngology Head and Neck Surgery,* Vol. 10, No. 3 (September),1999:184–191. Copyright 1999 by W.B. Saunders Company.)

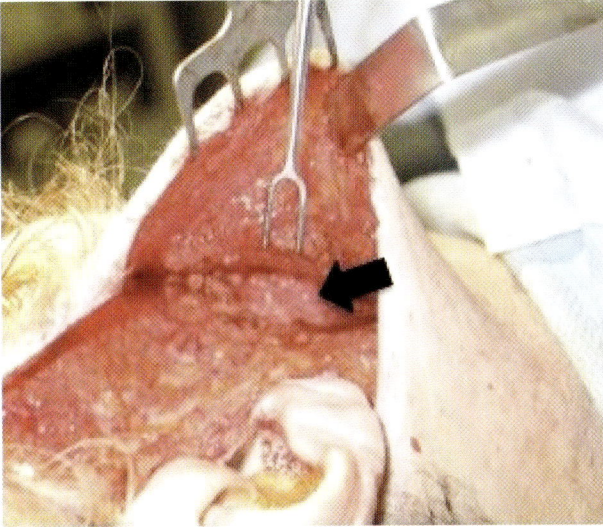

FIGURE 74.10 In the deep plane rhytidectomy, the subcutaneous dissection is extended only up to the SMAS flap (held up by the two-pronged forceps). The deep cervical fascia (arrow) is seen as a loose areolar tissue covering the branches of the facial nerve.

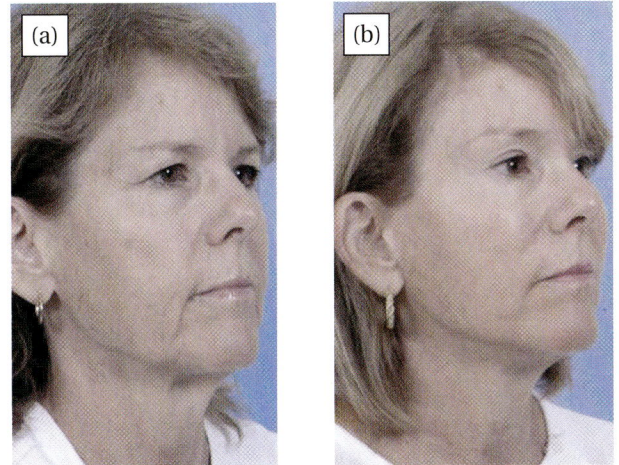

FIGURE 74.11 Preoperative (a) and postoperative (b) oblique views of a patient who underwent brow lift, midface lift and deep plane facial rhytidectomy. Oblique views demonstrate improved brow and midface positions, and reduced jowling and marionette lines.

Short Incision Technique

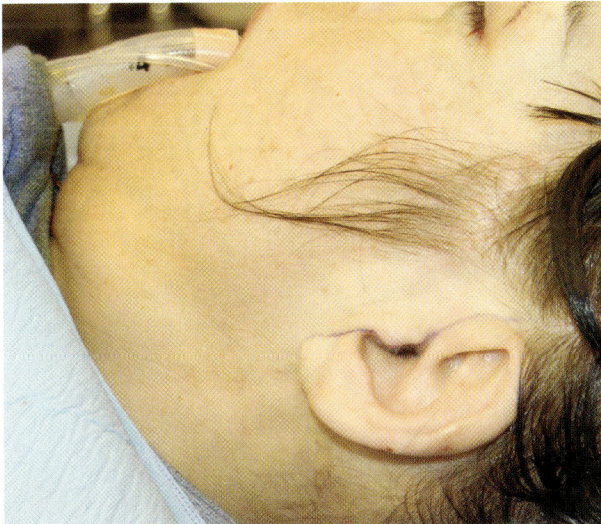

FIGURE 74.12 Skin marking. Preauricular retrotragal incision marked with marking pen extending from top of helix to bottom of ear lobe.

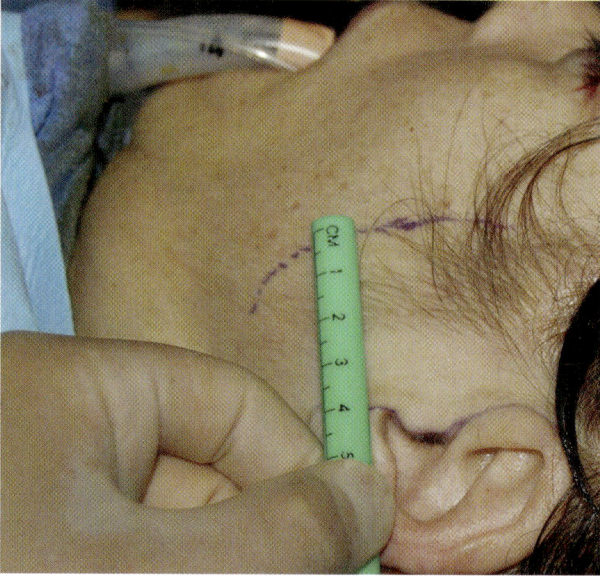

FIGURE 74.13 Extent of skin undermining marked to 4 cm from incision.

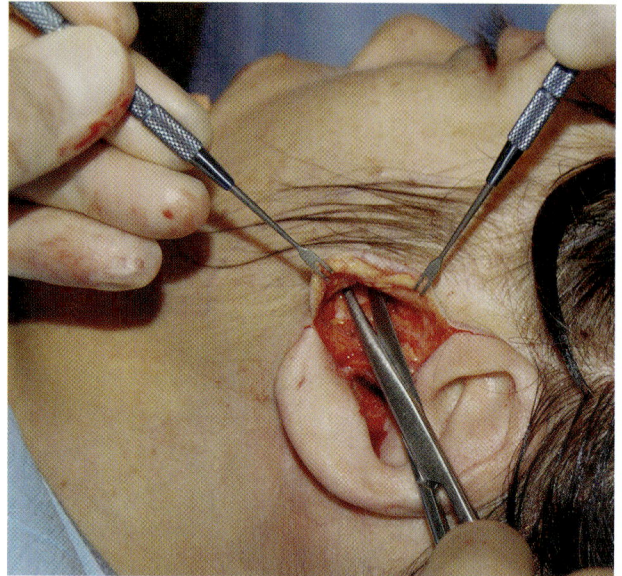

FIGURE 74.14 Subcutaneous undermining within subdermal fat plexus, superficial to the SMAS.

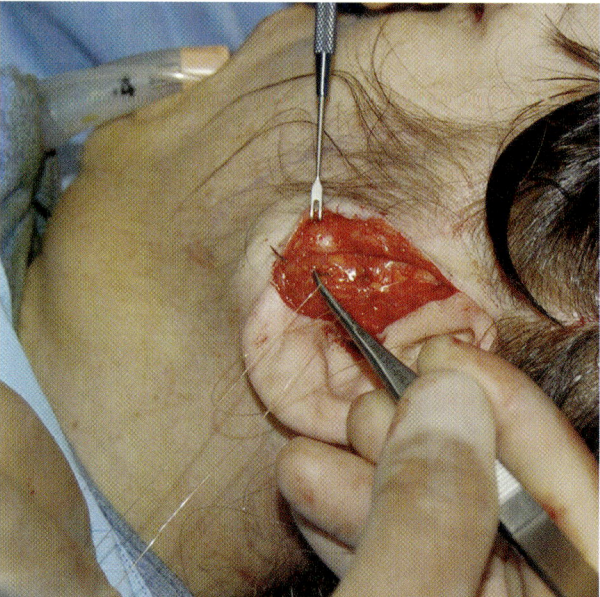

FIGURE 74.15 Needle pass through SMAS just above mandibular angle using 2-0 monofilament polyglyconate (Maxon) suture.

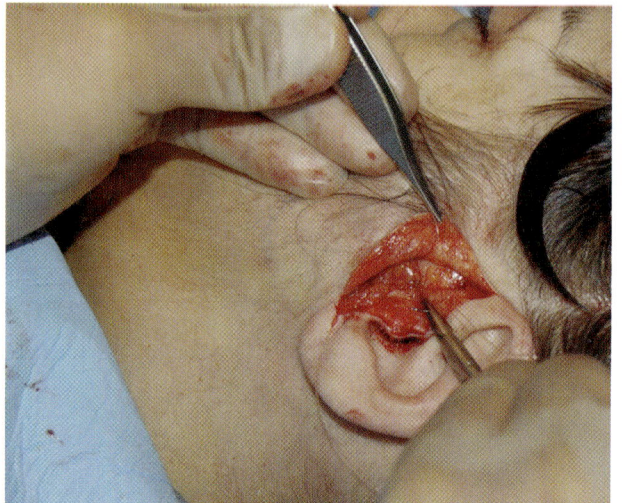

FIGURE 74.16 Needle pass of same suture superiorly to pretragal periosteum.

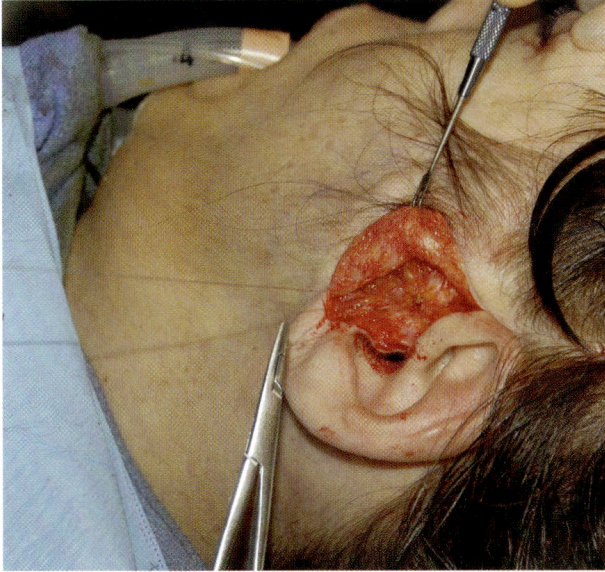

FIGURE 74.17 The suture is then tied with firm tension.

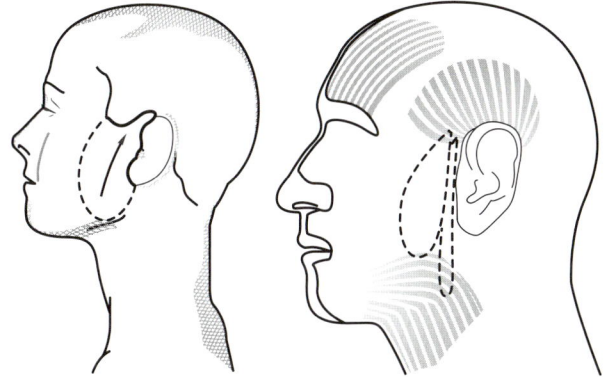

FIGURE 74.18 A second, more medial suture is also placed. (Credit: Tonnard P, Verpaele A, Monstrey S, Van Landuyt K, Blondeel P, Hamdi M, Matton G. Minimal access cranial suspension lift: a modified S-lift. *Plast Reconstr Surg.* 2002 May;109(6):2074–2086.)

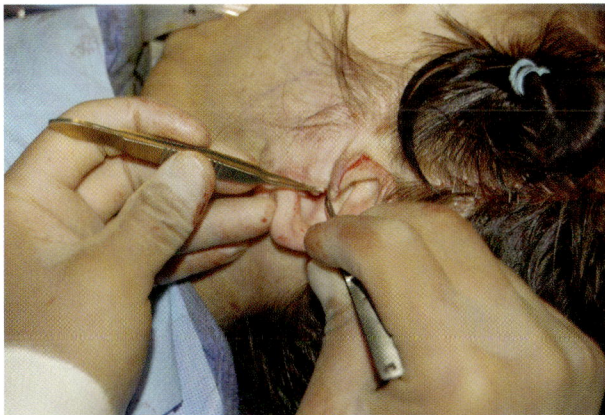

FIGURE 74.19 Excess skin is then redraped and conservatively excised.

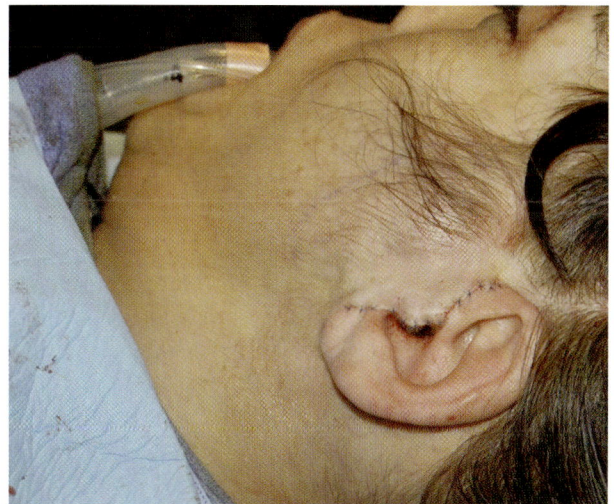

FIGURE 74.20 Skin closure is then performed using interrupted 6-0 polypropylene sutures. They are removed at the one week postoperative visit.

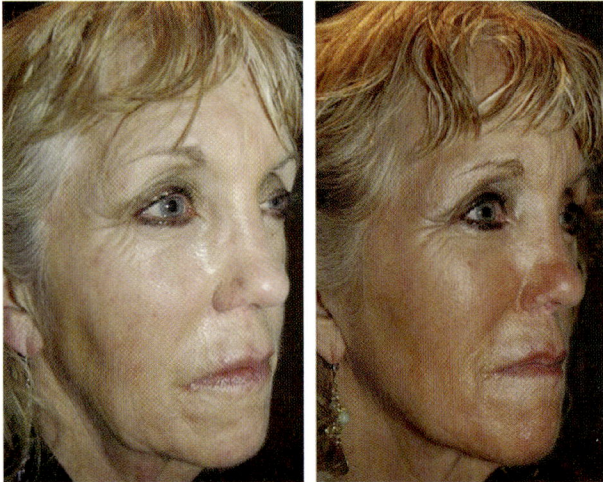

FIGURE 74.21 Before and after oblique views of patient one year after short incision facelift technique.

TABLE 74.4 *Potential Complications of Face-lifting*

Hemorrhage/Hematoma

Facial nerve damage

Skin Flap necrosis

Hypertrophic scarring

Hypesthesia/Paresthesia

Early recurrence of facial aging

Ear lobe malposition

Alopecia/Hairline deformity

Asymmetry or facial contour issues

SELECTED REFERENCES

Baker DC. Minimal incision rhytidectomy (short scar facelift) with lateral SMASectomy: evolution and application. *Aesthet Surg J.* 2001;21(1):68–79.

Hamra ST. The deep plane rhytidectomy. *Plast Reconstr Surg.* 1990;86(1): 53–61.

Johnson CM, Godin MS. The anterior extension face-lift. *Arch Otolaryngol Head Neck Surg.* 1995;121:613–616.

Stuzin JM, Baker TJ, Gordon HL. The relationship of the superficial and deep facial fascias: relevance to rhytidectomy and aging. *Plast Reconstr Surg.* 1992;89(3):441–449.

Tonnard P, Verpaele A, Monstrey S, Van Landuyt K, Blondeel P, Hamdi M, Matton G. Minimal access cranial suspension lift: a modified S-lift. *Plast Reconstr Surg.* 2002;109(6):2074–2086.

75 Ptosis Surgery

Srinivas S. Iyengar, MD and Steven C. Dresner, MD

TABLE 75.1 *Indications for Ptosis Surgery*

Symptomatic visual field loss
Palpebral fissure asymmetry
Cosmetic concerns
Abnormal head positioning
Amblyopia/Risk of amblyopia in children

TABLE 75.2 *Preoperative Considerations*

Identifying type of ptosis—myogenic, involutional, neurogenic, or mechanical

Rule out myasthenia

Assess levator function

Perform phenylephrine testing to help decide option for repair

Is the degree of ptosis mild, moderate, or severe?

Is concurrent dermatochalasis or brow ptosis present?

TABLE 75.3 *Comparison of Surgical Options*

	Levator Function	Degree of ptosis	Phenylephrine response
Conjunctival Muellerectomy	Good	Mild-moderate	Positive
Modified Fasanella Servat	Good	Mild-moderate	Positive
External levator resection	Good	Severe	Negative
Frontalis suspension	Poor	Severe	N/A

Conjunctival Muellerectomy

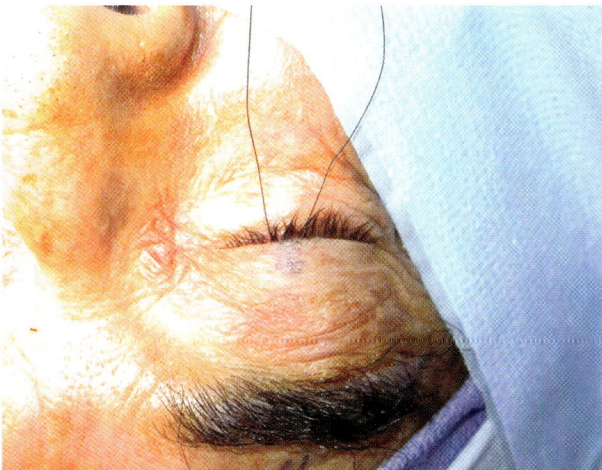

FIGURE 75.1 The pupillary axis is marked, and a 4-0 silk traction suture is placed.

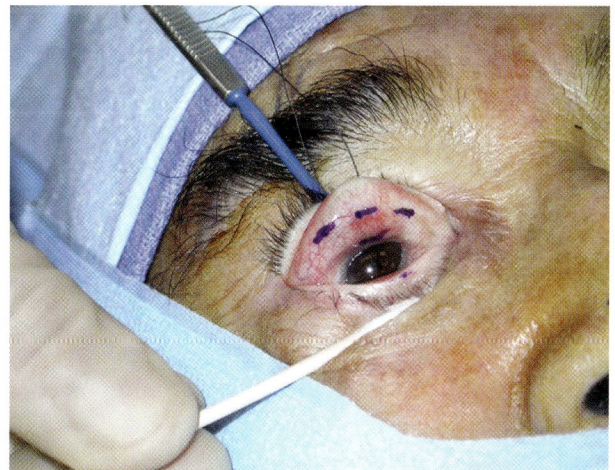

FIGURE 75.2 The eyelid is everted and a marking pen used to delineate half the amount (in mm) of the total resection laterally, centrally, and nasally. An additional mark is made at the full resection amount. In an 8 mm resection, the three marks would be 4 mm from the superior tarsal border.

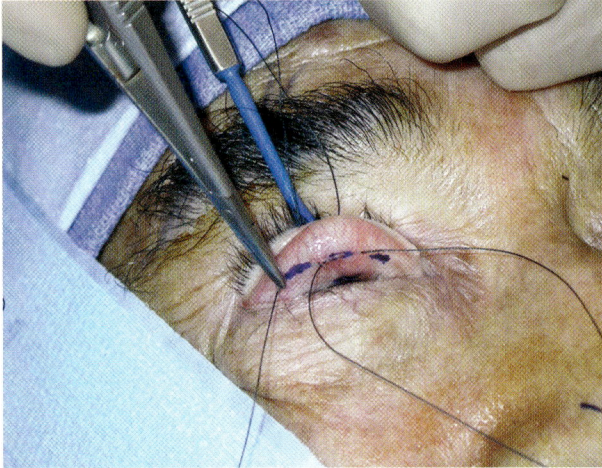

FIGURE 75.3 Three 4-0 silk sutures are placed through the 3 horizontal markings (at half the distance of the total resection) engaging Mueller's muscle and conjunctiva.

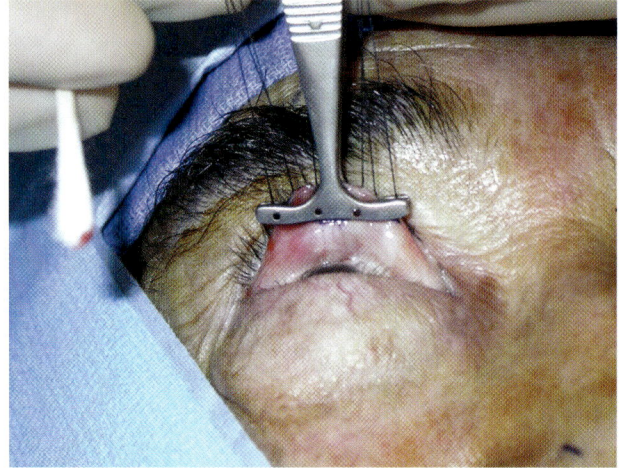

FIGURE 75.4 The silk sutures are placed on tension, grouped in two, and a Putterman clamp applied.

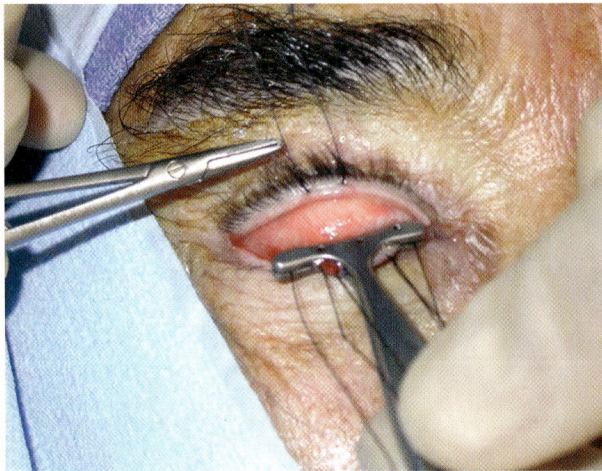

FIGURE 75.5 A 6-0 polypropylene suture is then passed, backhanded, through the skin, then under the clamp. This suture is then passed back and forth, under the clamp, in a horizontal fashion, and then externalized through the skin.

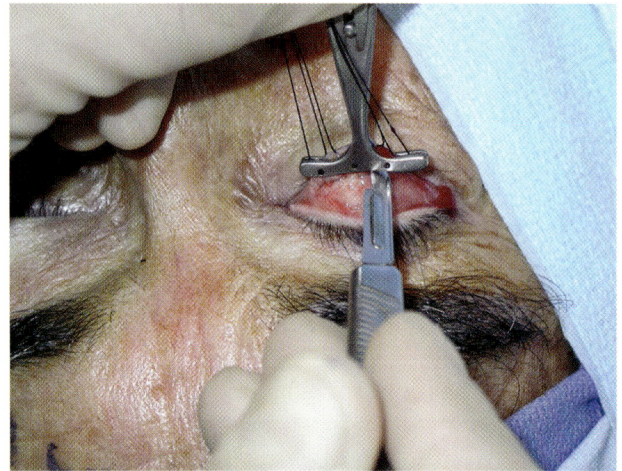

FIGURE 75.6 The polypropylene suture, now externalized, is placed on tension, as a No. 15 Bard-Parker blade is used to cut the clamped tissue keeping metal on metal.

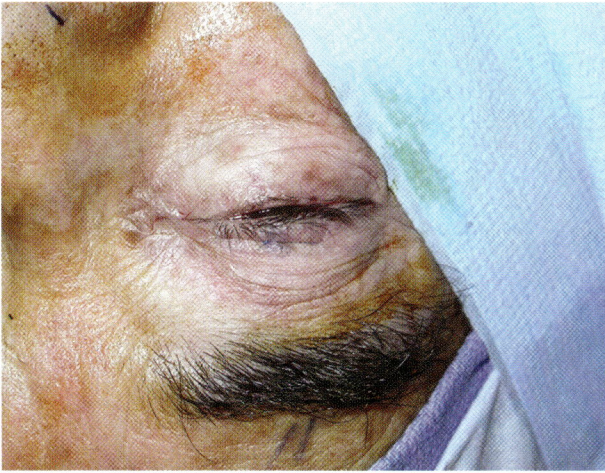

FIGURE 75.7 The 6-0 polypropylene suture is then gently tied on the anterior surface of the eyelid.

Modified Fasanella-Servat

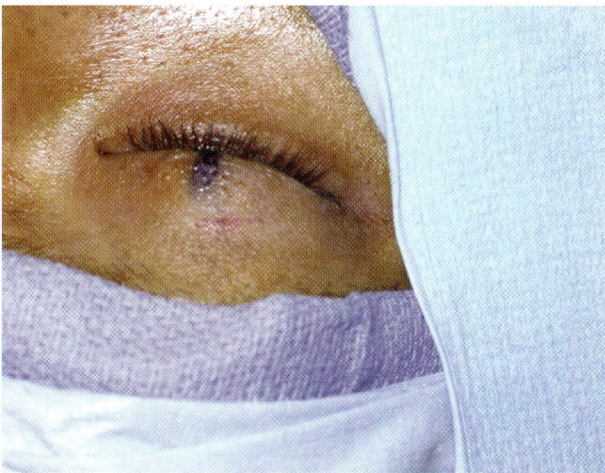

FIGURE 75.8 The central pupillary axis is marked on the upper eyelid.

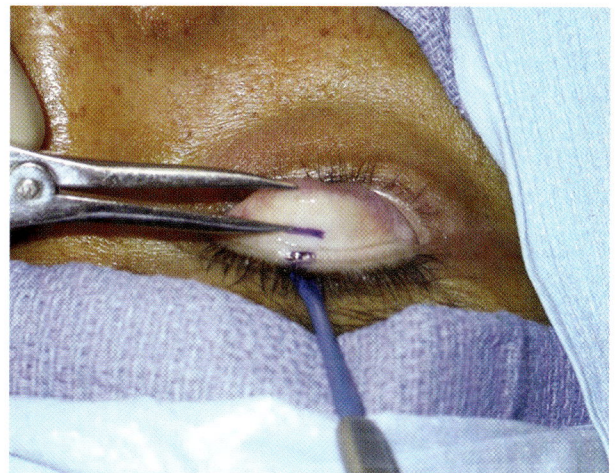

FIGURE 75.9 A Desmarres retractor is placed, everting the upper eyelid, and the amount of tarsus to be removed is measured and marked with a caliper. A 2:1 ratio for marking is used (i.e., 2 mm of tarsus is removed for 1 mm of expected eyelid lift).

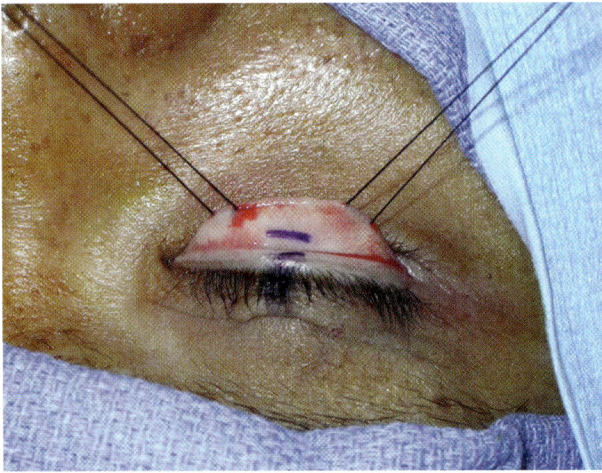

FIGURE 75.10 Two 4-0 silk sutures are then placed at the tarsal edge and placed under tension to elevate the tarsus.

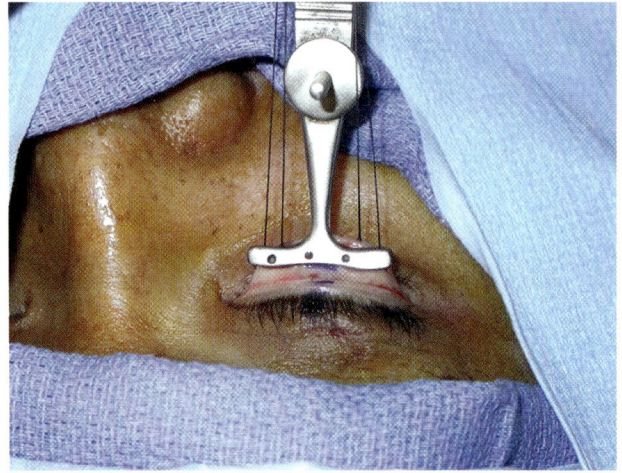

FIGURE 75.11 A ptosis clamp is then applied at the previously measured marking.

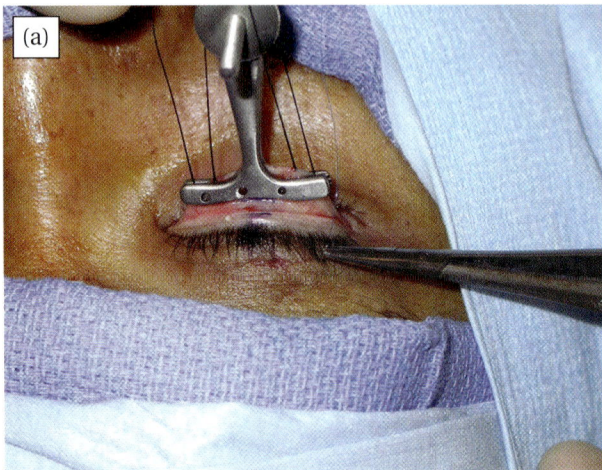

(a)

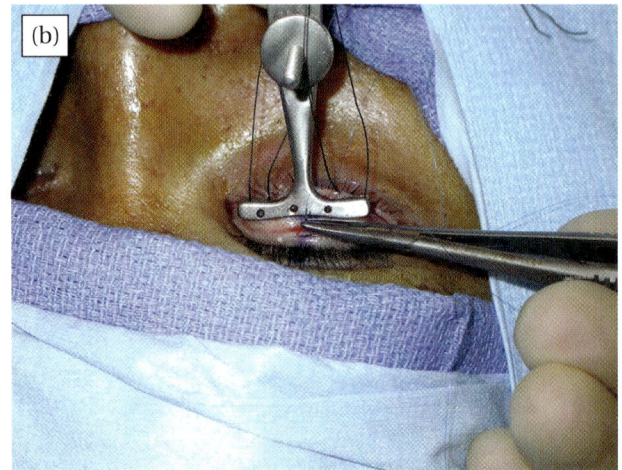

(b)

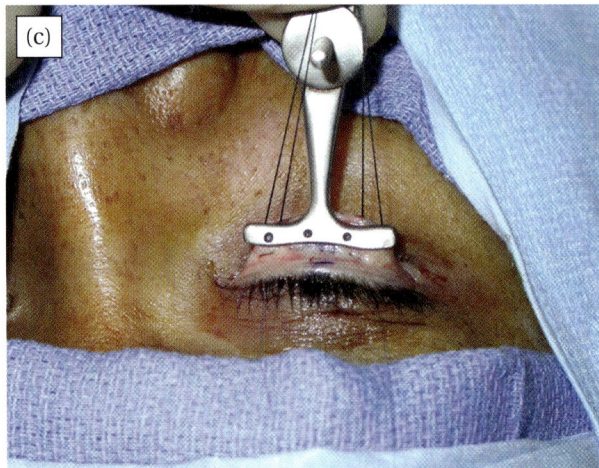

(c)

FIGURE 75.12 (a, b, c) A 6-0 polypropylene suture is then placed through the skin, under the clamp, and passed in a horizontal mattress fashion, with the last pass being again externalized through the skin.

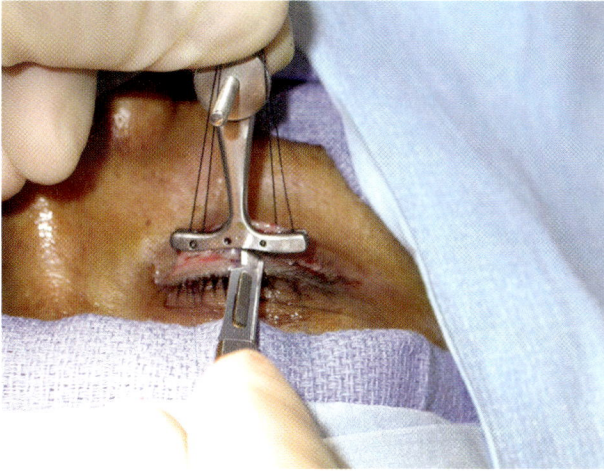

FIGURE 75.13 The polypropylene suture, now externalized, is placed on tension, as a No. 15 Bard-Parker blade is used to cut the clamped tarsal tissue keeping metal on metal.

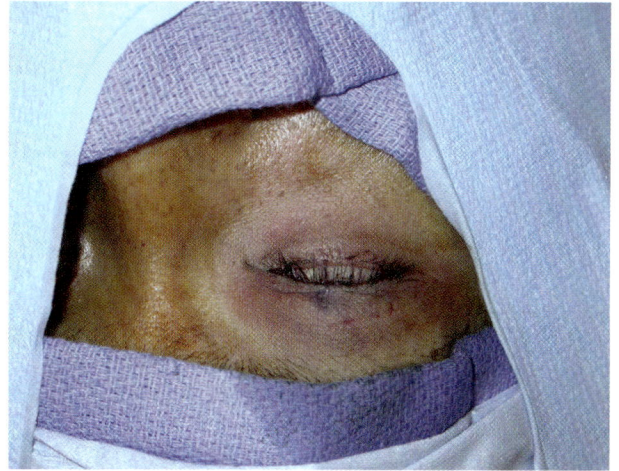

FIGURE 75.14 The 6-0 polypropylene suture is then gently tied on the anterior surface of the eyelid.

External Levator Resection

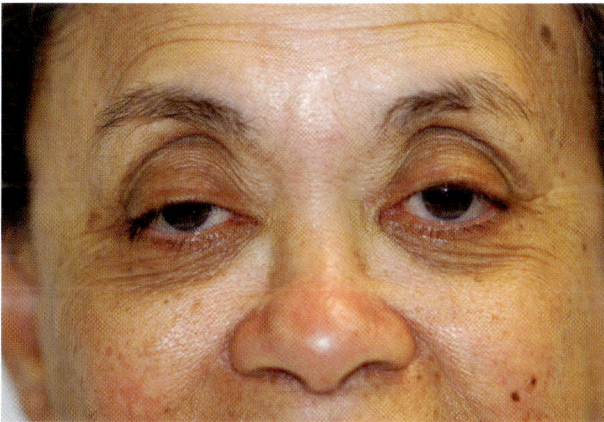

FIGURE 75.15 Significant ptosis, right upper eyelid greater than left, with minimal response to 2.5% phenylephrine.

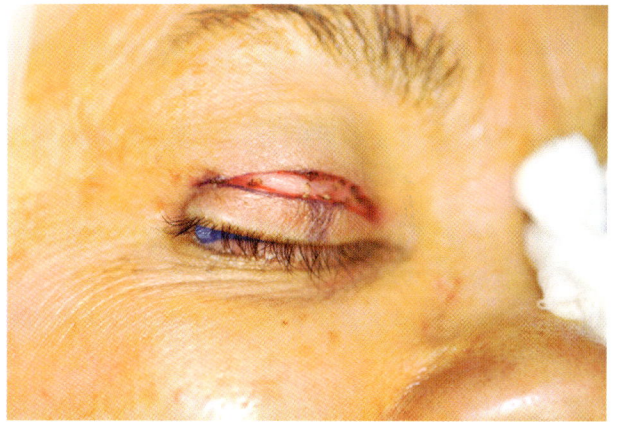

FIGURE 75.16 The pupillary axis is marked, a corneal shield is placed, and a lid crease incision is made with a No. 15 Bard-Parker blade.

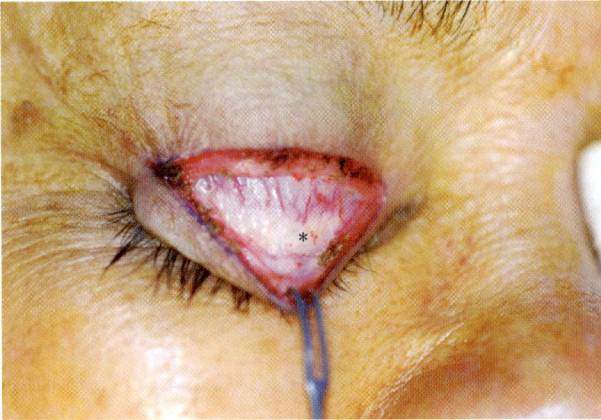

FIGURE 75.17   Dissection is carried down to expose the tarsal plate*.

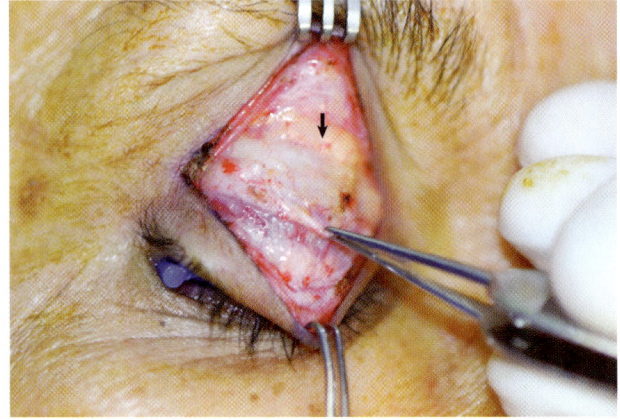

FIGURE 75.18   After identifying the preaponeurotic fat landmark (arrow head), the free levator (held by forceps) is identified.

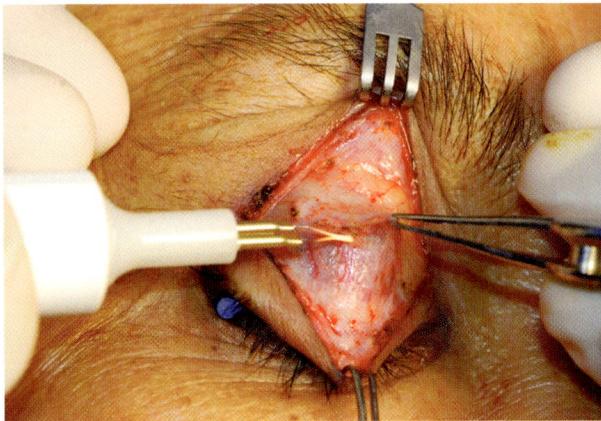

FIGURE 75.19   A handheld hot-temp cautery is used to free the levator aponeurosis from underlying attachments.

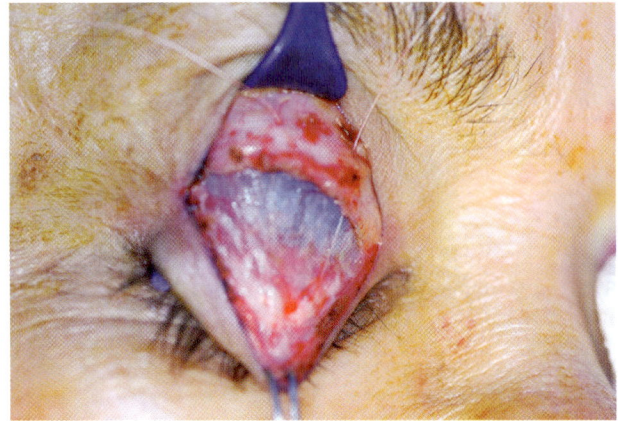

FIGURE 75.20   Two lamellar passes are made through the tarsus, with a double-armed single 5-0 vicryl S-14 suture. The suture is then passed through the levator aponeurosis.

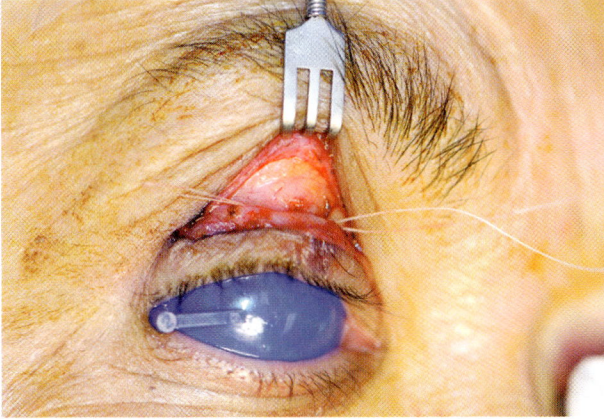

FIGURE 75.21 The 5-0 Vicryl suture is then tied, securing the levator aponeurosis to the anterior tarsus. Editor's note: Many surgeons favor a non-absorbable suture (i.e., 6-0 polypropylene) for external levator repair.

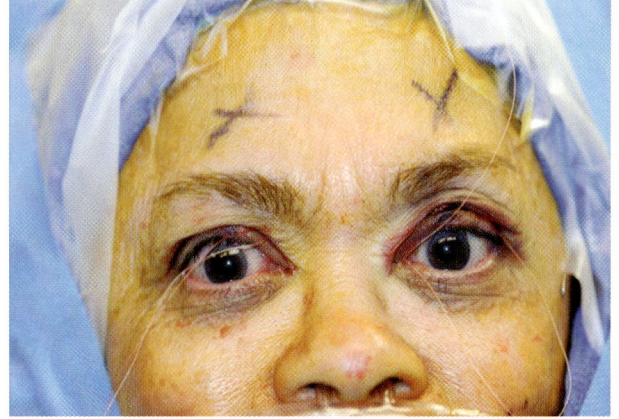

FIGURE 75.22 After performing the same steps on the left side, the patient is examined in the seated position. The lids are assessed for contour and position.

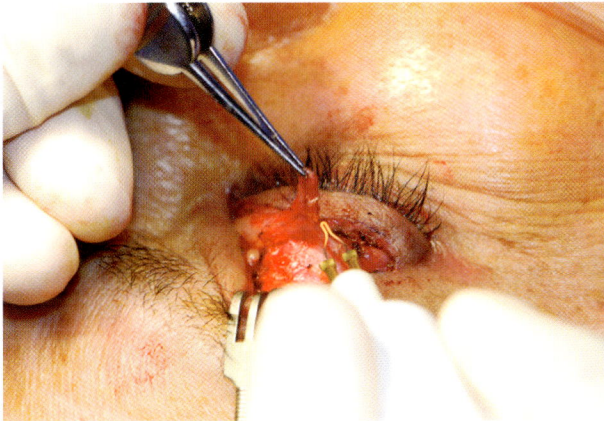

FIGURE 75.23 The excess levator aponeurosis is excised using high-temp cautery.

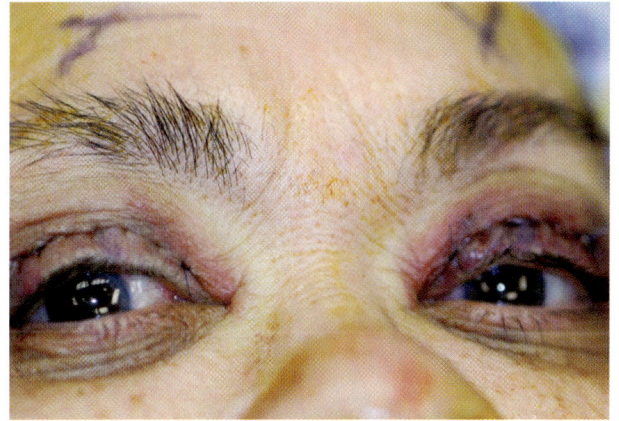

FIGURE 75.24 6-0 polypropylene suture is used to close the skin in a running fashion with supratarsal fixation of skin to levator.

Frontalis Suspension Procedure

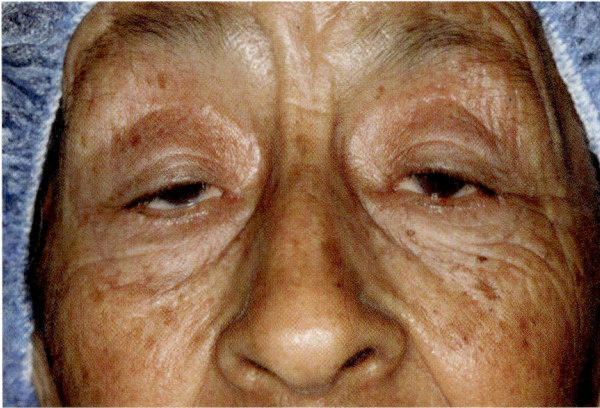

FIGURE 75.25   Severe bilateral ptosis with poor levator function.

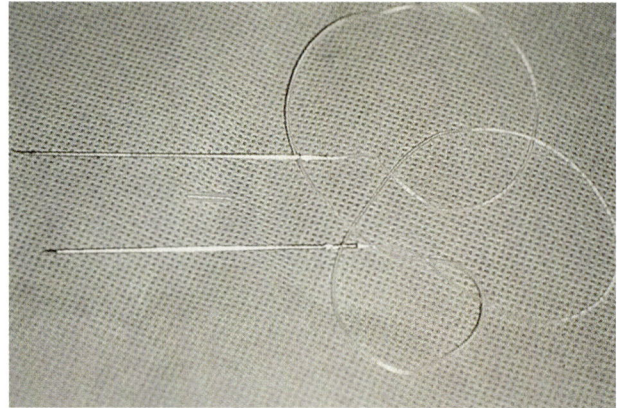

FIGURE 75.26   Silicone rod (BD Visitec Frontalis Suspension Set).

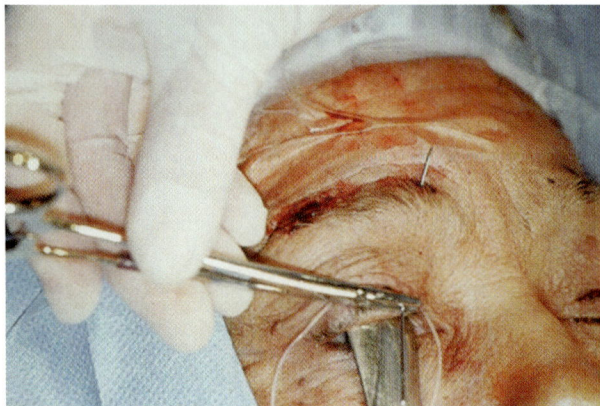

FIGURE 75.27   Following a lid crease incision, a metal Jaeger lid plate is placed below the upper lid before passing the silicone rods through the post-septal plane, and out the suprabrow stab incisions. A No. 15 Bard-Parker blade is used to make the stab incisions down to periosteum, with care to avoid the supraorbital neurovascular bundle. The rods are externalized through the suprabrow incisions before making a final pass to the superior incision, completing the pentagon. The external lid crease incision allows for direct visualization to secure the rods to the tarsus with 4-5 interrupted 6-0 neurilon or polypropylene suture.

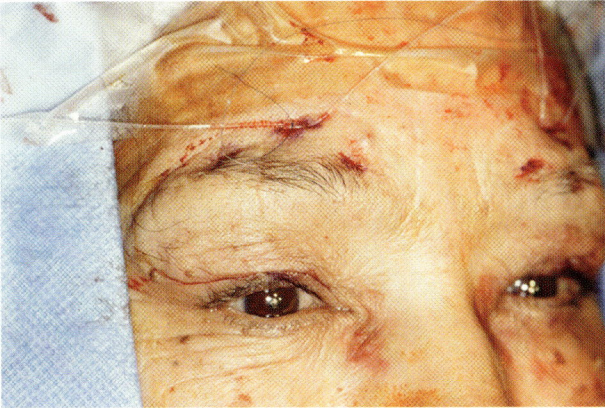

FIGURE 75.28 The silicone rods are finally externalized through the superior incision, and passed through a Watzke sleeve. Lid contour and position is then assessed.

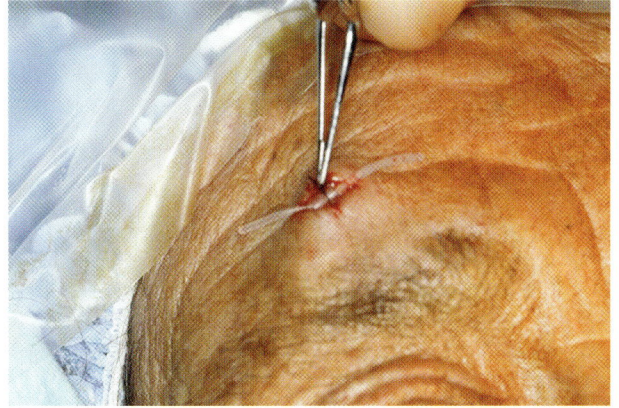

FIGURE 75.29 The rods are secured with 6-0 Neurilon suture, then cut short, leaving some redundant length for possible future adjustment. Ophthalmic ointment is applied to both eyes at the conclusion of the case. Skin incisions are all closed with 5-0 fast-absorbing plain gut suture.

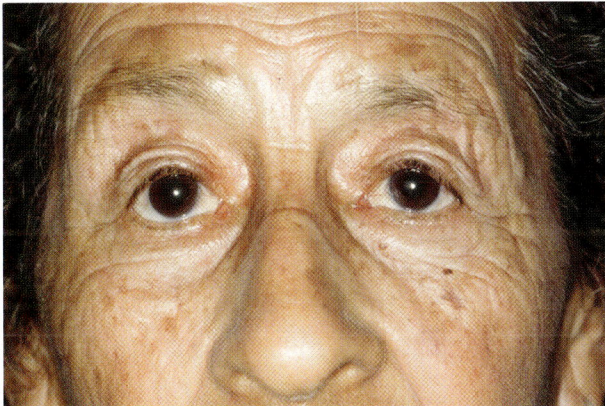

FIGURE 75.30 Use of the frontalis to elevate the eyelids following bilateral frontalis suspension procedure with silicone rod placement.

Preoperative and Postoperative Photos

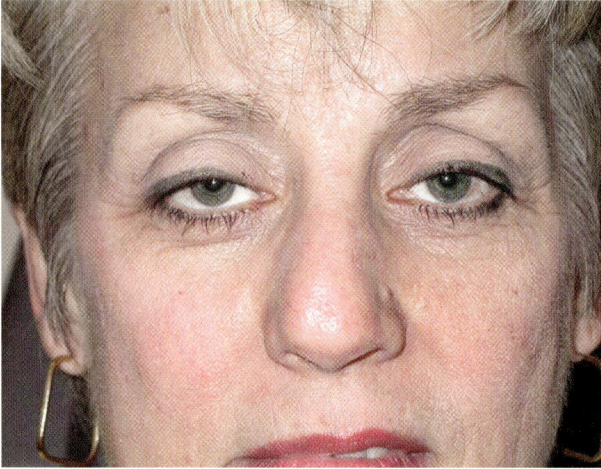

FIGURE 75.31   Bilateral involutional ptosis.

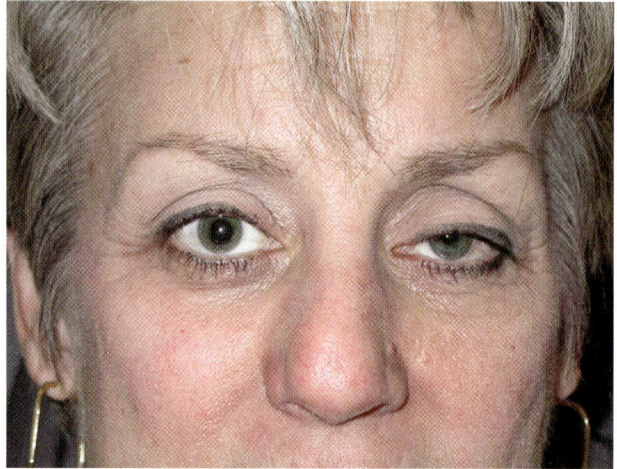

FIGURE 75.32   Positive response to phenylephrine 2.5%, after placement in the right eye.

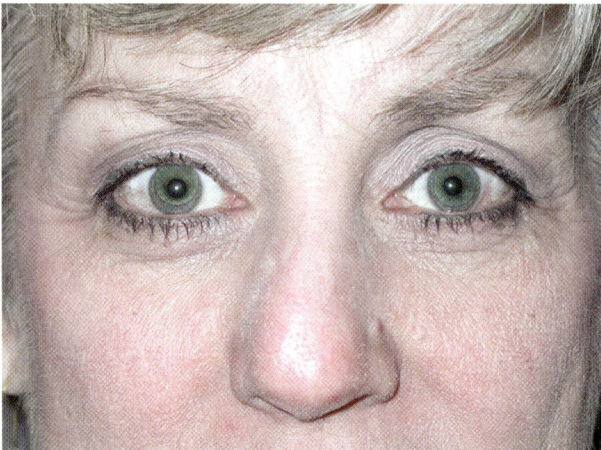

FIGURE 75.33   After undergoing bilateral Mueller's muscle conjunctival resections.

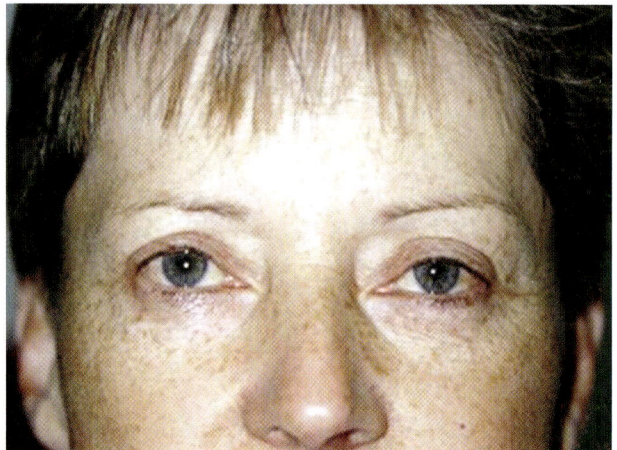

FIGURE 75.34   Patient with mild left upper eyelid ptosis before undergoing modified Fasanella-Servat procedure.

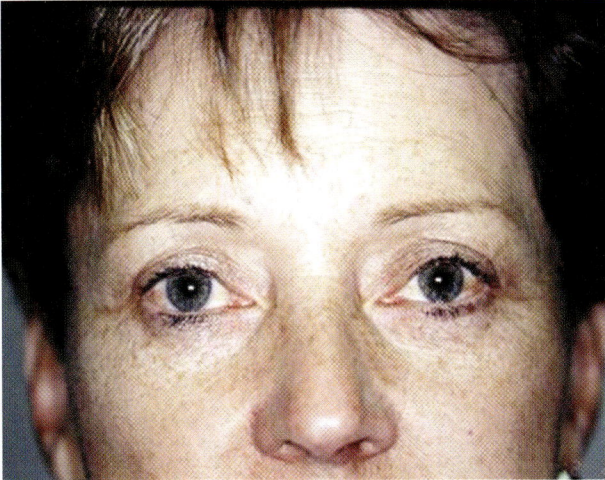

FIGURE 75.35 Same patient after modified Fasanella-Servat procedure on left upper lid.

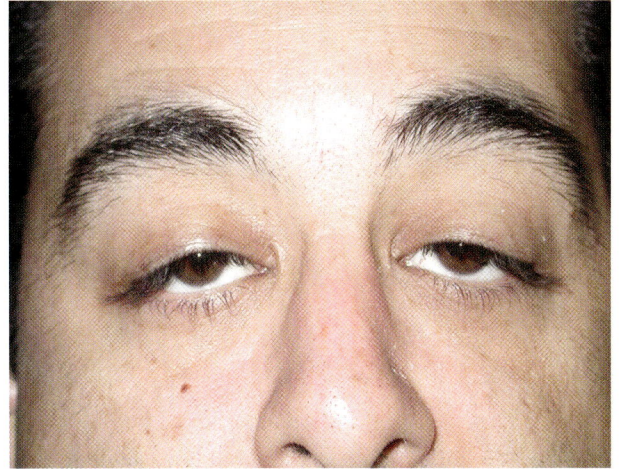

FIGURE 75.36 Severe congenital ptosis with poor levator function.

FIGURE 75.37 After frontalis sling placement on both sides.

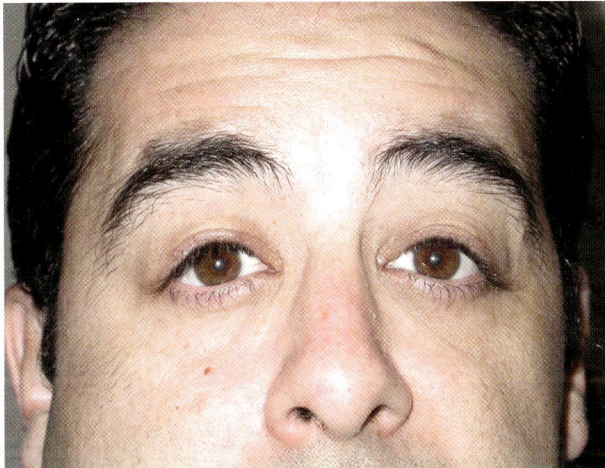

TABLE 75.4 *Complications of Ptosis Surgery*

Undercorrection

Overcorrection

Corneal abrasion

Lagophthalmos/Exposure keratopathy

Contour abnormality

SELECTED REFERENCES

Dresner SC. Further modifications of the Mueller's muscle conjunctival resection procedure for blepharoptosis. *Ophthalmic Plast Reconstr Surg.* 1991;7:114–122.

Dresner SC. Ptosis management: A practical approach. In Chen WP, *Oculoplastic Surgery*, Theime, 2001.

Putterman AM, Urist MJ. Mueller muscle–conjunctival resection. Technique for treatment of blepharoptosis. *Arch Ophthalmol.* 1975;93:619–623.

76 Entropion

Dale R. Meyer, MD, FACS and Mohit A. Dewan, MD

TABLE 76.1 *Indications for Entropion Repair*

Entropion of the eyelid margin

Symptomatic foreign body sensation (pain, tearing and/or discharge)

Corneal epithelial breakdown (ulcers in severe cases)

TABLE 76.2 *Preoperative Considerations*

Confirmation of type of entropion (congenital, cicatricial, spastic, involutional)

Systemic work-up if autoimmune condition (ocular cicatricial pemphigoid)

Use of glaucoma medications

Thermal or chemical injury

History of trachoma

Upper and/or lower lid involvement

Unilateral or bilateral

Consider posterior lamellar grafting in cases of more severe cicatrical conjunctival disorders

Involutional Entropion

Temporizing Procedures (Quickert Sutures)

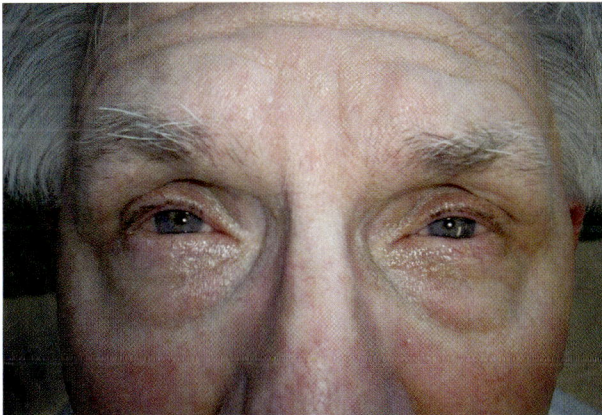

FIGURE 76.1 Preoperative presentation. Note bilateral lower lid entropion.

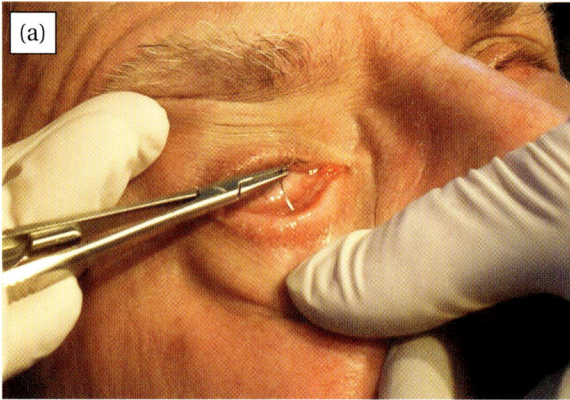

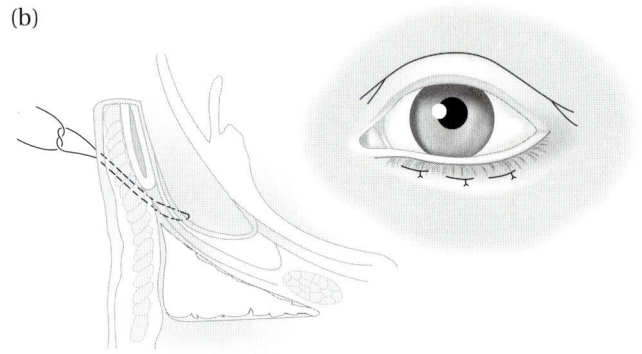

FIGURE 76.2 (a) Passage of needle (double-armed 5-0 chromic suture) from just below the tarsal plate, exiting 2–4 mm below the lash line. The second arm of the suture is passed similarly 3–4 mm adjacent to the first needle. (b) Diagram of Quickert suture placement.

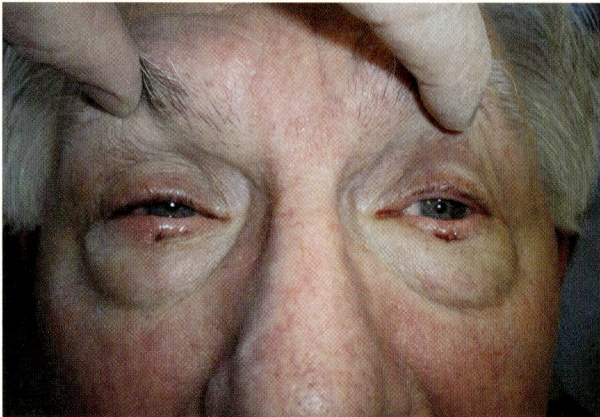

FIGURE 76.3 The two arms of the suture are tied to produce a slight eversion of the lid margin.

Horizontal Tightening with Retractor Plication and Orbicularis Excision via Transconjunctival Approach

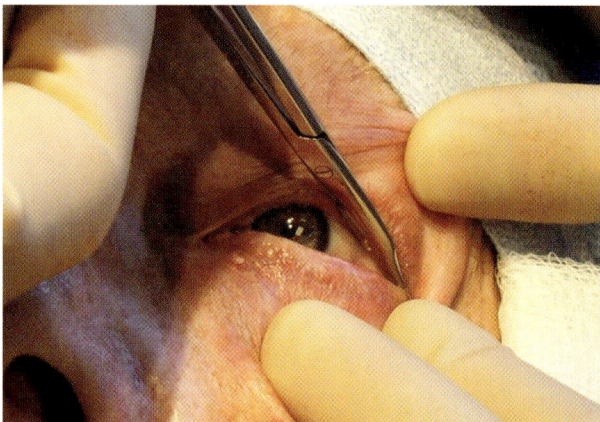

FIGURE 76.4 Lateral canthotomy and cantholysis.

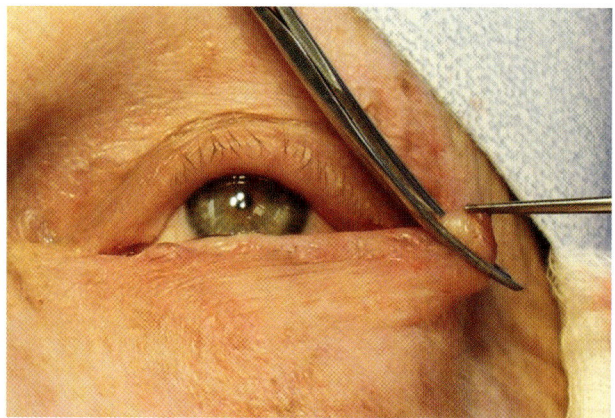

FIGURE 76.5 Removal of adequate lateral tarsus to achieve the desired amount of horizontal tightening.

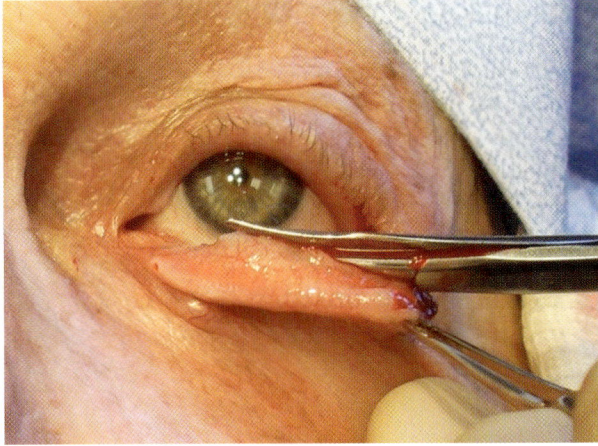

FIGURE 76.6 Undermining of the lower lid retractors.

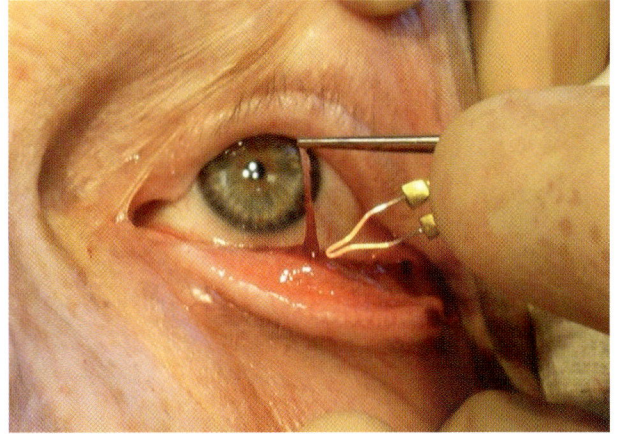

FIGURE 76.7 Orbicularis excision using high temperature cautery.

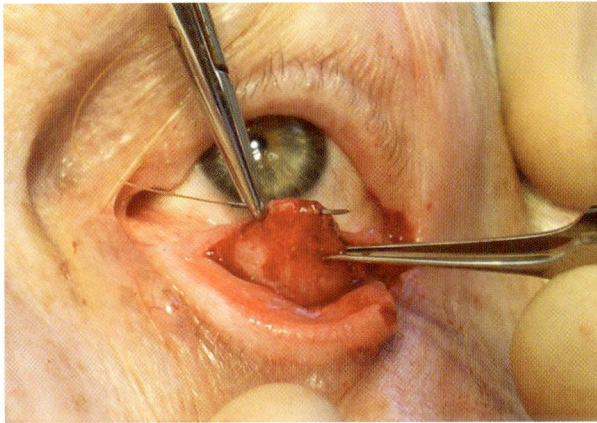

FIGURE 76.8 Plication of lower lid retractors using mattress sutures. After engaging the lower lid retractors, the double-armed suture is then passed through the skin, exiting just beneath the lash line in a horizontal mattress fashion.

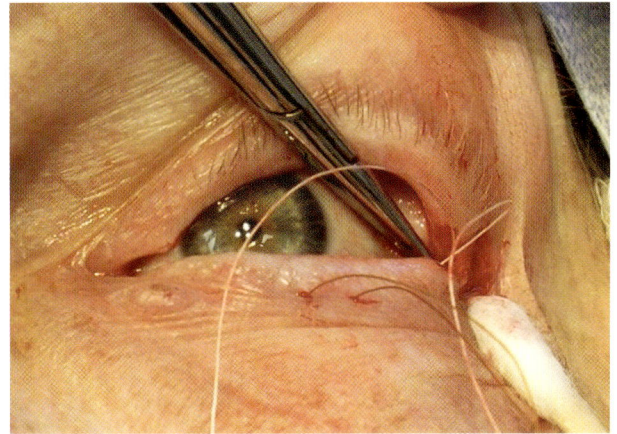

FIGURE 76.9 Insertion of lateral tarsal strip to lateral orbital periosteum. This suture is tied to the desired level of tightness. Note the lower lid retractor sutures have been passed full thickness through the lid and are to be tied after insertion of the lateral tarsal strip.

FIGURE 76.10 Postoperative appearance.

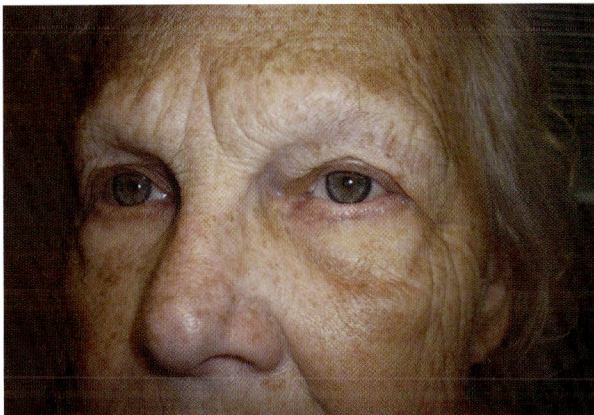

Cicatricial Entropion

Transverse Tarsotomy or Blepharotomy (Wies Procedure)

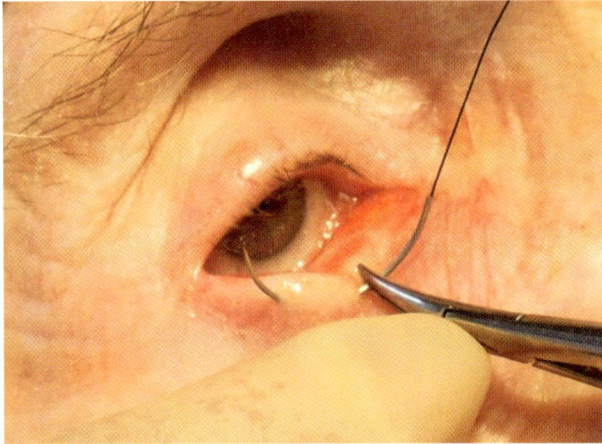

FIGURE 76.11 A 4-0 silk traction suture passed through the gray line.

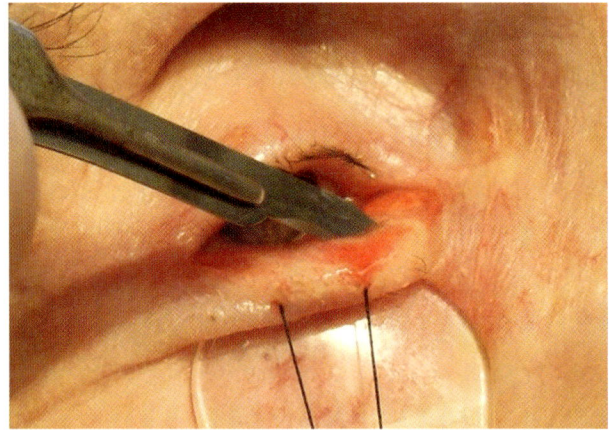

FIGURE 76.12 Lower lid everted over lid plate and incision made through tarsus.

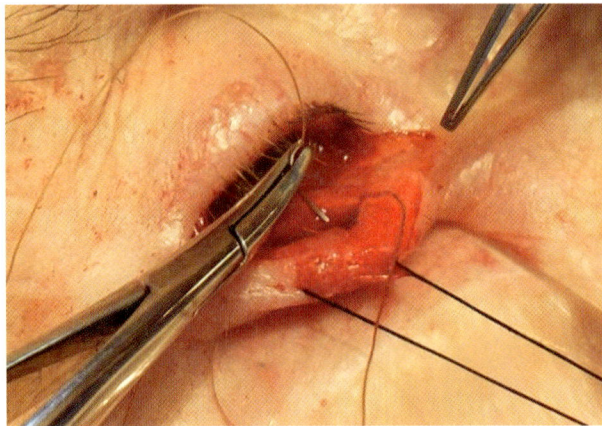

FIGURE 76.13 A double armed 5-0 absorbable suture is passed through the conjunctiva and lower lid retractor layer.

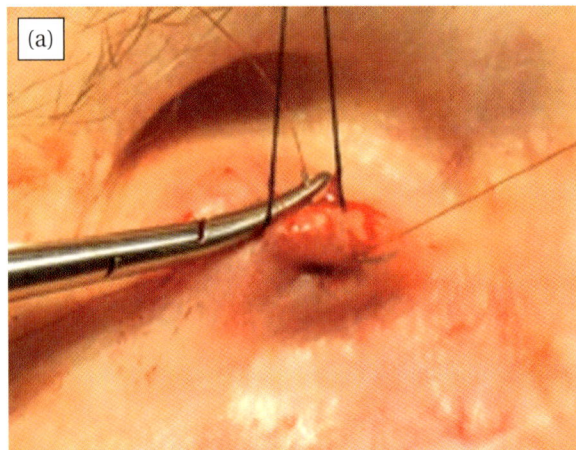

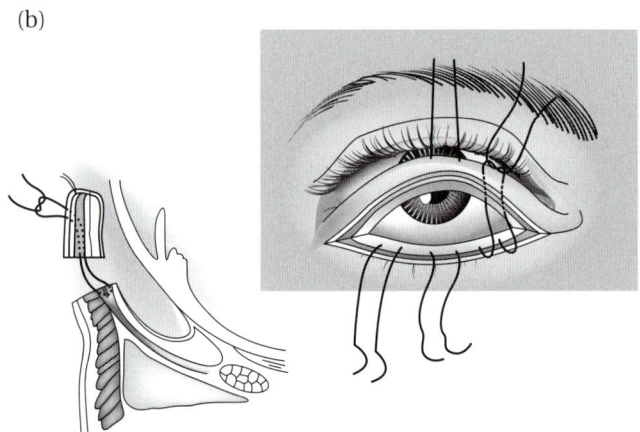

FIGURE 76.14 (a) The sutures are passed into the orbicularis muscle layer anterior to the tarsal plate and out through the skin 2–3 mm inferior to lashes. (b) Diagram of Wies suture placement.

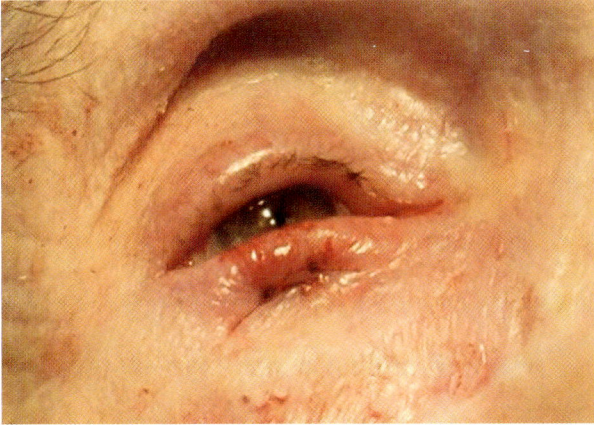

FIGURE 76.15 Sutures are tied externally, creating a slight eversion of the lid margin.

Posterior Lamellar Grafts

used for more severe cicatricial conjunctival disease with entropion: conjunctiva, mucous membrane, amniotic membrane, acellular matrix.

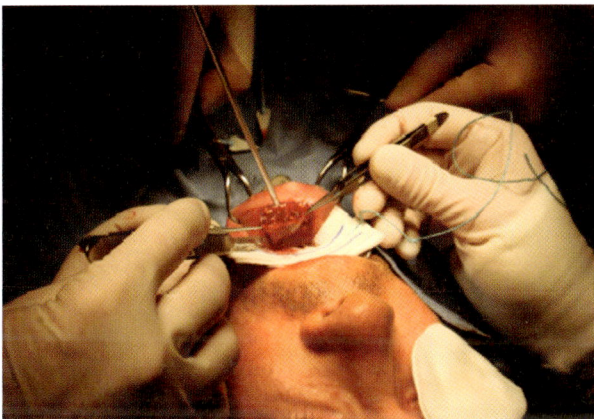

FIGURE 76.16 Harvesting full-thickness mucous membrane graft from lower lip.

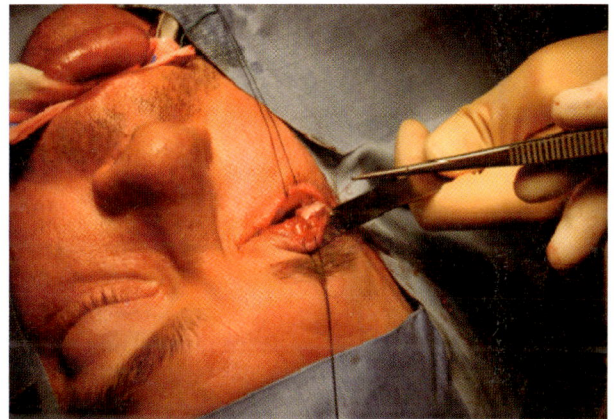

FIGURE 76.17 Suturing of mucous membrane graft into posterior lamella of right upper lid for cicatricial entropion.

TABLE 76.3 *Treatment for Trichiasis/Distichiasis*

Epilation—simple removal of lashes using forceps at the slit lamp

Electrolysis (Radiofrequency unit with partially insulated needle tip inserted along shaft of cilia, with energy delivered for 1–2 sec at low power cut/coagulation mode to destroy follicle)

Cryotherapy—nitrous oxide probe double freeze–thaw for approximately 30 sec with temperature monitoring (–20°C)

Argon Laser (1–2 watts with 50–100 um spot size for 0.1–0.2 sec directed down to lash follicle)

Surgical excision (Focal pentagonal excision, or more complex reconstructive procedures— please refer to Chapter 81 on eyelid reconstruction)

Distichiasis—lid splitting at gray line with one of modalities above, or with excision of distal tarsus with mucous membrane graft to margin

Electrolysis Surgical Series

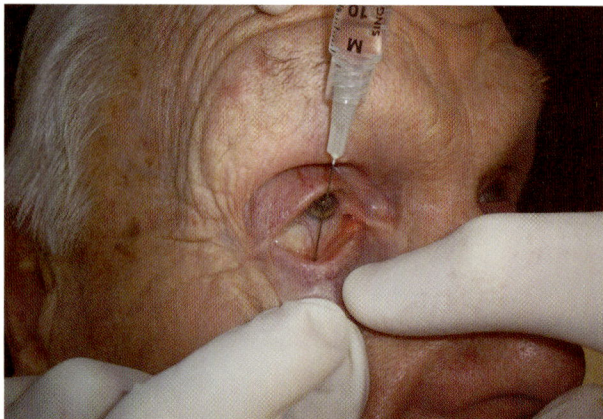

FIGURE 76.18 Injection of local anesthetic into conjunctiva adjacent to trichiasis lashes.

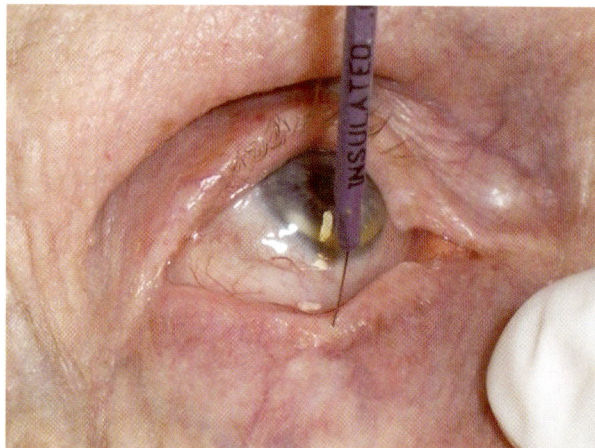

FIGURE 76.19 Insertion of electrolysis needle into base of lash follicle. The needle is activated until the follicle blanches, 1–2 sec.

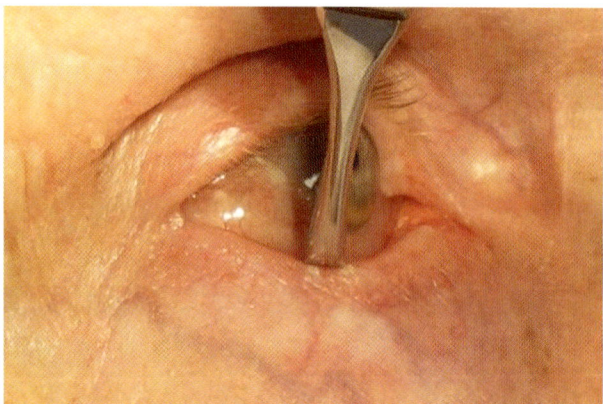

FIGURE 76.20 The treated eyelash is epilated with forceps without any possible resistance.

TABLE 76.4 *Complications of Entropion Repair and Trichiasis/Distichiasis Treatment*

Undercorrection

Overcorrection

Eyelid contour deformity

Recurrence

Eyelid scarring/atrophy

Depigmentation from cryotherapy

SELECTED REFERENCES

Bartley GB, Bullock JD, Olsen TG, et al. An experimental study to compare methods of eyelash ablation. *Ophthalmology*. 1987;94:1286–1289.

Bartley GB, Lowry JC. Argon laser treatment of trichiasis. *Am J Ophthalmol*. 1992;113:71–74.

Dresner SC, Karesh JW. Transconjunctival entropion repair. *Arch Ophthalmol*. 1993;111:1144–1148.

Elder MJ, Bernauer W. Cryotherapy for trichiasis in ocular cicatricial pemphigoid. *Br J Ophthalmol*. 1994;78:769–771.

Kersten RC, Kleiner FP, Kulwin DR. Tarsotomy for the treatment of cicatricial entropion with trichiasis. *Arch Ophthalmol*. 1992;110:714–717.

Khan SJ, Meyer DR. Transconjunctival lower eyelid involution entropion repair: long-term follow-up and efficacy. *Ophthalmology*. 2002;109:2112–2117.

Shore JW, Foster S, Westfall CT, et al. Results of buccal mucosal grafting for patients with medically controlled ocular pemphigoid. *Ophthalmology*. 1992;99:383–385.

77 Lower Eyelid Epiblepharon

Sang In Khwarg, MD and Min Joung Lee, MD

TABLE 77.1 *Clinical Features of Epiblepharon*

Normal position of eyelid margin

Horizontal fold of skin and underlying orbicularis oculi muscle causing inversion of eyelashes rubbing against the cornea

More common and severe at the medial aspect of the eyelid

Accentuated in downgaze

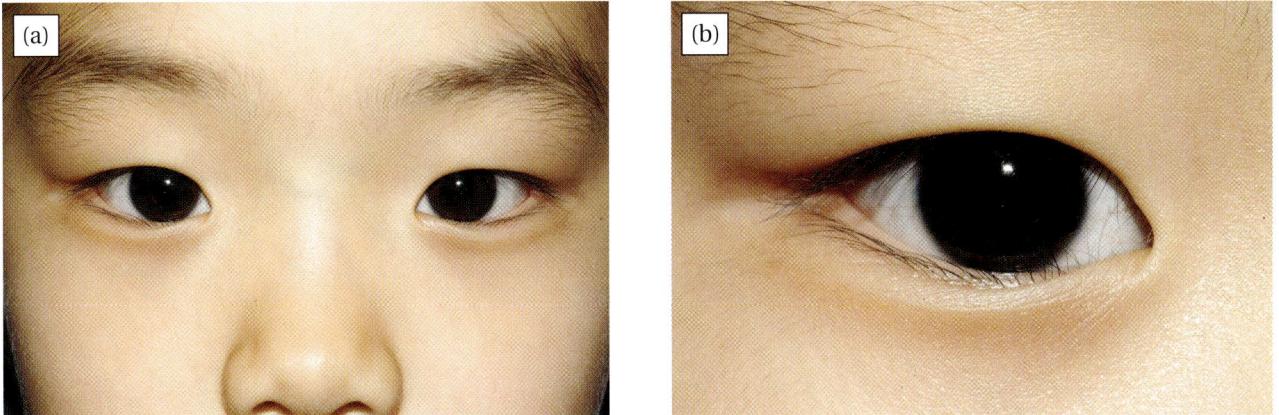

FIGURE 77.1 (a, b) Typical appearance of lower eyelid epiblepharon.

TABLE 77.2 *Indications for Epiblepharon Repair Surgery*

Symptomatic ocular surface irritation: Eye rubbing, photophobia, foreign body sensation, discharge, frequent blinking

Signs of keratopathy: Conjunctival injection, punctate corneal erosion corresponding to area of lash inversion

TABLE 77.3 *Preoperative Considerations*

Age of the patient: Surgical repair can be usually postponed to the age of 3 years or later if signs and symptoms are not severe

Severity of epiblepharon is judged by the extent of epiblepharon and the degree of corneal erosion. Mild epiblepharon is typically observed.

Height of skin fold: The vertical extent of the skin fold should be measured preoperatively to determine the amount of skin excision

Lower Eyelid Epiblepharon Repair by Cilia-everting Suture Technique

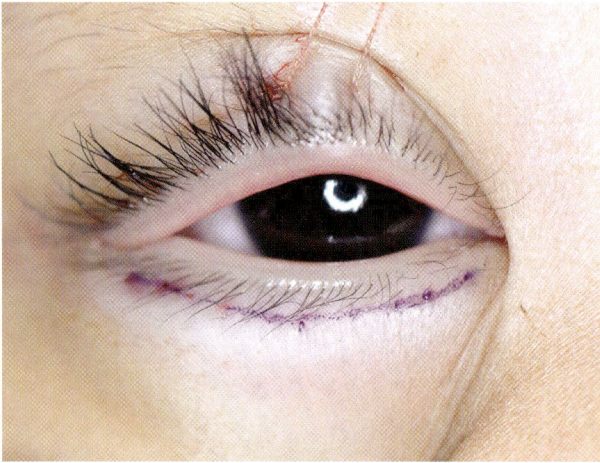

FIGURE 77.2 A subciliary incision is marked from just temporal to the inferior punctum along the whole lid length, 1–2 mm below the cilia line. 2% lidocaine mixed with epinephrine at a ratio of 1:100,000 is infiltrated subcutaneously along the marked line. A 4-0 silk traction suture is applied to the upper eyelid to assist with exposure.

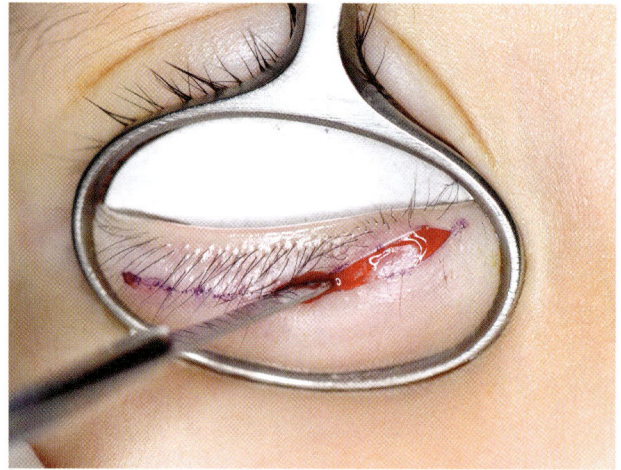

FIGURE 77.3 The skin and orbicularis muscle are incised using a #15 blade along the previous mark while the lid is immobilized with the chalazion clamp.

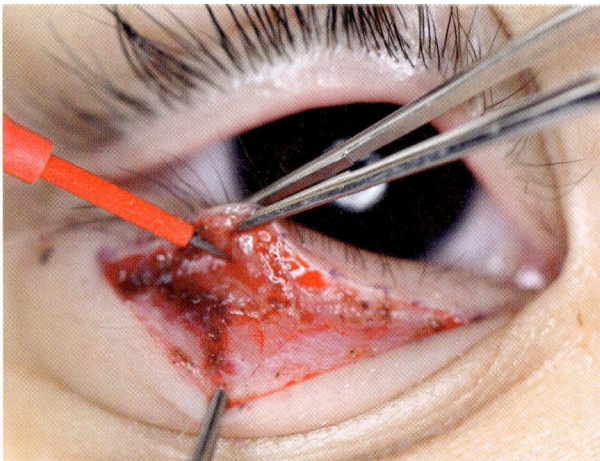

FIGURE 77.4 Dissection is performed, separating the pretarsal orbicularis oculi muscle and the tarsus using a monopolar cautery until the lower margin of the tarsus is exposed.

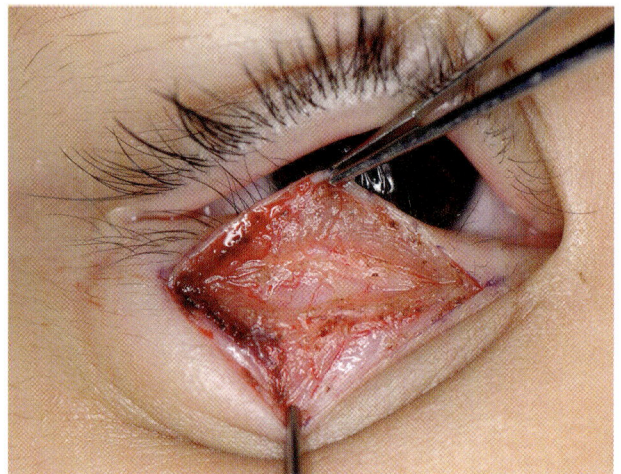

FIGURE 77.5 Inferior extent of orbicularis oculi dissection.

(a)

(b)

Tarsal plate

Lower eyelid
retractor

Orbital
septum

Orbicularis
muscle

Tarsal
plate

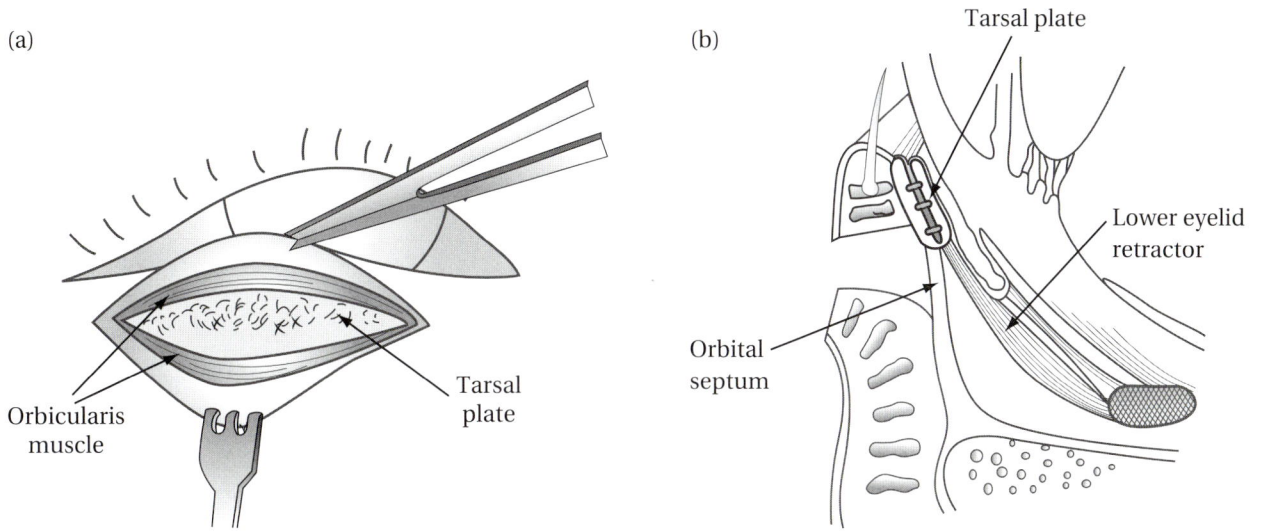

FIGURE 77.6 Frontal (a) and sagittal (b) view diagrams showing plane of dissection.

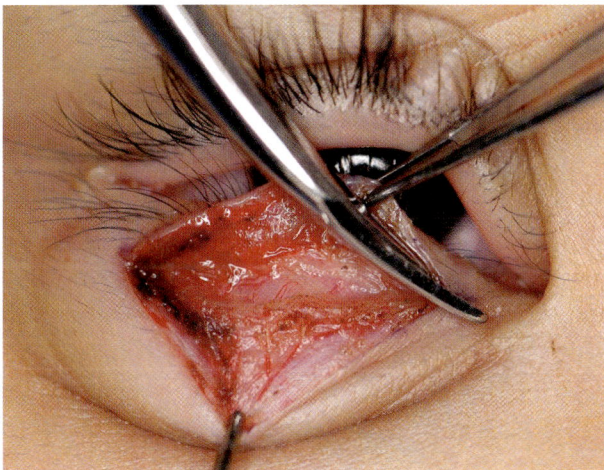

FIGURE 77.7 The skin incision is extended medially to the level of epicanthal fold using Stevens tenotomy scissors. This step aims to correct the most medial aspect of the epiblepharon. The incision should be made parallel to the lid margin to avoid the injury to the inferior canaliculus.

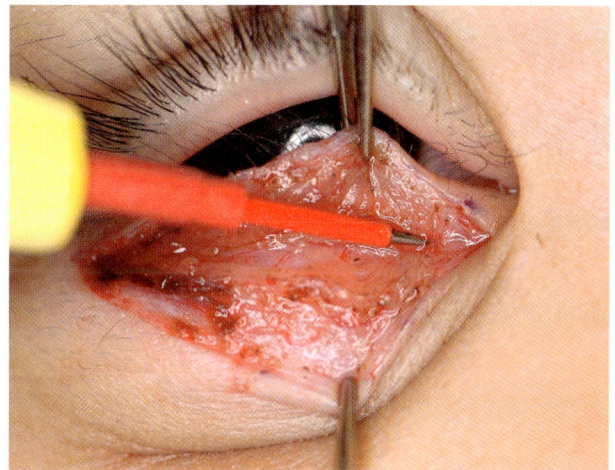

FIGURE 77.8 Further pretarsal orbicularis oculi dissection performed along the medial extent of the incision.

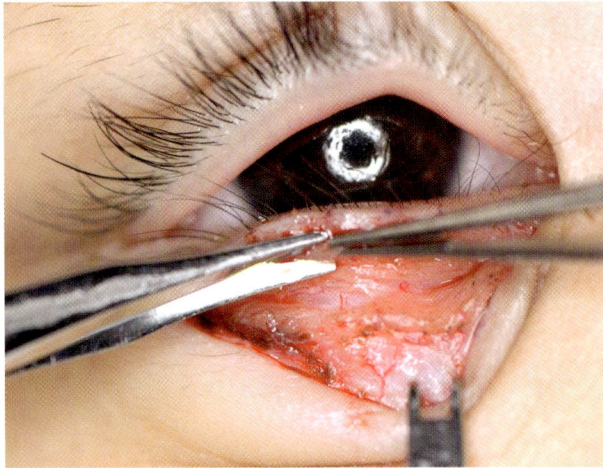

FIGURE 77.9   The pretarsal orbicularis muscle just inferior to the upper edge of the skin incision is excised using Wescott scissors. Care must be taken to avoid damage to the cilia follicles.

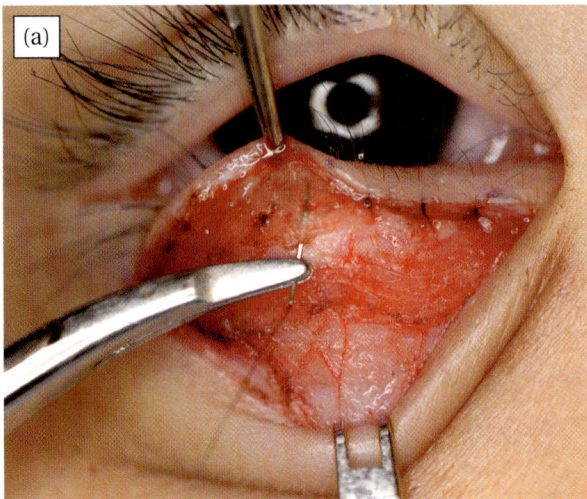

(a)

(b)

Upper edge of skin

Lower margin of tarsus

(c)

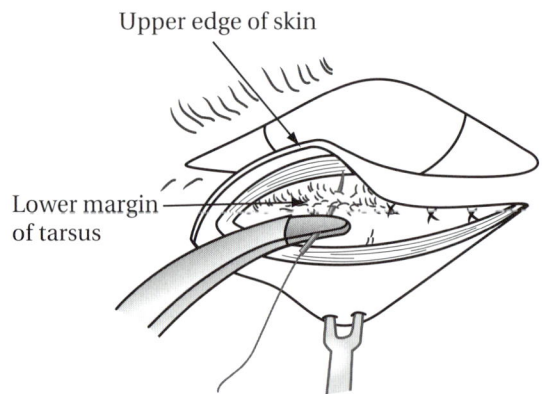

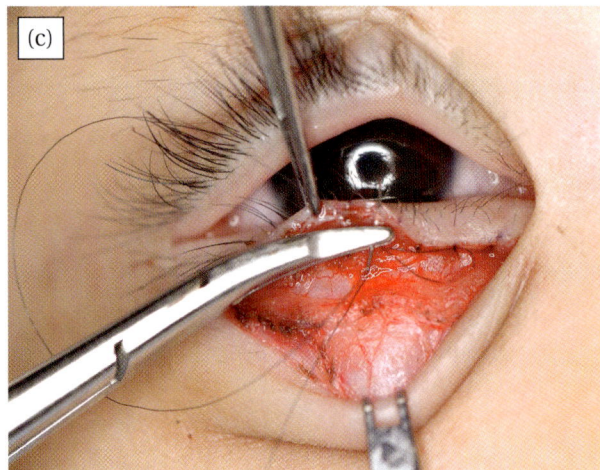

FIGURE 77.10   8-0 nylon fixation sutures are placed between the tarsal plate and the upper skin edge. Figures (a) and (b) show the needle passing through the lower margin of the tarsus. Figure (c) subsequently shows the needle passing through the subcutaneous tissue of the upper skin edge.

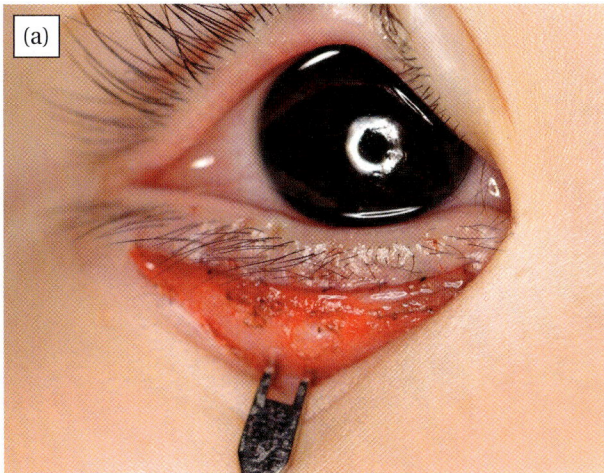

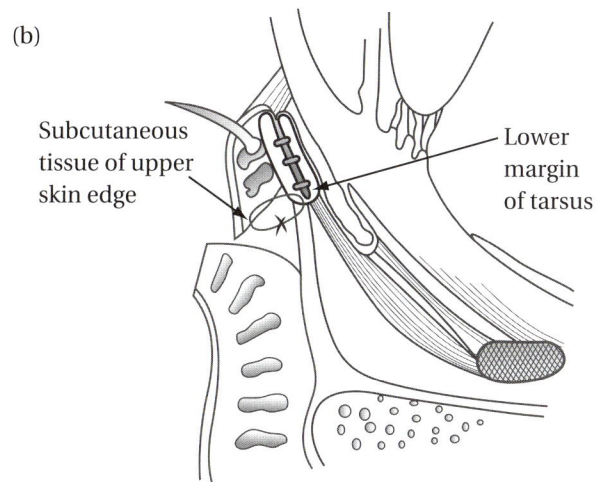

FIGURE 77.11 (a) A total of seven interrupted fixation sutures are placed using 8-0 nylon. Note the excellent eversion of the cilia. Figure (b) shows a sagittal section diagram of the suture placement.

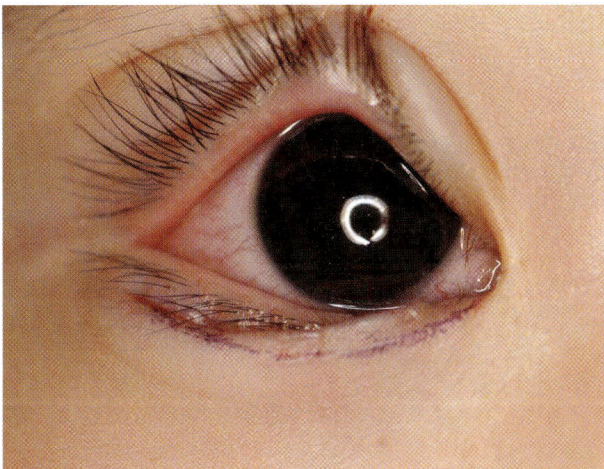

FIGURE 77.12 The lower edge of the incised skin is advanced to the upper skin edge, and the redundant skin is excised.

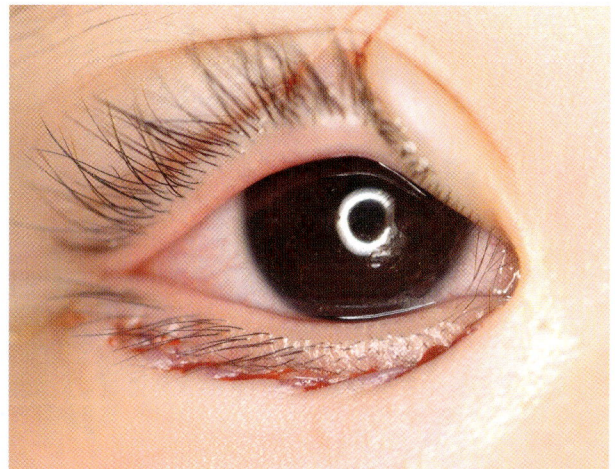

FIGURE 77.13 The skin is closed with 6-0 fast-absorbing plain gut suture.

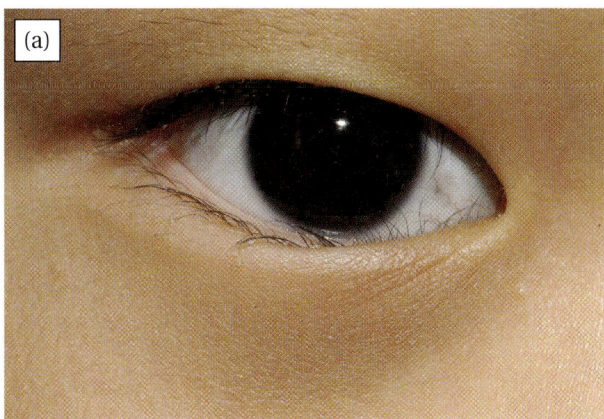

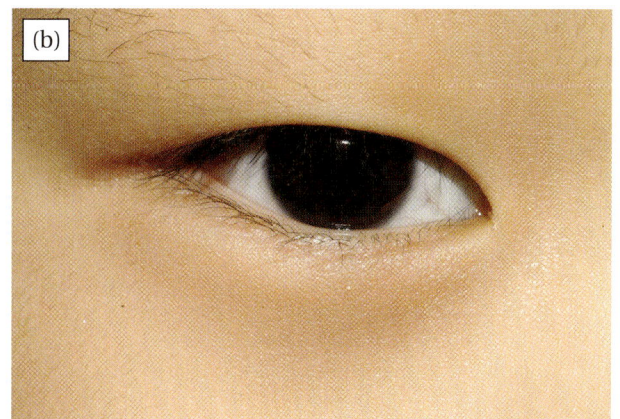

FIGURE 77.14 (a) Preoperative photo of a 3-year-old with lower eyelid epiblepharon. (b) Postoperative photo taken two months after surgical repair. Note excellent lash eversion and lid crease formation.

TABLE 77.4   *Potential Complications*

Recurrence in approximately 3% of cases
Abnormal oblique crease on downgaze
Suture abscess or exposure

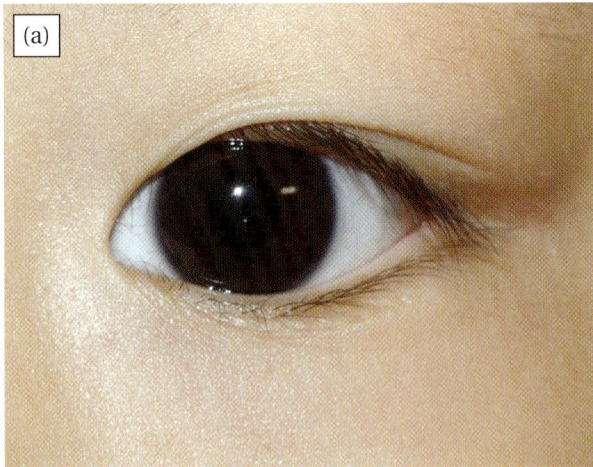

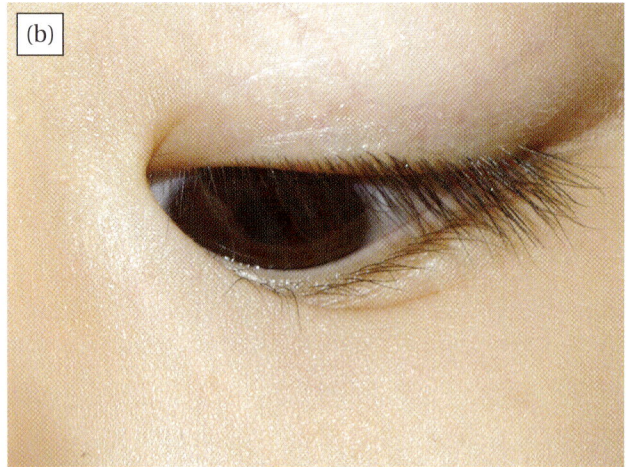

FIGURE 77.15   Abnormal lid crease formation after surgical epiblepharon repair. It is more prominent in downgaze (b) than primary gaze (a). This abnormal crease may arise from unexpected scar formation below skin incision at the medial eyelid, or from loose tarsal fixation of the subcutaneous tissue of the upper skin edge at the lateral eyelid. It typically becomes less apparent or disappears, but may occasionally persist in few cases.

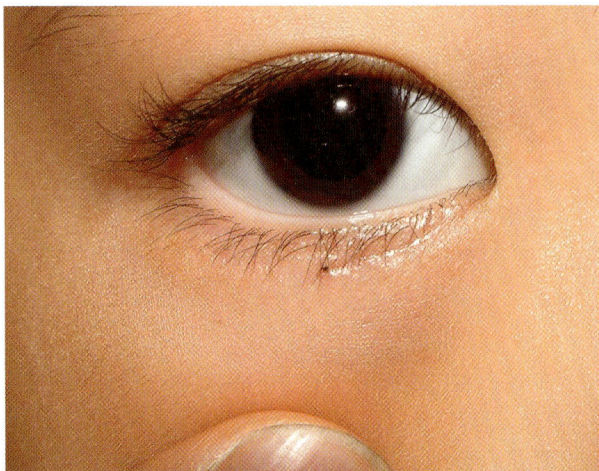

FIGURE 77.16   Central suture knot exposure noted 3 months after surgery.

SELECTED REFERENCES

Khwarg SI, Lee YJ. Epiblepharon of the lower eyelid: classification and association with astigmatism. *Korean J Ophthalmol.* 1997;11(2):111–117.

Khwarg SI, Choung HK. Epiblepharon of the lower eyelid: technique of surgical repair and quantification of excision according to the skin fold height. *Ophthalmic Surg Lasers.* 2002;33:280–287.

Woo KI, Yi K, Kim YD. Surgical correction for lower lid epiblepharon in Asians. *Br J Ophthalmol.* 2000;84:1407–1410.

Ectropion

Bryan J. Winn, MD and Bryan S. Sires, MD, PhD, FACS

TABLE 78.1   *Types of Ectropion*

Involutional Ectropion
Punctal ectropion
Medial ectropion in the absence of horizontal lid laxity
Medial ectropion with horizontal lid laxity
Medial ectropion with medial canthal tendon laxity
Lateral canthal tendon laxity/tear pump dysfunction
Tarsal ectropion

Paralytic Ectropion
Cicatricial Ectropion
Congenital Lower Eyelid Ectropion
Congenital Upper Eyelid Ectropion
Mechanical Ectropion

TABLE 78.2   *Indications for Surgery*

Epiphora
Foreign body sensation
Photophobia
Corneal punctate epithelial erosions
Corneal ulceration
Tarsal conjunctival keratinization

TABLE 78.3   *Patient Evaluation*

Evaluate orbicularis oculi tone—history of facial nerve palsy?
Floppy eyelid syndrome
Surgical or traumatic facial scars
Infiltrating cutaneous lesions
Systemic skin disorders (ichthyosis, atopic dermatitis, scleroderma, etc.)
Assess lower eyelid laxity (distraction test, snap test)
Punctal position
Punctal stenosis
Lateral canthal tendon laxity (canthal rounding, horizontal palpebral fissure shortening)
Medial canthal tendon laxity (lateral punctal pull test)
Disinsertion of lower-lid retractors

TABLE 78.4 *Preoperative Considerations/Surgical Options*

Preoperative Considerations

Condition/Finding	Surgical Options/Considerations
Punctal ectropion	• Medial spindle operation
	• Medial posterior lamella cautery
Punctal stenosis	• One-snip, two-snip, or three-snip punctoplasty
	• Silicone intubation
Medial ectropion in the absence of horizontal lid laxity	• Medial spindle operation
Medial ectropion in the presence of horizontal lid laxity	• Medial spindle operation with lateral tarsal strip procedure
	• Medial spindle operation with full thickness wedge resection (Smith "lazy T")
Medial ectropion with medial canthal tendon laxity	• Anterior medial canthal tendon plication ± medial spindle operation
	• Transcaruncular medial canthal tendon plication
	• Medial full thickness wedge resection with reconstitution of the posterior limb of the medial canthal tendon (for severe medial ectropion and non-functioning canaliculus)
	• Shortening of anterior limb of the medial canthal tendon, posterior fixation of the posterior limb of the medial canthal tendon to the posterior lacrimal crest, marsupialization of the cut inferior canaliculus to the fornix
Lateral canthal tendon laxity/tear pump dysfunction	• Lateral tarsal strip procedure
	• Canthus-sparing lateral canthopexy (for mild to moderate laxity)
	• Trans-upper eyelid blepharoplasty approach to lateral canthopexy
Tarsal ectropion (disinsertion of lower lid retractors)	• Advancement of lower lid retractors to inferior tarsal border ± lateral tarsal strip procedure
	• Suture repair (Reverse Quickert technique)
Paralytic ectropion	• Temporary tarsorrhaphy
	• Reversible "tarsal pillar" tarsorrhaphy
	• Permanent (tarsal transposition) tarsorrhaphy
	• Reinnervation surgery/facial nerve grafting
	• Temporalis muscle transfer
	• Temporalis fascia sling + horizontal lid tightening
	• Gold weight (upper eyelid)
	• Palpebral spring (upper eyelid)
Cicatricial ectropion	• Steroid injection into scar
	• Full thickness wedge resection
	• Soft tissue rearrangement (Z-plasty, V-Y plasty)
	• Full thickness skin graft + horizontal lid tightening
	• Myocutaneous cheek flap advancement + tarsal strip procedure ± posterior lamellar graft
Congenital lower-eyelid ectropion	• Horizontal lid tightening + skin grafting
Congenital upper-eyelid ectropion	• Pressure patch over repositioned lids
	• Temporary fornix forming sutures
	• More extensive eyelid reconstruction as needed
Mechanical ectropion	• Address underlying cause

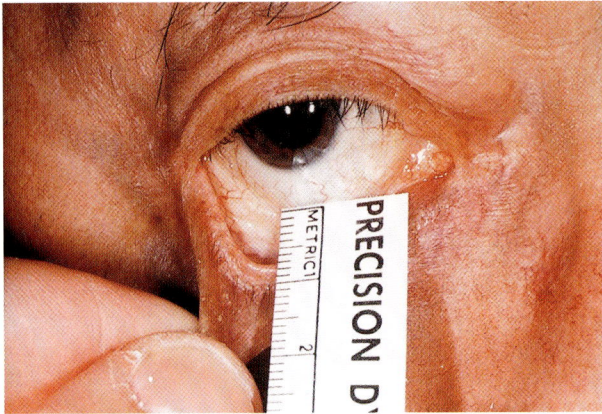

FIGURE 78.1   The distraction test demonstrates lower eyelid laxity. The lower eyelid is gently grasped between the index finger and thumb and pulled away from the globe. If the eyelid can be gently distracted more than 6 mm from the globe, significant horizontal eyelid laxity is present. (From Murphy ML and Nerad JA. Chapter 72: Ectropion. In: Albert DM. *Ophthalmic surgery: Principles and techniques.* Malden, MA: Blackwell Science; 1999, p. 1176.)

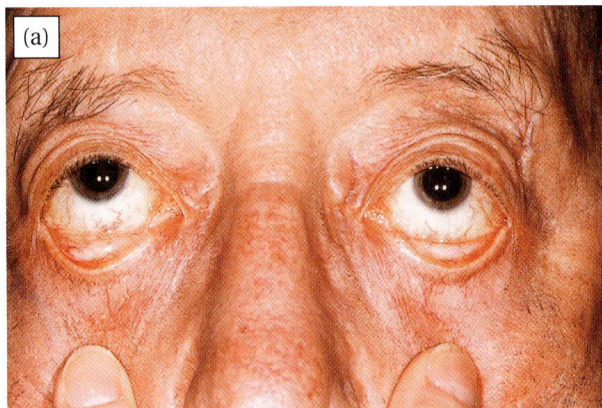

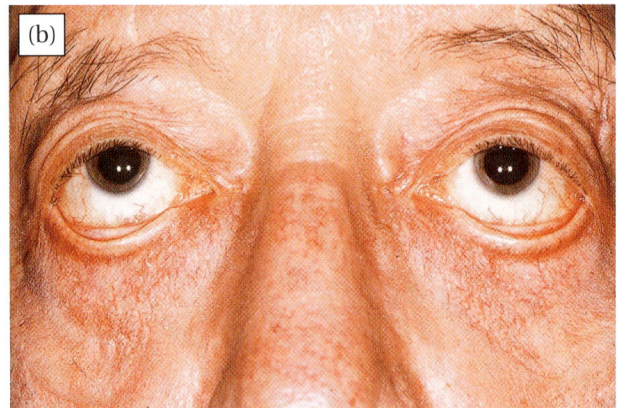

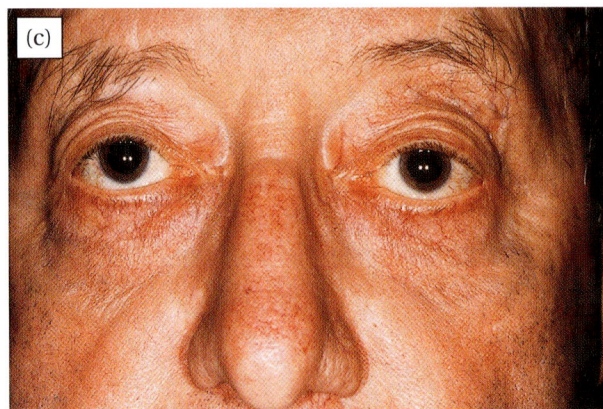

FIGURE 78.2   The snap-back test demonstrates horizontal eyelid laxity. (a)The central portion of each lower eyelid is gently pulled away from the globe. (b) When the eyelids are released, they remain retracted from the globe. (c) After 2 blinks, both lower eyelids return to their normal position. (From Murphy ML and Nerad JA. Chapter 72: Ectropion. In: Albert DM. *Ophthalmic surgery: Principles and techniques.* Malden, MA: Blackwell Science; 1999, p. 1176.)

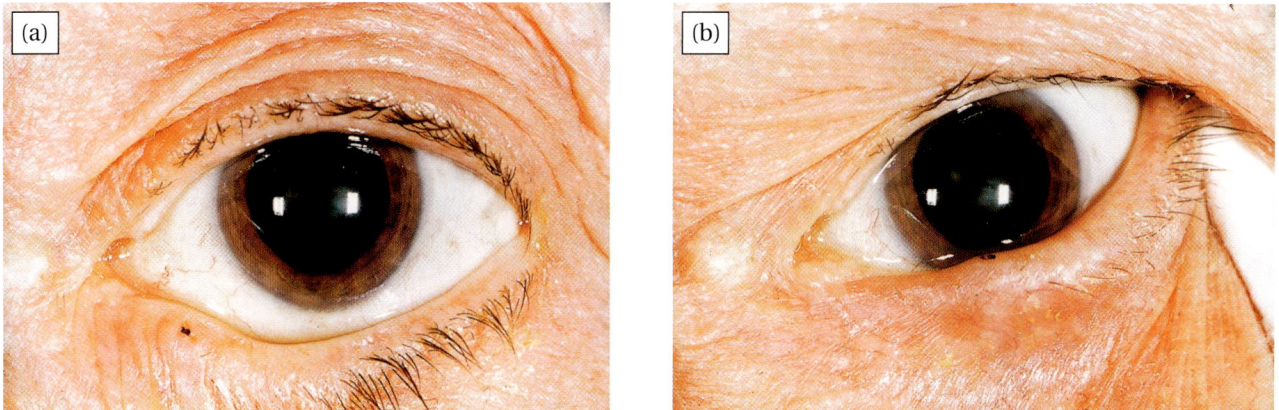

FIGURE 78.3 The lateral punctal pull test. (a) The left lower punctum has been marked with gentian violet to indicate its position at rest. Note that the punctum is directed anteriorly, away from the globe. (b) A cotton-tipped applicator is used to apply lateral traction to the lower eyelid at the lateral canthus. Note how the punctum has moved far laterally to the nasal limbus, indicating significant laxity of the medial canthal tendon. (From Murphy ML and Nerad JA. Chapter 72: Ectropion. In: Albert DM. *Ophthalmic surgery: Principles and techniques.* Malden, MA: Blackwell Science; 1999, p. 1177.)

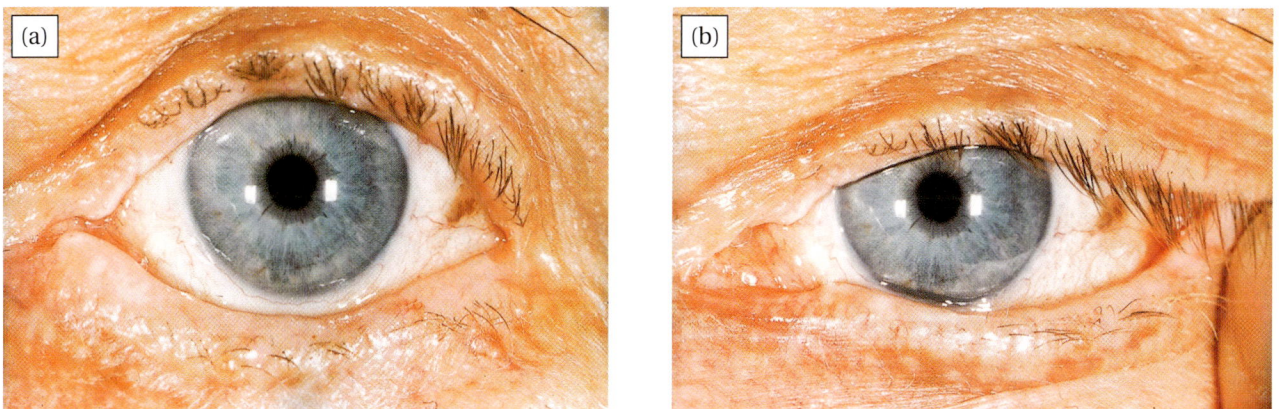

FIGURE 78.4 A patient with left lower eyelid punctal eversion. (a) Note how the medial one-third of the eyelid is not apposed to the globe, and the punctum is directed vertically and anteriorly. (b) As lateral traction is applied to the eyelid, note how the ectropion and punctal eversion are improved in this case, but not completely corrected. A medial spindle procedure would further invert the punctum against the globe. This simple test demonstrates how horizontal tightening at the lateral canthus will, in many cases, improve medial and punctal ectropion. (From Murphy ML and Nerad JA. Chapter 72: Ectropion. In: Albert DM. *Ophthalmic surgery: Principles and techniques.* Malden, MA: Blackwell Science; 1999, p. 1181.)

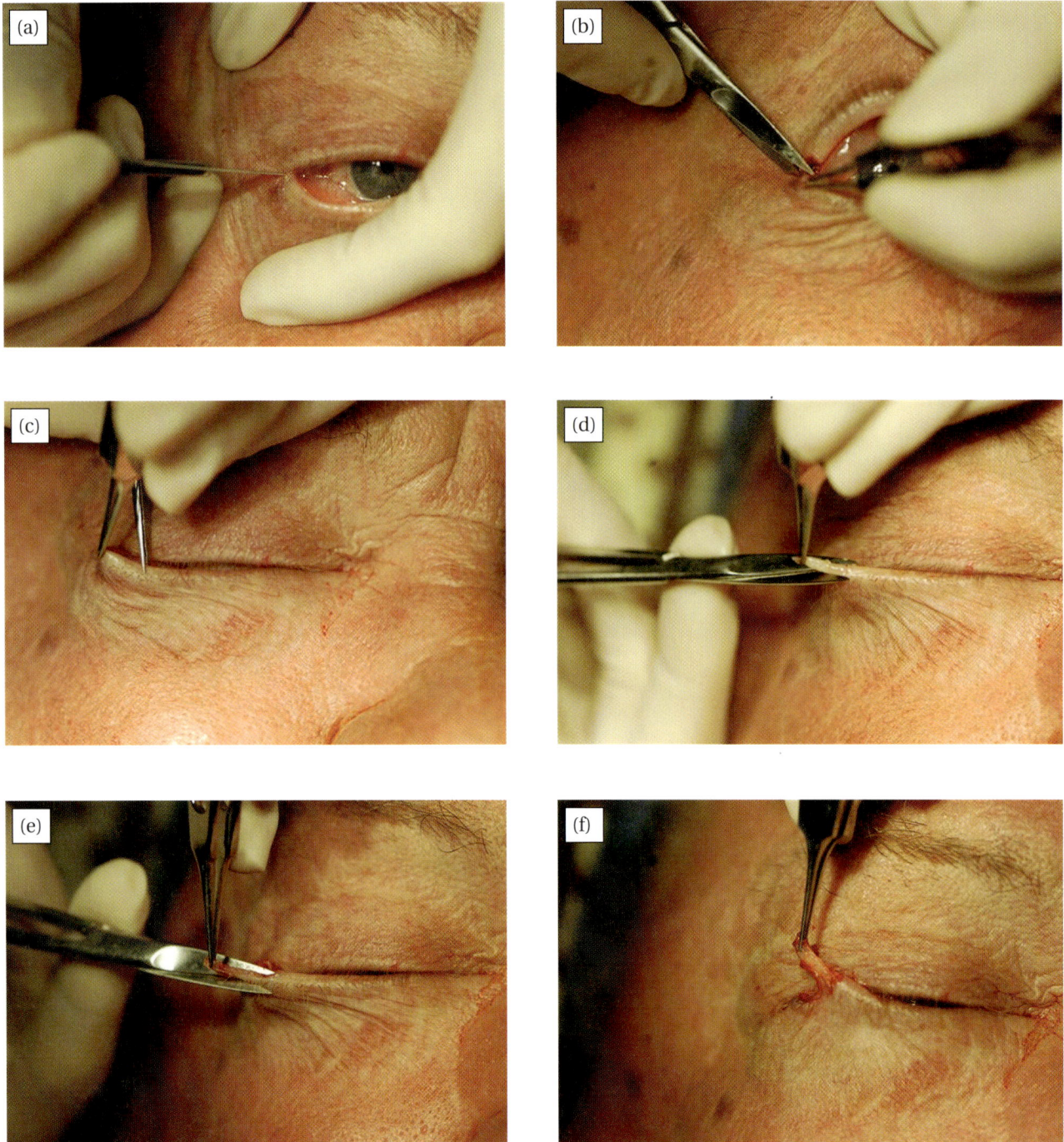

FIGURE 78.5 A patient with punctal eversion, punctal stenosis, and lateral canthal tendon laxity requiring a combined procedure including a medial spindle, 3-snip punctoplasty, and tarsal trip. (a) The tarsal strip procedure is begun. A 5mm incision is made in the skin above the horizontal raphe just lateral to the canthus with a #15 blade followed by a lateral canthotomy. (b) An inferior crus cantholysis is completed with straight iris scissors (c) The extent of horizontal shortening is determined. Lateral tension is applied to the lower lid. A mark then is made on the margin with the scissors where the cut edge of the upper lid margin meets the lower lid margin. (d) The lower lid margin is denuded with straight iris scissors to the previously made mark on the margin. (e) The lash follicles are removed for the length of the strip. (f) The conjunctiva, retractors and orbicularis muscle are trimmed to leave a squared-off tarsal strip. The pretarsal conjunctiva on the strip may be denuded with cautery to avoid the possibility of conjunctival inclusion cysts. (*For tarsal strip procedure only, skip to Figure 78.5n.*)

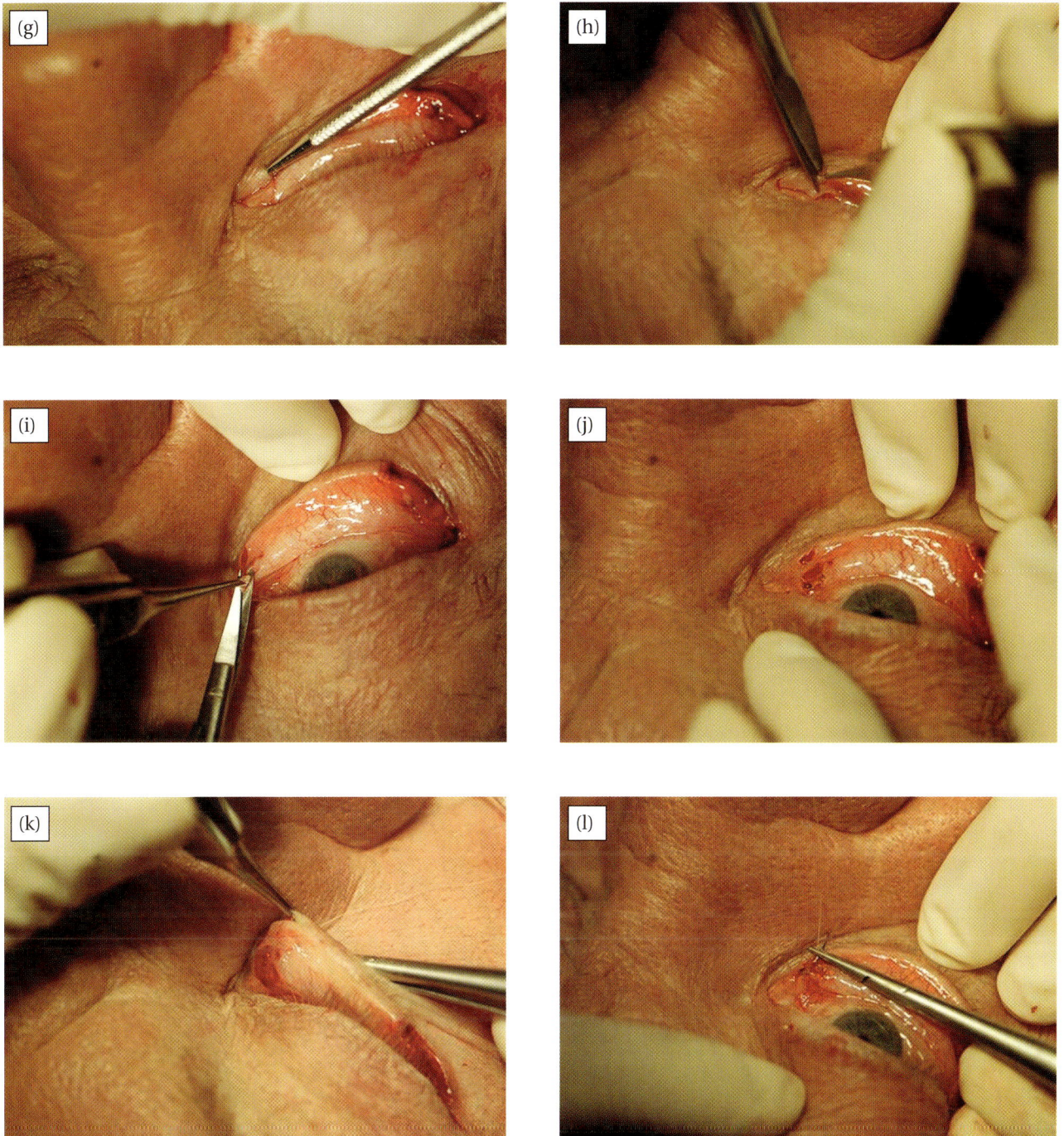

FIGURE 78.5 (*continued*) (g) The 3-snip punctoplasty is then performed to open the stenotic punctum. The punctum is dilated. (h) One edge of a sharp dissecting scissor is placed in the punctal vault. A 2 mm vertical incision is made through the conjunctiva and posterior punctal vault (1st snip). The medial aspect of this incision is picked up with a fine-toothed forceps, and a similar vertical incision is made approximately 2 mm medial to the first (2nd snip). The base of this flap is then trimmed (3rd snip). The punctum is re-dilated to ensure adequate patency (i) The medial spindle procedure is then performed to vertically shorten the posterior lamella to correct punctal eversion. A horizontal ellipse of conjunctiva and lower lid retractors 4 mm to 6 mm inferior to the punctum is created with Westcott scissors. (j) Gentle cautery is the applied to the base and edges of the ellipse. Note there is approximately 2–3 mm of intact conjunctiva between the base of the punctoplasty and the ellipse, to avoid symblepharon. (k) A single-armed 6-0 plain gut suture is passed percutaneously through the center of the ellipse. (l) The suture is then passed through the conjunctiva and retractors of the superior edge of the ellipse, and then through the retractors and conjunctiva of the inferior edge.

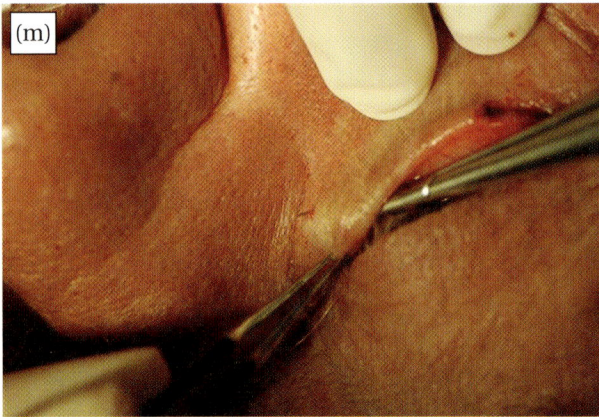

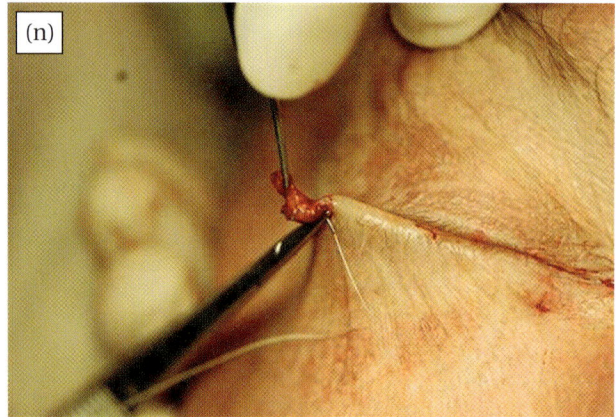

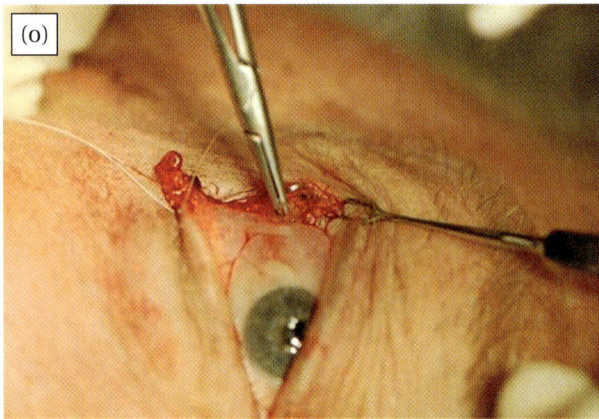

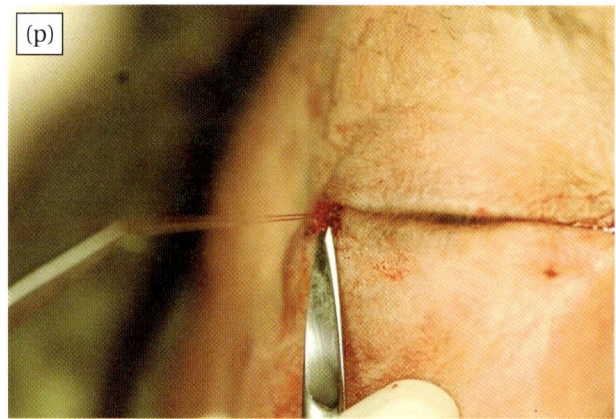

FIGURE 78.5 (*continued*) (m) The suture is then passed through the center of the ellipse out to the skin and tied. This completes the medial spindle procedure. Alternatively, a double-armed suture technique can be used to achieve the same effect. (n) The tarsal strip procedure is then completed. A 4-0 or 5-0 polyglycolic acid suture on a semicircular needle (e.g., P2) is passed twice through the tarsal strip to imbricate it. (o) A small bi-prong retractor is used to expose the periosteum of the lateral canthus. The suture is passed through the periosteum just inside the lateral orbital rim at the level of Whitnall's orbital tubercle. (p) A 6-0 plain gut cerclage stitch can then be passed through the cut edge of the lower lid margin and out through the grey line, then into the grey line of the upper lid margin and out through the cut edge of the margin, and tied. This creates a sharp lateral canthal angle and prevents lateral eyelid imbrication. The 5-0 polyglycolic acid suture is then tied with enough tension to allow the lower lid to be distracted manually approximately 1 mm from the globe. The skin is then closed with interrupted 6-0 plain gut suture.

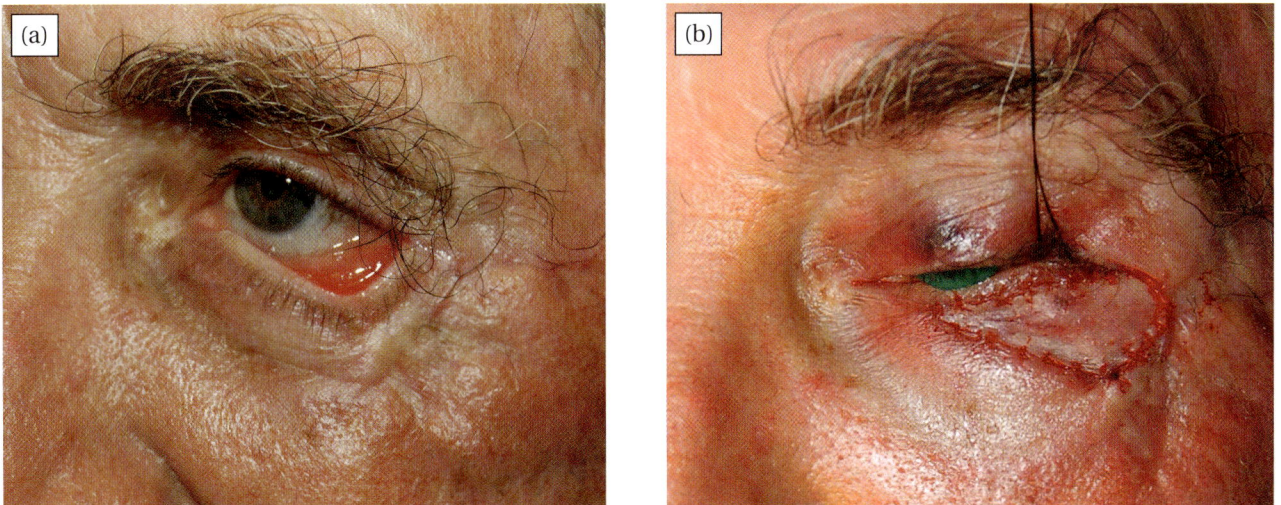

FIGURE 78.6 A patient with cicatricial ectropion of the left lower eyelid. (a) Preoperative photograph. Note the separation of the lateral portion of the lower eyelid from the globe. (b) Immediate postoperative photograph after excision of scar and placement of a full-thickness skin graft to lengthen the anterior lamella and temporary frost suture.

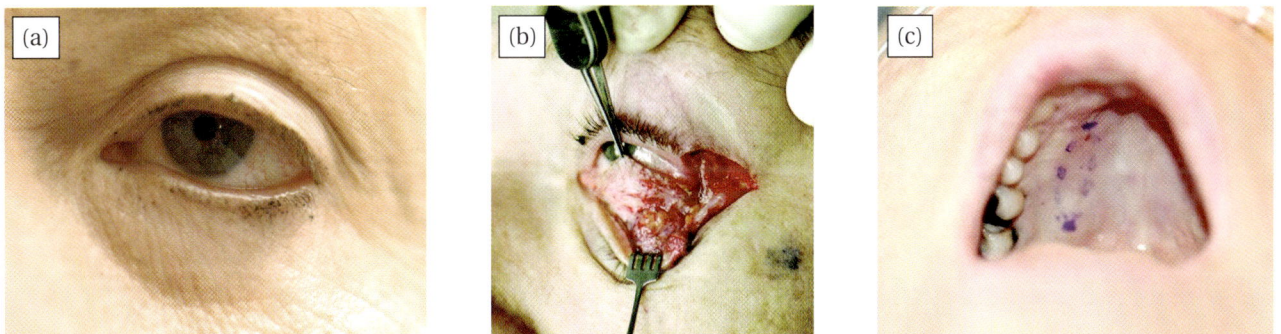

FIGURE 78.7 A patient with cicatricial ectropion with lateral lower lid retraction following lower lid blepharoplasty. The correction involves lateral canthal tightening, posterior lamellar augmentation with a hard palate graft and cheek resuspension to support the anterior lamella via a myocutaneous advancement flap of the suborbicularis oculi fibro-fatty layer (SOOF) and overlying skin and orbicularis. (a) Preoperative photograph. (b) Following a skin incision through the horizontal raphe, lateral canthotomy and cantholysis, and creation of a conservative tarsal strip (as in Figures 78.5a–f), a dissection through conjunctiva and lower lid retractors is accomplished. (c) The length and width for the posterior lamella graft are determined and then outlined with a marking pen on the hard palate. The posterior edge of the hard palate can be palpated. Care is taken to avoid midline anterior dissection into the incisive foramen and posterior extension into the soft palate, where the greater and lesser palatine arteries may be encountered and the pharyngeal muscles damaged. Monopolar cautery is used to outline the graft perimeter, and Westcott scissors or a #15 blade are used to remove the graft. The underlying periosteum is left intact. After gentle cautery, a gauze sponge can be held in place by the patient's tongue for hemostasis.

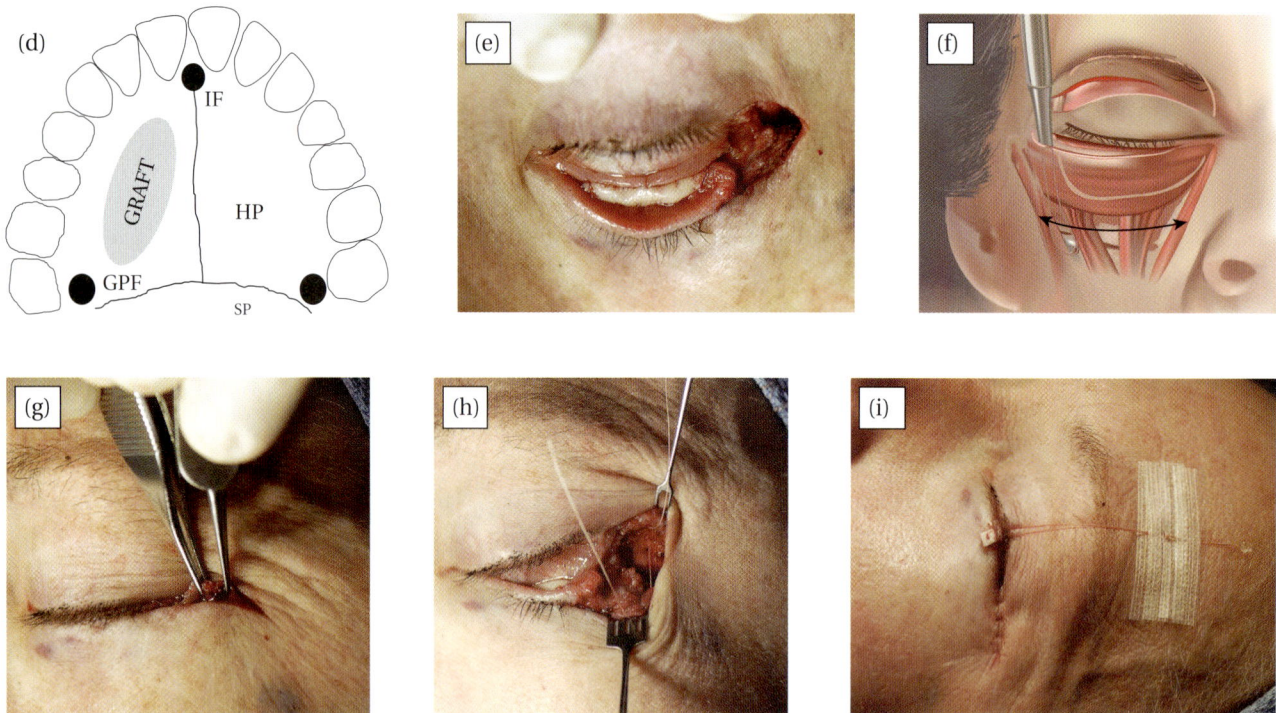

FIGURE 78.7 (*continued*) (d) Diagram of the hard (HP) and soft (SP) palate demonstrating the positions of the incisive foramen (IF), the greater palatine foramen (GPF) and optimum area for graft harvest posterior to the second incisors and anterior to the third molars. (e) The graft is then sewn inferiorly to the conjunctiva/retractors and superiorly to the inferior tarsal border with buried 6-0 plain gut suture. The mucosal side of the graft faces the eye. (f) Attention is then turned to the cheek. A periosteal elevator is used to bluntly dissect between the suborbicularis oculi fibro-fatty layer (SOOF) and the underlying periosteum. The nasal border is the infraorbital neurovascular bundle, the temporal border is the zygomaticofacial neurovascular bundle, and the inferior border is the malar eminence. (g) The SOOF is then retracted superiorly with forceps to determine if dissection is adequate to support the lower lid. (h) A baseball stitch is then used to imbricate the SOOF and then anchor it to the periosteum, lateral to the orbital rim and superior to the canthus. (i) The lateral tarsus is then anchored to the periosteum at the level of Whitnall's orbital tubercle, and the canthal angle reformed with an absorbable cerclage stitch, as in the standard tarsal strip procedure. The orbicularis is closed with buried interrupted absorbable suture, and the skin with 6-0 non-absorbable suture. A Frost suture is then placed in the lower lid and anchored to the forehead, to place the lower lid on superior tension. The Frost suture may be removed in several days. (Figure [f] originally published in Korn BS, Kikkawa DO, Cohen SR. Transcutaneous lower eyelid blepharoplasty with orbitomalar suspension: Retrospective review of 212 consecutive cases. *Plas Reconst Surg.* 125(1):315–323.)

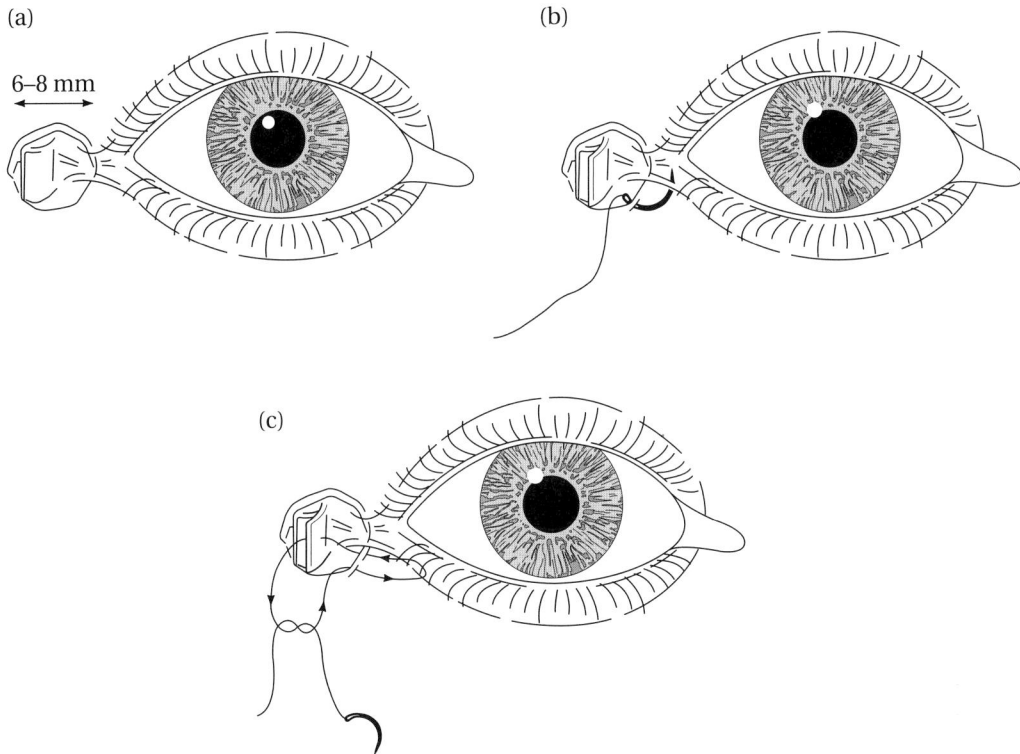

FIGURE 78.8 Canthus-sparing lateral canthopexy. (a) Diagrammatic representation of incision lateral to right lateral canthus. (b) Diagram shows how the inferior crus of the right lateral canthal tendon is grasped before the needle is passed through periosteal flap. (c) Passage of needle and suture through periosteal flap. (Images from Lucarelli MJ. Eyelid surgery. In: Albert DM, Lucarelli MJ. *Clinical atlas of procedures in ophthalmic surgery*. Chicago: American Medical Association, 2003; p. 256.)

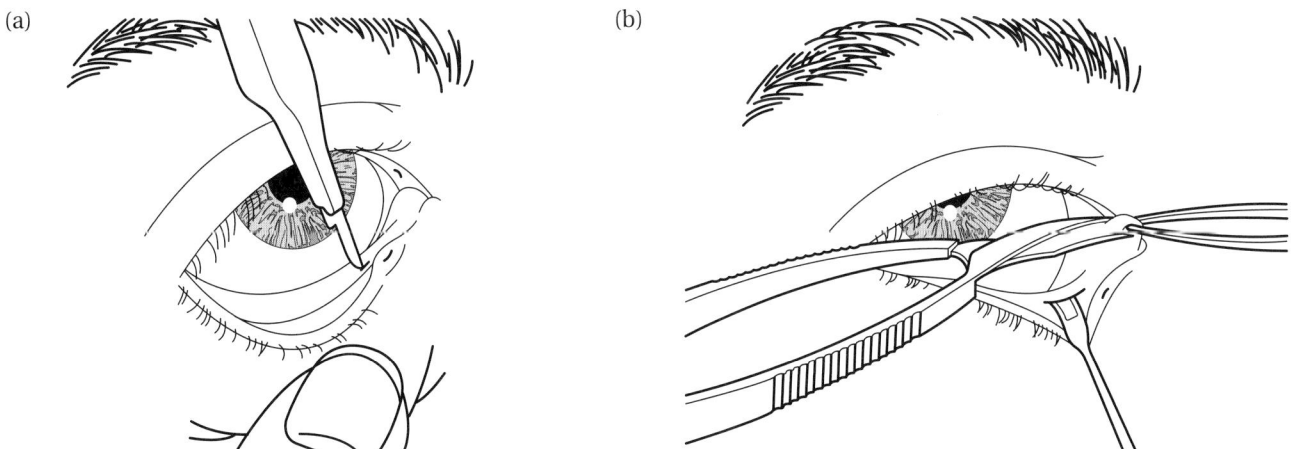

FIGURE 78.9 Transcaruncular medial canthal tendon plication. (a) A horizontal conjunctival incision is made at the base of the medial tarsus. (b) A second conjunctival incision is made in the medial fornix, just posterior to the caruncle. Blunt dissection proceeds to the medial periorbita.

(c)

(d)

(e)

(f)

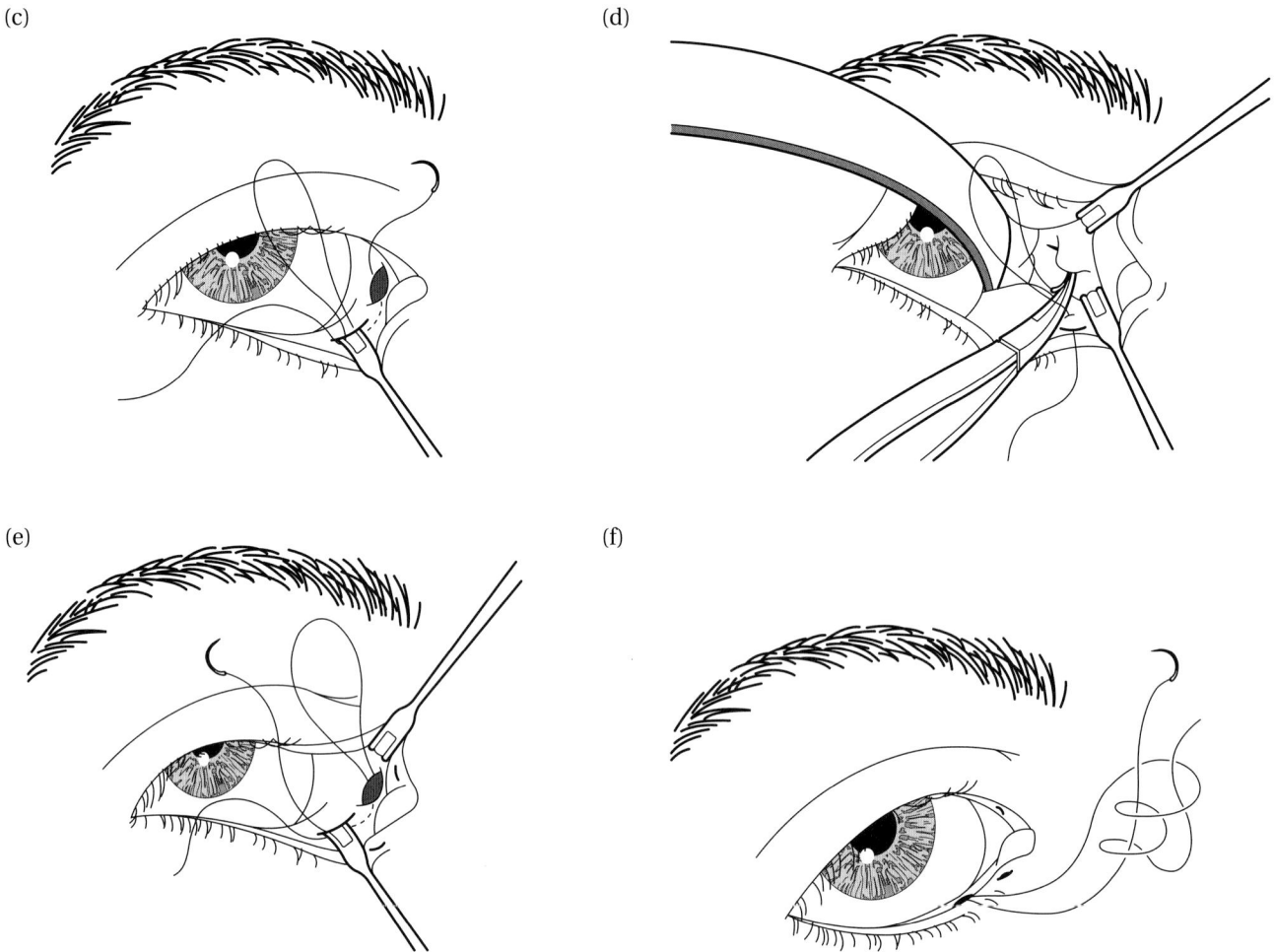

FIGURE 78.9 (*continued*) (c) The medial end of the tarsus is engaged by 4-0 polypropylene suture, which is then passed subconjunctivally from the lower eyelid incision to the medial fornix incision. (d) Periorbita at or above the posterior lacrimal crest is secured with the suture under direct headlamp observation, while an assistant provides exposure. (e) The needle is passed subconjunctivally from the medial fornix incision to the lower eyelid incision. At this point, both ends of the suture exit from the lower eyelid incision. (f) A fisherman's knot is tied to achieve appropriate tension. Once permanently tied, the ends are cut, and the knot is rotated into the medial orbit. (Images from Lucarelli MJ. Eyelid surgery. In: Albert DM, Lucarelli MJ. *Clinical atlas of procedures in ophthalmic surgery*. Chicago: American Medical Association, 2003; p. 255.)

TABLE 78.5 *Potential Complications*

Orbital hematoma

Wound infection

Suture granuloma

Excessive horizontal eyelid shortening with lower eyelid retraction

Canalicular laceration/scarring (with medial canthal surgery)

Facial anesthesia (with myocutaneous cheek advancement)

Symblepharon

Canthal dystopia

Lateral eyelid imbrication

Lateral canthal dehiscence

Dry eye

Recurrent ectropion

SELECTED REFERENCES

Anderson RL, Gordy DD. The tarsal strip procedure. *Arch Ophthalmol.* 1979;97(11):2192–2196.

Anderson RL. Tarsal strip procedure for correction of eyelid laxity and canthal malposition in the anophthalmic socket. *Ophthalmology.* 1981;88(9):895–903.

Becker FF. Lateral tarsal strip procedure for the correction of paralytic ectropion. *Laryngoscope.* 1982;92(4):382–384.

Ben Simon GJ, Lee S, Schwarcz RM, et al. Subperiosteal midface lift with or without a hard palate mucosal graft for correction of lower eyelid retraction. *Ophthalmology.* 2006;113(10):1869–1873.

Benger RS, Frueh BR. Involutional ectropion: a review of the management. *Ophthalmic Surg.* 1987;18(2):136–139.

Crawford GJ, Collin JR, Moriarty PA. The correction of paralytic medial ectropion. *Br J Ophthalmol.* 1984;68(9):639–641.

Demirci H, Hassan AS, Elner SG, et al. Comprehensive, combined anterior and transcaruncular orbital approach to medial canthal ligament plication. *Ophthal Plast Reconstr Surg.* 2007; 23(5):384–388.

Fong KC, Mavrikakis I, Sagili S, Malhotra R. Correction of involutional lower eyelid medial ectropion with transconjunctival approach retractor plication and lateral tarsal strip. *Acta Ophthalmol Scand.* 2006;84(2):246–249.

Fox SA. Marginal (tarsal) ectropion. *Arch Ophthalmol.* 1960;63:660–662.

Frueh BR, Schoengarth LD. Evaluation and treatment of the patient with ectropion. *Ophthalmology.* 1982;89(9):1049–1054.

Frueh BR, Su CS. Medial tarsal suspension: a method of elevating the medial lower eyelid. *Ophthal Plast Reconstr Surg.* 2002;18(2):133–137.

Kostakoglu N, Ozcan G. Orbicularis oculi myocutaneous flap in reconstruction of postburn lower eyelid ectropion. *Burns.* 1999;25(6):553–557.

Lemke BN, Cook BE, Jr., Lucarelli MJ. Canthus-sparing ectropion repair. *Ophthal Plast Reconstr Surg.* 2001;17(3):161–168.

Lemke BN, Sires BS, Dortzbach RK. A tarsal strip-periosteal flap technique for lateral canthal fixation. *Ophthalmic Surg Lasers.* 1999;30(3):232–236.

Loeffler M, Hornblass A. Surgical management of congenital upper-eyelid eversion. *Ophthalmic Surg.* 1990;21(6):435–437.

Manku K, Leong JK, Ghabrial R. Cicatricial ectropion: repair with myocutaneous flaps and canthopexy. *Clin Experiment Ophthalmol.* 2006;34(7):677–681.

McGraw BL, Adamson PA. Postblepharoplasty ectropion. Prevention and management. *Arch Otolaryngol Head Neck Surg.* 1991;117(8):852–856.

Nowinski TS, Anderson RL. The medial spindle procedure for involutional medial ectropion. *Arch Ophthalmol.* 1985;103(11):1750–1753.

Pelletier CR, Jordan DR, Konzuk PJ, Pashby RC. Tarsal eversion: a dramatic form of ectropion at birth. *Can J Ophthalmol.* 1996;31(6):313–314.

Periman LM, Sires BS. Floppy eyelid syndrome: a modified surgical technique. *Ophthal Plast Reconstr Surg.* 2002;18(5):370–372.

Putterman AM. Ectropion of the lower eyelid secondary to Muller's muscle-capsulopalpebral fascia detachment. *Am J Ophthalmol.* 1978; 85(6):814–817.

Shore JW. Changes in lower eyelid resting position, movement, and tone with age. *Am J Ophthalmol.* 1985;99(4):415–423.

Smith B. The "lazy-T" correction of ectropion of the lower punctum. *Arch Ophthalmol.* 1976;94(7):1149–1150.

Sullivan TJ, Collin JR. Medical canthal resection: an effective long-term cure for medial ectropion. *Br J Ophthalmol.* 1991;75(5):288–291.

Tenzel RR, Buffam FV, Miller GR. The use of the "lateral canthal sling" in ectropion repair. *Can J Ophthalmol.* 1977;12(3):199–202.

Tenzel RR. Treatment of lagophthalmos of the lower lid. *Arch Ophthalmol.* 1969;81(3):366–368.

Tse DT. Surgical correction of punctal malposition. *Am J Ophthalmol.* 1985;100(2):339–341.

Wesley RE, Collins JW. McCord procedure for ectropion repair. *Arch Otolaryngol.* 1983;109(5):319–322.

79 Eyelid Retraction

David B. Lyon, MD

TABLE 79.1 *Indications for Eyelid Retraction Surgery*

Inadequate globe coverage and protection

Lagophthalmos—paralytic or cicatricial

Symptomatic dry eyes unresponsive to medical therapy

Exposure keratitis

Asymmetric lid position

Aesthetic

TABLE 79.2 *Preoperative Considerations*

Margin reflex distance (upper and lower)

Lid contour

Exophthalmometry

Lateral canthal position

Upper lid crease

Lagophthalmos

Downward traction test (upper lid)

Upward traction test (lower lid)

Lid and canthal ligament laxity—distraction and snapback tests

Skin adequacy

Orbicularis function

History of prior lid, orbital, or strabismus surgery

Strabismus

Bell's phenomenon

Tear film adequacy

Corneal integrity

Surgical Procedures

Upper Lid Retraction Repair via Graded Full-Thickness Blepharotomy

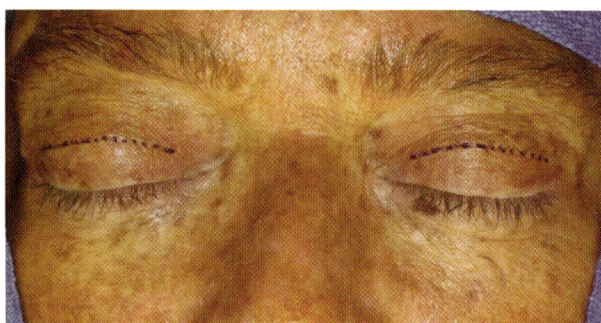

FIGURE 79.1 The upper lid creases are marked within the patient's preexisting eyelid crease. Local anesthetic is infiltrated. Local or monitored anesthetic care is employed for upper lid surgery to enable intraoperative adjustment with patient cooperation.

(a)

1. Orbicularis oculi m.
2. Muller's m.
3. Aponeurosis of levator palpebral m.
4. Palpebral conjunctiva
5. Superior tarsal plate

1

2
3
4
INCISION
5

(b)

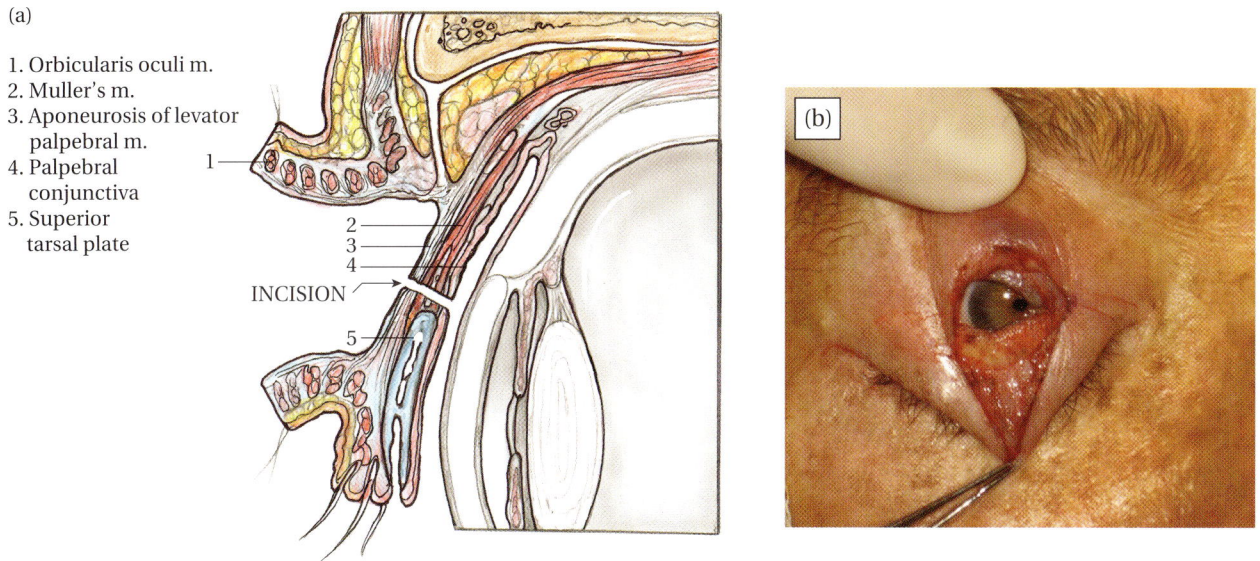

FIGURE 79.2   (a, b) Skin incisions are made with a #15 blade. After dissection through the orbicularis oculi muscle and levator aponeurosis, the superior tarsal border is exposed. Müeller's muscle and conjunctiva at the superior tarsal border are incised, creating a full-thickness blepharotomy.

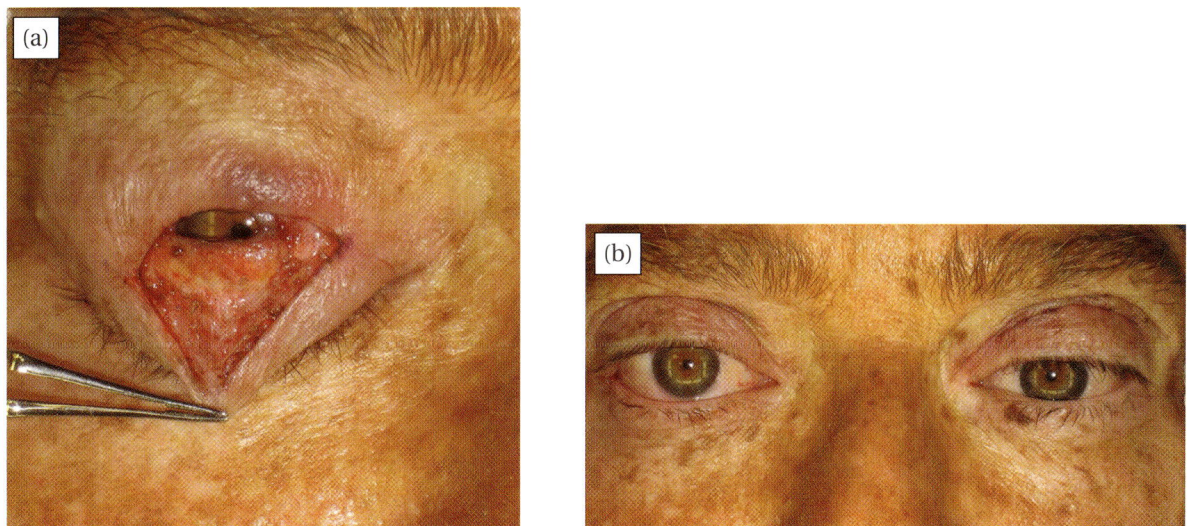

(a)

(b)

FIGURE 79.3   This can then be titrated as needed (a) and extended medially and laterally to achieve the desired lid height and contour determined with the patient sitting and looking in primary gaze (b). The skin is then closed with a 6-0 running absorbable suture.

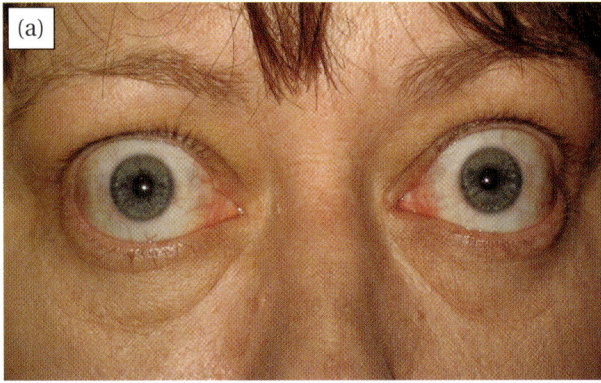

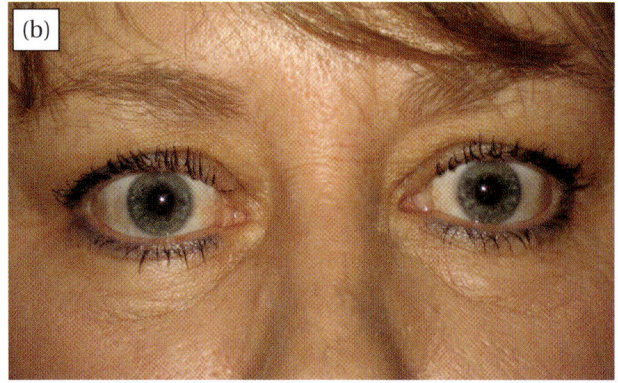

FIGURE 79.4 (a) Patient with thyroid related orbitopathy, showing proptosis, upper lid retraction and lower lid retraction. (b) Same patient after undergoing bilateral balanced medial and lateral wall orbital decompression, followed by upper lid retraction repair with graded full thickness blepharotomy.

Gold or Platinum (if gold allergy) Weight Placement: Pretarsal and Intraorbital Locations

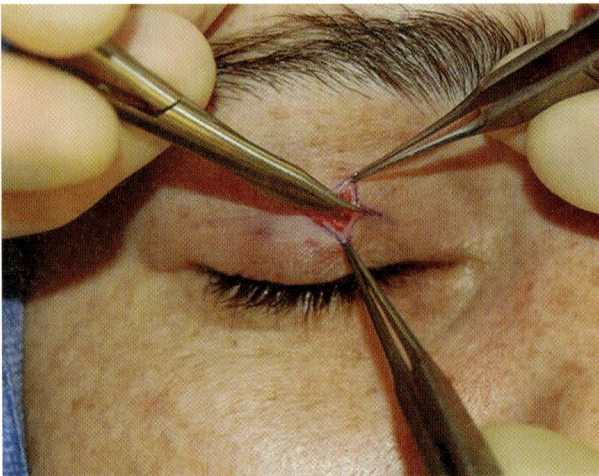

FIGURE 79.5 The lid crease is marked and the skin is then incised. (Photo courtesy of Don O. Kikkawa, MD.)

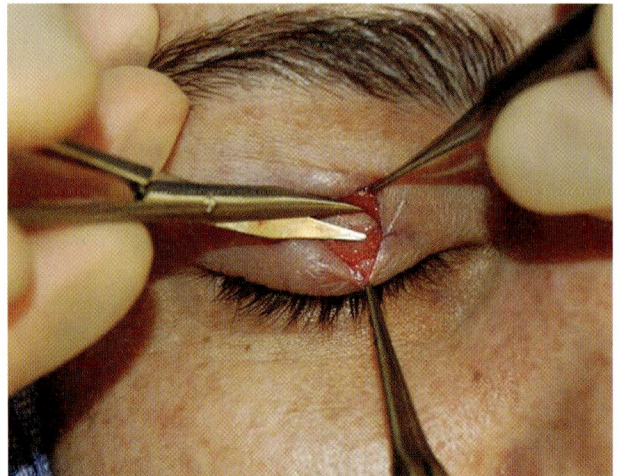

FIGURE 79.6 Dissection is then performed through the orbicularis muscle. A pretarsal suborbicularis pocket is then created, and the anterior tarsal surface is exposed. (Photo courtesy of Don O. Kikkawa, MD.)

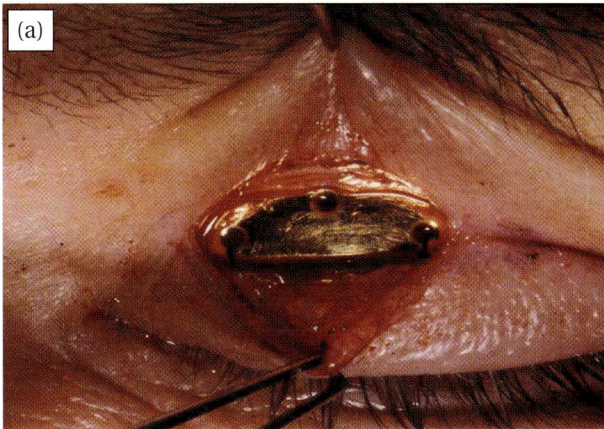

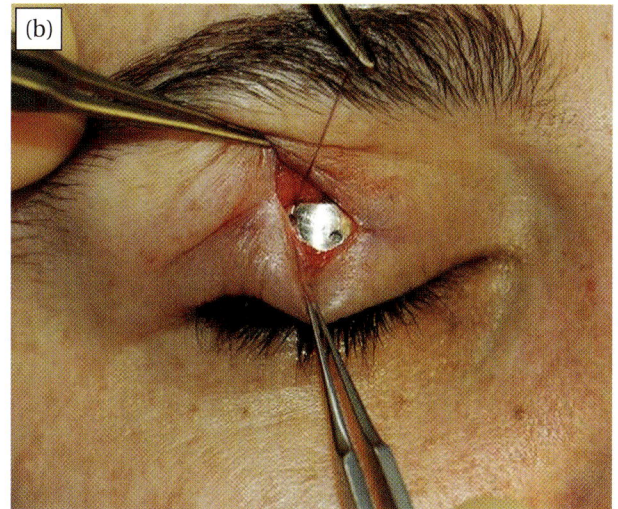

FIGURE 79.7 The weight (usually 1.2–1.4 gram) is then inserted in the pretarsal pocket (a) and secured with permanent sutures to the tarsus using the holes in the weight (b). An alternative placement is intraorbital (not depicted). The orbital septum is incised above its fusion with the levator aponeurosis, and the preaponeurotic fat pad is separated. The weight (usually 1.6–2.0 gram) is then sutured to the levator aponeurosis with permanent sutures, using the holes in the weight. The weight function is then assessed with the patient in the sitting position, opening and closing the eyes. The weight and position are adjusted as needed. Many surgeons favor selection of the weight preoperatively, using a sizer set of external weights. (Photos courtesy of Don O. Kikkawa, MD.)

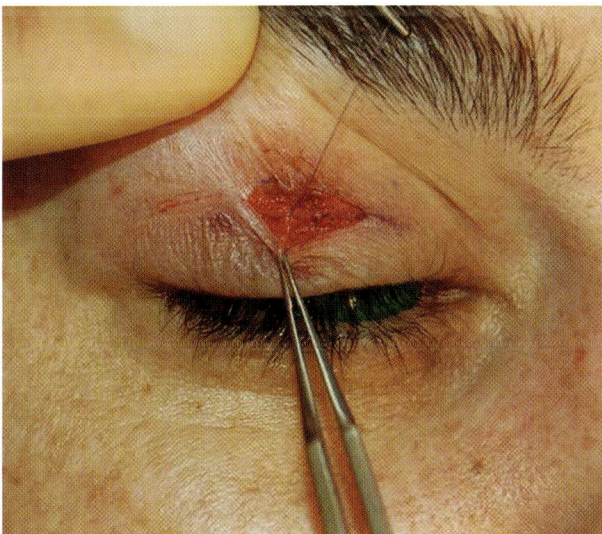

FIGURE 79.8 The orbicularis oculi and skin are then closed in separate layers.

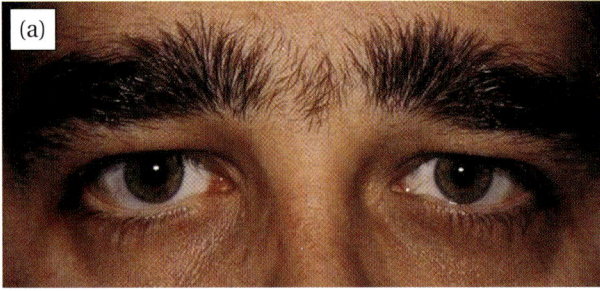

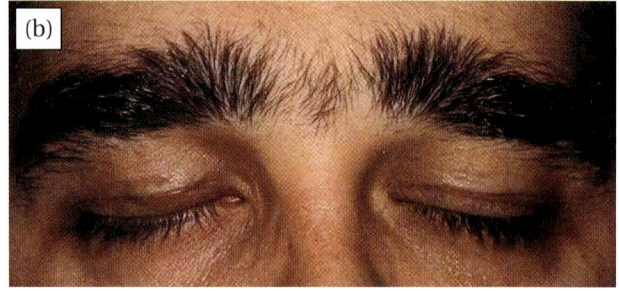

FIGURE 79.9 Patient with right facial nerve palsy after resection of acoustic neuroma, following pretarsal gold weight implant in right upper lid. Eyes open (a) and eyes closed showing complete closure (b).

Lower Lid Retraction Repair with Hard Palate Mucosal Graft

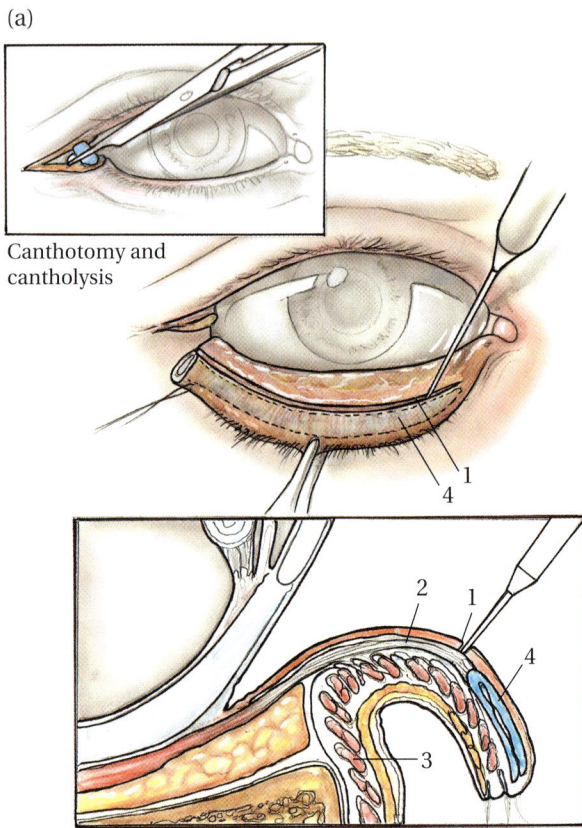

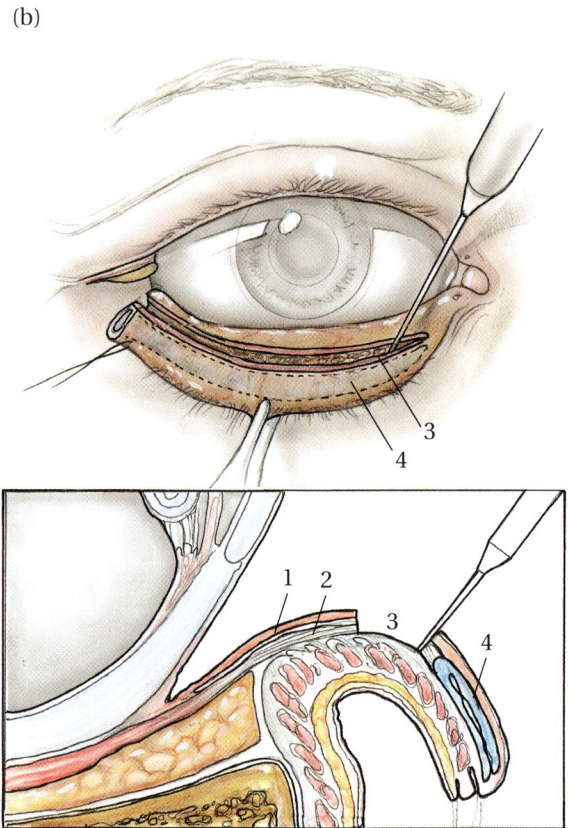

(a)

Canthotomy and
cantholysis

1. Palpebral conjunctive incised   3. Orbicularis oculi m.
2. Lower lid retractors   4. Inferior tarsal plate

(b)

1. Palpebral conjunctiva   3. Create gap
2. Lower lid retractors   4. Inferior tarsal plate

FIGURE 79.10 (a, b) A lateral canthotomy and inferior cantholysis is performed to swing the lid outward. The conjunctiva and lower lid retractors are divided from the inferior tarsal border and separated from the orbital septum and mid-lamellar scar tissue.

* Lower lid retraction repair with midface lift ± hard palate spacer (post-bleph, facial nerve palsy). Refer to Chapter 73.

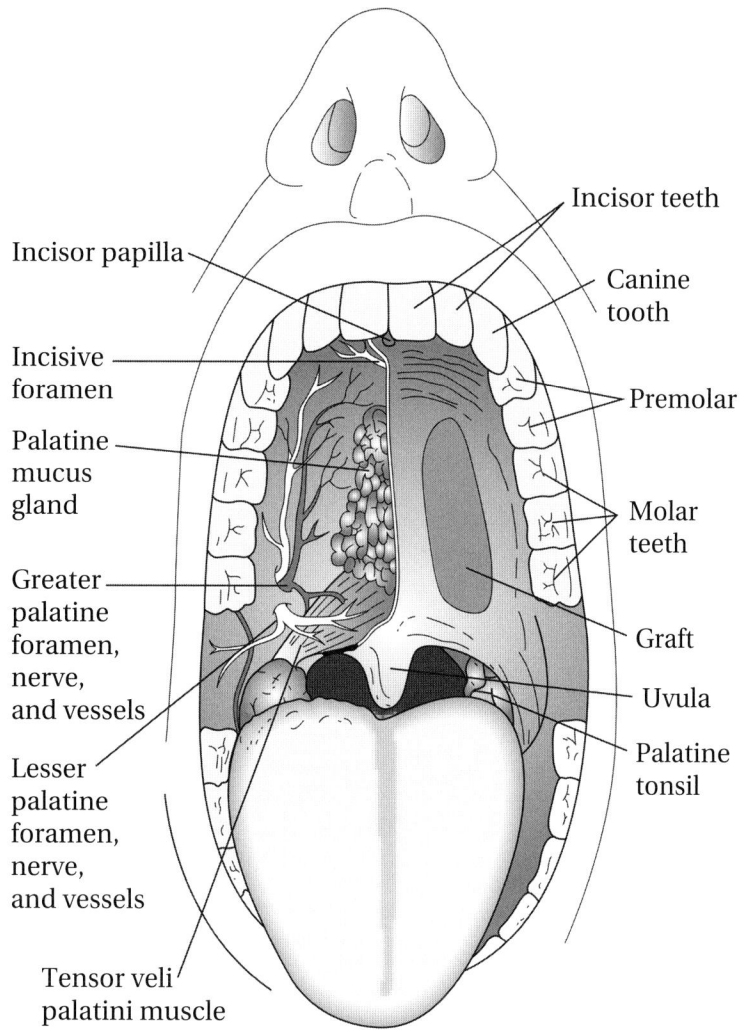

FIGURE 79.11 Anatomy of the hard palate. The graft is harvested lateral to the midline.

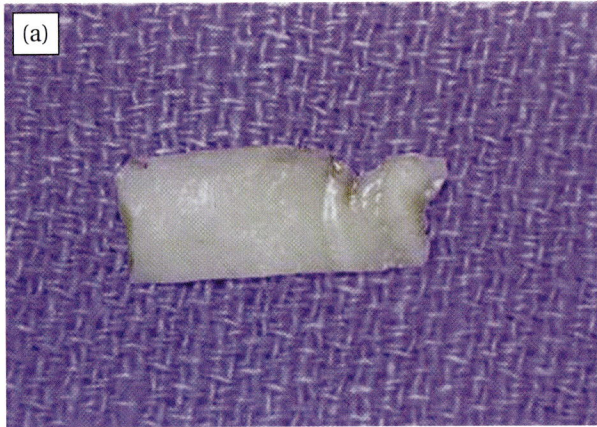

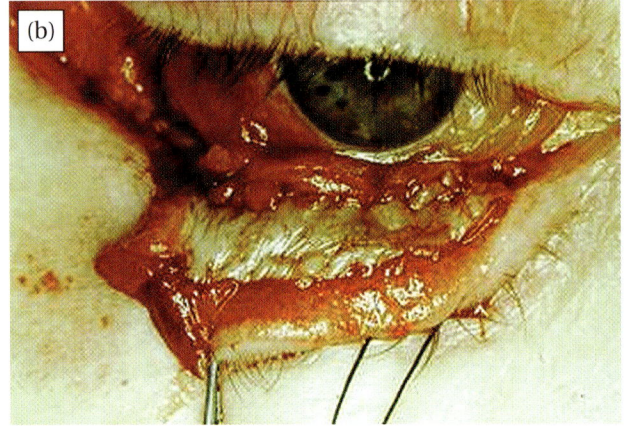

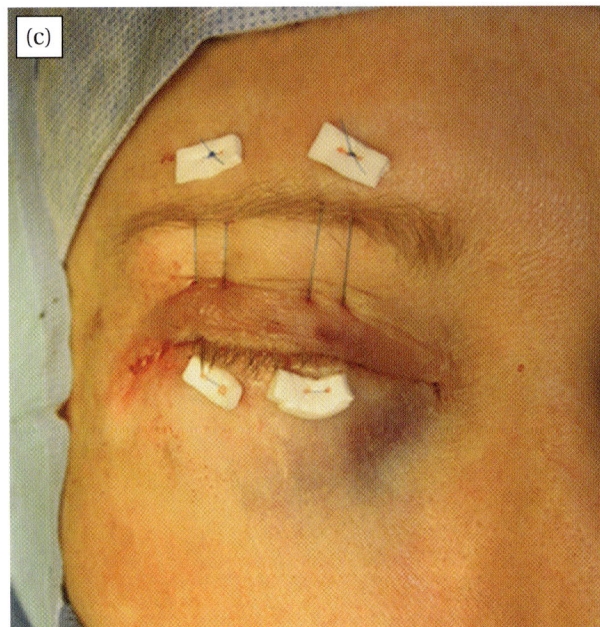

FIGURE 79.12 Hard palate graft is harvested of desired size (typically 8–10 mm wide) and thinned of submucosal tissue (a). The graft is then sutured to the inferior tarsal border superiorly, and the recessed conjunctiva and lower lid retractors inferiorly, using a 6-0 fast absorbing gut suture (b). A canthoplasty is then performed with horizontal tightening and repositioning as needed. Frost sutures are then placed for 3–5 days postoperatively (c). (Photos courtesy of Don O. Kikkawa, MD.)

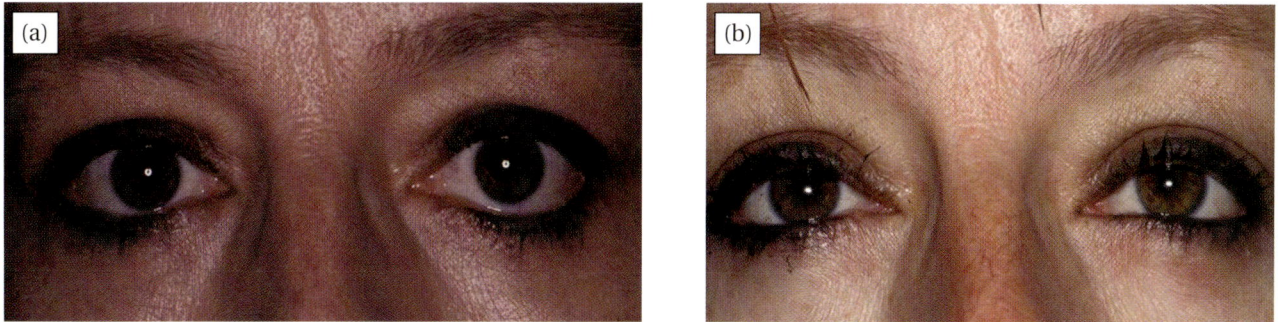

FIGURE 79.13 (a) Preoperative photo of patient with bilateral lower lid retraction, left worse than right, following transcutaneous lower blepharoplasty. (b) Postoperative view of same patient after undergoing lower lid retraction repair with hard palate mucosal grafts and lateral canthoplasty.

TABLE 79.3 *Complications*

Upper lid
- Overcorrection (ptosis)
- Undercorrection (residual lid retraction)
- Lid margin contour abnormalities
- Lid crease abnormalities
- Persistent lagophthalmos and exposure keratitis
- Gold weight migration, exposure, allergy, or infection
- Eyelid fistula (if full thickness blepharotomy)

Lower lid
- Overcorrection (lid too high)
- Undercorrection (residual lid retraction)
- Ectropion or entropion
- Lid margin contour abnormalities
- Graft problems—necrosis, keratinization, lid thickening
- Persistent lagophthalmos and exposure keratitis
- Oral pain and bleeding from graft donor site

SELECTED REFERENCES

Ben Simon GJ, Lee S, Schwarcz RM, McCann JD, Goldberg RA. Subperiosteal midface lift with or without a hard palate mucosal graft for correction of lower eyelid retraction. *Ophthalmology.* 2006;113(10):1869–1873.

Demirci H, Hassan AS, Reck SD, Frueh BR, Elner VM. Graded full-thickness anterior blepharotomy for correction of upper eyelid retraction not associated with thyroid eye disease. *Ophthalmic Plast Reconstr Surg.* 2007;23:39–45.

Elner VM, Hassan AS, Frueh BR. Graded full thickness anterior blepharotomy for upper eyelid retraction. *Arch Ophthalmol.* 2004; 122:55–60.

Kersten RC, Kulwin DR, Levartovsky S, Tiradellis H, Tse DT. Management of lower-lid retraction with hard-palate mucosa grafting. *Arch Ophthalmol.* 1990;108:1339–1343.

Tower RN, Dailey RA. Gold weight implantation: a better way? *Ophthal Plast Reconstr Surg.* 2004; 20:202–206.

80 | Management of Periocular Skin Cancer

Gregg S. Gayre, MD, Seaver L. Soon, MD, Daniel E. Zelac, MD, Bita Esmaeli, MD, FACS and Geva Mannor, MD, MPH

TABLE 80.1 *Indications for Periocular Skin Cancer Excision*

- Basal Cell Carcinoma
- Squamous Cell Carcinoma
- Malignant Melanoma (including *in situ* and lentigo subtypes)
- Sebaceous (Meibomian) Gland Adenocarcinoma
- Merkel Cell Carcinoma (Neuroendocrine or Trabecular carcinoma)
- Kaposi Sarcoma
- Sweat Gland Carcinoma
- Malignant Syringoma
- Other unusual or rare malignancies

* Some of above cancers may benefit from additional techniques and/or treatment (i.e., permanent section histological margin control for melanoma, cryotherapy and/or conjunctival mapping for sebaceous gland adenocarcinoma, radiation for Merkel cell carcinoma and Kaposi sarcoma, topical (ocular or cutaneous) or systemic chemotherapy, radioactive plaque brachytherapy, etc).

TABLE 80.2 *Possible Contraindications for Periocular Skin Cancer Excision*

- Extension of periocular skin cancers into and/or beyond orbit, brain, nose, sinuses, etc
- Concomitant spread of periocular skin cancer to lymph node(s)
- Concomitant metastatic spread of periocular skin cancer
- Cancer that is metastatic to periocular skin

TABLE 80.3 *Preoperative Considerations*

- Confirm histopathologic diagnosis with preoperative biopsy
- Check biopsy for perineural or vascular invasion, ulceration and skip lesions (pagetoid)
- Examination for possible perineural spread (cranial nerve or sensory neuropathy)
- Evaluate spread to brain, lymph node(s), orbit, sinonasal region, tear sac, and metastasis
- CT and/or MRI to assess bone destruction and/or extension beyond eyelid
- Otolaryngology, Neurosurgery, Oncology, and/or Radiotherapy Consult(s) as needed
- Standard assessment of medical status and anticoagulation medication history

TABLE 80.4 *Additional Preoperative Work-Up*

- If tumor tethered to deeper structures or bone or immobile, consider imaging of orbit
- Evert eyelids to assess spread to conjunctival fornices
- Lacrimal probing and irrigation for tumors near medial canthus
- Examine orbit for proptosis, palpable mass, globe dystopia or increased resistance
- Examine head & neck skin for prior cancers and their treatment (i.e., scars, radiotherapy)
- Examine head & neck for prior surgery, trauma, cosmetic rejuvenation or surgery
- Examine head & neck lymph node(s), cranial nerves, and central nervous system
- Evaluate mouth, nose, and sinuses as suggested by history and physical examination

Mohs Excision and Modified En Face Frozen Section, Margin-Controlled Periocular Skin Cancer Excision

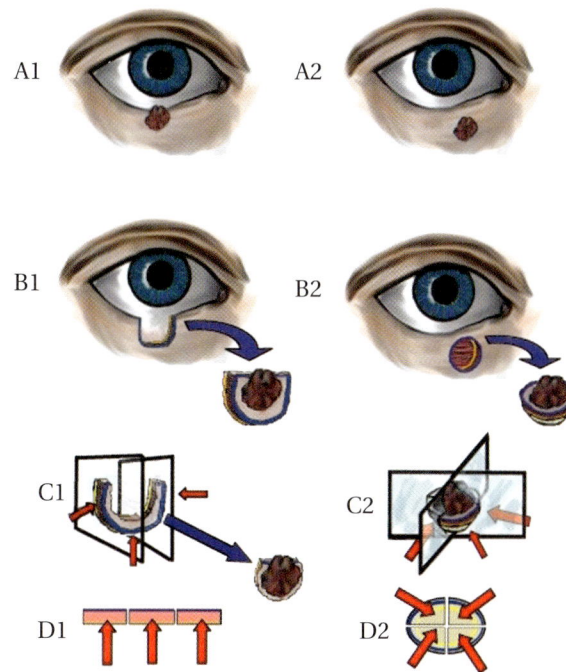

FIGURE 80.1 Mohs Micrographic or Modified En Face Frozen Section, Margin-Controlled Excision of Eyelid Margin and other Periocular Tissues. A1 & A2: Skin cancer present on the lid margin (A1, left panel) or on periocular tissue away from the lid margin (A2, right panel). B1 & B2: Demonstration of a first (Stage I) removal of clinically evident tumor and surrounding tissues. B1 diagrams a full-thickness wedge that may be employed if the tumor appears clinically to involve both cutaneous and conjunctival surfaces. B2 diagrams a saucerization of the cutaneous and subcutaneous tissue where the depth and breadth is based on the clinical impression. C1: Sectioning of the excised tissue from B1, including the debulking of central clinically evident tumor. C2: Sectioning of the excised tissue from B2. D1: The en face examination of the outermost surgical margins of the Stage I sections. D2: The en face examination of the deep and peripheral tissue edges representing the outermost surgical margins of the Stage I sections.

A clinical tumor excision map of size, shape, and location of the excision is drawn with precise and meticulous correlation to the surgical specimen(s). Colors are used to indicate certain landmarks. Although there is some variation among practitioners, blue highlights usually identify the cutaneous margin. Yellow highlights identify the mucosal or deep dermal margin. Red arrows depict the plane of the surgical margins that are microscopically examined.

In the first stage, up to four sections are circumferentially harvested, color coded, and processed as inverted (en face), horizontal frozen section(s). This maximizes amount of surgical margin(s) that can be histologically evaluated. Should tumor be observed on the outer margin in any or all of the sections of Stage 1, an additional stage will be performed that will address areas of positive tumor presence by continuing the surgical procedure only in areas of known residual tumor. Additional stages will be performed until a tumor-free margin is obtained in each plane.

A specialist specifically trained in Mohs micrographic excision or an oculoplastic surgeon removes the clinical tumor. The Mohs surgeon or a pathologist (if oculoplastic surgeon excises tissue) is responsible for histological analysis to confirm that all tumor is removed. Repair may then be performed by an oculoplastic surgeon.

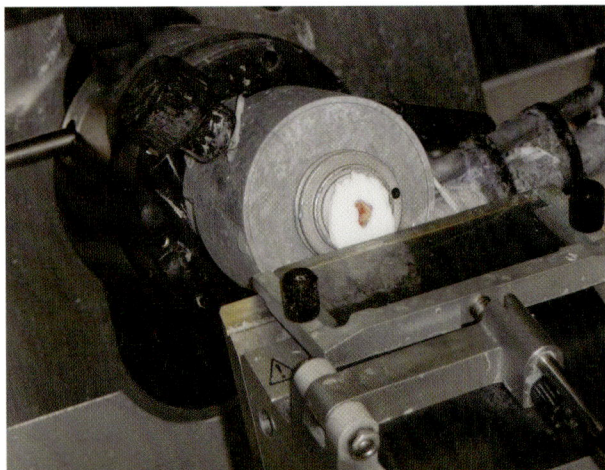

FIGURE 80.2 This photograph shows a clinical surgical margin specimen embedded in a block mounted on cryostat, ready for sectioning.

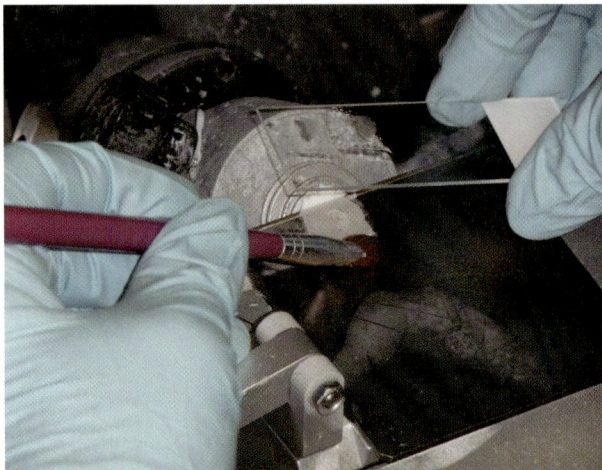

FIGURE 80.3 The histopathology technician delicately and precisely cuts thin, inverted (en face) horizontal sections (layers) of the specimen onto a microscope slide, with good cryostat technique to avoid problems such as artifacts, rips, tears, folds, bubbles, chips, fragments, and incomplete margin(s).

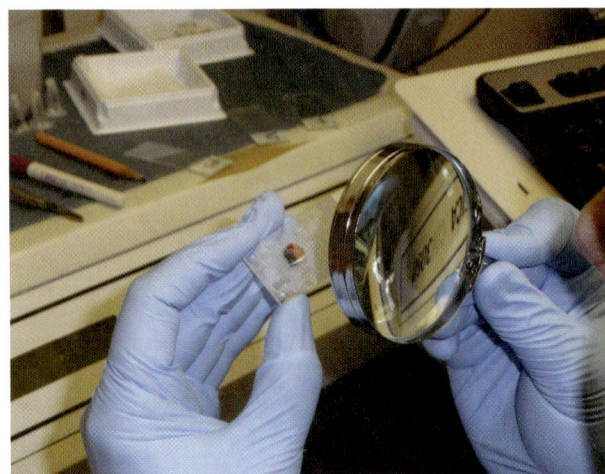

FIGURE 80.4 The histopathology technician closely examines (with magnification) the thin tissue layer on microscope slide to confirm appropriate tissue processing and thickness with inverted (en face) horizontal orientation and adequate quality control of specimen. The slide is then stained with hematoxylin and eosin (H & E) and analyzed. If residual tumor cells are visible at any margin, further stages (and sections) are taken until no tumor is visible at all final margins. The wound is then redraped, re-prepped, and reconstructed with new sterile instruments by the reconstructive surgeon.

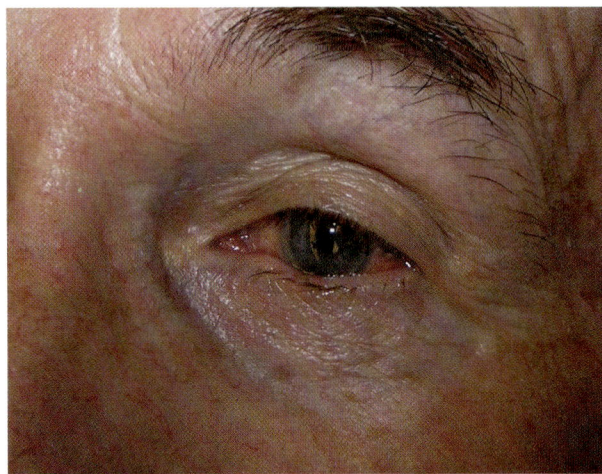

FIGURE 80.5 Basal cell carcinoma located in central third of left lower eyelid (mucocutaneous) margin.

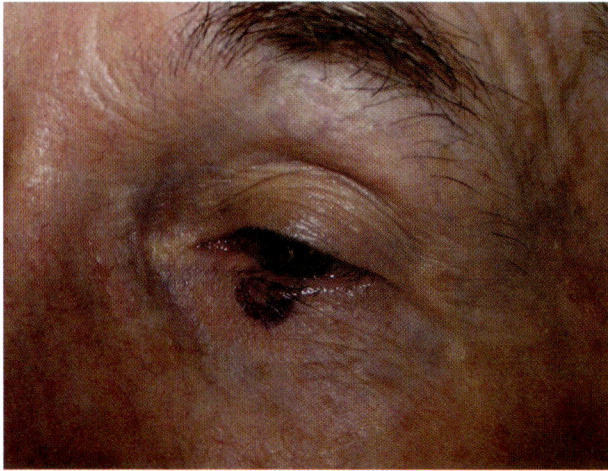

FIGURE 80.6 The left lower lid lesion with clinical excision margins is now marked.

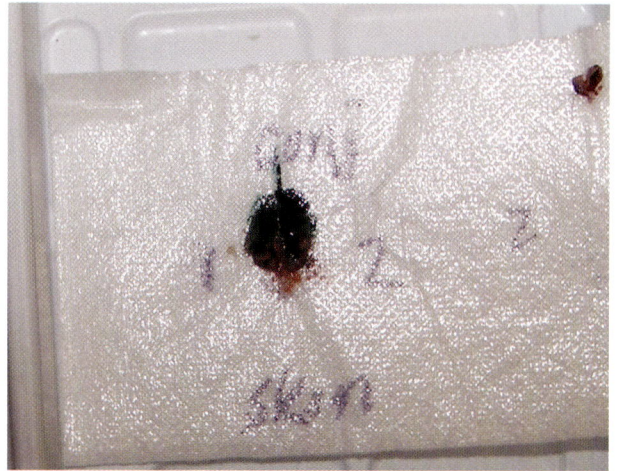

FIGURE 80.7 Clinical margins from Stage I comprising 2 separate sections (layers) after marking with color dyes prior to histological processing.

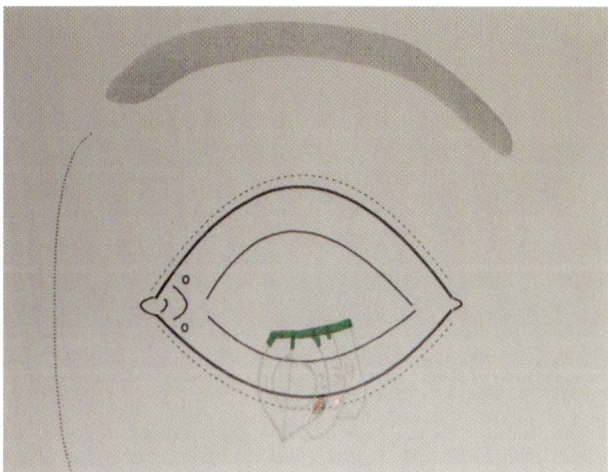

FIGURE 80.8 Final tumor map after three stages with mucocutaneous lid margin labeled in green and residual tumor marked in red. Stage I comprises (two) sections 1 and 2, with residual tumor cells (marked red in map) identified histologically in the inferior-lateral (lower right in map) portion of the margin of section. Stage II comprises (one) section 3, excised just lateral (right in map) to section 2 of Stage I; it still contains residual tumor cells (red) in the inferior-lateral (lower right in map) portion of margin. Stage III comprises (one) section 4, without any residual tumor cells at margin, indicated by absence of red markings; it is the final stage.

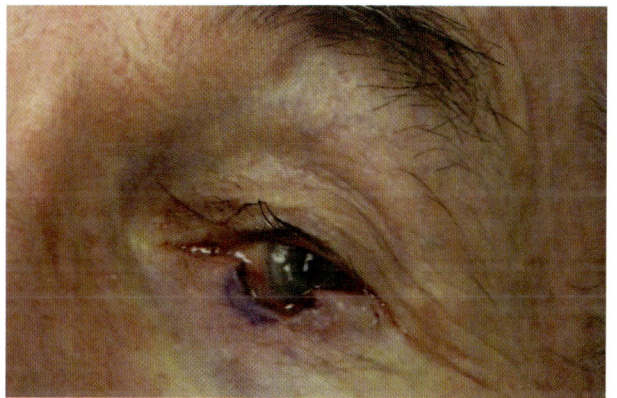

FIGURE 80.9 Final left lower lid defect after Stage III modified, inverted (en face) horizontal frozen section, margin-controlled tumor excision. The reconstructive surgeon can now reconstruct the defect after re-prepping, redraping, and using new sterile surgical instruments.

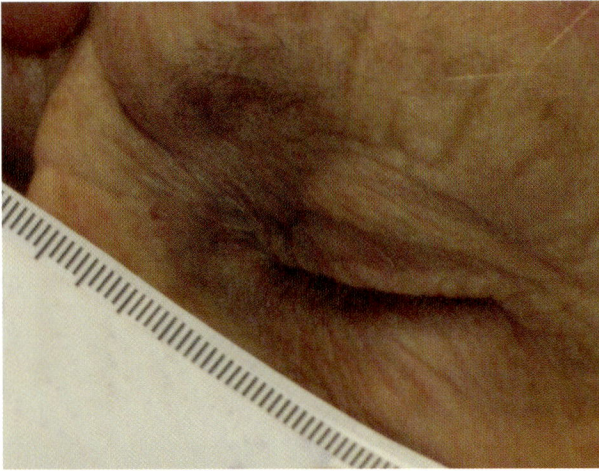

FIGURE 80.10   Subtle left medial canthal skin tumor prior to marking and excision.

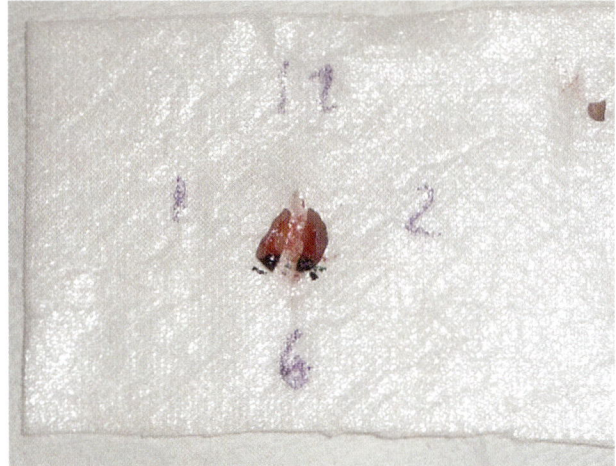

FIGURE 80.11   Clinical surgical margins of left medial canthal cancer Stage I excision, comprising two sections marked with dye, in their inferior portions.

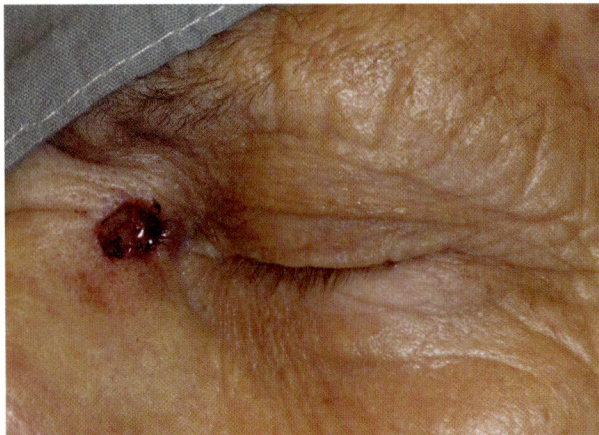

FIGURE 80.12   Left medial canthal defect after Stage I cancer excision.

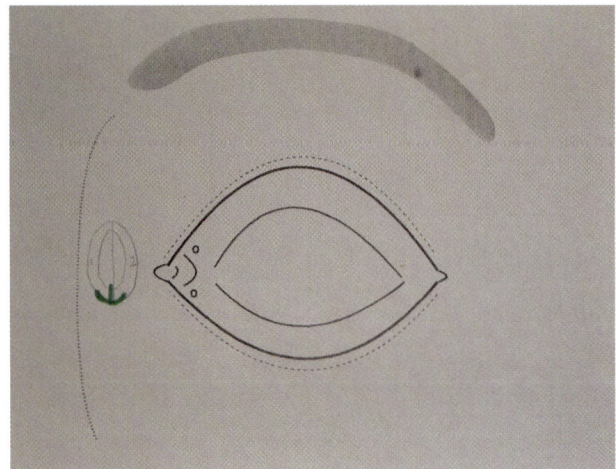

FIGURE 80.13   Final tumor map showing Stage I clinical margin excision comprising two sections (1 and 2) whose inferior border is marked with green dye. Absence of positive tumor margins is indicated by absence of red dye where residual tumor cells would be. Stage I is final stage representing complete tumor excision.

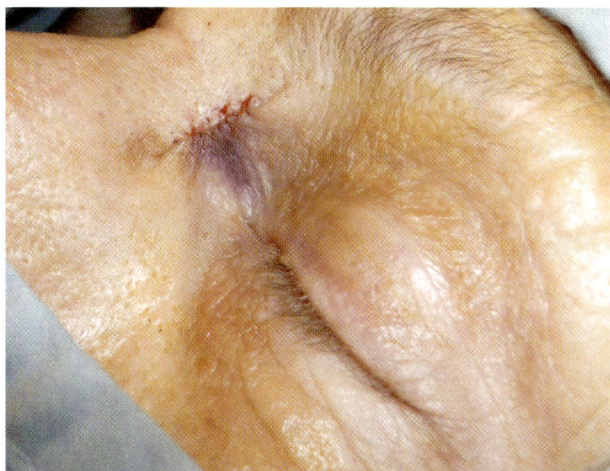

FIGURE 80.14   Left medial canthal defect repaired after complete tumor excision.

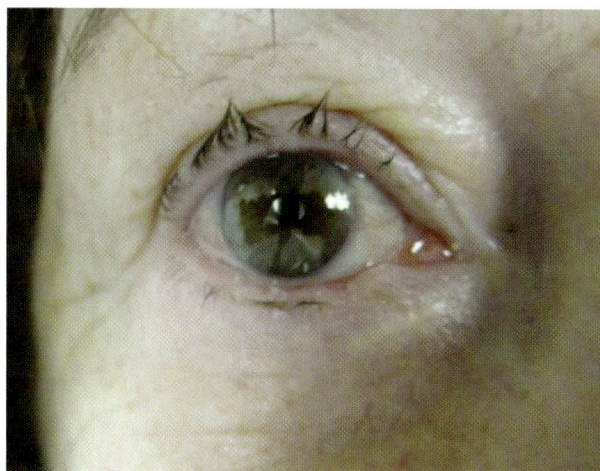

FIGURE 80.15   Right lower lid margin basal cell carcinoma as a small focus with erythema.

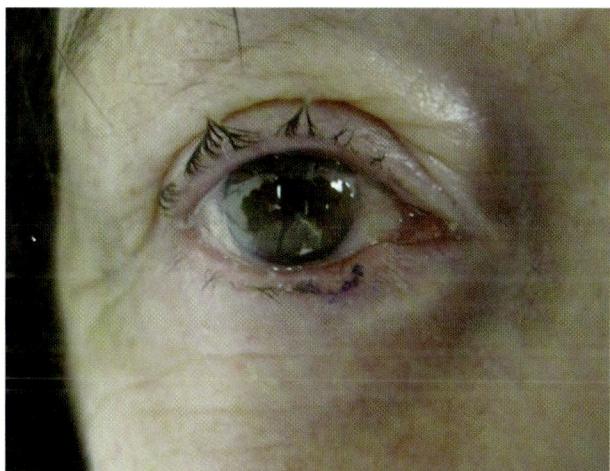

FIGURE 80.16   Clinical tumor and Mohs excision margins now marked on lower lid margin.

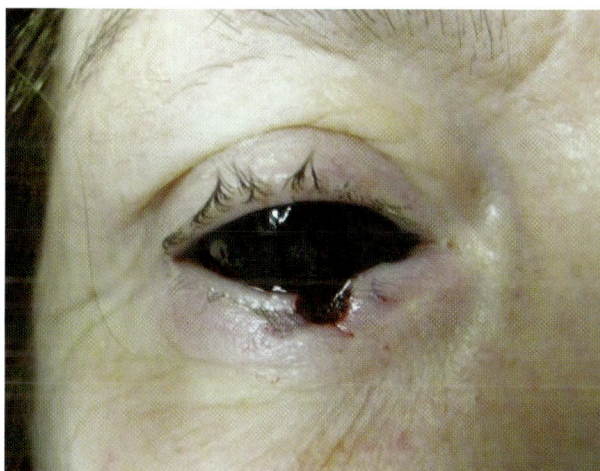

FIGURE 80.17   Right lower lid after Stage I Mohs tumor excision; black corneal protector is in place.

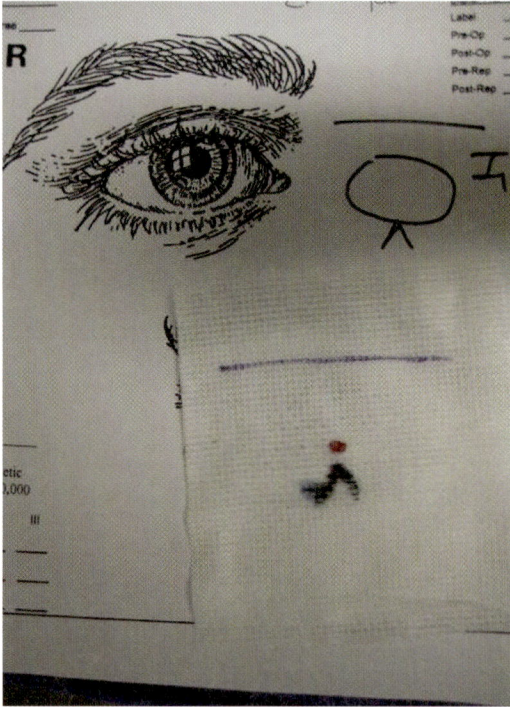

FIGURE 80.18 Clinical excision map with Stage I Mohs tissue below the circular unlabeled map.

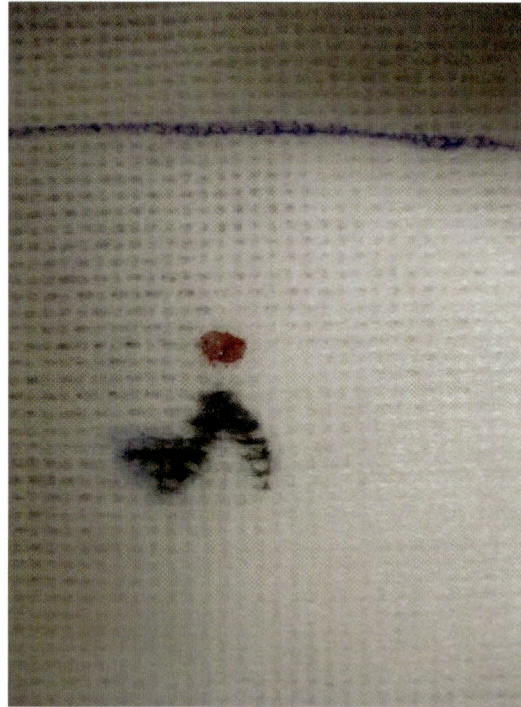

FIGURE 80.19 Close-up of initial Stage I Mohs tissue containing clinical surgical margins.

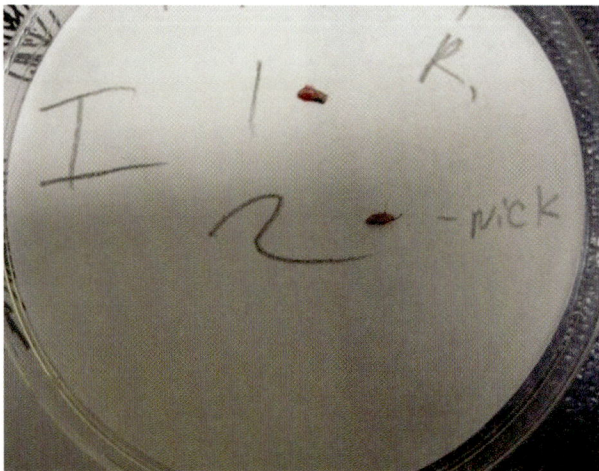

FIGURE 80.20 Initial Stage I Mohs tissue margins divided into two separate sections (layers).

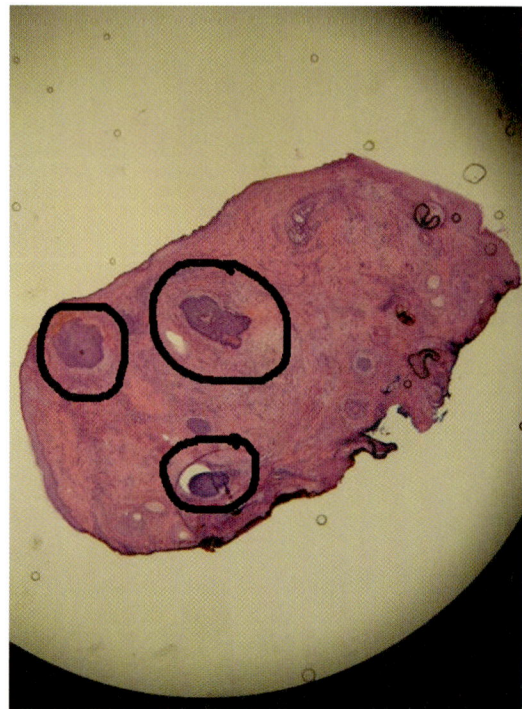

FIGURE 80.21 Stage I Mohs histologic slide of surgical margin of lid excision (epidermis oriented superiorly) demonstrating islands of invading basophilic (bluish) tumor cells circled in black.

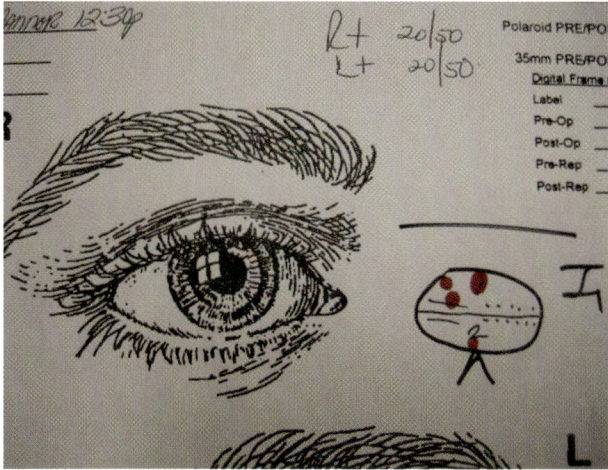

FIGURE 80.22 Stage I Mohs completed histologic tumor map with tumor cells marked in red in (both) sections 1 and 2.

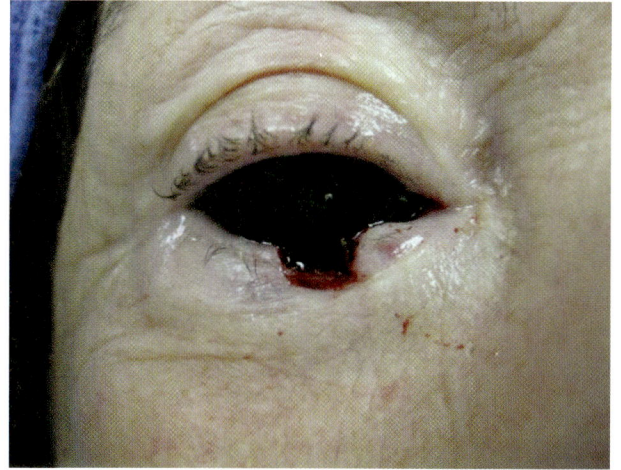

FIGURE 80.23 Right lower lid after Stage II Mohs excision; black eye shield in place.

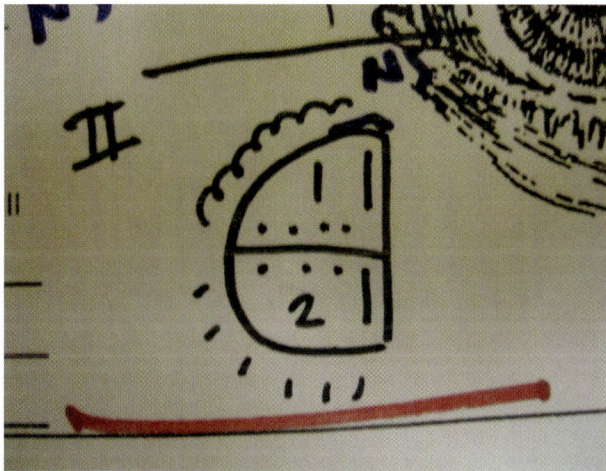

FIGURE 80.24 Close up of completed Stage II Mohs histopathologic tumor map with no tumor cells present (red ink absent). Stage II comprises two separate sections (1 and 2) taken from the lateral (left in map of figure 80.22) half of initial Stage I Mohs clinical margin (see map in Figure 80.22, compare Figures 80.17 and 80.23).

Sentinel Lymph Node Biopsy in Periocular Skin Cancer Excision

TABLE 80.5 *Possible Indications for Sentinel Lymph Node Biopsy in Periocular Skin Cancers*

- Malignant Melanoma with tumor thickness greater or equal to 2 mm
- Malignant Melanoma with histopathologic presence of ulceration
- Merkel Cell Carcinoma
- Large or advanced Sebaceous Gland Adenocarcinoma (Stage greater than or equal to T2)
- Large or advanced Squamous Cell Carcinoma (Stage greater than or equal to T2)

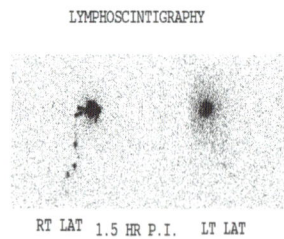

FIGURE 80.25 Preoperative lymphoscintigraphy before planned sentinel lymph node biopsy. 0.2 cc volume of radioactive tracer was injected into subconjunctival space.

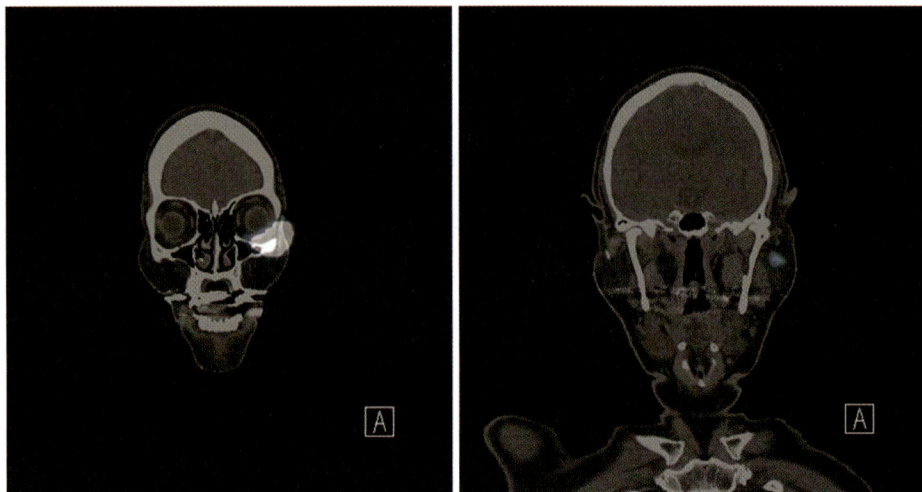

FIGURE 80.26 SPECT/CT scans provide greater anatomic detail than traditional lymphoscintigraphy (compare to Figure 80.25).

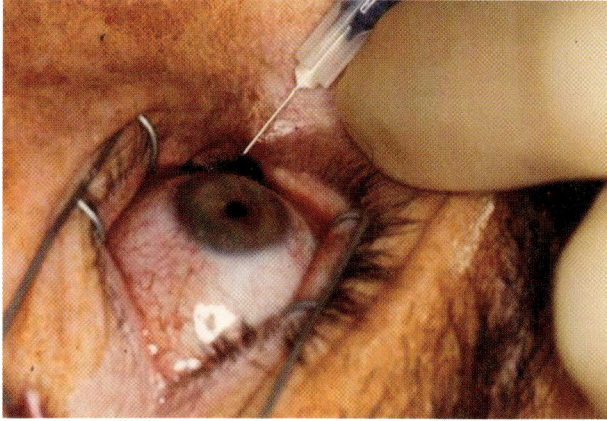

FIGURE 80.27 Close up of periocular injection of isosulfan blue dye with possible tracer.

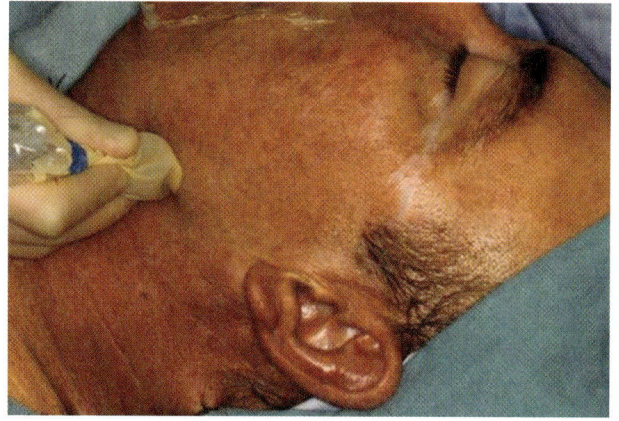

FIGURE 80.28 Perioperative gamma probe tracing radioactivity to localize sentinel lymph node.

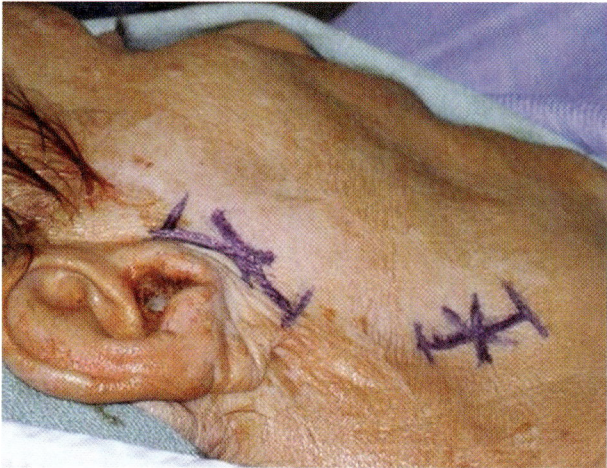

FIGURE 80.29 Incisions for planned pre-auricular (parotid) and cervical lymph node exploration in a different patient.

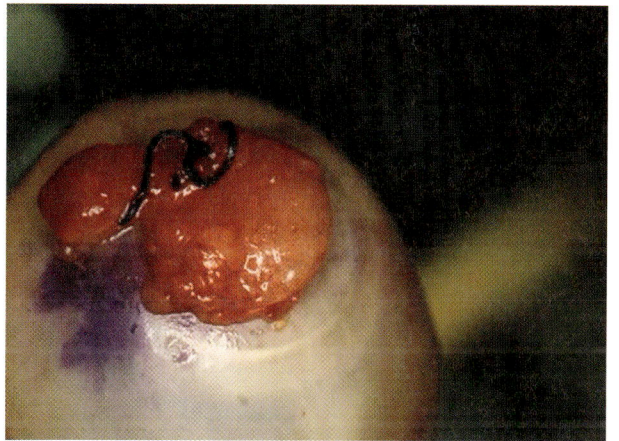

FIGURE 80.30 Close-up of excised sentinel lymph node. (Image from Esmaeli B. Advances in the management of malignant tumors of the eyelid and conjunctiva: The role of sentinel lymph node biopsy. *Int Ophthalmol Clin.* 2002;42(2):151–162, with permission of Wolters Kluwer Health.)

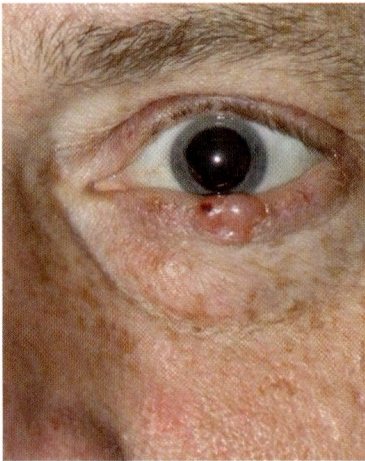

FIGURE 80.31 Left lower lid margin amelanotic melanoma (Breslow thickness 3.8 mm, Clark level IV) with systemic work-up negative, including no palpable lymph nodes, and no suspicious lymph nodes on ultrasound and MRI testing. (Image from Sanchez R, Ivan D, Esmaeli B. Eyelid and periorbital cutaneous malignant melanoma. *Int Ophthalmol Clin.* 2009;49(4):25–43, with permission of Wolters Kluwer Health.)

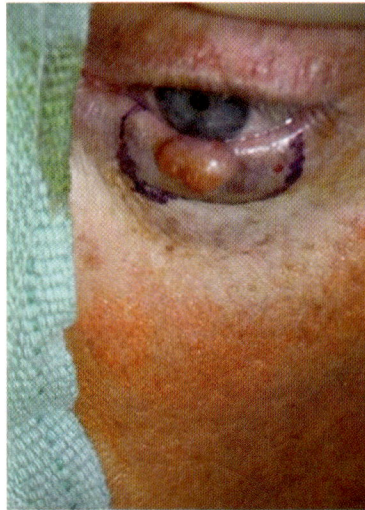

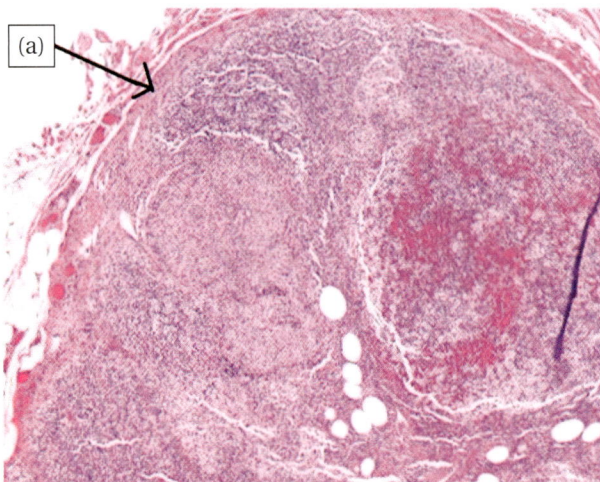

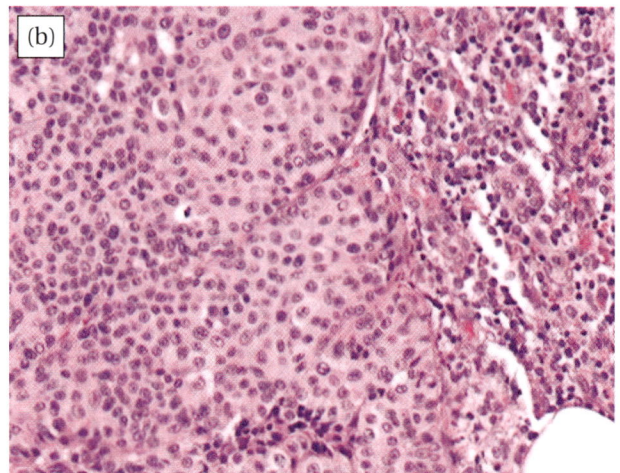

FIGURE 80.32 Wide local excision of left lower lid amelanotic melanoma with margins marked. One positive lymph node each was detected via sentinel lymph node biopsy in both the parotid tail and in lower jugular chain. (Image from Sanchez R, Ivan D, Esmaeli B. Eyelid and periorbital cutaneous malignant melanoma. *Int Ophthalmol Clin.* 2009;49(4):25–43, with permission of Wolters Kluwer Health.)

FIGURE 80.33 Histologic slides of left parotid sentinel lymph node showing 0.8 × 0.5 mm malignant melanoma without extracapsular extension (arrow in Figure [a] marks capsule). Figure (b) shows high-power magnified view. During left parotidectomy and completion neck dissection, no additional positive nodes were found (other than 2 sentinel lymph nodes with micrometastasis). (Image from Sanchez R, Ivan D, Esmaeli B. Eyelid and periorbital cutaneous malignant melanoma. *Int Ophthalmol Clin.* 2009;49(4):25–43, with permission of Wolters Kluwer Health.)

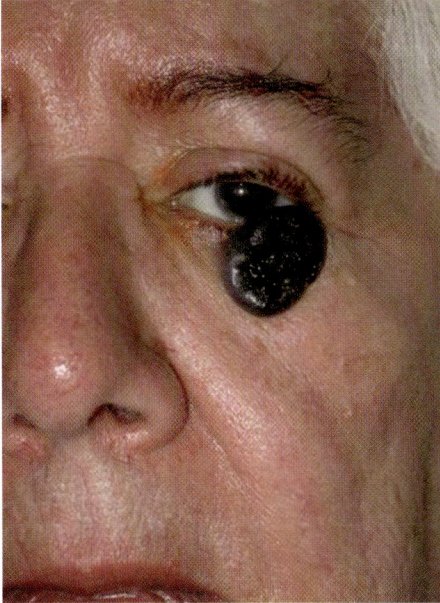

FIGURE 80.34 Left lower lid and cheek malignant melanoma (Breslow thickness 7.2 mm plus ulceration, Clark level II) with clinically negative evaluation for lymph node spread. Patient had wide local excision with one pre-auricular sentinel lymph node positive for metastatic disease. (Image from Savar A, Ross MI, Prieto VG et al. Sentinel lymph node biopsy for ocular adnexal melanoma: Experience in 30 patients. *Ophthalmology.* 2009;116(11):2217–2223, with permission of Elsevier, Inc.)

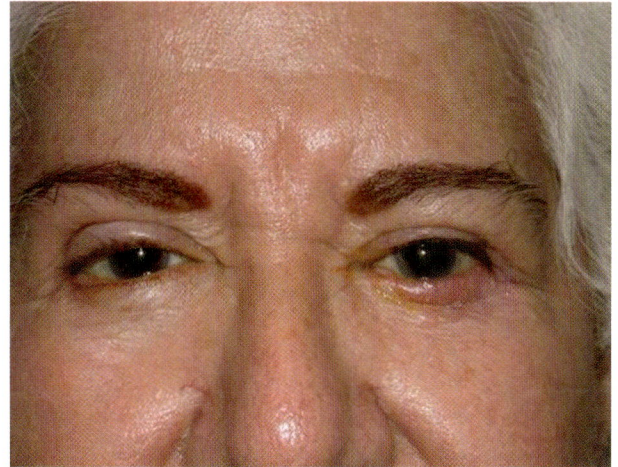

FIGURE 80.35 Postoperative close up of same patient after repair using multiple flaps and grafts. Left lower lid margin demonstrates proper contour, position, symmetry with excellent aesthetic outcome.

TABLE 80.6 *Potential Complications of Periocular Skin Cancer Excision*

- Cancer recurrence, lymph node spread, and/or metastasis
- Cancer extension to globe, lacrimal sac, orbit, brain, nose, sinuses, oral cavity, etc.
- Unrecognized perineural invasion
- Vision loss
- Lacrimal obstruction with tearing and dacryocystitis
- Irreplaceable loss of critical periocular tissues such as conjuctiva or tarsus
- Facial palsy
- Cranial neuropathy
- Sensory disturbance
- Dry eye and lagophthalmos
- Exposure keratopathy
- Eyelid malposition
- Aesthetic concerns

* Above are also complications of delayed, partial, or absence of periocular skin cancer excision.

TABLE 80.7 *Potential Complications of Sentinel Lymph Node Biopsy in Periocular Skin Cancer Excision*

- Facial nerve weakness
- Blue discoloration of globe or skin from dye
- Anaphylactic reaction to dye

SELECTED REFERENCES

Barrett RV, Meyer DR. Eyelid and periocular cutaneous Merkel cell carcinoma (aka. neuroendocrine or trabecular carcinoma). *Int Ophthalmol Clin.* 2009;49(4):63–76.

Chan FM, O'Donnell BA, Whitehead K, et al. Treatment and outcomes of malignant melanoma of the eyelid: a review of 29 cases in Australia. *Ophthalmology.* 2007;114:187–192.

Conway RM, Themel S, Holbach LM. Surgery for primary basal cell carcinoma including the eyelid margins with intraoperative frozen section control comparative interventional study with a minimum clinical follow up of 5 years. *Br J Ophthalmol.* 2004;88:236–238.

Cook BE, Bartley GB. Treatment options and future prospects for the management of eyelid malignancies: an evidence-based update. *Ophthalmology.* 2001;108:2088–2100.

Esmaeli B, Wang B, Deavers M, et al. Prognostic factors for survival in malignant melanoma of the eyelid skin. *Ophthal Plast Reconstr Surg.* 2000:16:250–257.

Esmaeli B. Sentinel lymph node mapping for patients with cutaneous and conjunctival malignant melanoma. *Ophthal Plast Reconstr Surg.* 2000;16:170–172.

Gayre GS, Hybarger CP, Mannor G, et al. Outcomes of excision of 1750 eyelid and periocular skin basal cell and squamous cell carcinomas by modified en face, frozen section margin-controlled technique. *Int Ophthalmol Clin.* 2009,49(4):97–110.

Kim JW, Lee DK. Unusual eyelid, periocular, and periorbital cutaneous malignancies. *Int Ophthalmol Clin.* 2009;49(4):77–96.

Leshin B, Yeats RP. Management of periocular basal cell carcinoma: I. Mohs micrographic surgery. *Surv Ophthalmol* 1993;38:193–203.

Malhotra R, Huilgol SC, Huynh NT, et al. The Australian Mohs database, part II: periocular basal cell carcinoma outcome at 5 year follow up. *Ophthalmology.* 2004;111:631–636.

Mannor GE, ed. Eyelid, periocular and periorbital skin cancer: therapy & oculofacial plastic surgery repair. *Int Ophthalmol Clin* Philadelphia: 2009; 49(4):i-250.

Mannor GE, Chern PL, Barnette D. Eyelid and periorbital skin basal cell carcinoma. Oculoplastic management and surgery. *Int Ophthalmol Clin.* 2009;49(4):1–16.

Mohs FE. Micrographic surgery for microscopically controlled excision of eyelid tumors. *Arch Ophthalmol.* 1986;104:910–919.

Moul DK, Chern PL, Shumaker PR, Zelac DE, et al. Mohs micrographic surgery for eyelid and periorbital skin cancer. *Int Ophthalmol Clin.* 2009;49(4):111–128.

Nemet AY, Deckel Y, Martin PA, et al. Management of periocular basal cell and squamous cell carcinoma: a series of 453 cases. *Am J Ophthalmol.* 2006;142:293–297.

Satchi K, McNab AA. Orbital spread of eyelid and periocular cutaneous cancer. *Int Ophthalmol Clin.* 2009;49(4):223–236.

Shields JA, Demirci H, Marr BP, et al. Sebaceous carcinoma of the eyelids. Personal experience with 60 cases. *Ophthalmology.* 2004;111:2151–2157.

81 Eyelid Reconstruction

D.J. John Park, MD and Andrew Harrison, MD

SELECTED REFERENCES

TABLE 81.1 *Indications for Surgery*

Eyelid defects from tumors, trauma, or congenital processes impairing function or cosmesis, and that are not amenable to healing by secondary intention.

TABLE 81.2 *Preoperative Considerations*

Ensure tumor-free excision of the lesion prior to definitive reconstruction.

Determine if defect is full or partial thickness.

Measure dimensions and extent of defect, length of marginal involvement, and horizontal laxity.

Preoperative photography of the defect is valuable.

Evaluate whether canaliculi and canthal tendons are intact.

Assess for risks of local flap or free graft loss, such as a history of smoking or radiation.

Pertinent Surgical Anatomy

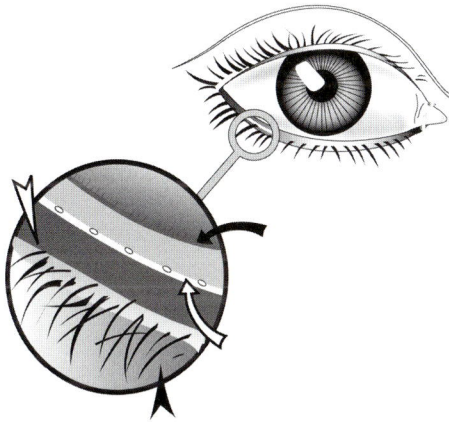

Anterior Lamella
• Skin
• Orbicularis

Middle Lamella
• Tarsus*
• Septum
• Levator aponeurosis/ Müller's muscle (upper eyelid)
• Capsulopalpebral fascia/ inferior tarsal muscle (lower eyelid)

Posterior Lamella
• Tarsus*
• Conjunctiva

* Because the conjunctiva is so adherent to the tarsus, there is an inseparable confluence between them, and the middle and posterior lamellas should be considered as one unit.

FIGURE 81.1 Topographical anatomy of the eyelid margin. The posterior eyelid margin (black arrow) abuts the ocular surface. The gray line (white arrow) is a light reflex formed by the muscle of Riolan. It lies just anterior to the line of Meibomian gland orifices and demarcates the junction of the anterior and posterior lamella. The posterior and anterior lash lines are demarcated by the white and black arrowheads, respectively. With age or chronic inflammation, these features become less distinct and the margin becomes rounded.

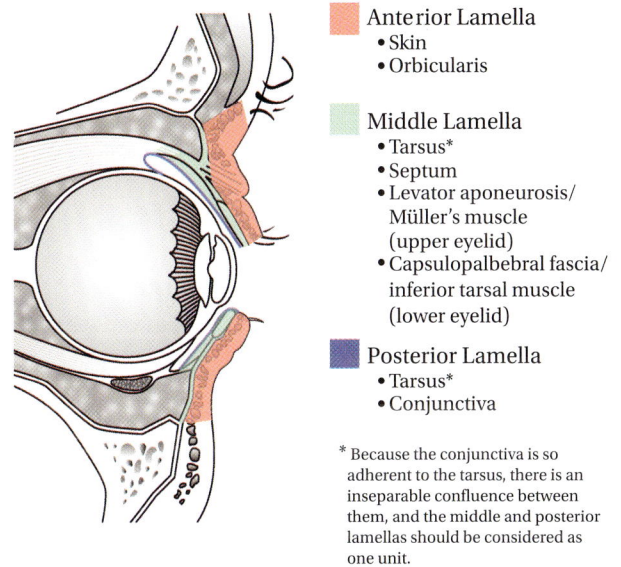

FIGURE 81.2 Sagittal cross-section of the upper and lower eyelids. Deficiency in the middle lamella will cause eyelid retraction, whereas deficiencies in the anterior and posterior lamella will produce ectropion and entropion, respectively.

Step-by-Step Surgical Series

TABLE 81.3 *Primary Closure ± Canthotomy*

Preoperative Considerations

Are the tarsal edges of the defect sharp and perpendicular to the eyelid margin?

Is there sufficient horizontal laxity to allow closure with limited tension?

In general, defects less than 25% of the horizontal dimension can easily be closed primarily. However, with preexistent horizontal laxity, larger defects can be closed in this manner as well.

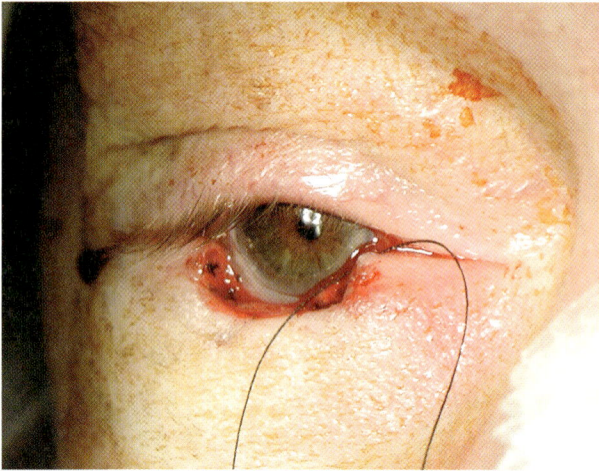

FIGURE 81.3 Full-thickness pentagonal defect involving just over 25% of horizontal dimension of the lower eyelid. In this case, a lateral canthotomy/cantholysis was performed to recruit additional horizontal length.

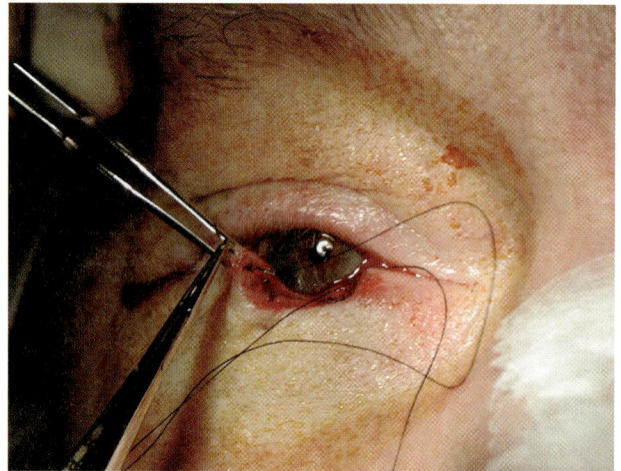

FIGURE 81.4 A single interrupted 6-0 silk suture is placed at the gray line and left long for use as traction. The margin edges should line up in three dimensions once the suture is secured. An additional suture is placed at the posterior lash line after the tarsal sutures are placed.

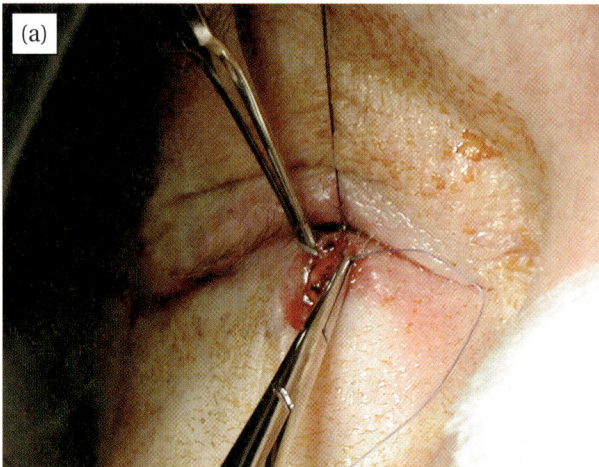

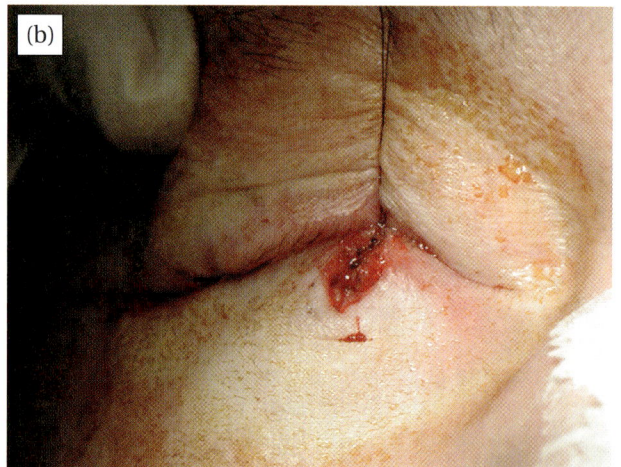

FIGURE 81.5 (a, b) The tarsus is re-approximated with two partial-thickness interrupted 6-0 polyglactin sutures on a spatulated needle. For analogous defects involving the upper eyelid, three such sutures should be placed to account for the taller tarsus.

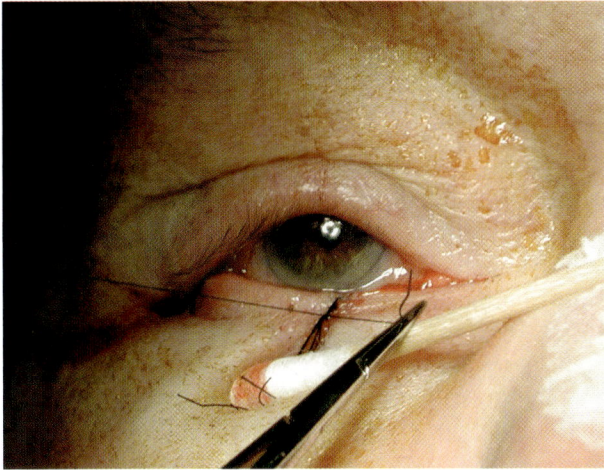

FIGURE 81.6 The ends of the two 6-0 silk sutures at the margin are trimmed, after being folded away from the globe, and tied into the knot of a third 6-0 silk suture placed at the anterior lash line.

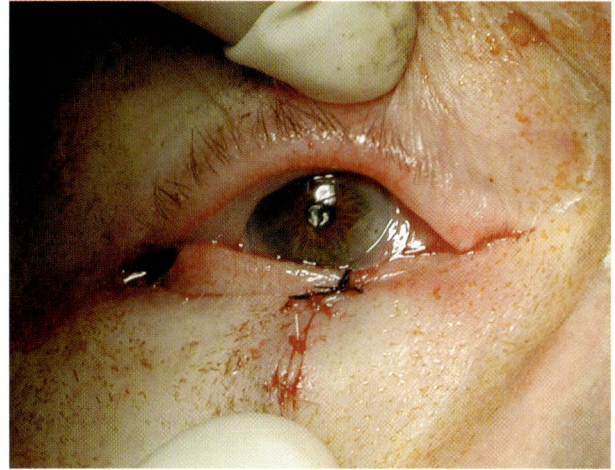

FIGURE 81.7 The remaining skin defect can be closed with a fine absorbable or non-absorbable suture. If a dog-ear is present, a Burrow's triangle can be excised. In corresponding defects of the upper eyelid, the dog-ear can be managed by making horizontal relaxing incisions at the upper eyelid crease, medially and laterally, forming a "T" with the vertical closure.

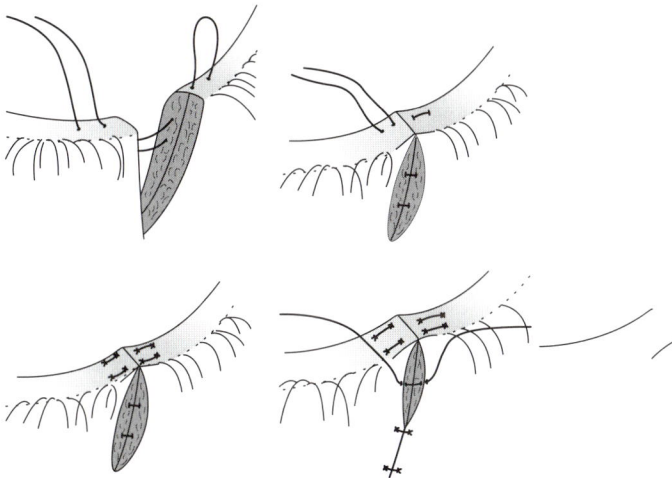

FIGURE 81.8 Alternatively, for the lid margin closure, two interrupted 6-0 chromic gut sutures can be placed as a vertical mattress at the gray line and posterior lash line to evert the edges of the lid margin. With secondary wound contraction, the eversion settles down to create a smooth contour. (Adapted from Nerad JA. The requisites in Ophthalmology: *Oculoplastic Surgery*. Philadelphia, Mosby 2001:319.)

TABLE 81.4 *Tenzel Semicircular Flap for Upper/Lower Lid*

Preoperative Considerations

Full thickness defects of approximately 50% of the horizontal dimensions can be closed with a Tenzel flap.

A thin Tenzel flap may require augmentation of the posterior lamella with a concurrent periosteal flap.

It is crucial to reconstruct the lateral support of the eyelid as well as to redefine the lateral palpebral commissure.

(a)

(b)

Reconstructed margin

(c)

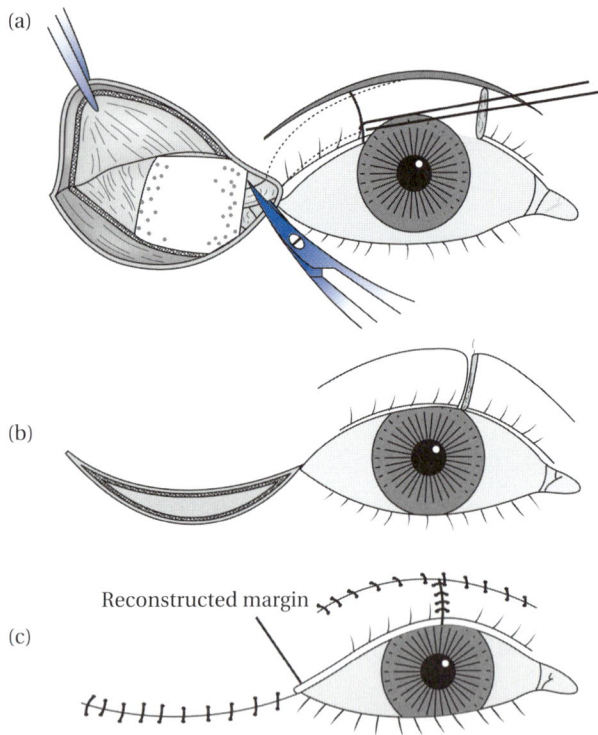

FIGURE 81.9 For upper eyelid defects, the Tenzel flap is designed with the arc convex inferiorly. For corresponding defects of the lower eyelid, the arc should curve superiorly. (a) The flap is undermined in the suborbicularis preperiosteal plane. A complete upper lateral cantholysis is required for maximal mobilization into the defect. (b) The flap is rotated into the defect medially. (c) The eyelid margin is closed primarily as described previously, and the donor site closed with simple running or interrupted sutures. The flap should be secured to the periosteum at the lateral orbital rim, and the commissure redefined with a single 6-0 plain gut suture. Because the Tenzel flap tends to be thinner than the eyelid margin, it can be combined with a periosteal flap to add bulk in the posterior lamella. (Adapted from Basic and Clinical Science Course Section 7, *American Academy of Ophthalmology*, San Francisco, CA 2003:186)

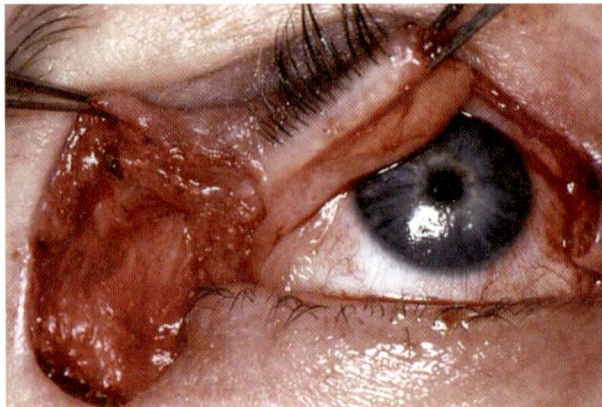

FIGURE 81.10 Right upper lid defect between 25% and 50% of the lid margin. A Tenzel semicircular flap elevated and lateral canthal tendon transected. Note medial distraction of the eyelid with disinsertion of the canthal tendon. (Courtesy of Mark J. Lucarelli MD, FACS.)

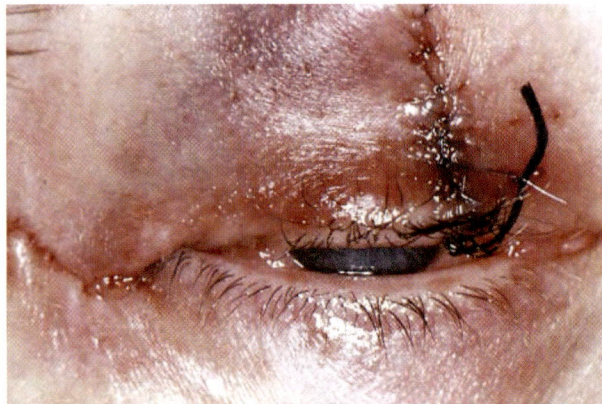

FIGURE 81.11 Appearance immediately following reconstruction of the lid margin and closure of the lateral canthal defect. (Courtesy of Mark J. Lucarelli MD, FACS.)

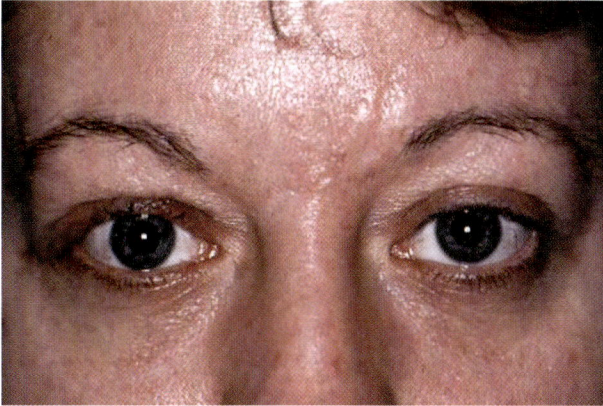

FIGURE 81.12 Appearance several months following right upper lid reconstruction with Tenzel semicircular flap. (Courtesy of Mark J. Lucarelli MD, FACS.)

TABLE 81.5 *Periosteal Flap*

Preoperative Considerations

The maximal length of the periosteal flap is up to 10 mm. For defects greater than this, a periosteal flap alone is likely not suitable.

This flap is a random flap and its inherent vascularity is typically insufficient to support an overlying skin graft. Therefore, it is usually combined with a Tripier myocutaneous flap from the ipsilateral upper eyelid.

This flap can be combined with a Hughes tarsoconjunctival flap for large defects with complete loss of the lateral lower eyelid.

TABLE 81.6 *Medial Canthal Reconstruction*

Preoperative Considerations

Does the defect involve the medial canthal tendon or the canaliculus?

Does the defect span both the aesthetic subunits of the lateral nasal wall and the medial eyelids?

Is there adequate redundancy in the glabella?

Will the planned local flap reconstruction cause distortion in eyebrow position or webbing of the medial canthal skin?

Is this defect amenable to healing by secondary intention?

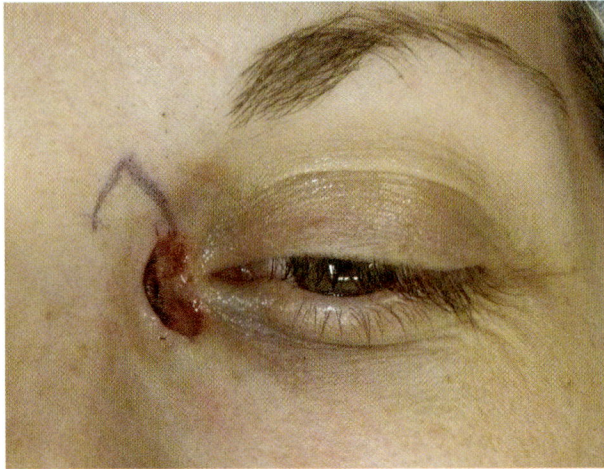

FIGURE 81.13   Planned rhomboid (Limberg) flap for reconstruction of a left medial canthal defect not involving the canaliculus, medial canthal tendon, or eyelid skin. Bilobed flaps may also be used for larger defects to distribute the tension and transposition across two lobes. If the defect spans both the lateral nasal wall and the medial eyelids, these flaps from the glabella can be combined with horizontal eyelid advancement flaps.

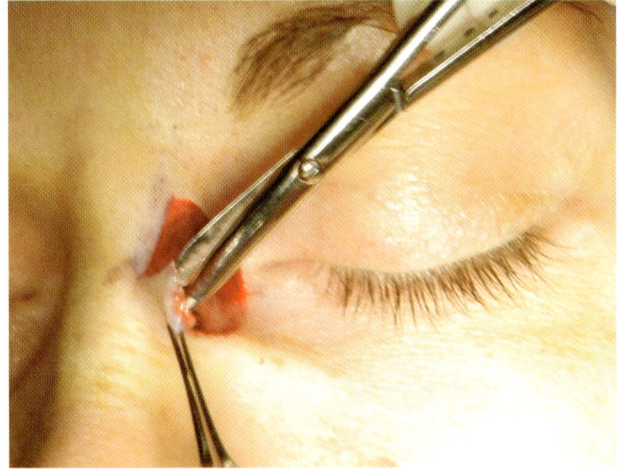

FIGURE 81.14   The flap is undermined in the subcutaneous plane.

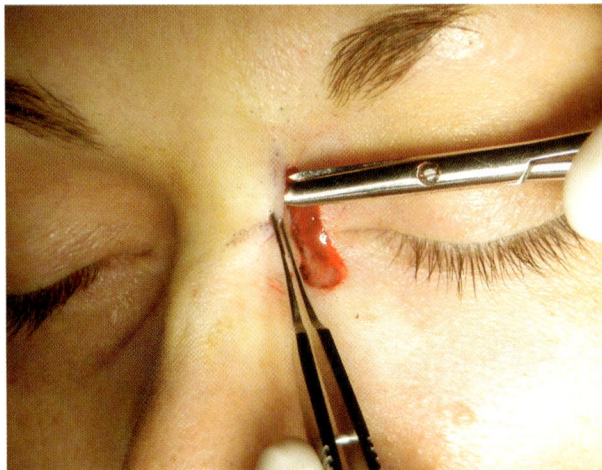

FIGURE 81.15   A sufficient area around the defect should be undermined to allow for approximation of the edges under minimal tension.

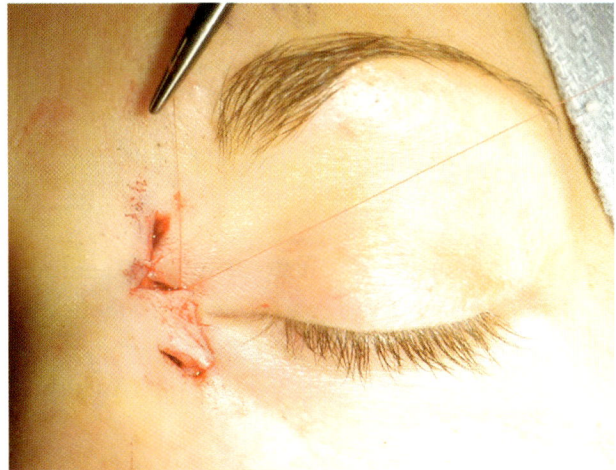

FIGURE 81.16   Several subcutaneous interrupted 5-0 or 6-0 polyglactin sutures are placed to secure the flap after it has been transposed to fill the defect. Securing the flap to the medial canthal tendon helps assure proper medial canthal contour.

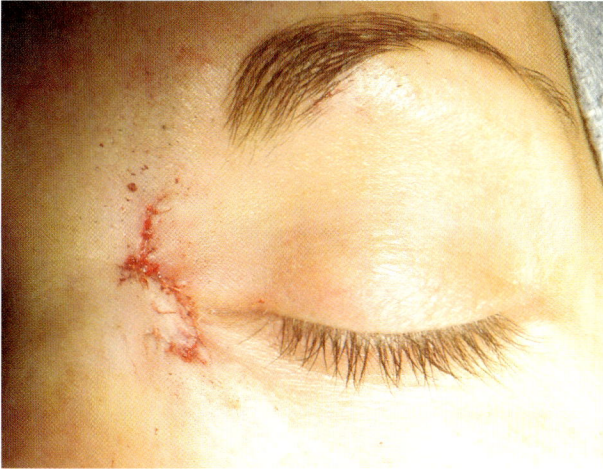

FIGURE 81.17 The skin edges are then re-approximated and is then closed with a fine absorbable or non-absorbable suture of the surgeon's preference.

Greater than 50% Defects of Upper and Lower Eyelids

TABLE 81.7 *Hughes Tarsoconjunctival Interpolation Flap for Lower Lid Reconstruction*

Preoperative Considerations

Can the defect be reconstructed in one stage with a Tenzel flap?

What is the visual capacity of the contralateral eye?

Can the patient tolerate occlusion of the ipsilateral eye between first and second stage reconstruction? This flap should be avoided in young children due to amblyogenic potential.

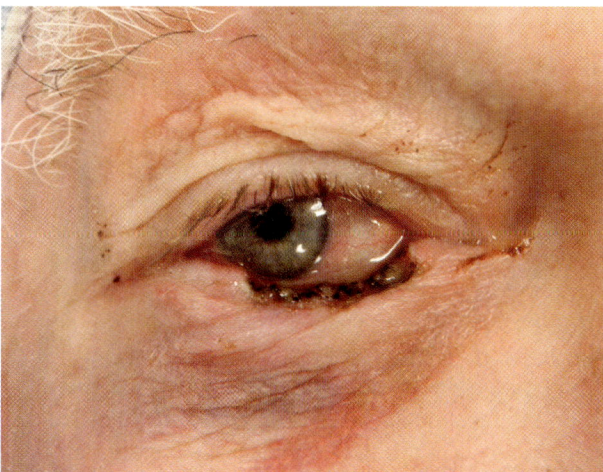

FIGURE 81.18 Hughes Stage I. Full-thickness defect of the lower eyelid involving well over 50% of its horiztonal length. The canthal tendons and canaliculus are intact.

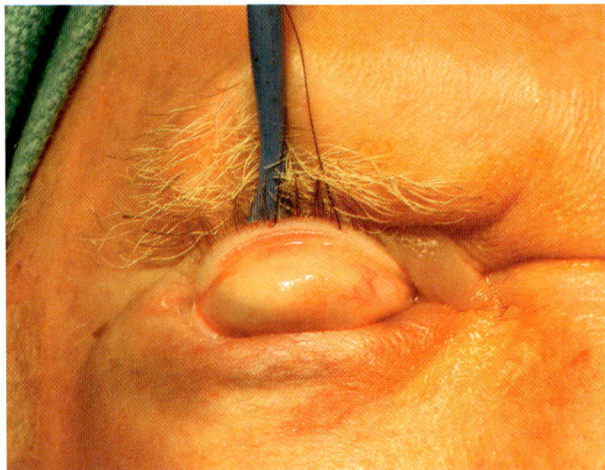

FIGURE 81.19 A 4-0 silk suture is place at the upper eyelid margin for traction. The conjunctival surface of the tarsus is exposed by everting the upper eyelid over a Desmarres retractor.

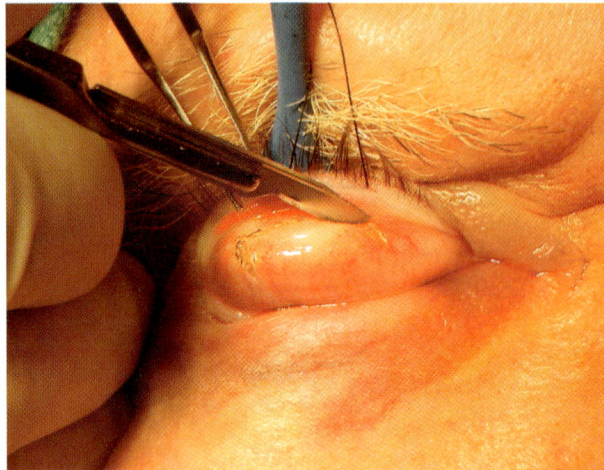

FIGURE 81.20 The tarsal portion of the flap is incised with a #15 blade. The horizontal dimension is determined by the horizontal dimension of the defect. At least 4 mm of vertical tarsal height should be preserved in the upper eyelid to prevent instability of the upper eyelid margin. As a result of the curved contour of the upper tarsus, the tarsal portion of the flap is tallest at its center.

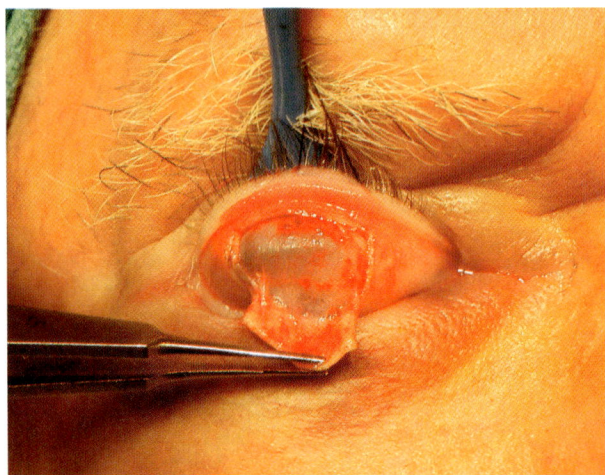

FIGURE 81.21 The tarsal flap is sharply elevated from its underlying attachments consisting of the orbicularis oculi muscle and the confluence of the septum and levator aponeurosis.

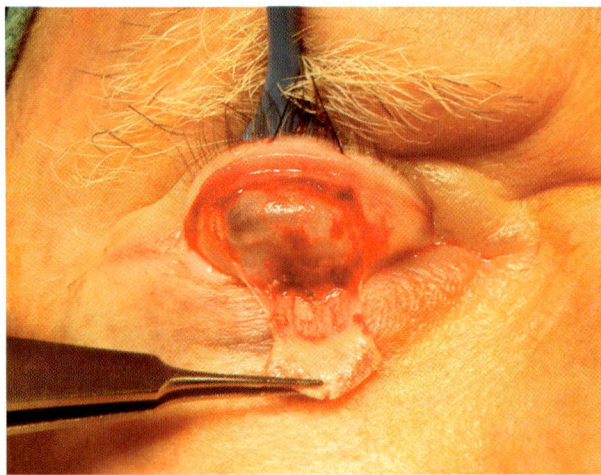

FIGURE 81.22 Flanking vertical relaxing incisions are made in the conjunctiva as the flap is sharply developed between the plane of the conjunctiva and Mueller's muscle. Saline or local anesthetic can be injected to hydrodissect between the planes and facilitate dissection. It is essential to remove Mueller's muscle from the flap to help prevent upper lid retraction after the second stage division of the flap.

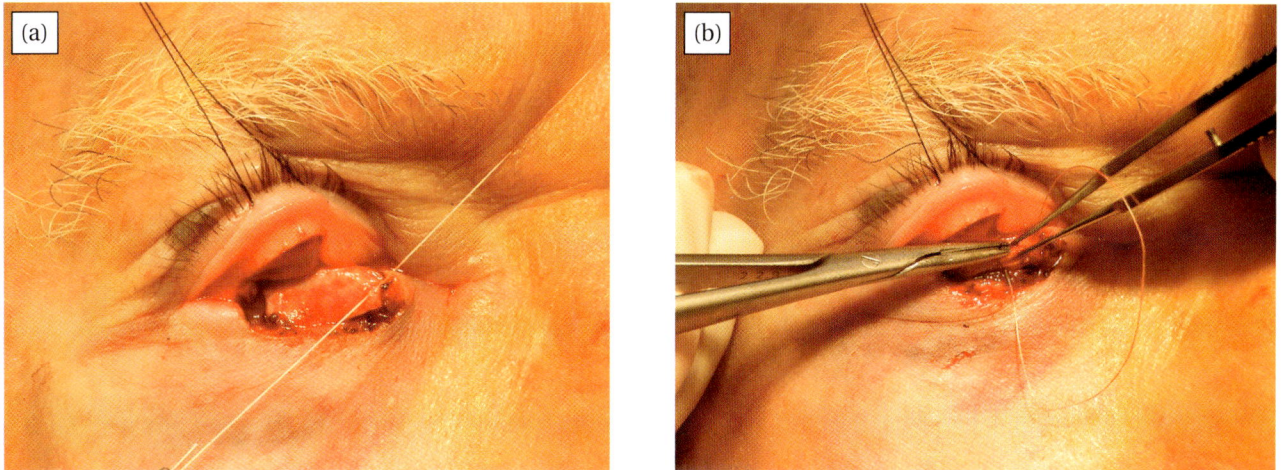

FIGURE 81.23 (a) Two partial-thickness interrupted 5-0 or 6-0 polyglactin sutures on a spatulated needle are used to approximate the tarsal portion of the flap to the tarsal edge of the recipient defect. The superior limit of the tarsal portion of the flap should be in line with, or 1 mm superior to, the eyelid margin of the defect. (b) An additional 5-0 or 6-0 polyglactin suture is used in a running fashion to approximate the inferior edge of the tarsoconjunctival flap to the edge of the conjunctiva and lower eyelid retractors of the defect.

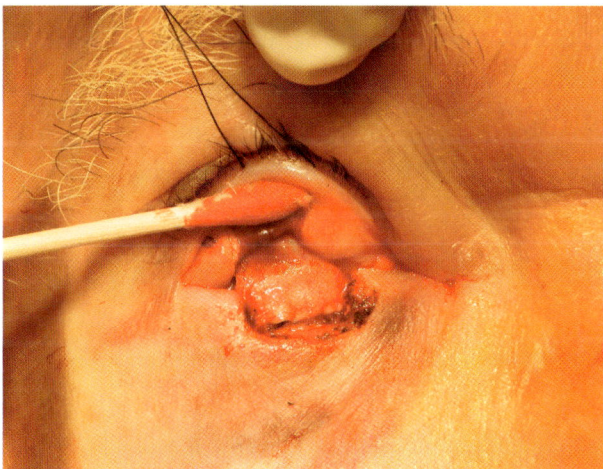

FIGURE 81.24 After inset of the Hughes flap into the defect, there should be minimal tension.

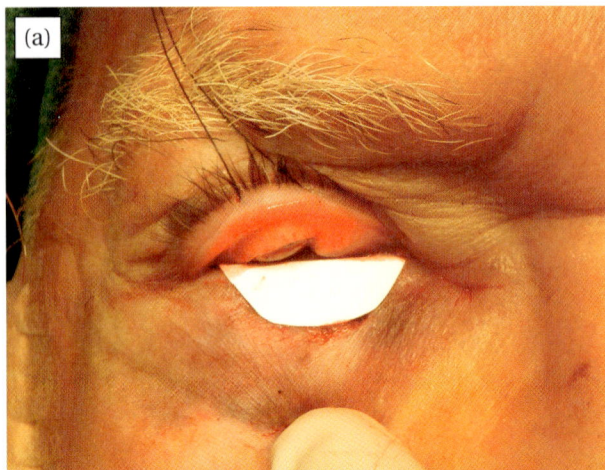

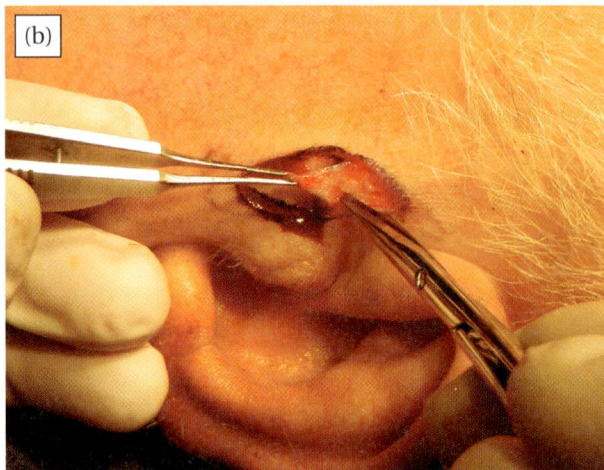

FIGURE 81.25   (a, b) A template should be used to determine the size and shape of the full-thickness skin graft, which can be harvested from the preauricular skin, as in this case, or from the postauricular areas.

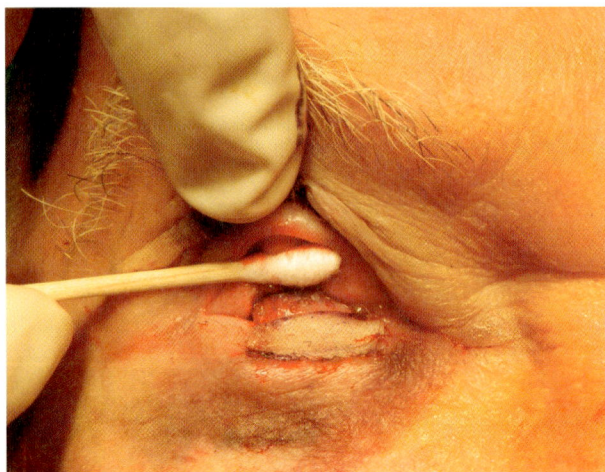

FIGURE 81.26 The full-thickness skin graft is approximated to the edge of the recipient skin defect with fine absorbable or non-absorbable sutures.

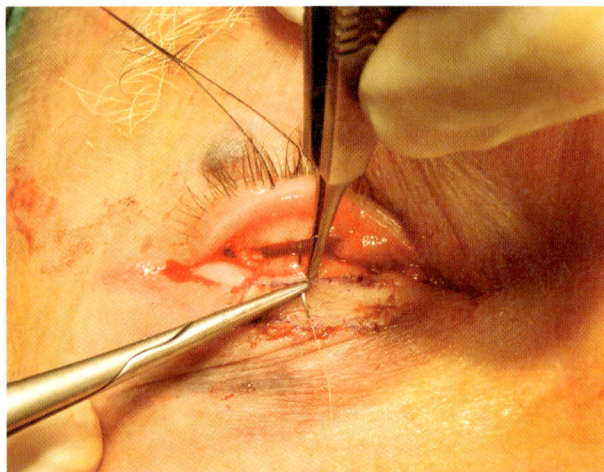

FIGURE 81.27 The superior edge of the skin graft is secured to the conjunctival flap with 6-0 fast-absorbing gut in an interrupted fashion with partial-thickness bites.

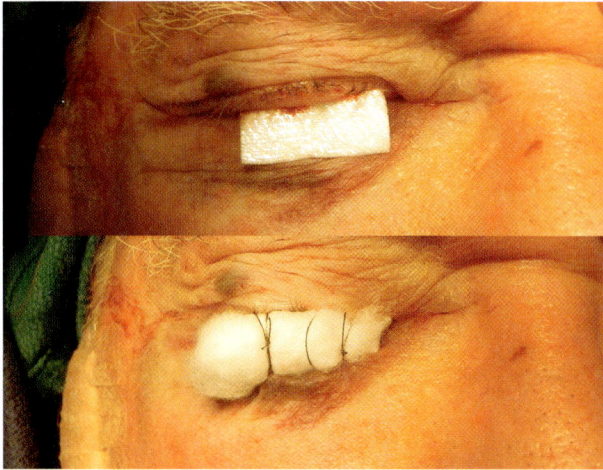

FIGURE 81.28 A bolster dressing with first Telfa, and then cotton balls, is tied over the skin graft with several 5-0 silk sutures.

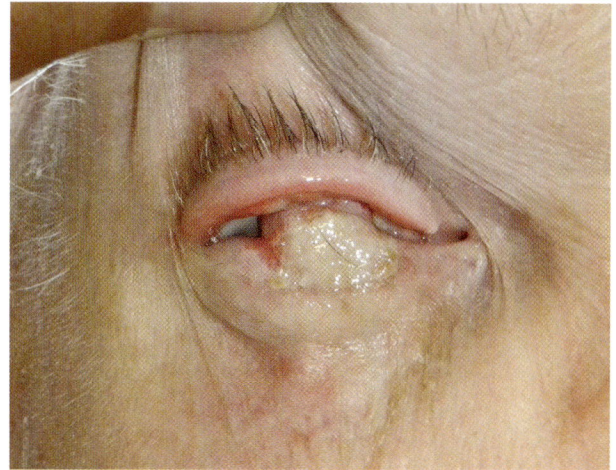

FIGURE 81.29 Hughes Stage II. Appearance six weeks after first stage reconstruction with a Hughes flap. Notice how the margin of keratinized epithelium has migrated proximally on the flap.

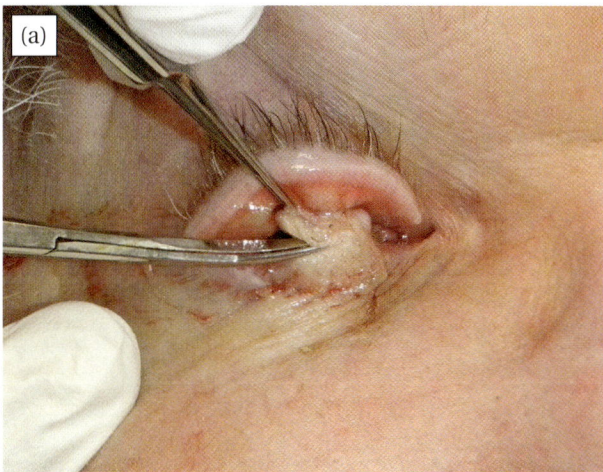

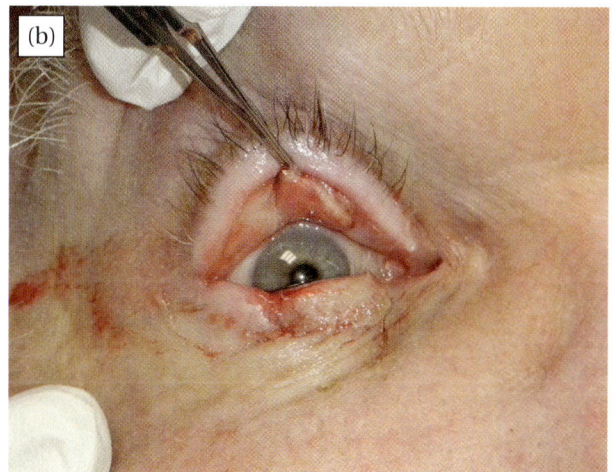

FIGURE 81.30 (a) The Hughes flap is released just slightly above the planned eyelid margin. With further healing, the flap contracts to be in line with the native eyelid margin. (Some surgeons prefer to release the flap from its origin prior to determining the position of the new margin.) (b) The remaining proximal portion of the flap is severed from the upper eyelid and hemostasis achieved with cautery.

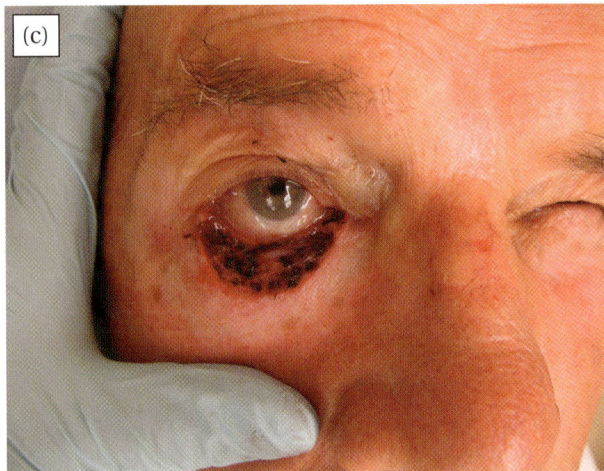

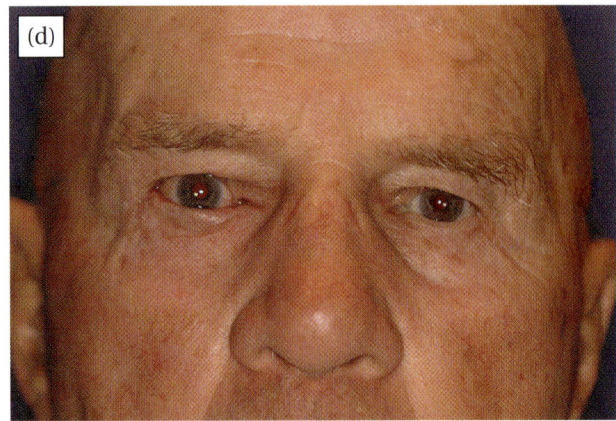

FIGURE 81.30 (*continued*) (c) Patient with total right lower lid defect following Mohs surgery. (d) Patient following right lower lid reconstruction with Hughes procedure. (Images c and d courtesy Mark J. Lucarelli, MD.)

TABLE 81.8 *Hewes Tarsoconjunctival Rotational Flap*

Preoperative Considerations

Can the posterior lamella be reconstructed with a periosteal flap from the lateral orbital rim?

Is there sufficient redundancy in the ipsilateral upper eyelid for reconstruction of the anterior lamella, or is a full-thickness skin graft required?

Useful when lid sharing procedures are to be avoided.

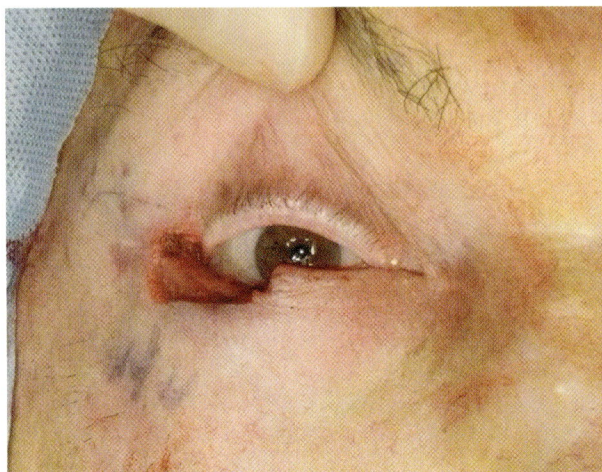

FIGURE 81.31 Full-thickness defect of the right lateral lower eyelid including the canthus, with no residual of eyelid laterally.

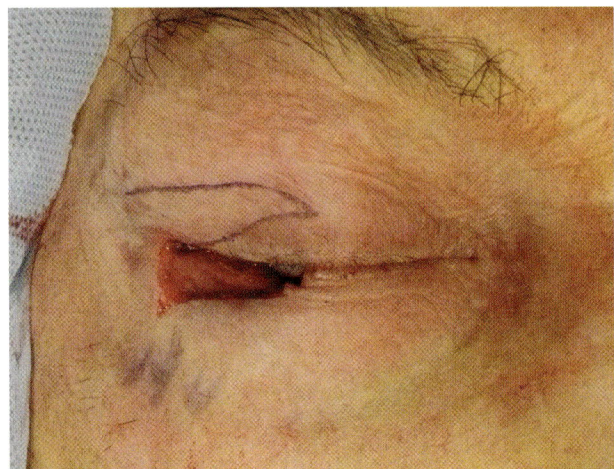

FIGURE 81.32 The anterior lamella is reconstructed with a Tripier flap, which is a myocutaneous transposition flap from the upper eyelid.

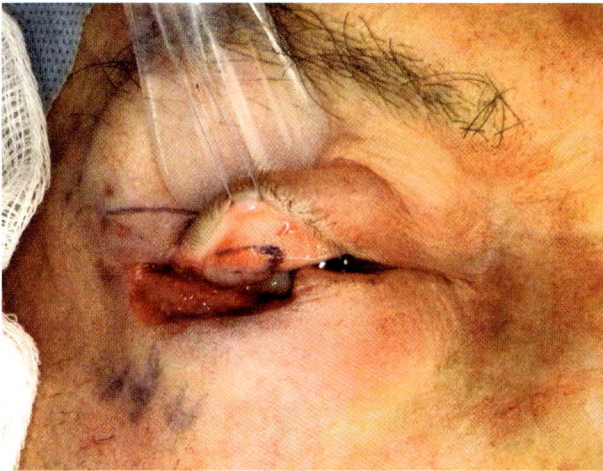

FIGURE 81.33 The posterior lamella is reconstructed with the Hewes flap, a tarsoconjunctival transposition flap with a laterally based pedicle. At least 4 mm of vertical tarsal height should remain in the upper eyelid centrally.

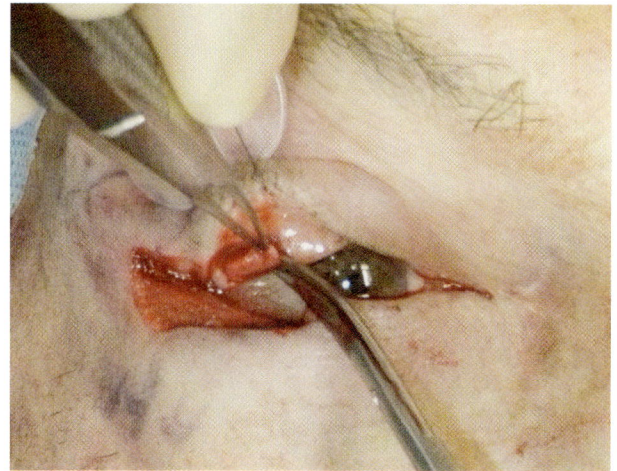

FIGURE 81.34 The flap is elevated with sharp dissection, taking care to presevere its laterally hinged base.

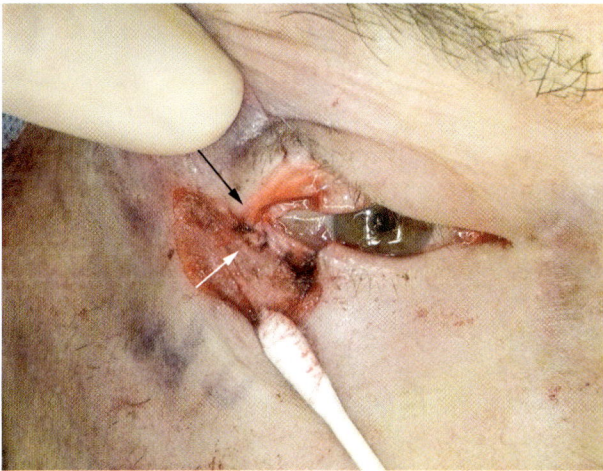

FIGURE 81.35 The flap is secured to the recipient defect with 5-0 or 6-0 polyglactin sutures. To reconstitute support laterally, the Hewes flap is secured to the remnant of the lateral canthal tendon (white arrow). A thin bridge of conjunctiva from the lateral upper eyelid should be de-epithelialized (black arrow).

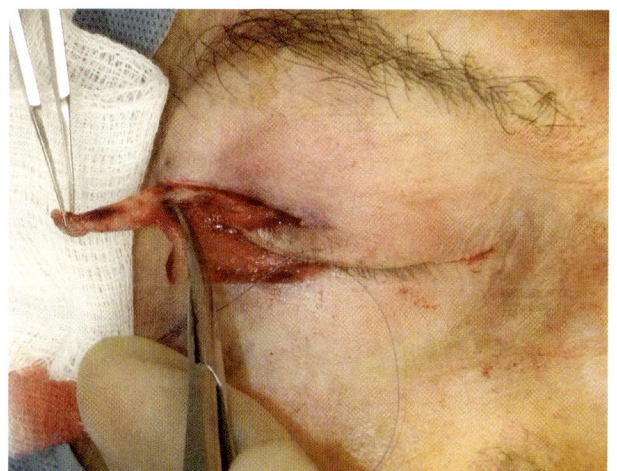

FIGURE 81.36 The Tripier flap is then elevated in the suborbicularis plane.

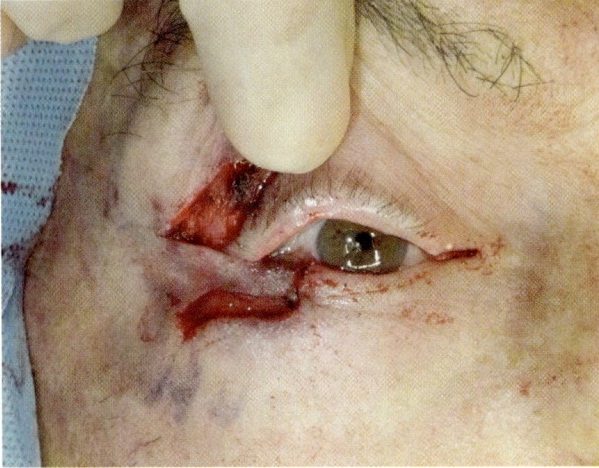

FIGURE 81.37 The Tripier flap is trimmed and transposed to fill the cutaneous defect. The skin can be closed with fine absorbable or non-absorbable sutures. A single interupted 6-0 plain gut suture is used to define the new lateral commissure.

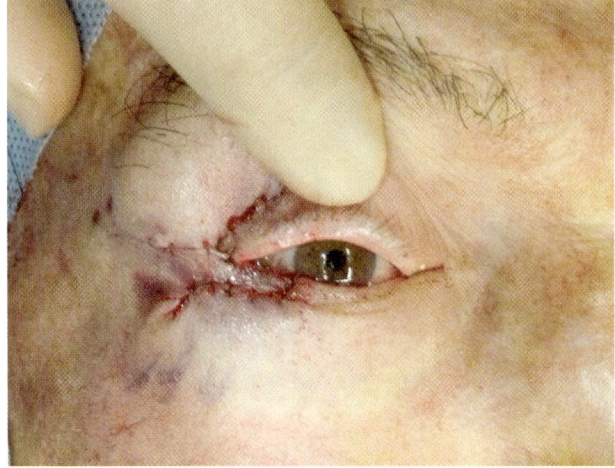

FIGURE 81.38 Appearance immediately following reconstruction with Hewes tarsoconjunctival flap.

TABLE 81.9 *Cutler-Beard Tarsoconjunctival Interpolation Flap for Upper Lid Defects*

Preoperative Considerations

Can the patient tolerate occlusion of the ipsilateral eye until division of the flap in the second stage?

Consider donor autologous cartilage as a tarsal substitute when much of the tarsus is missing. Alloplastic dermal matrix may be used as well.

Contralateral free tarsal grafts are limited by the size of the graft available.

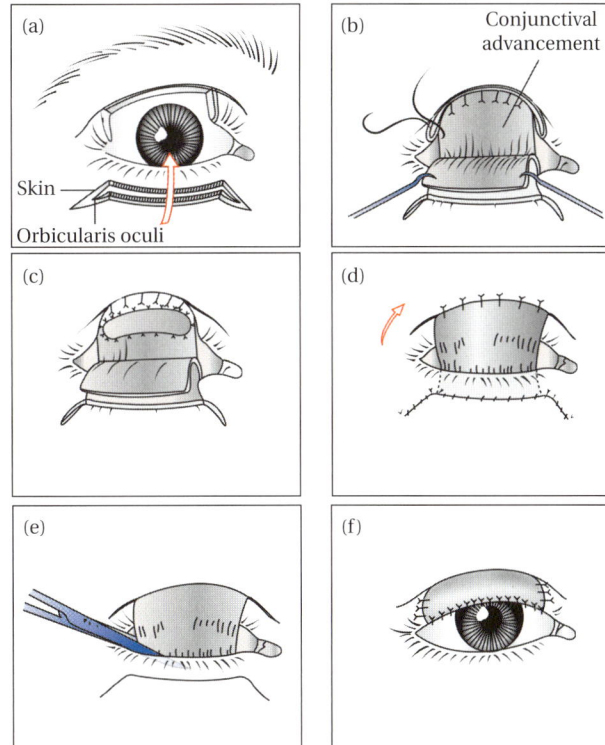

FIGURE 81.39 Large full-thickness defects of the upper eyelid can be closed with a Cutler-Beard flap, a cross-eyelid flap advanced under a bridge of intact lower eyelid margin. (a) A full-thickness transverse blepharotomy is made 5–6 mm below the eyelid margin, leaving the lower palpebral arcade intact. Relaxing incisions are made extending inferiorly. (b, c) The flap is split between the conjunctiva and the lower lid retractors to prepare a bed for a free graft with contralateral tarsus, cartilage, or alloplastic dermal matrix. (d) The anterior layer of the flap is draped over the free graft and secured to approximate the defect. (e, f) At 4–6 weeks, the flap is divided, the eyelid margin contoured, and the donor site in the lower eyelid reconstructed as needed. (Adapted from Basic and Clinical Science Course Section 7, American Academy of Ophthalmology, San Francisco, CA 2003:186)

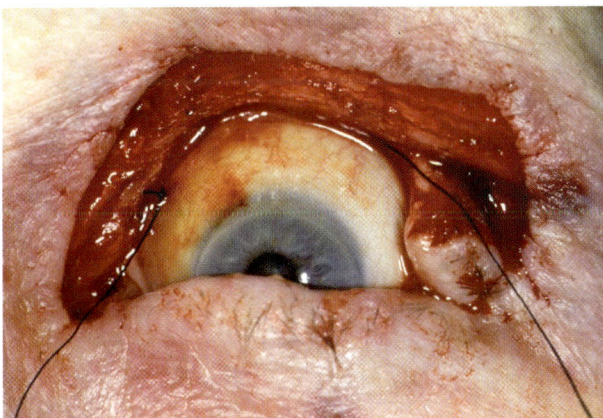

FIGURE 81.40 Culter-Beard Stage I. Near total full-thickness defect of the left upper eyelid. Some residual eyelid is present laterally.

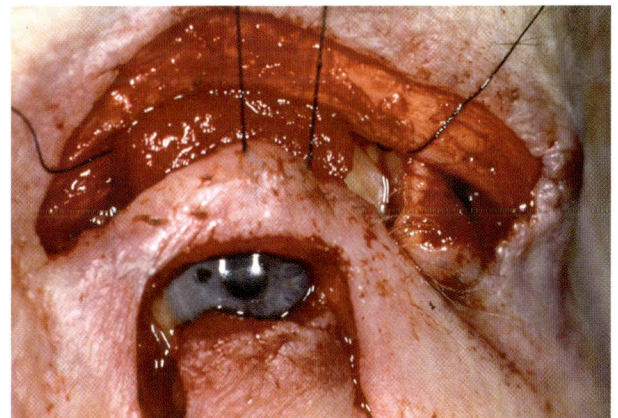

FIGURE 81.41 A full-thickness transverse blepharotomy with relaxing incisions is made to develop the Cutler-Beard flap. The transverse incision is made below the vascular arcade, so as to preserve perfusion to the marginal bridge.

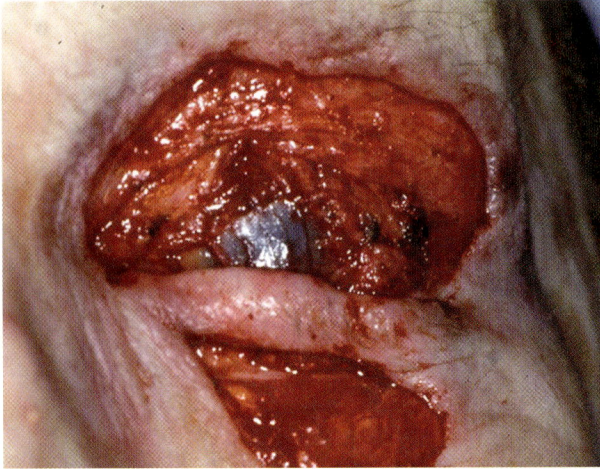

FIGURE 81.42 The flap is split between the conjunctiva and the retractors. The posterior component is advanced to close the defect. It is secured with running 6-0 plain gut sutures. The anterior layer of the flap is reflected inferiorly here.

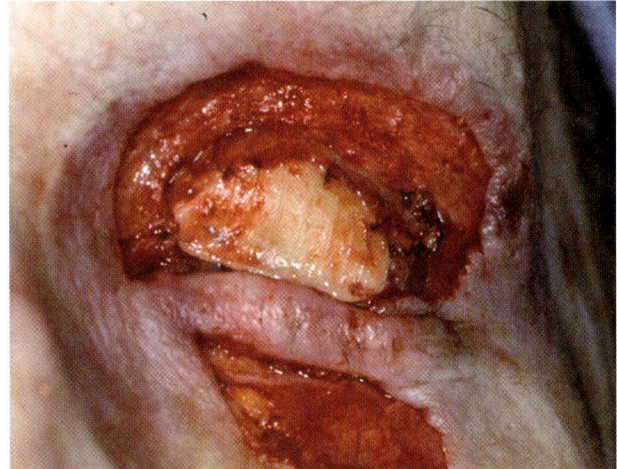

FIGURE 81.43 A free cartilage graft is fashioned and secured superiorly to the residual levator aponeurosis, laterally to the tarsal edge, and medially to the medial canthal tendon, with interrupted partial thickness 6-0 polyglactin sutures.

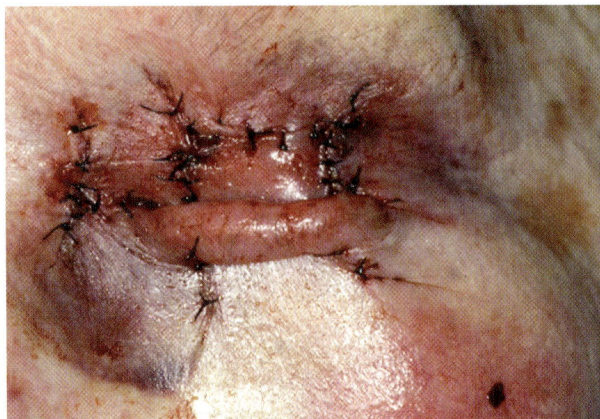

FIGURE 81.44 Appearance at the conclusion of first stage reconstruction. The anterior layer of the flap has been advanced under the lower marginal bridge and secured with 5-0 polyglactin sutures and 6-0 silk sutures.

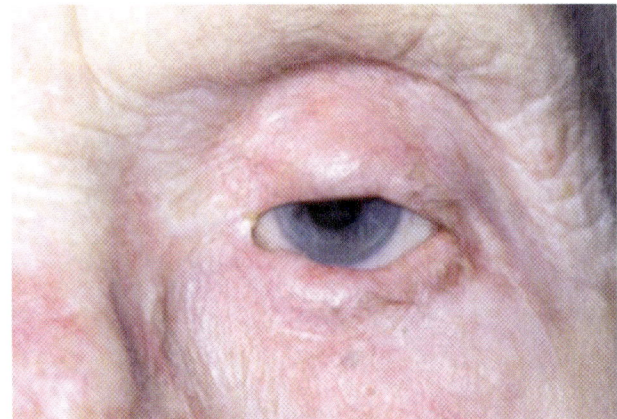

FIGURE 81.45 Cutler-Beard Stage II. Appearance two months following second stage division of the Cutler-Beard flap.

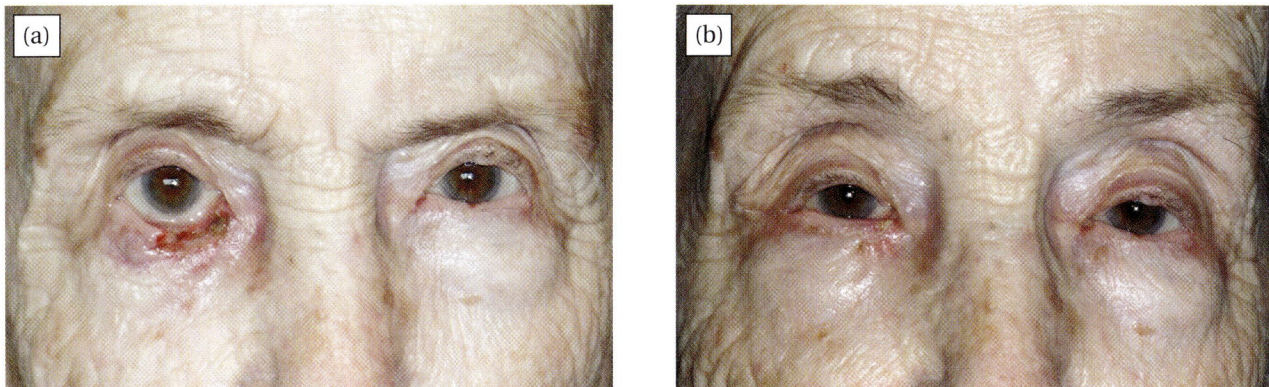

FIGURE 81.46   (a, b) Before and after color photos of patient who underwent right lower lid reconstruction with a Tenzel semicircular flap.

TABLE 81.10   *Complications of Eyelid Reconstruction*

Wound dehiscence
Partial or complete flap/graft loss
Eyelid retraction or malposition
Impaired eyelid movement
Lagophthalmos
Ptosis

SELECTED REFERENCES

Cutler NL, Beard C. A method for partial and total upper lid reconstruction. *Am J Ophthalmol.* 1955 Jan;39(1):1–7.

Fischer, T., Noever, G., Langer, M., & Kammer, E. (2001). Experience in upper eyelid reconstruction with the Cutler-Beard technique. *Ann Plast Surg.* 47(3):338–342.

Hewes EH, Sullivan JH, Beard C: Lower eyelid reconstruction by tarsal transposition. *Am J Ophthalmol.* 1976;81:512–514.

Hughes WL. A new method for rebuilding a lower lid: Report of a case. *Arch Ophthalmol.* 1937;17:1008.

Leone CR Jr. Periosteal flap for lower eyelid reconstruction. *Am J Ophthalmol.* 1992 Oct 15;114(4):513–514.

Lowry JC, Bartley GB, Garrity JA. The role of second-intention healing in periocular reconstruction. *Ophthalmol Plast Reconstr Surg.* 1997 Sep;13(3):174–188.

Rohrich RJ, Zbar RI. The evolution of the Hughes tarsoconjunctival flap for the lower eyelid reconstruction. *Plast Reconstr Surg.* 1999 Aug;104(2):518–522.

Tenzel RR, Stewart WB: Eyelid reconstruction by the semi-circle flap technique. *Ophthalmology.* 1978;85: 1164–1169.

Management of Oculofacial Dystonias

Michael T. Yen, MD

TABLE 82.1 *Indications for Botulinum Toxin Injections*

TABLE 82.1 *Indications for Botulinum Toxin Injections*

- Uncontrolled eyelid or facial spasms
- Inadequate relief with oral or other noninvasive therapies
- In patients with hemifacial spasm who are unwilling or unable to undergo surgical decompression of the facial nerve root

TABLE 82.2 *Indications for Protractor Myectomy*

- Uncontrolled eyelid or facial spasms
- Inadequate response to botulinum toxin injections and/or oral medications
- Unable or unwilling to undergo serial injections with botulinum toxin
- Presence of eyelid malpositions requiring surgical correction

TABLE 82.3 *Preoperative Considerations*

- Inject botulinum toxin at lowest dose and with longest interval between injections
- Consider upper eyelid myectomy and corrugator excision if patient has some response to botulinum toxin
- Consider upper and lower eyelid myectomy if patient truly unresponsive to botulinum toxin
- Address eyelid malpositions concurrently at the time of surgical myectomy
- Avoid anticoagulation prior to surgery to minimize risk of hematoma formation

Botulinum Toxin Injections

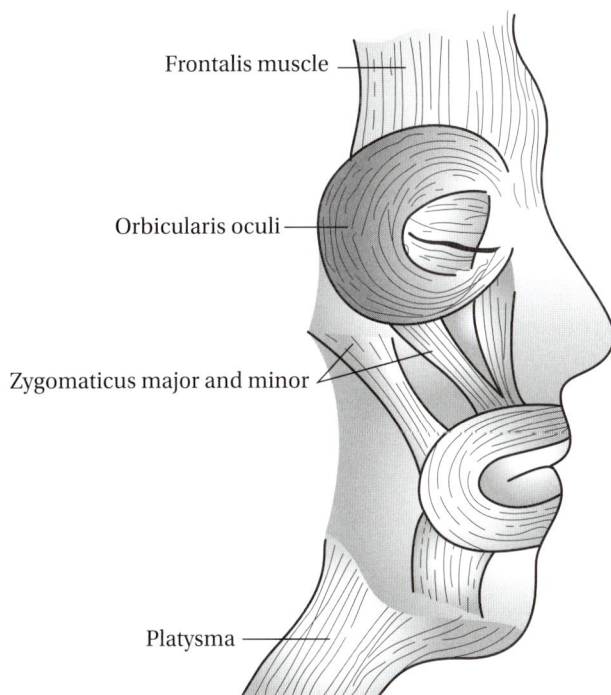

FIGURE 82.1 Anatomy of pertinent facial muscles of expression.

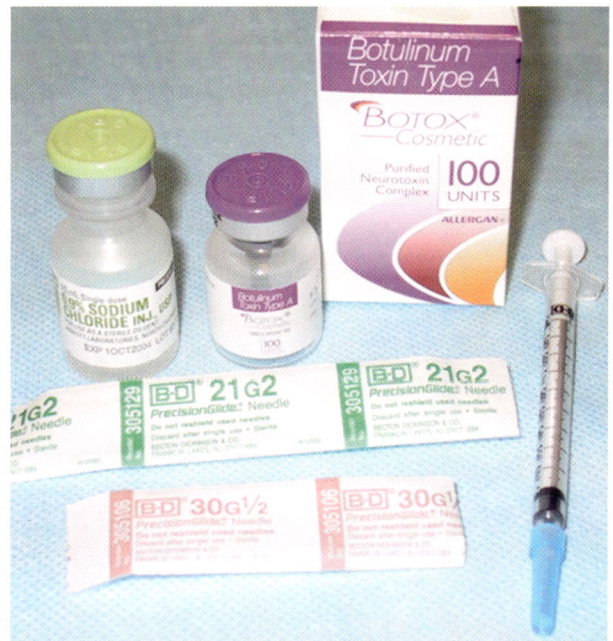

FIGURE 82.2 Supplies needed for botulinum toxin injection include syringe, needles, and normal saline for injection.

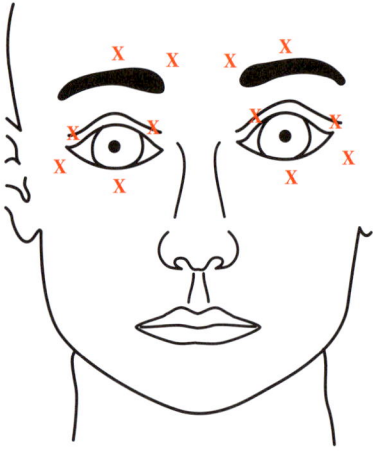

FIGURE 82.3 Schematic for injection of blepharospasm. The central upper eyelid is avoided to minimize the risk of levator palpebrae muscle paralysis. The medial lower eyelid is avoided to minimize the risk of inferior oblique paralysis. Two injections in the corrugator provide additional protractor weakening.

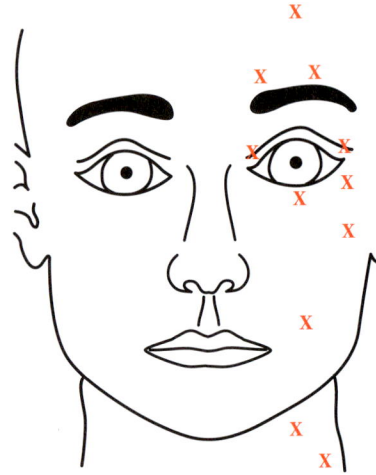

FIGURE 82.4 Schematic for injection of hemifacial spasm. In addition to injections in the corrugator and orbicularis muscles, the zygomaticus major and minor, frontalis, and platysma may also be treated. Special care must be taken when injecting the zygomaticus major and minor to avoid drooping of the oral commissure and the lateral upper lip.

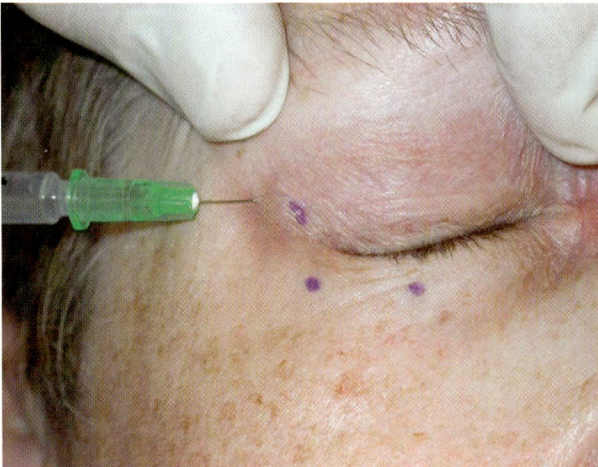

FIGURE 82.5 Injection of botulinum toxin to the eyelids should be very superficial, just below the skin surface.

Eyelid Myectomy

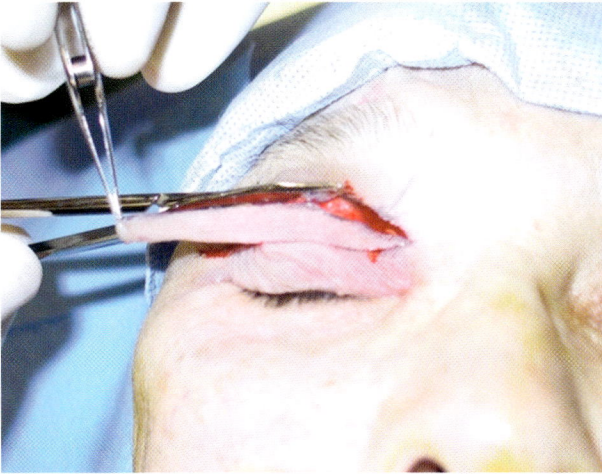

FIGURE 82.6 Upper eyelid myectomy. A standard blepharoplasty is used with excision of a skin and orbicularis muscle flap.

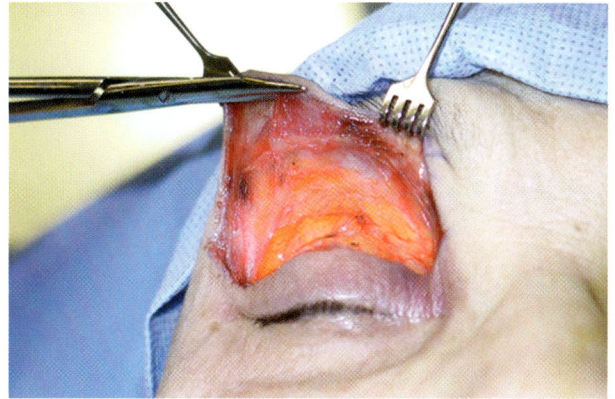

FIGURE 82.7 While elevating the skin above the eyelid crease incision, the orbicularis muscle is dissected away from the overlying skin.

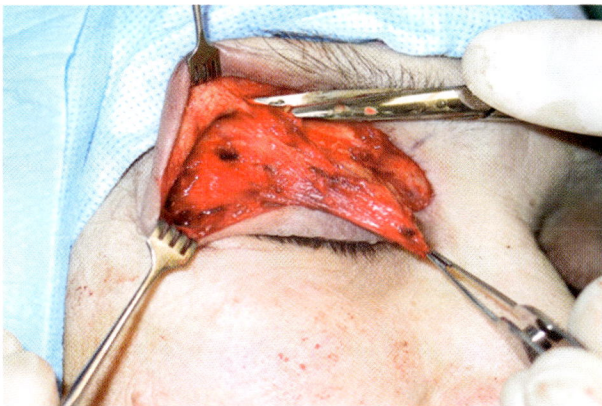

FIGURE 82.8 The orbicularis oculi muscle is dissected from the overlying skin, up underneath the brow, and extending from medial canthus to lateral canthus.

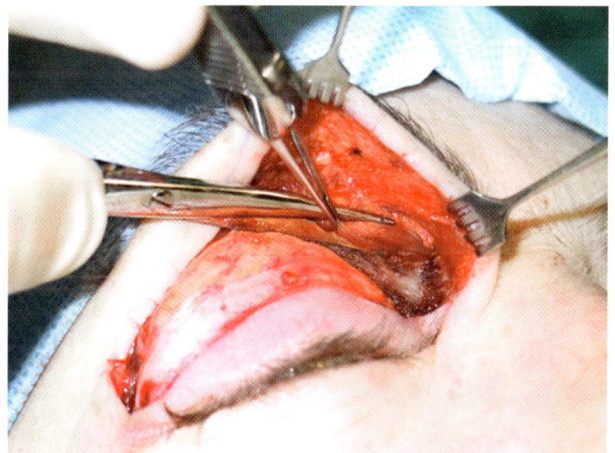

FIGURE 82.9 Once the orbicularis oculi muscle has been excised, the corrugator muscle can be identified and excised.

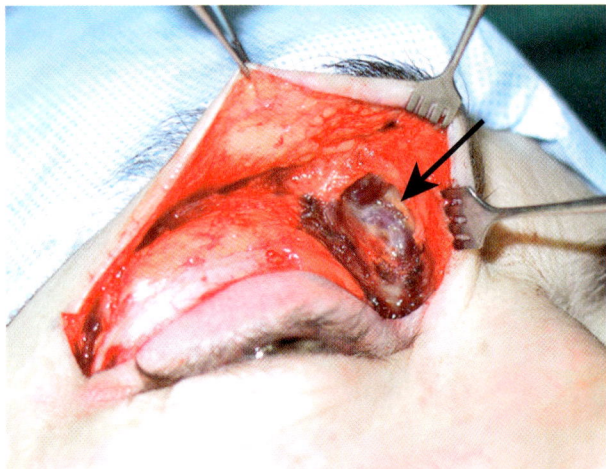

FIGURE 82.10 Caution should be used when excising the corrugator muscle, as the supraorbital vascular structures (arrowhead) are located just posterior to the muscle.

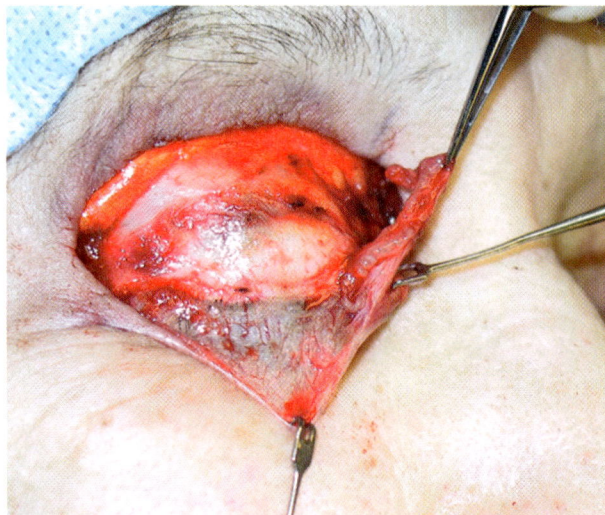

FIGURE 82.11 Using a similar technique, the pretarsal orbicularis oculi muscle is dissected away from the overlying skin, inferior from the eyelid crease incision to the eyelid margin.

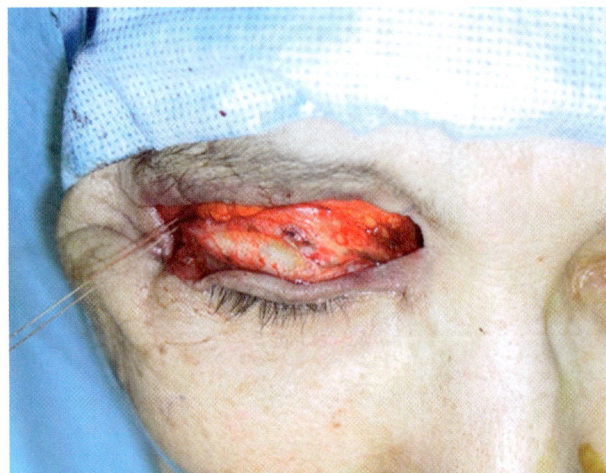

FIGURE 82.12 If necessary, a lateral canthopexy should be performed to correct horizontal phimosis.

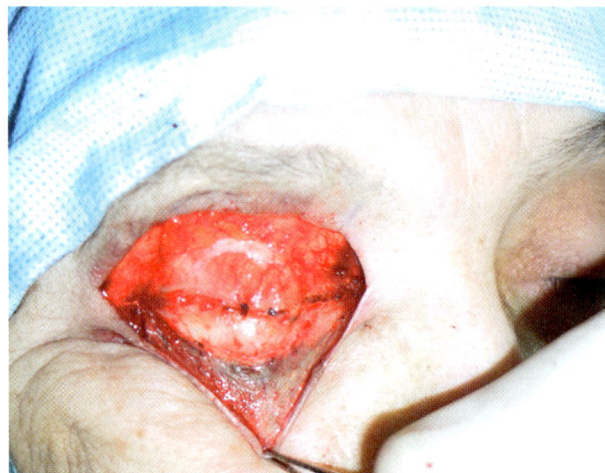

FIGURE 82.13 Levator aponeurosis advancement can also be performed to correct blepharoptosis.

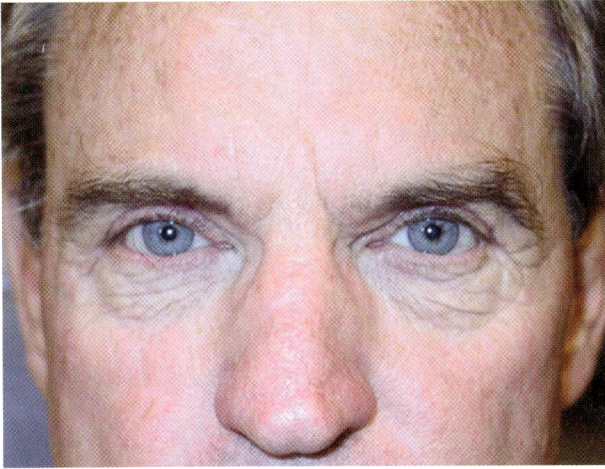

FIGURE 82.14 One month postoperative. This patient has some contour asymmetry of the upper eyelid, but otherwise has a good appearance and excellent control of his eyelid spasms after upper eyelid myectomy.

TABLE 82.4 *Potential Complications of Botulinum Toxin Injections*

- Inadequate dosage may lead to suboptimal response
- Excessive dosage may lead to temporary lagophthalmos and dry eyes
- Upper eyelid ptosis
- Diplopia

TABLE 82.5 *Potential Complications of Eyelid Myectomy*

- Eyelid retraction
- Lagophthalmos
- Dry eye
- Chronic lymphedema
- Contour deformities due to debulking of muscle
- Necrosis or atrophy of eyelid skin

SELECTED REFERENCES

Anderson RL, Patel BCK, Holds JB, Jordan DR. Blepharospasm: past, present, and future. *Ophthal Plast Reconstr Surg.* 1998;14:305–317.

Callahan A. Blepharospasm with resection of part of the orbicularis nerve supply. *Arch Ophthalmol.* 1963;70:508–511.

Frueh BR, Musch DC, Bersani TA. Effects of eyelid protractor excision for the treatment of benign essential blepharospasm. *Am J Ophthalmol.* 1992;113:681–686.

Gillum WN, Anderson RL. Blepharospasm surgery. *Arch Ophthalmol.* 1981;99:1056–1062.

Jankovic J, Schwartz K. Response and immunoresistance to botulinum toxin injections. *Neurology.* 1995;45:1743–1746.

Lucci LM, Yen MT, Anderson RL, Hwang IP, Black RE. Orbicularis myectomy with levator advancement in Schwartz-Jampel syndrome. *Am J Ophthalmol.* 2001;132:799–801.

McCord CD, Coles WH, Shore JW, et al. Treatment of essential blepharospasm: comparison of facial nerve avulsion and eyebrow-eyelid muscle stripping procedure. *Arch Ophthalmol.* 1984;102:266–273.

Scott AB, Kennedy RA, Stubbs HA. Botulinum-A toxin injection as a treatment for blepharospasm. *Arch Ophthalmol.* 1985;103:347–350.

Yen MT, Anderson RL. Orbicularis oculi muscle graft augmentation after protractor myectomy in blepharospasm. *Ophthal Plast Reconstr Surg.* 2003;19:287–296.

83 Enucleation

Philip L. Custer, MD and Adam G. Buchanan, MD

TABLE 83.1 *Indications*

Blind painful eye

Recent trauma with total vision loss and risk of sympathetic ophthalmia

Advanced endophthalmitis

Intraocular tumor

Phthisical globe with cosmetic deformity

TABLE 83.2 *Preoperative Considerations*

Evisceration is avoided when the risk of sympathetic ophthalmia is of significant concern, or when intraocular tumor cannot be ruled out.

Preserve conjunctiva and fornices for future prosthesis fitting.

Restore adequate orbital volume with appropriate implant.

Good layered closure to prevent implant migration/exposure.

Promote motility of implant-prosthesis unit.

Implant Materials

1. Nonporous spherical implants made from inert materials such as silicone, acrylic, or PMMA may be used in cases at high risk of infection with porous implants.

2. Hydroxyapatite is an inorganic salt of calcium phosphate used in buried integrated orbital implants. Its porous form is similar to human cancellous bone, with interconnecting canals approximately 500 microns in size.

3. Porous polyethylene implant with an interconnecting pore structure greater than 150 microns. The open and multidirectional pore structure allows ingrowth of the patient's tissues and vascular network. Many surgeons choose to wrap the anterior surface with banked sclera or fascia.

Enucleation Technique

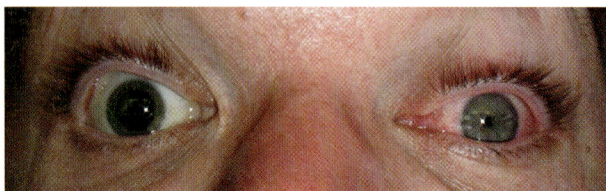

FIGURE 83.1   A preoperative phenylephrine drop "marks" the operative eye by dilation and constricts conjunctival blood vessels to limit hemorrhage during peritomy. Pathologic findings are visualized and confirmed before proceeding with surgery.

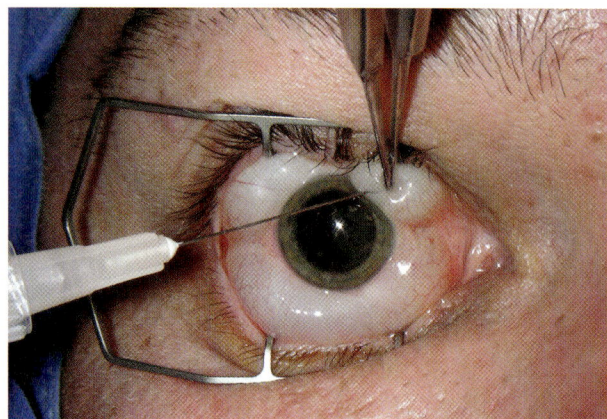

FIGURE 83.2   Subconjunctival anesthesia is administered with a combination of short- and long-acting local anesthetics with epinephrine.

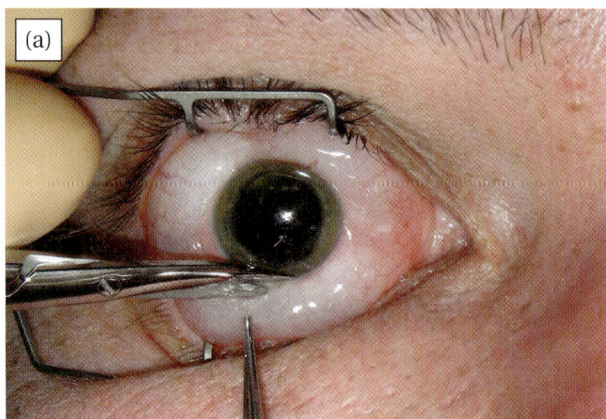

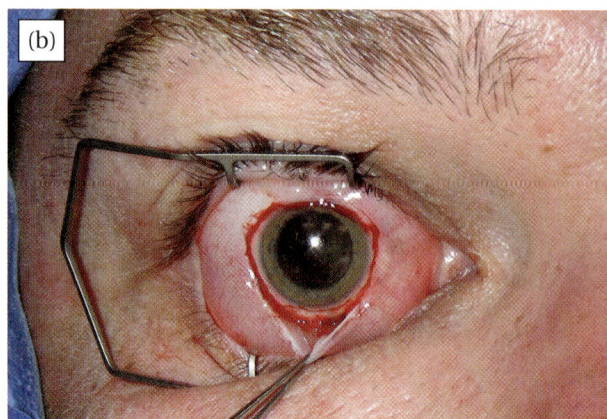

FIGURES 83.3   (a, b) A 360-degree limbal peritomy is performed with Westcott scissors, taking care to preserve all viable conjunctiva and Tenon's fascia.

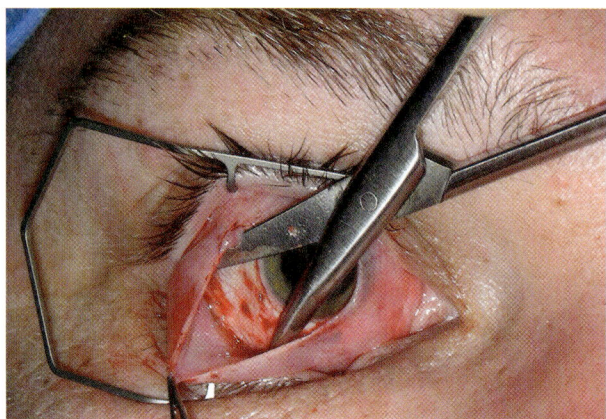

FIGURE 83.4   The four quadrants are cleared in a subTenon's plane by spreading with blunt tip scissors.

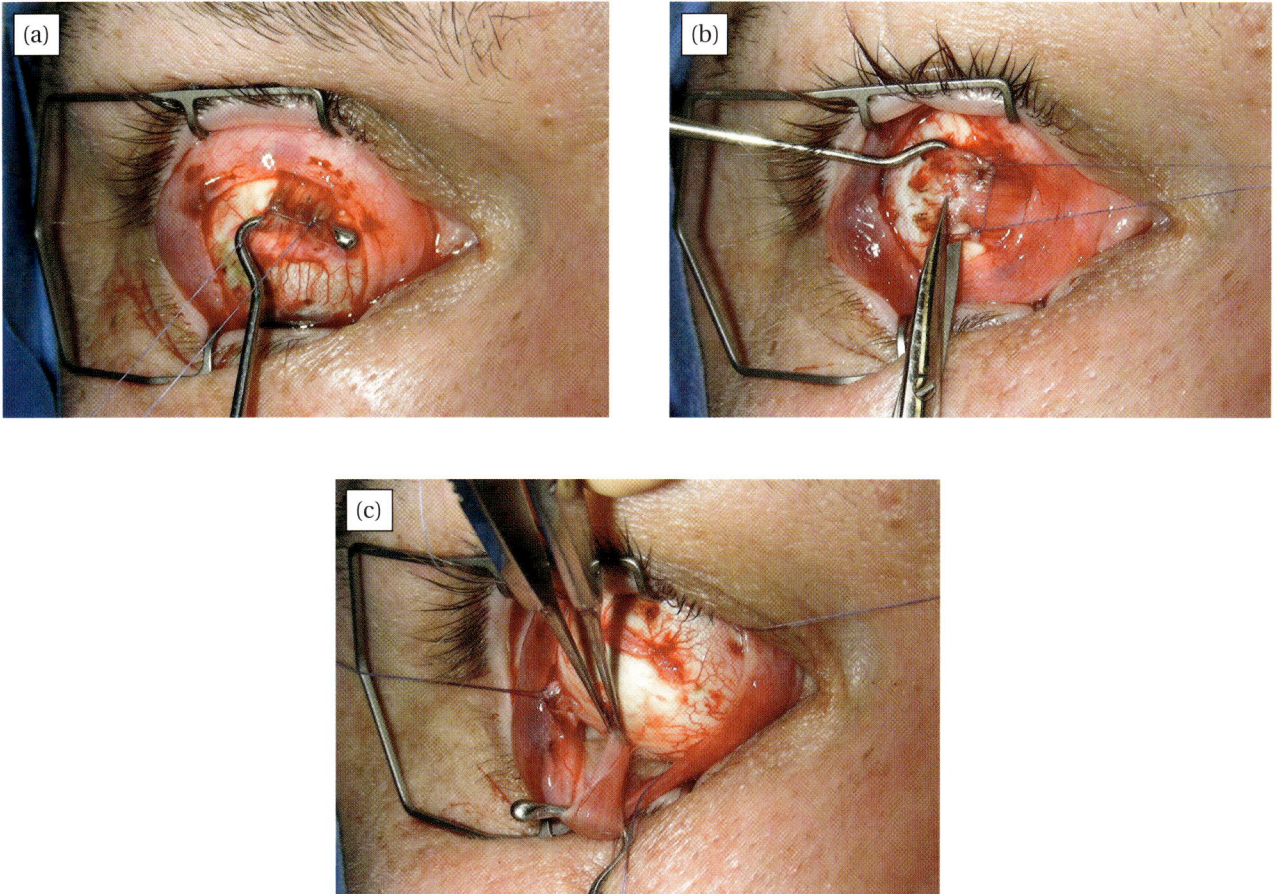

FIGURES 83.5 (a, b, c) The horizontal and vertical rectus muscles are isolated with muscle hooks and secured with double-armed 6-0 polyglactin sutures prior to disinsertion from the globe. A locking bite on the muscle is recommended. If desired, the inferior and superior oblique muscles may be isolated in a similar fashion and tagged with sutures if they are to be reattached to the implant.

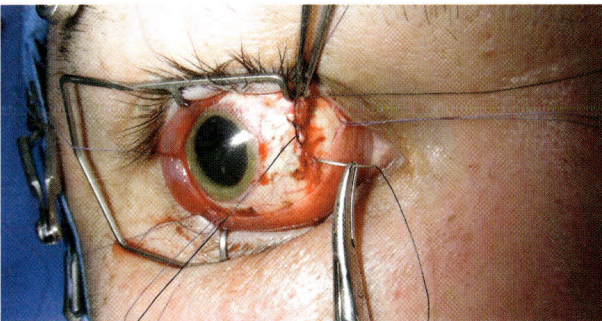

FIGURE 83.6 Silk traction sutures are woven through the medial and lateral rectus muscle stumps to facilitate manipulation of the globe.

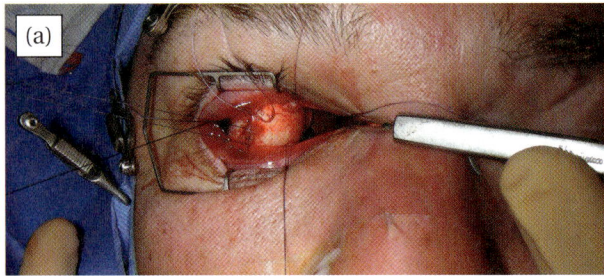

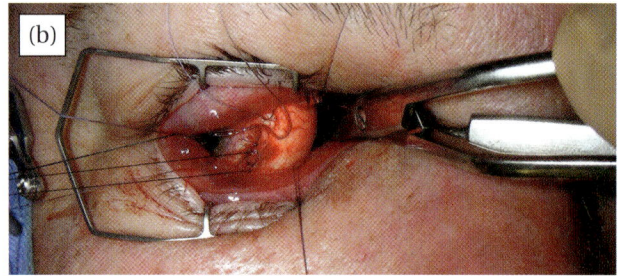

FIGURES 83.7 (a, b) An enucleation "spoon" retractor is placed nasally to aid in visualization. The spoon is best used to protect and retract the orbital soft tissues posteriorly, thereby facilitating direct visualization of the optic nerve. Once all soft tissue attachments to the globe have been lysed, and after careful efforts at hemostasis, including bipolar cautery to the optic nerve sheath, the optic nerve is transected with blunt, curved enucleation scissors.

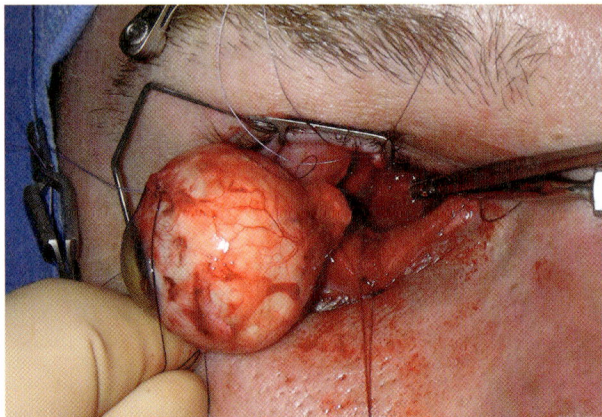

FIGURE 83.8 Gross appearance of removed globe with stump of optic nerve.

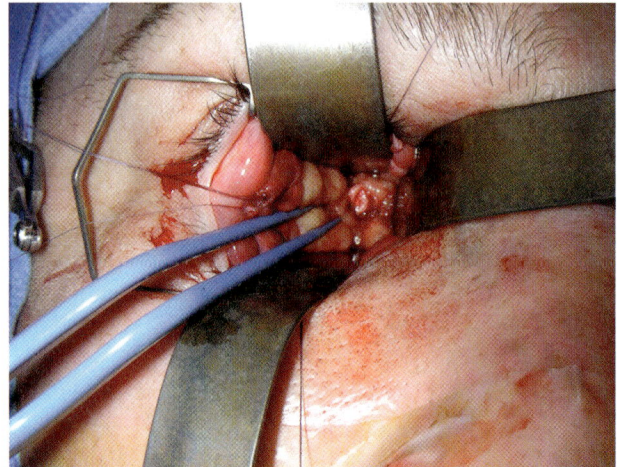

FIGURE 83.9 Cautery of the optic nerve stump, using a bipolar bayonet forceps, may be necessary to limit hemorrhage and prevent hematoma formation.

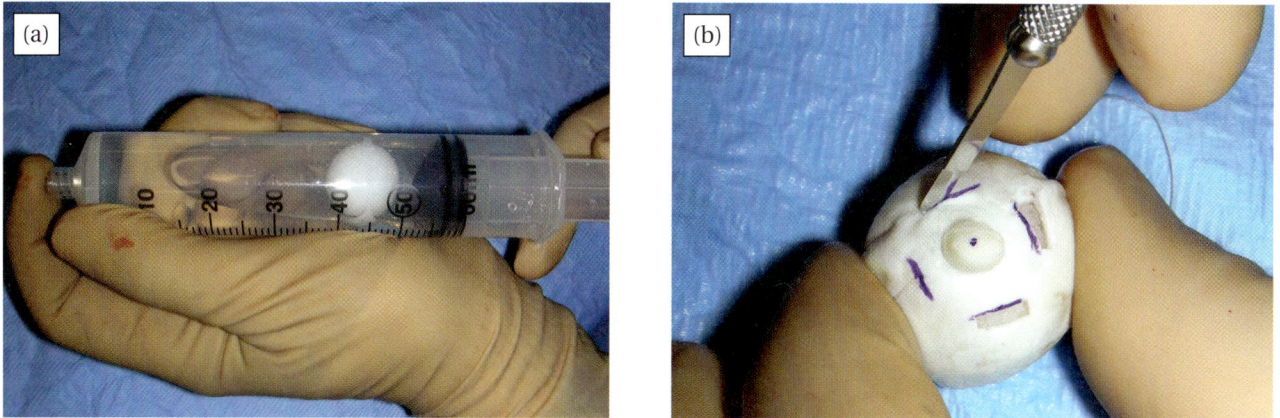

FIGURE 83.10   (a, b) A porous polyethylene implant is prepared by soaking in a dilute gentamicin solution (note use of syringe to create negative pressure, saturating the porous spaces with the solution), and suturing a donor scleral wrap. The posterior aspect of the spherical implant is left open to enhance vascularization. Slots or windows may be cut into the wrap anteriorly to facilitate anatomic placement of the extraocular muscles and vascular ingrowth.

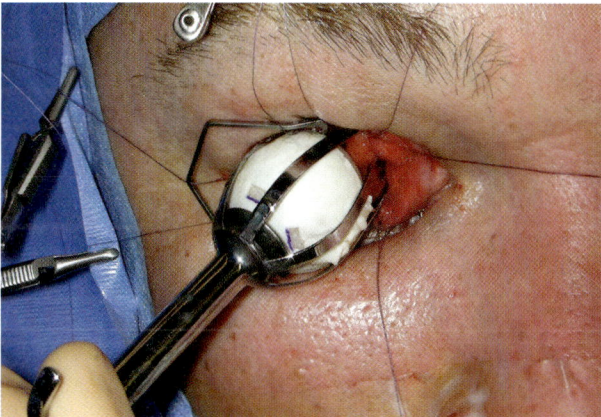

FIGURE 83.11 The implant is inserted deep into the intraconal space using a metal Carter sphere introducer or plastic tube inserter.

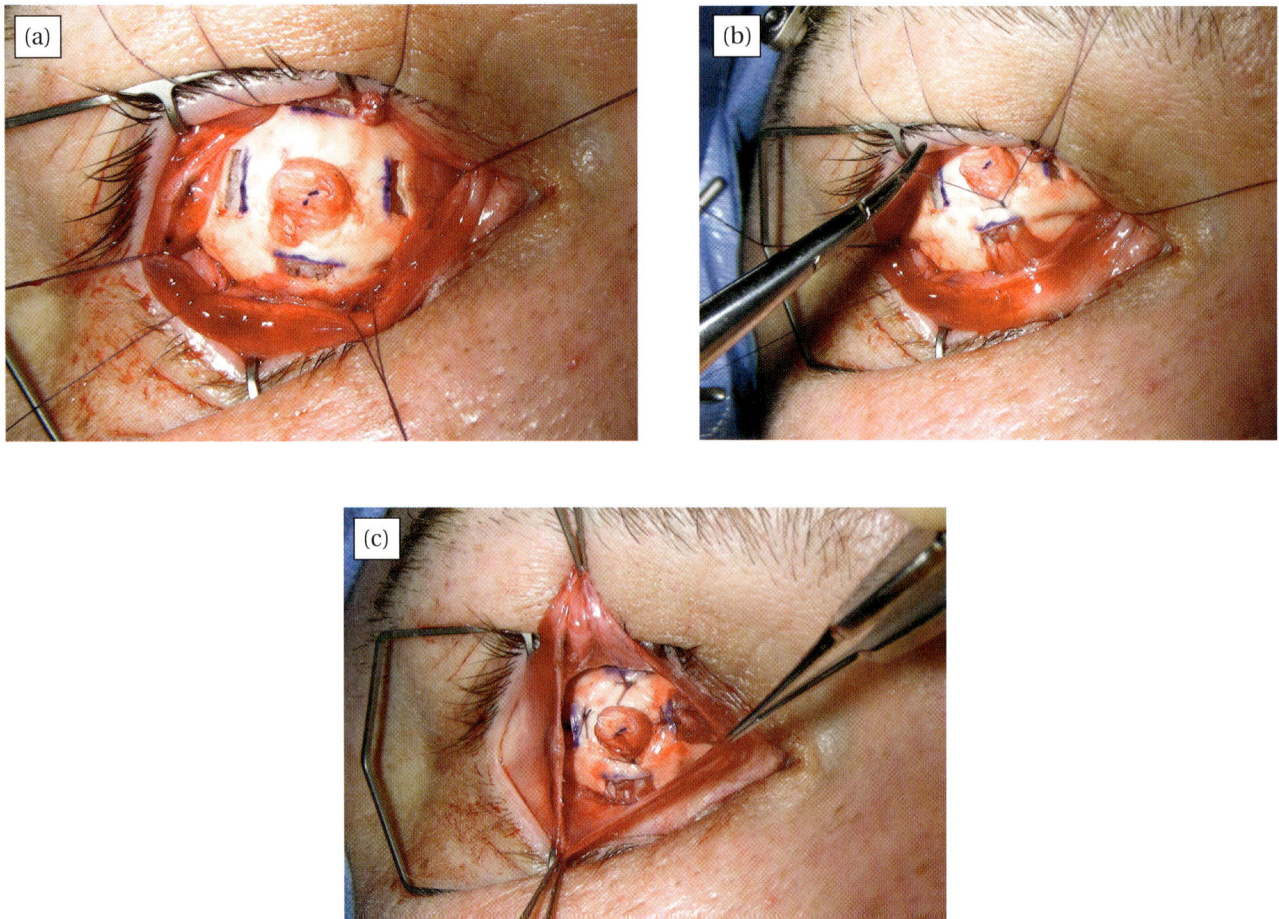

FIGURES 83.12 (a, b, c) The rectus muscles are sutured to the sclerotomies using the double-armed 6-0 polyglactin sutures. The inferior oblique may be re-approximated to its anatomical position with the thought that anatomic attachment of the inferior oblique may help maintain the inferior fornix.

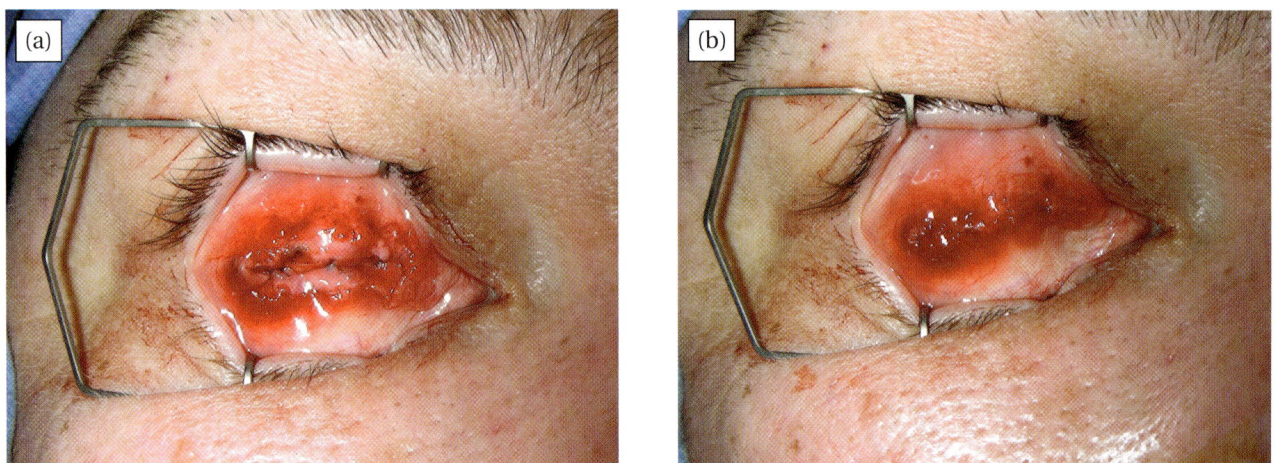

FIGURES 83.13 (a, b) Tenon's fascia is closed in two layers with deep interrupted and a more superficial running 6-0 polyglactin sutures. Conjunctiva is sutured with a running 7-0 chromic suture.

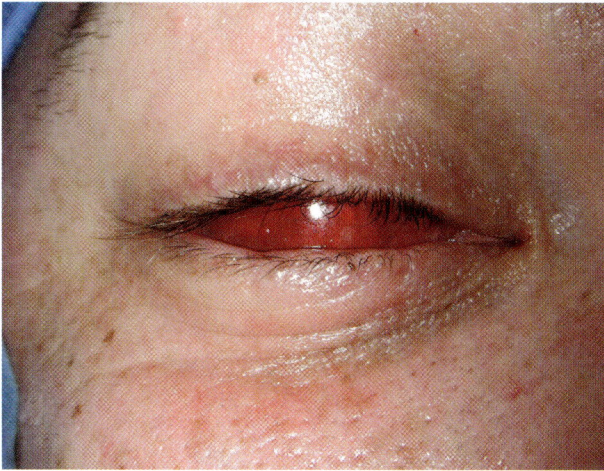

FIGURE 83.14 An appropriately sized plastic conformer is placed to maintain the conjunctival fornices. In cases with conjuctival chemosis, a temporary tarsorrhaphy may be placed to facilitate conformer retention.

TABLE 83.3 *Complications*

Removal of wrong eye

Orbital hemorrhage

Orbital volume deficit

Conjunctival loss with shortened fornices

Implant migration, exposure, or extrusion

Infection of orbit or implant

Socket contraction

Eyelid malposition (i.e., ptosis or ectropion)

Poor prosthesis fit

SELECTED REFERENCES

Custer PL, Trinkaus KM. Porous implant exposure: incidence, management, and morbidity. *Ophthal Plast Reconstr Surg.* 2007;23:1–7.

Kaltreider SA, Lucarelli MJ. A simple algorithm for selection of implant size for enucleation and evisceration. *Ophthal Plast Reconstr Surg.* 2002;18:336–341.

Massry GG, Holds JB. Evisceration with scleral modification. *Ophthal Plast Reconstr Surg.* 2001;17:42–47.

Migliori ME. Enucleation versus evisceration. *Curr Opin Ophthal.* 2002;13:298–302.

Moshfeghi DM, Moshfeghi AA, Finger PT. Enucleation. *Surv Ophthalmol.* 2000;44:277–301.

Sami D, Young S, Petersen R. Perspective on orbital enucleation implants. *Surv Ophthalmol.* 2007;52:244–265.

84 Evisceration

Brenda L. Bohnsack, MD, PhD, Christine C. Nelson, MD, FACS
and Alon Kahana MD, PhD

Preoperative Evaluation

Surgical Procedure

Complications

SELECTED REFERENCES

Preoperative Evaluation

TABLE 84.1 *Indications for Evisceration*

- Blind, painful eyes in which removal of the sclera is not indicated.
- Requires **<u>complete</u>** preoperative evaluation of the globe, including **<u>imaging</u>**, to assess for occult intraocular tumors (Eagle et al., 2009; Perry et al., 2009; Rosner 2009; Kahana and Dutton, 2010).
- Advantages over enucleation:
  - Orbital stability—minimal risk of implant exposure/extrusion with the transscleral approach
  - Implant motility
  - Psychologically easier on patients than enucleation
  - Faster
  - Easier to perform under local anesthesia

TABLE 84.2 *Preoperative Considerations*

- Traditional surgery placed the orbital implant within the scleral shell.
- Long et al. described a modification that placed larger orbital implants behind the posterior sclera and created a more secure double-layered closure, allowing for better volume replacement (see References). This technique has been used successfully by the senior authors for years and is described below.

Surgical Procedure

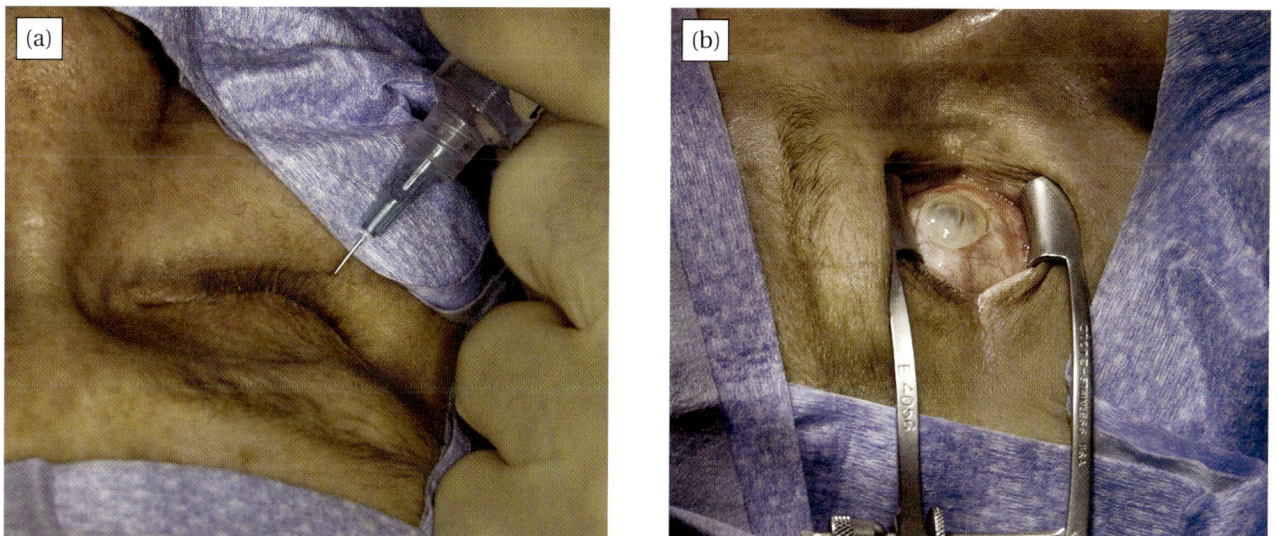

FIGURE 84.1 (a) Local anesthetic (a mixture of 1% lidocaine and 0.25% bupivacaine with 1:100,000 dilution of epinephrine) is given in a retrobulbar fashion. (b) A lid retractor is placed in the palpebral fissure to expose the globe.

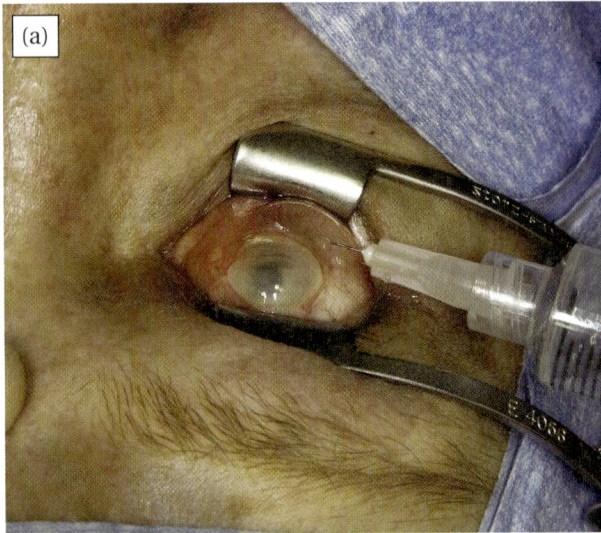

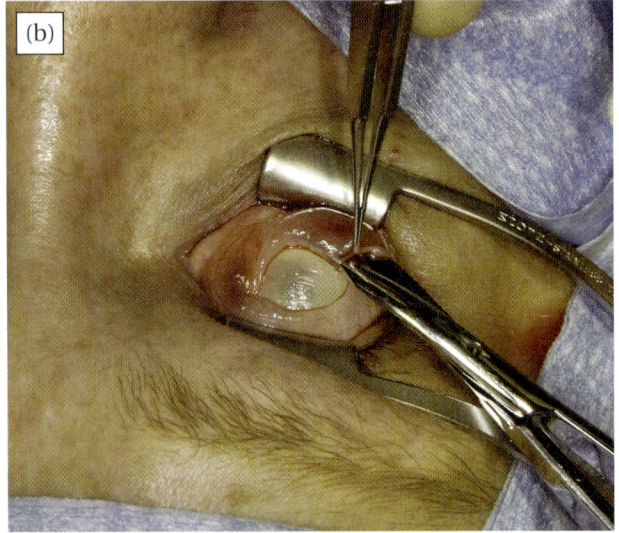

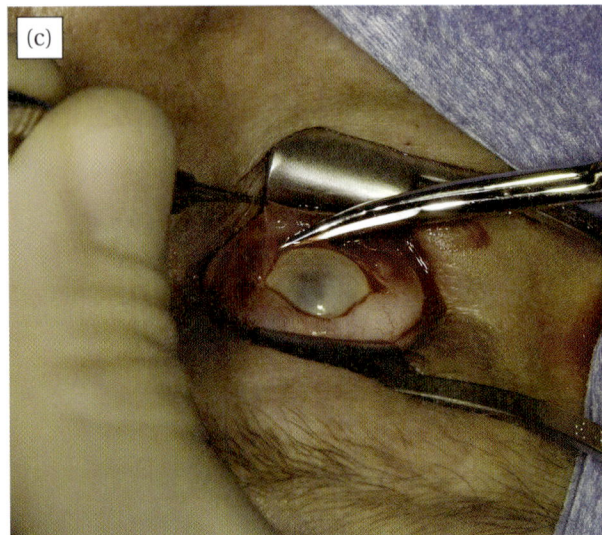

FIGURE 84.2 (a, b, c) Local anesthetic is used to elevate the conjunctiva around the cornea. A 360-degree peritomy is then performed.

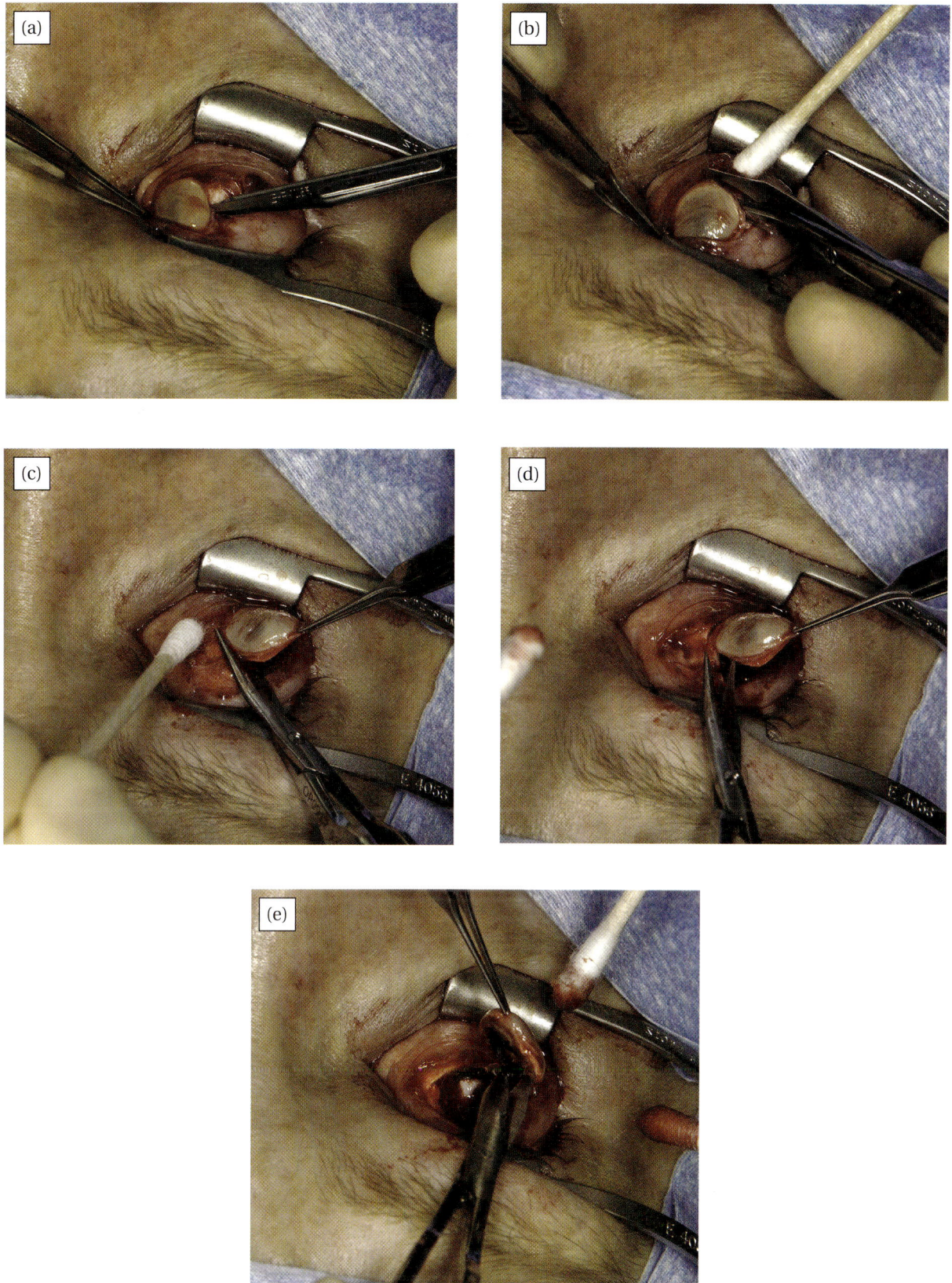

FIGURE 84.3 (a, b, c, d, e) Wescott scissors are used to excise the cornea at (or just beyond) the limbus. Care is taken to preserve the sclera, but the entire cornea must be removed in order to reduce the risk of epithelial inclusion cysts.

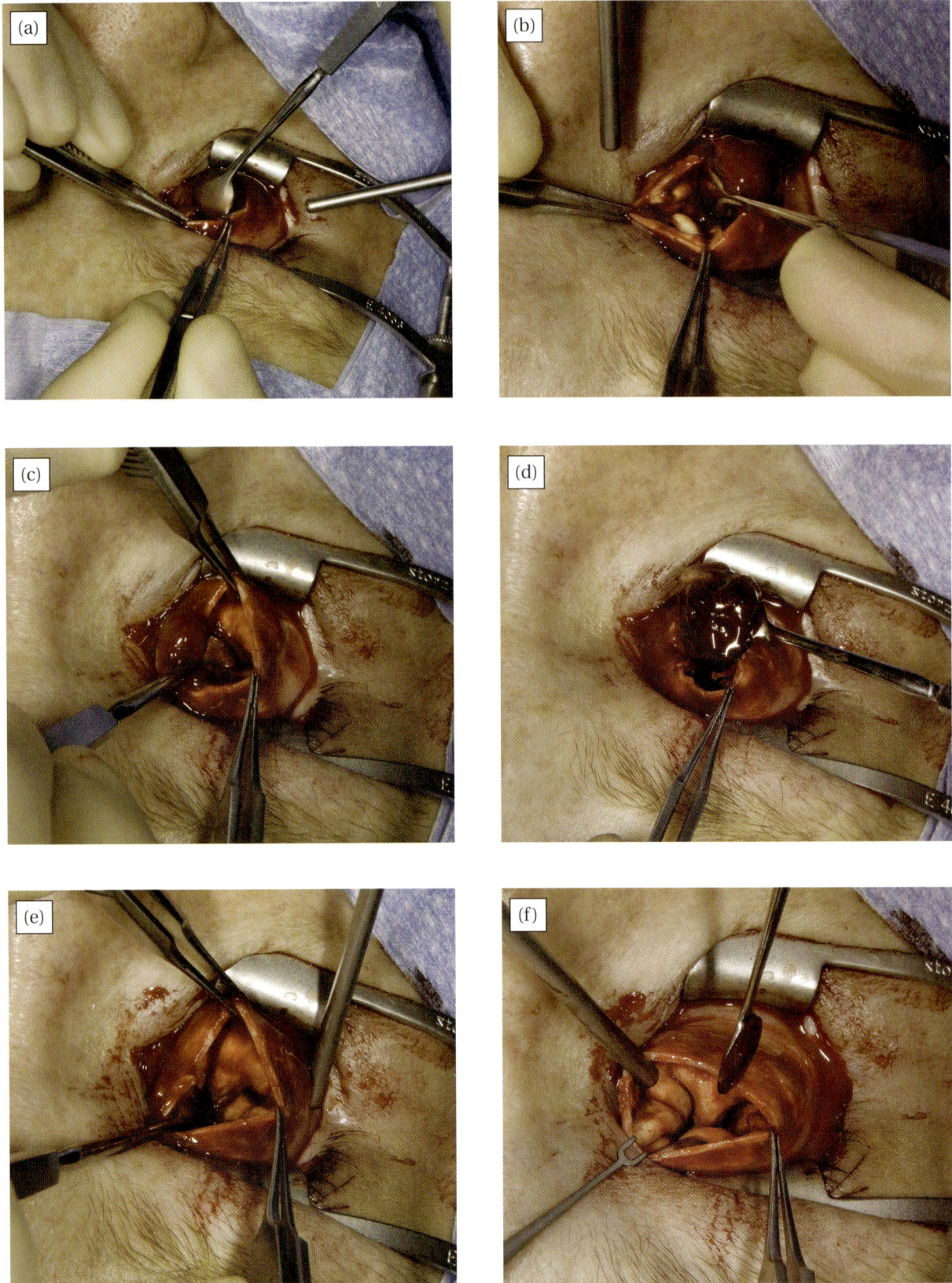

FIGURE 84.4 (a, b, c, d, e, f) The intraocular contents, including the lens and uvea, are carefully removed with an evisceration scoop. The evisceration scoop is used to scrape the inner scleral surface to remove adherent uveal tissue.

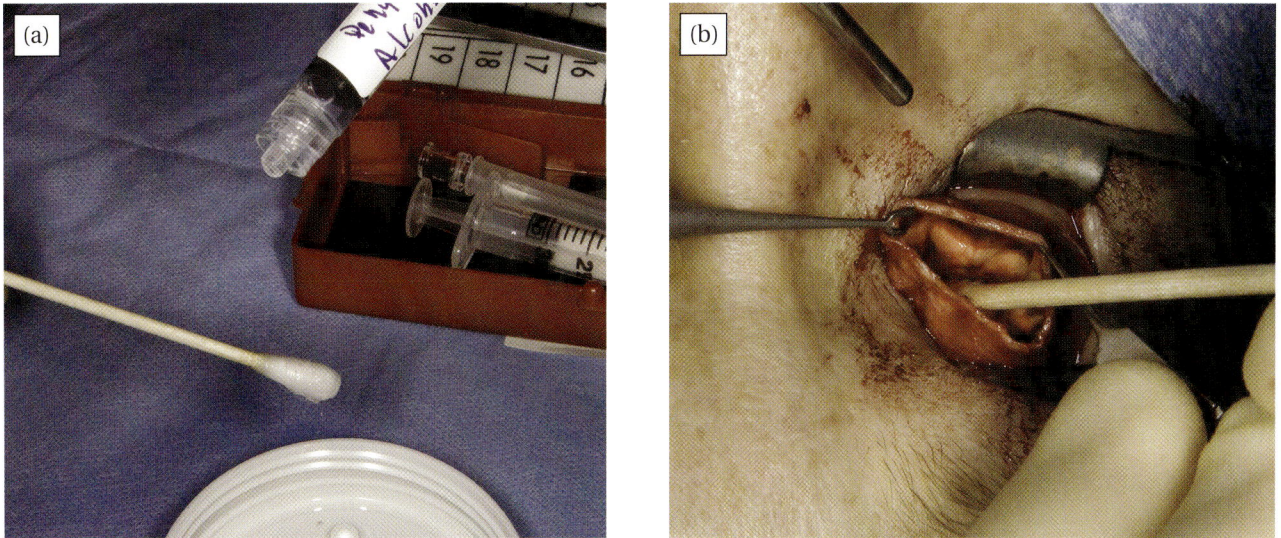

FIGURE 84.5 (a, b) A cotton-tipped applicator is soaked with absolute ethyl alcohol. The inner scleral surface is swabbed with the cotton-tipped applicator to remove and denature residual uveal tissue.

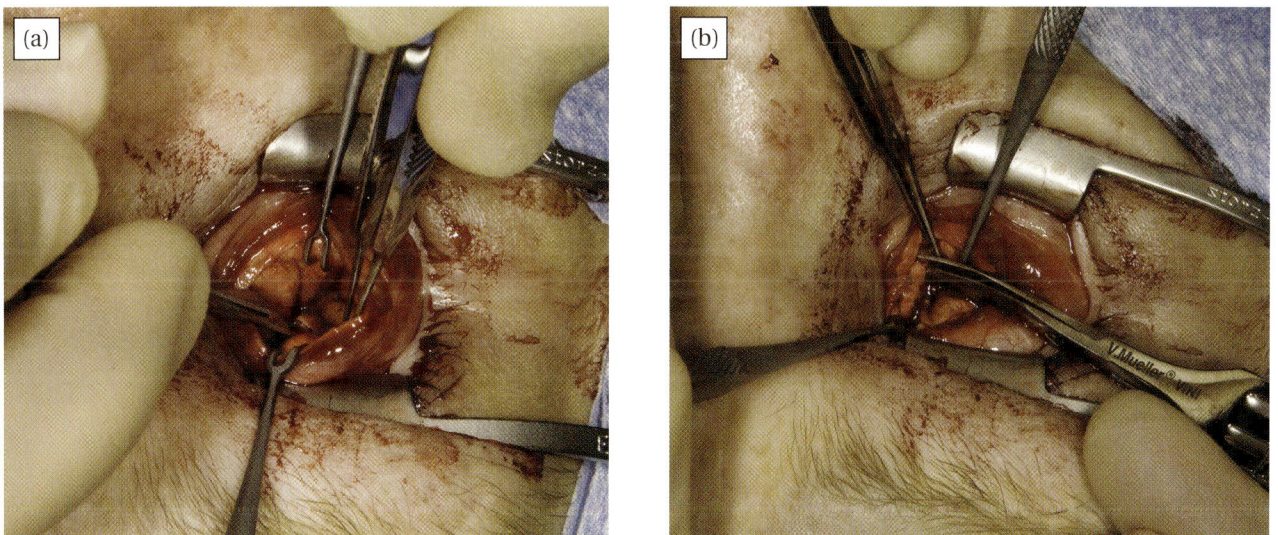

FIGURE 84.6 (a, b, c) The posterior sclera is opened with Wescott scissors to expose the retrobulbar space. The optic nerve is detached from the posterior sclera, to allow anteriorization of the posterior sclera and maximal space for the implant. The nerve can be cauterized with bipolar cautery to reduce the risk of bleeding. A diagonal incision is made in the posterior sclera to expose the intraconal space.

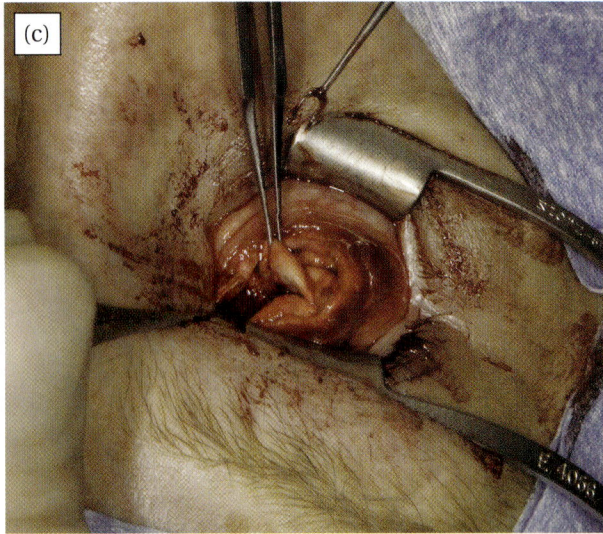

FIGURE 84.6 (*continued*)

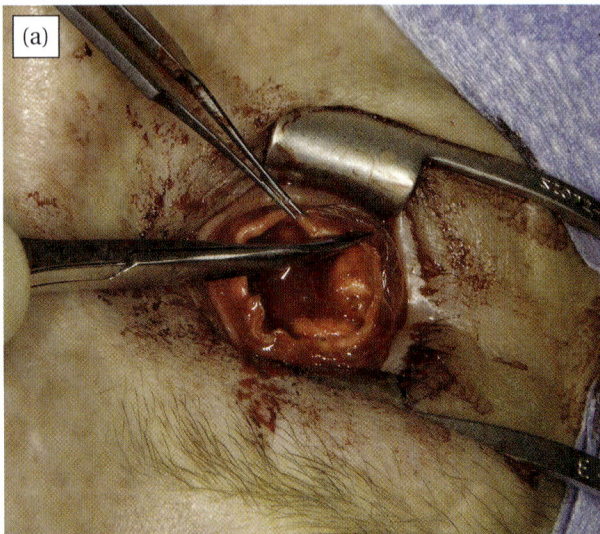

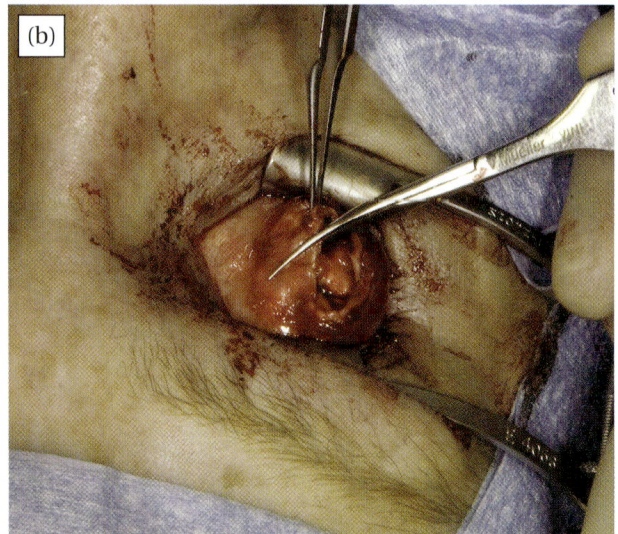

FIGURE 84.7 (a, b) Two relaxing incisions are made in the anterior sclera. These incisions should be perpendicular to the posterior scleral opening in order to create a layered cross configuration. This will allow for a secure closure.

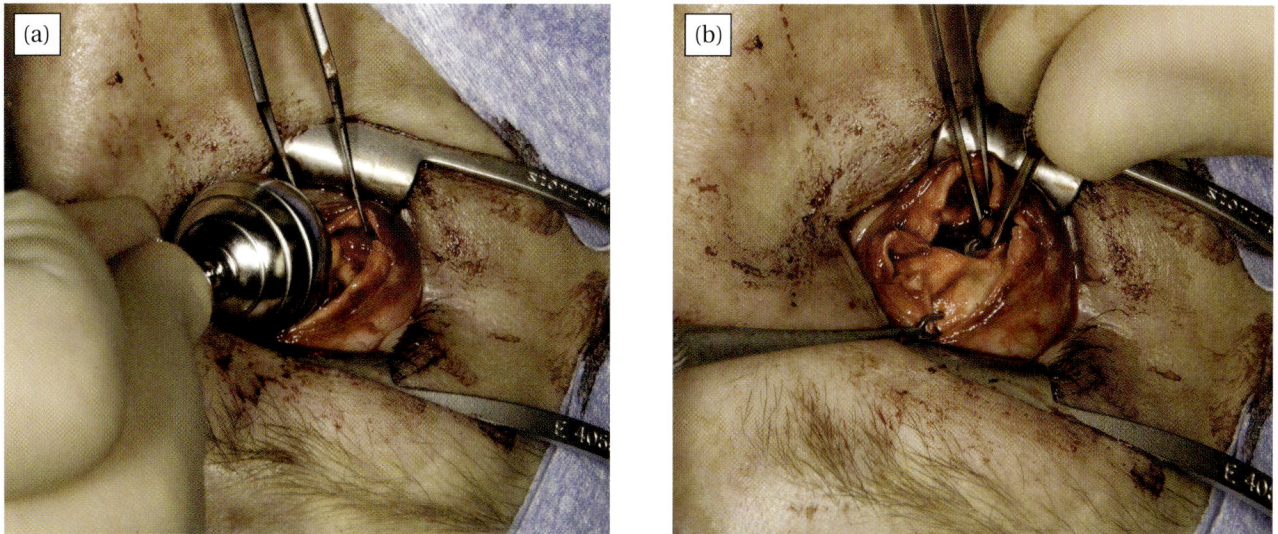

FIGURE 84.8 (a, b) An orbital implant sizer is passed through both layers of the sclera and inserted into the retroscleral space. Alternatively, the desired size of the orbital implant can be calculated from the axial length (AL) of the fellow eye using a formula described by Kaltreider and Lucarelli (see References). If a preoperative CT scan is available, it can be used to estimate the axial length for use in the Kaltreider-Lucarelli (KL) formula. KL formula: Evisceration implant size = AL – 3; Enucleation implant size = AL – 2.

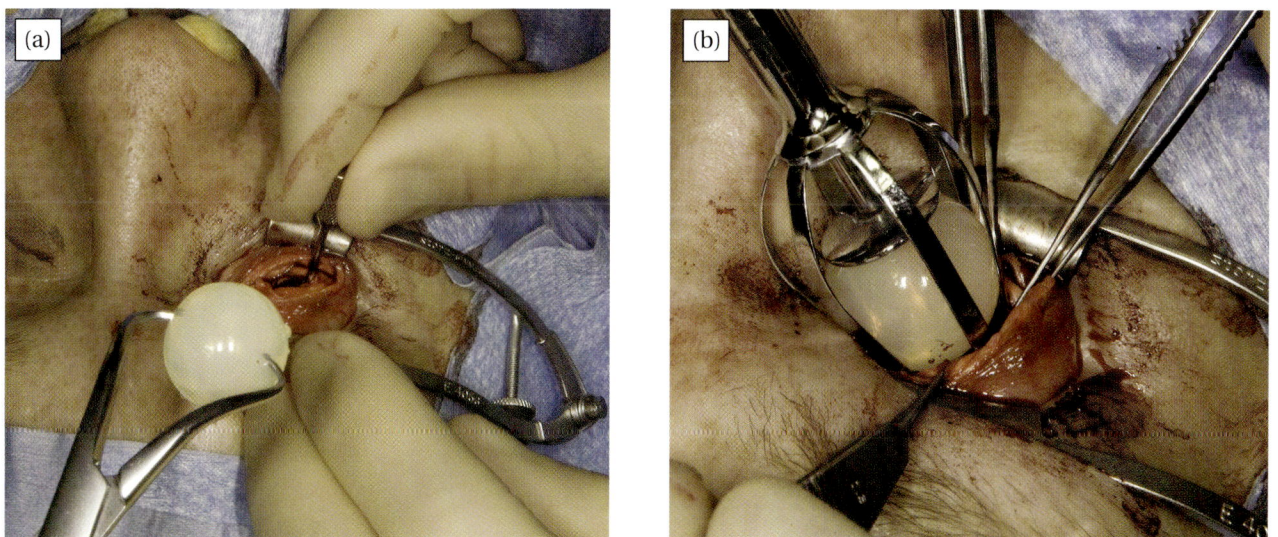

FIGURE 84.9 (a, b) The properly sized orbital implant is placed behind the posterior sclera using either an implant introducer or a plastic drape sleeve. In order to place a large implant in the cone, it is often helpful to remove the lid speculum.

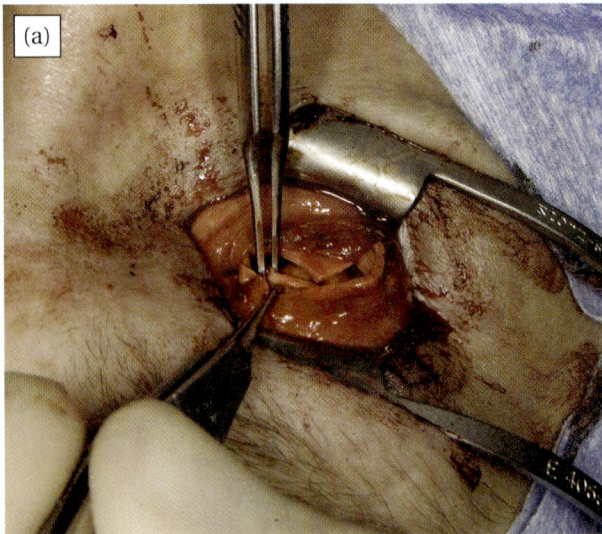

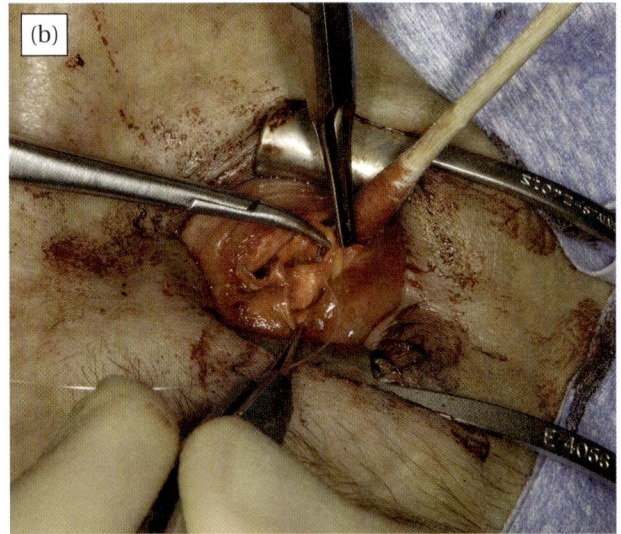

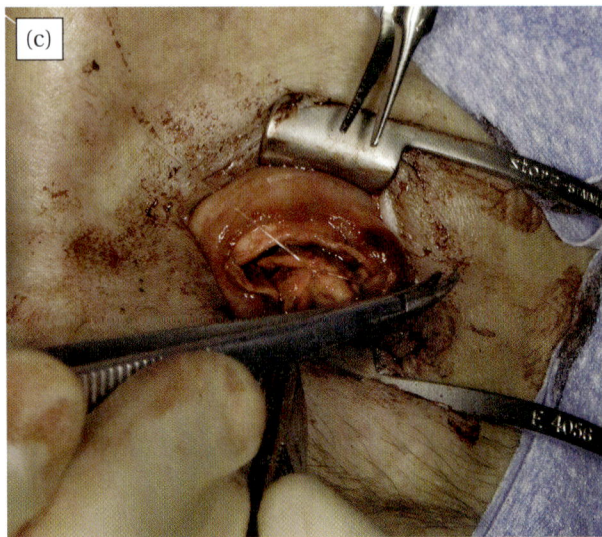

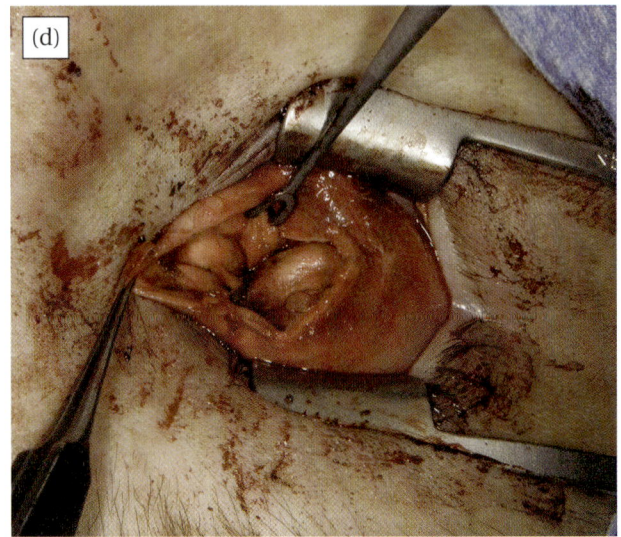

FIGURE 84.10 (a, b, c, d) The posterior sclera is closed with interrupted sutures using 4-0 or 5-0 polyglactin or PDS.

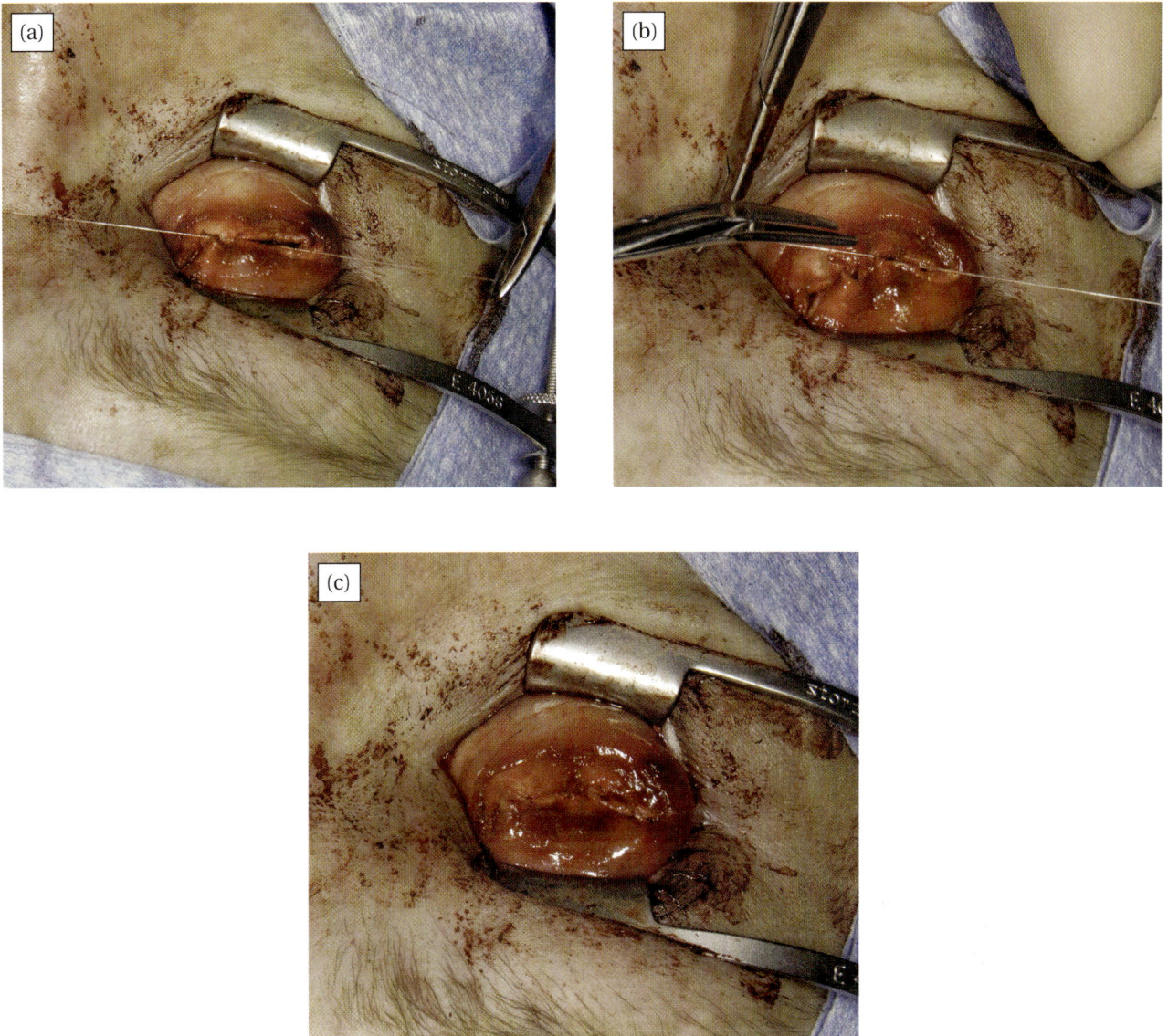

FIGURE 84.11 (a, b, c) The anterior sclera is then closed with a buried-interrupted and/or running 5-0 polyglactin suture. Tenon's layer is then closed in one or two layers, using buried-interrupted sutures.

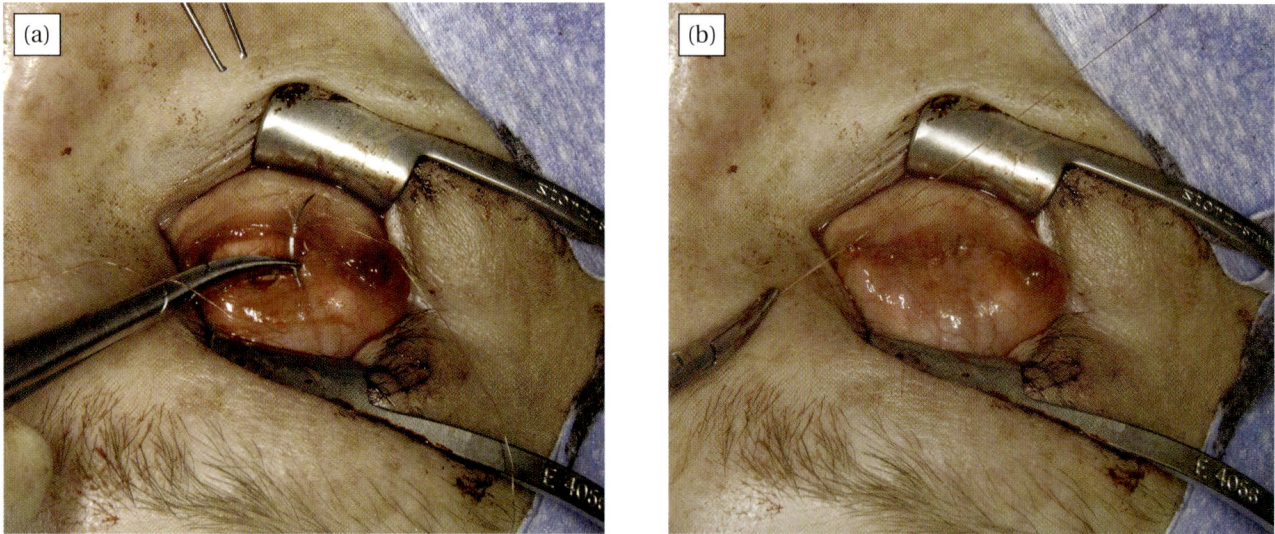

FIGURE 84.12   (a, b) The conjunctiva is closed with a running 6-0 plain gut suture.

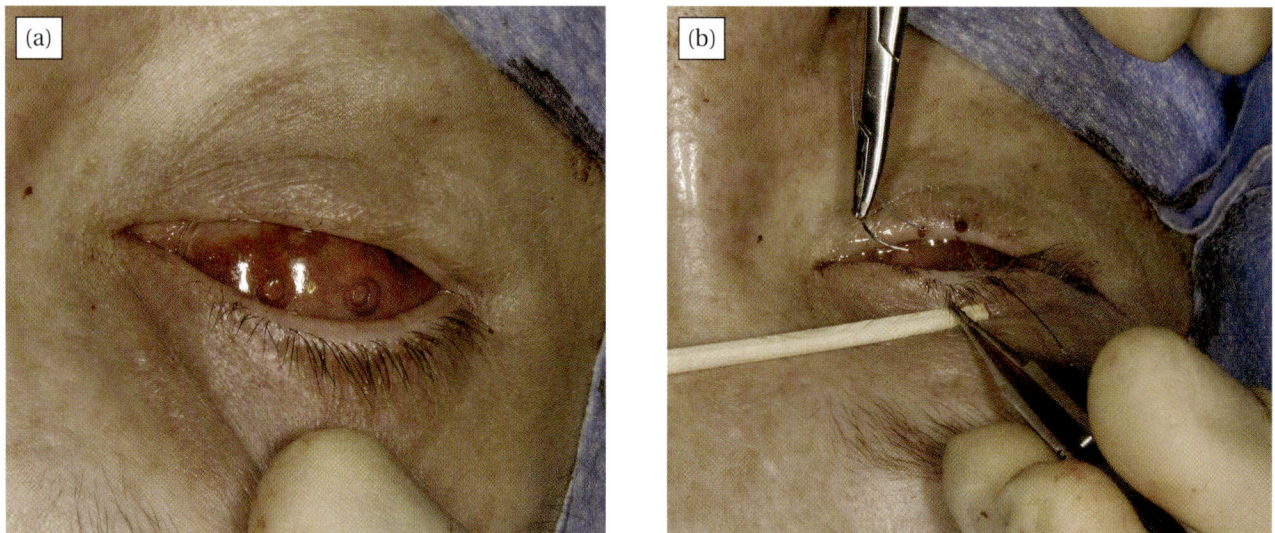

FIGURE 84.13   (a, b) After antibiotic ointment is placed in the socket, a conformer is placed in the palpebral fissure. The eyelids are then closed with a temporary tarsorrhaphy to avoid conjunctival prolapse. We often place a pressure patch for 3 days post-evisceration. The patients will be given 8–12 mg of dexamethasone by anesthesia to reduce postoperative swelling and nausea.

Complications

TABLE 84.3 *Potential Complications*

- Risk of sympathetic ophthalmia
- Risk of occult malignancy
- Implant exposure or extrusion
- Implant infection
- Fornix shortening with overaggressive Tenon overlap or oversized implant

---

SELECTED REFERENCES

Eagle RC, Grossniklaus HE, Syed N, Hogan RN, Lloyd WCI, Flberg R. Inadvertent evisceration of eyes containing uveal melanoma. *Arch Ophthalmol.* 2009;127:141–145.

Kahana A, Dutton JD. Evisceration is a useful option in certain situations. *Arch Ophthalmol.* 2010;128(11):1496.

Kaltreider SA, Lucarelli MJ. A simple algorithm for selection of implant size for enucleation and evisceration: A prospective study. *Ophthal Plast Reconstr Surg.* 2002;18:336–341.

Long JA, Tann TMI, Girkin CA. Evisceration: A new technique of trans-scleral implant placement. *Ophthal Plast Reconstr Surg.* 2000;16:322–325.

Perry JD, Lewis CD, Levine M. Evisceration after complete evaluation is an acceptable option. *Arch Ophthalmol.* 2009;127:1227–1228.

Rosner M. Blind eyes with occult malignant melanoma. *Arch Ophthalmol.* 2009;127:1227.

85 Exenteration of the Orbit

Thomas E. Johnson, MD and Chrisfouad Alabiad, MD

Preoperative Assessment

TABLE 85.1 *Indications for Orbital Exenteration*

- Malignant tumors invading the orbit
- Cutaneous malignancies
- Sinus malignancies
- Intracranial malignancies
- Primary orbital malignancies with chance of cure
- Malignant epithelial lacrimal gland tumors
- Invasive malignant lacrimal sac tumors
- Aggressive infectious processes
- Mucormycosis with advanced orbital disease
- Invasive aspergillosis with visual loss
- Necrotizing fasciitis with orbital involvement
- Disfiguring orbital diseases with total loss of vision
- Advanced neurofibromatosis
- Sclerosing idiopathic orbital inflammatory disease unresponsive to medical therapy with blind frozen globe

TABLE 85.2 *Preoperative evaluation*

History and physical exam

Complete ophthalmic evaluation

Imaging (CT and/or MRI)

Metastatic workup if indicated

Informed consent

Discontinue blood thinners under direction of primary physician

Type and cross-match red blood cells (if high risk for bleeding)

TABLE 85.3 *Preoperative Considerations*

Technique

- Lid-sparing (subtotal exenteration)
- Non-lid-sparing technique

Need for bone removal

Need for combined procedure with otorhinolaryngology or neurosurgery

Need for postoperative radiation and/or chemotherapy

Psychological counseling

Operative Technique

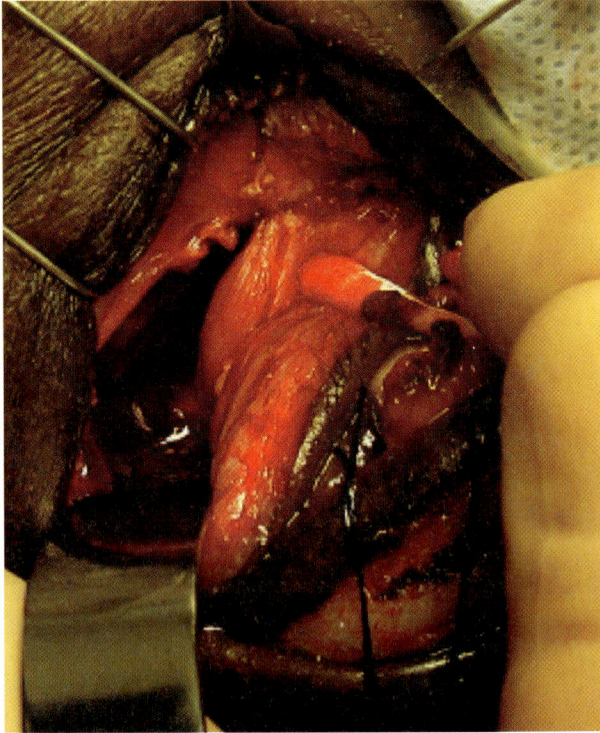

FIGURE 85.1 Exenteration using a lid-sparing (subtotal) technique. Skin incisions are made just above the eyelashes in the upper lid, and just below the lashes in the lower lid. A skin-muscle flap is dissected to the orbital rim.

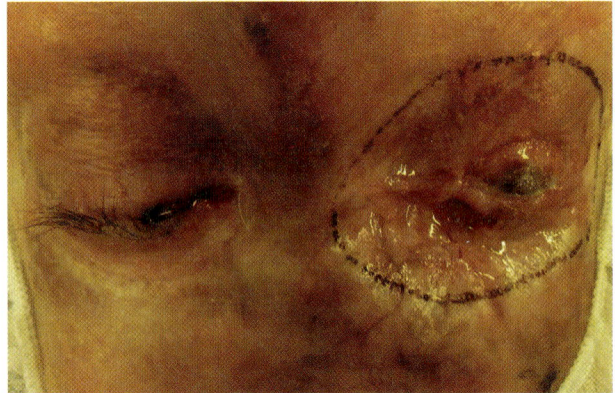

FIGURE 85.2 Classic exenteration technique uses a skin incision made over the orbital rim 360 degrees, and the eyelid tissue is not spared. This is especially useful when the procedure is performed for eyelid malignancies that secondarily invade the orbit.

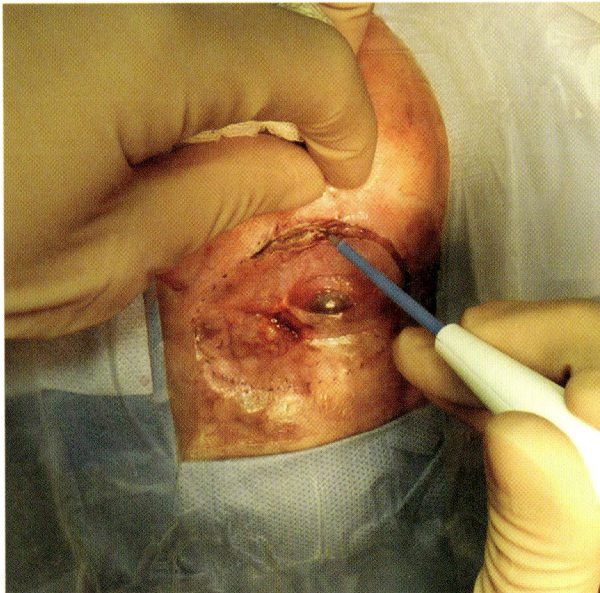

FIGURE 85.3 A monopolar cutting cautery is used to dissect down to the bony orbital rim and aid in hemostasis.

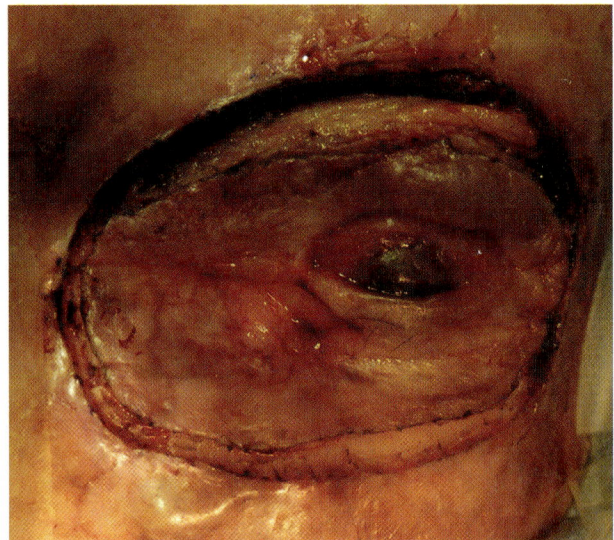

FIGURE 85.4 The incision is made through skin and muscle to the bony orbital rim 360 degrees.

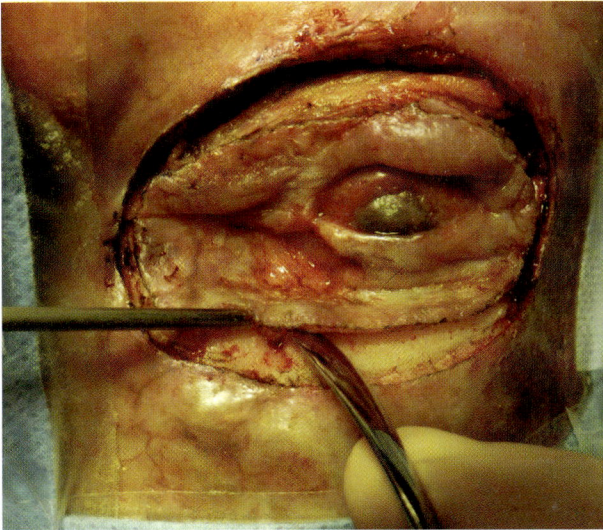

FIGURE 85.5 A Freer periosteal elevator is used to cut the periosteum, reflect it off the orbital rim, and gently lift it off the orbital walls.

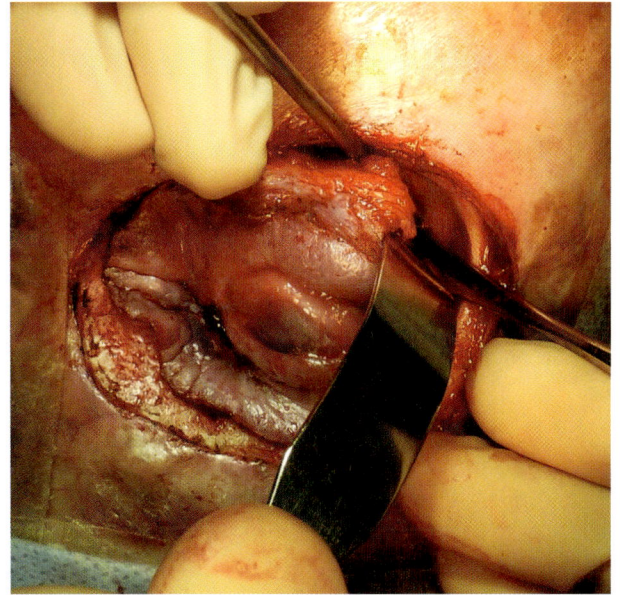

FIGURE 85.6 Inferotemporally, malleable retractors are used to identify the inferior orbital fissure. Sharp dissection is performed to lyse the tissues entering the fissure and release the orbital tissues.

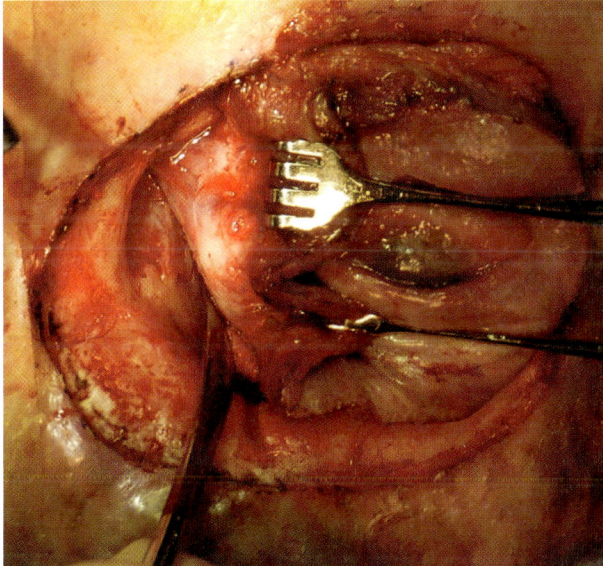

FIGURE 85.7 The lacrimal sac fossa is visualized, and the lacrimal sac is transected as it enters the nasolacrimal duct.

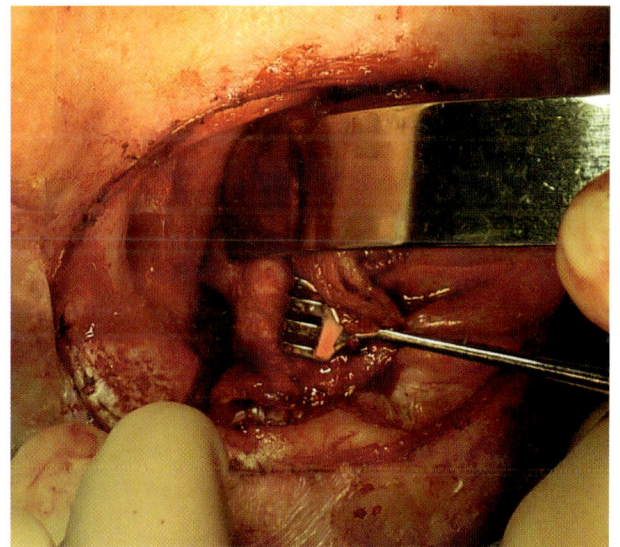

FIGURE 85.8 Malleable and rake retractors distract the tissues away from the orbital walls, allowing visualization of intraorbital structures. Medial dissection is carried down to the anterior and posterior ethmoidal neurovascular bundles, which are cauterized and cut.

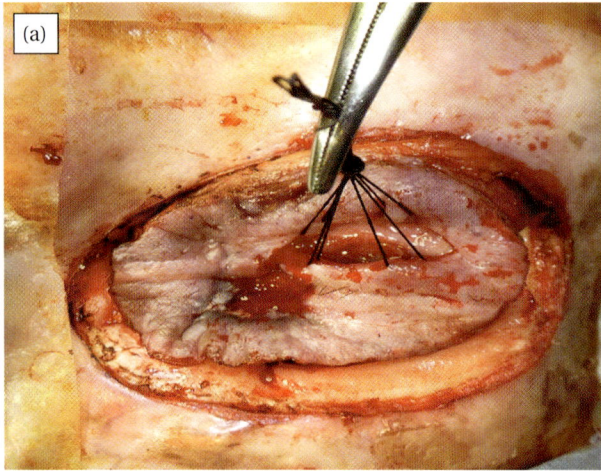

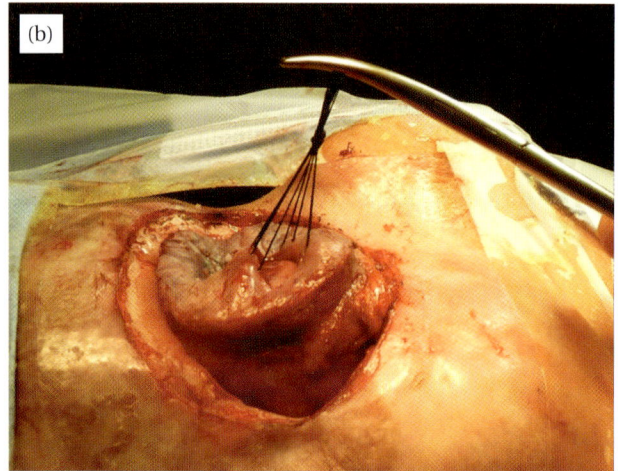

FIGURE 85.9 (a, b) 4-0 silk traction sutures are used for upward traction.

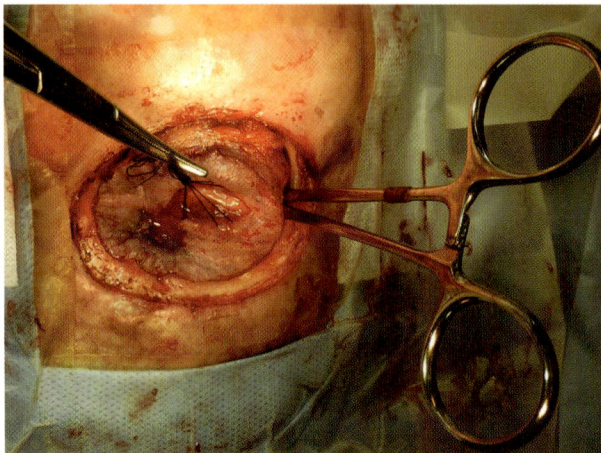

FIGURE 85.10 Once the dissection is complete to the orbital apex 360 degrees, the orbital apical tissues are clamped with a hemostat. The hemostat is left in place for one minute for hemostasis.

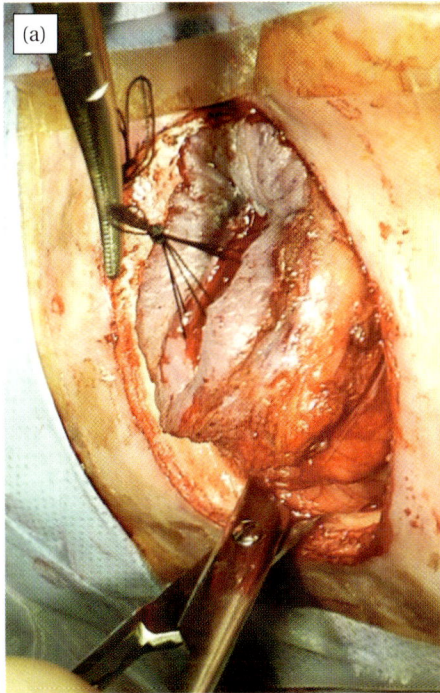

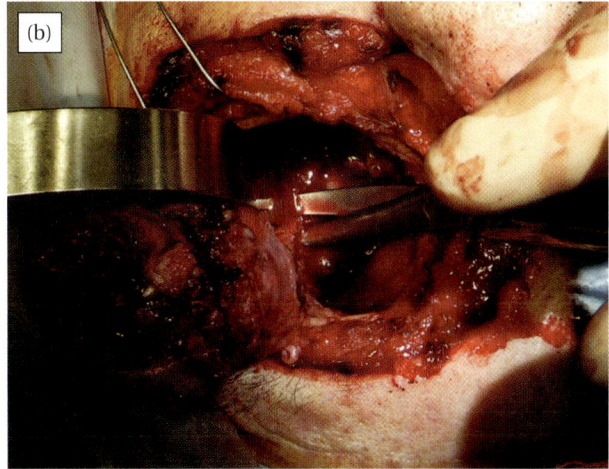

FIGURE 85.11 (a, b) Orbital tissues are gently retracted as apical structures are cut with enucleation scissors.

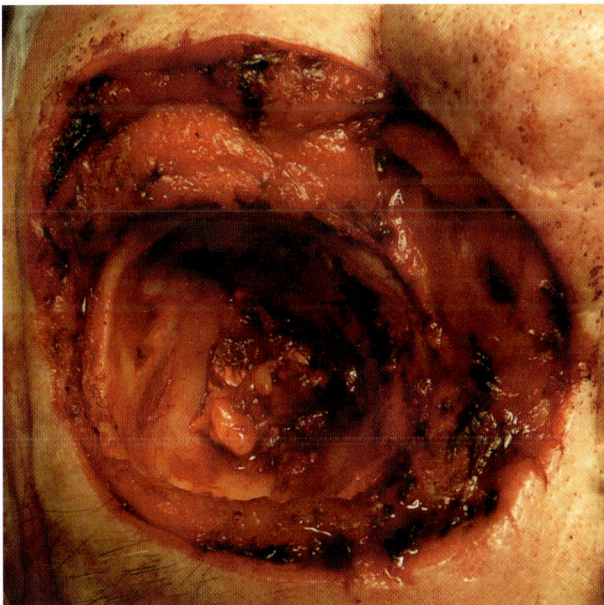

FIGURE 85.12 The apical stump (left orbit) aids in socket healing and graft vascularization; however, care is taken to amputate the stump in cases of deep orbital disease.

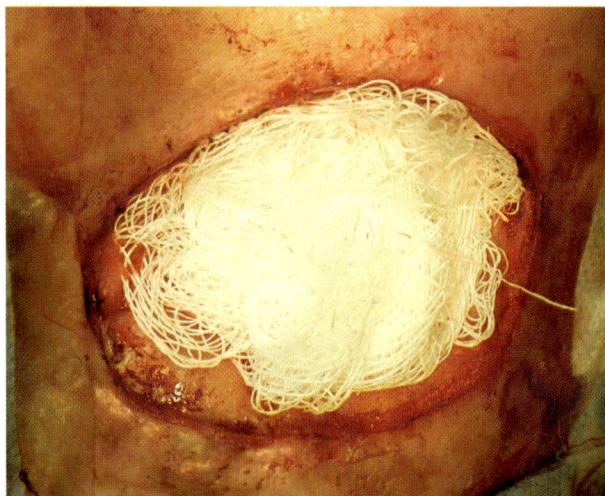

FIGURE 85.13 The socket is firmly packed with gauze to ensure hemostasis after the orbital contents are removed.

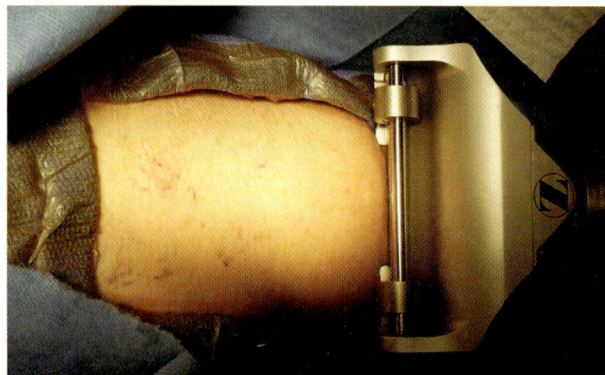

FIGURE 85.14 The anterior thigh is prepped and draped in preparation for split-thickness skin grafting. The leg may need to be shaved, and a thin layer of mineral oil is applied.

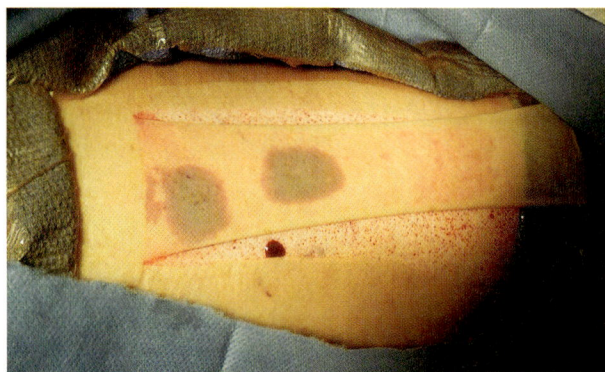

FIGURE 85.15 A dermatome is used to make a split thickness skin graft 0.14–0.18 mm thick and 2–3 inches wide. The assistant carefully manages the graft as it exits the dermatome.

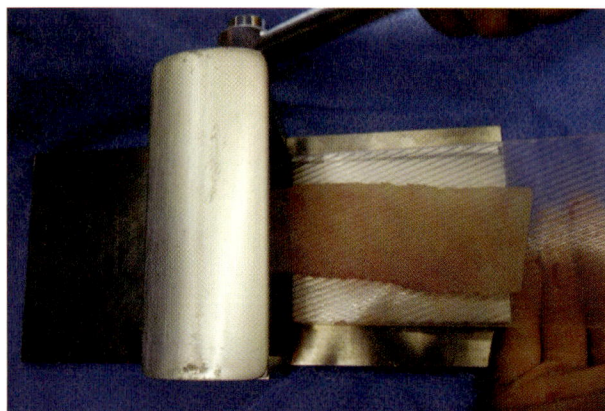

FIGURE 85.16 The split thickness graft is passed through a mesher to create more surface area.

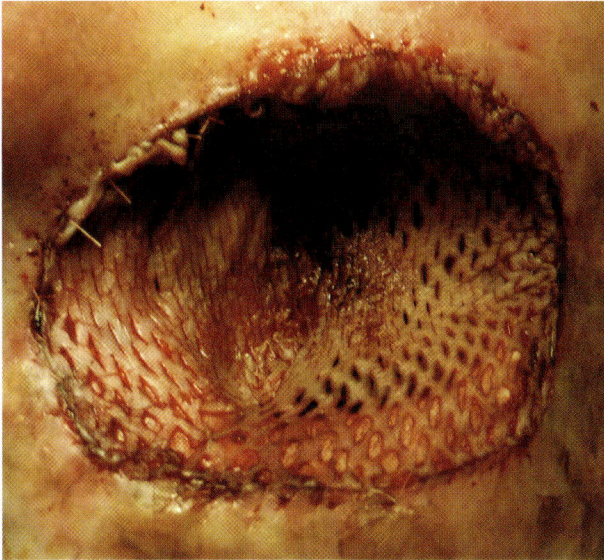

FIGURE 85.17 The socket is lined with the meshed split-thickness skin graft, and is sutured into position with 7-0 polyglactin 910 sutures.

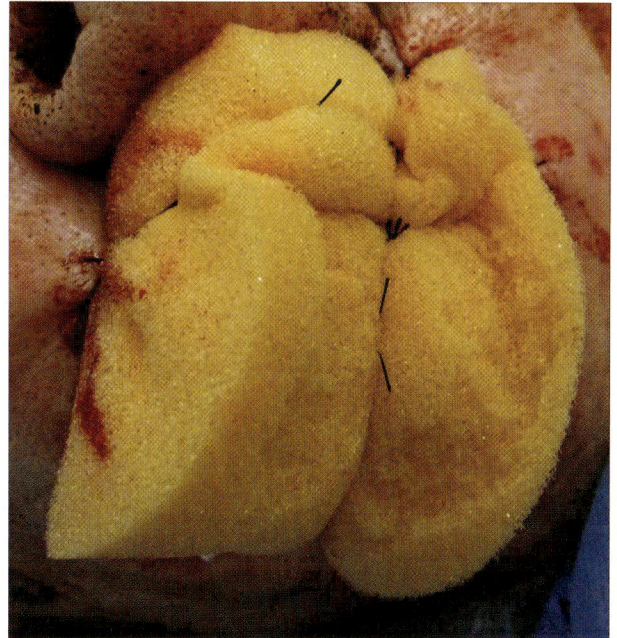

FIGURE 85.18 A firm pressure patch is placed in the socket using a combination of nonstick dressing, antibiotic ointment, and surgical scrub brushes, and held in position with 4-0 silk sutures.

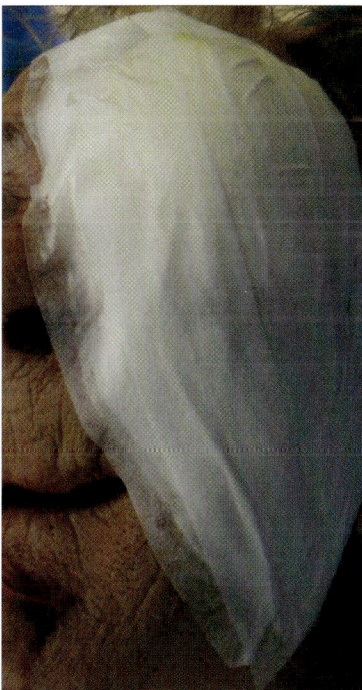

FIGURE 85.19 A firm outer dressing is applied with benzoin, gauzes, eyepads, and paper tape, and is left in place for one week.

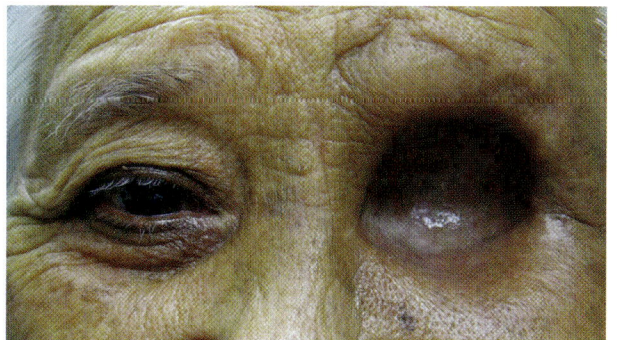

FIGURE 85.20 Exenteration socket that was lined with patients own eyelid skin (subtotal technique). The advantage of the technique is rapid healing and a smooth, thick skin lining.

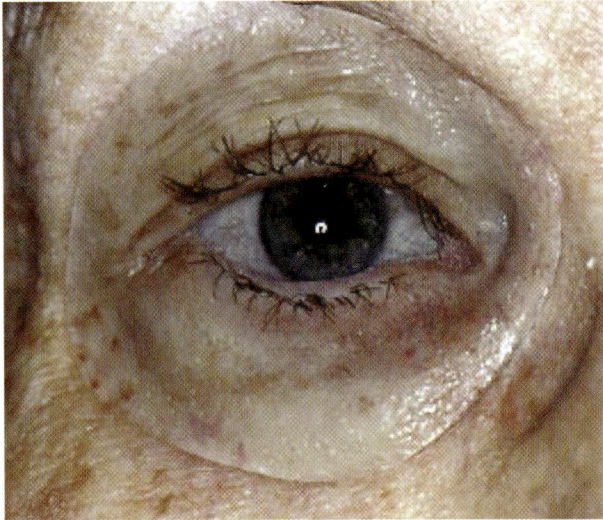

FIGURE 85.21 An orbital/facial prosthesis is created by an anaplastologist approximately 4 months after the procedure.

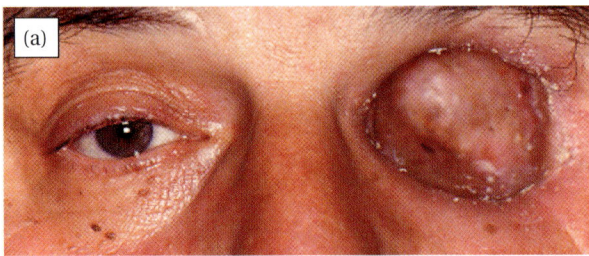

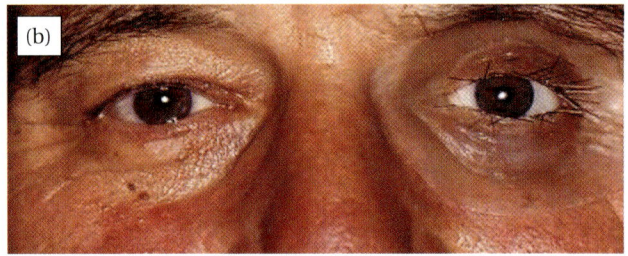

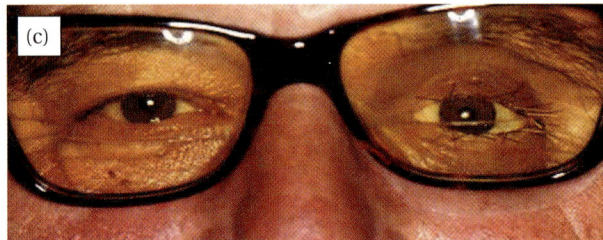

FIGURE 85.22 Socket with skin graft after exenteration (a). Same patient with orbital/facial prosthesis in place (b). Tinted glasses help camouflage the prosthesis (c).

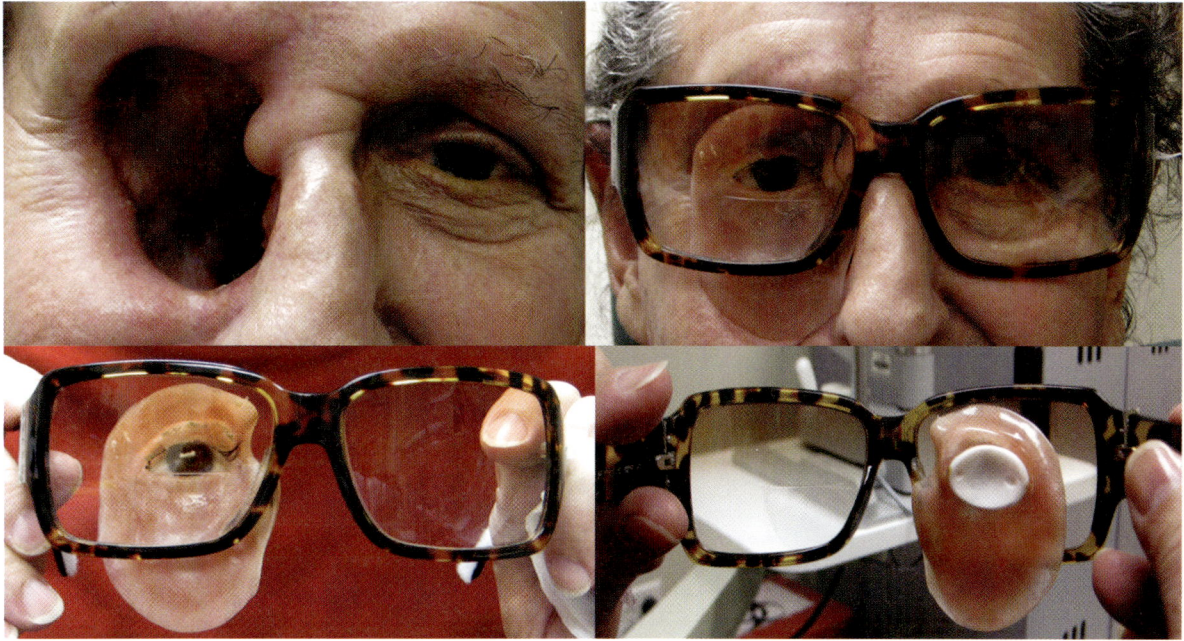

FIGURE 85.23 A spectacle-mounted prosthesis is useful in patients with absent bony orbital walls.

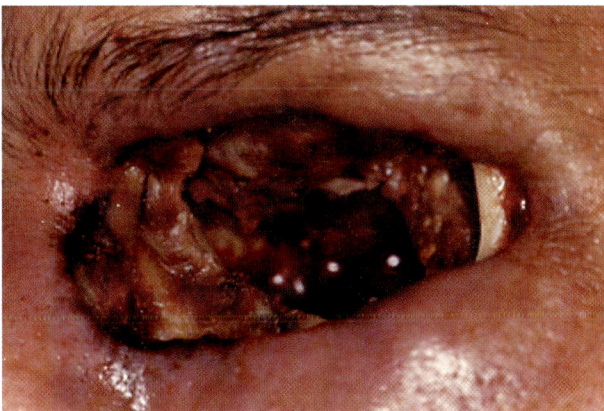

FIGURE 85.24 Socket and sinus exenteration for mucormycosis does not permit skin grafting.

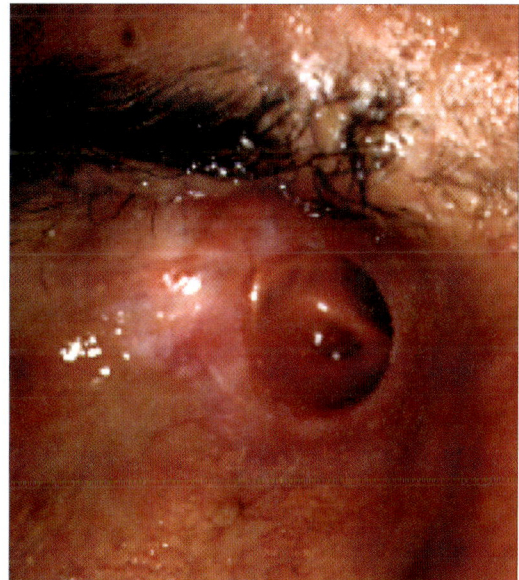

FIGURE 85.25 Sino-orbital fistula.

Postoperative Considerations

TABLE 85.4 *Postoperative Care*

Systemic antibiotics for one week

Pressure patch for one week

Dressing changes

Daily wet to dry povidone-iodine dressings to orbit after first week

Leg dressing changes weekly (if skin graft taken)

Orbital/facial prosthesis fitting after four months if desired, otherwise black patch

TABLE 85.5 *Potential Complications*

Infection

Bleeding

Fistula formation

CSF leak

Psychological adjustment

SELECTED REFERENCES

Bartley GB, Garrity JA, Waller RR, et al. Orbital exenteration at the Mayo Clinic 1967–1986. *Ophthalmology.* 1989;96:468–474.

Goldberg RA, Kim JW, Shorr, N. Orbital exenteration: Results of an individualized approach. *Ophthal Plast Reconstr Surg.* 2003;19:229–236.

Gunalp I, Gunduz K, Duruk K. Orbital exenteration: a review of 429 cases. *Int Ophthalmol.* 1996;19:177–184.

Levin PS, Dutton JJ. A 20 year series of orbital exenteration. *Am J Ophthalmol.* 1991;112:496–501.

Levin PS, Ellis DS, Stewart WB, Toth BA. Orbital exenteration: the reconstructive ladder. *Ophthal Plast Reconstr Surg.* 1991;7:84–92.

Mohr C, Esser J. Orbital exenteration: surgical and reconstructive strategies. *Graefe's Arch Clin Exp Ophthalmol.* 1997;235:288–295.

Putterman AM. Orbital exenteration with spontaneous granulation. *Arch Ophthalmol.* 1986;104:139–140.

Shields JA, Shields, CL, Demirci H, et al. Experience with eyelid-sparing orbital exenteration: The 2000 Tullos O. Coston Lecture. *Ophthal Plast Reconstr Surg.* 2001;17:355–361.

86

Socket Reconstruction

Morris E. Hartstein, MD, FACS

Implant Exposure

SELECTED REFERENCES

TABLE 86.1 *Indications for Surgery*

Superior sulcus deformity

Lid malposition

• Ptosis, lower lid retraction

Implant exposure

TABLE 86.2 *Preoperative Considerations*

• Superior sulcus deformities may be addressed by several approaches used alone or in combination, such as subperiosteal volume augmentation, implant exchange, ptosis repair, and/or direct filler injection.

• Lid malpositions, such as ptosis and lower lid retraction, may contribute to superior sulcus deformities, and treating the lid malpositions may be sufficient to improve the sulcus.

• Implant exposures should be treated first with oral antibiotics in order to quiet down the socket. Some small exposures may even heal spontaneously. Initial surgical treatment may involve patch grafting. Autologous grafts such as fascia or dermis fat are preferred.

• In some cases of implant exposure, especially with porous implants, a patch graft may not be successful, and an implant exchange may be required.

• When planning socket surgery, it is often useful to stage the procedures sequentially, instead of trying to accomplish several procedures together at once.

Orbital Volume Augmentation: Subperiosteal Approach

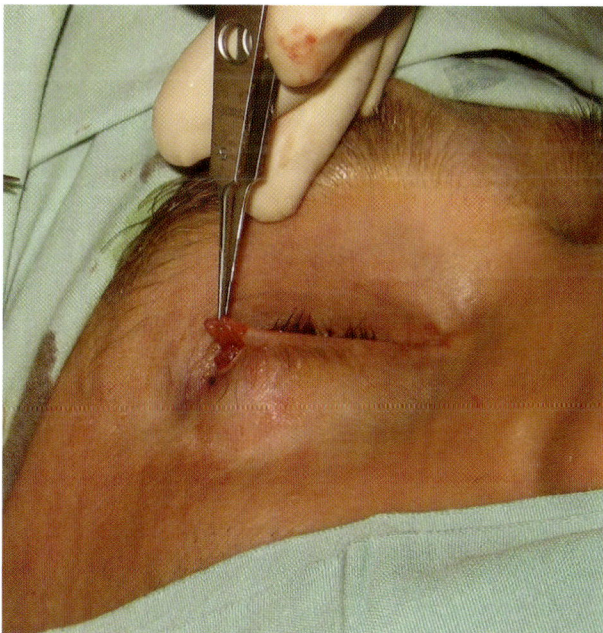

FIGURE 86.1 The approach to the orbital floor begins with a lateral canthotomy/cantholysis and the fashioning of a tarsal strip.

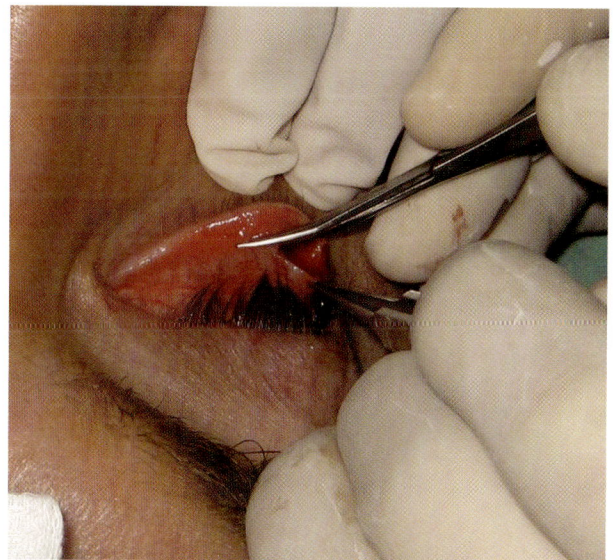

FIGURE 86.2 A transconjunctival incision is made across the lid at the inferior tarsal border. This incision may also be made with a cutting cautery.

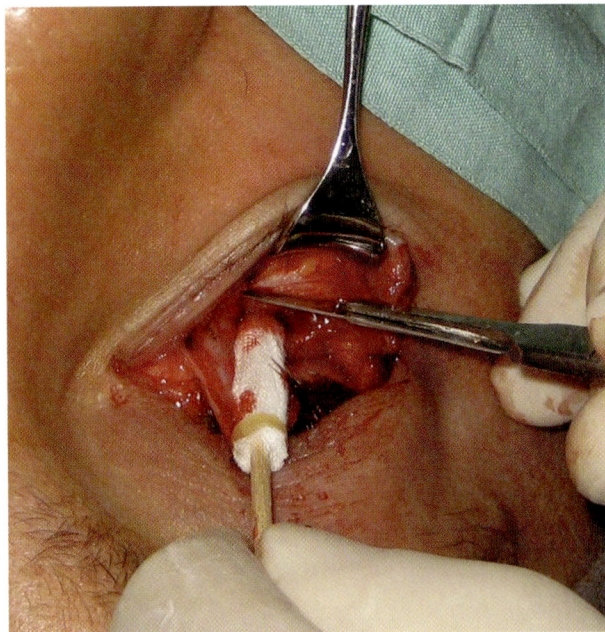

FIGURE 86.3   The periosteum at the inferior orbital rim is incised along the length of the rim.

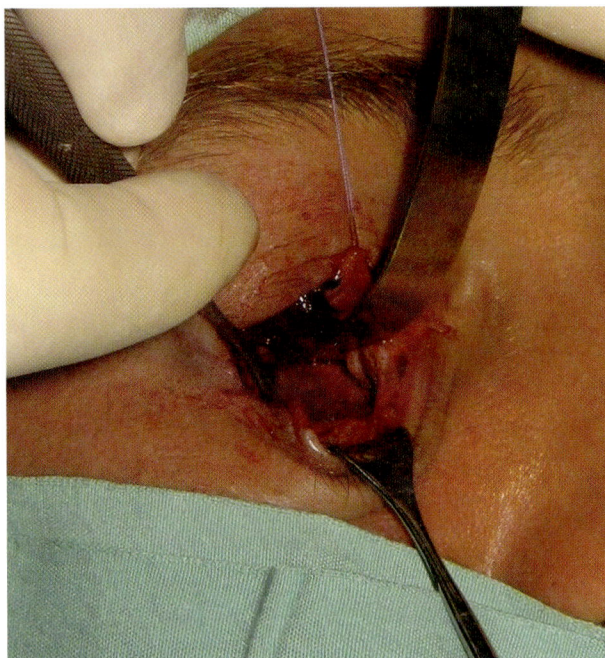

FIGURE 86.4   Using a freer elevator and malleable retractors, the periosteum is elevated off the orbital floor.

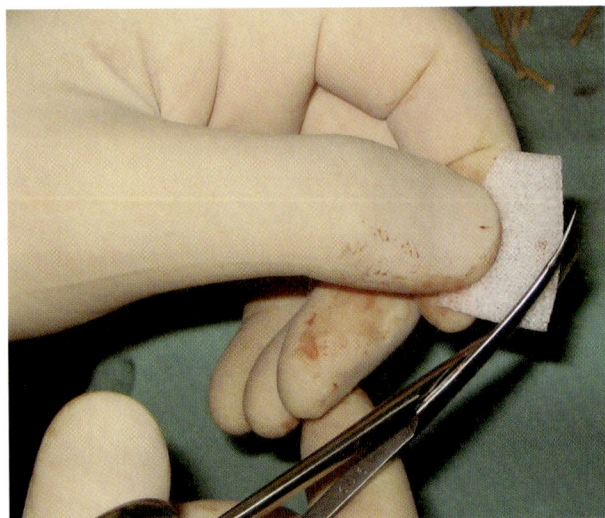

FIGURE 86.5   1.5mm thickness porous polyethylene (Medpor Sheets, Porex Surgical, Atlanta, GA) sheets are then trimmed to fit over the orbital floor.

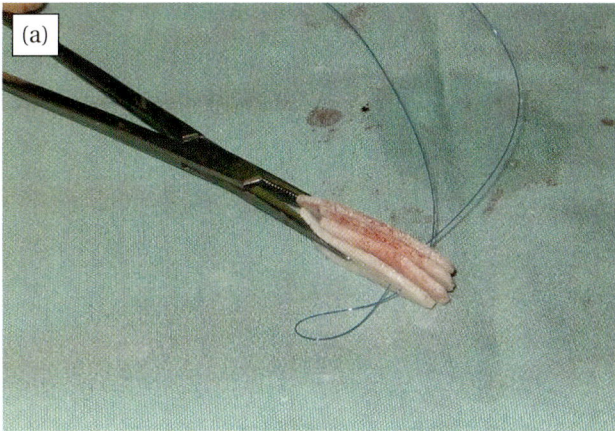

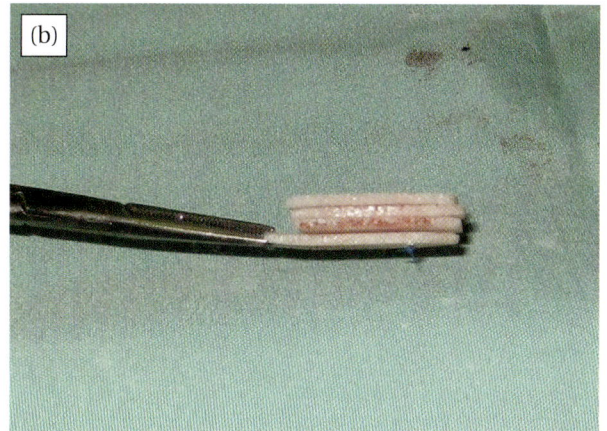

FIGURE 86.6 (a) The sheets are stacked and held together by a 4-0 polypropylene suture passed in a mattress fashion. (b) The suture is tied with the knot on the underside of the stack to rest on bone.

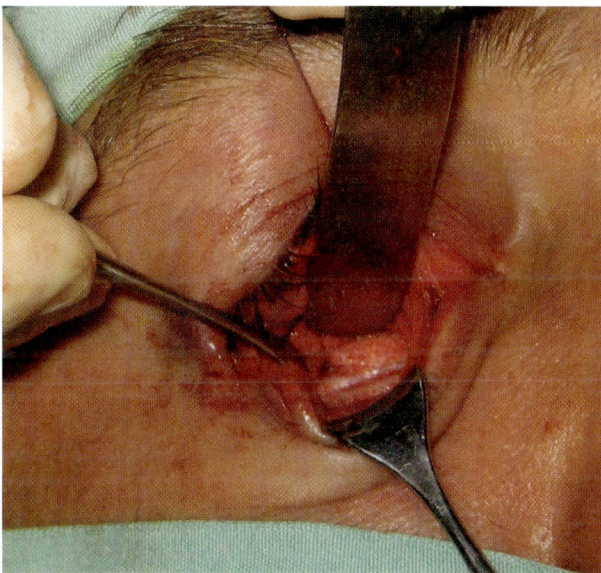

FIGURE 86.7 The stacked sheets are placed along the floor. It is important to place the stack posteriorly to get the full volume-augmenting effect.

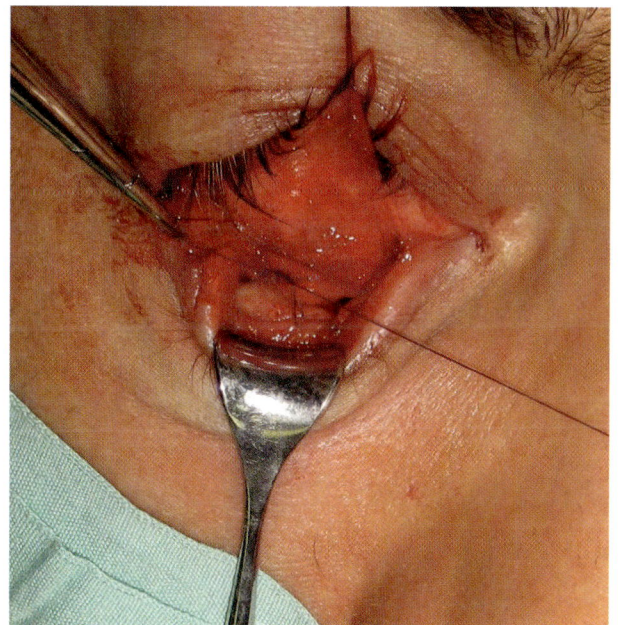

FIGURE 86.8 The periosteum is closed using 5-0 polyglactin sutures, securing the implant in place. The conjunctiva is then closed with interrupted and running 6-0 plain gut suture.

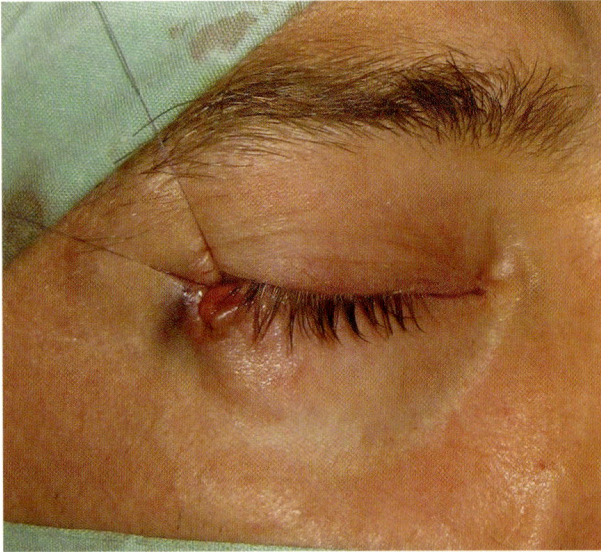

FIGURE 86.9 The tarsal strip is then secured to the lateral orbital rim periosteum. A conformer is placed and the lids closed with a suture tarsorrhaphy.

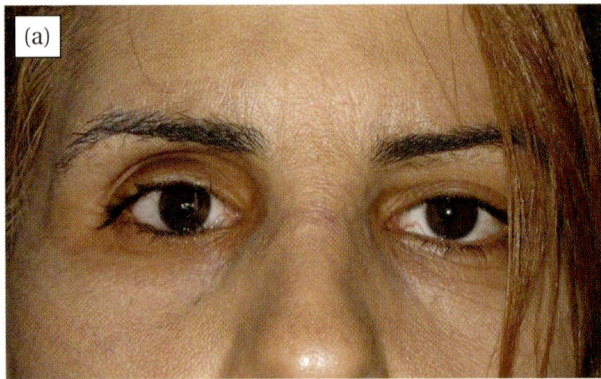

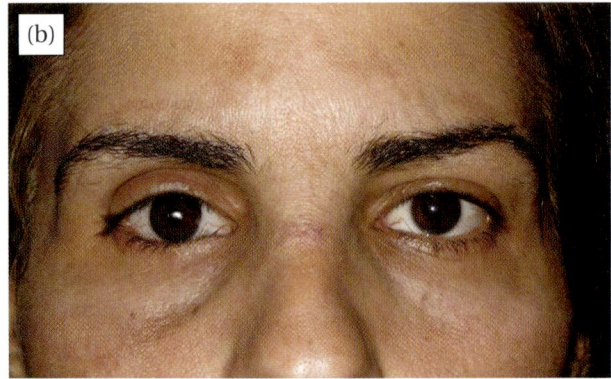

FIGURE 86.10 Before (a) and after (b) orbital volume augmentation of right socket to correct a deep superior sulcus.

Orbital Volume Augmentation with Filler

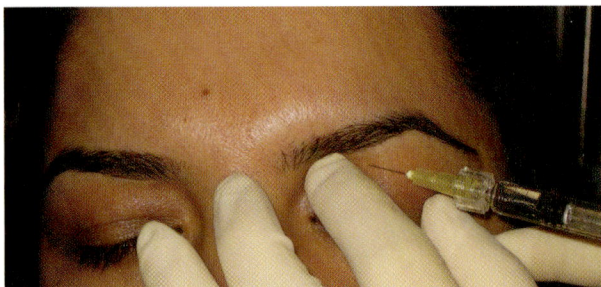

FIGURE 86.11 Superior sulcus deficits may also be addressed in the office using filler injections. Hyaluronic acid (HA; e.g., Restylane or Perlane, Medicis Pharmaceutical, Scottsdale, AZ) is injected while palpating along the superior orbital rim. Filler should not be placed deep as it will not correct the defect. Other fillers can be used as well, but the HAs are well tolerated and reversible.

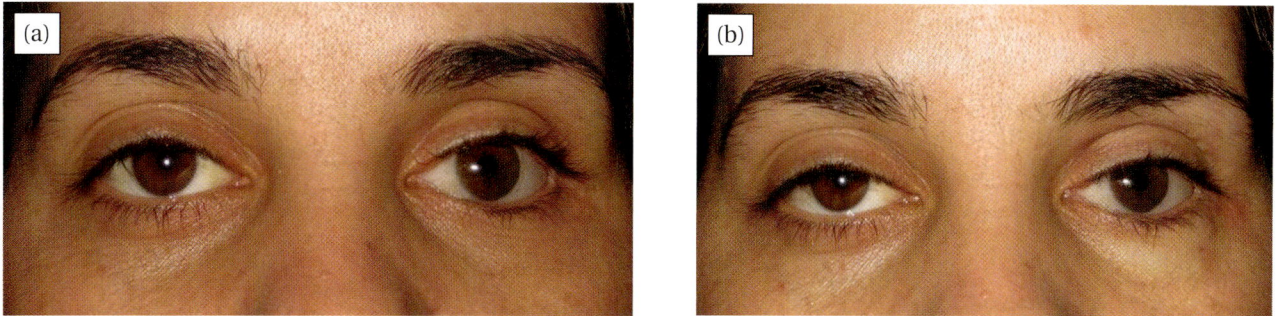

FIGURE 86.12   Before (a) and after (b) volume augmentation with HA filler to left superior sulcus.

Correcting a Deep Superior Sulcus with Eyelid Repair

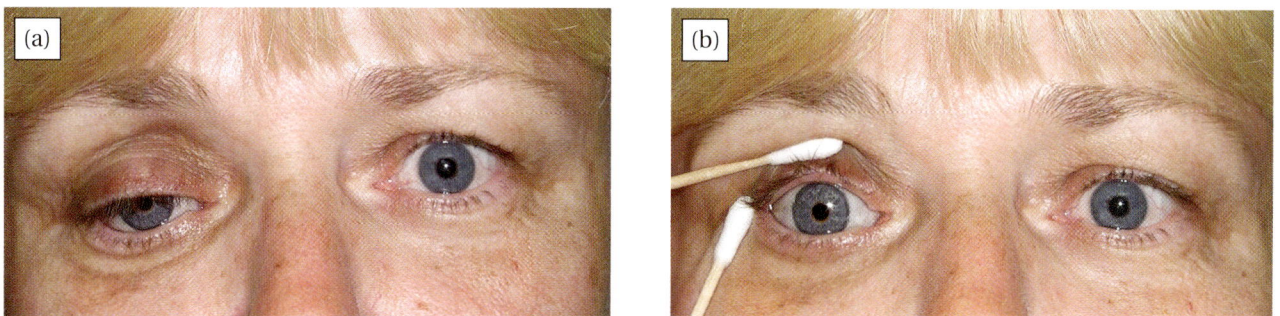

FIGURE 86.13   (a) Example of a typical patient with dystopic right socket demonstrating deep superior sulcus, ptosis, and lower lid retraction. (b) Demonstration for the patient using cotton tipped applicators of how correction of the lid malposition will improve overall socket appearance.

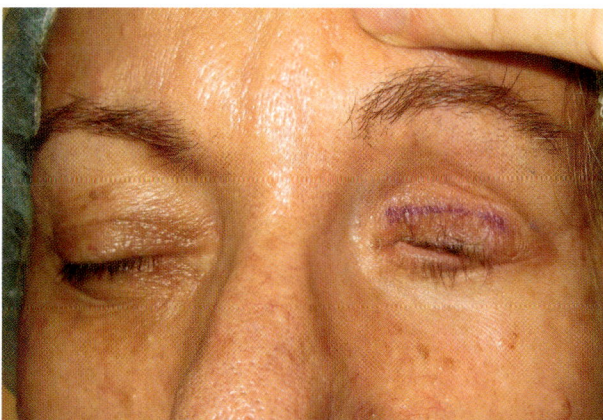

FIGURE 86.14   Lid crease marked in standard fashion—no additional skin is removed.

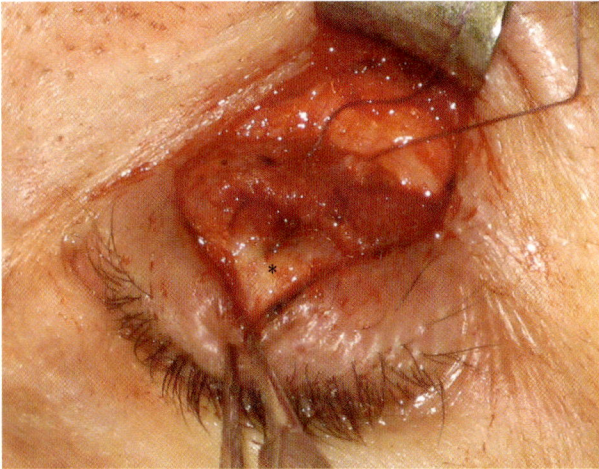

FIGURE 86.15 After exposing levator and tarsus in standard fashion, a 5-0 polyglactin suture is passed through the anterior surface of the tarsus* and then through the levator complex in a horizontal mattress fashion.

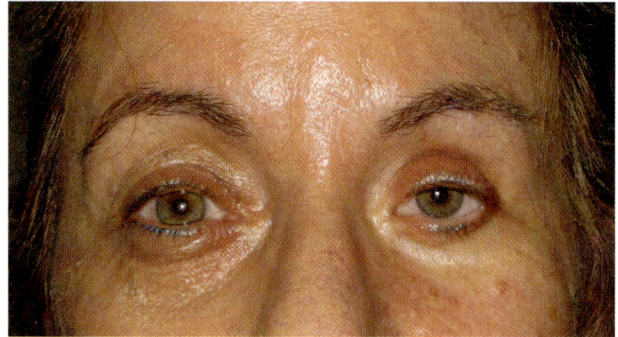

FIGURE 86.16 Preoperative photo of patient with deep superior sulcus and ptosis on the left side. This patient did not wish to undergo volume augmentation of the orbit.

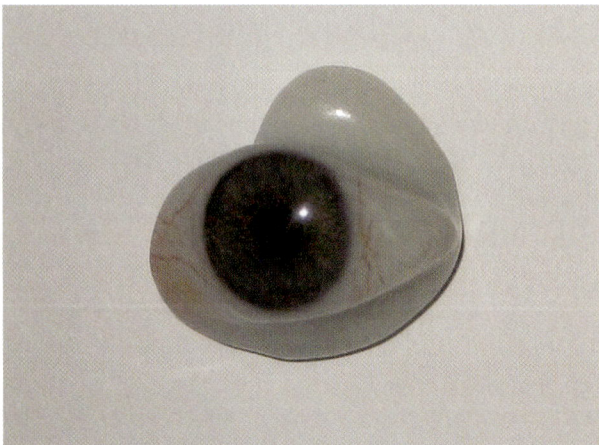

FIGURE 86.17 Prosthesis of patient in previous figure with significant buildup of superior aspect of prosthesis in an attempt to fill the deep superior sulcus.

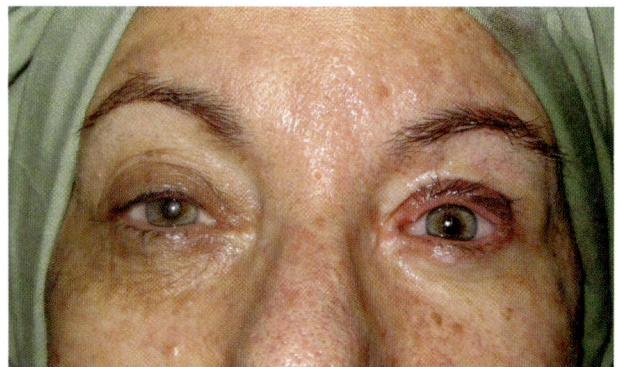

FIGURE 86.18 Immediate postoperative appearance of patient after undergoing ptosis repair. In addition to correction of the ptosis, note the improvement in superior sulcus defect.

Implant Exposure

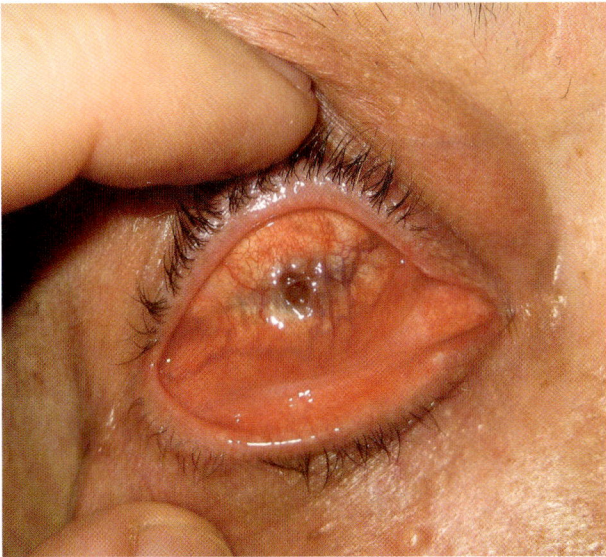

FIGURE 86.19 Patient with exposed polymethylmethacrylate implant.

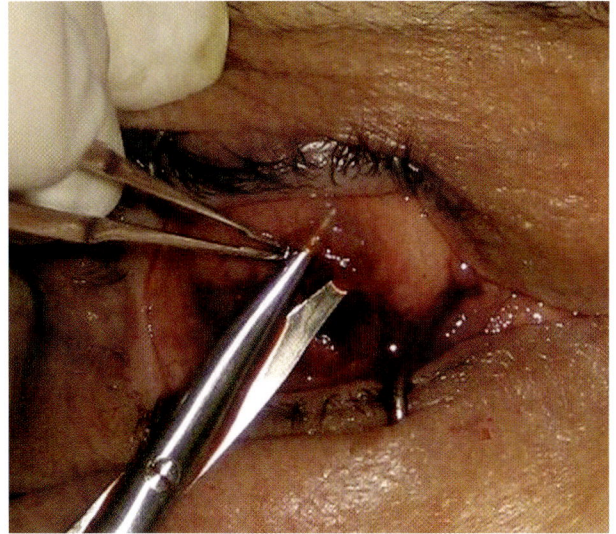

FIGURE 86.20 Subconjunctival dissection to mobilize conjunctiva around the exposure and to identify healthy Tenon's and sclera.

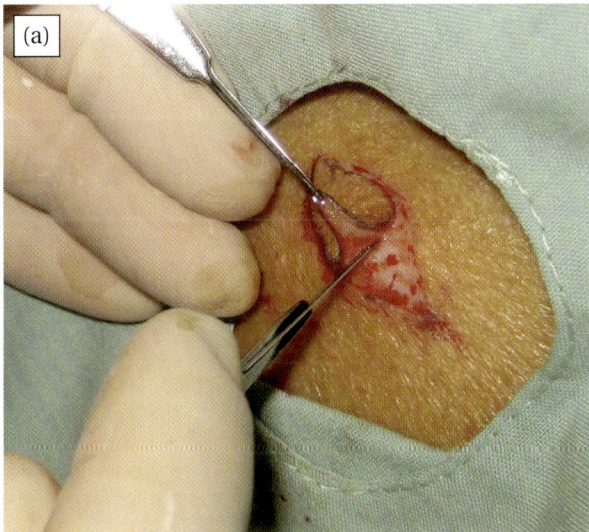

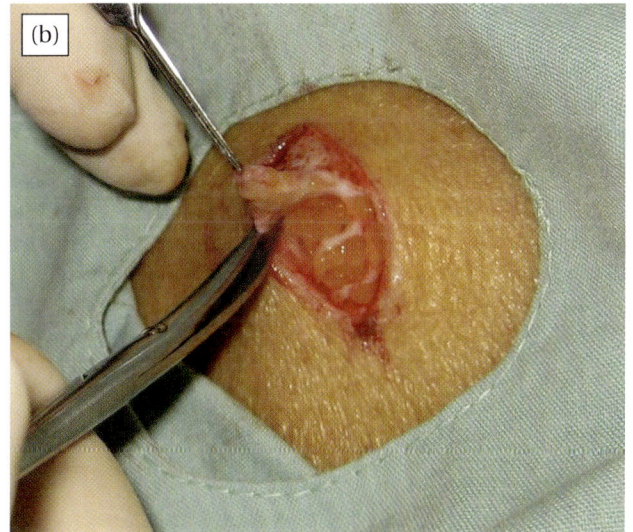

FIGURE 86.21 Dermis fat graft harvesting. (a) Epidermis is removed with a 15 blade to prepare dermis fat graft. A dermabrader may also be used. (b) Very thin dermis fat graft is harvested. Other materials can be used for patching such as fascia or donor sclera.

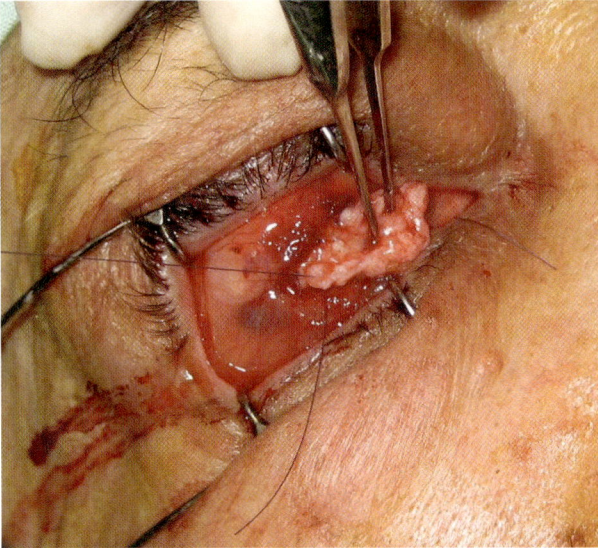

FIGURE 86.22 The dermis fat graft is sutured to edges of the defect using multiple interrupted 6-0 polyglactin sutures.

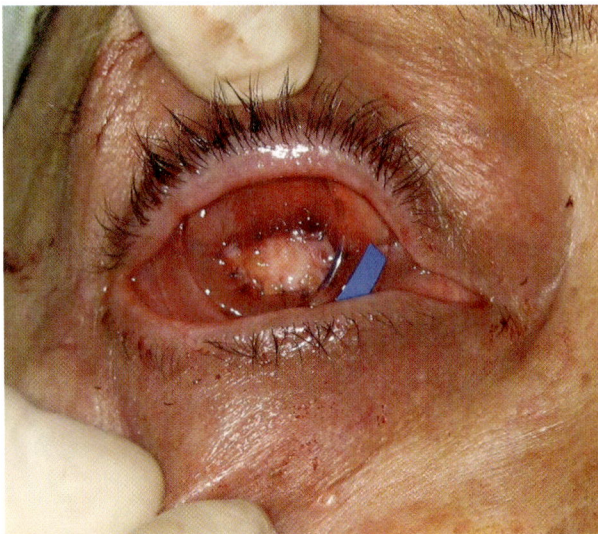

FIGURE 86.23 The conjunctiva is advanced over the edges of the graft and sutured to the graft surface using 6-0 polyglactin suture. At the completion of the procedure, a ring conformer is placed to preserve the fornices without putting pressure on the graft site. Antibiotic ointment is used postoperatively.

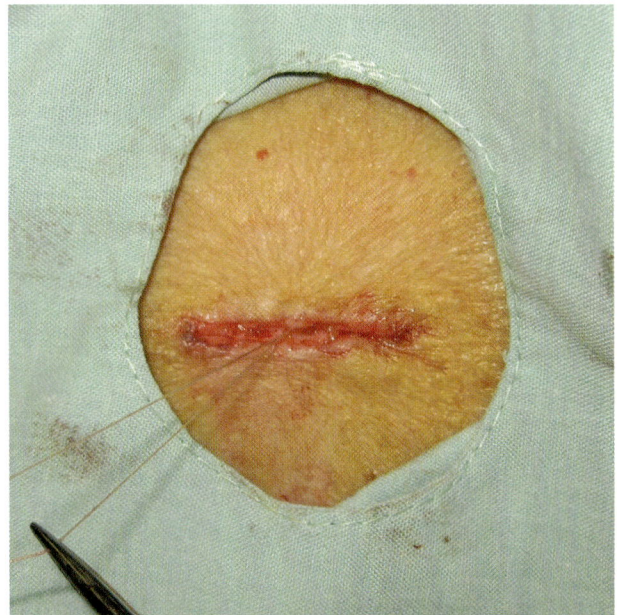

FIGURE 86.24 Multilayered closure of donor site.

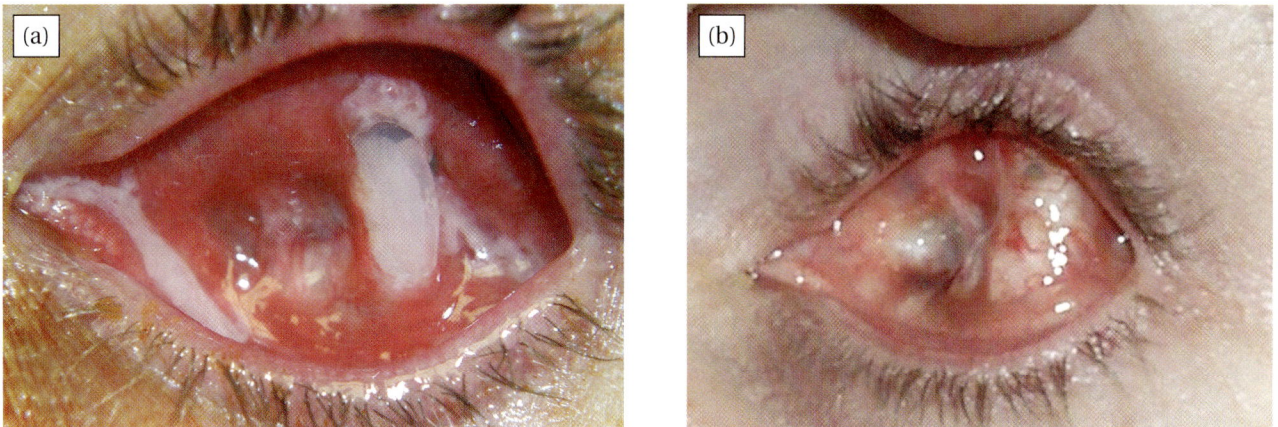

FIGURE 86.25 (a) Exposed Allen type orbital implant. (b) After repair with dermis fat graft patch, which acts as a scaffold for conjunctival growth.

TABLE 86.3 *Potential Complications*

- Volume deficits in the socket are often more significant than they appear, and there may be a tendency to undercorrect.
- Patch grafts for implant exposure may fail due to chronic socket infection and/or poor socket vascularity.
- Our experience suggests that autologous grafts shrink less than synthetic materials, and thus are better suited for reconstruction where conjunctival shortage is a concern.
- Symblepharon and shortening of the fornices can lead to an inability to retain a prosthesis. Care should be taken when performing surgery on the conjunctiva, or even when horizontally shortening the lid, to ensure that adequate fornix remains for the prosthesis.
- Often, more than one procedure may be required to achieve successful rehabilitation of the socket, and this should be discussed with the patient preoperatively.

SELECTED REFERENCES

Beaver HA, Patrinely JR, Holds JB, Soper MP. Periocular autografts in socket reconstruction. *Ophthalmology.* 1996;103(9):1498–1502.

Conn H, Tenzel D, Schou K. Subperiosteal volume augmentation of the anophthalmic socket with RTV silastic. *Adv Ophthalmic Plast Reconstr Surg.* 1990;8:220–228. Review.

Custer PL, Trinkaus KM. Porous implant exposure: Incidence, management, and morbidity. *Ophthal Plast Reconstr Surg.* 2007;23(1):1–7. Review.

Dolphin KW. Complications of postenucleation/evisceration implants. *Curr Opin Ophthalmol.* 1998;9(5):75–77. Review.

Hardy TG, Joshi N, Kelly MH. Orbital volume augmentation with autologous micro-fat grafts. *Ophthal Plast Reconstr Surg.* 2007 Nov-Dec;23(6):445–449.

Holck DE, Foster JA, Dutton JJ, Dillon HD. Hard palate mucosal grafts in the treatment of the contracted socket. *Ophthal Plast Reconstr Surg.* 1999;15(3):202–209.

Kotlus BS, Dryden RM. Correction of anophthalmic enophthalmos with injectable calcium hydroxylapatite (Radiesse). *Ophthal Plast Reconstr Surg.* 2007;23(4):313–314.

Kumar S, Sugandhi P, Arora R, Pandey PK. Amniotic membrane transplantation versus mucous membrane grafting in anophthalmic contracted socket. *Orbit*. 2006;25(3):195–203.

Massry GG, Hornblass A, Rubin P, Holds JB. Tarsal switch procedure for the surgical rehabilitation of the eyelid and socket deficiencies of the anophthalmic socket. *Ophthal Plast Reconstr Surg*. 1999;15(5):333–340.

Mazzoli RA, Raymond WR 4th, Ainbinder DJ, Hansen EA. Use of self-expanding, hydrophilic osmotic expanders (hydrogel) in the reconstruction of congenital clinical anophthalmos. *Curr Opin Ophthalmol*. 2004;15(5):426–431. Review.

Nunery WR, Heinz GW, Bonnin JM, Martin RT, Cepela MA. Exposure rate of hydroxyapatite spheres in the anophthalmic socket: histopathologic correlation and comparison with silicone sphere implants. *Ophthal Plast Reconstr Surg*. 1993;9(2):96–104.

Quaranta-Leoni FM. Treatment of the anophthalmic socket. *Curr Opin Ophthalmol*. 2008;19(5):422–427. Review.

Shoamanesh A, Pang NK, Oestreicher JH. Complications of orbital implants: a review of 542 patients who have undergone orbital implantation and 275 subsequent peg placements. *Orbit*. 2007 Sep;26(3):173–182.

Shore JW, McCord CD Jr, Bergin DJ, Dittmar SJ, Maiorca JP, Burks WR. Management of complications following dermis-fat grafting for anophthalmic socket reconstruction. *Ophthalmology*. 1985;92(10):1342–1350.

Weiss RA, McCord CD Jr, Ellsworth RM. Reconstruction of the anophthalmic socket: lower eyelid malposition and canthal tendon laxity. *Adv Ophthalmic Plast Reconstr Surg*. 1990;8:192–208. Review.

Yoon JS, Lew H, Kim SJ, Lee SY. Exposure rate of hydroxyapatite orbital implants a 15-year experience of 802 cases. *Ophthalmology*. 2008;115(3):566–572.

87

Anterior Orbitotomy

Karim G. Punja, MD

TABLE 87.1 *Indications for Anterior Orbitotomy*

1. Diagnostic biopsy
2. Removal of lesion
3. Orbital decompression
4. Orbital reconstruction

TABLE 87.2 *Preoperative Considerations*

1. High resolution axial and coronal orbital imaging is a prerequisite for devising a sound surgical plan.
2. CT imaging is superb for bony detail, as well as soft tissue delineation.
3. MRI imaging with contrast is ideal for soft tissue detail and for vascular lesions.
4. The surgical approach into the orbit is dependent upon the quadrant of interest: superior/lateral, inferior, medial, central. Lateral orbitotomy is covered in Chapter 88. The choice of surgical approach should balance function with the aesthetic result, with the former always taking precedence.
5. Superior orbitotomy
   a. Upper eyelid crease incision
6. Inferior orbitotomy
   a. Transconjunctival incision
   b. Infraciliary incision
   c. Lower eyelid skin crease incision (not preferred approach)
7. Medial orbitotomy
   a. Transcaruncular incision
   b. Perilimbal incision
   c. Lynch incision (not preferred approach)
8. Adequate exposure is critical, and is facilitated by traction sutures, proper instrumentation, a surgical assistant, and a head light.

Surgical Approaches to Anterior Orbitotomy

Superior Orbitotomy through Upper Eyelid Crease Incision

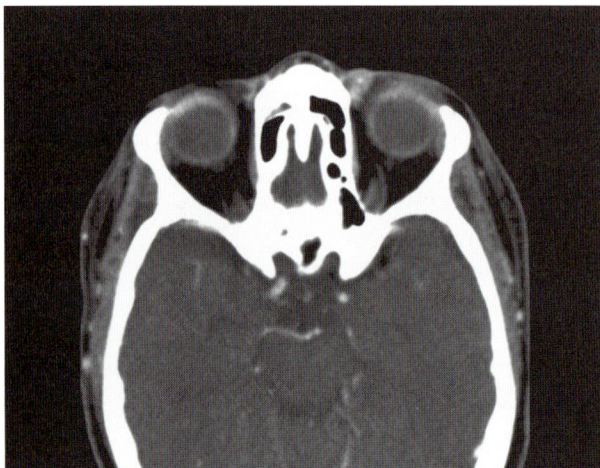

FIGURE 87.1 Preoperative Imaging. The patient presented with a left superonasal orbital mass. This mobile, firm, nontender mass had been progressively enlarging for 1 year.

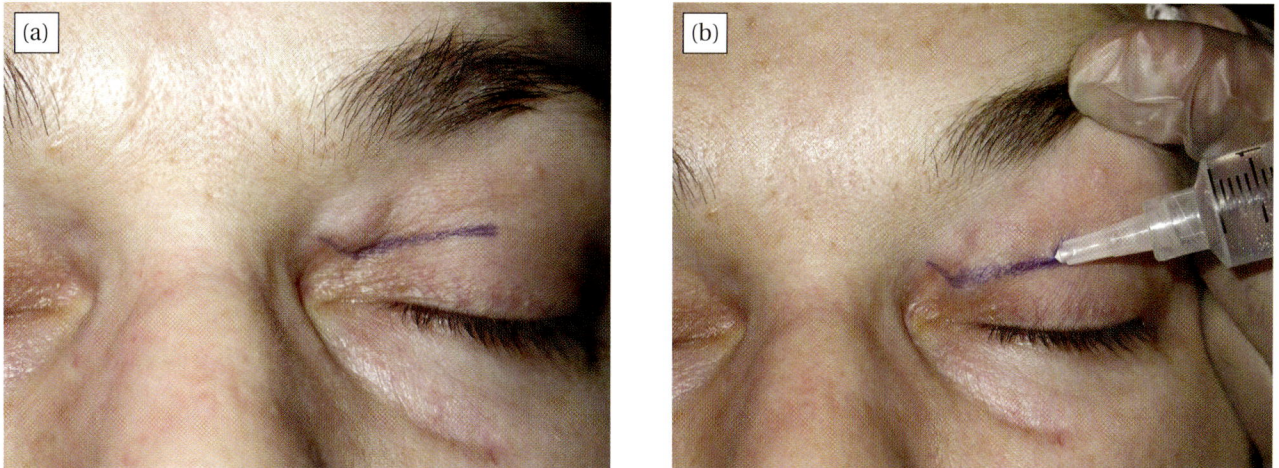

FIGURE 87.2 Eyelid Crease Marking and Local Anesthetic. A medial upper eyelid crease incision is delineated with the marking pen overlying the orbital mass (a). Local anesthetic is infiltrated into the superior orbit around the mass. Lidocaine 2% with 1:100,000 epinephrine, mixed with 0.75% bupivacaine in a 50:50 solution, is injected using a short (1/2 inch) 30 gauge needle (b).

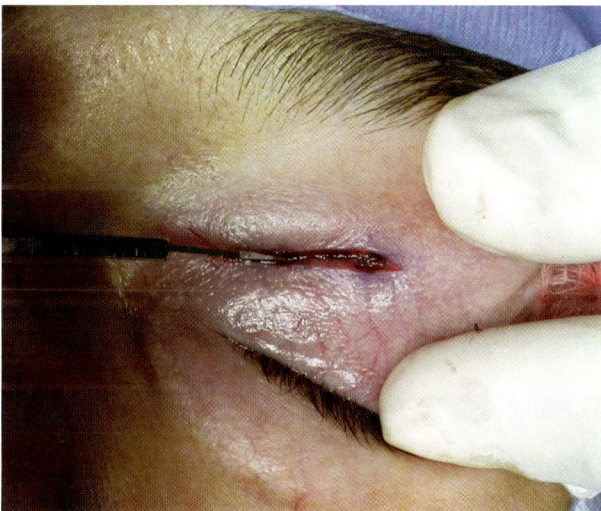

FIGURE 87.3 Eyelid Crease Incision. A #15 Bard Parker blade is used to make an incision through skin and orbicularis.

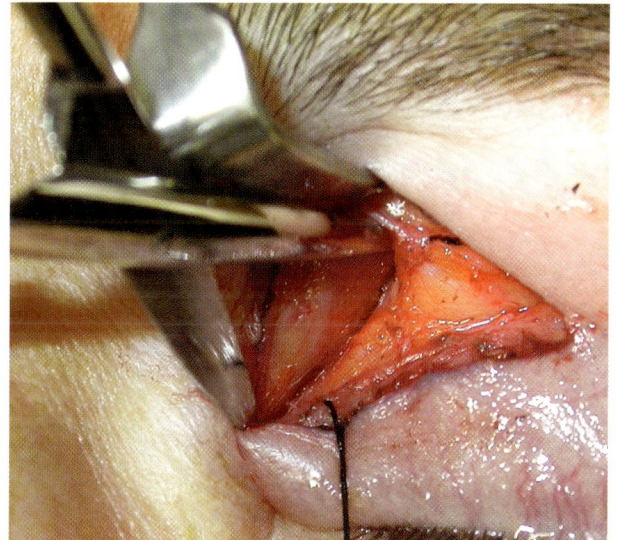

FIGURE 87.4 Blunt Dissection in Anterior Orbit. The orbital septum is divided with careful dissection using blunt tipped Westcott scissors and curved iris scissors. A 4-0 silk suture is placed along the preseptal orbicularis for retraction inferiorly.

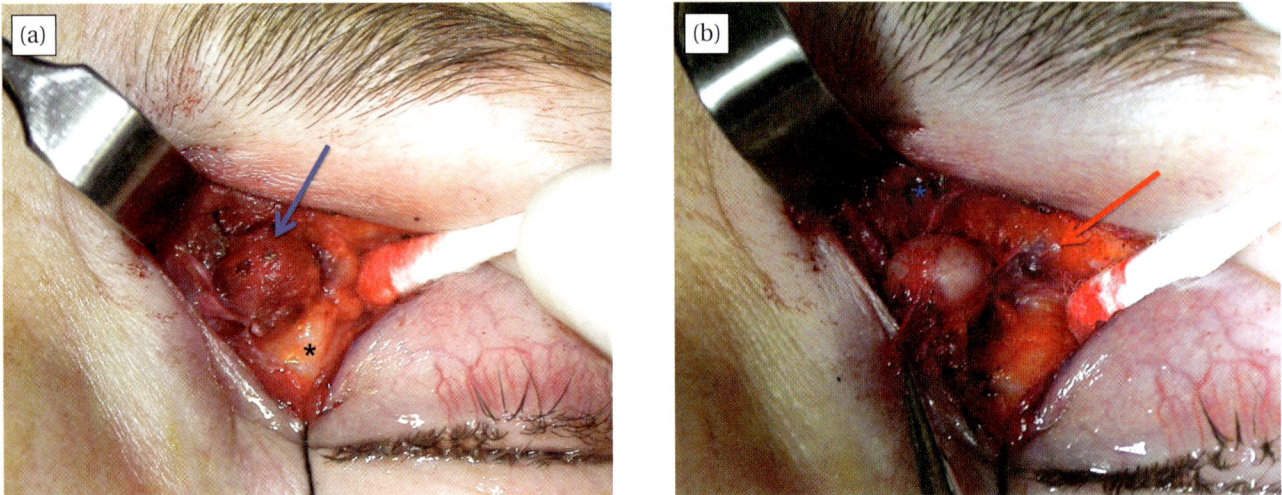

FIGURE 87.5 Delineation of Orbital Mass. (a, b) The mass (blue arrow) is visible just posterior to the orbital septum and superior to the preaponeurotic fat pad (black asterisk). The superior ophthalmic vein (b; red arrow) is identified and avoided. Cotton-tipped applicators keep the surgical field dry, and are a useful adjunct for blunt dissection. The trochlea (blue asterisk) is located in this superonasal quadrant. Injury can result in an acquired Brown's syndrome.

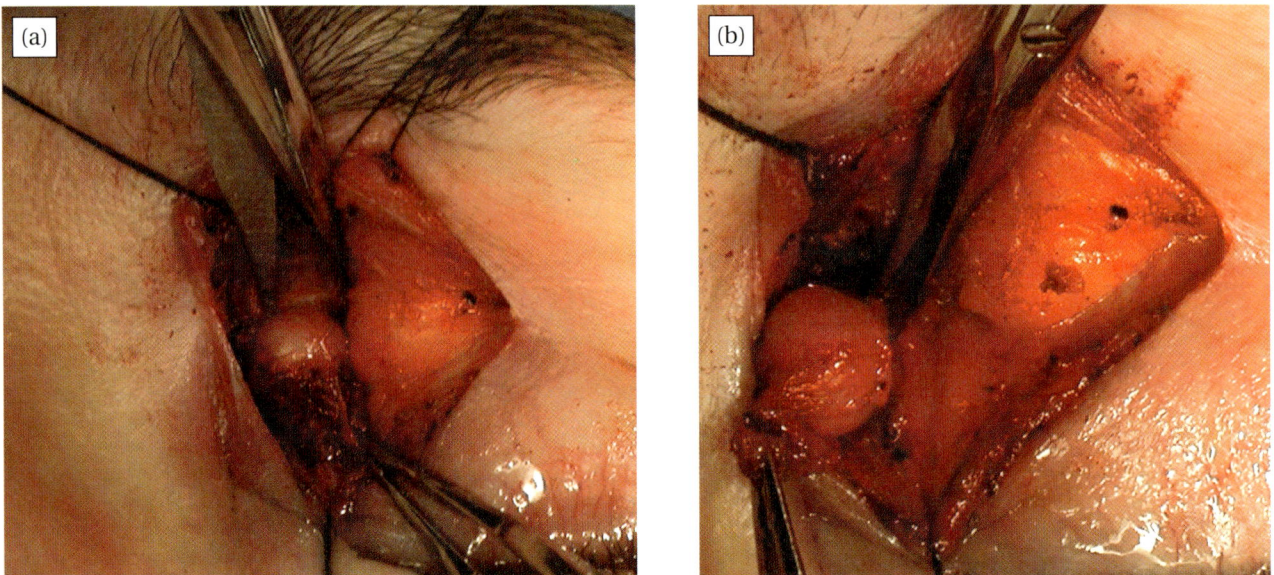

FIGURE 87.6 Removal of Orbital Mass. Blunt and sharp dissection is performed around the mass with blunt tipped Westcott scissors (a). Gentle traction is placed on the lesion by grasping the soft tissue adherent to the anterior aspect of the lesion (b). Note that additional traction sutures are placed superiorly, enhancing exposure.

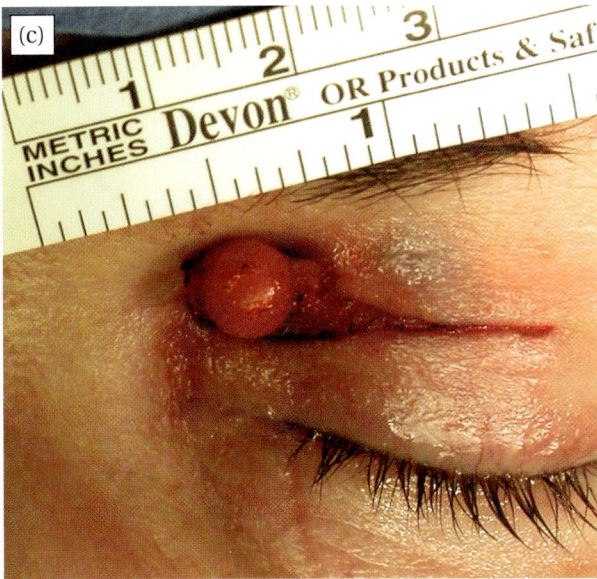

FIGURE 87.6 (*continued*) The intact cystic lesion is removed and measures 9 mm in diameter (c). Histopathology of the lesion revealed a thrombosed varix.

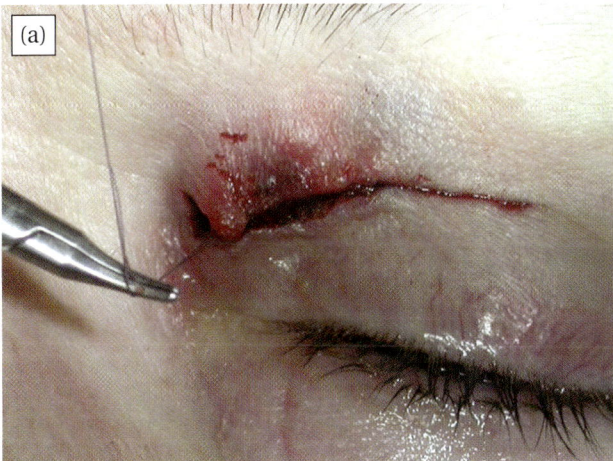

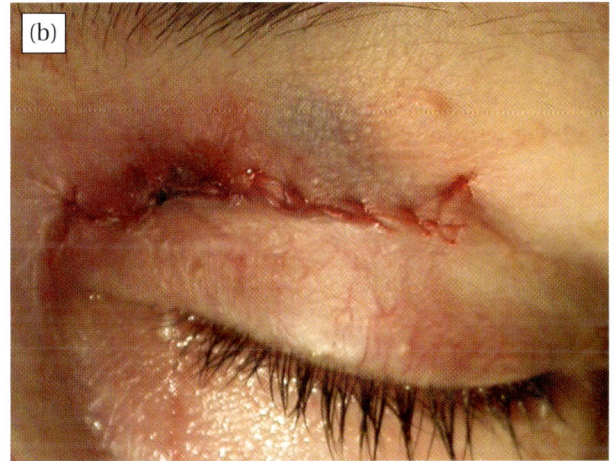

FIGURE 87.7 Closure. (a, b) The orbicularis is closed with buried, interrupted 6-0 polyglactin sutures. The orbital septum is not closed, as this can result in eyelid retraction. The skin is closed with 6-0 poliglecaprone (Monocryl).

Inferior Orbitotomy through Transconjunctival Incision

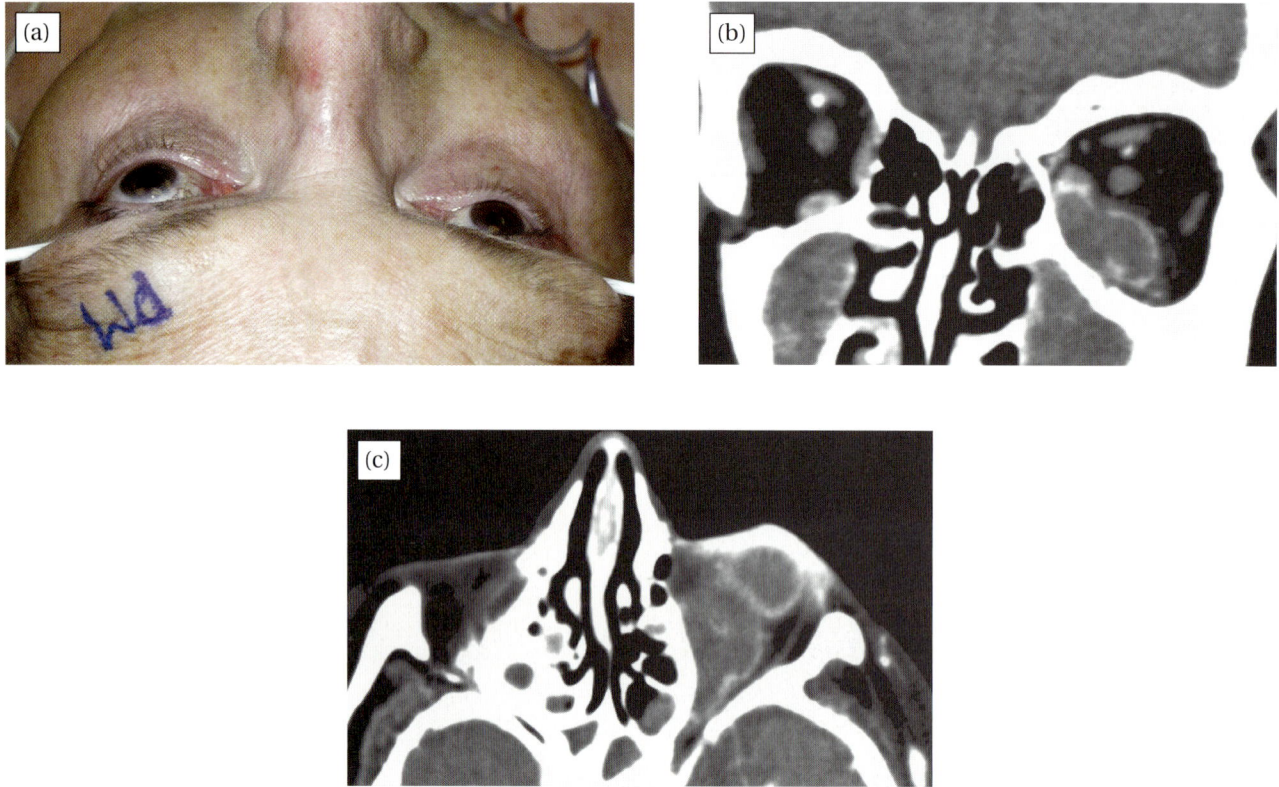

FIGURE 87.8   (a, b, c) Subperiosteal abscess along inferomedial wall left eye. Note left eye proptosis.

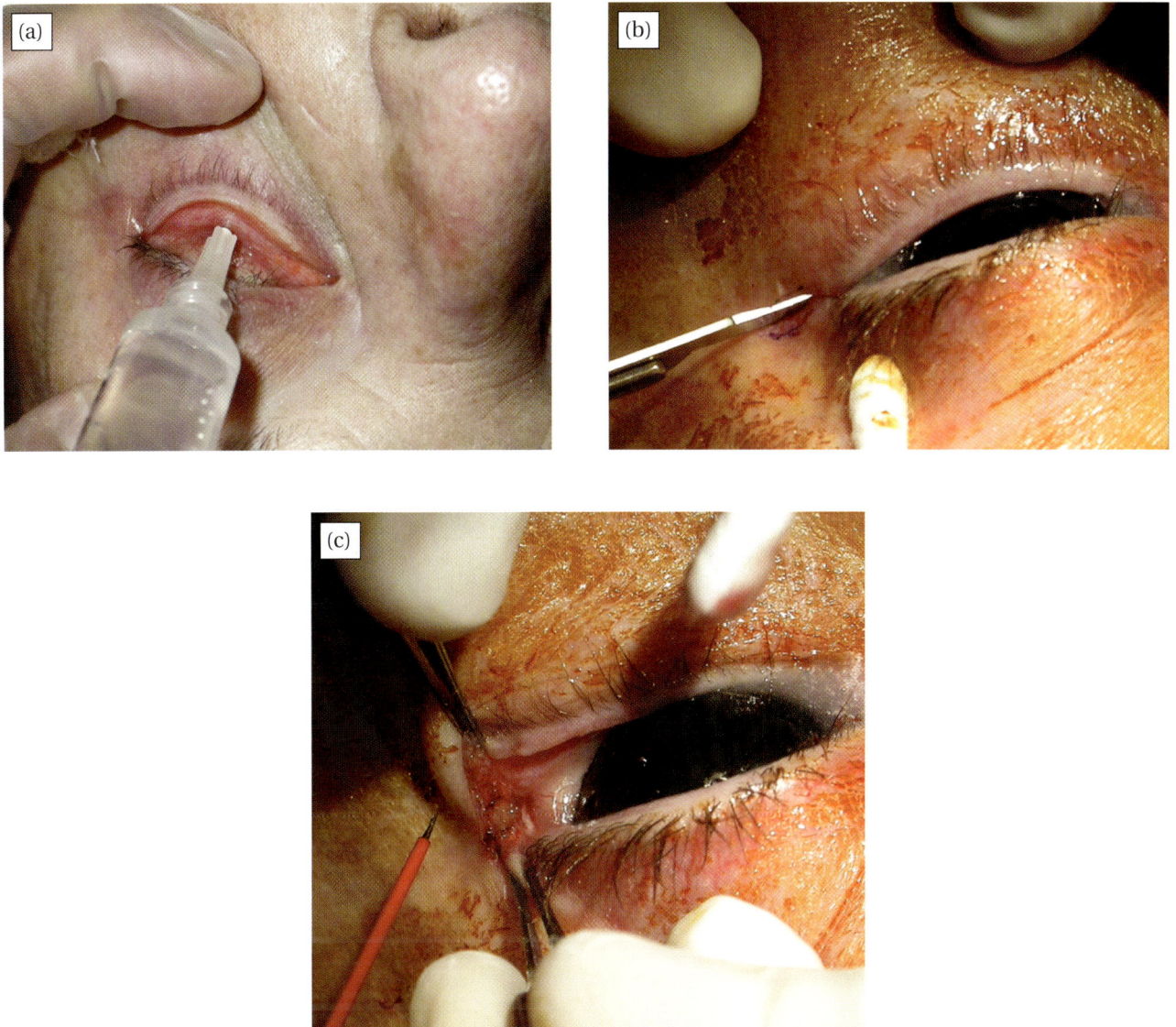

FIGURE 87.9 Lateral Canthotomy. Local anesthetic is given through a transconjunctival injection (a). A #15 blade is used to make a lateral canthotomy (b). Monopolar cautery is used to perform the inferior cantholysis (c).

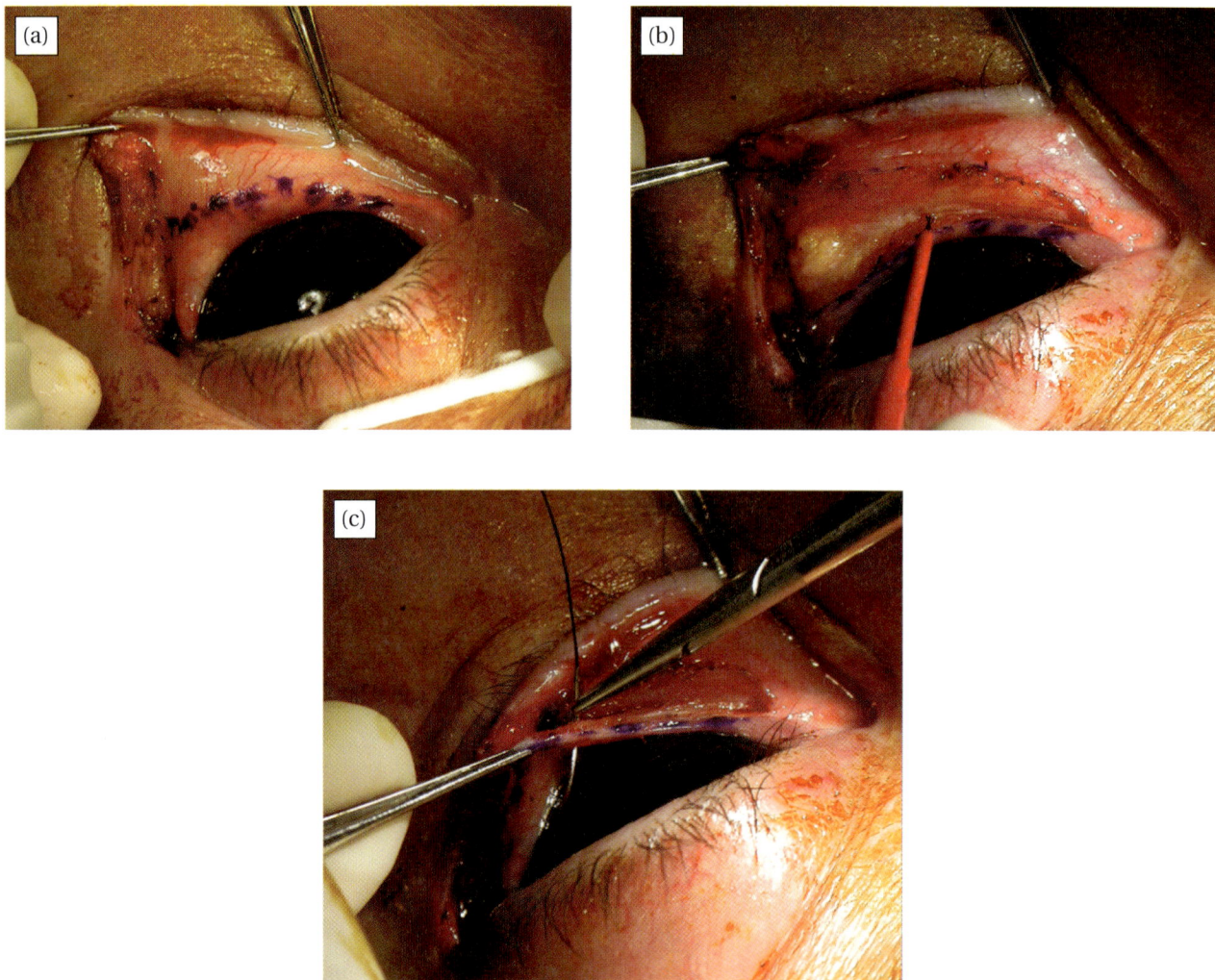

FIGURE 87.10 Transconjunctival Incision. A transconjunctival incision is performed with the cutting monopolar (a, b). The swinging eyelid approach provides improved access particularly when the orbit is congested. A 4-0 silk suture is placed through the conjunctiva and lower eyelid retractors for traction (c).

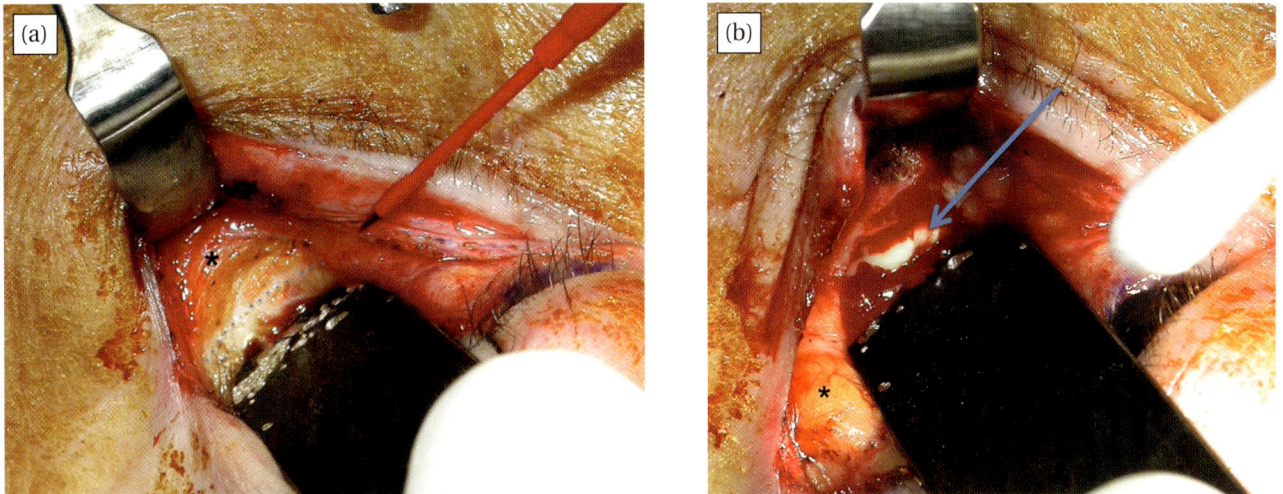

FIGURE 87.11 Subperiosteal Dissection. The lower eyelid is retracted inferiorly with the Senn retractor. The Senn and the malleable retractors straddle the inferior orbital rim (a) guiding the correct plane of dissection along the inferior orbital rim temporal to nasal. The malleable retractor protects the globe from injury. Inferior orbital rim periosteum is the glistening white tissue along the dashed line. The orbicularis oculi is marked with an asterisk (a). Once the subperiosteal plane is entered along the orbital floor, purulent discharge immediately drains out (Figure [b], blue arrow). Cultures are taken of the discharge. The asterisk in figure (b) indicates the lower eyelid temporal fat pad.

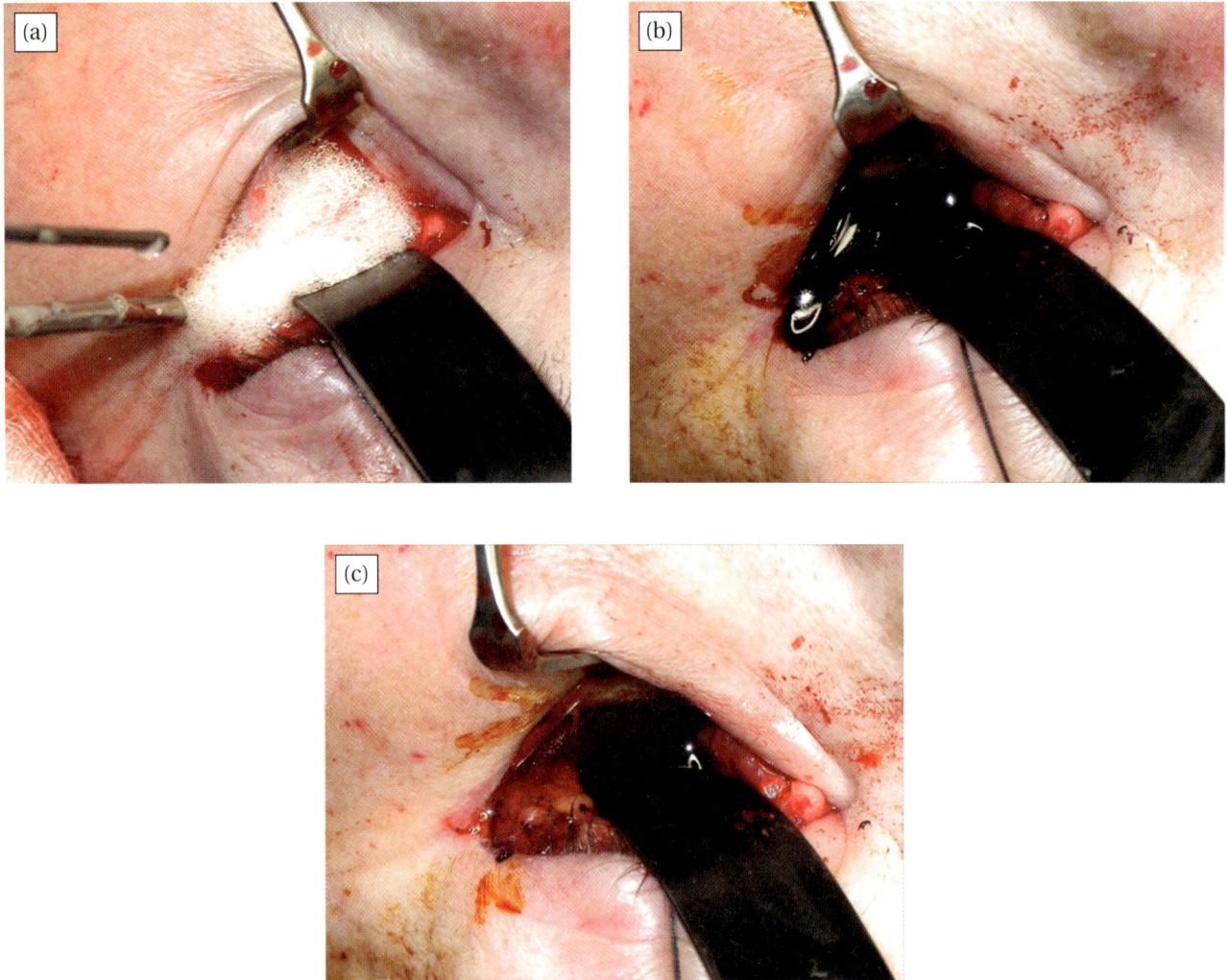

FIGURE 87.12 Drainage of Abscess. The subperiosteal abscess is then drained, and hydrogen peroxide is irrigated along the inferior orbit (a). Povidone iodine solution is irrigated subsequently (b), and this is followed by a copious normal saline wash (c).

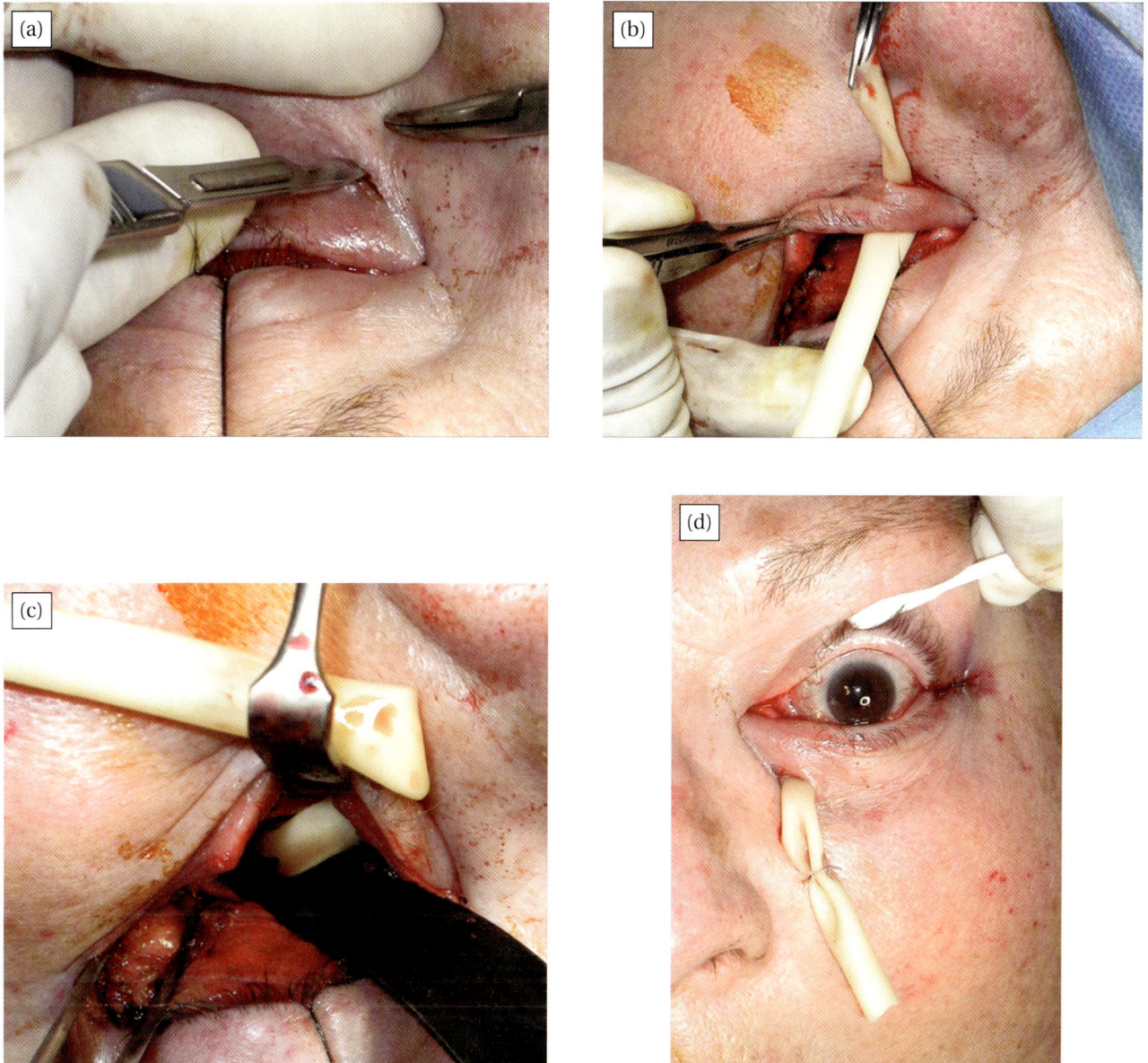

FIGURE 87.13 Placement of Penrose Drain. A small incision is made in the lower eyelid with a #15 blade (a). A Penrose drain is drawn through this incision and placed along the orbital floor (b, c). The drain is then secured anteriorly to the skin for removal in 24–48 hours (d). Concurrent endoscopic sinus surgery may be performed to address the underlying sinusitis.

Medial Orbitotomy through Transcaruncular Incision

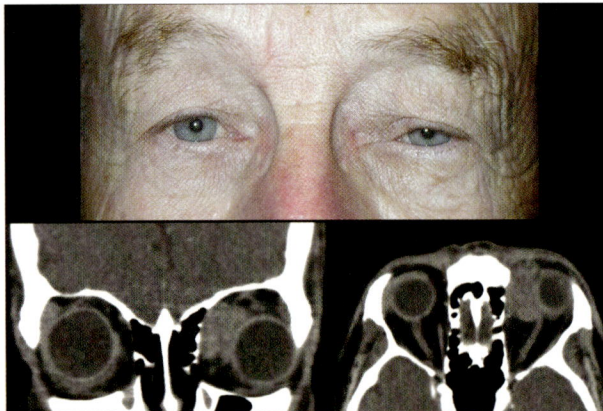

FIGURE 87.14 Medial Orbital Mass. This elderly patient presented with diplopia and left orbital pressure. CT imaging shows a vascular malformation in the left medial orbit.

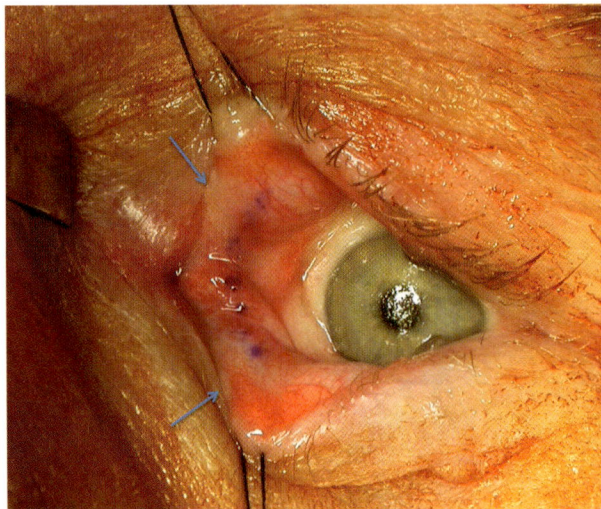

FIGURE 87.15 Transcaruncular Approach. Traction sutures with 4-0 silk are placed along the lid margins just temporal to the lacrimal puncta (arrows). The plane of incision is between the medial 3/4 and the lateral 1/4 of the caruncle, extending to the superior and inferior fornices nasally. The canaliculi are adjacent to the incision, and care must be taken to avoid injuring these structures. Exposure can be improved by making an inferior transconjunctival incision first, and extending the mouth of the internal incision.

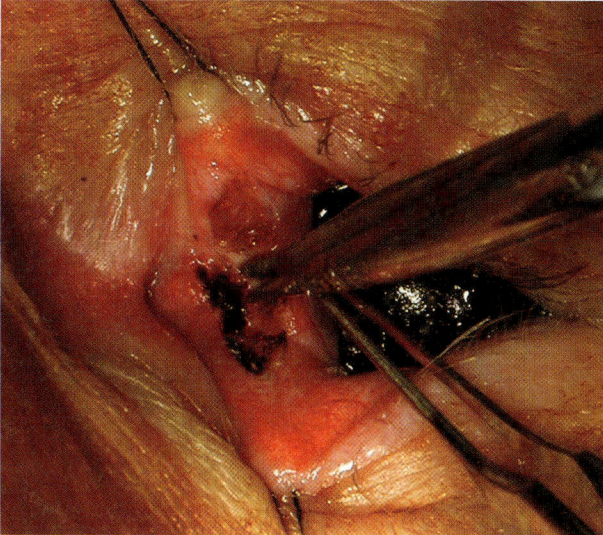

FIGURE 87.16 Transcaruncular Incision. Using the blunt tipped Westcott scissors, sharp and blunt dissection proceeds posteriorly through Tenon's capsule in the direction of the posterior lacrimal crest. Note that a corneal protector is necessary to protect the anterior surface of the globe. The periosteum is incised and dissection proceeds posteriorly.

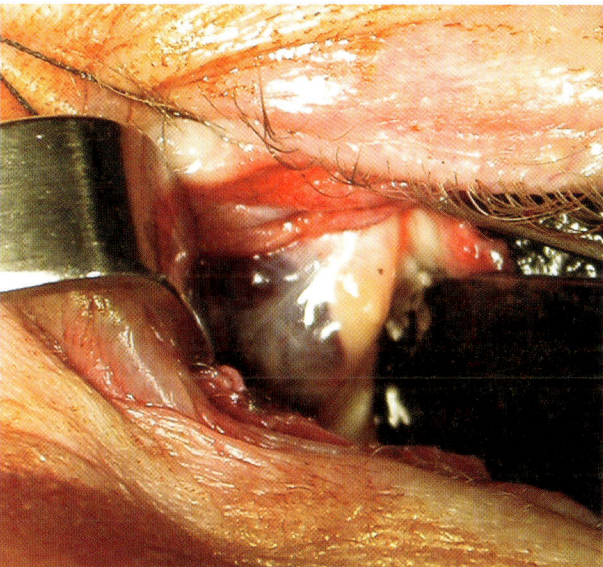

FIGURE 87.17 Dissection to Mass. Blunt dissection with cotton-tipped applicators and malleable retractors reveals the dark blue color of the vascular malformation medial to the intraconal fat. Note the plane of dissection: the medial retractor is extraconal. The mass is protruding anteriorly from the intraconal space between the globe and the medial rectus muscle. The medial rectus muscle is being displaced inferiorly by the more lateral malleable retractor.

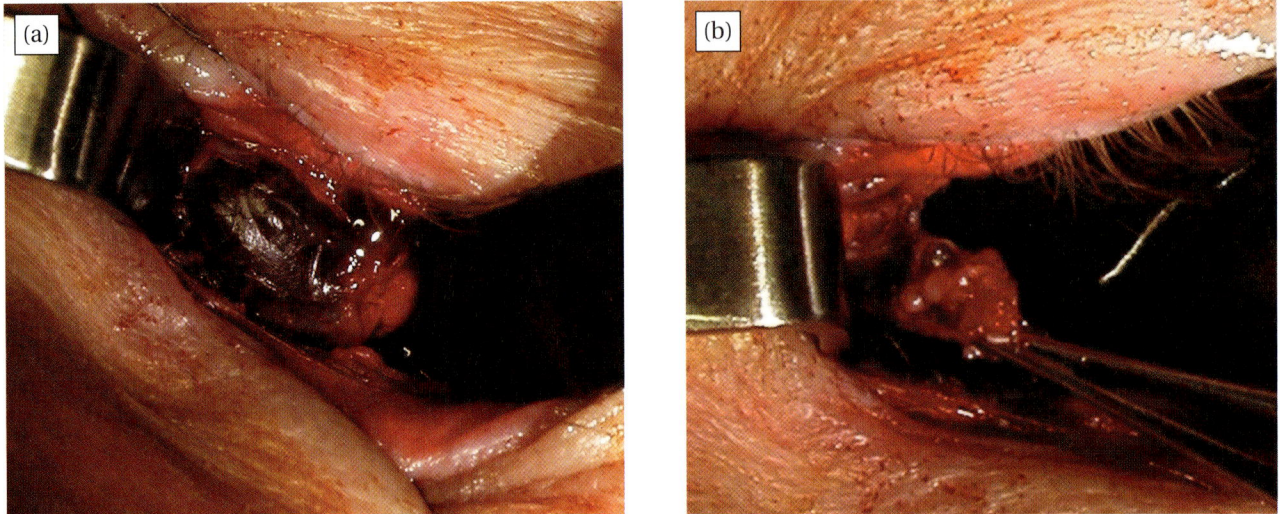

FIGURE 87.18 Excision of Mass. The malleable retractor moves the globe and intraconal fat laterally. With careful blunt dissection, the posterior boundaries of the vascular malformation are identified between the superior rectus, medial rectus, and the optic nerve. Potential feeding vessels are meticulously addressed with bipolar cautery (a). As this was a very low-flow malformation, exsanguination of the malformation was performed. By decompressing this large-volume lesion, better exposure of the central orbital space was achieved, allowing complete dissection of the posterior aspect of lesion (b).

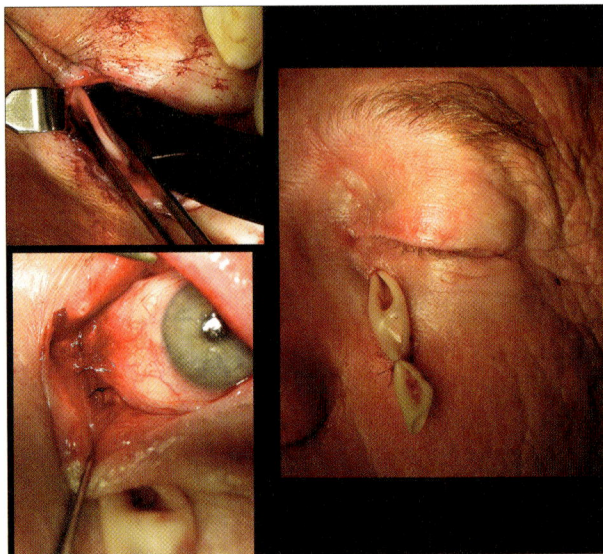

FIGURE 87.19 Placement of Penrose Drain. A drain is placed in the medial intraconal space. The transcaruncular incision is closed with a running 6-0 mild chromic suture.

TABLE 87.3 *Potential Complications of Anterior Orbitotomy*

1. Retrobulbar hemorrhage
2. Orbital cellulitis
3. Damage to cranial nerves, ciliary ganglion, or sensory nerves
4. Traumatic optic neuropathy
5. Globe rupture/retinal detachment
6. Ptosis
7. Incomplete tumor removal

SELECTED REFERENCES

Dortzbach RK, Kronish JW. Orbital disease. In: Dortzbach RK (ed). *Ophthalmic plastic surgery: Prevention and management of complications.* (pp. 307–361). New York: Raven Press, Ltd.; 1994.

Leone CR. Surgical approach to the medial retrobulbar space. *Am J Ophthalmol.* 1983;96:1–5.

Rootman J. Regional approach to anterior, mid, and apical orbit. In: Rootman J, Stewart B, Goldberg RA (eds). *Orbital surgery: a conceptual approach.* (pp. 151–175) Philadelphia: Lipincott-Raven; 1995.

Shore JW. The fornix approach to the inferior orbit. In: Bosniak SL (ed) *Advances in Ophthalmic plastic reconstructive surgery* (pp. 377–385). New York: Pergamon Press; 1987.

Shorr N, Baylis HI, Goldberg RA, Perry JD. Transcaruncular approach to the medial orbit and orbital apex. *Ophthalmology.* 2000;107:1459–1463.

Westfall CT, Shore JW, Nunery WR, Hawes MJ, Yaremchuk MJ. Operative complications of the transconjunctival inferior fornix approach. *Ophthalmology.* 1991;98:1525–1528.

88 | Lateral Orbitotomy

Roberta E. Gausas, MD

TABLE 88.1 *Indications for Orbital Surgery*

Identification of disease:
  – *Biopsy*
Treatment of disease:
  – *Resection of tumor*
  – *Abscess drainage*
Restoration of ocular function:
  – *Repair of orbital fracture*
  – *Thyroid-related orbital decompression*
Functional and Social Orbital Rehabilitation:
  – *Following head & neck cancer removal*

TABLE 88.2 *Goals of Orbital Surgery*

Gain access to specific location in orbit safely:
  – *selection of appropriate surgical approach based on evaluation of preoperative imaging*
Achieve optimum aesthetic outcome without compromising exposure:
  – *balance choice of surgical approach with risks specific to orbital surgery*

TABLE 88.3 *Historical Evolution of Lateral Orbitotomy and Modifications*

Kronlein 1888
  pioneered lateral bone flap to access retrobulbar space
Berke 1953
  modified incision for improved exposure & cosmesis
Stallard-Wright 1960
  alternative lateral approach with improved exposure
Modification of Stallard-Wright
Extended Lid Crease Approach
  allows for hidden scar without compromising exposure
Modification of Berke approach
Lateral Canthotomy/Cantholysis with/without Bone Flap
  minimizes incision, appropriate for lesions located in antero-lateral orbit
Combined Lateral Orbitotomy and Medial Transconjunctival Incision
  allows improved access to lesions located in medial orbit

Surgical Approach to Lateral Orbitotomy

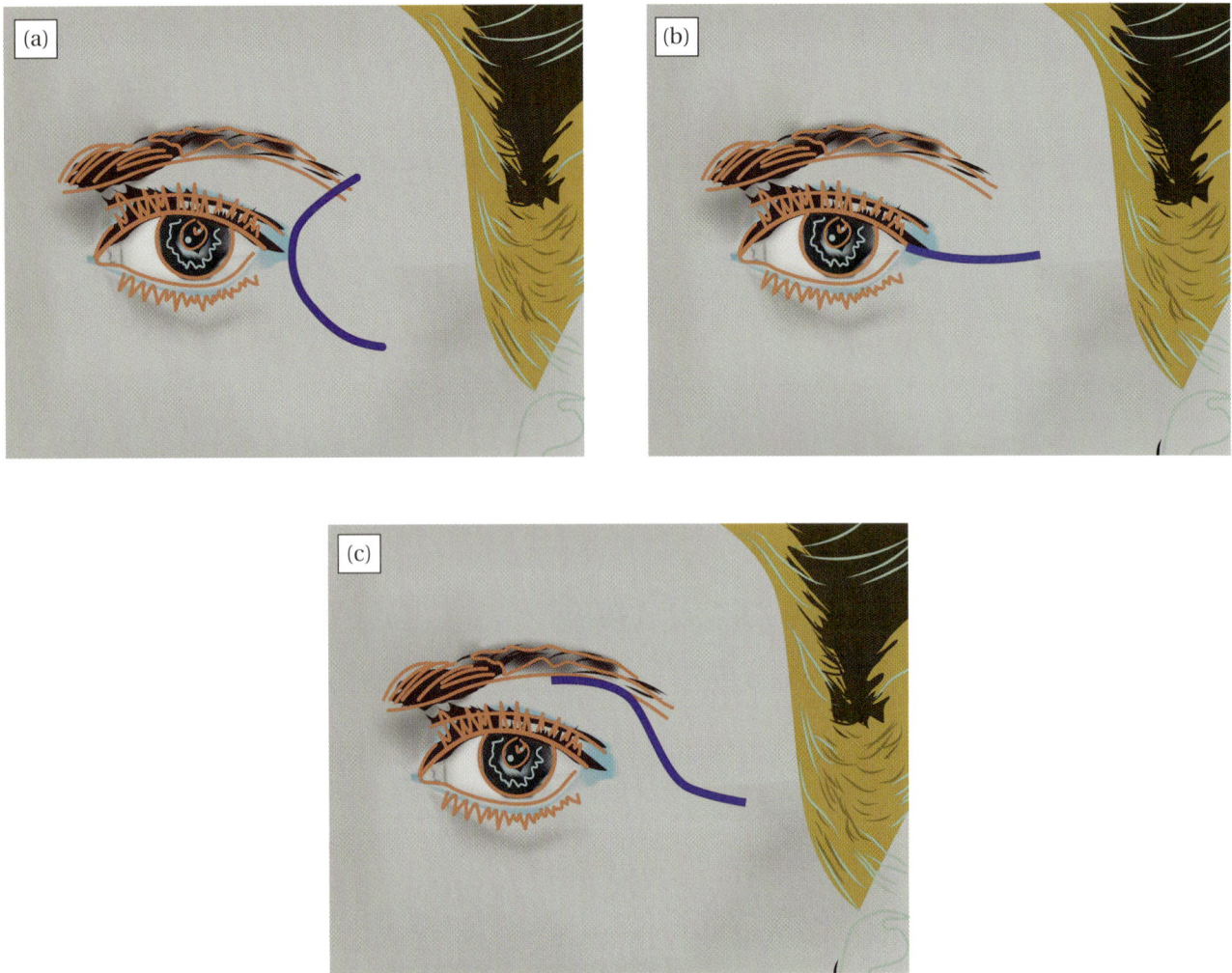

FIGURE 88.1 Summary of Surgical Approaches (incisions depicted in blue). (a) Kronlein approach; (b) Berke approach; (c) Stallard-Wright approach.

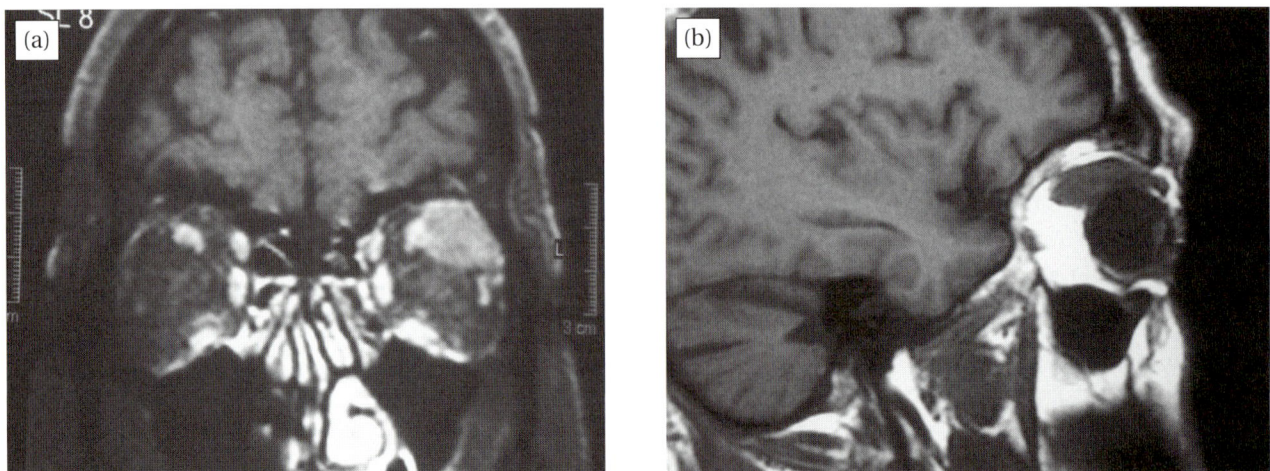

FIGURE 88.2 (a) Coronal MRI of left postero-lateral orbital lesion. (b) Sagittal MRI of same patient.

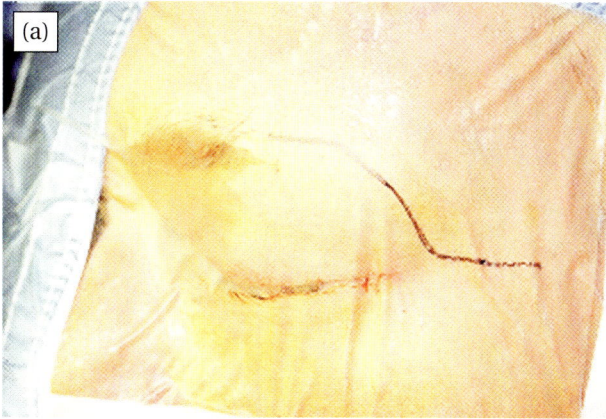

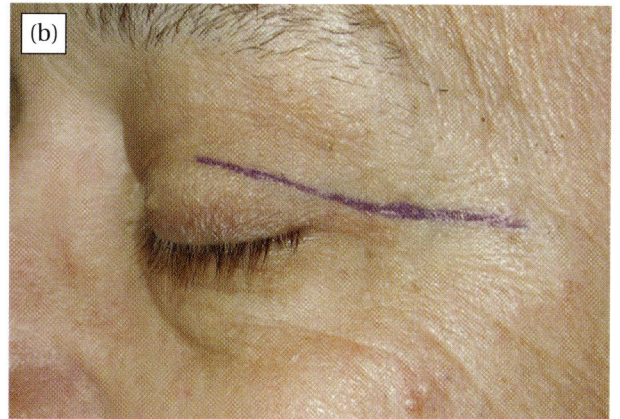

FIGURE 88.3 (a) Patient preparation for Stallard-Wright incision. (b) Patient preparation for extended eyelid incision.

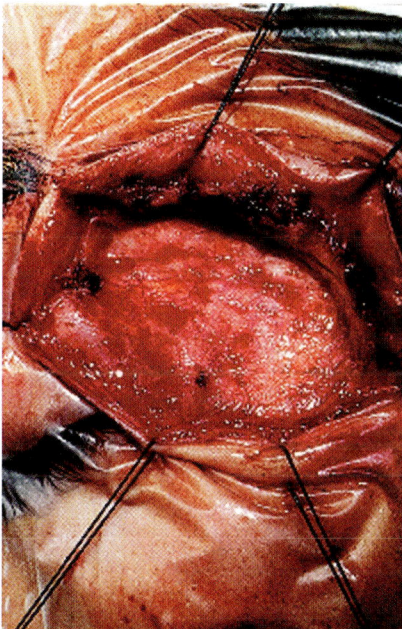

FIGURE 88.4 Exposure of temporalis fascia and periosteum of right lateral orbital wall after elevation of skin-muscle flap.

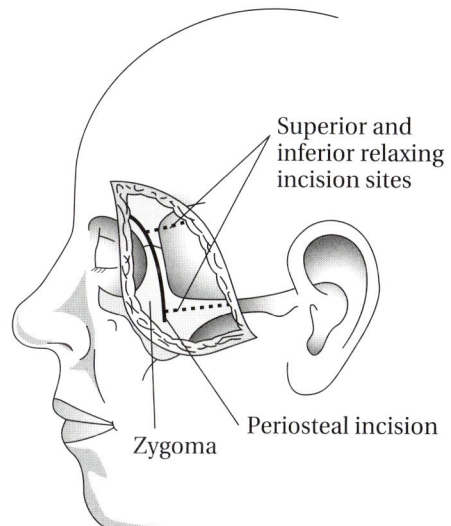

FIGURE 88.5 Incision of periosteum along anterior edge of lateral orbital rim. Relaxing incisions above zygomatic arch and at upper limit of temporal fossa.

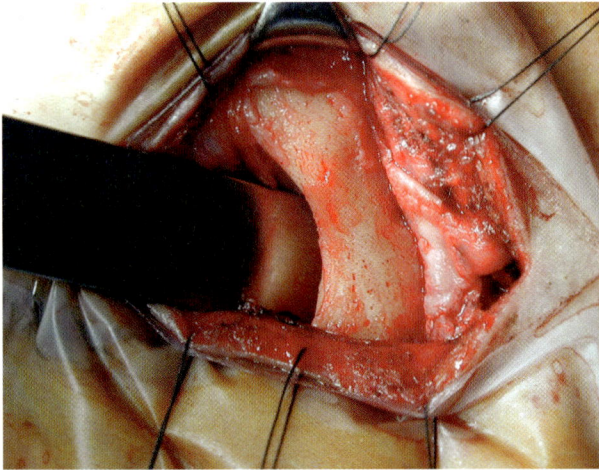

FIGURE 88.6 Exposure of left lateral orbital rim and wall after elevation of periosteum.

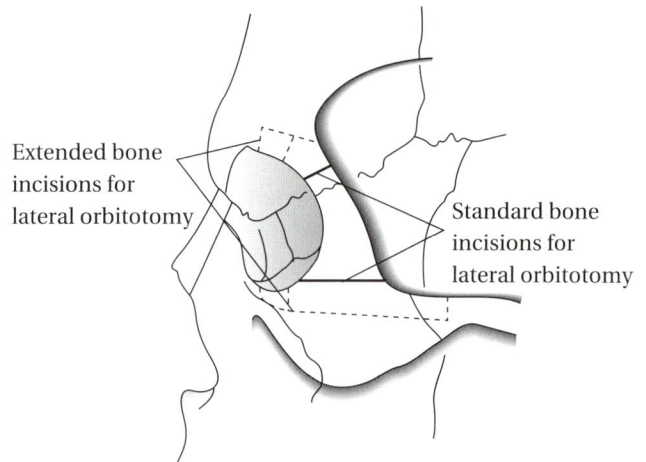

FIGURE 88.7 Coronal and lateral anatomical placement of standard bony orbital incisions demonstrated by bold lines. Dotted lines indicate alternative extended bony cuts as dictated by location of lesion.

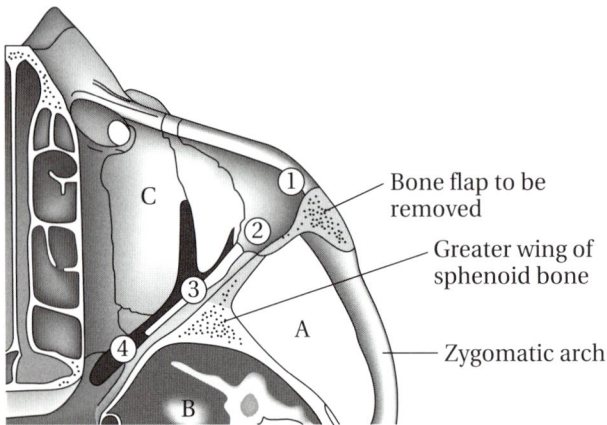

FIGURE 88.8 The lateral orbital wall has varying thicknesses. It is thick at the orbital rim (1); thin adjacent to the temporal fossa (2); thick at the junction with cranium (3); and thin adjacent to the middle cranial fossa (4). A indicates temporal fossa; B, middle cranial fossa; and C, orbit.

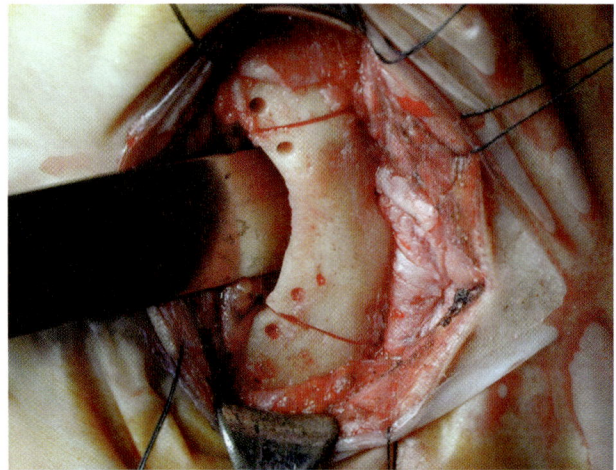

FIGURE 88.9 Pre-drill holes before placement of final bone cuts (left orbit).

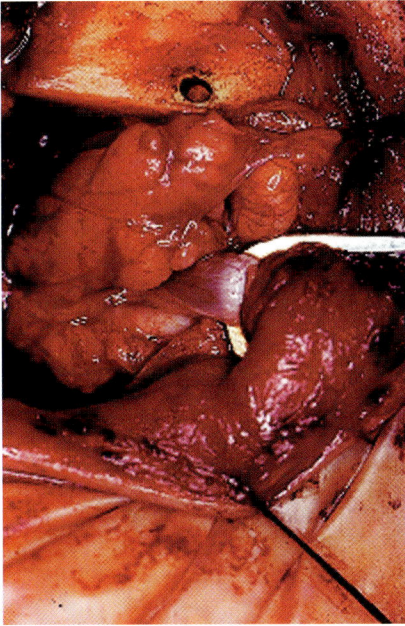

FIGURE 88.10 Opening of orbital periosteum and identification of lateral rectus muscle with muscle hook, immediately inferior to lacrimal gland.

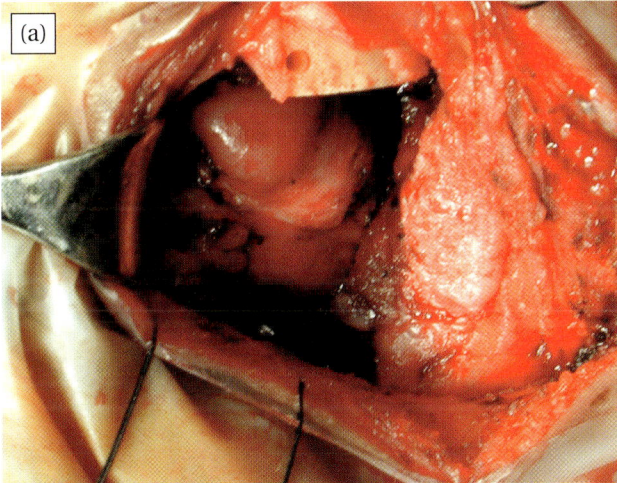

(a)

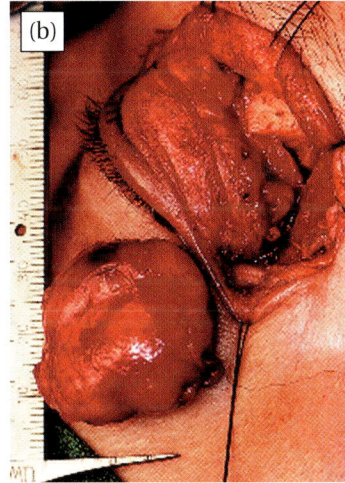

(b)

FIGURE 88.11 (a) Orbital dissection exposes mass. (b) Completed resection of mass through osteotomy.

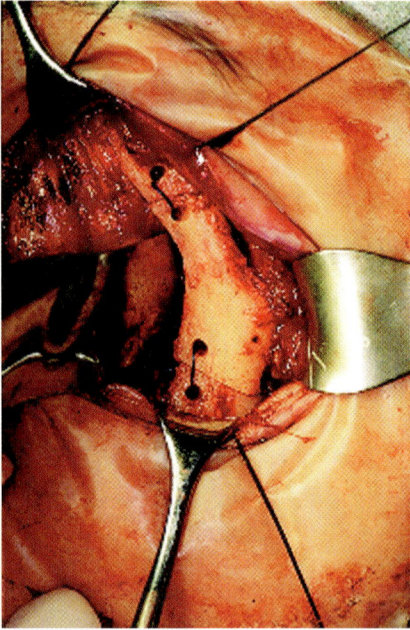

FIGURE 88.12 Replacement of lateral rim bone fragment with 2-0 polypropylene suture through predrilled holes.

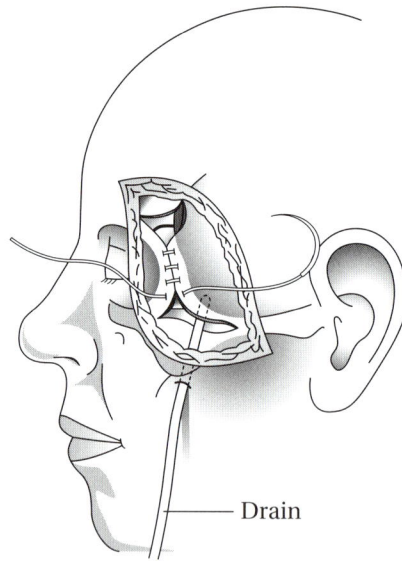

FIGURE 88.13 Closure of deep layers achieved by re-approximating periosteum over bone with 5-0 polyglactin suture. Close inferior relaxing incision loosely to allow egress of possible hemorrhage. Drain is placed deep to the periosteum within temporalis fossa but not within orbit.

FIGURE 88.14 Closure of superficial layers achieved by re-approximating muscle and skin. Drain secured lateral to orbit.

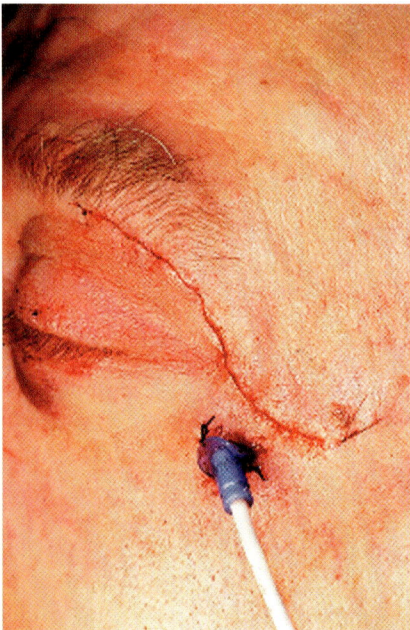

TABLE 88.4 *Potential Complications of Orbital Surgery*

Optic Nerve Injury
  visual loss
Extraocular Muscle Injury
  diplopia
Cranial Nerve III, IV or VI Injury
  ptosis and/or diplopia
CSF leak
  meningitis
Orbital Hemorrhage
Incomplete Excision of Lesion

SELECTED REFERENCES

Harris GJ, Logani SC. Eyelid crease incision for lateral orbitotomy. *Ophthal Plast Reconstr Surg.* 1999;15:916.
Rootman J, Kao SC, Graeb DA. Multidisciplinary approaches to complicated vascular lesions of the orbit. *Ophthalmology.* 1992;99:1440–1446.

Rootman J, Stewart B, Goldberg RA. *Orbital surgery. A conceptual approach.* 1st ed. Philadelphia: Lippincott-Raven; 1995.

Optic Nerve Sheath Fenestration

Timothy J. McCulley, MD

TABLE 89.1 *Indications for Optic Nerve Sheath Fenestration*

Intracranial hypertension refractory to maximum medical therapy causing optic neuropathy

Cryptococcal optic neuropathy

TABLE 89.2 *Preoperative Considerations*

Maximize medical therapy prior to consideration of surgery

General anesthesia considerations with respect to patient habitus (idiopathic intracranial hypertension)

Surgical approaches:

Limbal, transcaruncular, supramedial eyelid crease, or lateral canthotomy

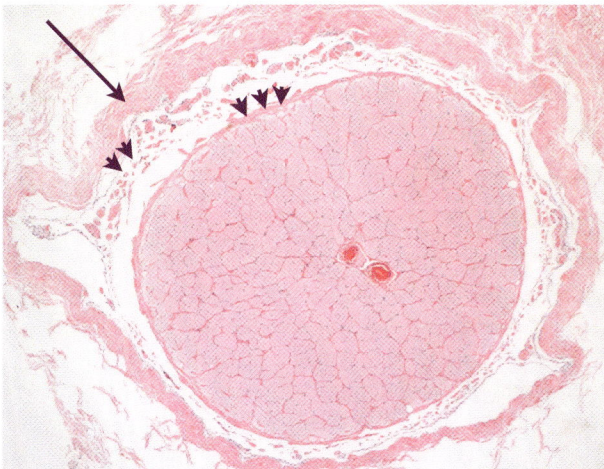

FIGURE 89.1 Cross section of the optic nerve (stain, hematoxylin-eosin; original magnification, 20×). Optic nerve sheath fenestration (ONSF) or decompression creates a window through the dural and arachnoid meningeal layers of the optic nerve sheath. Note the thicker outer dural layer (arrow). A thinner arachnoid layer (two arrowheads) surrounds the subarachnoid space, which contains the cerebral spinal fluid (CSF). To effectively decompress the optic nerve, the fenestration must continue through the dura and arachnoid layers. When reached, a "rush" of CSF is often observed, especially in cases with marked elevations in intracranial pressure. Care must be taken not to injure the underlying pial layer (three arrowheads), which contains blood vessels supplying the optic nerve. Direct injury to the nerve should also be avoided.

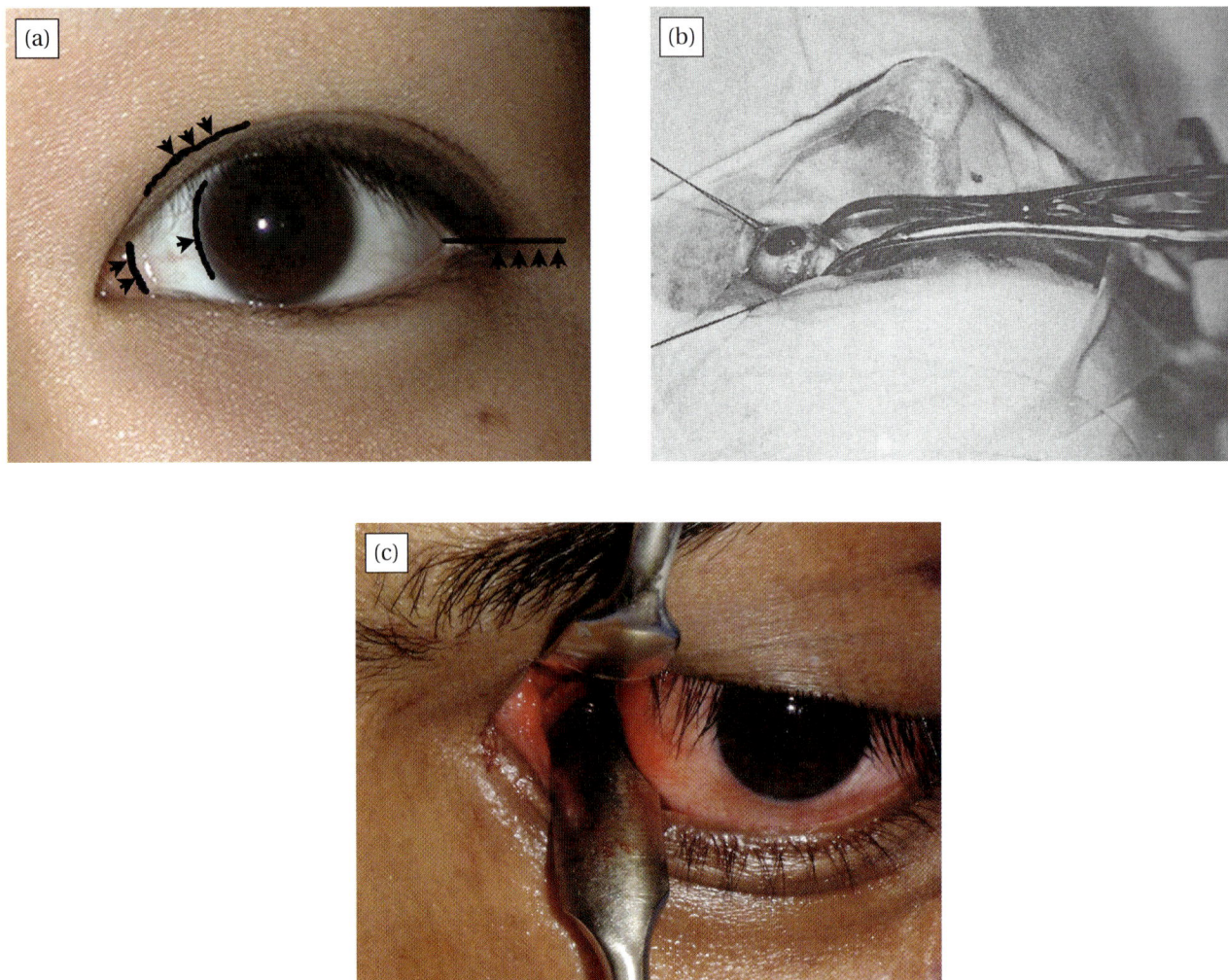

FIGURE 89.2 Exposing the optic nerve. There are numerous approaches to the optic nerve. Panel (a) illustrates various incisions sites: limbal (single arrowhead), transcaruncular (two arrowheads), supramedial eyelid crease (three arrowheads) and lateral canthotomy (four arrowheads). The medial approach was popularized following the 1973 description by Galbraith and Sullivan, through a conjunctival incision (b). This requires detaching the medial rectus muscle. Cutting of a rectus muscle can be avoided with several modified techniques, such as a transcaruncular (c) or supramedial eyelid crease incisions. A "lateral" ONSF also avoids detachment of a rectus and is described in detail in Figure 89.4. (Figure [b] reprinted from Galbraith JE, Sullivan JH: Decompression of the perioptic meninges for relief of papilledema. *Am J Ophthalmol.* 1973;76: 687–692. With kind permission of Elsevier, Inc.)

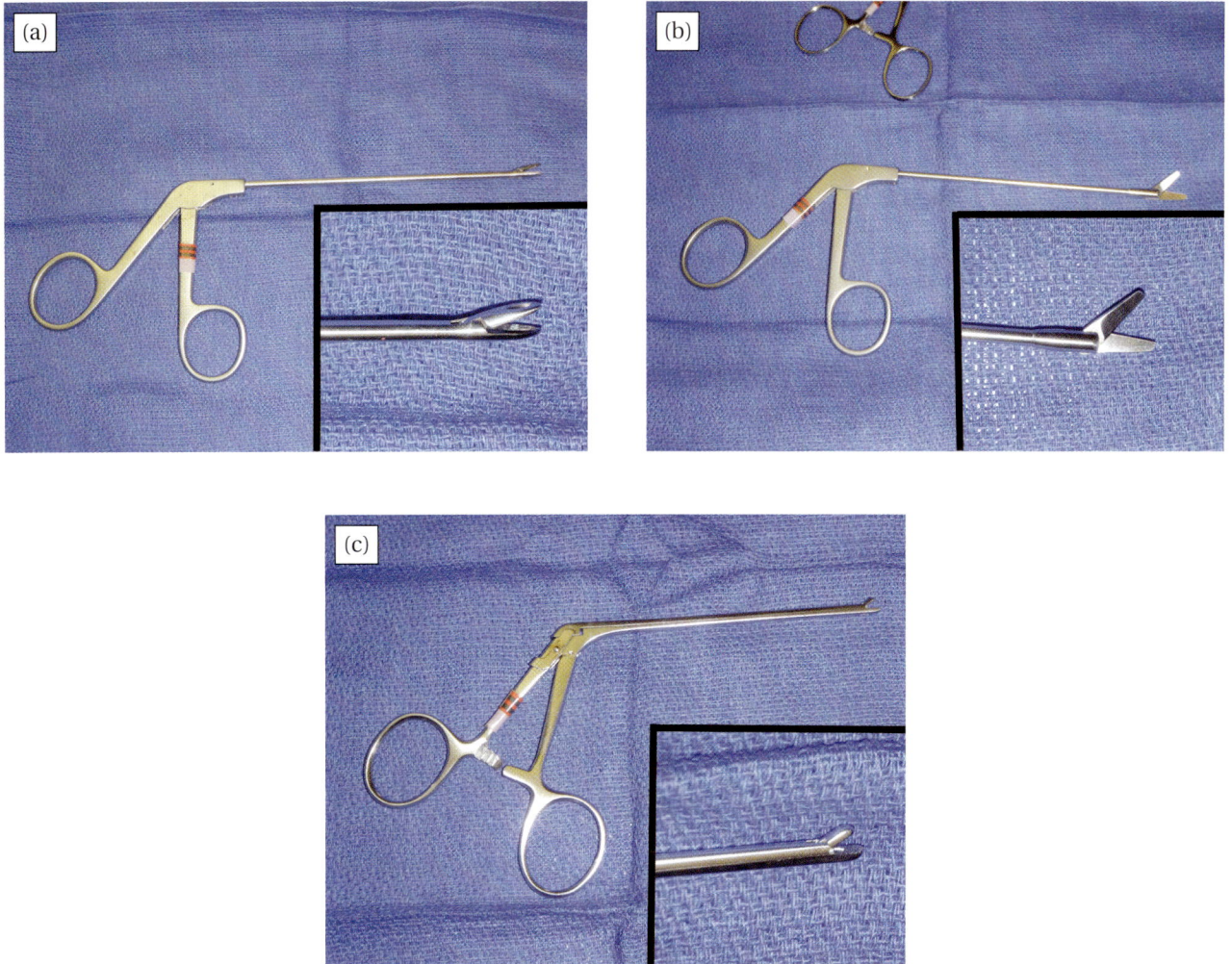

FIGURE 89.3 Instrumentation for lateral approach ONSF. In addition to equipment common to oculoplastic surgery, such as basic forceps, scissors and retractors a few specialized instruments are required. (a) Endoscopic *forceps* are used for grasping the dura and arachnoid layers. (b) *Fine endoscopic scissors* are necessary to ensure that surrounding and underlying structures are not inadvertently injured. (c) *Endoscopic needle drivers*, although designed for suturing, can also be used to grasp soft tissue.

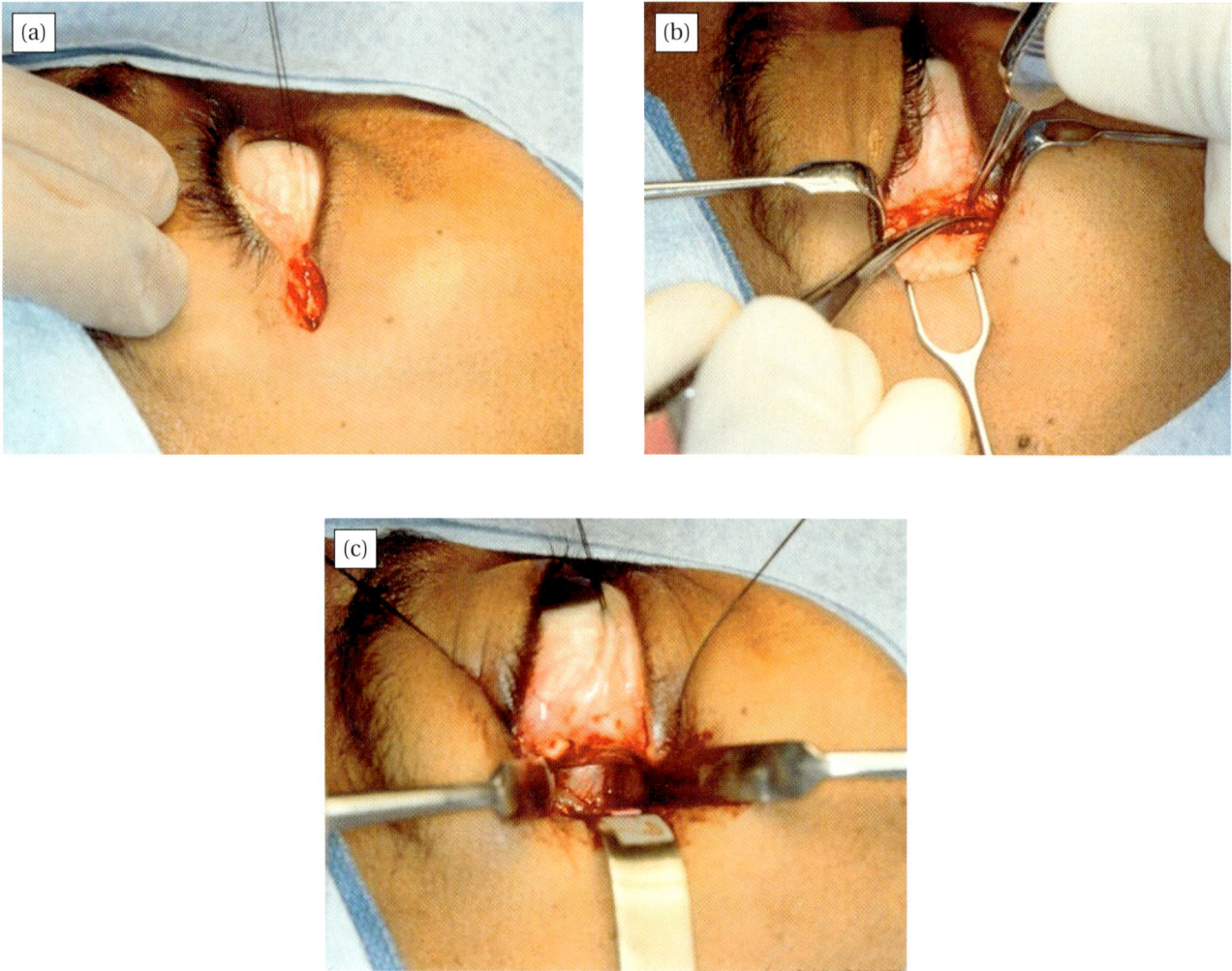

FIGURE 89.4   Lateral ONSF, right orbit. The original descriptions of ONSF from the late 1800s were of a lateral approach. Since then numerous modifications have been advocated. The author's preferred approach is performed as follows. A lateral canthotomy incision (a) is made with straight iris scissors. Dissection is then continued through the extraconal fat, intermuscular septum and intraconal fat (b). Dissection through fibrous septum is best achieved with by blunt dissection with scissors, whereas orbital fat can be separated with cotton tip applicators or retractors. By dissecting inferior to the lateral rectus muscle, the lacrimal gland, accompanying nerves and blood vessels are avoided. Once the optic nerve is reached (c), surgery does not differ significantly from other approaches.

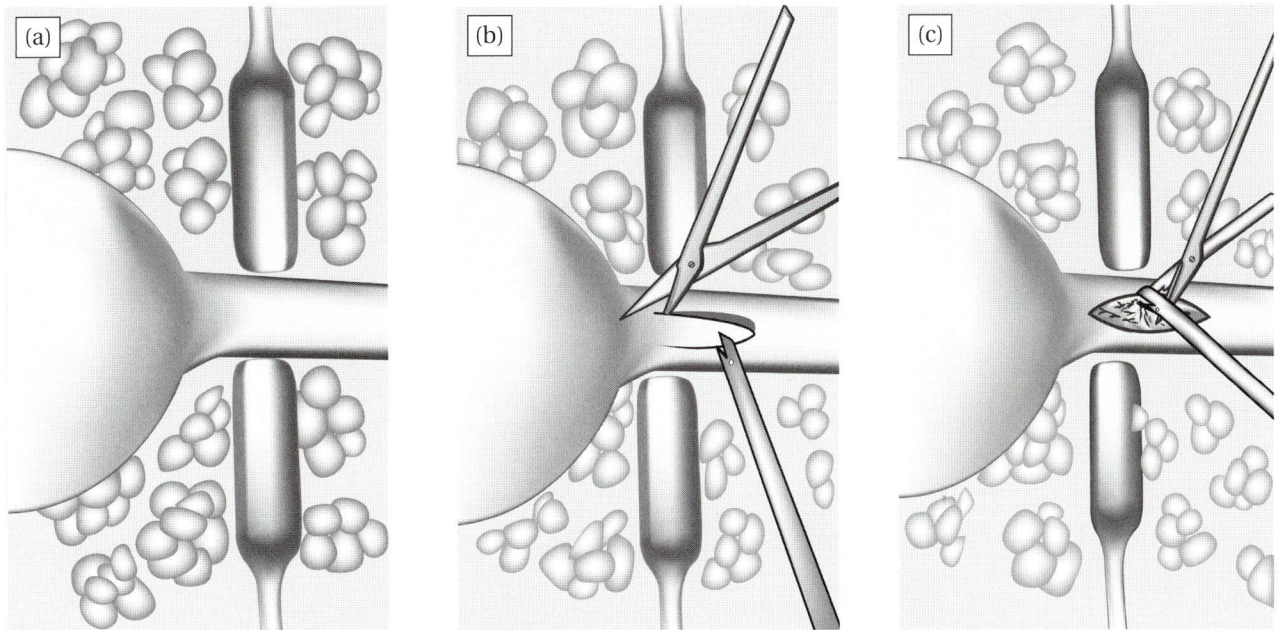

FIGURE 89.5 Fenestration of the optic nerve sheath through lateral approach. Although some surgeons prefer loops, most perform the actual fenestration with a binocular operating microscope. Greater magnification allows for the short ciliary nerve, posterior ciliary arteries, and the vascular network from the ophthalmic artery to more readily be identified and preserved. Sewell retractors are useful to retract the fat surrounding the optic nerve (a). Choose an area relatively devoid of vessels. In some cases the arachnoid is adherent to the dura and excised at the same time. Following creation of a dural window (b), if the arachnoid remains, this meningeal layer must also be incised (c). Care should be taken to avoid damaging the underlying optic nerve or pial vasculature. (Illustrations courtesy of Lynda V. McCulley, PharmD.)

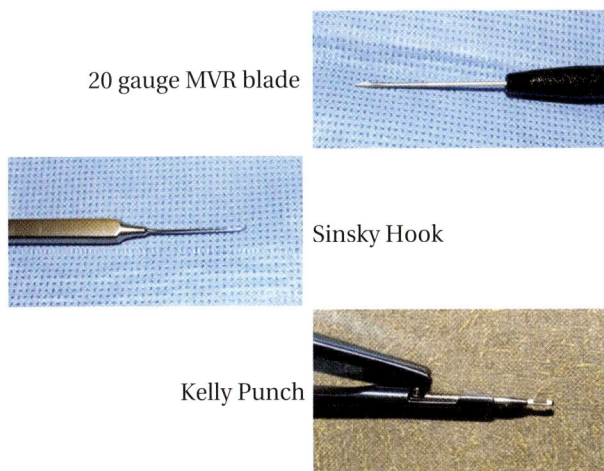

20 gauge MVR blade

Sinsky Hook

Kelly Punch

FIGURE 89.6 Instrumentation for supramedial lid crease approach ONSF. When performing the supramedial lid crease technique, the optic nerve is approached from a different angle and utilizes additional ophthalmic instrumentation. A 20 gauge microvitreoretinal (MVR) blade, Sinsky hook and Kelly Descemet's punch are used for nerve sheath fenestration.

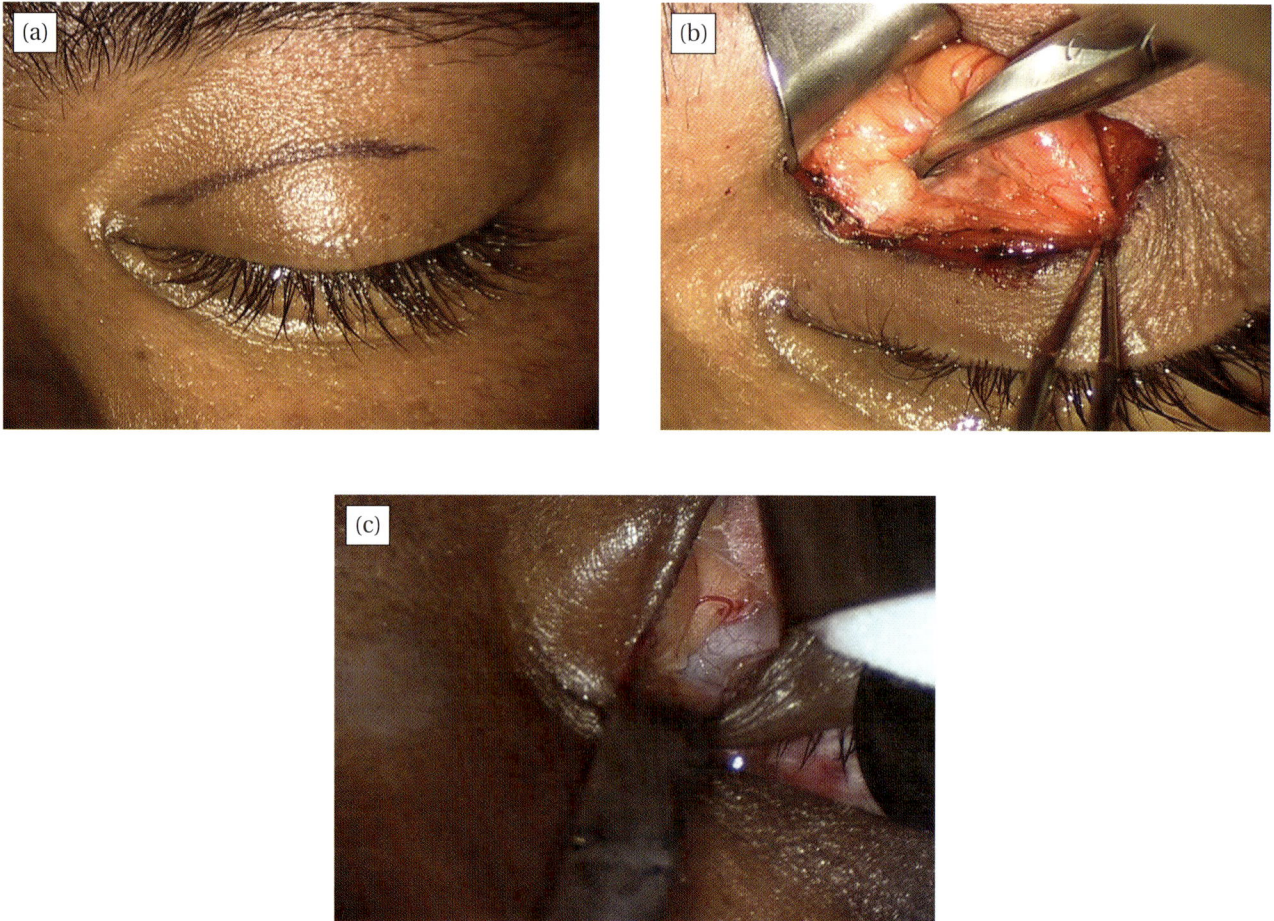

FIGURE 89.7 Supramedial lid crease approach. A medial 1/3 eyelid crease incision is performed and blunt dissection is performed in the superomedial orbit between the nasal and central fat pads (a). The dissection is continued inferior to the trochlea and superior oblique tendon while the medial horn of the levator is reflected laterally (b). Using the sclera and ciliary vessels as landmarks, the optic nerve is identified (c).

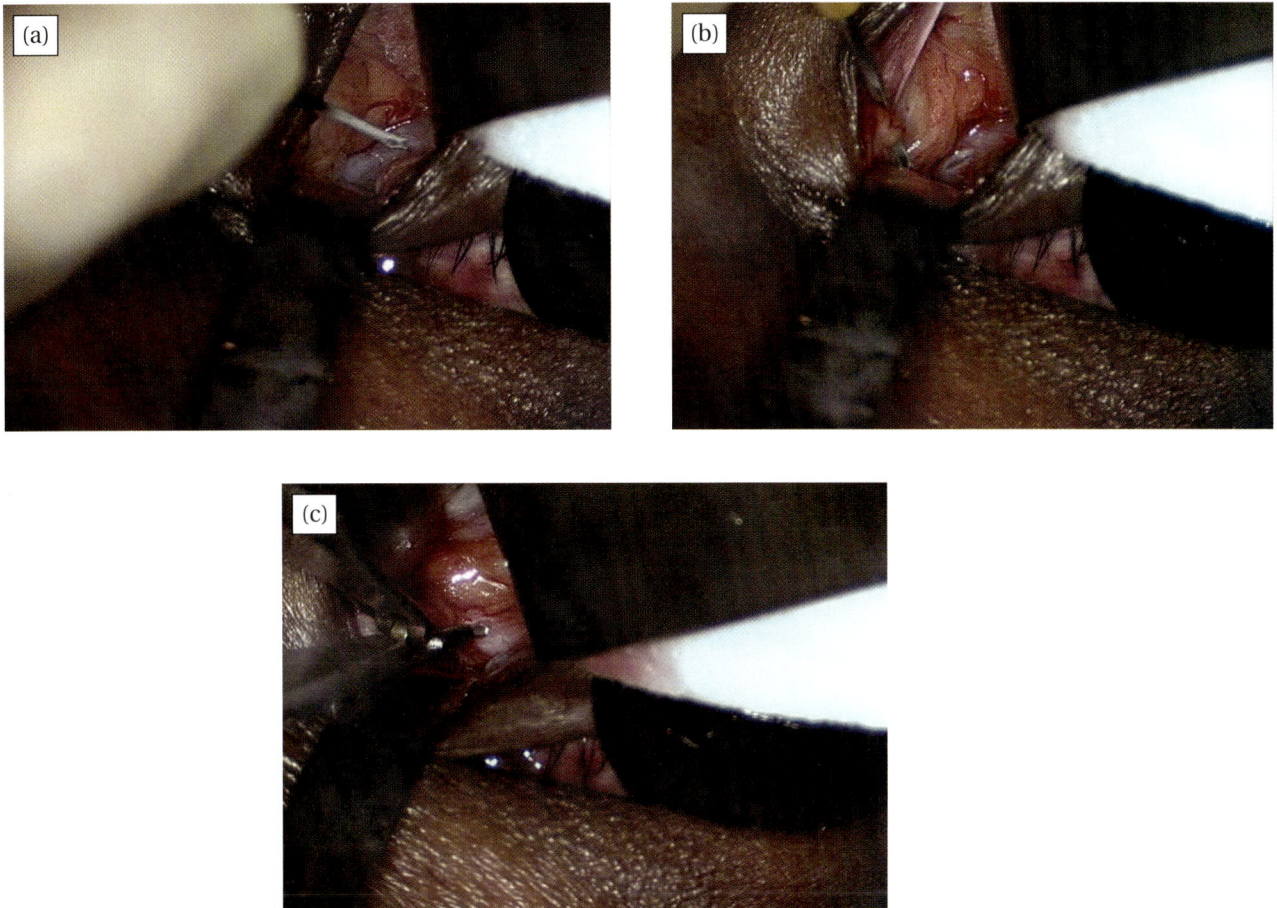

FIGURE 89.8 Fenestration of the optic nerve sheath through supramedial approach. The MVR blade is used to incise the dural sheath (a). Once a burst of cerebrospinal fluid is noted, a Sinskey hook is used to tent the dura and arachnoid from the underlying pia (b). A Kelly punch is then used to widen the dural window (c).

TABLE 89.3 *Potential Complications*

Direct trauma to optic nerve fibers

Trauma to pial vasculature

Retrobulbar/subdural sheath hemorrhage

Diplopia/ocular misalignment

Ptosis

Persistent subconjunctival CSF leak

Damage to ciliary ganglion

Central retinal artery occlusion

SELECTED REFERENCES

Carter RB. On retrobulbar incision of the optic nerve in cases of swollen disc. *Brain.* 1887;10:199–209.

Carter RB. Operation of opening the sheath of the optic nerve for the relief of pressure. *Br Med J.* 1889;1:399–401.

Davidson SI. A surgical approach to plerocephalic disc edema. *Eye.* 1969;89:669–690.

Davidson SI. The surgical relief of papilloedema. In: Cant JS, ed. *The Optic Nerve. Proceedings of Second William Mackenzie Memorial Symposium, Glasgow.* 1971. London: Kimpton; 1972;3:174–179.

DeWecker L. On incision of the optic nerve in cases of neuroretinitis. *Int Ophthalmol Congr Rep.* 1872;4:11–14.

Galbraith JE, Sullivan JH. Decompression of the perioptic meninges for relief of papilledema. *Am J Ophthalmol.* 1973;76:687–692.

Kersten RC, Kulwin DR. Optic nerve sheath fenestration through a lateral canthotomy incision. *Arch Ophthalmol.* 1993;111(6):870–874.

Pelton RW, Patel BC. Superomedial lid crease approach to the medial intraconal space: a new technique for access to the optic nerve and central space. *Ophthal Plast Reconstr Surg.* 2001;17(4):241–253.

Tse DT, Nerad JA, Anderson RL, et al. Optic nerve sheath fenestration in pseudotumor cerebri. A lateral orbitotomy approach. *Arch Ophthalmol.* 1988;106:1458–1462.

Orbitofacial Fracture Repair

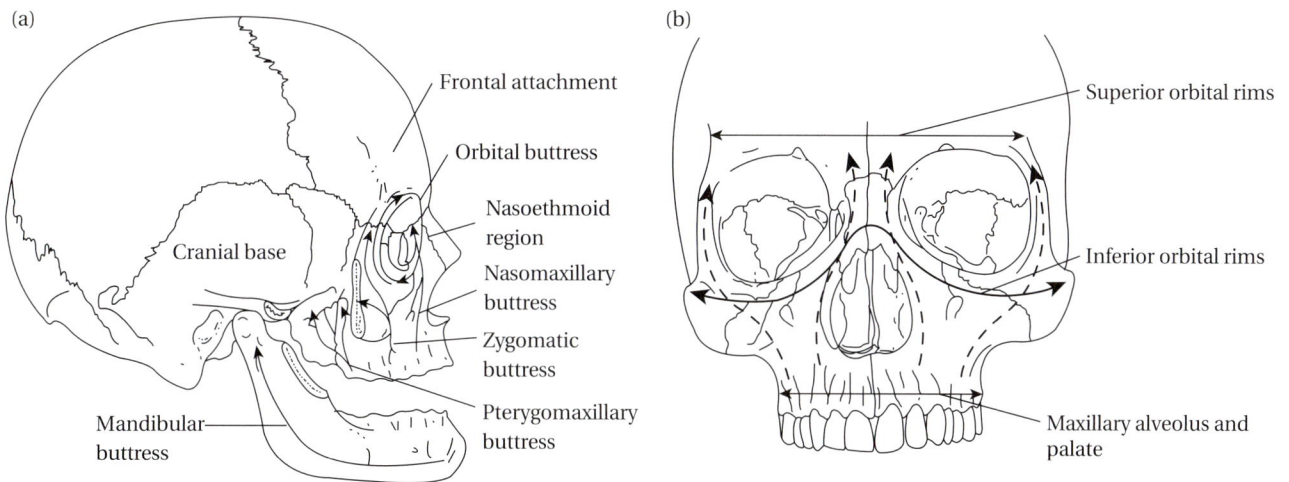

(a)

Frontal attachment

Orbital buttress

Nasoethmoid region

Nasomaxillary buttress

Zygomatic buttress

Pterygomaxillary buttress

Cranial base

Mandibular buttress

(b)

Superior orbital rims

Inferior orbital rims

Maxillary alveolus and palate

FIGURE 90.1 Structural pillars of the facial and orbital skeleton. (a) The major vertical buttresses are the nasomaxillary, zygomatic, and pterygomaxillary. The mandibular buttress is another vertical pillar of bone. (b) The horizontal buttresses are the superior orbital rims, the inferior orbital rims, and the maxillary alveolus and palate. The dashed lines represent the vertical buttresses.

Isolated Orbital Floor Fractures

TABLE 90.1 *Indications for Orbital Floor Fracture Repair*

Immediate Repair (24–72 hours)

Entrapped muscle or periorbital tissue with or without motility restriction and diplopia, oculocardiac reflex (bradycardia, heart block), nausea, vomiting, or syncope

Repair in 5–14 days

Persistent diplopia in primary gaze (central 30 degrees)

Large orbital floor fractures (>50% of surface area)

Enophthalmos greater than 2 mm

Complex trauma involving orbital rim and with displacement

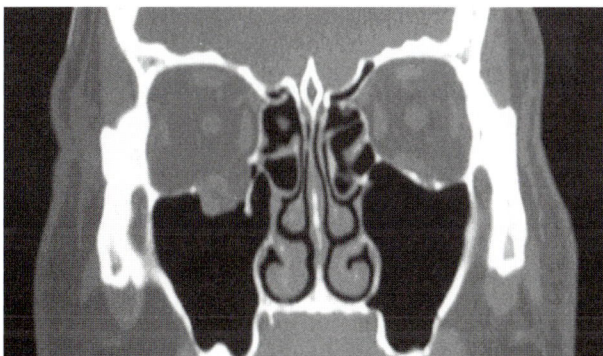

FIGURE 90.2 Coronal CT of an isolated right orbital floor fracture with herniation of periorbital tissue.

Lateral Canthal and Transconjunctival Approach to the Inferior Orbit (and midface, if necessary)

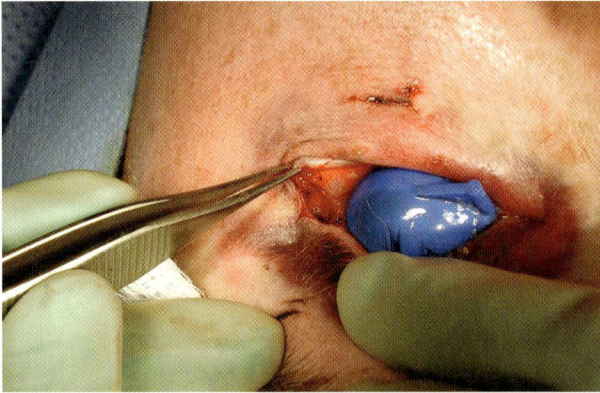

FIGURE 90.3 Lateral canthotomy, followed by cantholysis of the inferior ramus of the lateral canthal tendon.

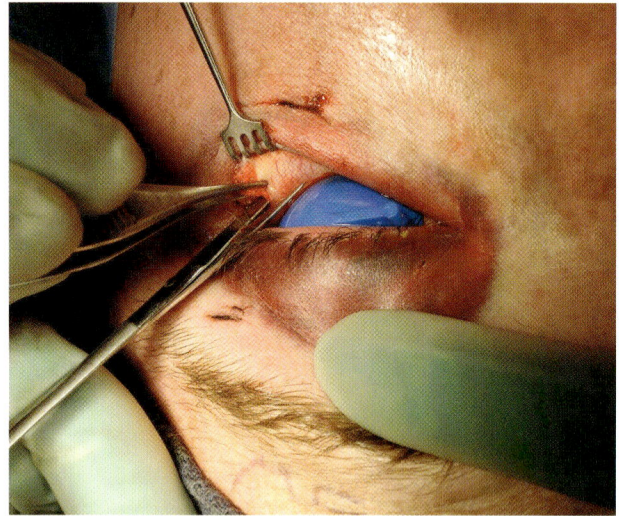

FIGURE 90.4 Incision of the conjunctiva and lower eyelid retractors at the inferior one-quarter, upper three-quarter line between the fornix and inferior tarsus.

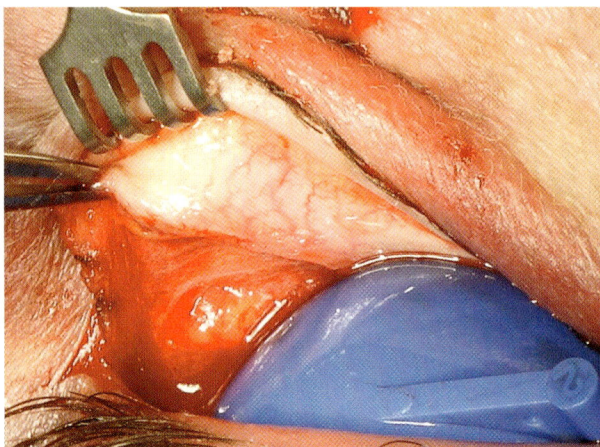

FIGURE 90.5 Eversion of the lower eyelid and dissection in the septal plane, avoiding both the orbicularis (anterior) and orbital fat (posterior), down to the inferior orbital rim.

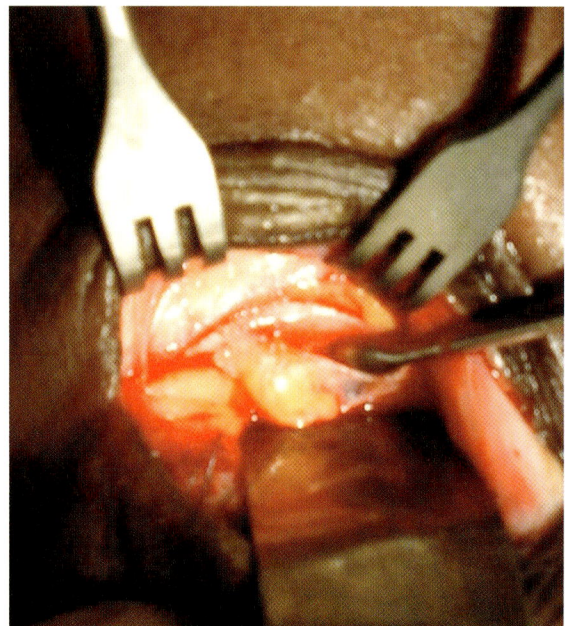

FIGURE 90.6 Incision of the periosteum of the inferior orbital rim, followed by periosteal elevation.

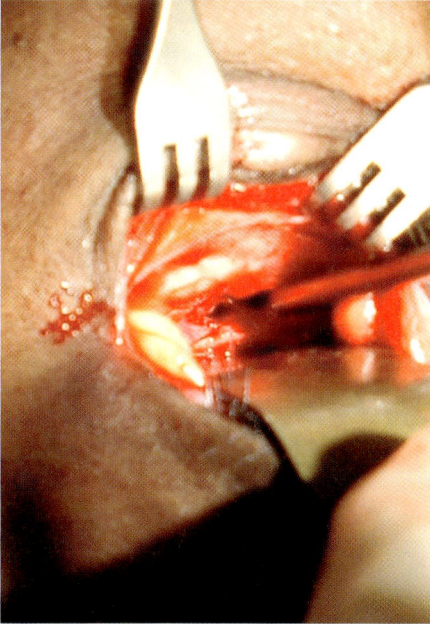

FIGURE 90.7 Identification of the fracture, with removal of incarcerated periorbital tissue until the entire perimeter of the fracture (including lateral and posterior) is exposed.

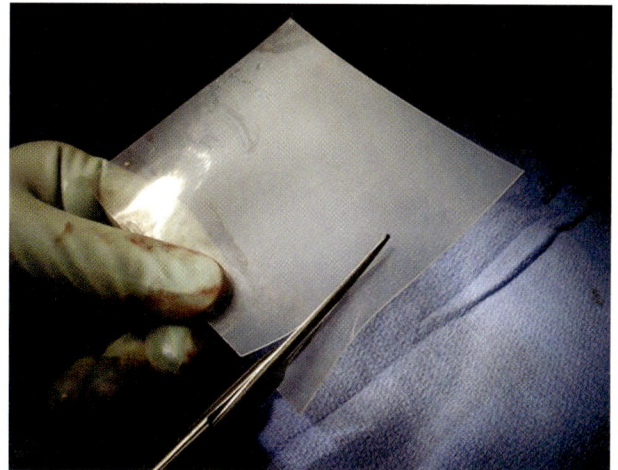

FIGURE 90.8 The authors prefer 0.4 mm nylon foil, which is cut to a custom size adequate to span entire fracture.

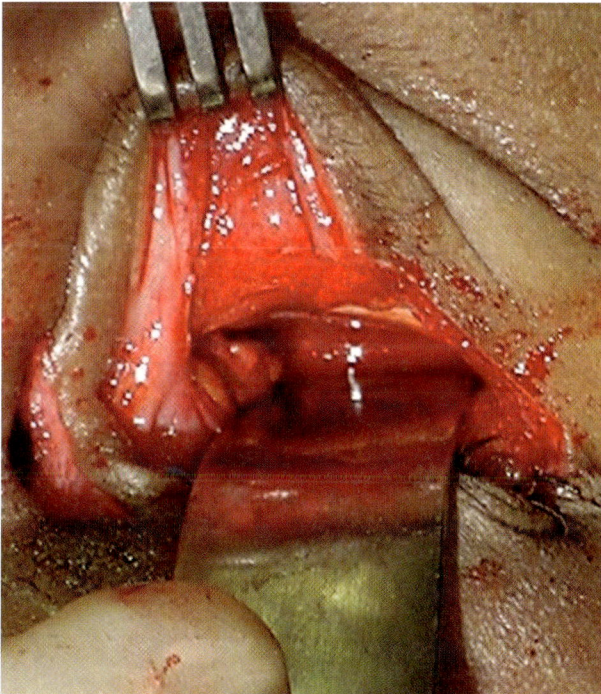

FIGURE 90.9 The implant is introduced through the inferior transconjunctival approach with positioning of the implant over the perimeter of the fracture site. The authors do not fix nylon foil with screws, sutures, or tabbing since migration has not been observed.

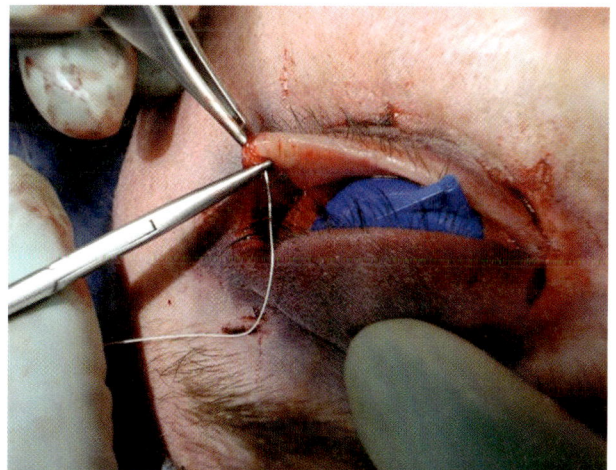

FIGURE 90.10 Conjunctiva is closed with 6-0 chromic sutures and reattachment, and the lateral canthus is reformed by attaching the free lateral tarsus to the lateral orbital tubercle using a 4-0 polyglactin suture.

Isolated Medial Orbital Wall Fractures

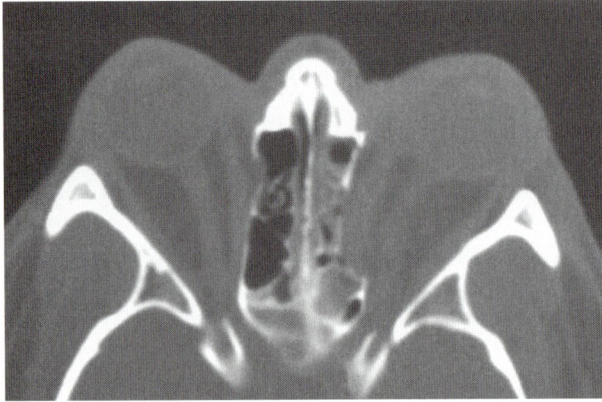

FIGURE 90.11 Axial CT of an isolated left medial orbital wall fracture with herniation of orbital contents (including medial rectus muscle) into the defect.

Transcaruncular Approach to the Medial Wall

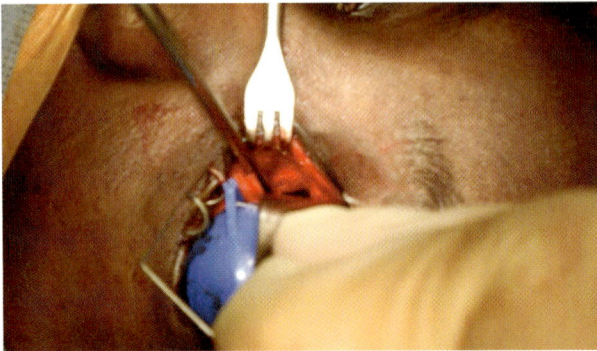

FIGURE 90.12 The conjunctiva is incised between the plica and caruncle. Stevens tenotomy scissors are used to bluntly dissect posterior to the lacrimal drainage apparatus to the left medial wall, where periosteum is elevated to expose the fracture. Orbital tissues are elevated from fracture and an implant is seated across the perimeter of the fracture.

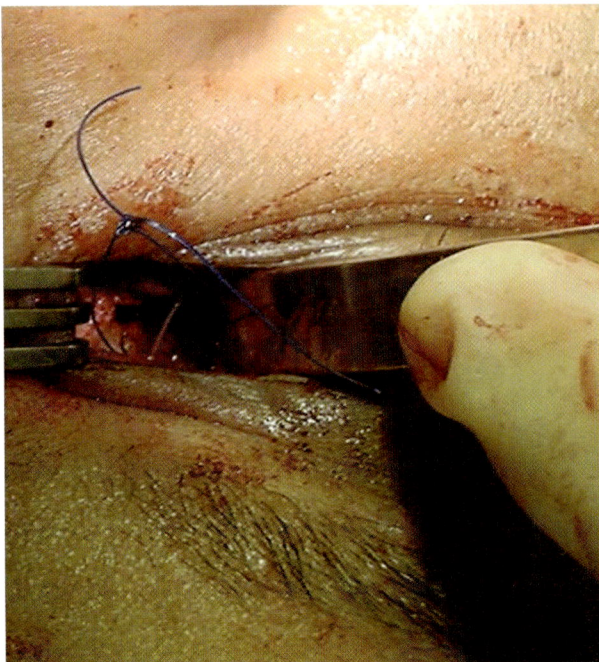

FIGURE 90.13 Nylon foil implant placed across perimeter of right medial wall fracture site.

Combined Orbital Floor and Medial Wall Fractures

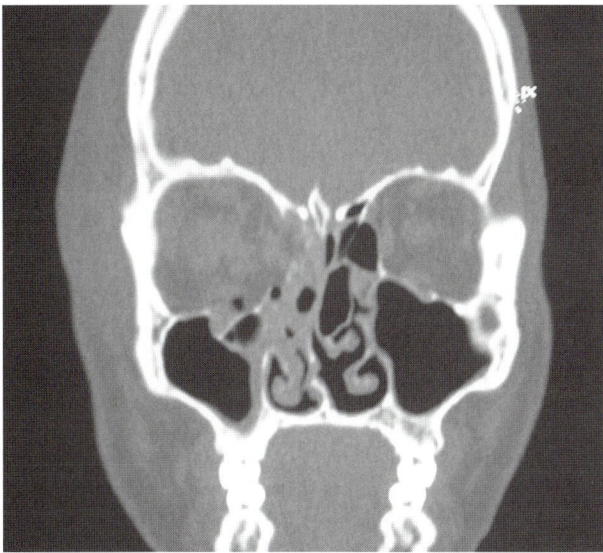

FIGURE 90.14 Coronal CT scan demonstrating a combined right orbital floor and medial wall fractures.

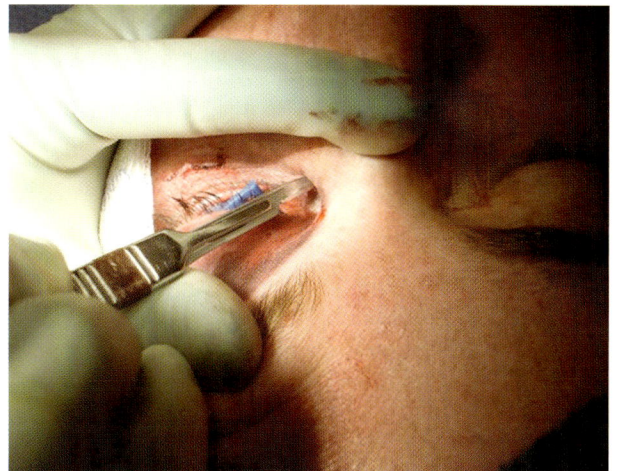

FIGURE 90.15 A transconjunctival approach exposes the left orbital floor to expose the fracture site (see isolated orbital floor fracture approach images). The medial wall is approached using a 1 cm vertical incision just anterior to the medial canthal tendon. (Also known as a "Nunery" incision; not to be confused with a Lynch incision—a longer, more anterior, and angled, L-shaped incision. A transcaruncular approach may be utilized, but the transcutaneous approach achieves wider exposure aids in developing a continuous subperiosteal plane, in the authors' hands).

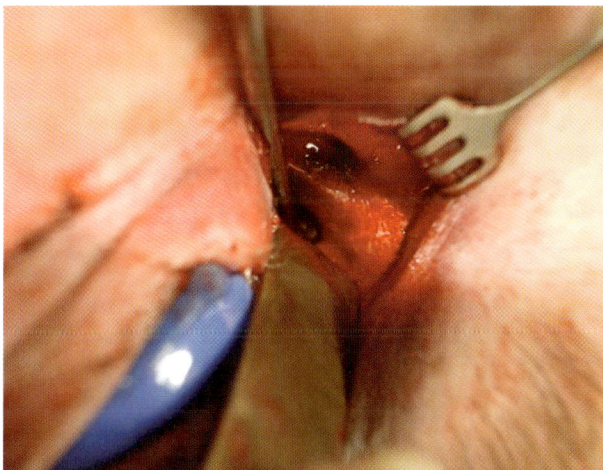

FIGURE 90.16 Dissection is continued down to periosteum, with care to preserve the nasolacrimal outflow system and medial canthal tendon. The medial canthal tendon remains attached to elevated periosteum, but is otherwise undisturbed. The perimeter of the medial wall fracture is exposed, and soft tissue is extracted from the defect.

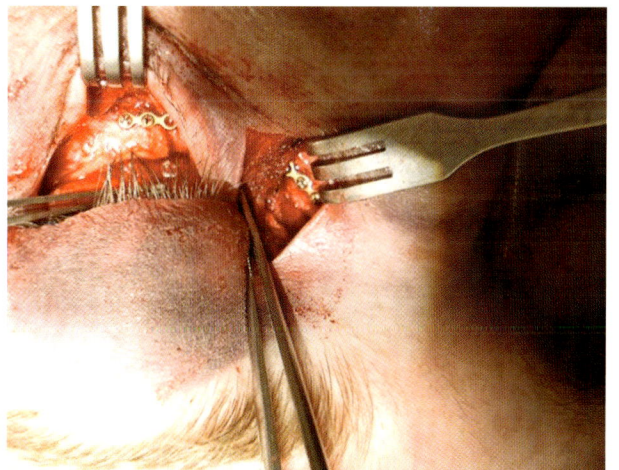

FIGURE 90.17 Subperiosteal plane dissection is performed inferotemporally until continuous with the previous transconjunctival orbital floor approach. (Note: this patient had concomitant orbital rim fractures; plate fixation is otherwise not necessary in orbital wall fracture repair.)

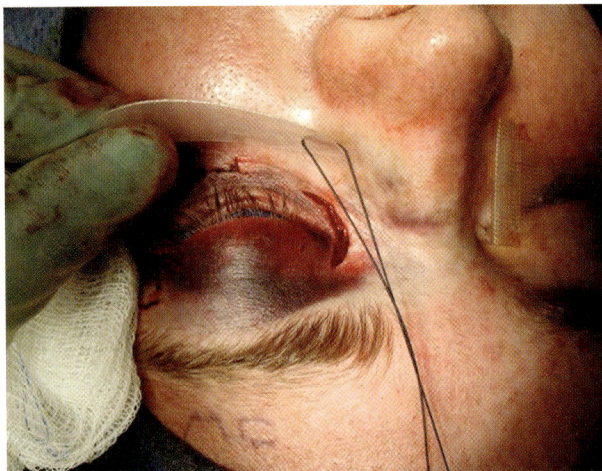

FIGURE 90.18 A 0.4 mm nylon foil implant is cut in an ovoid pattern that adequately spans all fractures as a single unit, and a temporary suture lariat is placed.

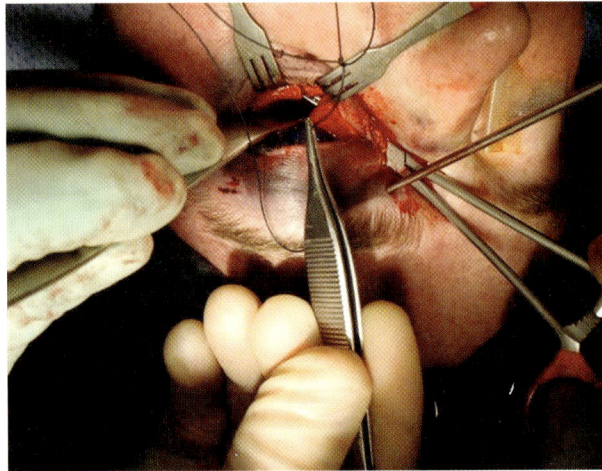

FIGURE 90.19 The implant is advanced through the transconjunctival route in the subperiosteal plane, and a curved hemostat is used to pull the implant superomedially.

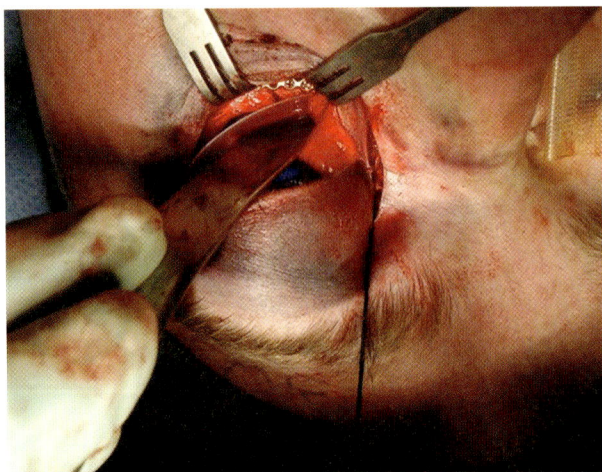

FIGURE 90.20 Implant is introduced through the inferior transconjunctival approach with positioning of the implant over all fractures (medial wall and floor) as a single plate.

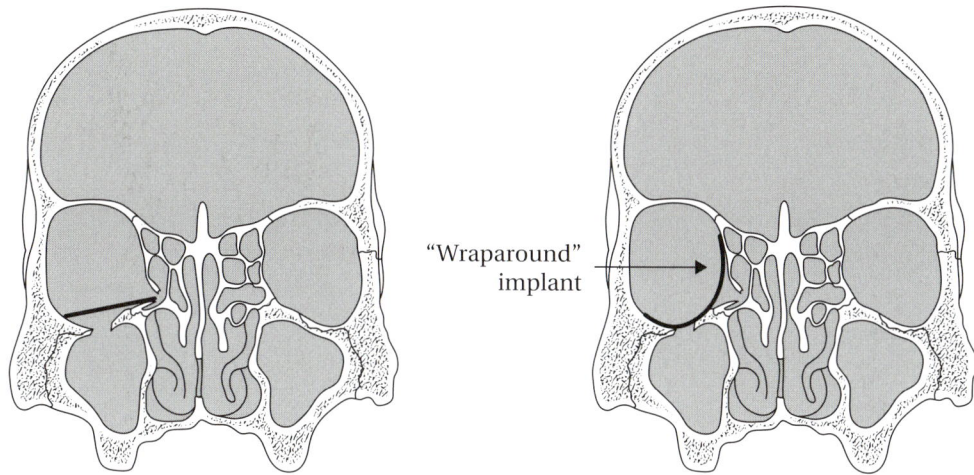

FIGURE 90.21 Left: Suboptimal repair of a two wall fracture with resultant poor orbital contour and implant herniation in the ethmoid sinus. Right: "Wraparound" implant with complete coverage of the 2-wall fracture, with reestablishment of more normal orbital contour.

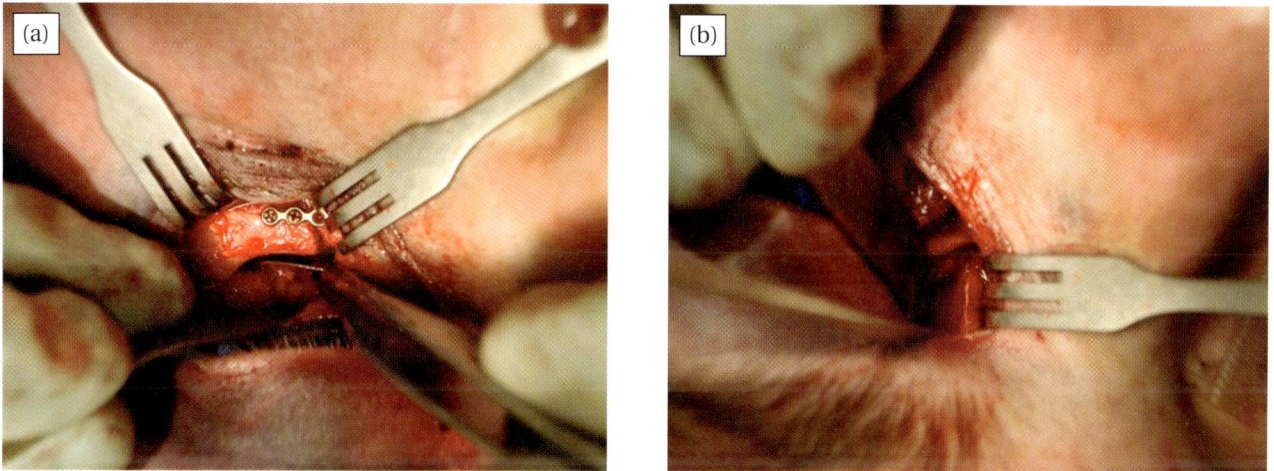

FIGURE 90.22 The "wraparound" implant is verified to be in position across the perimeter of both floor (a) and medial wall fractures (b).

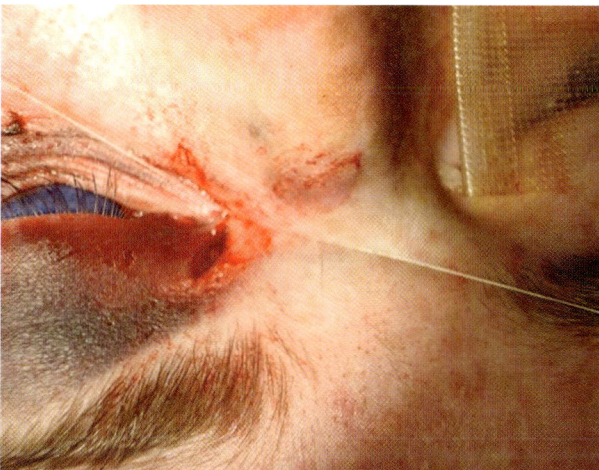

FIGURE 90.23 The medial canthus is closed with a 5-0 polyglactin suture that engages periosteum on the central pass which returns the tendon to the desired anatomic position and avoids telecanthus. The skin is closed with 6-0 sutures.

Zygomaticomaxillary (ZMC) Complex Fractures

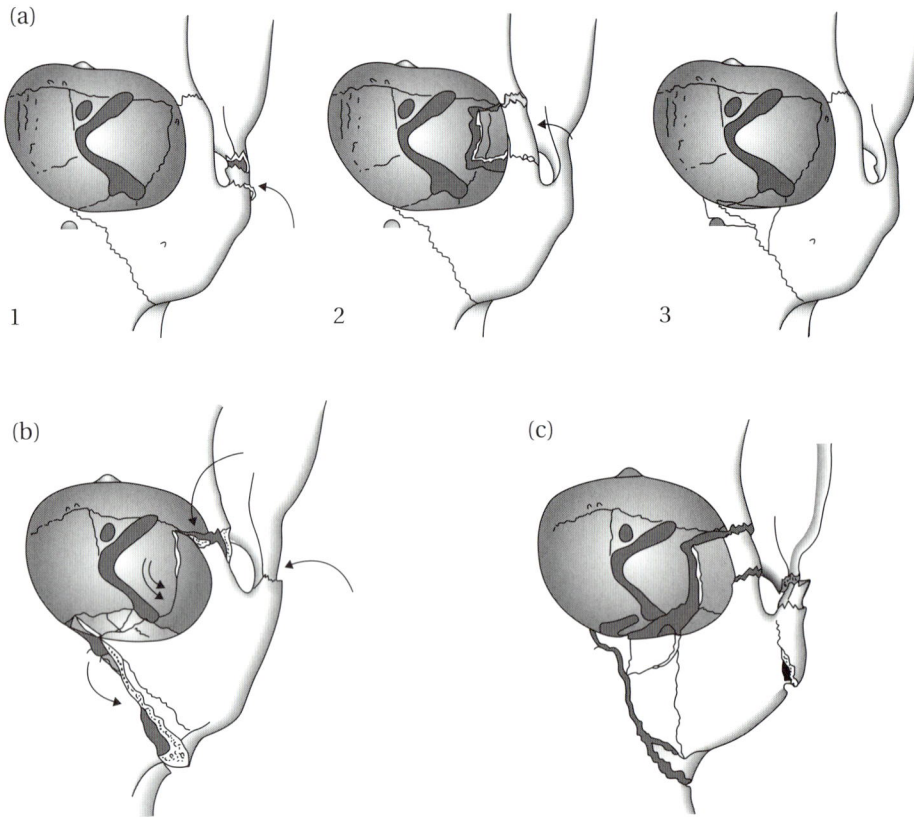

FIGURE 90.24 ZMC fracture classification. A: Low-energy injuries to the ZMC can result in segmental fractures of the zygomatic arch (1), lateral orbital wall (2), and inferior orbital rim (3). B: Middle-energy fractures cause a classic ZMC fracture. C: High-energy injuries result in severe displacement and fragmentation of the ZMC. (Image Credit: *Clinical Atlas of Procedures in Ophthalmic Surgery*, 1st ed.)

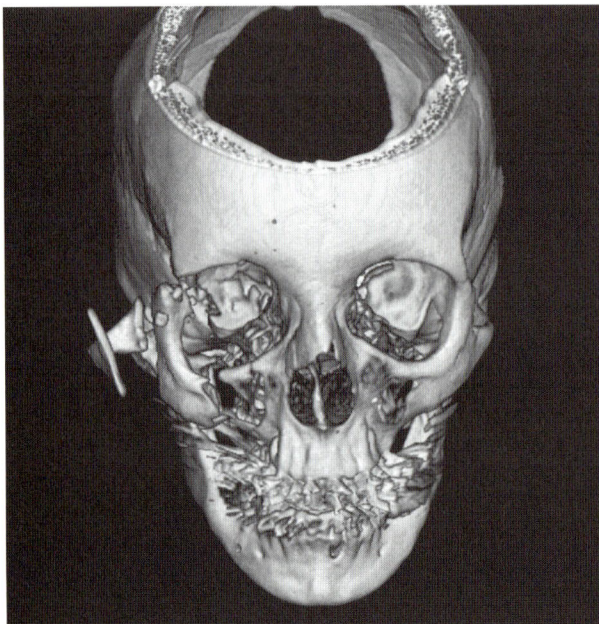

FIGURE 90.25 3D-CT reconstruction of a right zygomaticomaxillary complex fracture (ZMC or tripod fracture) occurring at lateral orbital rim, inferior orbital rim, zygomatic arch and lateral wall of the maxillary sinus.

TABLE 90.2 *Indications for ZMC Fracture Repair*

Enophthalmos
Globe Ptosis
Lid Retraction
Lateral canthal dystopia
Flattening of the malar eminence
Diplopia
Trismus

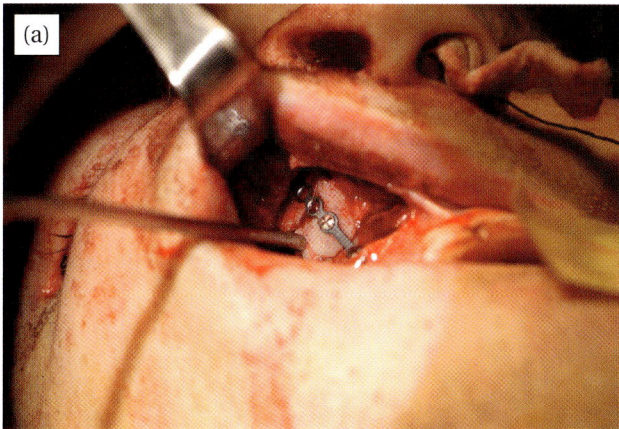

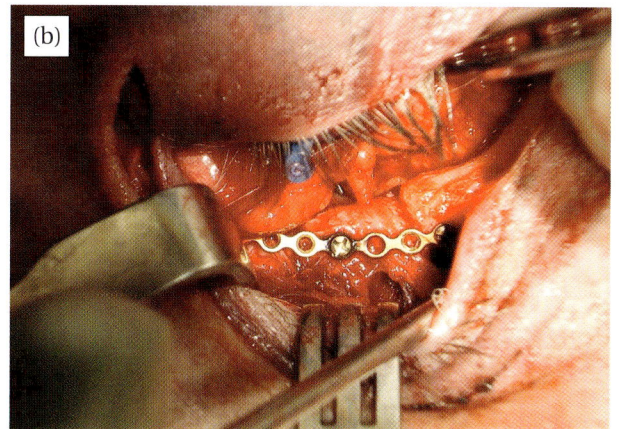

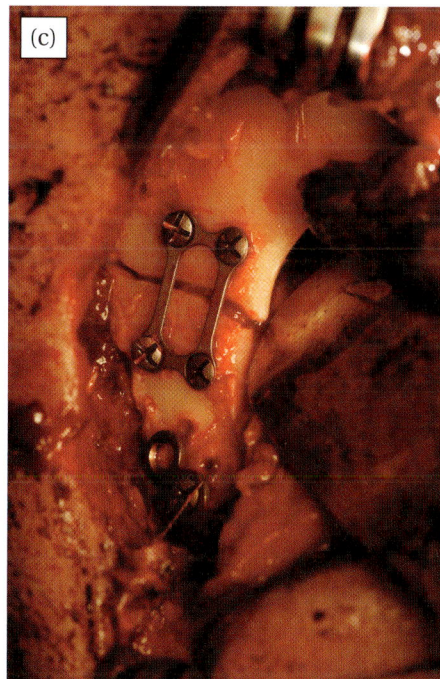

FIGURE 90.26 (a, b, c) Open reduction and internal fixation of zygomatic fractures. Exposure to the fracture can be achieved with incisions at the lateral canthal, inferior fornix, and through the gingival sulcus. Bone is replaced to the normal anatomic position and then fixated with titanium microplates. Brow or coronal scalp incisions may be excessive and provide less optimal exposure for most ZMC fractures. (Photo courtesy of H.B. Harold Lee, MD.)

Nasoorbitoethmoid (NOE) Fractures

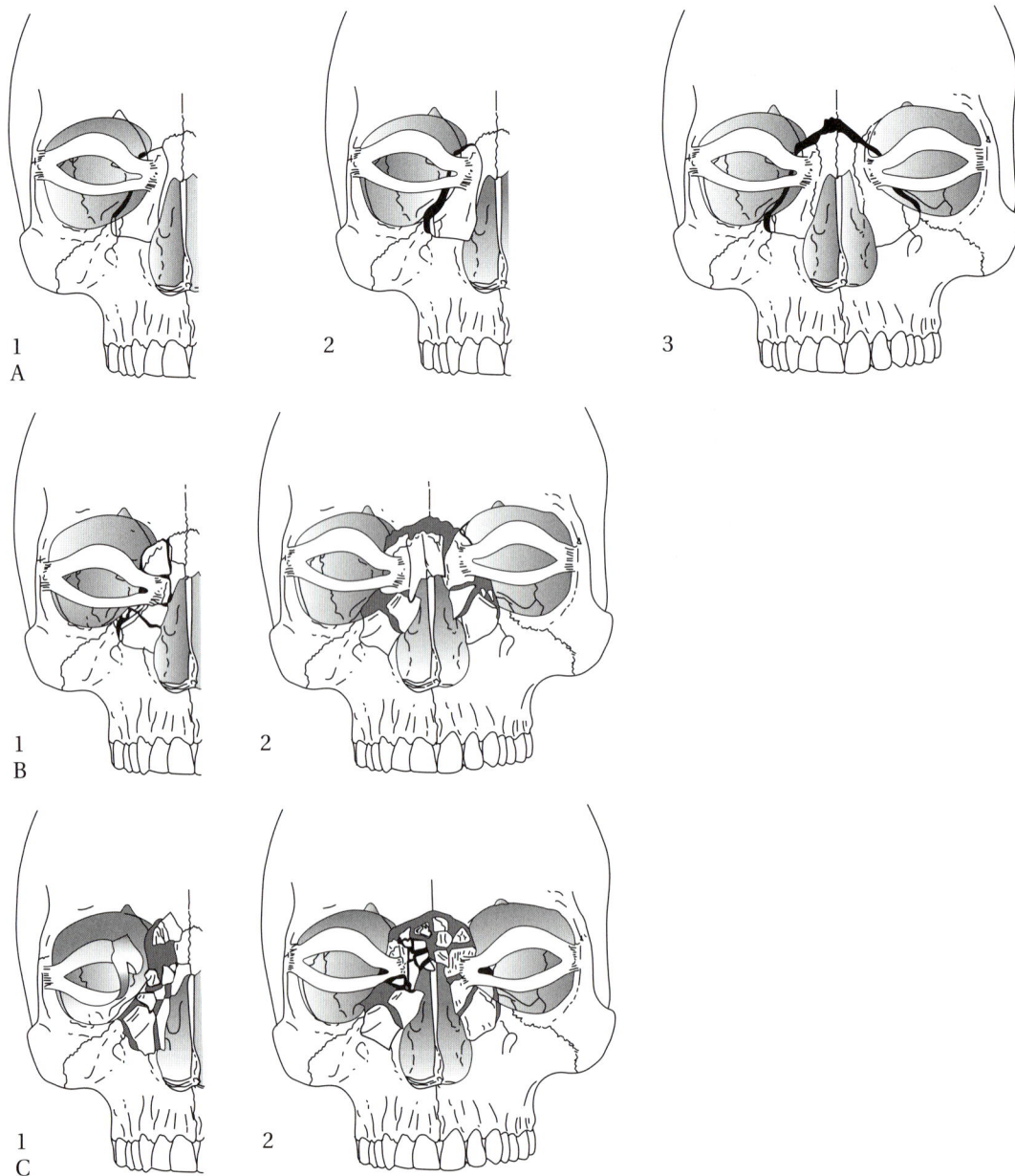

FIGURE 90.27 NOE fracture classification. A: Type 1 fractures may be incomplete (1) or complete (2). Bilateral injuries may result in the "monoblock" fracture (3). B: Type 2 fractures involve the central fragment but spare the medial canthal tendon insertion. The fractures may be unilateral (1) or bilateral (2). C: Type 3 injuries cause severe fragmentation with fracture extension beneath the medial canthal tendon insertion. Again, these may be unilateral (1) or bilateral (2). (Image Credit: *Clinical Atlas of Procedures in Ophthalmic Surgery,* 1st ed.)

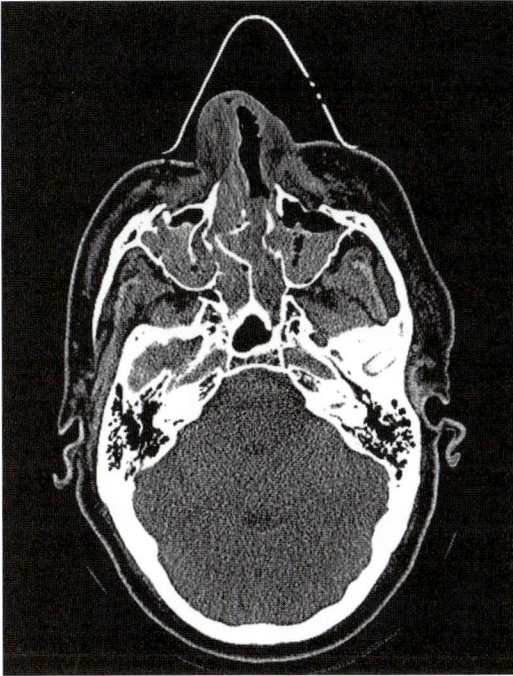

FIGURE 90.28 Axial CT scan demonstrates a bilateral nasoorbitoethmoid (NOE) fracture. The NOE complex is comprised of the frontal bone, nasal bone, maxillary bone, lacrimal bone, and sphenoid bone.

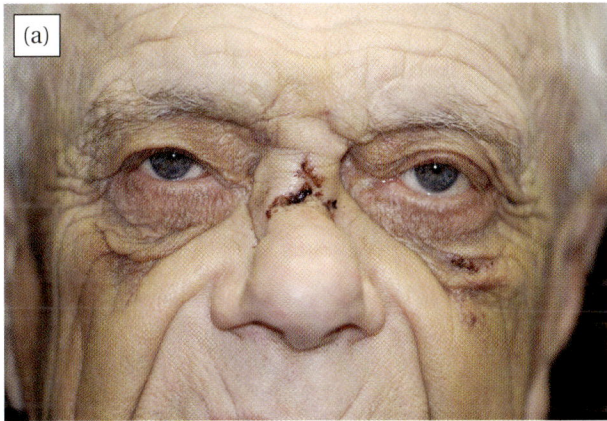

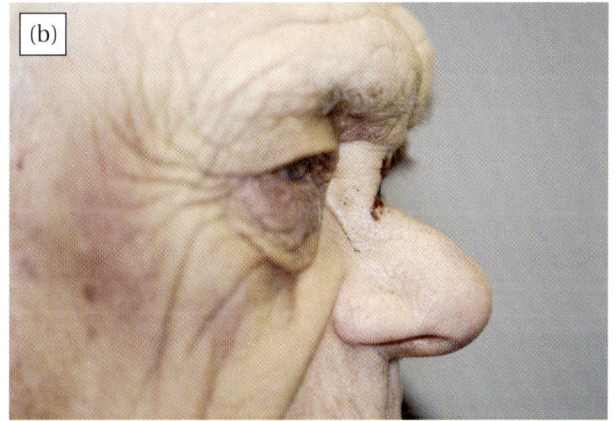

FIGURE 90.29   (a, b) Telescoping bilateral NOE fracture with mild telecanthus and severe flattening of the nasal bridge. (Photos courtesy of H.B. Harold Lee, MD.)

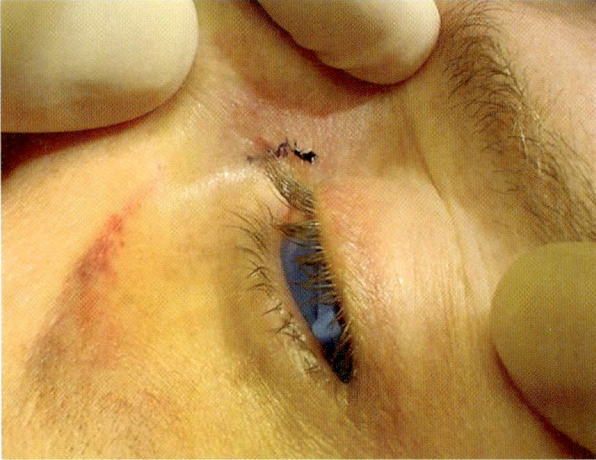

FIGURE 90.30 NOE complex is approached through small medial canthus incisions (not Lynch incisions, which are more anterior).

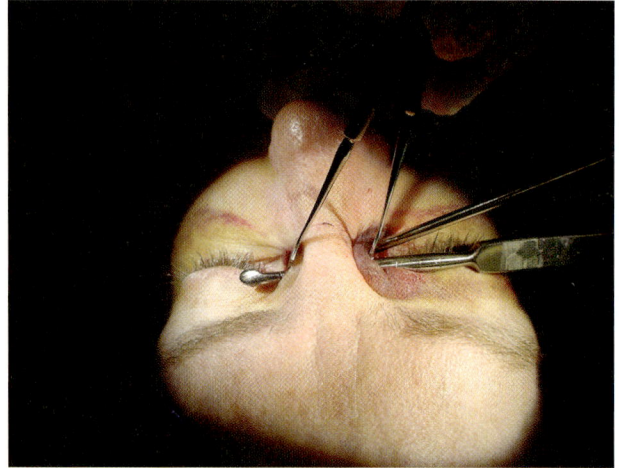

FIGURE 90.31 If bilateral involvement, bilateral medial canthus incisions are created and wide subperiosteal dissection is achieved, exposing fractures.

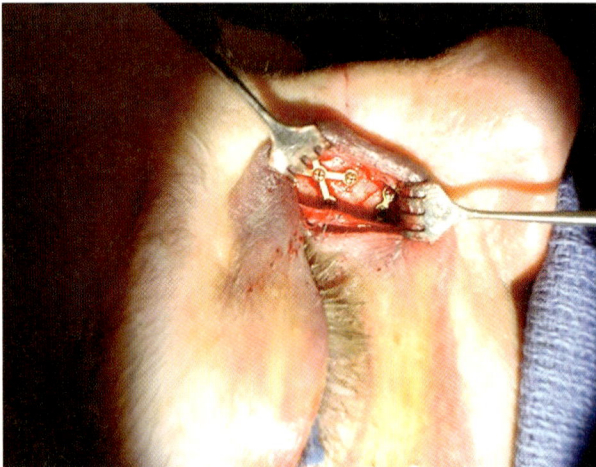

FIGURE 90.32 Titanium microplate fixation of fractured bones to the normal anatomic position.

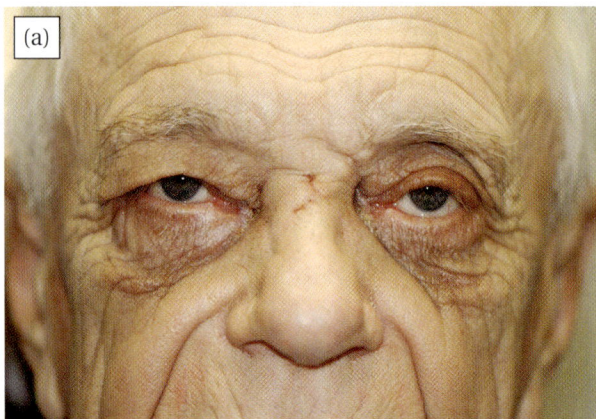

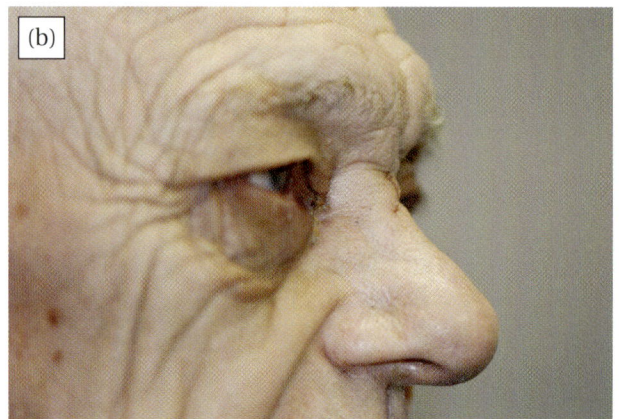

FIGURE 90.33 (a, b) Postoperative images of the patient above after nasoorbitoethmoid fracture repair. Improvement of telecanthus and the depressed nasal bridge. (Photos courtesy of H.B. Harold Lee, MD.)

TABLE 90.3 *Implant Options**

Nylon foil implants

Porous polyethylene implants

Silicone implants

Titanium alloy mesh implants

Allografts (calvarial or ear cartilage)

Xenograft implants

*The authors prefer nylon foil for its long-term integrity, low tissue reactivity, customizable shape, and minimization of fibrosis and orbital restriction. Porous grafts, including titanium mesh, porous polyethylene, and grafts may be associated with greater orbital restriction, in our experience. Rigid implants, may not recapture the natural orbital contours.

SELECTED REFERENCES

American Academy of Ophthalmology: *Basic and clinical science course: Orbit, eyelids, and lacrimal system.* San Francisco: Author; 2006; pp. 97–117.

Burnstine M. Clinical recommendations for repair of orbital facial fractures. *Curr Opin Ophthalmol.* 2003;14(5):236–240.

McCord CD, Tanenbaum M, Nunery W. *Oculoplastic surgery.* 3rd ed. New York: Raven Press, 1995; pp. 515–551.

Nerad JA. *Oculoplastic surgery: The requisites in ophthalmology.* Chapter 12. St. Louis: Mosby, 2001; pp. 327–347.

Nunery WR, Tao J, Johl S. Nylon foil wraparound repair of combined orbital floor and medial wall fractures. *Ophthal Plast Reconstr Surg.* 2008;24(4):271–275.

Nunery W, Tao J. Medial canthal open nasal fracture repair. *Ophthal Plast Reconstr Surg.* 2008;24(4):276–279.

Nunery WR. Lateral canthal approach to repair of trimalar fractures of the zygoma. *Ophthal Plast Reconstr Surg.* 1985;1(3):175–183.

91 Orbital Decompression

Sang-Rog Oh, MD, Don O. Kikkawa, MD, and Bobby S. Korn, MD, PhD

TABLE 91.1 *Indications for Orbital Decompression*

Optic neuropathy

Corneal exposure

Disfiguring proptosis

Deep orbital pain and pressure

In preparation for planned strabismus surgery (large muscle recessions usually cause worsening of proptosis)

TABLE 91.2 *Preoperative Considerations*

Euthyroid state desirable unless emergent decompression necessary—consult with endocrinologist as needed

Obtain high-resolution CT scan of orbits with coronals images—assess sinuses and bony volume of greater wing of sphenoid; also assess if soft tissue involvement is more increased fat volume (type I disease) or muscle enlargement (type II disease)

Assess amount of proptosis reduction desired to formulate the surgical plan (see Table 91.3)

Advise patient of risk of diplopia, hypesthesia, need for possible subsequent strabismus and eyelid surgery, remote risk of blindness

Look at old photos to assess prominence of eyes in pre-disease state

Preoperative Evaluation and Surgical Planning

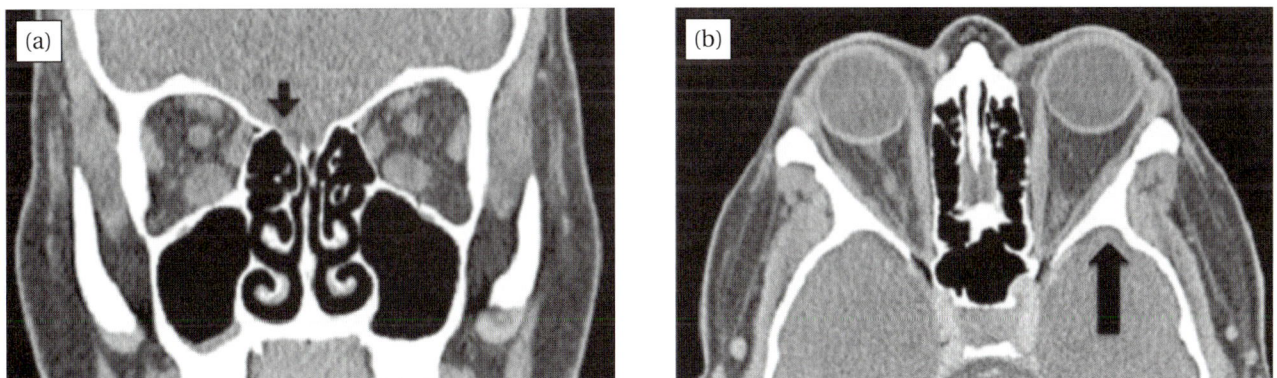

FIGURE 91.1 CT scan of orbits. Coronal view (a) is useful for assessing ethmoid sinus and orbital floor. Skull base (short arrow) is clearly visible and is avoided during medial wall decompression. Axial view (b) is useful for assessing amount of bony volume of the greater wing of the sphenoid (long arrow).

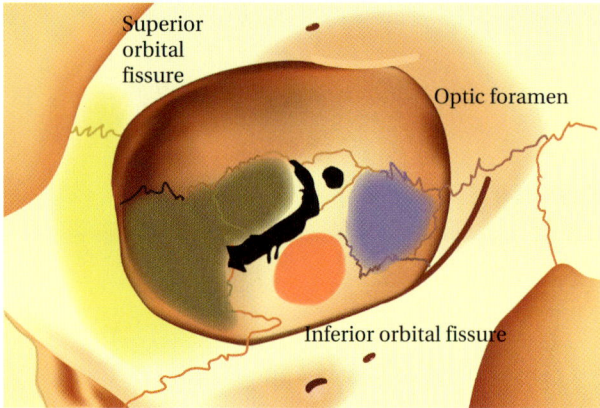

FIGURE 91.2 Diagram of areas of bone removal during decompression. Gray-green = lateral wall, Blue = medial wall, Red = posterior floor, and Yellow = lateral rim removal. (Credit: Bobby S Korn MD PhD, Don Kikkawa MD. *Video Atlas of Oculofacial Plastic and Reconstructive Surgery*: DVD with text. Elsevier; 2010.)

TABLE 91.3 *Average Proptosis Reduction Effect of Different Areas of Bone Removal*

Area of decompression	Amount of reduction
Orbital fat	2 mm
Orbital fat + lateral wall	4 mm
Orbital fat + lateral wall + medial wall	6 mm
Orbital fat + lateral wall + medial wall + floor	8 mm
Orbital fat + lateral wall + medial wall + floor + lateral rim	10 mm

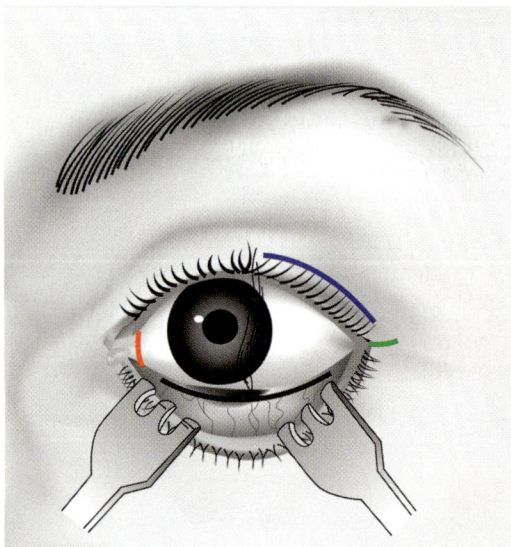

FIGURE 91.3 Common incisions. Blue = eyelid crease. Green = lateral canthotomy. Black = transconjunctival. Red = transcaruncular. (Credit: Bobby S. Korn MD PhD, Don Kikkawa MD. *Video Atlas of Oculofacial Plastic and Reconstructive Surgery*: DVD with text. Elsevier; 2010.)

TABLE 91.4 *Incision for Different Areas of Decompression*

Incision	Area to be decompressed
Lid crease or lateral canthotomy	Lateral wall
Transconjunctival	Orbital floor
Transcaruncular	Medial wall

Lateral Wall Decompression with Rim Removal

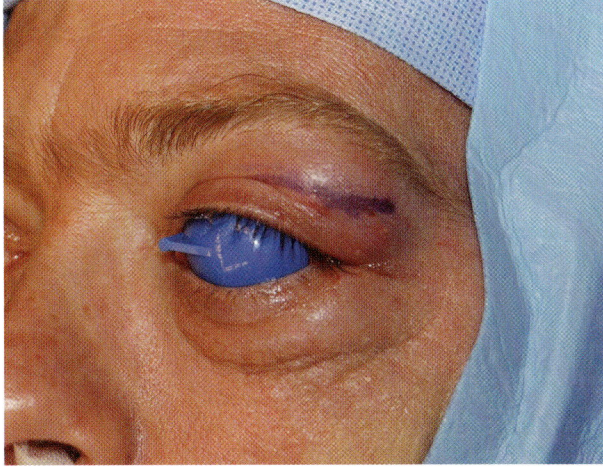

FIGURE 91.4 Upper eyelid crease incision.

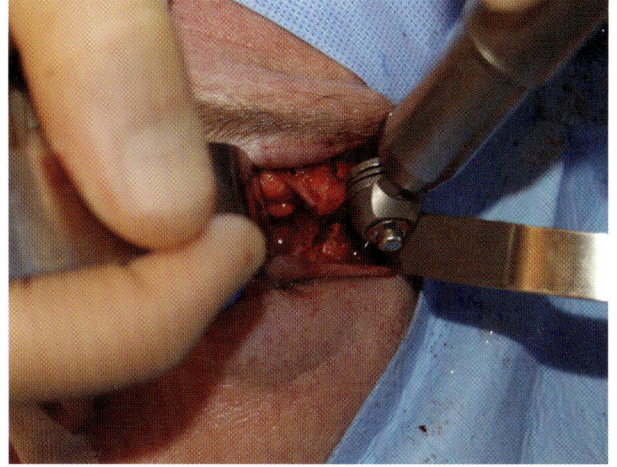

FIGURE 91.5 Superior osteotomy at level of frontozygomatic suture.

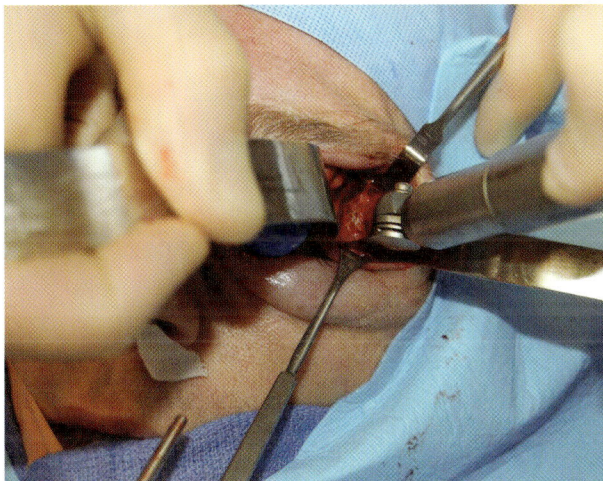

FIGURE 91.6 Inferior osteotomy just above level of zygomatic arch.

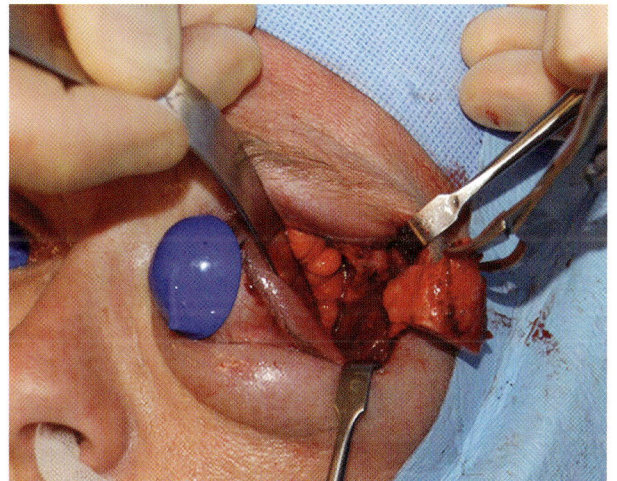

FIGURE 91.7 Lateral orbital rim removed with rongeur.

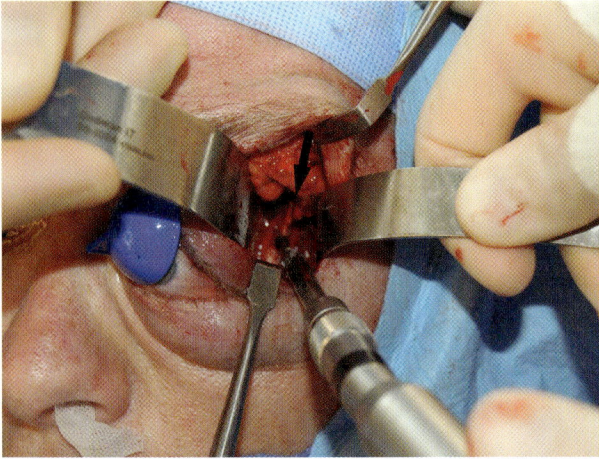

FIGURE 91.8 Removal of thinner portion of lateral orbital wall with high-speed diamond burr (4.0 mm Stryker TPS).

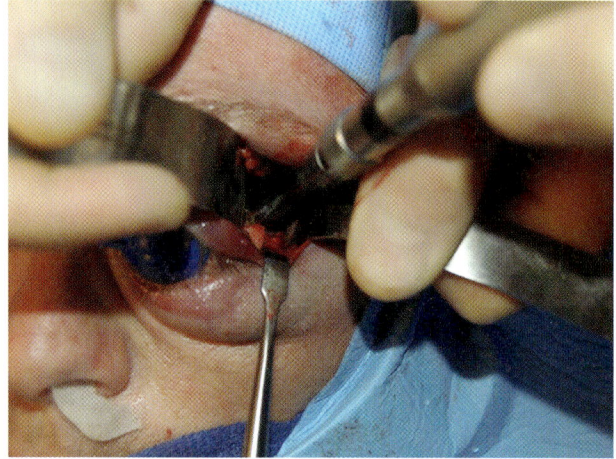

FIGURE 91.9 Removal of greater wing of sphenoid with diamond burr. Note relatively bloodless bone removal within marrow space due to coagulation from high drill speed (drill speed approaches 60,000 rpm).

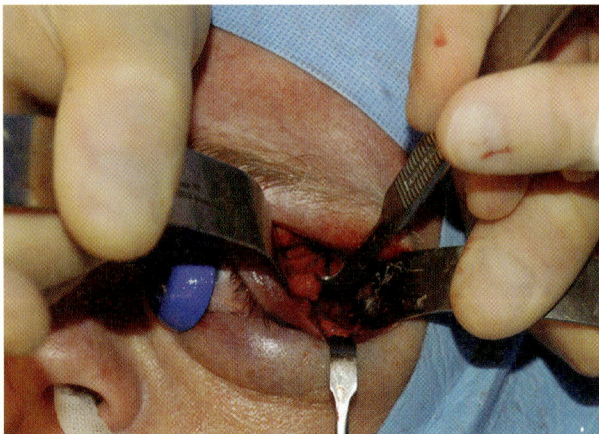

FIGURE 91.10 Opening of periorbita with # 12 (Bard Parker) blade. Note bulging orbital fat.

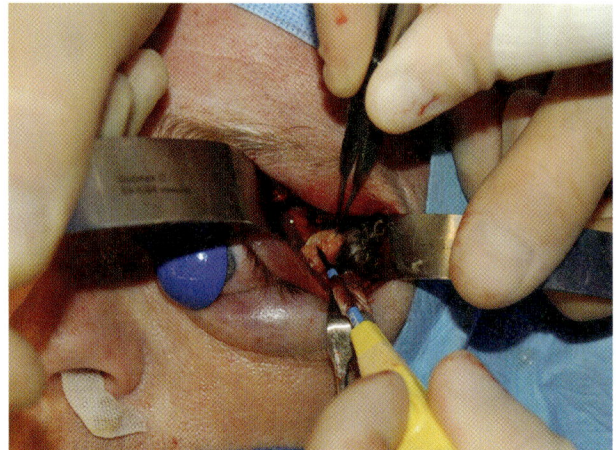

FIGURE 91.11 Removal of intraconal fat (between lateral and inferior rectus muscles) from opening in periorbita. Volume of fat removal ranges from 2 to 4 cc's.

Medial Wall Decompression

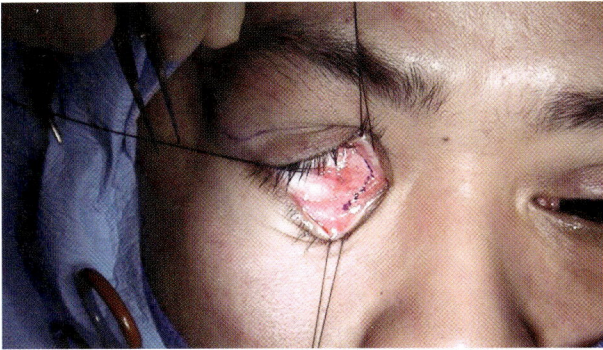

FIGURE 91.12 A transcaruncular incision is made (outlined by the marking pen). The upper and lower lids are retracted with 4-0 silk sutures for exposure.

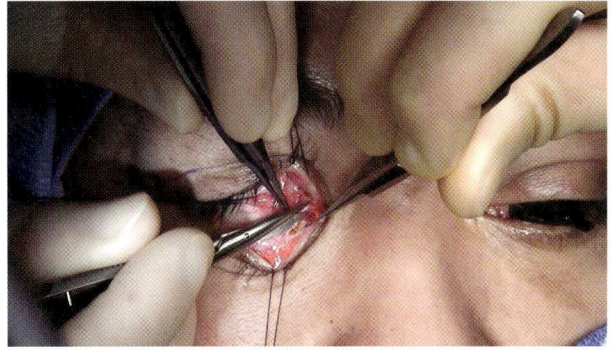

FIGURE 91.13 Posterior caruncular incision to access medial wall.

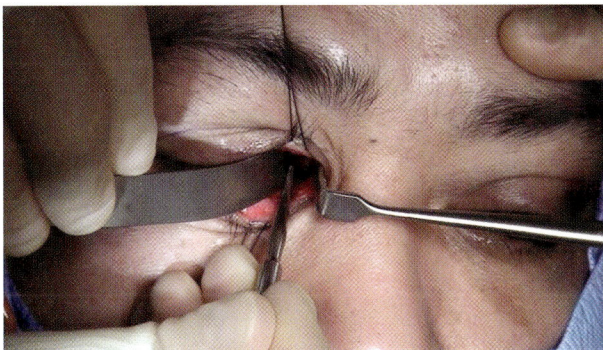

FIGURE 91.14 A subperiosteal dissection is performed to visualize lamina papyracea of medial orbital wall. The entire medial wall is exposed.

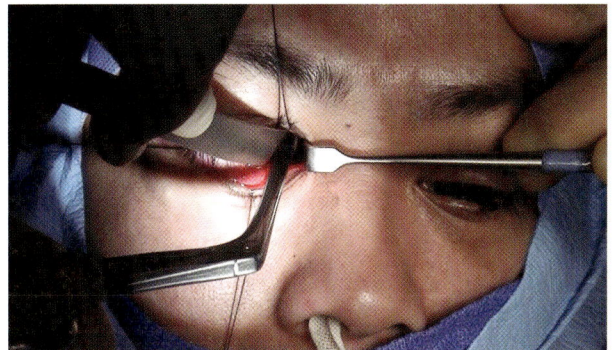

FIGURE 91.15 Takahashi forceps is used to remove the ethmoidal air cells.

Orbital Floor Decompression

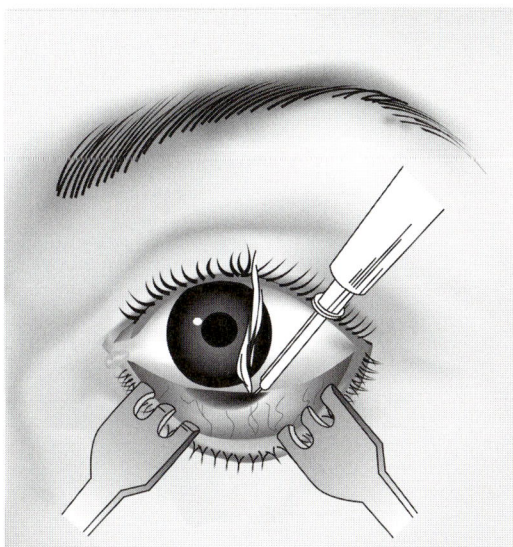

FIGURE 91.16 The orbital floor is accessed through a transconjunctival incision, in conjunction with a lateral canthotomy and cantholysis to assist with exposure.

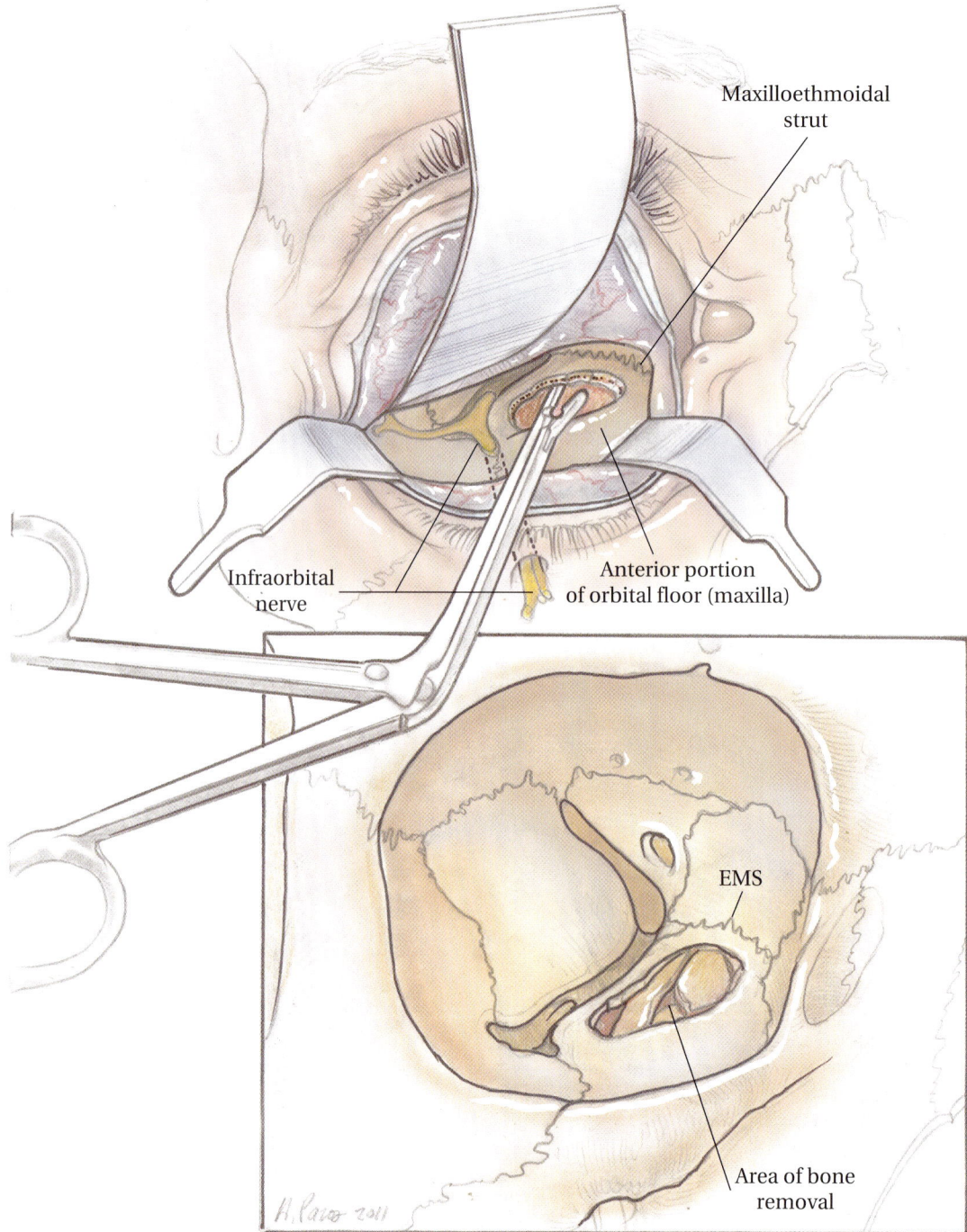

FIGURE 91.17 The posterior orbital floor is removed medial to the infraorbital nerve, with preservation of the maxilloethmoidal strut. Only the posterior one-half of orbital floor is removed. The anterior one-half is preserved to prevent globe ptosis and maintain patency of maxillary sinus ositum.

Preoperative and Postoperative Photograph

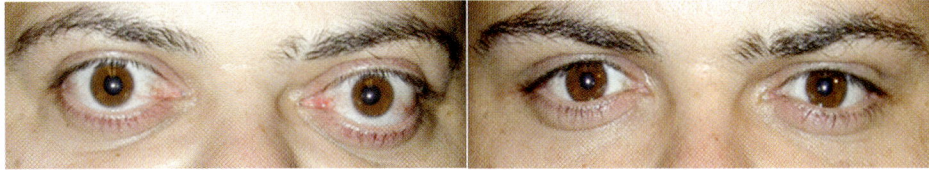

FIGURE 91.18 50-year-old male with bilateral thyroid related orbitopathy and right optic neuropathy (left). He underwent 3-wall bilateral orbital decompression, with reversal of his optic neuropathy and resolution of inflammatory symptoms (right).

TABLE 91.5 *Potential Complications of Orbital Decompression*

Sinusitis
Strabismus
Vision threatening orbital hemorrhage
Sensory nerve damage (hypesthesia)
Hypoglobus (floor removed to far anteriorly)
Reactivation of disease

SELECTED REFERENCES

Alper MG. Pioneers in the history of orbital decompression for Graves' ophthalmopathy. R.U. Kroenlein (1847–1910), O. Hirsch (1877–1965) and H.C. Naffziger (1884–1961). *Doc Ophthalmol* 1995;89:163–171.

Chang EL, Bernardino CR, Rubin PA. Transcaruncular orbital decompression for management of compressive optic neuropathy in thyroid-related orbitopathy. *Plast Reconstr Surg.* 2003;112(3):739–747.

Graham SM, Brown CL, Carter KD, Song A, Nerad JA. Medial and lateral orbital wall surgery for balanced decompression in thyroid eye disease. *Laryngoscope* 2003;113(7):1206–1209.

Kikkawa DO, Pornpanich K, Cruz RC Jr, Levi L, Granet DB. Graded orbital decompression based on severity of proptosis. *Ophthalmology.* 2002;109(7):1219–1224.

Kim JW, Goldberg RA, Shorr N. The inferomedial orbital strut: an anatomic and radiographic study. *Ophthal Plast Reconstr Surg.* 2002;18(5):355–364.

Lyons CJ, Rootman J. Orbital decompression for disfiguring exophthalmos in thyroid orbitopathy. *Ophthalmology* 1994; 101(2): 223–230.

Mourits MP, Bijl HM, Baldeschi L, et al. Outcome of orbital decompression for disfiguring proptosis in patients with Graves' orbitopathy using various surgical procedures. *Br J Ophthalmol.* 2009; 93:1518–1523.

Rootman J, Stewart B, Goldberg RA. *Orbital surgery: A conceptual approach.* Baltimore: Williams & Wilkins; 1995.

Shorr N, Baylis HI, Goldberg RA, Perry JD. Transcaruncular approach to the medial orbit and orbital apex. *Ophthalmology.* 2000;107(8):1459–1463.

92 Craniofacial Approaches for Orbital Osteotomies

Ryan C. Frank, MD, FRCSC and Steven R. Cohen, MD, FACS

TABLE 92.1 *Indications for Orbital Osteotomies*

Fronto-orbital Advancement	Supraorbital rim abnormalities as in metopic, unicoronal, and bicoronal craniosynostosis
Monobloc	Retrusion of supraorbital and infraorbital rims, along with retrusion of zygoma and maxilla (including dentition)
Facial Bipartition	Hypertelorbitism with narrow palatal width
LeFort III	Inferior orbital rim and nasomaxillary/midface retrusion
Periorbital Osteotomies	Orbital tumor access; removal of fibrous dysplasia; post-traumatic reconstruction

TABLE 92.2 *Preoperative Considerations*

Preoperative imaging with three-dimensional computed tomography scans are essential for operative planning

Computed tomography-derived, sterilizable models aid intraoperative decision making

Optimize all medical comorbidities before undergoing procedures

Type and cross-matching blood necessary for most orbital osteotomy procedures

Fronto-orbital Advancement

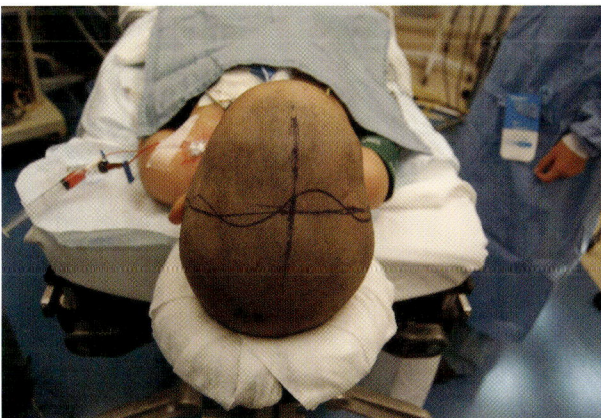

FIGURE 92.1 Bicoronal incision. The incision is planned as a curvilinear line from helical root to helical root. It can be extended in an inferior direction either anterior to the ear or posterior to it, depending on exposure requirements.

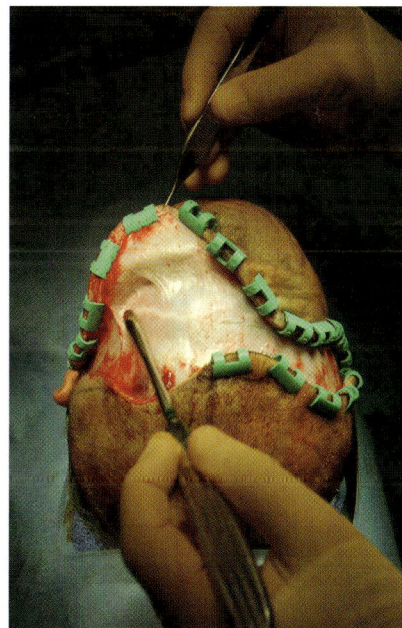

FIGURE 92.2 Dissection is first carried out in a subgaleal plane, as this is primarily avascular. Complete exposure of the frontal bone and supraorbital bar is performed. Dissection deepens to subpericranial 2 cm above the supraorbital rim, and continues in this plane until complete exposure of the supraorbital bar is obtained.

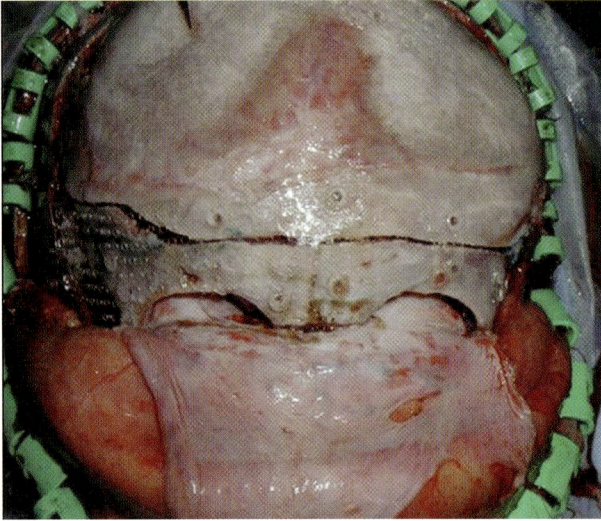

FIGURE 92.3 This figure demonstrates complete exposure of the supraorbital bar, following fixation with a resorbable plating system. The osteotomies performed to create this bar include the following: (a) Superiorly, 2 cm above the supraorbital rim. (b) Laterally, through the greater wing of the sphenoid. (c) Inferiorly, through the frontozygomatic suture and the nasofrontal suture. (d) Posteriorly, through the supraorbital roof. A frontal craniotomy is needed in conjunction with this procedure to properly gain access to complete all osteotomies. Notice the pericranial flap based inferiorly—this can be used to obliterate the frontal sinus, or to provide soft-tissue barrier between extracranial and intracranial contents.

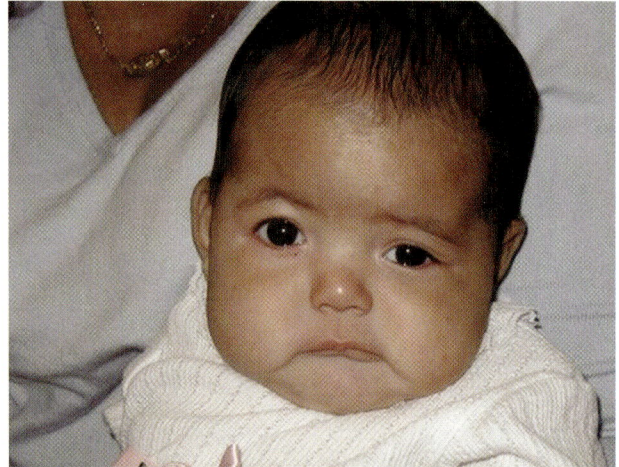

FIGURE 92.4 Preoperative photograph of a patient with right-sided unicoronal craniosynostosis. Notice the retruded supraorbital bar above the right eye, with an associated ipsilateral widened palpebral fissure. In conjunction with this deformity, there is contralateral frontal bossing.

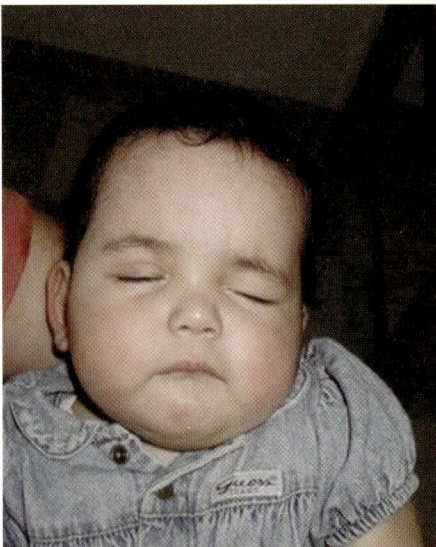

FIGURE 92.5 Postoperative photograph of the same patient 6 months later. Excellent supraorbital symmetry has been obtained with the fronto-orbital advancement.

Monobloc

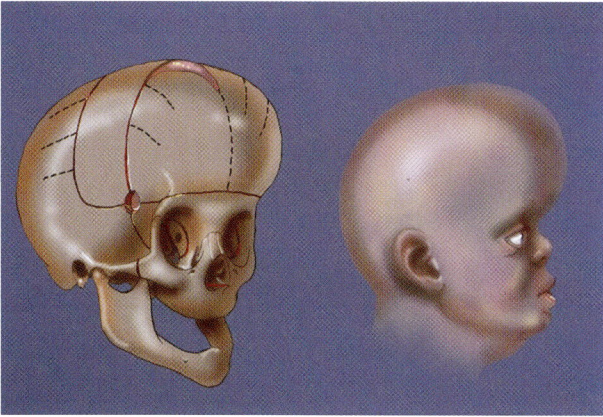

FIGURE 92.6   Planned osteotomies for monobloc advancement with cranial vault reshaping. The monobloc procedure is performed for children with combined supraorbital and infraorbital retrusion. It is an advancement of the entire frontal bone with zygoma, maxilla, and nasal bones. Access to these osteotomies is gained via a bicoronal incision, as well as an upper buccal sulcus (intraoral) incision.

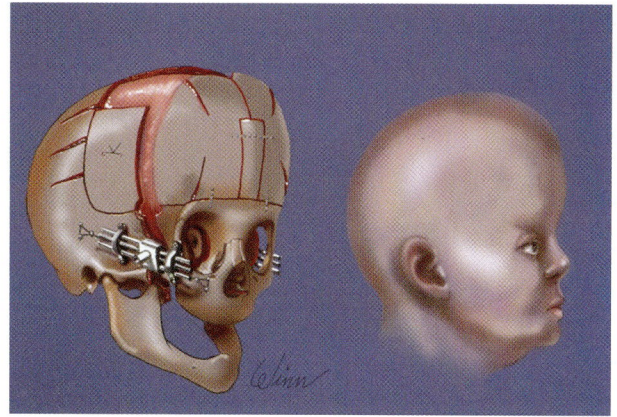

FIGURE 92.7   The monobloc procedure can be performed either as a one-time advancement procedure with bone graft insertion in the created gaps, or as a distraction type case. Internal distractors are placed at the time the osteotomies are made. Distraction of the monobloc segment anteriorly occurs at a rate of approximately 1 mm per day, until the desired displacement has occurred.

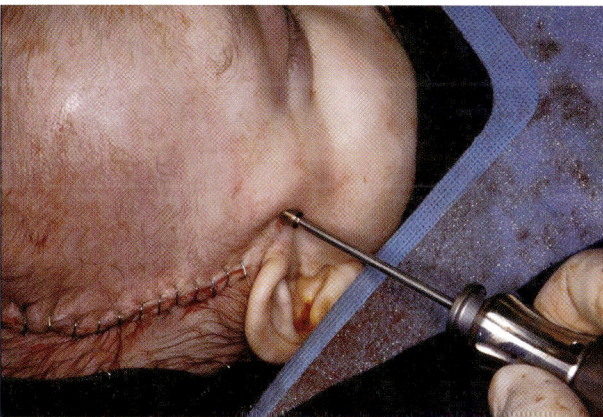

FIGURE 92.8   Through a small percutaneous site, access to the distractor mechanism can be gained.

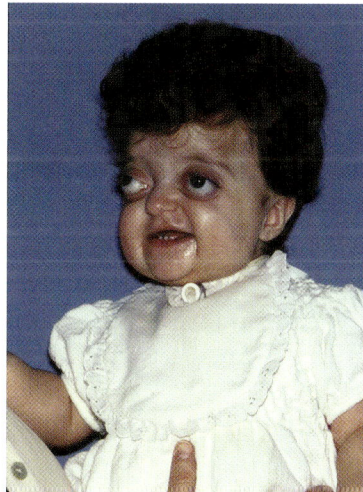

FIGURE 92.9   Preoperative photograph of a patient with Pfeiffer syndrome. Notice the proptosis in association with supraorbital and midface retrusion.

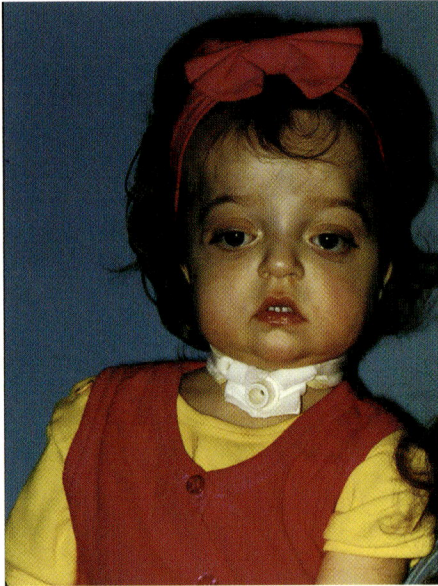

FIGURE 92.10 Postoperative view of the same patient 1 year following monobloc advancement. Notice the much-improved periorbital aesthetics.

Facial Bipartition

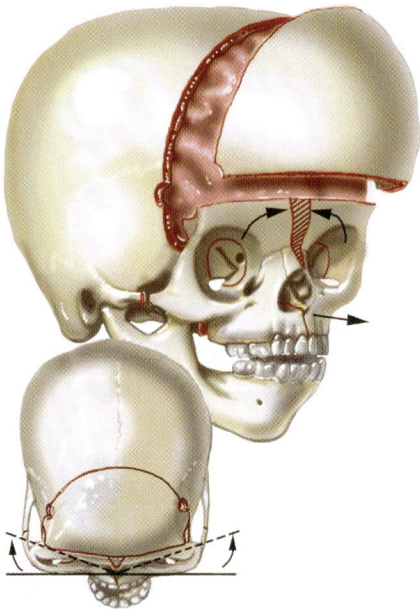

FIGURE 92.11 Hypertelorism is commonly found as an associated deformity in many of the craniofacial syndromes. The facial bipartition procedure removes a segment of excess midline bone (between the medial orbital walls). The split orbits are then translocated medially and stabilized to each other. The facial bipartition extends inferiorly to the hard palate, which is also split and subsequently widened. This procedure can be combined with a monobloc type advancement. The top illustration demonstrates the proposed medial movement of the orbits, along with the anterior movement of the maxilla. The bottom illustration demonstrates the desired anatomic facial profile with more anterior projection medially (dotted line). The facial deformity present in many of the craniofacial syndromes is one of poor facial contour, with a flattened medial facial projection (solid line).

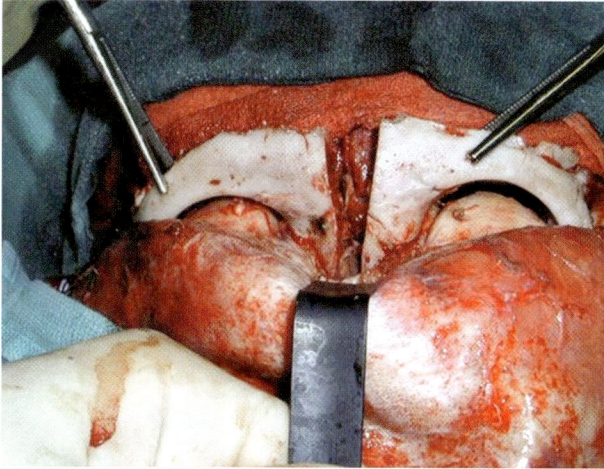

FIGURE 92.12 Intraoperative photograph of the facial bipartition procedure. Notice the resected bony gap present in the midline, between the orbits.

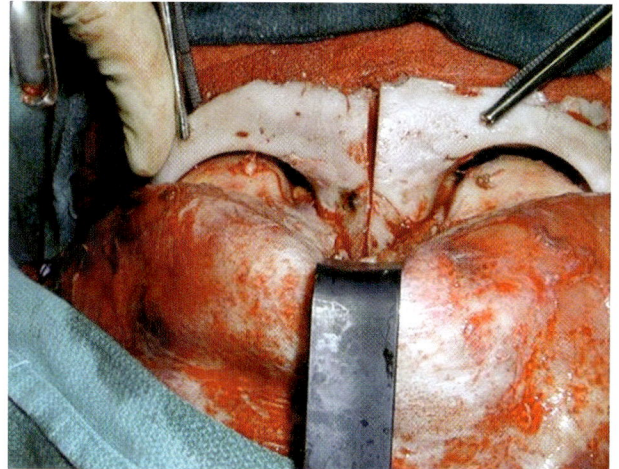

FIGURE 92.13 Intraoperative photograph of the facial bipartition procedure. The bony gap is now closed as the orbits are translocated medially, toward each other.

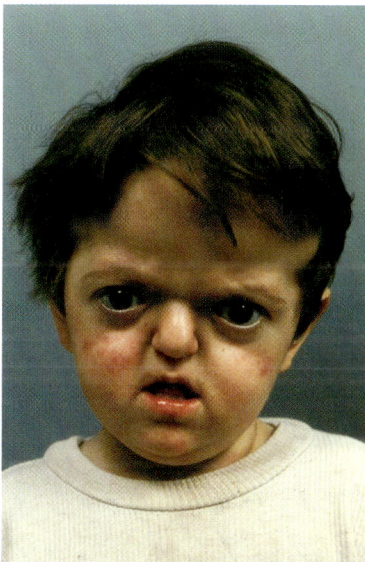

FIGURE 92.14 Preoperative photograph of a 4-year-old child with Apert syndrome. Notice the hypertelorbitism in association with the supraorbital and infraorbital retrusion.

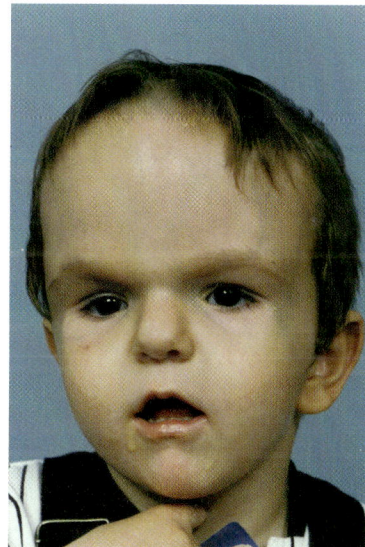

FIGURE 92.15 Postoperative photograph of the same patient one year following monobloc advancement with facial bipartition.

LeFort III Procedure

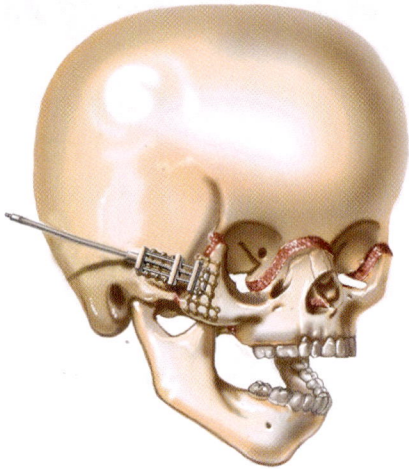

FIGURE 92.16 Moderate to severe midface retrusion and associated class III dental malocclusion (with normal supraorbital position) is best treated with the LeFort III advancement. This procedure is an advancement of the entire midface, including zygomatic bodies, maxillae, and nasal bones. Osteotomies are made through the frontozygomatic junction, zygomatic arch, posterior orbit (via infraorbital fissure), nasofrontal junction, and pterygomaxillary junction. The entire midface segment is then advanced and secured in place in its new anterior position.

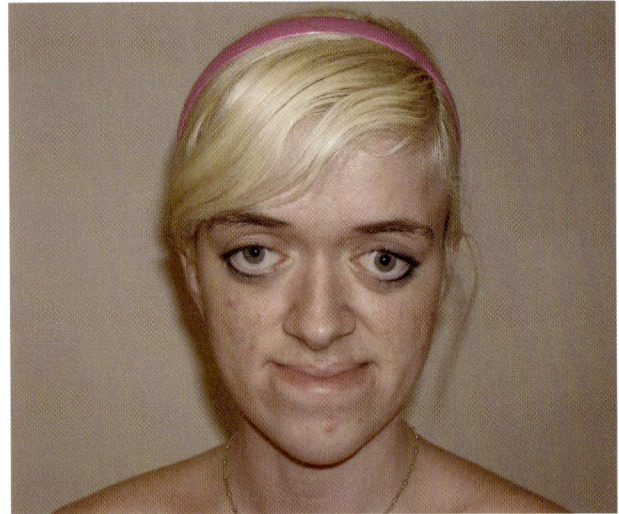

FIGURE 92.17 Preoperative photograph of a 17-year-old patient with Crouzon syndrome. Notice the retruded midface with excessive inferior scleral show.

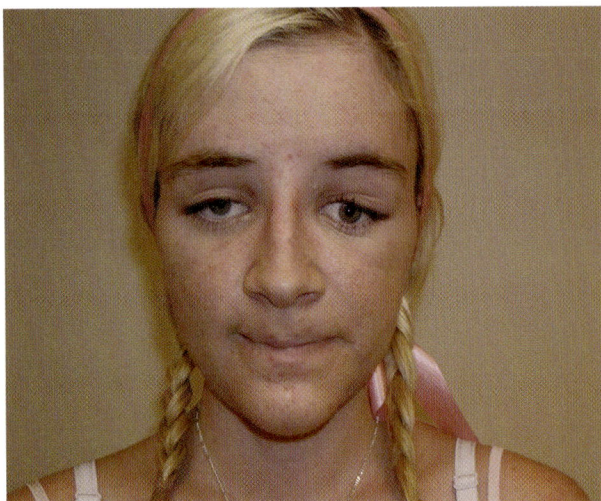

FIGURE 92.18 Two-week postoperative photograph of the patient in Figure 91.17. Notice the improved cheek contour and diminished scleral show.

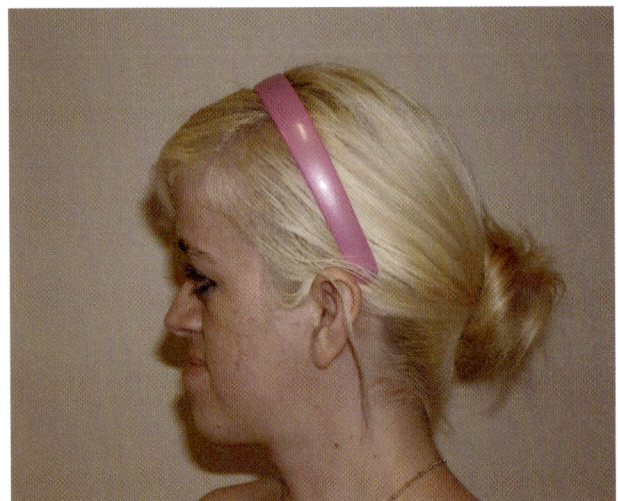

FIGURE 92.19 Preoperative side view of the same patient.

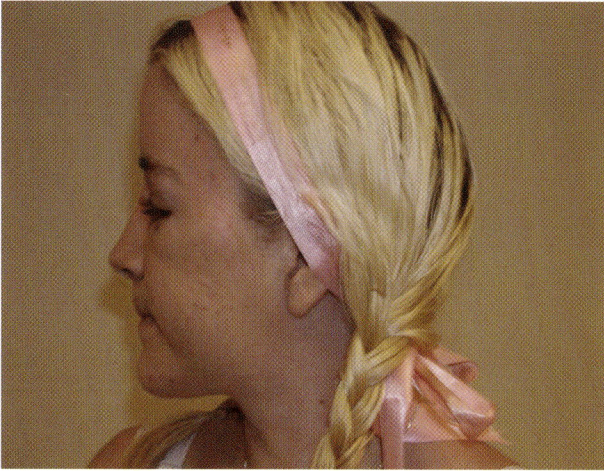

FIGURE 92.20 Two-week postoperative side view of the same patient.

Periorbital Osteotomies

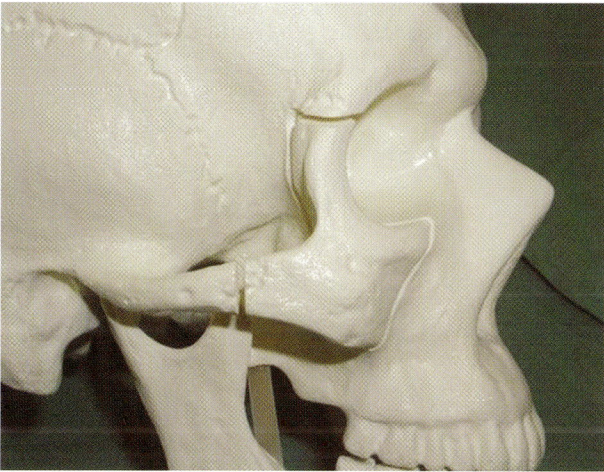

FIGURE 92.21 Creative orbital osteotomies are commonly required to reconstruct defects post-trauma, or to gain access to periorbital tumors. The orbitozygomatic osteotomy is commonly employed to expose intraorbital tumors. The frontozygomatic suture, zygomatic arch, lateral orbital wall, and orbital floor are all osteotomized in this approach.

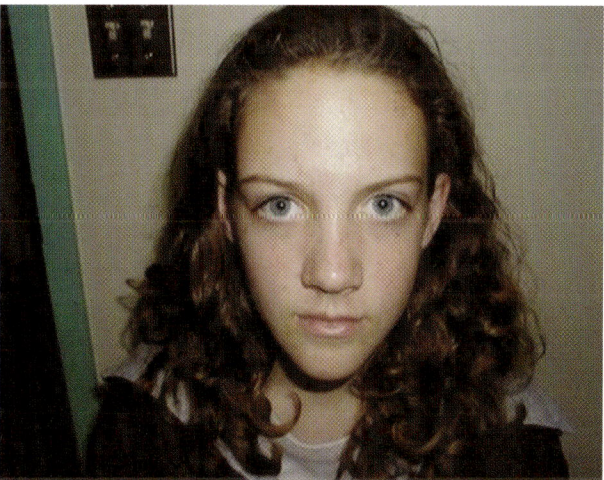

FIGURE 92.22 Preoperative photograph of a 15-year-old patient with fibrous dysplasia of the right orbit and frontal bone.

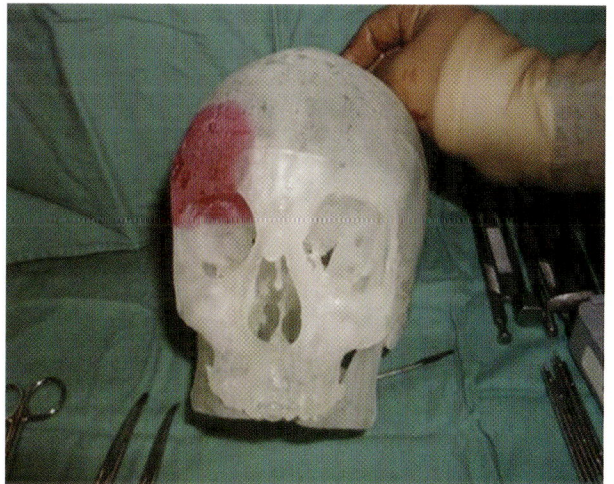

FIGURE 92.23 Three-dimensional model constructed via CT scan illustrating fibrous dysplasia location (red).

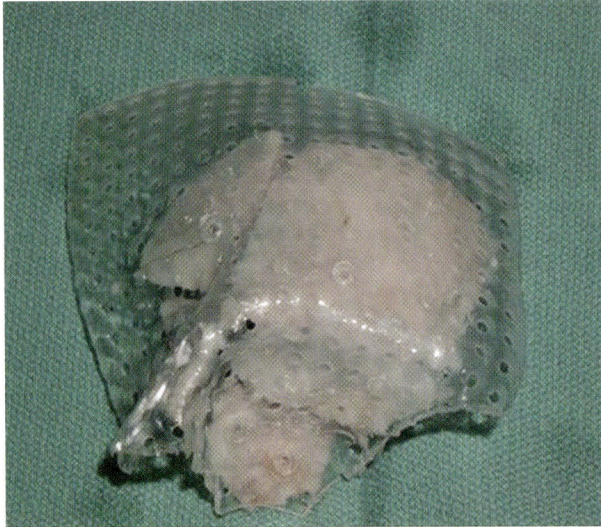

FIGURE 92.24 The affected bone is resected and the defect is reconstructed with split calvarial bone grafts. The grafts are secured in anatomic location using a resorbable plating system.

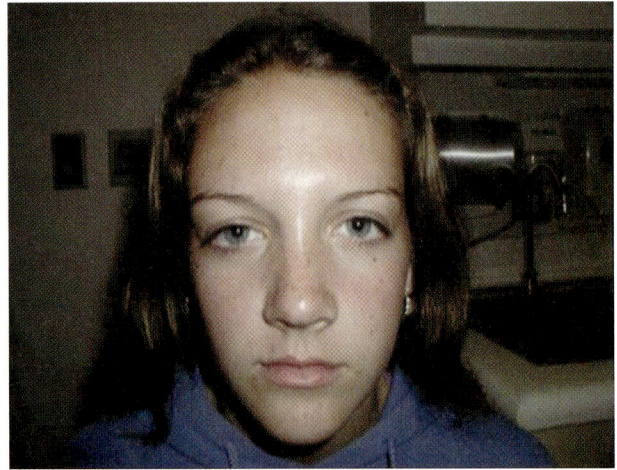

FIGURE 92.25 Postoperative photograph of same patient 3 months following resection of fibrous dysplasia and periorbital reconstruction.

TABLE 92.3 *Potential Complications of Orbital Osteotomies*

Over/under correction of deformity

Supra/infraorbital nerve damage

Hematoma/seroma

Infection of soft tissue, bone, brain

Diplopia, extraocular muscle dysfunction, blindness

SELECTED REFERENCES

Cohen SR. Craniofacial distraction with a modular internal distraction system: evolution of design and surgical techniques. *Plast Reconstr Surg.* 1999;103:1592.

Cohen SR, Boydston W, Hudgins R, Burstein FD: Monobloc and facial bipartition distraction with internal devices. *J Craniofac Surg.* 1999;10:244–251.

Converse JM et al. Ocular hypertelorism and pseudohypertelorism. Advances in surgical treatment. *Plast Reconstr Surg.* 1970;45:1.

Fearon JA. The Le Fort III osteotomy: to distract or not to distract? *Plast Reconstr Surg.* 2001;107:1091.

Gateno J, Teichgraeber JF, Aguilar E. Computer planning for distraction osteogenesis. *Plast Reconstr Surg.* 2000;105:873.

Kaban LB et al. Midface position after Le Fort III advancement. *Plast Reconstr Surg.* 1984;73:758.

McCarthy JG et al. The Le Fort III advancement osteotomy in the child under 7 years of age. *Plast Reconstr Surg.* 1990;86:633.

Van der Meulen JC, Vaandrager J. Surgery related to the correction of hypertelorism. *Plast Reconstr Surg.* 1983;71:6.

93 Lacrimal Probing and Intubation

Martin H. Devoto, MD

TABLE 93.1 *Indications for Surgery*

Condition	Timing	Procedure
Complete nasolacrimal duct obstruction	Preferably at 1 year of age	Probing and irrigation with or without inferior turbinate fracture
Complete nasolacrimal duct obstruction after failed probing and irrigation	After failed probing and irrigation	NLD Silicone Intubation
Congenital punctal occlusion	Elective	Membrane incision
Congenital punctal and canalicular agenesis	Elective Usually after 12 years old	CDCR with Jones Tube

TABLE 93.2 *Preoperative Considerations*

Careful preoperative examination to diagnose condition

Preoperative use of oxymetazoline for decongestion is very useful

Use loupes and fiberoptic headlight for good visualization

Endoscopically assisted procedures may enhance results

Pertinent Surgical Anatomy

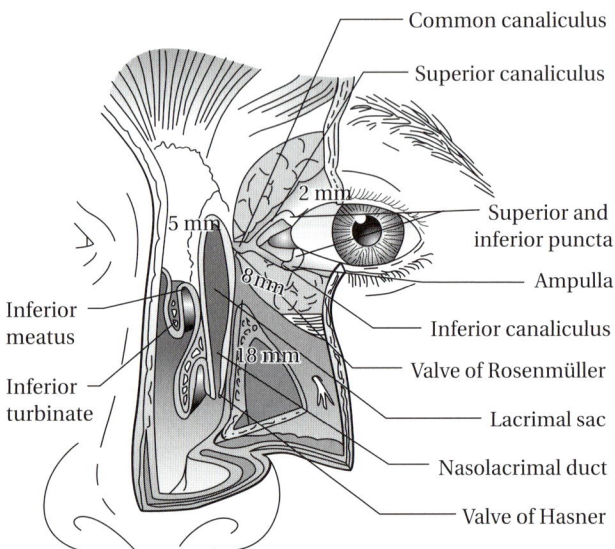

FIGURE 93.1 Nasolacrimal excretory system.

Step by Step Surgical Series

Probing

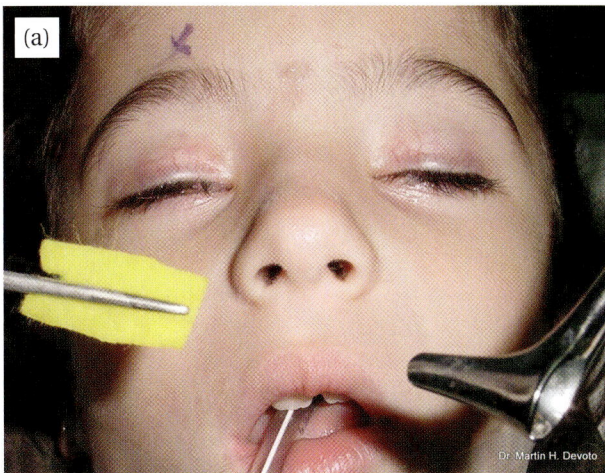

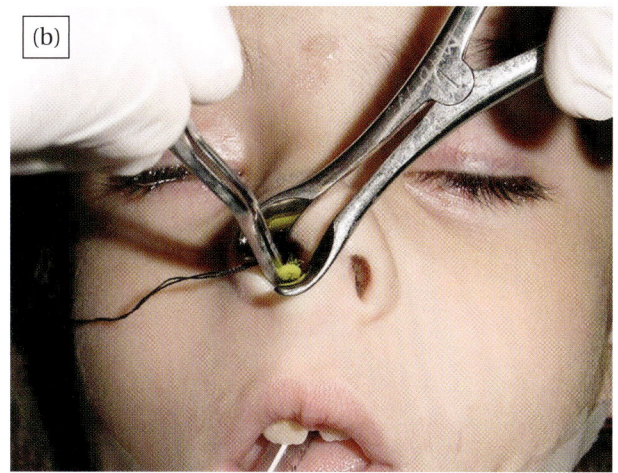

FIGURE 93.2 (a, b) Nasal packing with oxymetazoline. Place a cotton pledget under the inferior turbinate and a second one medial to the inferior turbinate. Note that the bayonet forceps is directed parallel to the floor of the nose.

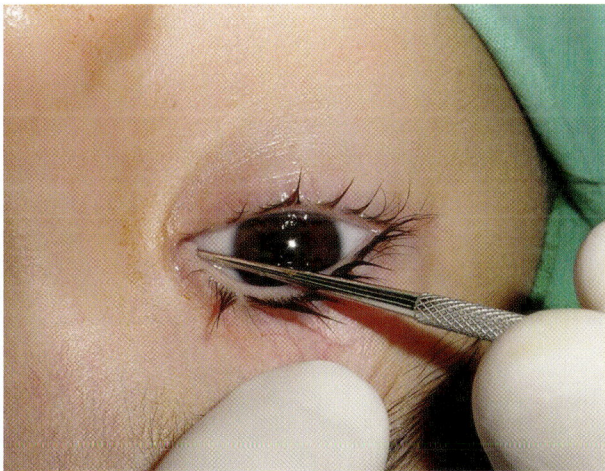

FIGURE 93.3 Dilation of upper punctum.

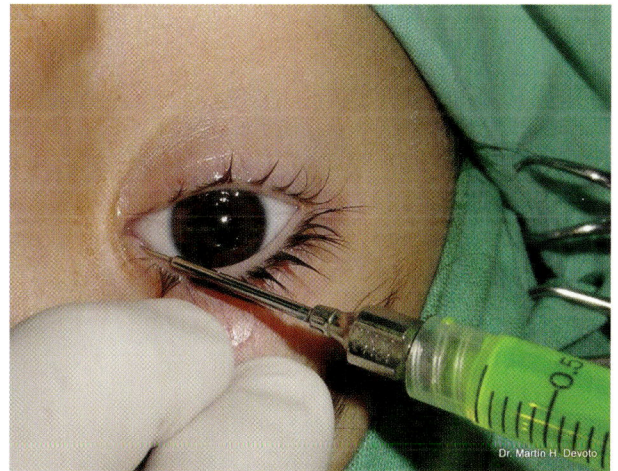

FIGURE 93.4 Irrigation with fluorescein through upper punctum.

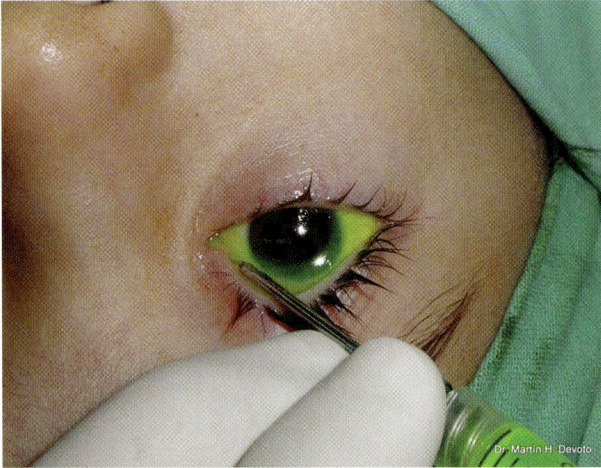

FIGURE 93.5 Complete fluorescein reflux confirms nasolacrimal duct obstruction.

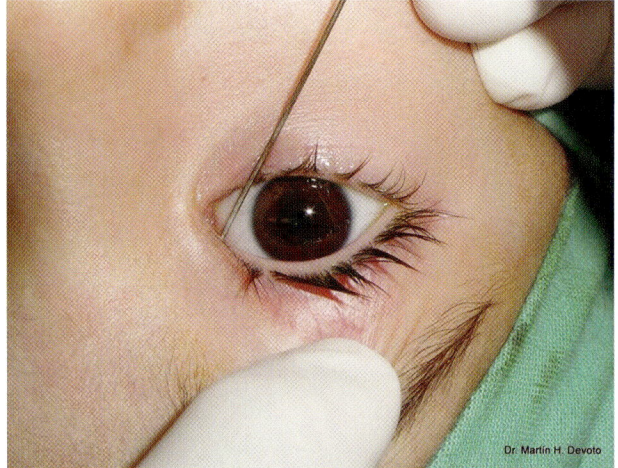

FIGURE 93.6 Placement of Bowman probe. Note that the placement is initially perpendicular to the eyelid border.

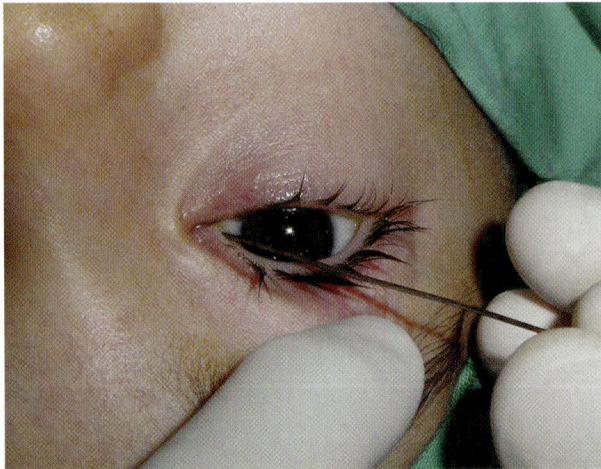

FIGURE 93.7 Probe is redirected medially towards the medial canthal tendon. A canalicular fold is observed in this case, accounting for a stop before the lacrimal sac. If the probe is forcefully passed at this step, a false way can be created.

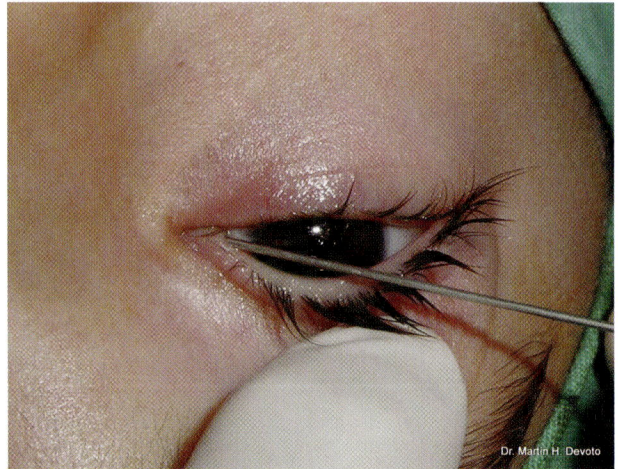

FIGURE 93.8 Gentle probing is done until a hard stop against bone is palpated at the medial lacrimal sac.

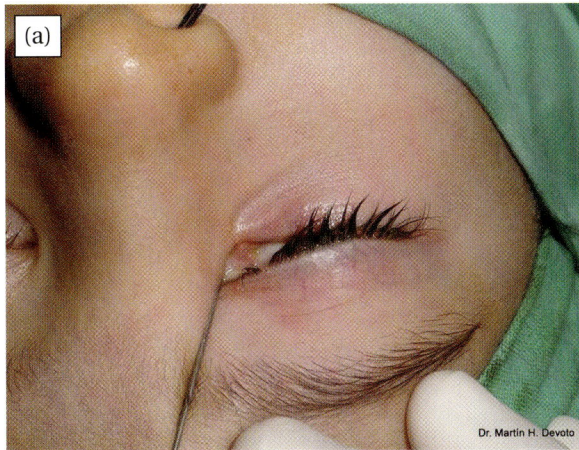

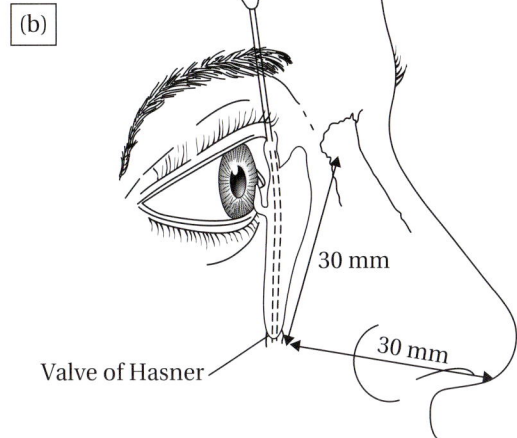

FIGURE 93.9 (a) The probe is then redirected toward the brow. Note that the probe is flush with the brow, and is angled slightly temporal to follow the nasolacrimal duct. Gentle pressure is applied after it stops. A soft pop is sometimes felt once Hasner's valve is opened. (b) This picture shows the correct placement of the lacrimal probe.

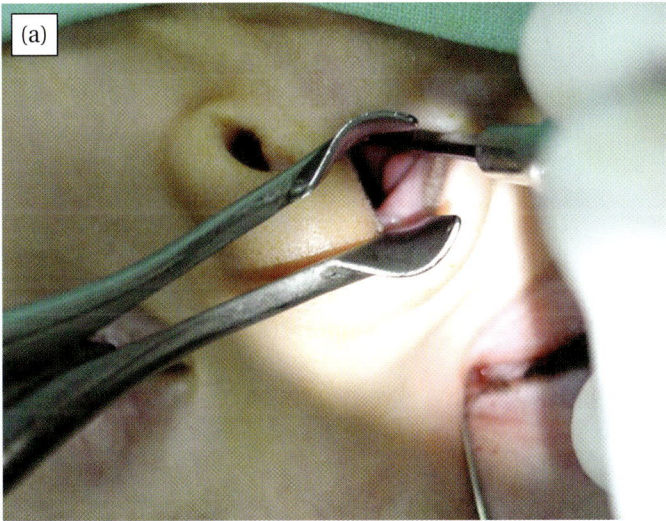

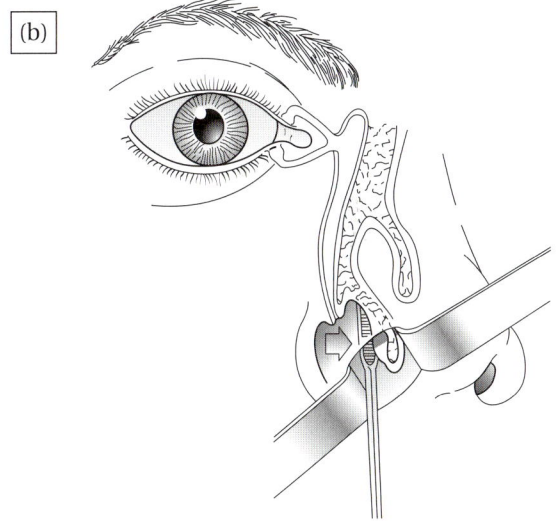

FIGURE 93.10 (a) Nasal visualization of the probe can be done directly with surgical loupes and a fiberoptic headlight, or with an endoscope. If the inferior turbinate obstructs the view, it can be fractured medially using the blunt end of a Freer periosteal elevator. Gentle pressure is applied medially until enough space is created to view the probe. (b) Schematic diagram of medial turbinate infracture.

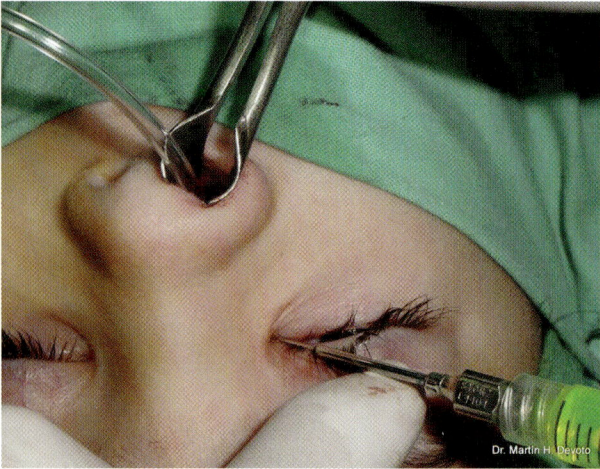

FIGURE 93.11   Lacrimal irrigation with fluorescein shows no reflux. Fluorescein can be seen within a clear aspiration cannula.

Intubation

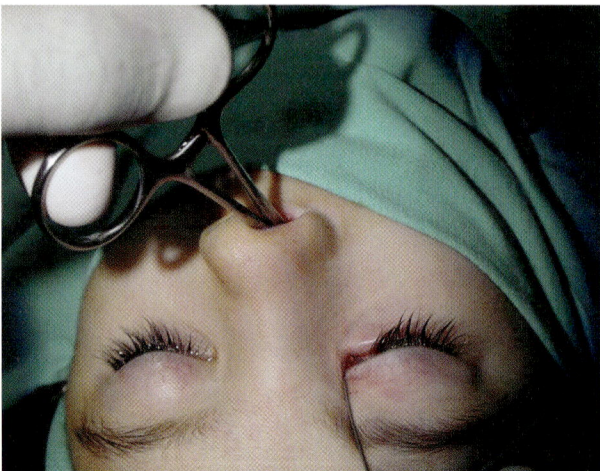

FIGURE 93.12   The preliminary steps are performed exactly as in a probing and irrigation (as above), but instead of a Bowman's probe, a silicone lacrimal stent set is used. Once the lacrimal probe is identified beneath the inferior turbinate, it is grasped with a small hemostat or a Crawford hook.

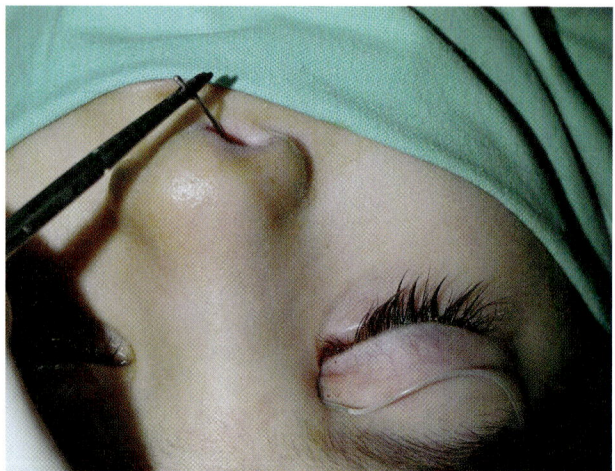

FIGURE 93.13   The probe is gently pulled out from the nose, making sure not to injure the nasal mucosa.

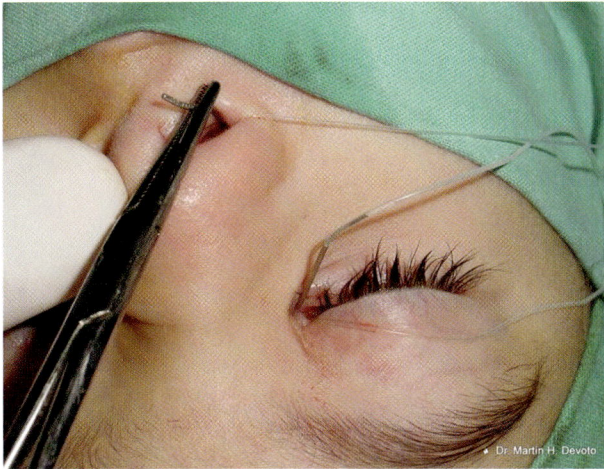

FIGURE 93.14 The second probe is passed in the same manner

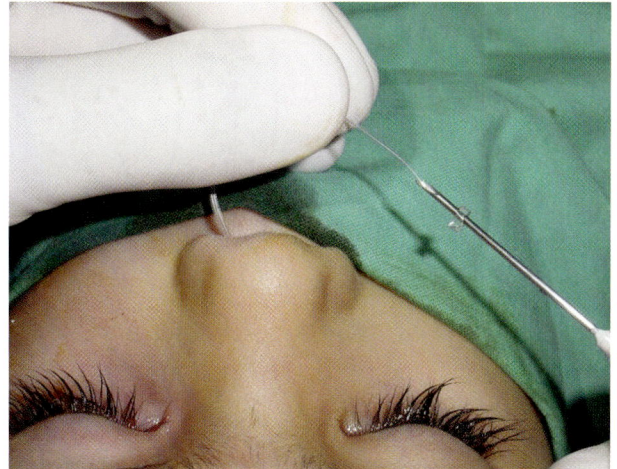

FIGURE 93.15 A small silicone block is useful to fix both ends of the stent together, to prevent the stent from migrating into the nasolacrimal duct if the patient pulls the eyelid loop in the medial canthus. To fixate the ends, a 16 G needle is passed through the silicone block, and one of the ends of the stent is threaded through the needle a few centimeters.

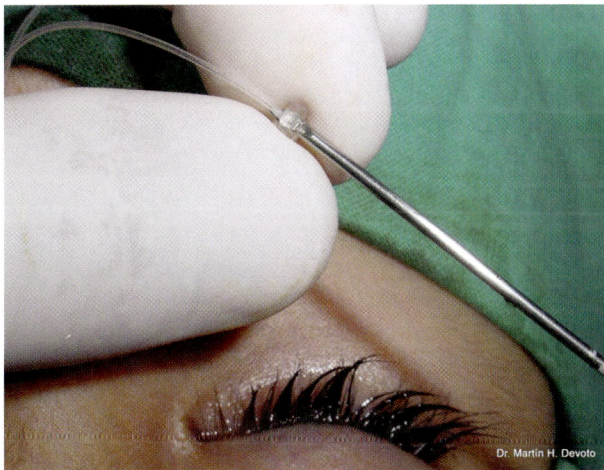

FIGURE 93.16 The silicone block is firmly grasped between the fingers, and the needle is pulled back, leaving the silicone firmly secured in the block. The second end of the stent is placed through the same block in the same fashion.

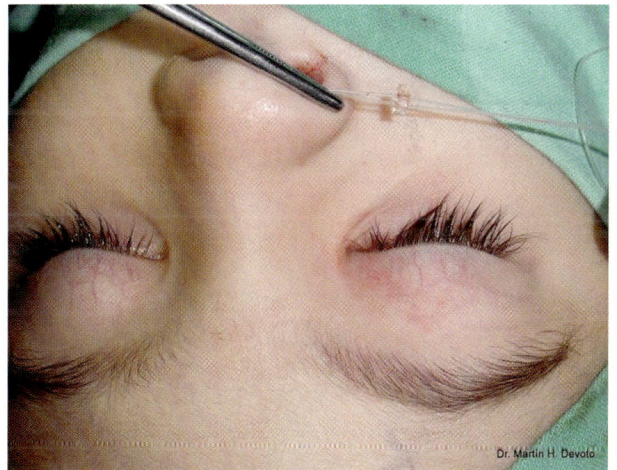

FIGURE 93.17 The block is adjusted and slid toward the nose. It is important to have the stents and silicone block inside the nasal vestibule, but not too tight, to avoid cheese-wiring of the punctum and canaliculus.

Before and After Examples

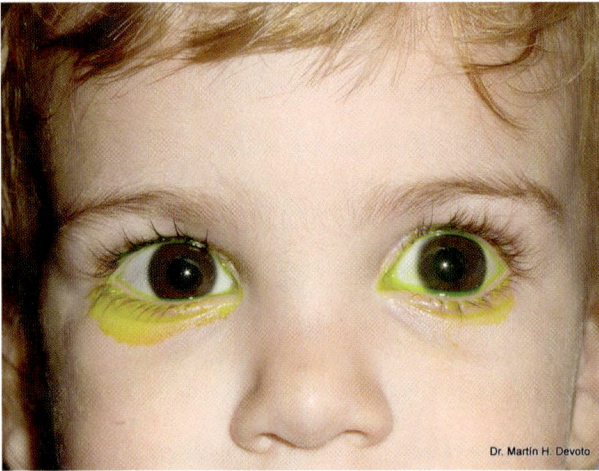

FIGURE 93.18 Patient with a delayed dye disappearance test (DDT) on both eyes.

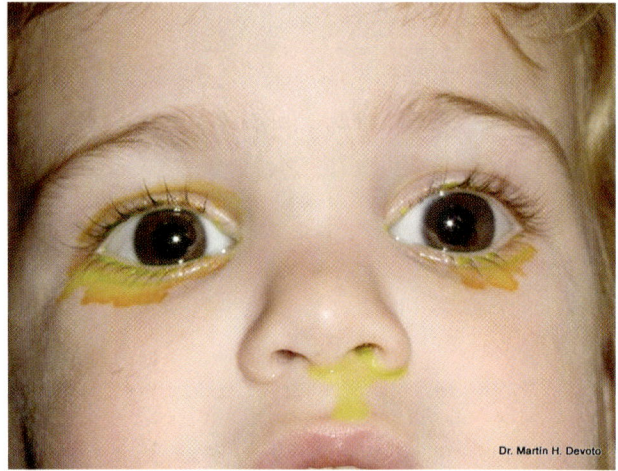

FIGURE 93.19 The same patient after successful probing and irrigation. Note the fluorescein dye now coming out of the left nostril.

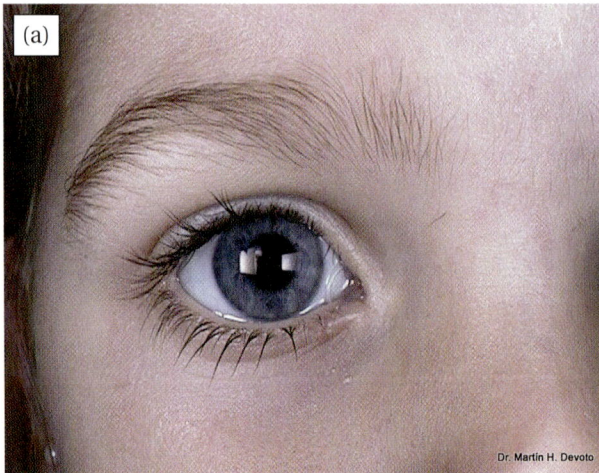

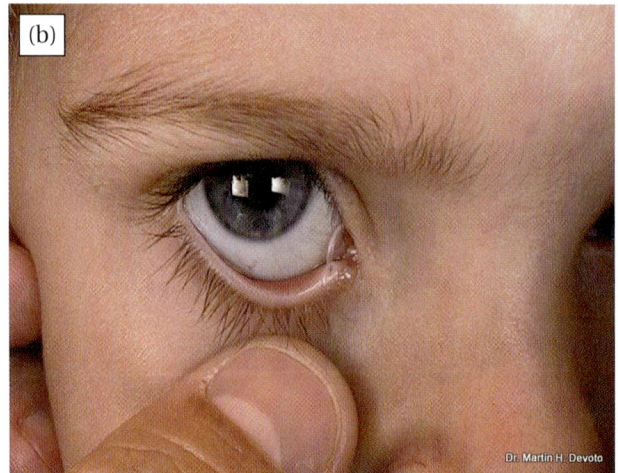

FIGURE 93.20 (a, b) Patient with lacrimal stent in place. Stents are left in place for 6 months before removal. A follow-up visit shows a round inferior punctum with no cheese-wiring.

TABLE 93.3 *Complications*

Complication	Procedure
Tearing after "successful probing"	Consider second probing
Tearing after 1 or 2 failed probings	Silicone intubation
Silicone stent prolapsed in the eye	Reposition stent or remove if near 6 months after placement

SELECTED REFERENCES

Dortzbach RK, France TD, et al. Silicone intubation for obstruction of the nasolacrimal duct in children. *Am J Ophthalmol.* 1982;94(5):585–590.

Katowitz JA, Welsh MG. Timing of initial probing and irrigation in congenital nasolacrimal duct obstruction. *Ophthalmology.* 1987;94(6):698–705.

Paul TO, Shepherd R. Congenital nasolacrimal duct obstruction: natural history and the timing of optimal intervention. *J Pediatr Ophthalmol Strabismus.* 1994;31(6):362–367.

94 Pediatric Nasolacrimal Intubation using the Ritleng Probe and Monoka Stent

Monte D. Mills, MD and William R. Katowitz, MD

TABLE 94.1 *Indications for Intubation of the Nasolacrimal System in Children*

Persistent or recurrent nasolacrimal obstruction after initial probing and irrigation procedure

Congenital nasolacrimal obstruction with risk factors for recurrence:

Age > 2 years

Associated with cleft palate or other facial anomaly

History of recurrent dacryocystitis or dacryocoele

Eyelid laceration with severed canaliculus

Canalicular or upper nasolacrimal system stenosis with epiphora

TABLE 94.2 *Preoperative Considerations for Intubation of the Nasolacrimal System in Children with Nasolacrimal Drainage Obstruction*

Severity of epiphora and other nasolacrimal obstruction symptoms

Prior history of nasolacrimal procedures, trauma, and infection

Associated craniofacial abnormalities including cleft palate, facial hypoplasia, Down syndrome, etc.

Patient age

Anesthetic risks

Site of expected or apparent obstruction within the nasolacrimal system

Parental and patient expectations

Surgical Anatomy of the Nasolacrimal System in Children

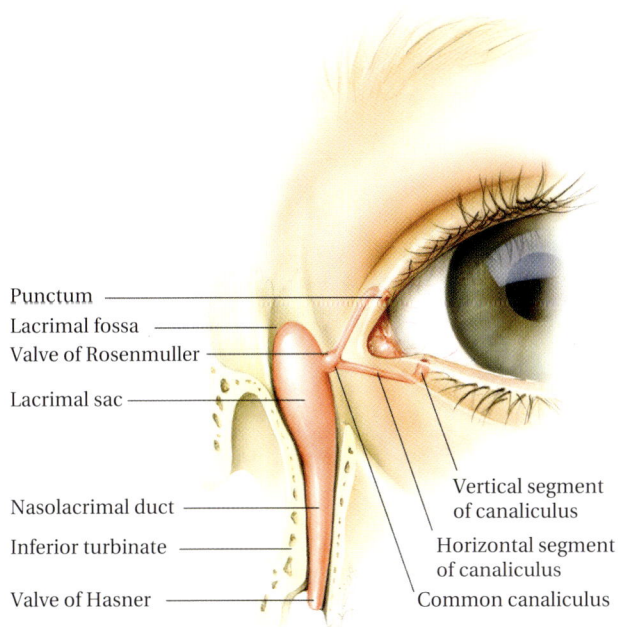

FIGURE 94.1 The upper and lower puncta open into the upper and lower canaliculi, which lead into a common canaliculus before entering the lacrimal sac. The nasolacrimal duct crosses into the bony nasolacrimal canal, passing between the maxilla and the ethmoid bones, into the nasal cavity where it opens into the inferior meatus beneath the inferior nasal turbinate. (From Katowitz JA ed, *Pediatric oculoplastic surgery*. New York: Springer-Verlag; 2002, p. 23. Reprinted with permission.)

Punctum
Lacrimal fossa
Valve of Rosenmuller
Lacrimal sac
Nasolacrimal duct
Inferior turbinate
Valve of Hasner
Vertical segment of canaliculus
Horizontal segment of canaliculus
Common canaliculus

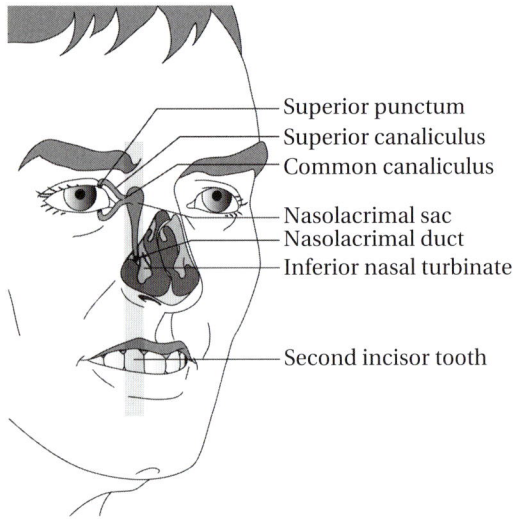

FIGURE 94.2 In a side view, the relationship of the nasolacrimal duct, the nasal floor (the upper surface of the palate) and the teeth can be seen. The trajectory of the nasolacrimal duct allows the teeth to serve as landmarks for probing, passing the probe downward in the direction of the second incisor. Instruments must be passed parallel to the palate under the inferior nasal turbinate, about 30–35 mm deep to the end of the nose, to retrieve nasolacrimal tubes.

Nasolacrimal Intubation Using the Ritleng System

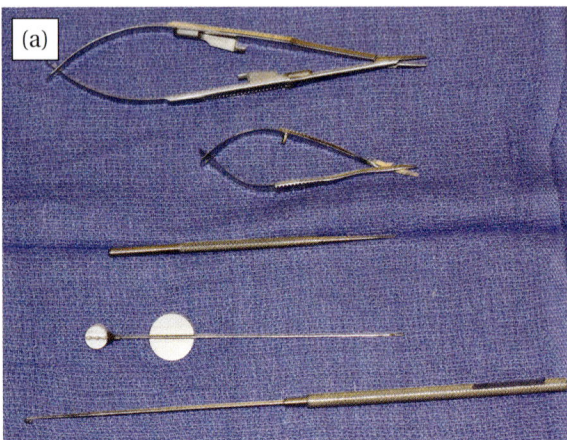

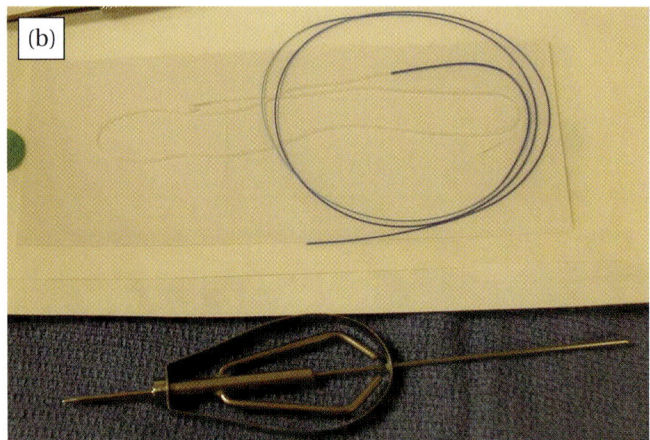

FIGURES 94.3 Surgical instrument set for nasolacrimal intubation using the Ritleng system. (a) Instruments include punctal dilator, Ritleng probe, Ritleng hook, Freer periosteal elevator, Van Ness scissors and needle holder. The Ritleng probe has a hollow shaft, and is designed to be used with intubation materials with flexible, stiff guide sutures attached to the silicone tubing. The Ritleng hook facilitates retrieval of the guide suture from the nose. (b) The self-threading monocanalicular stent (Monoka, FCI Ophthalmics) is designed with a polyethylene guide suture, to be used with the Ritleng probe. The self-retaining punctal footplate allows fixation without bicanalicular intubation or intranasal fixation. The inserter is shown below, which helps to seat the footplate into the punctum.

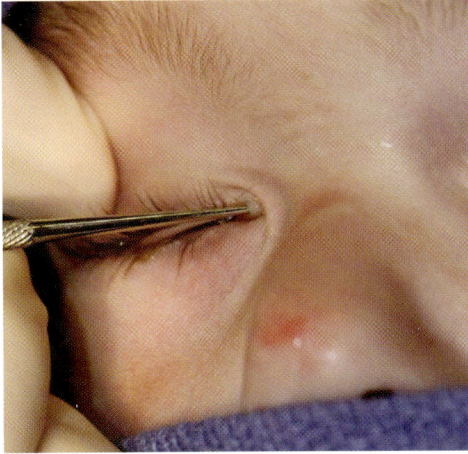

FIGURE 94.4 Punctal dilation. A punctal dilator is first passed vertically into the punctum for 2 mm then advanced horizontally until the punctum is dilated, with counter-traction on the eyelid.

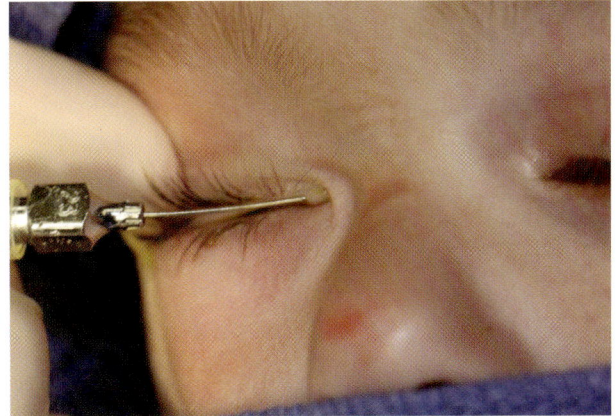

FIGURE 94.5 Probing of superior canaliculus and common canaliculus. Lateral traction manually is used on the upper eyelid to straighten the canaliculus. The Ritleng probe is first passed along the curvature of the upper canaliculus, then nasally into the lacrimal sac until a hard stop is felt.

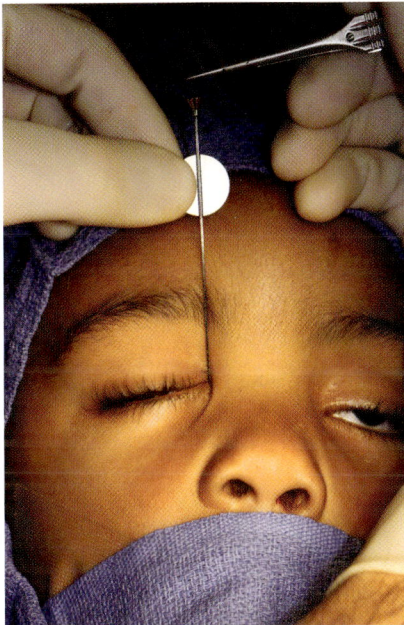

FIGURE 94.6 Probing of nasolacrimal sac and nasolacrimal duct and insertion of the Monoka stent. The Ritleng probe is rotated vertically, maintaining contact of the probe tip with the medial wall of the lacrimal sac. The probe is then advanced downward, using the second incisor tooth as a landmark, until the probe reaches the floor of the nose and stops. The Monoka monocanalicular stent guide suture is passed into the hollow Ritleng probe. Resistance may be encountered when the stiff guide suture reaches the end of the probe. Because of the stiffness of the guide suture, resistance may be felt when the suture end passes the end of the probe and contacts the floor of the nose. The suture can be advanced using a needle holder or other instrument until enough of the suture is in the nose that it will coil easily.

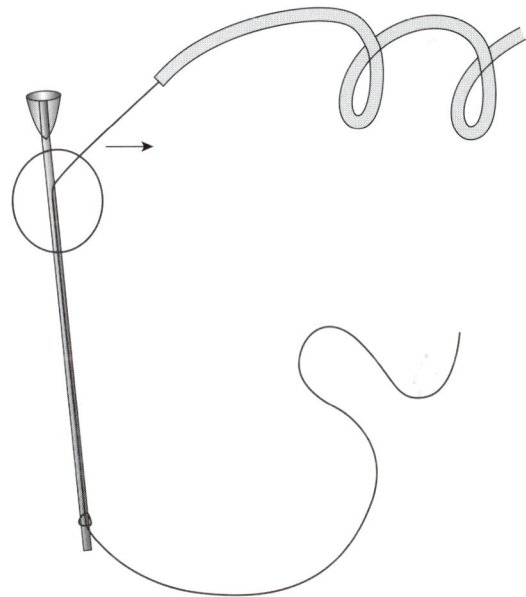

FIGURE 94.7 The suture is advanced until the lighter-colored, narrower segment is reached. The guide suture is then removed from the slot at the top of probe and the probe withdrawn from above, while stabilizing the guide suture from the nose.

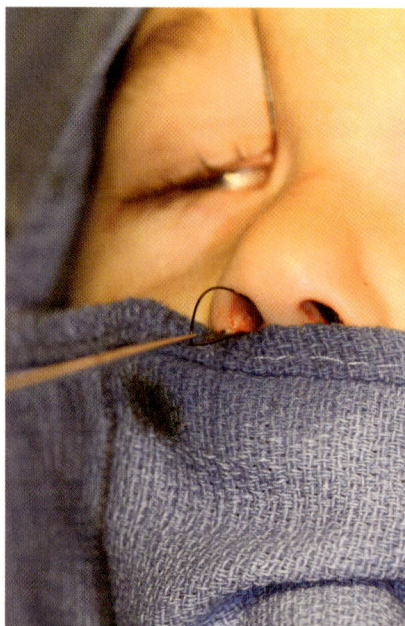

FIGURE 94.8 The suture is then used to pull the silicone tubing into the nasolacrimal system. After the silicone stent is visible outside the nose, the polypropylene suture is cut and removed from the tubing.

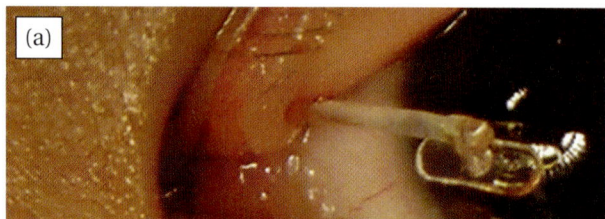

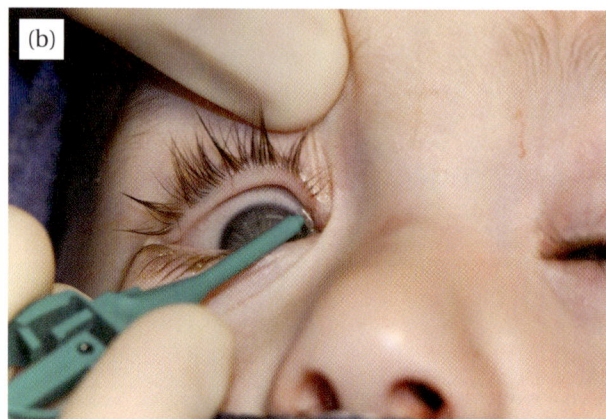

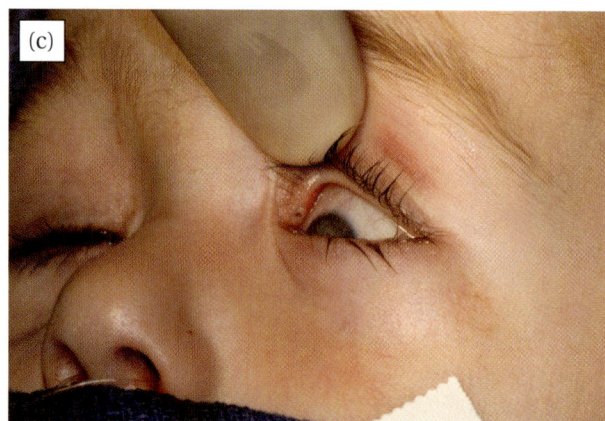

FIGURE 94.9 (a) The Monoka monocanalicular stent is in place in the upper canaliculus. (b) The Monoka punctal footplate is designed to fit tightly within the punctum and can be seated in the punctum using the special seating device, pressing and rotating the footplate into place before retracting the wire device. (c) The Monoka stent is now properly seated in the upper puncta. Intranasal fixation is not necessary, but the end of the stent is trimmed so as not to extrude from the nares.

TABLE 94.3 *Possible Complications of Probing and Irrigation of the Nasolacrimal System in Children*

Complication	Frequency	Associated Factors	Prevention and Treatment
Recurrent or persistent obstruction	uncommon	Chronic dacryocystitis Bony stenosis of nasolacrimal duct	Treatment of dacryocystitis with antibiotic Dacryocystorhinostomy
Nosebleed, damage or irritation of nasal mucosa	frequent	Inferior turbinate fracture	Atraumatic probing and tube retrieval Preoperative topical vasoconstriction (naphazoline, cocaine)
False passage with trauma to upper nasolacrimal system	uncommon	Inexperienced surgeon Upper system obstruction Lacrimal probe too fine	Careful probing with anatomic instrumentation 00-gauge probe or larger
False passage with trauma to nasolacrimal duct	uncommon	Inexperienced surgeon Anatomic anomaly	Intranasal exam with endoscope or speculum
Postoperative infection	rare	Chronic dacryocystitis	Topical ocular antibiotic
Enlargement/erosion of the punctum from stent (bicanalicular stent with excessive tension)	uncommon	Excessive tension on bicanalicular tube	Monocanalicular stent Loosen tension on stent
Migration/displacement of the tube	uncommon	Punctal plate too small or not seated properly Patient manipulation	Proper sizing of tube plate
Premature removal of tube	uncommon (monocanalicular)	Patient manipulation	Patient instructions
Retained tube	rare (monocanalicular)	Tube and footplate pulled past punctum into canaliculus or lacrimal sac Tube cut at proximal end	Remove monocanalicular tube from above

SELECTED REFERENCES

Engel JM, Hichie-Schmidt C, Khammar A, Ostfeld BM, Vyas A, Ticho BH. Monocanalicular silastic intubation for the initial correction of congenital nasolacrimal duct obstruction. *J AAPOS.* 2007;11:183–186.

Goldstein SM, Goldstein JB, Katowitz JA. Comparison of monocanalicular stenting and balloon dacryoplasty in secondary treatment of congenital nasolacrimal duct obstruction after failed primary probing. *Ophthal Plast Reconstr Surg.* 2004;20:352–357.

Lim CS, Martin F, Beckenham T, Cumming RG. Nasolacrimal duct obstruction in children: outcome of intubation. *J AAPOS.* 2004;8:466–472.

Repka MX, Melia BM, Beck RW, Atkinson CS, Chandler DL, Holmes JM, Khammar A, Morrison D, Quinn GE, Silbert DI, Ticho BH, Wallace KD, Weakley DR Jr., Pediatric Eye Disease Investigator Group. Primary treatment of nasolacrimal duct obstruction with nasolacrimal duct intubation in children younger than 4 years of age. *J AAPOS.* 2008;12:445–450.

95   Proximal Lacrimal System Surgery

Shubhra Goel, MD and Cat Nguyen Burkat, MD, FACS

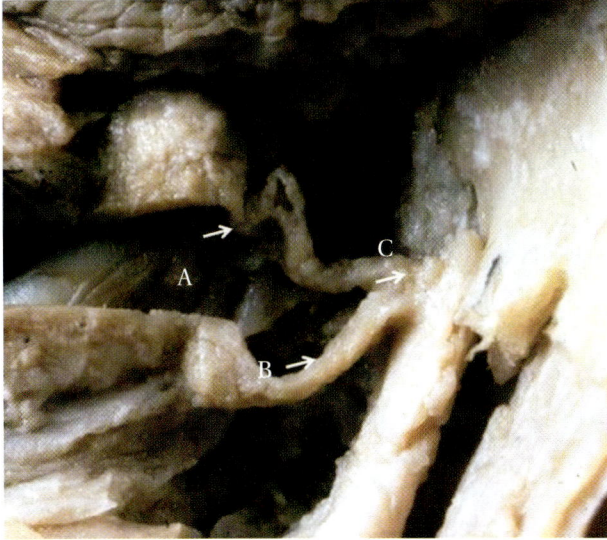

FIGURE 95.1 Cadaveric dissection illustrating the proximal lacrimal system anatomy. A: Upper punctum. B: Inferior canaliculus. C: Common canaliculus.

TABLE 95.1 *Indications for Surgery*

Punctal stenosis or occlusion
Punctal ectropion
Canalicular obstruction
Canaliculitis
Dry eyes (punctal occlusion)

TABLE 95.2 *Symptoms of Upper System Lacrimal Obstruction*

Epiphora
Irritation
Foreign body sensation
Mucus discharge
Mattering
Redness

TABLE 95.3 *Causes of Upper System Lacrimal Obstruction*

Allergic reactions
Blepharitis
Cicatrization secondary to burns, Stevens-Johnson syndrome, pemphigoid
Congenital
Canalicular tumors
Infections (Trachoma, herpes simplex and zoster, actinomyces)
Inflammations
Idiopathic
Involutional surface changes
Mechanical—kissing puncta, conjunctivochalasis
Medications (5-fluorouracil, docetaxel, idoxuridine, phospholine iodide, acyclovir, epinephrine)
Pyogenic granuloma
Punctal tumors (papilloma, nevi, skin tumors such as BCC)
Punctal ectropion
Postmenopausal hormonal changes
Radiation
Sjogren's syndrome
Trauma (iatrogenic and non-iatrogenic)

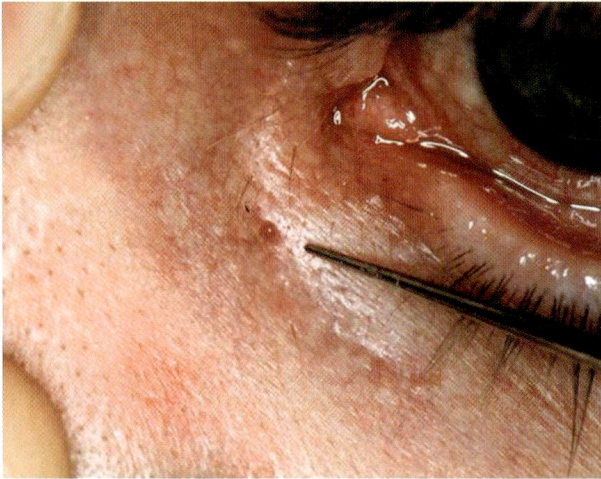

FIGURE 95.2 Photograph of patient with lacrimal anlage duct and supernumerary punctum in left lower eyelid.

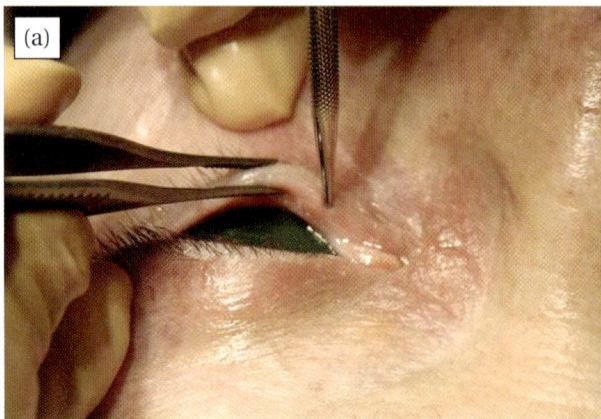

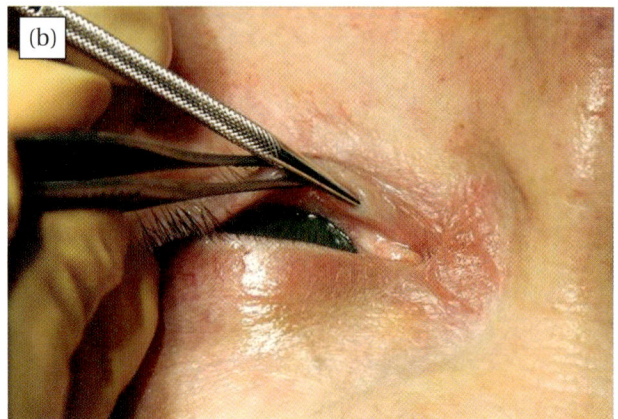

FIGURE 95.3 Punctal dilation. (a) The dilator is initially directed perpendicular to the eyelid margin. (b) With firm lateral traction on the eyelid, the dilator is advanced parallel to the eyelid margin in the direction of the canaliculus.

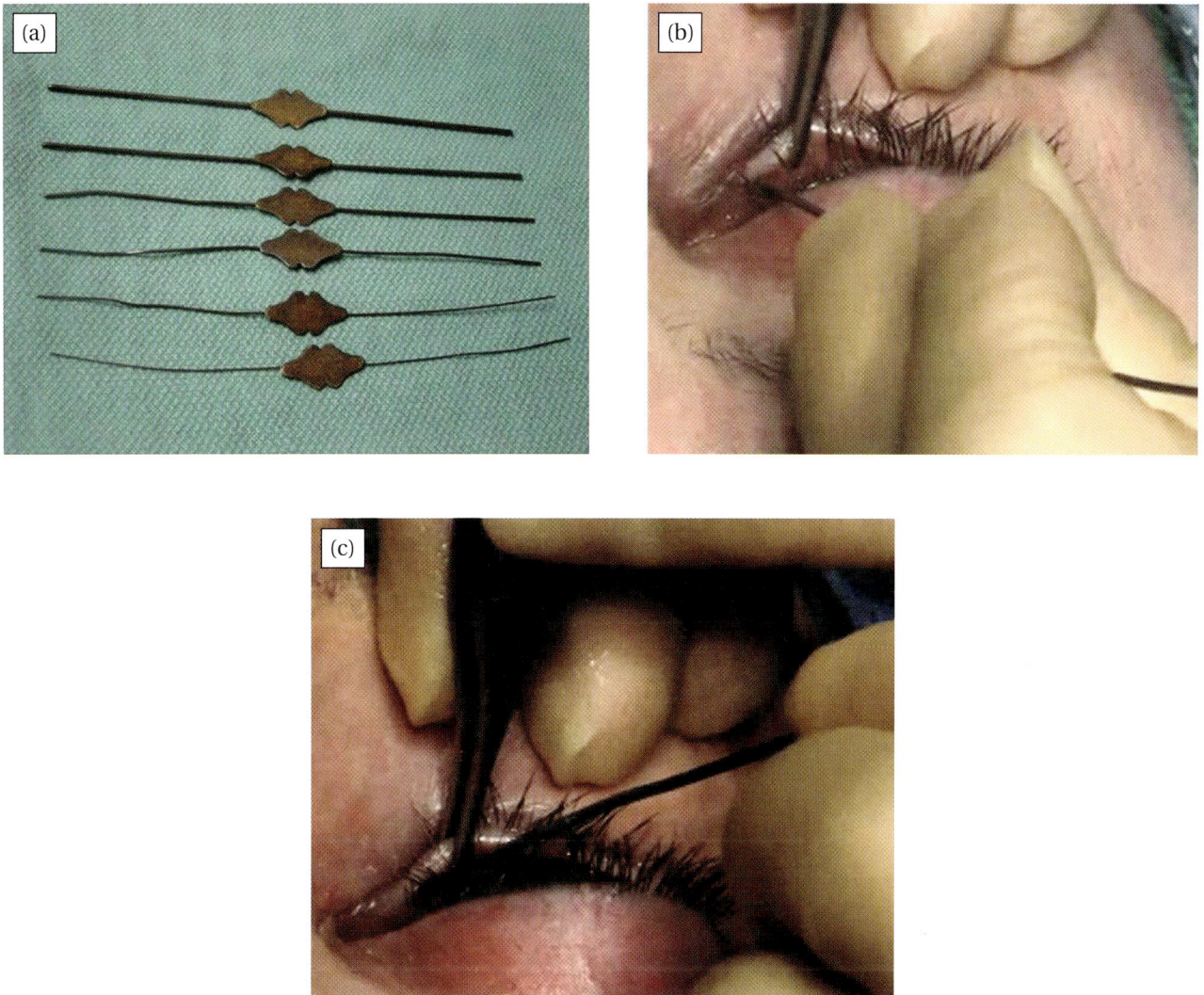

FIGURE 95.4 Probing of punctum and canaliculus. (a) Different sizes of Bowman lacrimal probes. (b) A Bowman lacrimal probe can be used to assess patency, with the probe being directed proximal perpendicular to the margin for the first 2 mm. (c) The horizontal canaliculus is next probed, while providing counter-traction to the eyelid to avoid creating a false passage. The location of any strictures is noted.

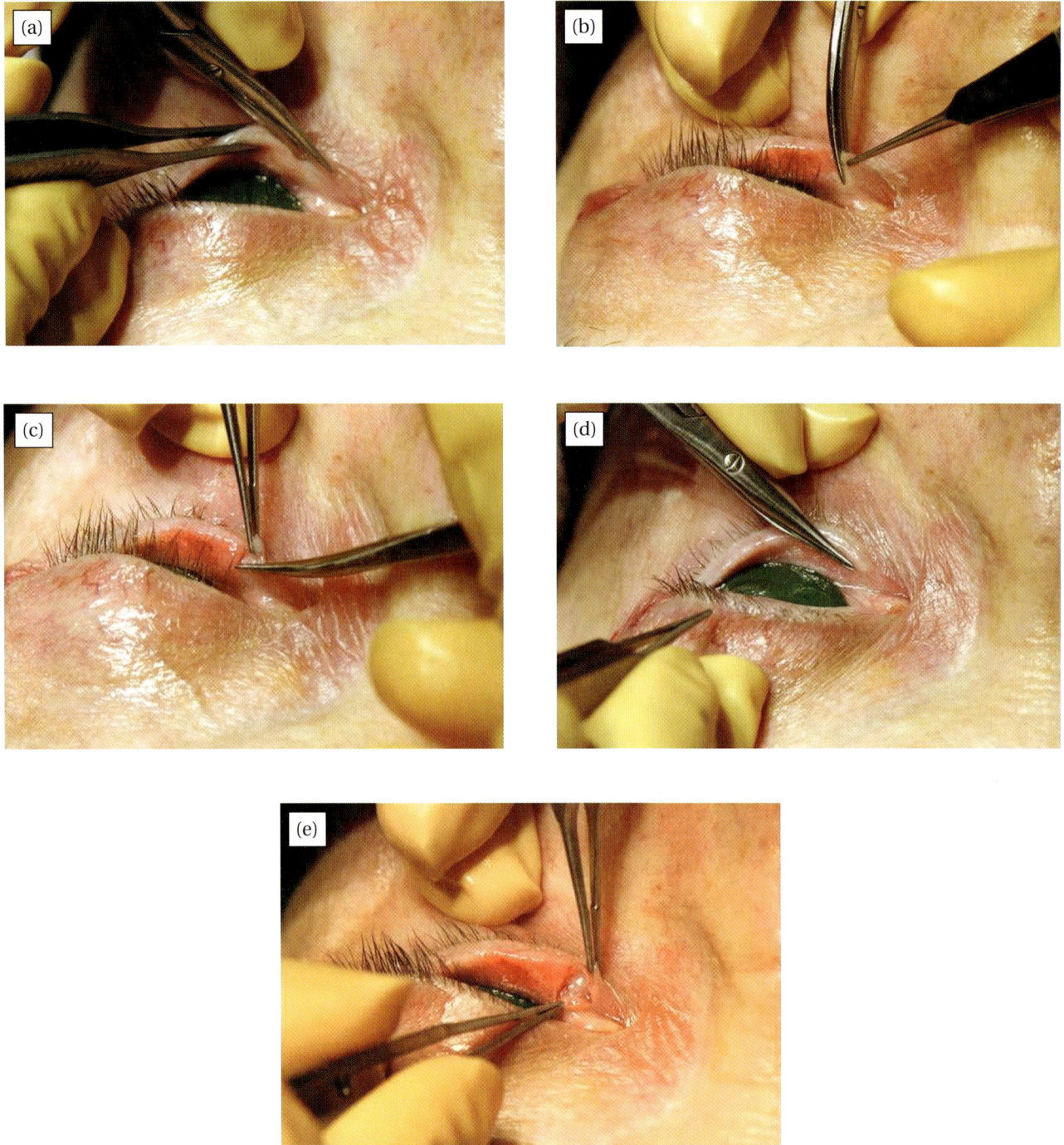

FIGURE 95.5 Three-snip punctoplasty. (a) The first snip is incised along the eyelid margin for approximately 2 mm medially from the punctum. (b) The second incision extends inferiorly through the ampulla, tarsus, and posterior conjunctiva. (c) The third snip connects the medial margin incision to the inferior extent of the second incision, to remove a triangular wedge of conjunctiva, tarsus, and posterior canaliculus to enlarge the punctum. (d) Closed scissor tips point to stenotic punctum prior to punctoplasty. (e) Enlarged punctal ostium and canalicular mucosa, visible following 3-snip punctoplasty.

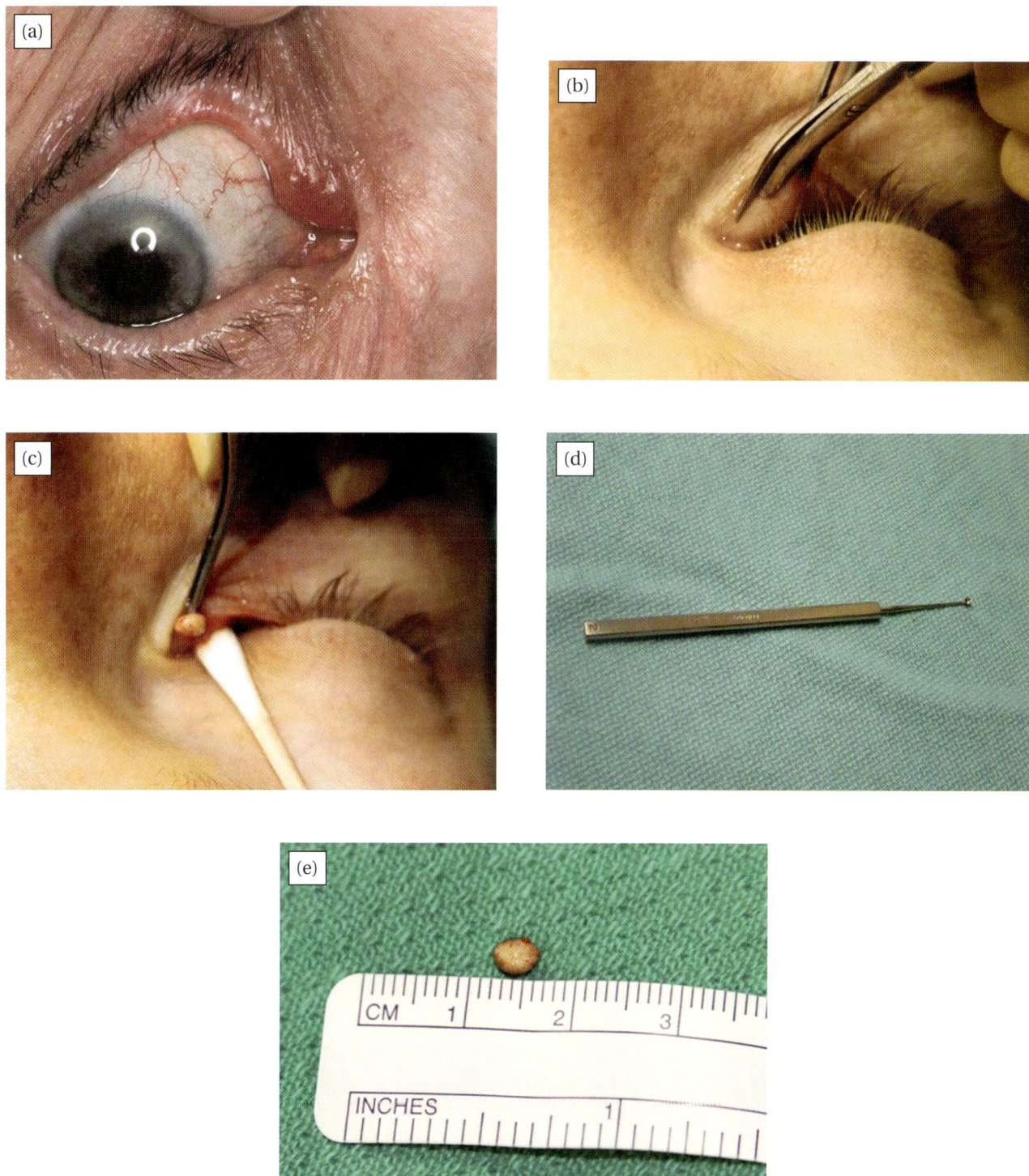

FIGURE 95.6 Canaliculotomy (a) Right upper lid canaliculitis demonstrating erythema and pouting punctum. (b) Canaliculotomy is performed by incising the eyelid margin and canaliculus medial to the punctum. (c) A dacryolith is expressed through the canaliculotomy. (d) A curette can be used to further remove any concretions. (e) Magnified view of the canalicular dacryolith.

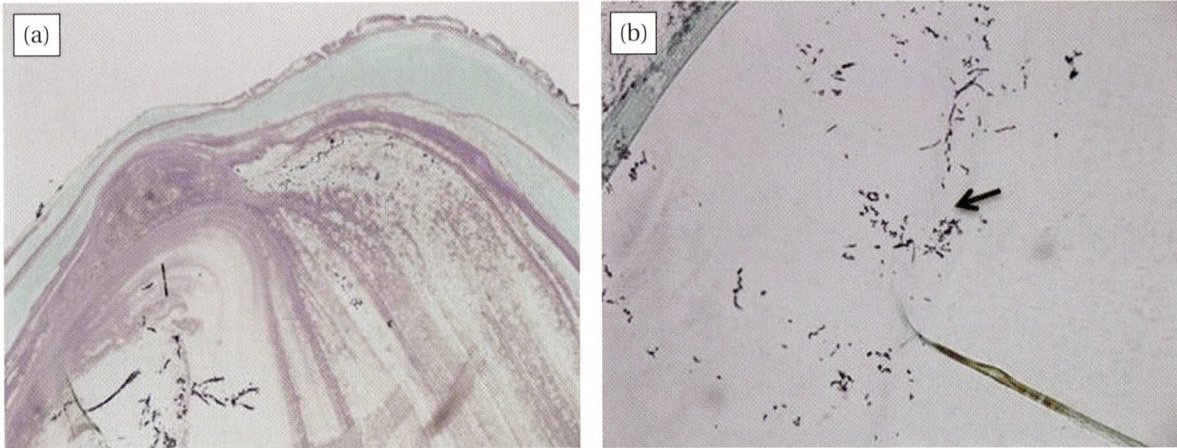

FIGURE 95.7   (a) Histopathology of the dacryolith demonstrating branching, filamentous Actinomyces israelii with Gomori methenamine silver stain (100×). (b) Arrow showing a higher magnification view (200×) of the hyphae.

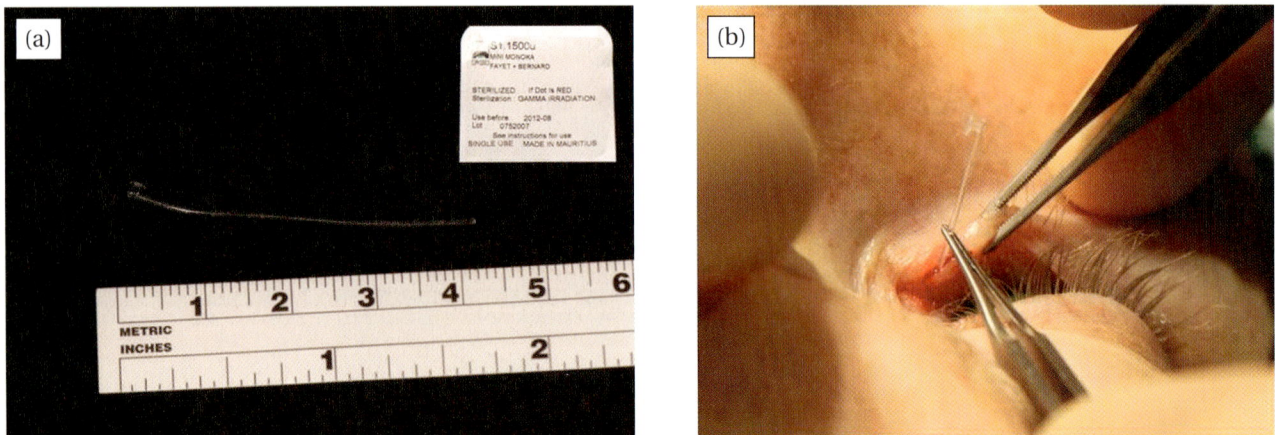

FIGURE 95.8   Monocanalicular intubation. (a) The mini-Monoka monocanalicular stent can be useful in cases of canaliculotomy, canalicular lacerations, or upper system lacrimal stenosis. (b) With lateral traction on the eyelid, a mini-Monoka stent is trimmed to the length of the canaliculus and inserted into position at the punctum.

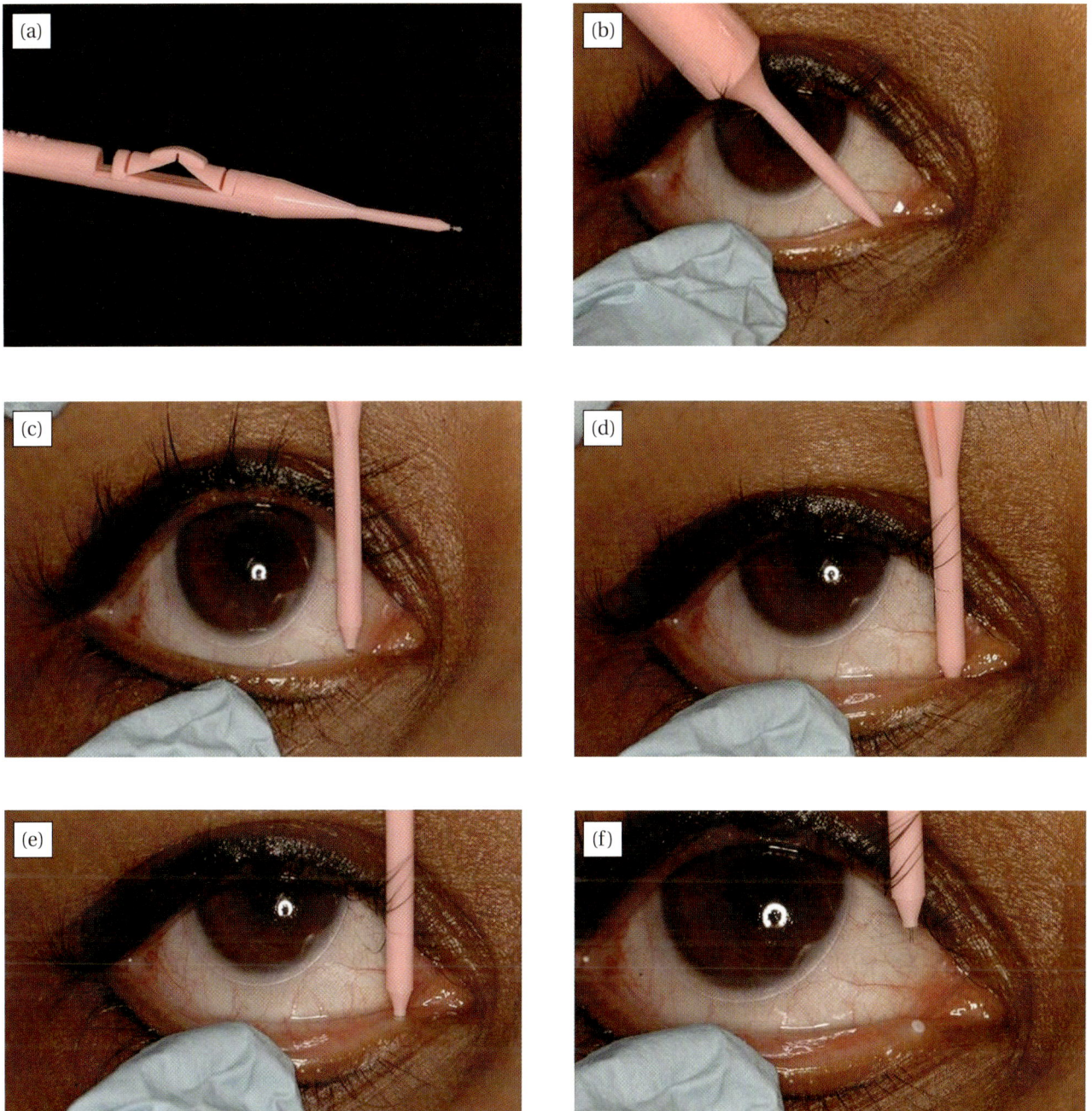

FIGURE 95.9 Punctal occlusion with a punctal plug. (a) Punctal plug on an inserter. These are commonly used for occluding the puncta in patients with symptomatic dry eyes. (b) The punctal dilator on the one end of the inserter can be used to dilate a stenotic punctum. Aggressive dilation that could result in the plug migrating into the canaliculus should be avoided. (c) The punctal plug is directed vertically through the punctal opening, while holding traction on the lid. (d) The punctal plug, including the flange, may occasionally snap completely into the ampulla. (e) The plug is retracted back until the flange rests above the punctum to avoid distal migration into the canaliculus. (f) The inserter is released and the punctal plug is in proper position.

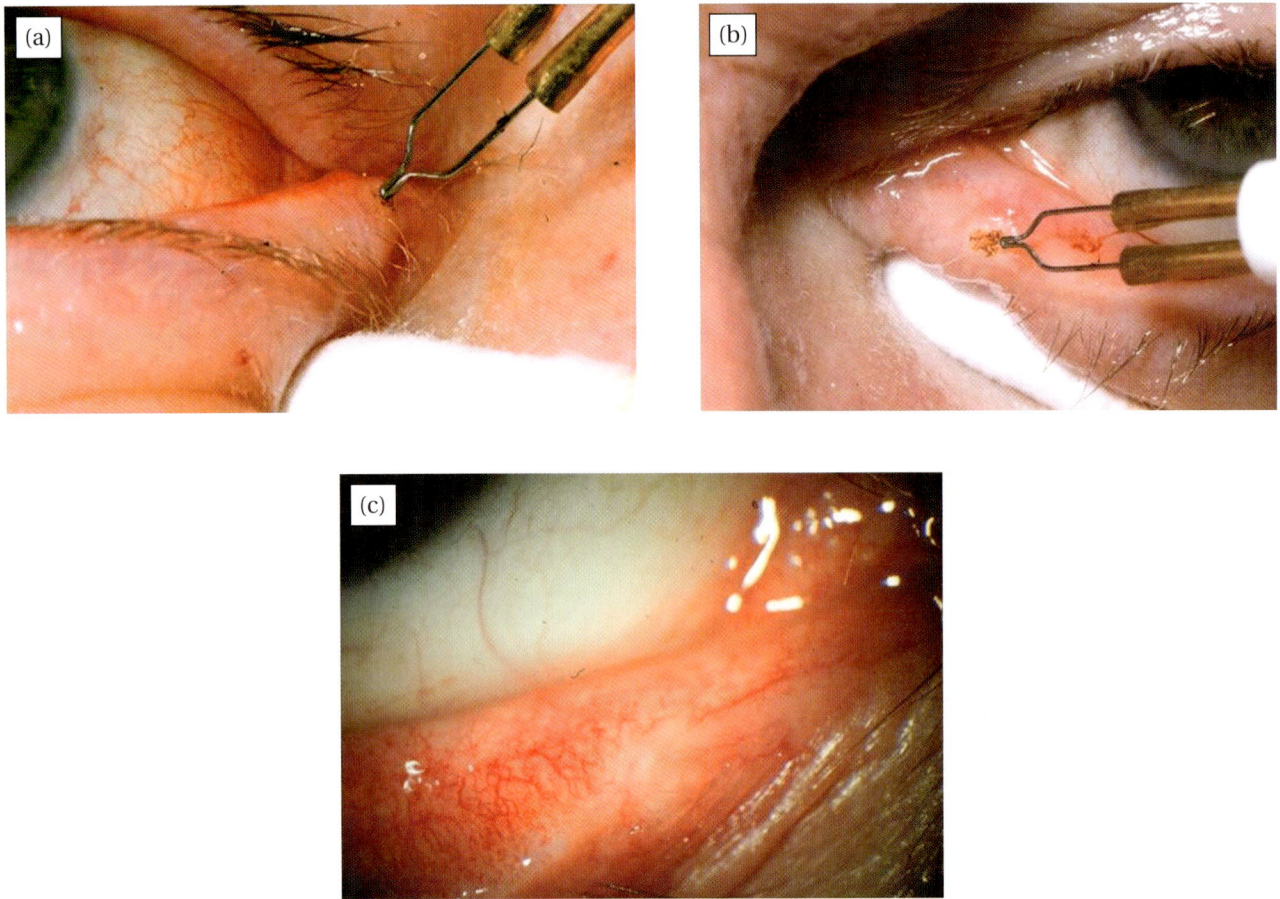

FIGURE 95.10 Punctal occlusion with thermal cautery. (a) Punctal occlusion with thermal cautery is performed for patients with severe symptomatic dry eyes, or those intolerant to punctal plugs. The punctal cautery tip is inserted into the punctum to cauterize the ampulla and punctum closed. (b) Occlusion of punctum following cautery. (c) Completely occluded punctum, right lower lid, 1 week following cauterization.

TABLE 95.4 *Potential Complications of Upper System Lacrimal Surgery*

Procedure	Potential Complications
Punctal dilatation, probing	False passage, canalicular injury, canalicular strictures if excessive manipulation
Three snip punctoplasty	Canalicular injury, larger opening at the puncta can lead to decreased sphincter action
Canaliculotomy	Injury to canaliculus, false passages, canalicular strictures if excessive manipulation
Punctal plugs	Punctal tear, migration of plugs, infection and granuloma formation, common canalicular obstruction due to migration

SELECTED REFERENCES

Bartley GB. Acquired lacrimal obstruction: an etiologic classification system, case report, and a review of literature. Part-3. *Ophthal Plast Reconstr Surg.* 1993;9:11–26.

Berlin AJ, Rath R, Rich L. Lacrimal system dacryoliths. *Ophthalmic Surg.* 1980;11:435–436.

Crawford JS. Intubation of the lacrimal system. *Ophthal Plast Reconstr Surg.* 1989;5:261–265.

Jones LT. The cure of epiphora due to canalicular disorders, trauma and surgical failures on the lacrimal passages. *Trans Am Acad Ophthalmol Otolaryngol.* 1962;66:506–524.

Latkany R. Dry eyes: etiology and management. *Curr Opin Ophthalmol.* 2008;19:287–291.

Liarakos VS, Boboridis KG, Mavrikakis E, Mavrikakis I. Management of canalicular obstructions. *Curr Opin Ophthalmol.* 2009;20:395–400.

Linberg JV, McCormick SA. Primary acquired nasolacrimal duct obstruction. A clinicopathologic report and biopsy technique. *Ophthalmology.*1986;93:1055–1063.

Paulsen FP, Thale AB, Maune S, Tillmann BN. New insights into the pathophysiology of primary acquired dacryostenosis. *Ophthalmology.* 2001;108:2329–2336.

Quickert MH, Dryden RM. Probes for intubation in lacrimal drainage. *Trans Am Acad Ophthalmol Otolaryngol.* 1970;74:431–433.

Repp DJ, Burkat CN, Lucarelli MJ. Lacrimal excretory system concretions: canalicular and lacrimal sac. *Ophthalmology.* 2009;116:2230–2235.

96

Eyelid and Canalicular Trauma

Cat Nguyen Burkat, MD, FACS, Karim G. Punja, MD, and
Nancy Kim, MD, PhD

TABLE 96.1 *Indications for Surgical Repair in Eyelid and Canalicular Trauma*

Full or partial thickness lacerating injury to the eyelids

Full or partial thickness laceration of the canaliculi

Avulsive injury to the medial or lateral canthal tendons

TABLE 96.2 *Preoperative Considerations*

Rule out any possible globe injury.

Perform careful wound exploration for orbital extension of the laceration and/or the presence of foreign bodies such as wood, which can be difficult to visualize on CT or MRI.

The goal is meticulous, layered, anatomic closure.

Avoid closing the orbital septum, to minimize the risk of retraction.

Avulsion of the lateral or medial canthal tendon (telecanthus) requires repair.

Exploration of Eyelid Wounds

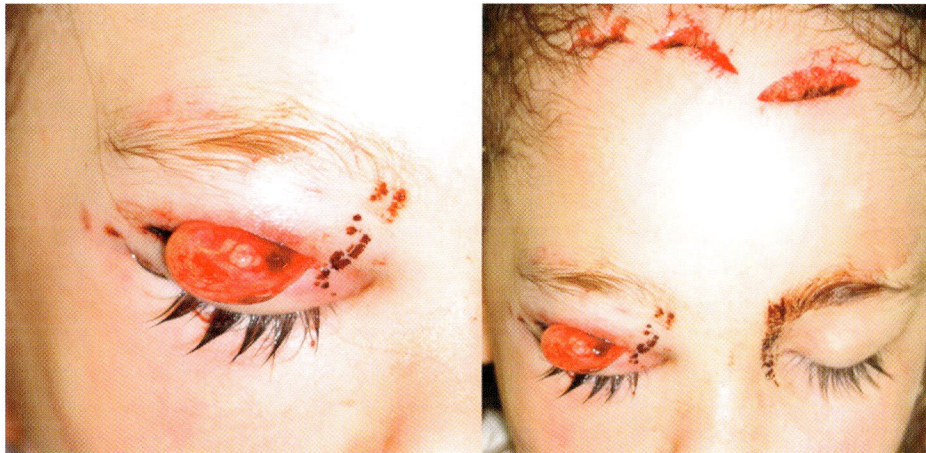

FIGURE 96.1 Orbital fat prolapse: This 5-year-old girl was bitten by a neighbor's dog. The presence of prolapsed orbital fat indicates violation of the orbital septum and possible injury to deeper structures. Exploration under anesthesia revealed an intact levator complex and no ocular injury. The laceration was closed anatomically by repositing viable fat, leaving orbital septum open, and reapproximating orbicularis muscle and skin with 7-0 polyglactin suture and 6-0 fast-absorbing plain gut suture, respectively.

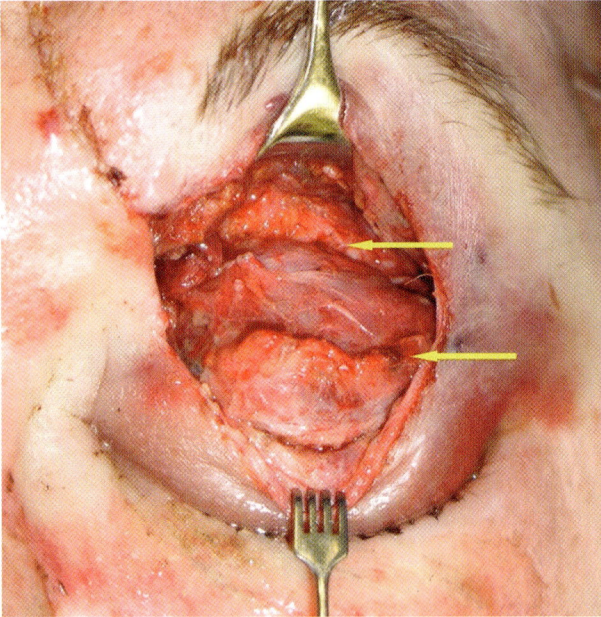

FIGURE 96.2 Levator muscle laceration: This 49-year-old female sustained extensive facial lacerations from a motorcycle accident, including a lacerated levator muscle in the left upper eyelid. Closure required identifying the split ends of the levator complex (yellow arrows) and re-approximating the ends with 6-0 prolene suture. The orbital septum was left open; the orbicularis muscle was closed with 6-0 polyglactin buried suture; and the skin edges were closed with 6-0 fast-absorbing plain gut suture.

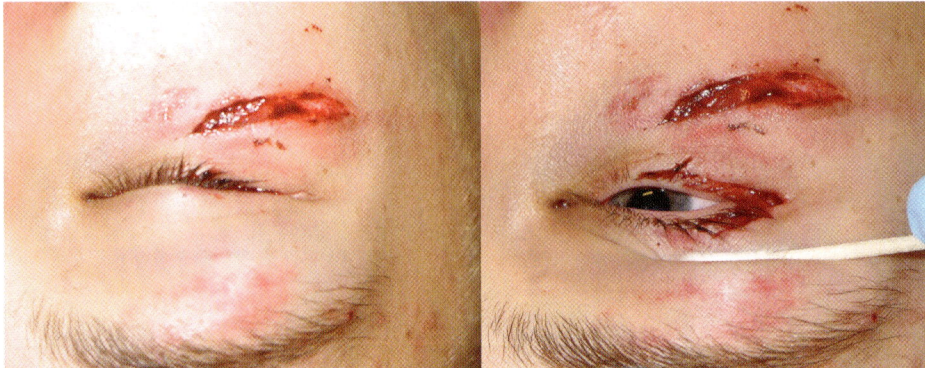

FIGURE 96.3 Careful preoperative exploration of a simple cheek laceration revealed an extensive right lateral canthal laceration with partial tendon avulsion that was not initially seen.

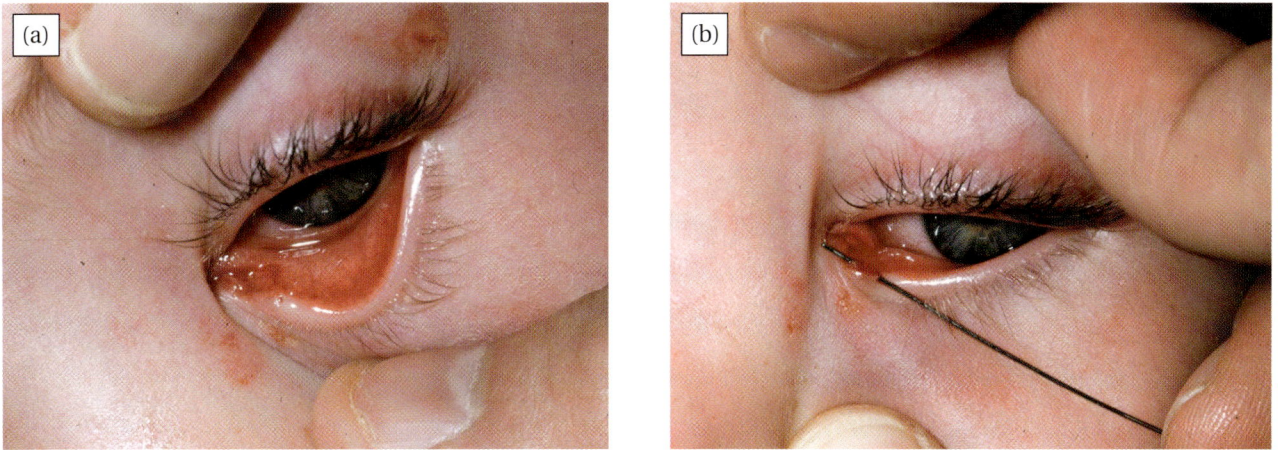

FIGURE 96.4 This 5-year-old boy fell and sustained trauma to the medial left lower eyelid (a). Evaluation of a medial eyelid laceration must include careful probing of the punctum, which may reveal the probe exiting through a torn canaliculus (b).

Overview of Common Eyelid Injuries and Repair

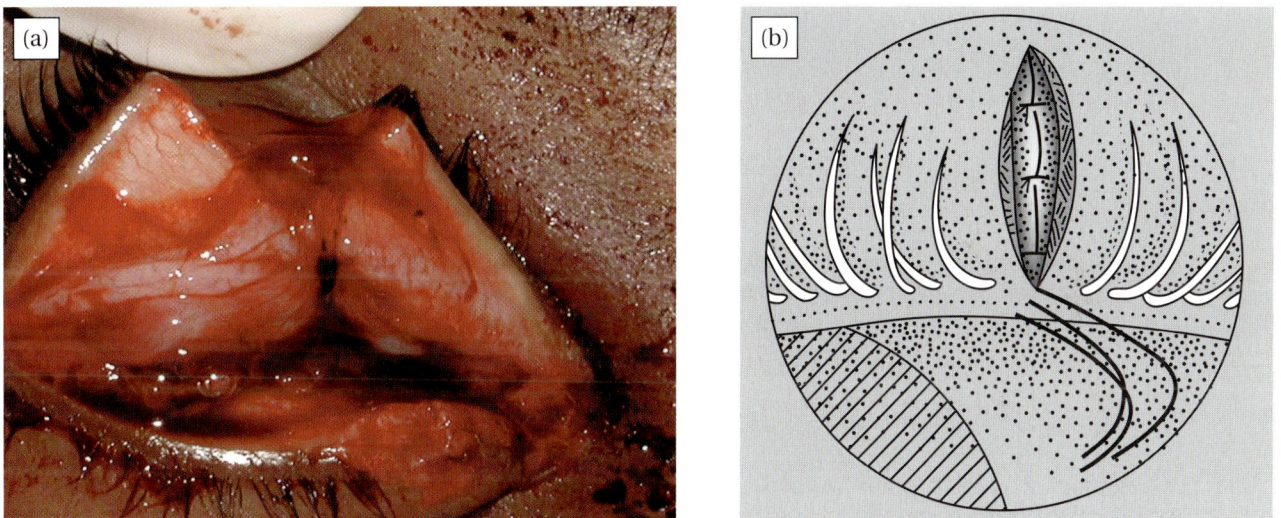

FIGURE 96.5 Lower eyelid full-thickness margin laceration (a). The eyelid margin is first closed at 3 sites with 6-0 silk suture along the lash line, posterior lid line, and gray line. The suture ends can be left long for superior traction to facilitate the rest of the closure. Tarsus is closed by placing 6-0 vicryl sutures in partial-thickness fashion along the height of the laceration. Placement of the suture closest to the eyelid margin is particularly important, as it imparts reinforcement to the marginal repair (b). The orbicularis muscle is closed with 6-0 polyglactin suture, followed by skin closure with 6-0 fast-absorbing gut suture. Finally, the marginal sutures are anchored to the eyelid skin away from the ocular surface.

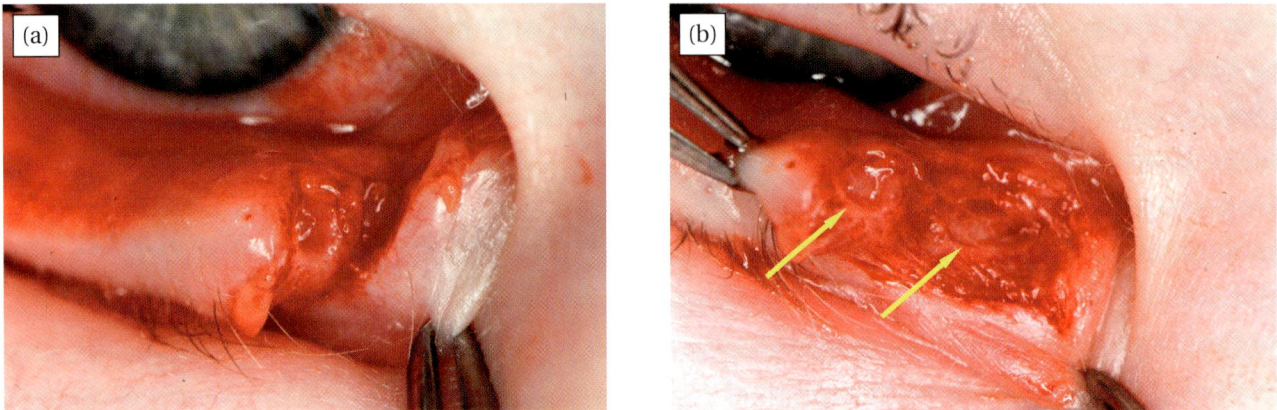

FIGURE 96.6 29-year-old patient with a right lower eyelid laceration involving full thickness margin and inferior canaliculus (a). Laceration held apart reveals the two ends (yellow arrows) of the canaliculus (b). Closure of the canalicular mucosa is necessary after placement of the silicone tube.

TABLE 96.3 *Steps for Canalicular Repair*

Repair within 24–48 hours of injury

Identify the cut ends of canaliculus (using cotton tips, irrigation through opposite punctum with fluorescein, pigtail probe)

Pass silicone stent through canalicular system

Re-approximate canaliculus

Re-establish medial canthal tendon support

Close eyelid margin

Close superficial tissues (orbicularis muscle, skin)

TABLE 96.4 *Options for Canalicular Intubation*

Bicanalicular + nasolacrimal duct intubation (Crawford stents, Quickert-Dryden stents)

Pigtail probe bicanalicular intubation

Monocanalicular intubation (mini-Monoka or long-Monoka stents)

TABLE 96.5 *Pigtail Probe Bicanalicular Intubation*

Advantages

General anesthesia not needed

Intubation of nasolacrimal duct not performed

Identifies the cut, proximal end of the canaliculus

Disadvantages

True common canaliculus required to avoid a false passage

Cannot use if lacerations of both upper and lower canaliculus are present

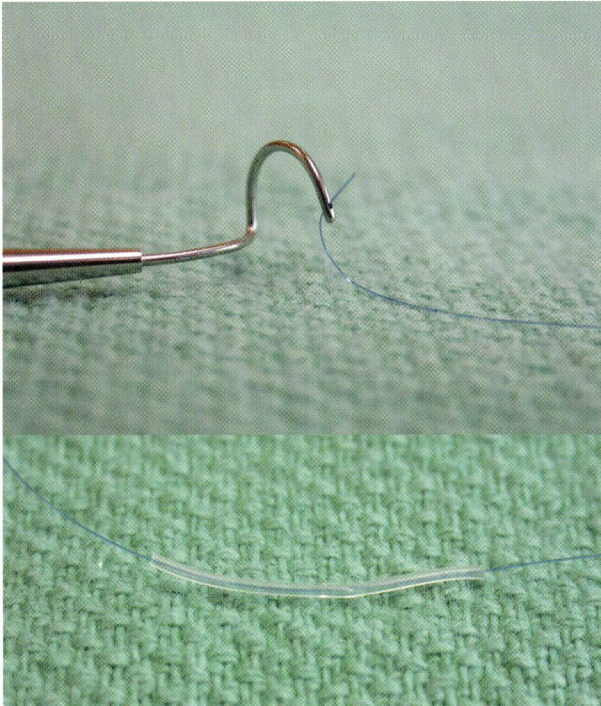

FIGURE 96.7 Pigtail probe bicanalicular intubation. Silicone tube segment is positioned at the medial canthus and within the canaliculi. Note the blunt, rather than sharp, tip of this pigtail probe.

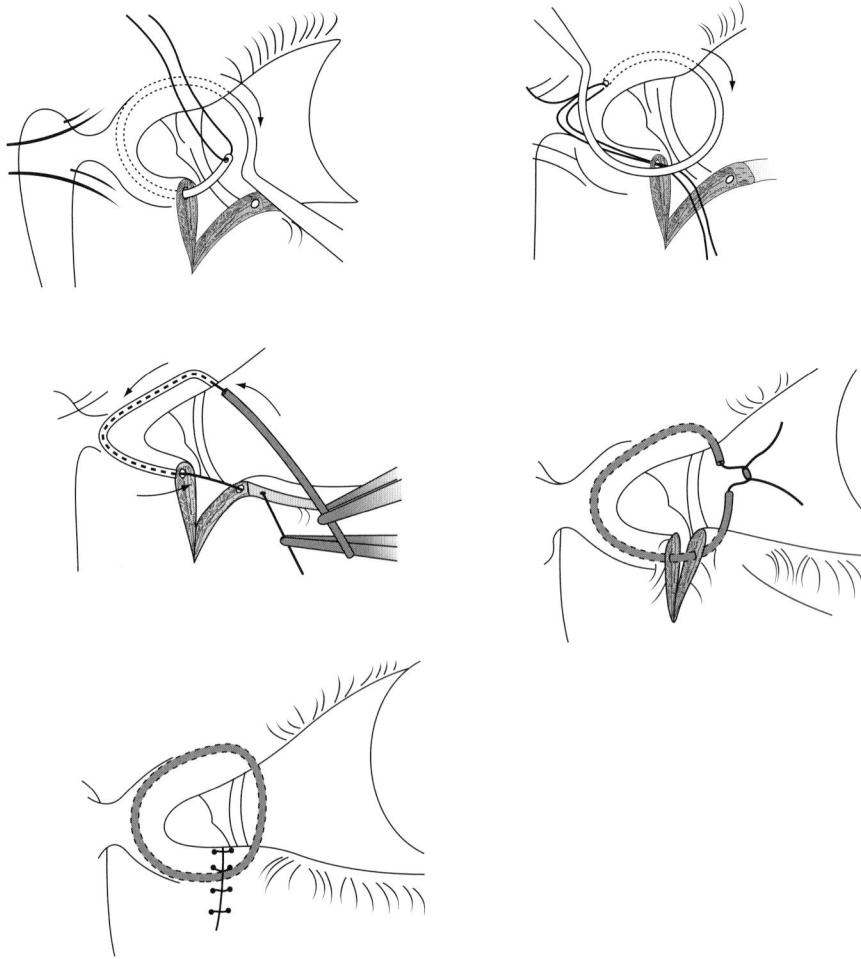

FIGURE 96.8 Schematic of stepwise bicanalicular intubation as part of a lower eyelid laceration repair corresponding to clinical photographs that follow.

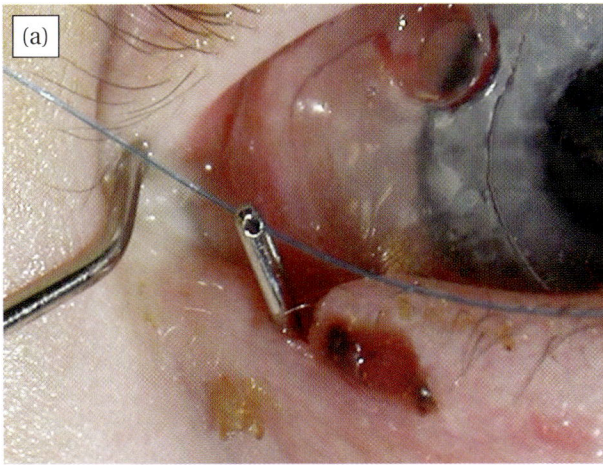

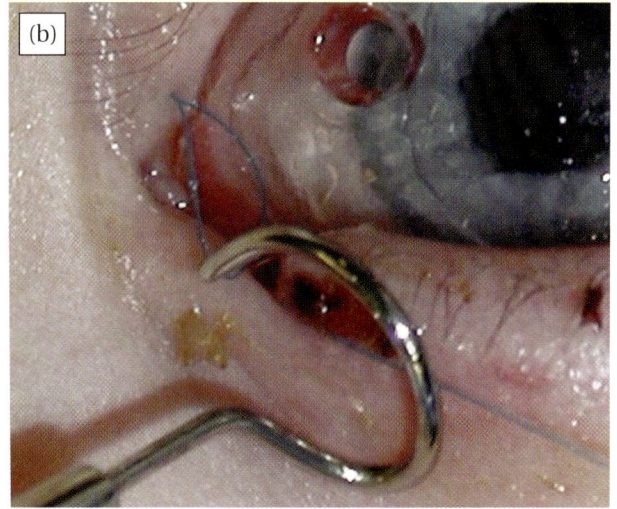

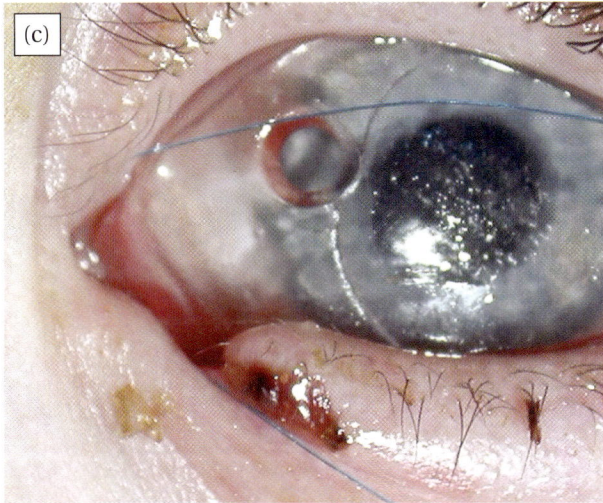

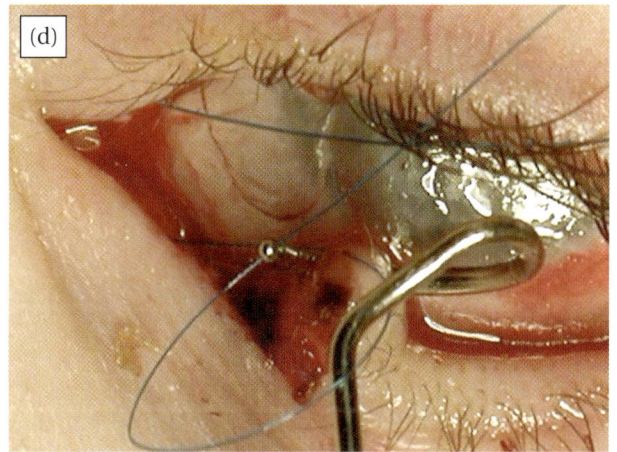

FIGURE 96.9 Clinical photographs of stepwise bicanalicular intubation as part of a left lower eyelid laceration repair in a 3-year-old boy with dog bite injury. The pigtail probe is inserted into the upper canaliculus and visualized through the proximal lacerated end. A 6-0 polypropylene suture is placed through the suture hole (a). The probe is then withdrawn through the upper lid with the polypropylene suture (b, c). The pigtail probe is then placed through the punctum and the distal lacerated edge (d) and retrieved (e). A silicone stent is then threaded over the polypropylene suture (f). The canalicular edges are then closed using 7-0 polyglactin at several sites. Medial canthal support is secured with 5-0 polyglactin suture if needed, followed by layered closure of the eyelid margin, orbicularis, and skin. The tube is tied and rotated to bury the knot away from the ocular surface (g).

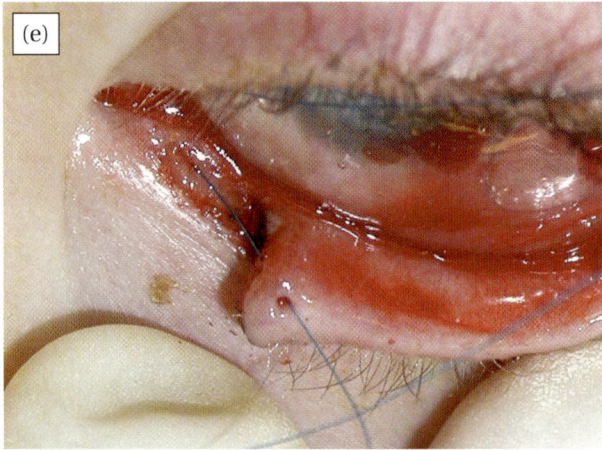

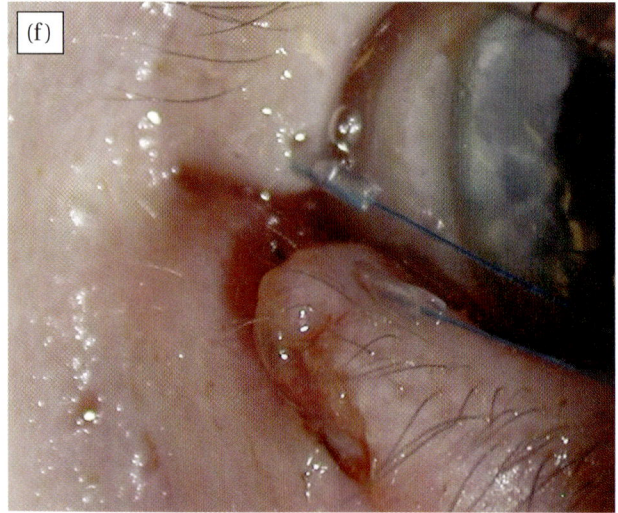

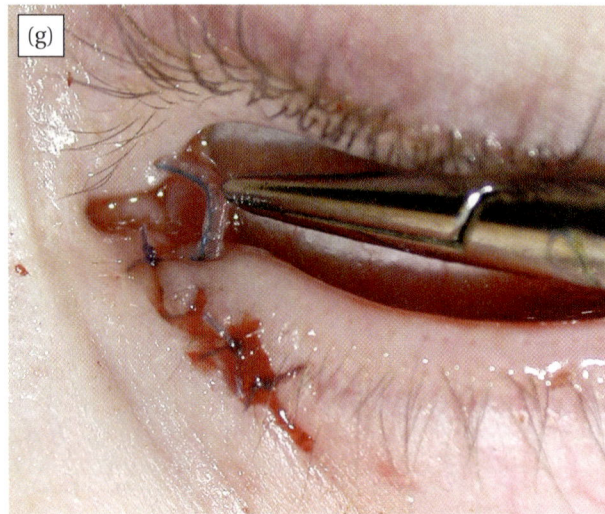

FIGURE 96.9 (*continued*)

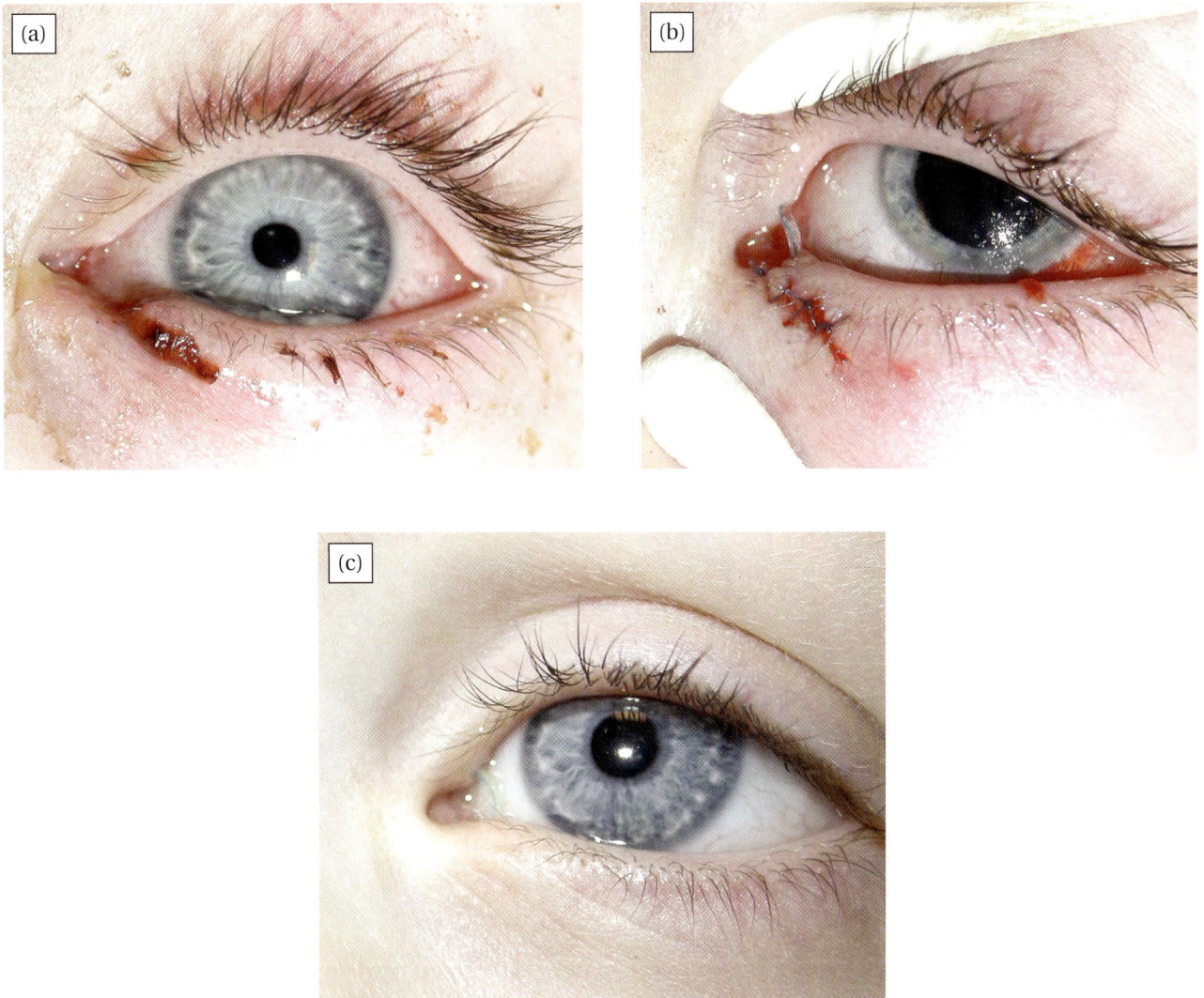

FIGURE 96.10 Pigtail probe intubation. (a) Before laceration repair. (b) Immediately after laceration repair and pigtail bicanalicular intubation. (c) Healed laceration with tube in place several months later.

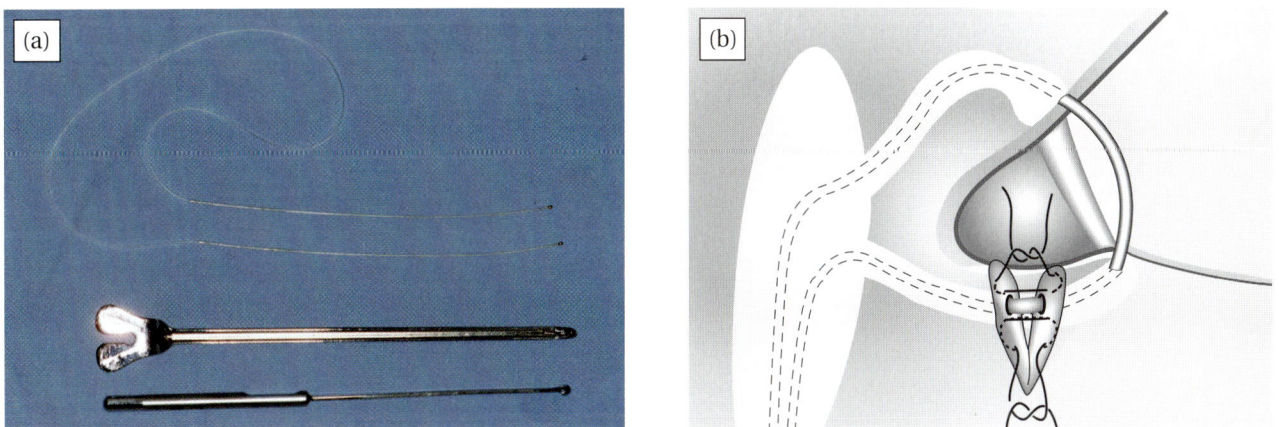

FIGURE 96.11 Bicanalicular intubation: Crawford or Quickert-Dryden stents are useful in both upper and lower canalicular lacerations (a). The nasolacrimal duct is also intubated; thus, this is typically difficult to perform under local anesthesia alone (b).

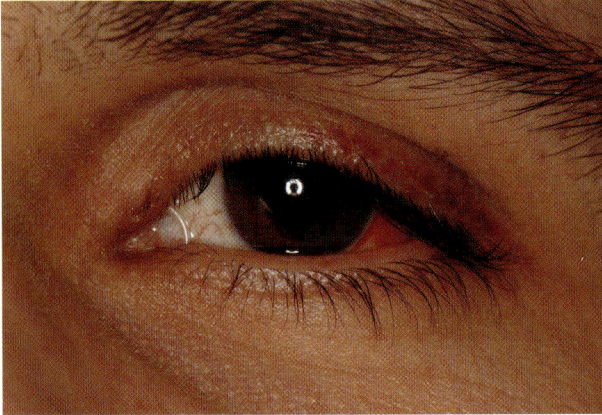

FIGURE 96.12 The bicanalicular silicone tube is left in place for 3–6 months after repair.

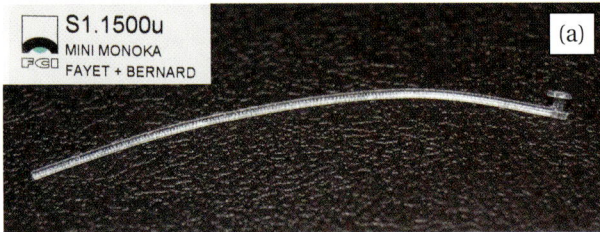

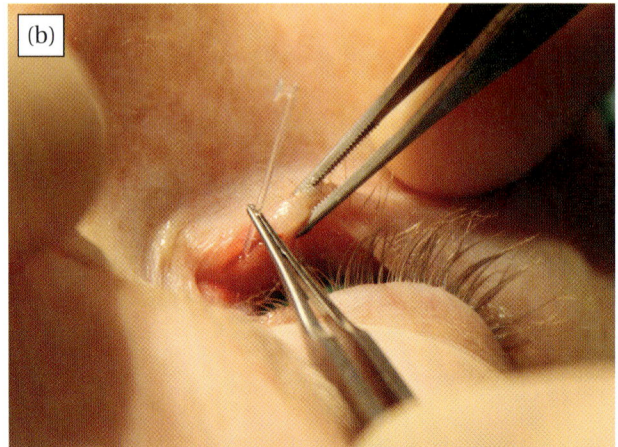

FIGURE 96.13 Monocanalicular intubation with a Mini-Monoka stent (a) can be easily performed in the office or emergency room under local anesthesia, and does not require intubation of the nasolacrimal duct (b).

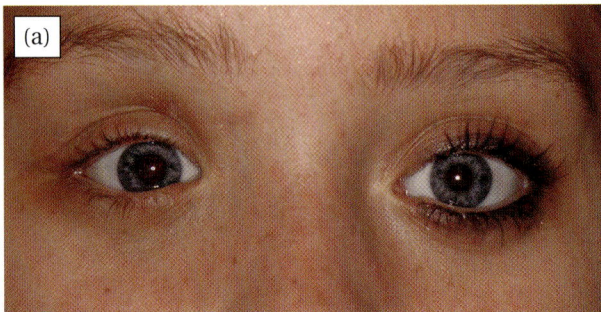

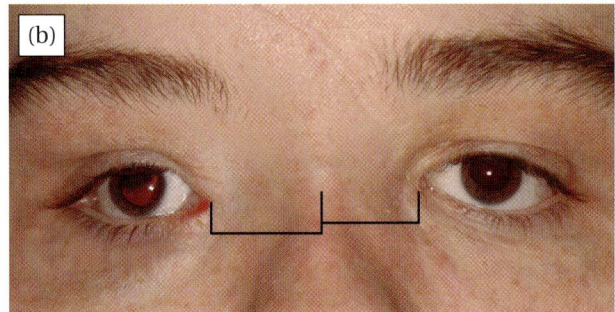

FIGURE 96.14 Traumatic telecanthus, or an abnormal widening of the distance between the medial canthi of both eyes (a, b) should be evaluated for with any medial orbital trauma and repaired primarily with plating or transnasal wiring.

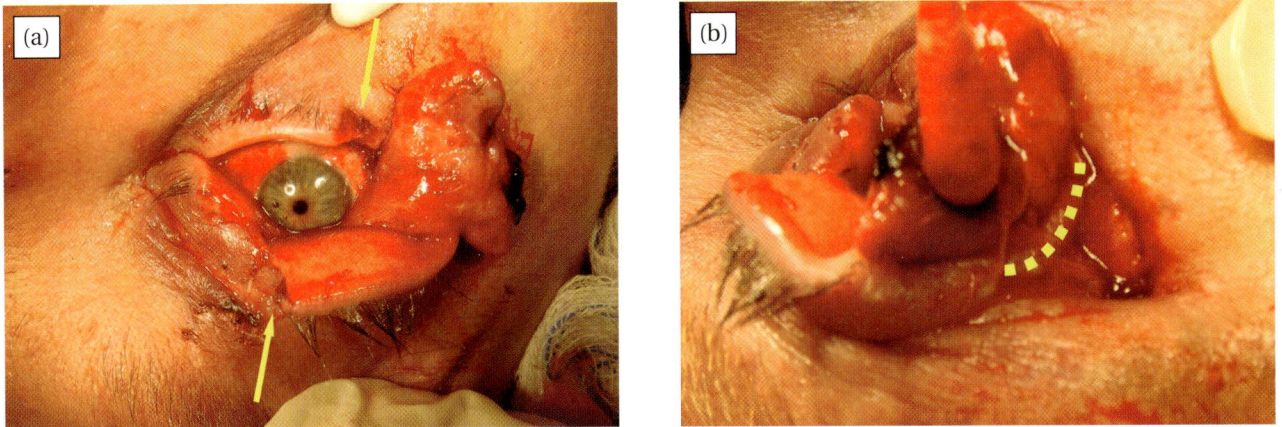

FIGURE 96.15 This patient had multiple lacerations including full thickness margin lacerations of the right upper and lower eyelids (a; yellow arrows), avulsion of the lateral canthal tendon and adjacent soft tissues, with extension into the lateral fornix. The lateral canthal tendon of both the upper and lower eyelid was completely dehisced from the orbital rim (b; dotted yellow line).

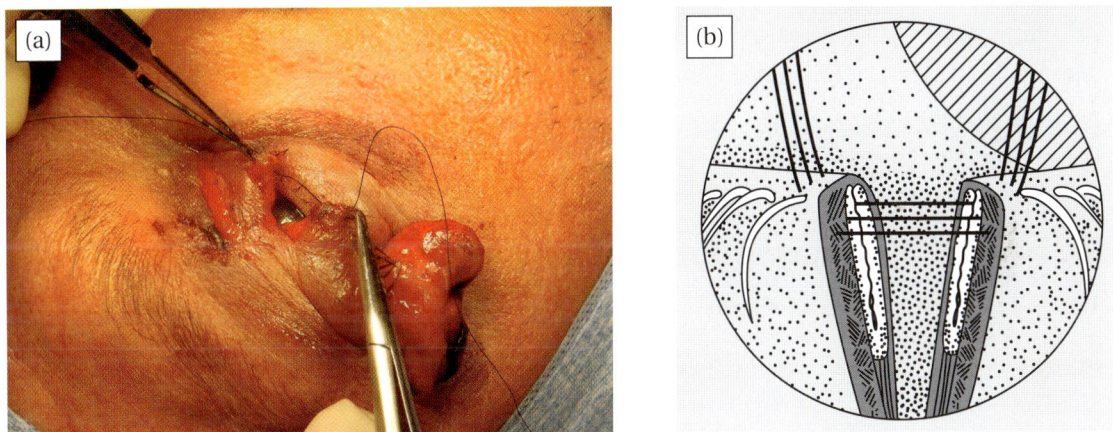

FIGURE 96.16 Repair of the right upper eyelid margin laceration was performed first, using a 3-suture technique with 6-0 silk (a). The first suture is passed through the posterior mucocutaneous margin along the meibomian glands. The second is passed anteriorly at the lash line. The third suture is passed between the first two, along the gray line. Note that the suture tails are left long to exert gentle traction on the lid to facilitate proper alignment and closure of the tarsus (b).

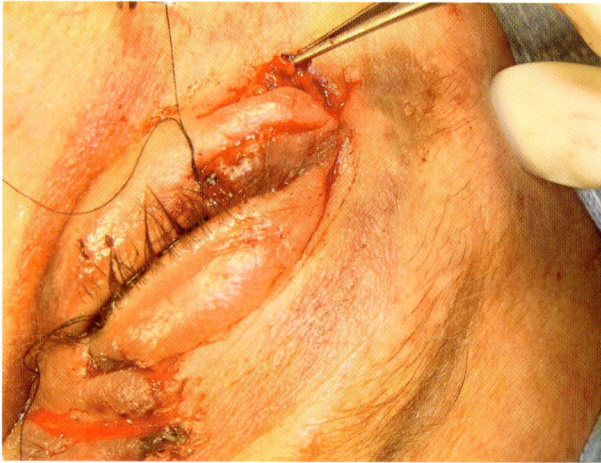

FIGURE 96.17 Following repair of the upper and lower marginal lacerations, the lateral canthal laceration was repaired by resuspension of the tendons to the lateral orbital periosteum with 5-0 suture and a lateral canthoplasty. Once eyelid support was restored, the orbicularis and skin were closed in layers.

TABLE 96.6 *Potential Complications of Surgical Repair of Eyelid Trauma*

Lid retraction (from anterior lamellar shortening or closure of orbital septum)

Notching of the lid margin

Corneal irritation from posterior marginal sutures (resolves with suture removal, ointment use, or placement of a bandage contact lens)

Lagophthalmos

Lid malposition

Lacrimal drainage system obstruction

Facial nerve damage

Sensory nerve damage (hypesthesia)

Tissue bunching (typically resolves with time)

Trichiasis

Cutaneous scarring

SELECTED REFERENCES

Burroughs JR, Soparkar CNS, Patrinely JR, Williams PD, Holck DEE. Periocular Dog Bite Injuries and Responsible Care. *Ophthal Plast Reconstr Surg.* 2002;18:416–419.

Hawes MJ, Dortzbach RK. Trauma of the lacrimal drainage system. In: Linberg J, ed. *Lacrimal Surgery.* New York: Churchill Livingstone; 1988, pp. 241–262.

Hawes MJ, Segrest DR. Effectiveness of bicanalicular silicone intubation in the repair of canalicular lacerations. *Ophthal Plast Reconstr Surg.* 1985;1(3):185–190.

Ho T, Lee V. National survey on the management of lacrimal canalicular injury in the United Kingdom. *Clin Experiment Ophthalmol.* 2006;34(1):39–43.

Jordan DR, Nerad JA, Tse DT. The pigtail probe, revisited. *Ophthalmology.* 1990;97(4):512–519.

Quickert MH, Dryden RM: Probes for intubation in lacrimal drainage. *Trans Am Acad Ophthalmol Otolaryngol.* 1970;74:431–433.

97

Balloon Dacryoplasty

Morris E. Hartstein, MD, FACS and Yair Morad, MD

TABLE 97.1 *Indications for Balloon Dacryoplasty*

Pediatric
- Primary congenital nasolacrimal duct obstruction
- Recurrent nasolacrimal duct obstruction

Adult
- Partial nasolacrimal duct obstruction
- Primary or failed dacryocystorhinostomy

TABLE 97.2 *Preoperative Considerations*

- Balloon catheter dacryoplasty (Quest Medical, Inc, Allen, TX) may be useful in pediatric cases of recurrent nasolacrimal duct obstruction, even after failed probing and failed silicone intubation.
- Balloon dacryoplasty may also be considered in primary cases of nasolacrimal obstruction.
- In children less than 30 months old, the 2 mm balloon is used. The 3 mm balloon is used in patients over the age of 30 months.
- Balloon dacryoplasty has been found to be useful in adults with partial obstruction (approximately <50% reflux through nose on irrigation).
- For failed dacryocystorhinostomy, a 5 mm balloon can be used with dilation occurring through the bony ostium and lacrimal sac.
- It is preferable to pass the balloon through the upper canaliculus in order to preserve the integrity of the lower canaliculus.
- Many surgeons prefer to use the balloon catheter in combination with silicone intubation.
- A key component of the procedure may be a preoperative and postoperative regimen of oral and topical antibiotics and steroids.
- An endoscope is not necessary for the procedure; however, one can be used to visualize the balloon beneath the inferior turbinate.

Surgical Series of Balloon Dacryoplasty

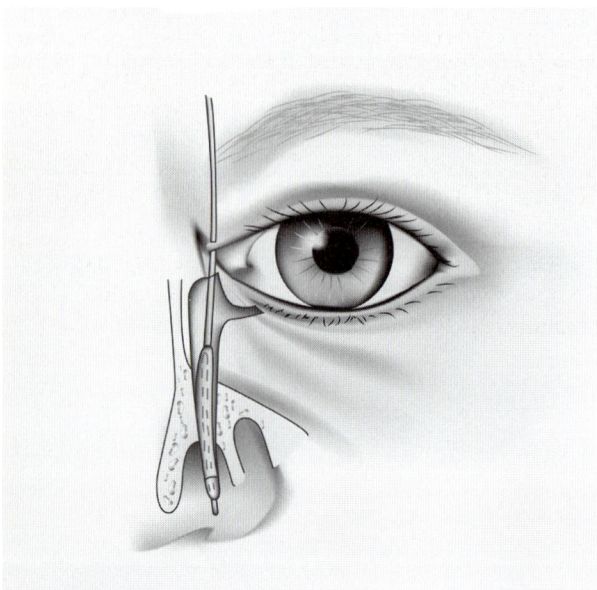

FIGURE 97.1 Diagram demonstrating proper positioning of inflated balloon in nasolacrimal duct. (Reprinted with permission from Quest Medical, Inc.)

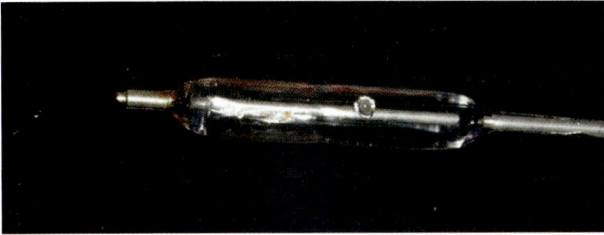

FIGURE 97.2 The balloon inflated.

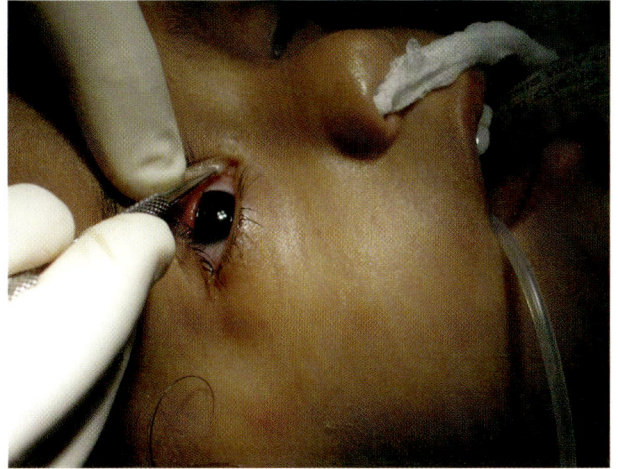

FIGURE 97.3 A punctal dilator is used to dilate the superior punctum.

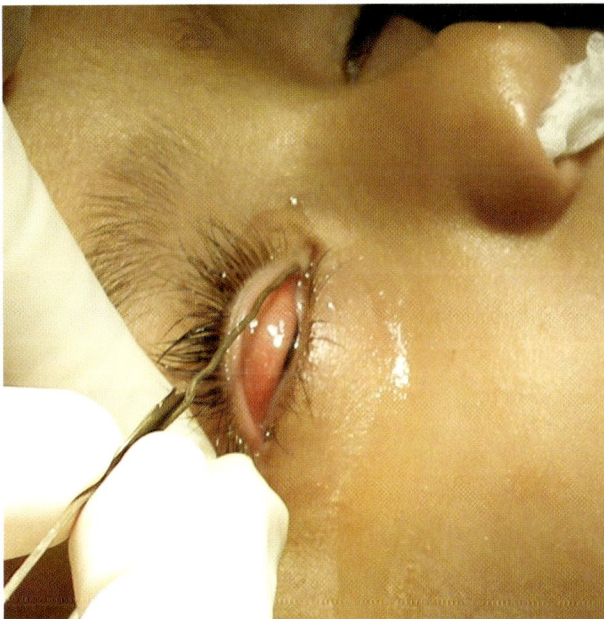

FIGURE 97.4 A standard Bowman probe is advanced into the punctum and canaliculus until a hard stop is encountered.

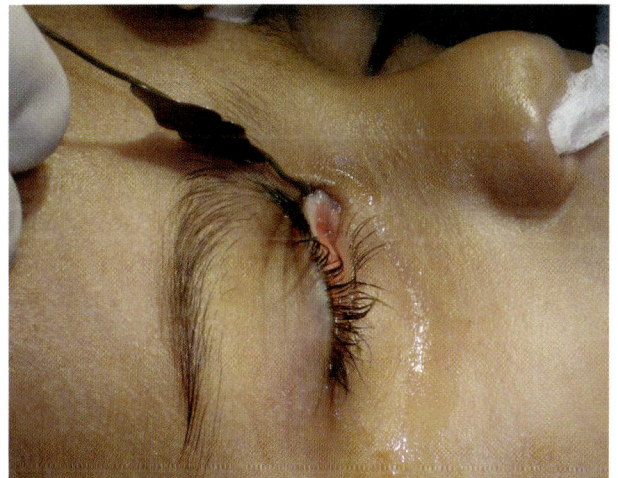

FIGURE 97.5 While maintaining pressure against the bone, the probe is rotated inferiorly into the nasolacrimal duct.

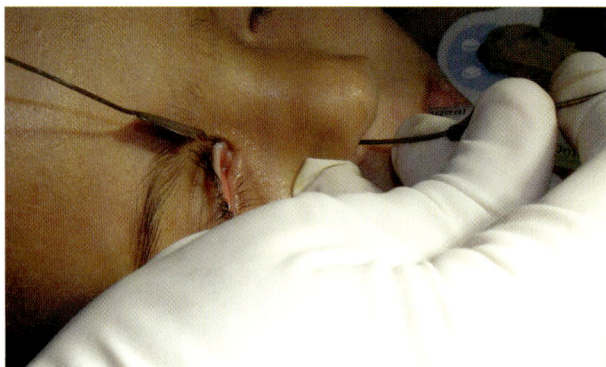

FIGURE 97.6 A second probe is used to confirm proper positioning of the probe under the inferior turbinate by metal-on-metal contact. If there is any doubt, the probe should be withdrawn and passed again.

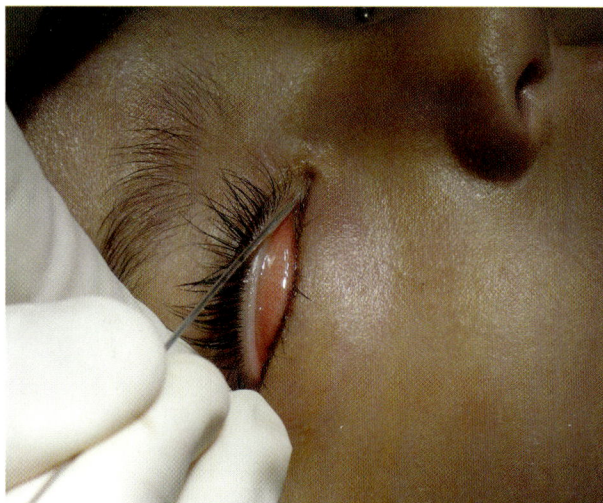

FIGURE 97.7 The plastic covering is removed from the balloon, and the balloon catheter is passed in similar fashion to the probe. The balloon is not inflated prior to insertion, as it will never return to the preinflation profile. The balloon catheter is more flexible than a probe, and can be slightly more difficult to pass. Metal-on-metal contact is again used to confirm the proper position of the balloon catheter in the nose.

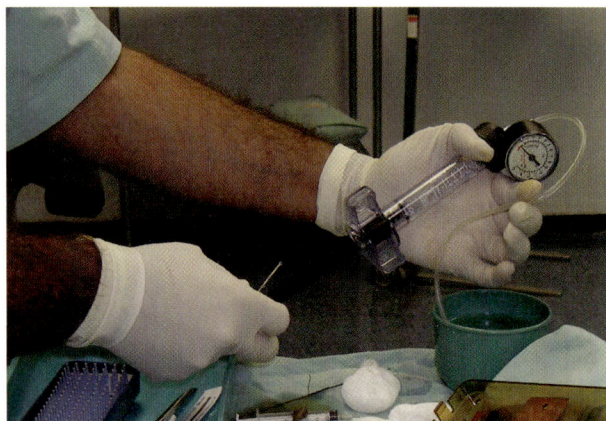

FIGURE 97.8 The pump is primed by filling it with 10 cc of saline and then locking the pump.

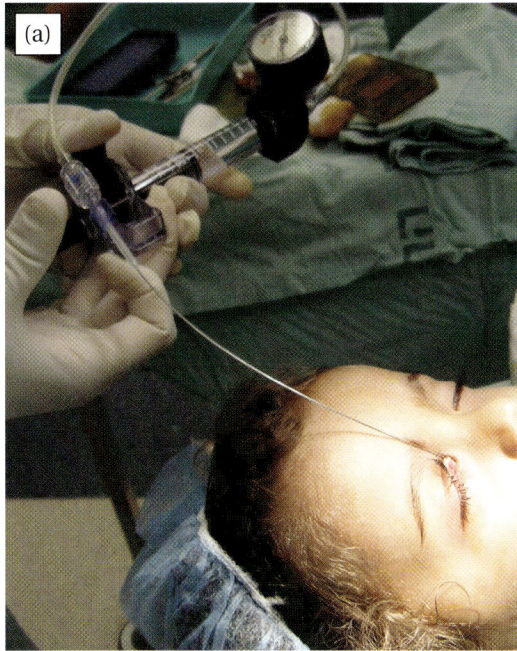

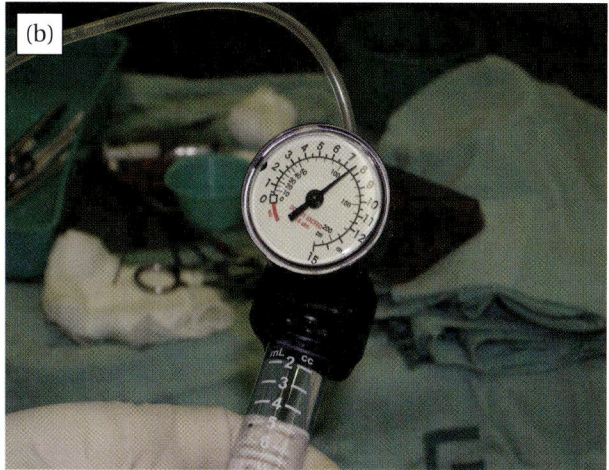

FIGURE 97.9 (a, b) The balloon is then attached to the pump and inflated to a pressure of 8 atmospheres for 90 seconds. Without withdrawing the balloon, the pressure is decreased to zero and reinflated to 8 atmospheres for 60 seconds. The catheter should be held in place during inflation, as it may tend to migrate.

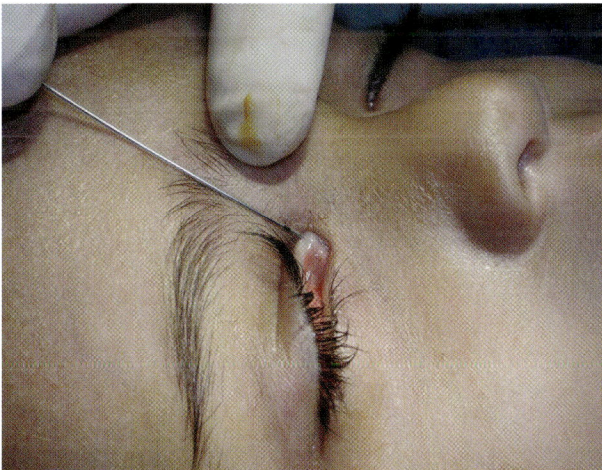

FIGURE 97.10 Using the markings on the catheter, the balloon is withdrawn more proximally, and two more inflations are carried out as previously described. The balloon is then completely deflated by decreasing the pressure to zero, withdrawing the plunger a bit to enable easier removal. Fluorescein can be irrigated and retrieved through the nose to confirm patency.

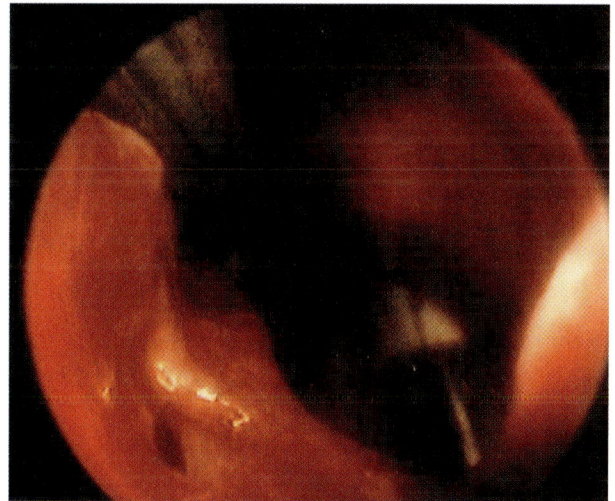

FIGURE 97.11 Endoscopic view of the inflated balloon beneath the inferior turbinate.

TABLE 97.3 *Potential Complications*

- Creation of false passage
- Epistaxis
- Balloon puncture (need backup on hand)
- Recurrent lacrimal obstruction

SELECTED REFERENCES

Becker BB, Berry FD. Balloon catheter dilatation in pediatric patients. *Ophthalmic Surg.* 1991;22(12):750–752.

Bleyen I, van den Bosch WA, Bockholts D, Mulder P, Paridaens D. Silicone intubation with or without balloon dacryocystoplasty in acquired partial nasolacrimal duct obstruction. *Am J Ophthalmol.* 2007;144(5):776–780.

Chen PL, Hsiao CH. Balloon dacryocystoplasty as the primary treatment in older children with congenital nasolacrimal duct obstruction. *J AAPOS.* 2005;9(6):546–549.

Couch SM, White WL. Endoscopically assisted balloon dacryoplasty treatment of incomplete nasolacrimal duct obstruction. *Ophthalmology.* 2004;111(3):585–589.

DeRespinis P, Coats D, Gold R. Management of nasolacrimal duct obstruction: balloons, tubes, and timing. *J Pediatr Ophthalmol Strabismus.* 2006;43(2):73–76.

Goldstein SM, Goldstein JB, Katowitz JA. Comparison of monocanalicular stenting and balloon dacryoplasty in secondary treatment of congenital nasolacrimal duct obstruction after failed primary probing. *Ophthal Plast Reconstr Surg.* 2004;20(5):352–357.

Goldstein SM, Katowitz JA, Syed NA. The histopathologic effects of balloon dacryoplasty on the rabbit nasolacrimal duct. *J AAPOS.* 2006;10(4):333–335.

Gunton KB, Chung CW, Schnall BM, Prieto D, Wexler A, Koller HP. Comparison of balloon dacryocystoplasty to probing as the primary treatment of congenital nasolacrimal duct obstruction. *J AAPOS.* 2001;5(3):139–142.

Huang YH, Liao SL, Lin LL. Balloon dacryocystoplasty and monocanalicular intubation with Monoka tubes in the treatment of congenital nasolacrimal duct obstruction. *Graefe's Arch Clin Exp Ophthalmol.* 2009;247(6):795–799.

Hutcheson KA, Drack AV, Lambert SR. Balloon dilatation for treatment of resistant nasolacrimal duct obstruction. *J AAPOS.* 1997;1(4):241–244.

Kashkouli MB, Beigi B, Tarassoly K, Kempster RC. Endoscopically assisted balloon dacryocystoplasty and silicone intubation versus silicone intubation alone in adults. *Eur J Ophthalmol.* 2006;16(4):514–519.

Konuk O, Ilgit E, Erdinc A, Onal B, Unal M. Long-term results of balloon dacryocystoplasty: success rates according to the site and severity of the obstruction. *Eye.* 2008;22(12):1483–1487.

Lachmund U, Ammann-Rauch D, Forrer A, Petralli C, Remonda L, Roeren T, Vonmoos F, Wilhelm K. Balloon catheter dilatation of common canaliculus stenoses. *Orbit.* 2005;24(3):177–183.

Lueder GT. Balloon catheter dilation for treatment of older children with nasolacrimal duct obstruction. *Arch Ophthalmol.* 2002;120(12):1685–1688.

Lueder GT. Balloon catheter dilation for treatment of persistent nasolacrimal duct obstruction. *Am J Ophthalmol.* 2002;133(3):337–340.

Maheshwari R. Balloon catheter dilation for complex congenital nasolacrimal duct obstruction in older children. *J Pediatr Ophthalmol Strabismus.* 2009;46(4):215–217.

Pediatric Eye Disease Investigator Group, Repka MX, Melia BM, Beck RW, Chandler DL, Fishman DR, Goldblum TA, Holmes JM, Perla BD, Quinn GE, Silbert DI, Wallace DK. Primary treatment of nasolacrimal duct obstruction with balloon catheter dilation in children younger than 4 years of age. *J AAPOS.* 2008;12(5):451–455.

Perry JD. Balloon dacryoplasty. *Ophthalmology.* 2004;111(9):1796–1797; author reply 1797.

Repka MX, Chandler DL, Holmes JM, Hoover DL, Morse CL, Schloff S, Silbert DI, Tien DR; Pediatric Eye Disease Investigator Group. Balloon catheter dilation and nasolacrimal duct intubation for treatment of nasolacrimal duct obstruction after failed probing. *Arch Ophthalmol.* 2009;127(5):633–639.

Tao S, Meyer DR, Simon JW, Zobal-Ratner J. Success of balloon catheter dilatation as a primary or secondary procedure for congenital nasolacrimal duct obstruction. *Ophthalmology.* 2002;109(11):2108–2111.

Vila-Coro AA, Al-Hussain H. Balloon catheter reuse in children with bilateral nasolacrimal duct obstruction. *Arch Ophthalmol.* 2003;121(12):1804; author reply 1804–1805.

Yazici Z, Yazici B, Parlak M, Erturk H, Savci G. Treatment of obstructive epiphora in adults by balloon dacryocystoplasty. *Br J Ophthalmol.* 199;83(6):692–696.

98 External Dacryocystorhinostomy

David H. Verity, MD, MA, FRCOphth and Geoffrey E. Rose, DSc, MS, MBBS, BSc, FRCOphth, FRCS, FRCP

TABLE 98.1   *Lacrimal Outflow Obstruction—A Polarization of Symptoms*

TABLE 98.2   *Preoperative Considerations*

TABLE 98.3   *Operative Considerations*

TABLE 98.4   *Postoperative Considerations*

TABLE 98.5   *Objectives of Surgery*

TABLE 98.6   *Indications for Surgery*

TABLE 98.7   *Creation of the Rhinostomy*

TABLE 98.8   *Creation of the Sutured Mucosal Anastomosis*

FIGURE 98.1   Flow symptoms and signs

FIGURE 98.2   Volume symptoms and signs

FIGURE 98.3   The lacrimal drainage apparatus—a three-compartment model

FIGURE 98.4   The objective of lacrimal drainage surgery: conversion of three compartments into two.

FIGURE 98.5   Anterior ethmoidal cells lie between the lacrimal sac and the nasal space in over 95% of patients.

FIGURE 98.6   Free, wide communication between the lacrimal sac and nasal

FIGURE 98.7   Anterior ethmoidectomy and trimming of the posterior lacrimal crest enables open communication between the lacrimal sac and nose.

FIGURE 98.8   Sutured flaps, which enable primary intention healing of the new soft-tissue union, avoid the marked granulation and contracture of secondary intention healing.

FIGURE 98.9   Desirable extent of a nasal osteotomy during external DCR (shaded area)

FIGURE 98.10   Nasal mucosal vasoconstriction is accomplished by positioning 3 cotton-tips, moistened in 1:1000 epinephrine.

FIGURE 98.11   A skin flap is created, exposing the medial canthal tendon (arrow) which inserts 2 3 mm in front of the anterior lacrimal crest.

FIGURE 98.12   The paranasal periosteum has been divided along the anterior lacrimal crest.

FIGURE 98.13   The lacrimal sac is displaced laterally, exposing the maxillo-lacrimal suture. This is infractured and the rhinostomy (arrow) is carried anteriorly before extending inferiorly.

FIGURE 98.14   All bone (arrow) lying alongside the level of the common canaliculus (dotted line) must be removed to allow the anterior nasal flaps to bridge the rhinostomy freely.

FIGURE 98.15   The lacrimal drainage system has been opened at the sac/duct junction with an E11 blade.

FIGURE 98.16   The sac is opened like a book, and the common canalicular opening is readily apparent (arrow).

SELECTED REFERENCES

TABLE 98.1 *Lacrimal Outflow Obstruction—A Polarization of Symptoms*

"Flow" Symptoms	"Volume" Symptoms
Due to lacrimal outflow impedance	*Due to retention and concentration of debris in the lacrimal sac, with backwash onto the ocular surface*
Wet sensation on eyelid margin	Gummy eyelids
"Watery vision," misty glasses	Matted eyelashes, particularly on waking
Aqueous overflow with irritation of eyelid skin	Mucus backwash onto the eye
Irritable outer canthus due to aqueous "wicking"	Recurrent conjunctivitis and/or dacryocystitis
Epiphora (frank aqueous overflow)	Medial canthal swelling—with discharge on lacrimal sac pressure—but later becoming firm and no longer expressible

TABLE 98.2 *Preoperative Considerations*

Consider CT imaging only in the presence of atypical clinical features, such as swelling *above* the medial canthal tendon, lateral displacement of the globe or a rocky-hard (or ulcerating) canthal mass.

Consider an endoscopic approach for patients unwilling to accept the small (3%) chance of a visible incision, but who are willing to accept a lower success rate.

Unless medically contraindicated, antiplatelet agents and spicy foods should be stopped at least 2 weeks prior to surgery.

In patients on warfarin, the INR should be approximately 2; low molecular weight heparin should be considered where anticoagulation cannot be stopped (as with metallic heart valves). The increased risk of major postoperative epistaxis in such patients should be weighed against the need for lacrimal surgery.

TABLE 98.3 *Operative Considerations*

In patients with a bleeding diathesis, having surgery under general anesthesia, consider infiltrating the operative site with local anesthetic containing adrenaline.

An intraoperative intravenous dose of a wide-spectrum antibiotic significantly reduces the rate of postoperative soft-tissue infection.

Position the patient head-up, with controlled hypotensive anesthesia.

Be meticulous with hemostasis at all stages.

TABLE 98.4 *Postoperative Considerations*

Instruct the patient not to drink hot fluids for 12 hours after surgery, as this increases nasal vasodilation and the risk of early epistaxis.

To reduce the chance of secondary hemorrhage, nose-blowing is discouraged for a week after surgery.

A short course of oral antibiotics might be considered for patients with gross sepsis or soft-tissue infection, or for patients undergoing bilateral simultaneous surgery.

Remove sutures at 7–10 days, and stenting at 3–6 weeks.

Advise the patient that lacrimal symptoms may continue to improve for many months after surgery, as postoperative edema settles.

TABLE 98.5 *Objectives of Surgery*

Reduction of lacrimal outflow resistance

Conversion of a three-compartment system to two compartments (Figures 98.4 and 98.24).

Total elimination of the lacrimal sac, with resolution of "volume" related symptoms and signs

The above objectives are met only with adequate anterior ethmoidectomy and a large rhinostomy, thereby permitting wide opening of the sac, whose mucosa becomes the lateral wall of the nose.

Drainage of mucocoele and removal of dacryoliths where present

To discourage the formation of a membrane over the entrance of the common canaliculus; for this reason *alone*, a silicone stent is placed for 3–6 weeks.

TABLE 98.6 *Indications for Surgery, Type of Surgery, and Prognosis for Symptoms*

Mucocoele of the nasolacrimal sac

    DCR and stent

    Excellent prognosis

Symptomatic nasolacrimal duct obstruction

    DCR and stent

    Excellent prognosis

Symptomatic nasolacrimal duct stenosis, in the absence of other treatable causes of lacrimal symptoms

    DCR and stent

    Good prognosis

Distal common canalicular membrane

    DCR, membranectomy, and stent

    Good prognosis

Patent nasolacrimal duct in the presence of significant lacrimal symptoms, after treating other identified causes for symptoms (so-called *functional epiphora*)

    DCR and stent

    Guarded prognosis

Canalicular block

    DCR, carunculectomy, retrograde canaliculostomy (examination of degree of canalicular patency *ab interno*), and stent

    Guarded prognosis, dependent upon the severity of canalicular occlusion. Subsequent Jones' canalicular bypass tube might be required.

TABLE 98.7 *Creation of the Rhinostomy*

The maxillolacrimal suture is exposed by lateral displacement of the lacrimal sac.

A periosteal elevator is moved along the suture line to allow entry of a small up-cutting rongeur into the bony infracture.

A large rhinostomy is created by crossing the anterior lacrimal crest close to the skull base, before continuing bone removal inferiorly, in front of the crest—thereby creating an "L-shaped" rhinostomy.

To enable large nasal mucosal flaps to be formed, the frontal process of the maxilla, along with the thin bone between the upper nasolacrimal duct and nose (the hamular process of the lacrimal bone), is removed.

Further removal of bone from the skull base (alongside the common canalicular opening), and posteriorly, to include a partial ethmoidectomy and trimming of the posterior lacrimal crest, facilitates suturing of the posterior mucosal flaps.

TABLE 98.8 *Creation of the Sutured Mucosal Anastomosis*

A "00" lacrimal probe is passed along the lower canaliculus to tent the medial wall of the sac, and a No.11 blade used to enter the lumen at the sac/duct junction (to avoid inadvertent damage to the common canalicular opening).

Spring scissors are used to open the medial wall of the sac, from the skull base to the nasolacrimal canal.

The tough union between the sac fundus and skull base should be divided to allow the sac to be opened widely ("like a book").

For a large posterior nasal flap, the primary incision should be ~3 mm in front of the arch formed by the anterior end of the middle turbinate attachment to the lateral nasal wall.

Horizontal (antero-posterior) incisions are fashioned at each end of this primary incision, to create a wide H-shaped incision and two large flaps.

The posterior flaps are sutured together, from the sac fundus to the upper duct, with a 6-0 absorbable suture placed as a locked, continuous suture.

The lacrimal probe is finally removed, a silicone stent placed and the knot reinforced with a 2-0 silk ligature, and the stent drawn from the nasal space.

The anterior flaps are sutured together, being "suspended" from the overlying orbicularis muscle closure, with a strand of orbicularis muscle being taken before the nasal mucosal flap and after the anterior sac flap "bites."

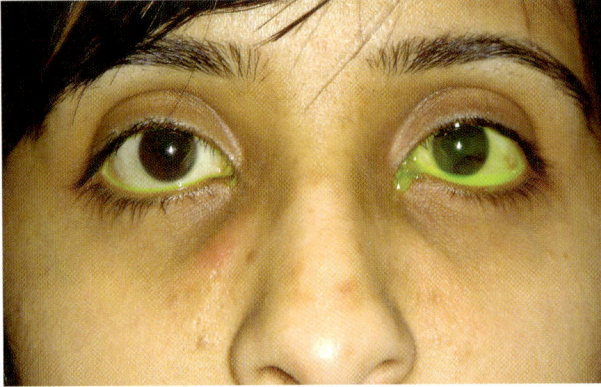

FIGURE 98.1 Flow symptoms and signs: note the raised marginal tear strip, delayed dye disappearance, and medial spillover (epiphora) on the left side.

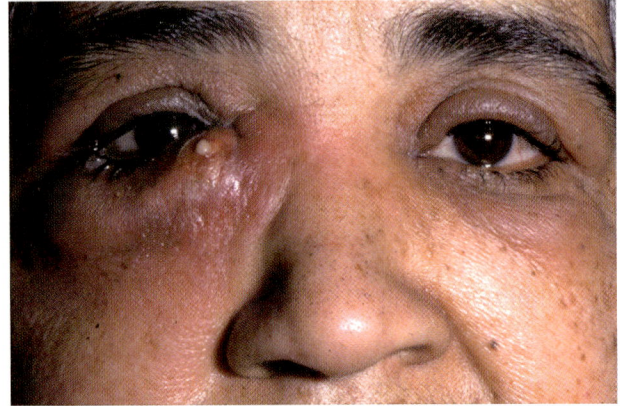

FIGURE 98.2 Volume symptoms and signs: Infected mucocoele of the lacrimal sac (dacryocystitis), with draining abscess.

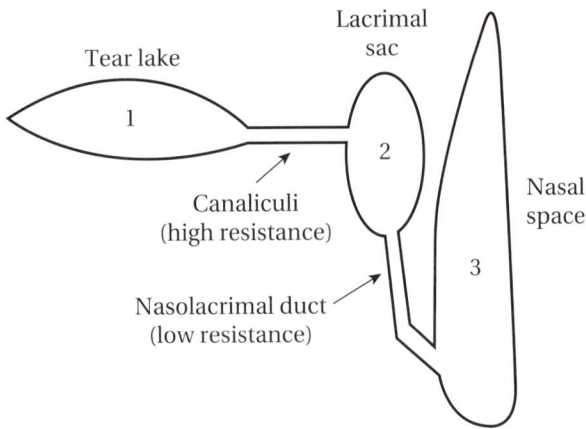

FIGURE 98.3 The lacrimal drainage apparatus—a three-compartment model.

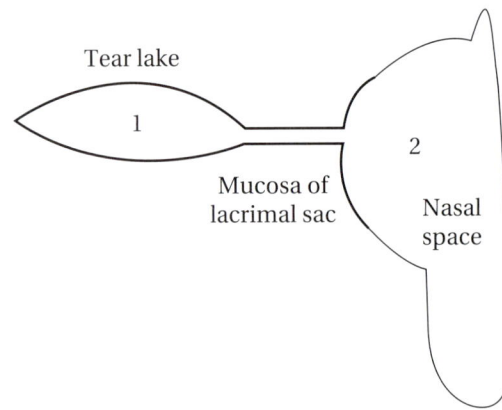

FIGURE 98.4 The objective of lacrimal drainage surgery: conversion of three compartments into two.

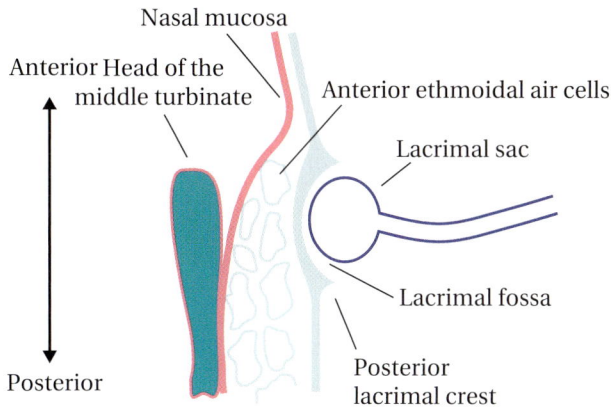

FIGURE 98.5 Anterior ethmoidal cells lie between the lacrimal sac and the nasal space in over 95% of patients.

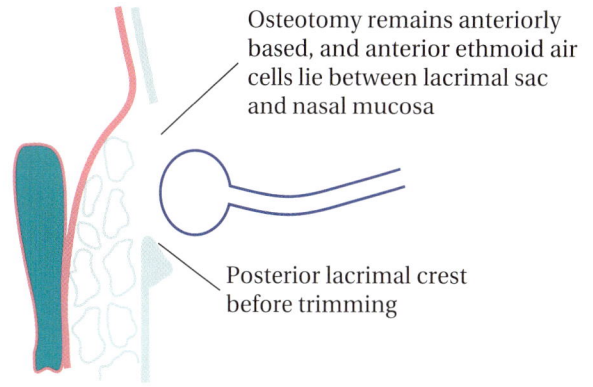

FIGURE 98.6 Free, wide communication between the lacrimal sac and nasal space generally requires anterior ethmoidectomy and trimming of the posterior lacrimal crest.

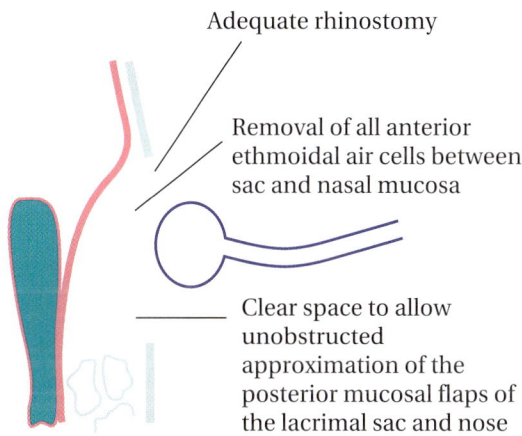

FIGURE 98.7 Anterior ethmoidectomy and trimming of the posterior lacrimal crest enables open communication between the lacrimal sac and nose.

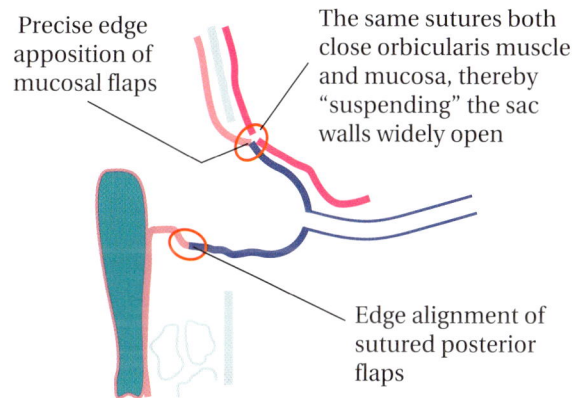

FIGURE 98.8 Sutured flaps, which enable primary intention healing of the new soft-tissue union, avoid the marked granulation and contracture of secondary intention healing. The continued "dead space," due to contracture of the ostium, leads to a persistence of volume symptoms and signs.

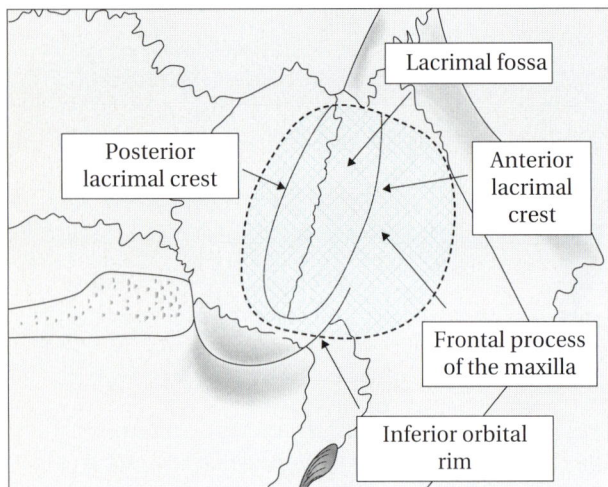

FIGURE 98.9 Desirable extent of a nasal osteotomy during external DCR (shaded area).

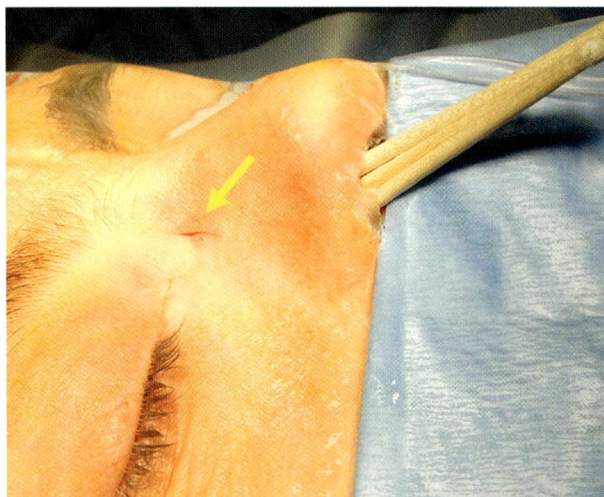

FIGURE 98.10 Nasal mucosal vasoconstriction is accomplished by positioning 3 cotton-tips, moistened in 1:1000 epinephrine, as far superiorly and anteriorly as possible within the nasal space. An incision (arrow) is made along the flat of the nose with a D15 blade.

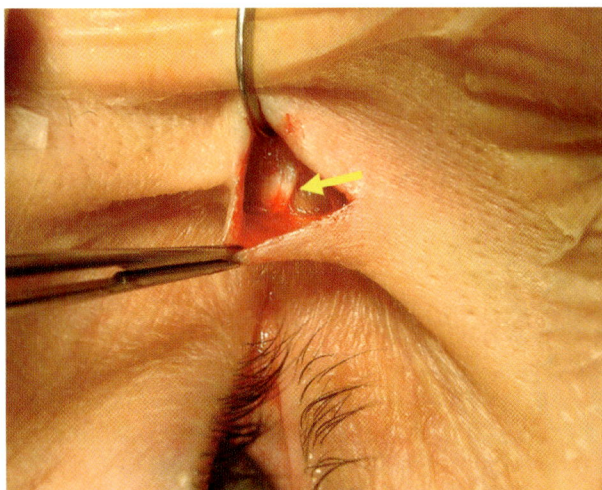

FIGURE 98.11 A skin flap is created, exposing the medial canthal tendon (arrow) which inserts 2–3 mm in front of the anterior lacrimal crest. Using a periosteal elevator, the tendon is separated from the periosteum, which is then reflected anteriorly away from the site of intended rhinostomy.

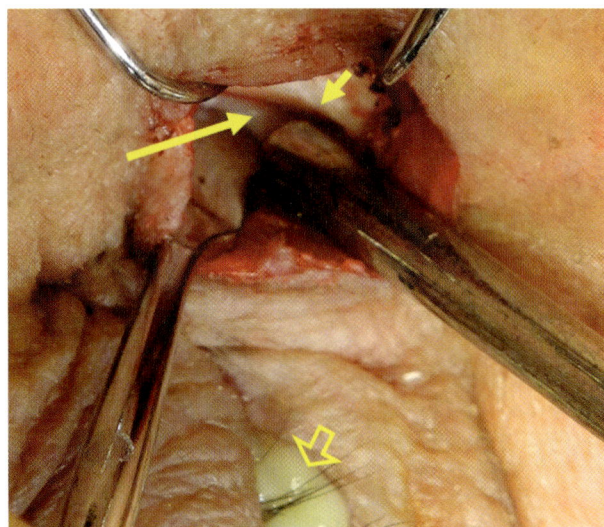

FIGURE 98.12 The paranasal periosteum has been divided along the anterior lacrimal crest (short arrow), and the lacrimal sac (long arrow) is being displaced laterally from its fossa, with mucopurulent backwash from the sac noted at the medial canthus (open arrow).

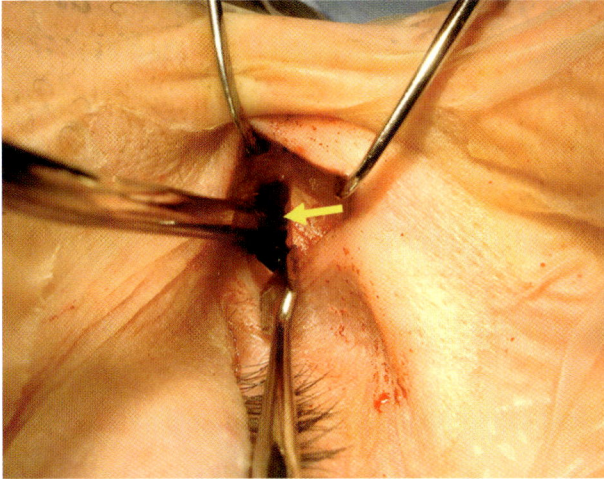

FIGURE 98.13 The lacrimal sac is displaced laterally, exposing the maxillolacrimal suture. This is infractured and the rhinostomy (arrow) is carried anteriorly before extending inferiorly.

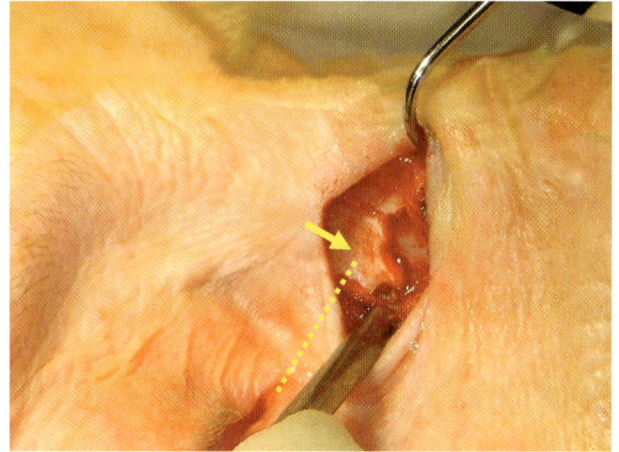

FIGURE 98.14 All bone (arrow) lying alongside the level of the common canaliculus (dotted line) must be removed, to allow the anterior nasal flaps to bridge the rhinostomy freely.

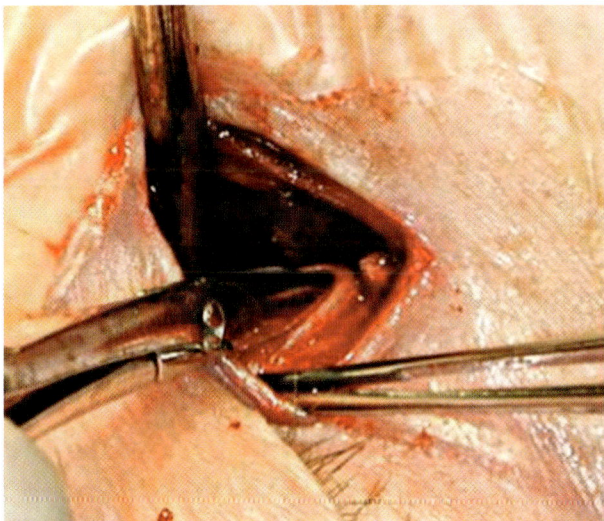

FIGURE 98.15 The lacrimal drainage system has been opened, at the sac/duct junction, with an E11 blade. The closed spring scissors are being used to "sound" the direction of the nasolacrimal duct, prior to opening the sac widely from its fundus to the duct.

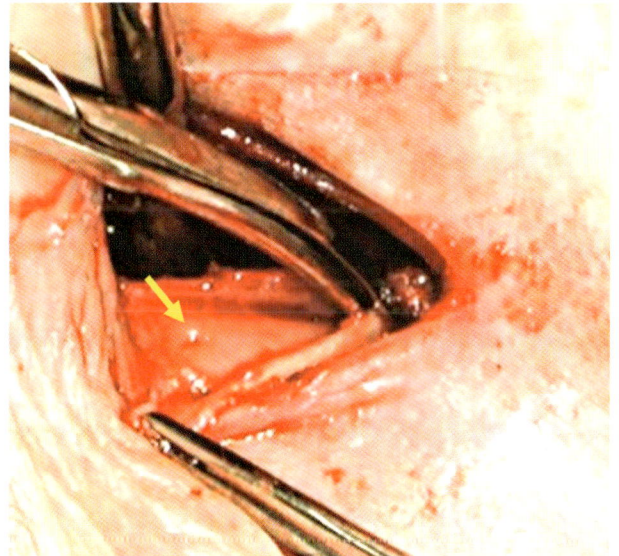

FIGURE 98.16 The sac is opened like a book, and the common canalicular opening is readily apparent (arrow).

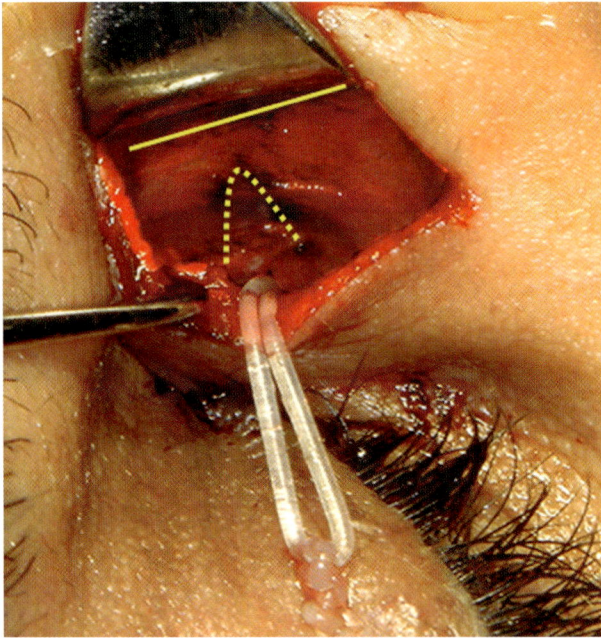

FIGURE 98.17 The bony rhinostomy is complete, the sac opened, and, in this example, intubated. The dotted line indicates the mucosal "arch" lining the uncinate process of the middle turbinate. Nasal flaps are created by making a horizontal incision 3 mm anterior to the arch (solid line).

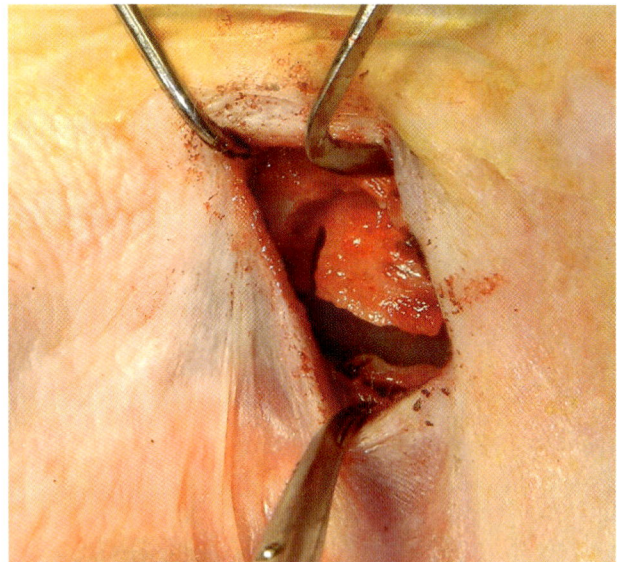

FIGURE 98.18 The anterior nasal flap is complete.

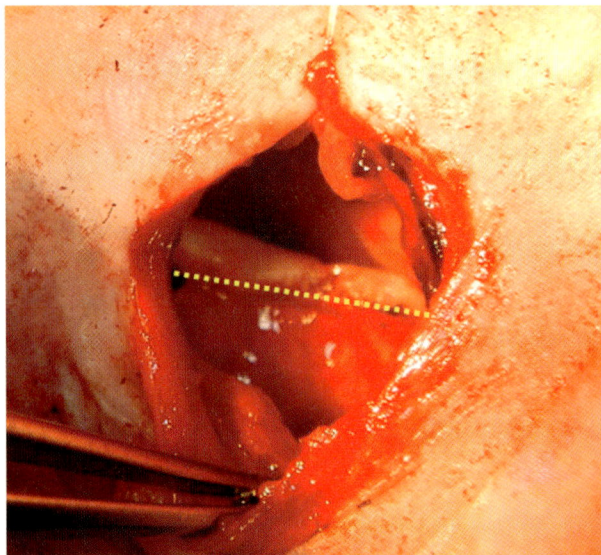

FIGURE 98.19 With adequate exposure and anterior ethmoidectomy, the posterior nasal and sac flaps are easily approximated: in this case, the flaps lie alongside each other (dotted line)—even prior to suturing.

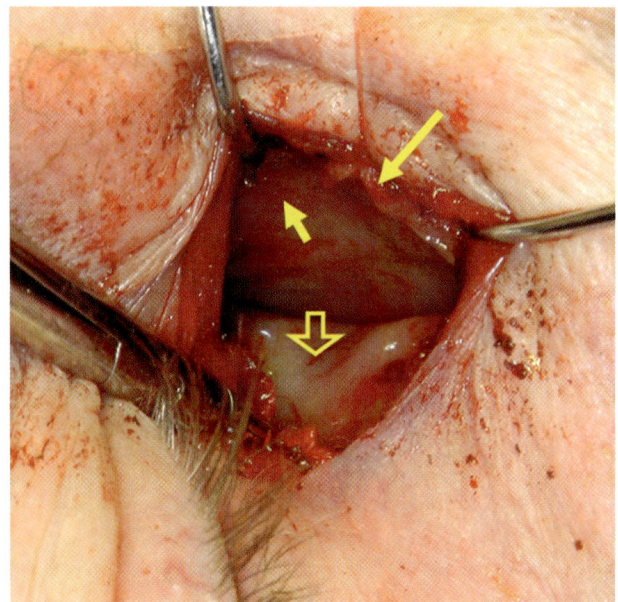

FIGURE 98.20 The posterior flaps are sutured, this figure showing the posterior nasal flap (open arrow), nasal septum (short arrow) and anterior nasal flap (long arrow), with the latter mucosa having been retracted anteriorly by a preplaced absorbable 6-0 suture.

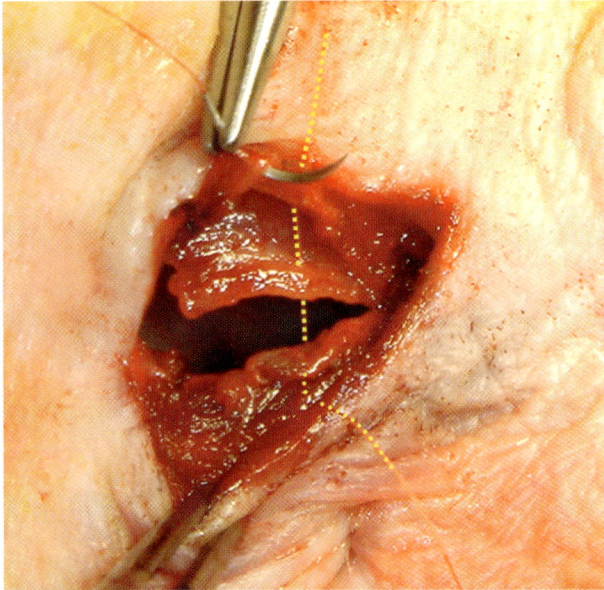

FIGURE 98.21 With the first of three "suspending" sutures placed through the orbicularis muscle, anterior nasal flap, anterior sac flap and orbicularis (dotted line), a second suture is being similarly placed 3–4 mm above the first—and this second suture will also pick up the anterior limb of the medial canthal tendon.

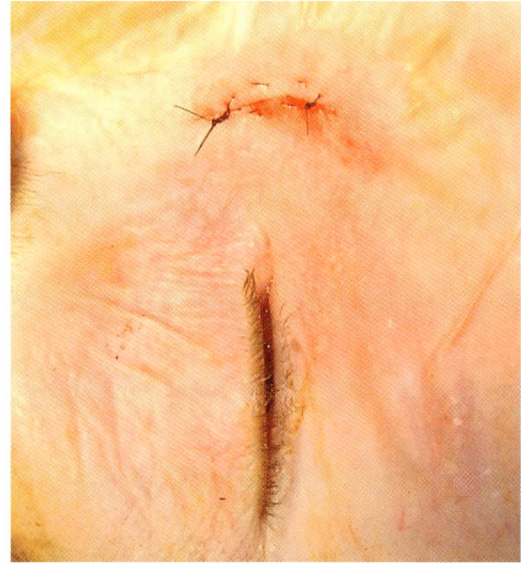

FIGURE 98.22 The skin is gently cleaned with a moist swab, and the incision closed using a horizontal mattress suture. The opposing edges of the incision should be kept flat, and not everted, such that the incision is tension-free along its axis.

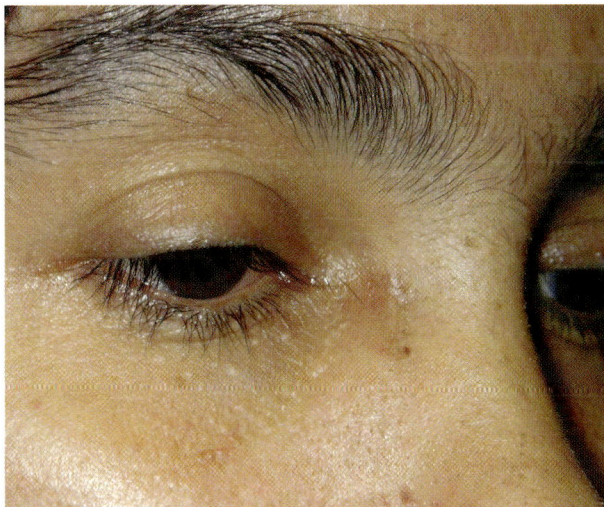

FIGURE 98.23 A typical example of the external incision at a month after surgery.

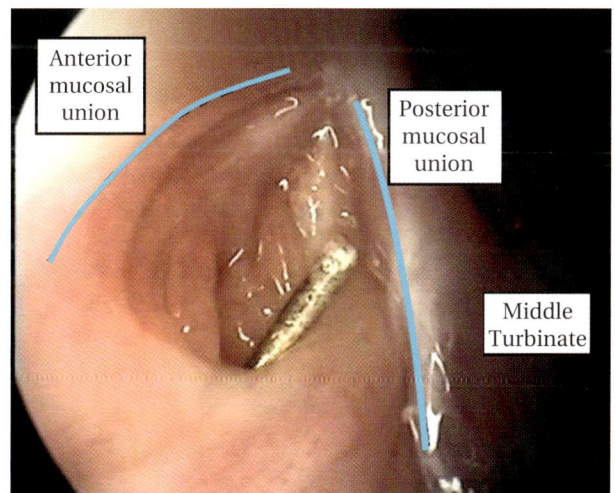

FIGURE 98.24 Endoscopic view of the DCR fistula: A probe passed through the inferior canaliculus identifies the wide opening of the sac into the nose, with no residual recess, and thus no residual volume symptoms.

SELECTED REFERENCES

Ezra EJ, Restori M, Mannor GE, Rose GE. Ultrasonic assessment of rhinostomy size following external dacryocystorhinostomy. *Brit J Ophthalmol.* 1998;82:786–789.

Hanna IM, Powrie S, Rose GE. Management outcome for daycase open lacrimal surgery, as compared to inpatient management. *Brit J Ophthalmol.* 1998;82:392–396.

Rose GE, Welham RAN. Jones' lacrimal canalicular bypass tubes: Twenty-five years' experience. *Eye.* 1991;5:13–19.

Rose GE. The lacrimal paradox: towards a greater understanding of success in lacrimal surgery. *Ophthalmic Plast Reconstr Surg.* 2004;20:262–265.

Vardy SJ, Rose GE. Prevention of cellulitis after open lacrimal surgery: a prospective study of three methods. *Ophthalmology.* 2000;107:315–317.

Walland MJ, Rose GE. Soft tissue infection after open lacrimal surgery. *Ophthalmology.* 1994;101:608–611.

Wearne MJ, Beigi B, Davis G, Rose GE. Retrograde intubation dacryocystorhinostomy for proximal and mid-canalicular obstruction. *Ophthalmology.* 1999;106:2325–2328.

Endonasal Dacryocystorhinostomy

Peter J. Dolman, MD, FRCSC

TABLE 99.1 *Indications for DCR Surgery*

- Epiphora, mucocoele, or dacryocystitis from acquired nasolacrimal duct (NLD) obstruction
- Congenital NLD obstruction refractory to probing and intubation
- Recurrent symptomatic dacryoliths

TABLE 99.2 *Contraindications for Endonasal Approach (EN DCR)*

The external approach may be preferred for:

- Trauma cases with medial canthal avulsion, where medial canthal reconstruction is planned, or where lacerations already expose the lacrimal sac
- Suspected lacrimal sac diverticuli or malignancies, where biopsy or removal of the lacrimal sac or duct is planned
- Patients with severe nasal anatomy disruption, making endonasal visualization of the surgical site too challenging
- Two or more failed endonasal DCR surgeries
- Cases in which pathology of the common canaliculus is present

TABLE 99.3 *Advantages of Endonasal DCR*

- No skin incision or wound complications (edema, hematoma, infections, discomfort and scarring)
- Visualization of nasal anatomy and possible surgical correction of abnormalities
- More rapid surgery compared to external approach
- More direct approach to surgical site, with less risk of collateral tissue injury
- Preferred by patients

TABLE 99.4 *Disadvantages of Endonasal DCR*

- Learning curve for ophthalmologists unfamiliar with intranasal anatomy and surgical tools
- Requirement for expensive equipment (endoscopes, video units) in the endoscopic EN DCR, and lasers in the laser EN DCR. These are *not* necessary for the non-endoscopic approach.
- May have limited view of lacrimal sac interior and common canalicular opening
- Nasal instrumentation may traumatize delicate lacrimal sac or nasal mucosa, promoting adhesions and failure of the ostium
- Potentially lower success rates compared with EX DCR (5%–10% lower, according to many clinicians). However, recent publications report success rates of 90%–95% for EN DCR, rivaling those of external DCR

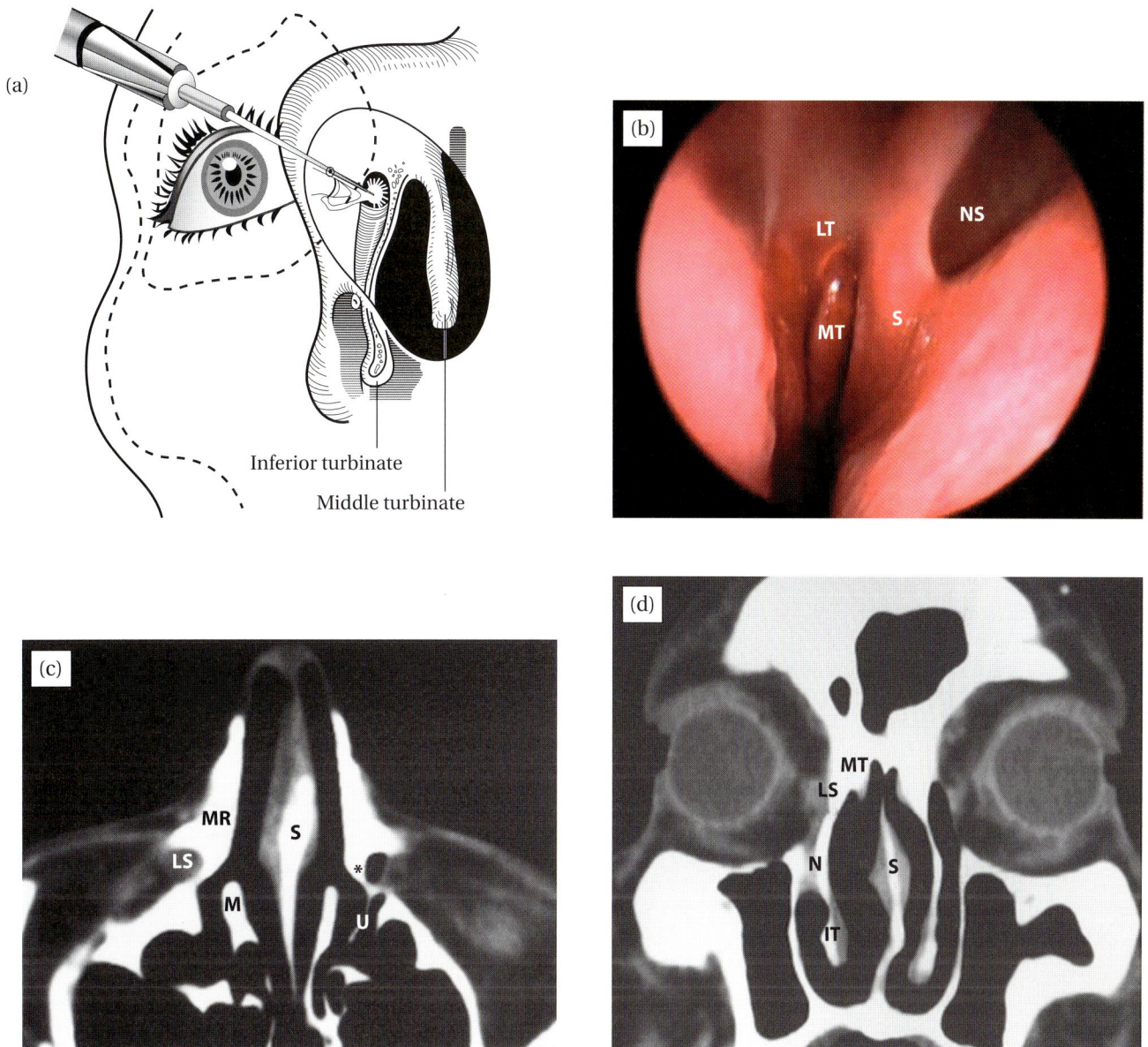

FIGURE 99.1 Surgical Anatomy. (a) Target light held parallel to lid margin through canaliculus and abutting medial bony wall of lacrimal sac. The view endonasally shows the position of the transilluminated light at the proposed ostium site, anterior to the middle turbinate. The nasolacrimal duct empties lateral to the inferior turbinate in the inferior meatus. (b) Endoscopic view of right nasal cavity with blades of the nasal speculum (NS) pressing on septum (S) and lateral wall of nose. The light target (LT) is visible, shining behind the internal maxillary ridge just lateral to the anterior tip of the middle turbinate (MT). (c) Axial CT Scan demonstrates the lacrimal sac (LS) shielded anteriorly by the thick maxillary ridge (MR) created by the frontal process of the maxilla, and forming the anterior lacrimal crest laterally and the internal maxillary ridge nasally. The lacrimal bone posterior to the internal ridge thins significantly, allowing the light target to be visualized intranasally, directly or with an endoscope between the nasal septum (S) and maxillary ridge. This thin bone is the site that can be penetrated most easily for creation of the ostium (*) anterior to the middle turbinate (M). The uncinate process (U) usually inserts posterior to the lacrimal sac, and typically does not need to be removed in an EN DCR, except for rare cases where its anterior insertion involves the medial bony wall of the sac. (d) Coronal CT Scan shows thick maxillary ridge bone anteriorly that must be removed at the right ostium site medial to the lacrimal sac (LS). The neck of the middle turbinate (MT) is just visible at this anterior view. The extent of the nasolacrimal duct (N) can be seen as it passes inferiorly and laterally to the inferior turbinate (IT).

TABLE 99.5 *Preoperative Evaluation*

- Exclude **lacrimation from irritative sources** (dry eyes, blepharitis, trichiasis, drops), eyelid malpositions, and lacrimal punctal abnormalities.

- Assess **anatomic patency** of the lacrimal outflow tract by irrigation through the canaliculi. Partial or complete obstruction causes reflux through the opposite canaliculus. Mucus or pus suggests acute/chronic dacryocystitis. Reflux along the same canaliculus, often associated with discomfort, suggests canalicular obstruction.

- **Functional testing** may be useful when anatomic blockage is not identified. Upper system failure may result in the inability of fluorescein dye to pass from the inferior cul-de-sac to the punctum. Nasolacrimal duct functional obstruction may be confirmed on a negative Jones 1 test: lack of spontaneous passage of fluorescein from the punctum to a cotton applicator placed under the inferior meatus. Dacryoscintigraphy may also confirm functional NLD obstruction.

- **Dacryocystography** may confirm dacryoliths or diverticuli, but is not routinely required.

- **CT Scans** are helpful if the clinical examination suggests neoplasm (bloody tears, epistaxis or an expanding lacrimal sac mass), or to assess bony and sinus anatomy in previous trauma, surgery, or reconstruction around the lacrimal sac and duct.

- An office **intranasal examination** with loupes and nasal speculum or endoscope may identify anatomic variations (septal deviation or prominent turbinates) or pathology (allergic rhinitis, necrotizing vasculitis, or polyps) that should be treated prior to or during surgery.

- Discontinue anticoagulants with approval of the patient's physician, cardiologist, or neurologist. Warfarin should be stopped 3 days preoperatively, and INR checked on surgical day (aim for INR < 2.0) Nonsteroidal anti-inflammatories, aspirin, vitamin C/E, and herbs with anticoagulant properties should be discontinued 1–2 weeks preoperatively.

- Ensure that blood pressure is controlled preoperatively. The anesthesiologist can also maintain relative hypotension intraoperatively.

Operative Series

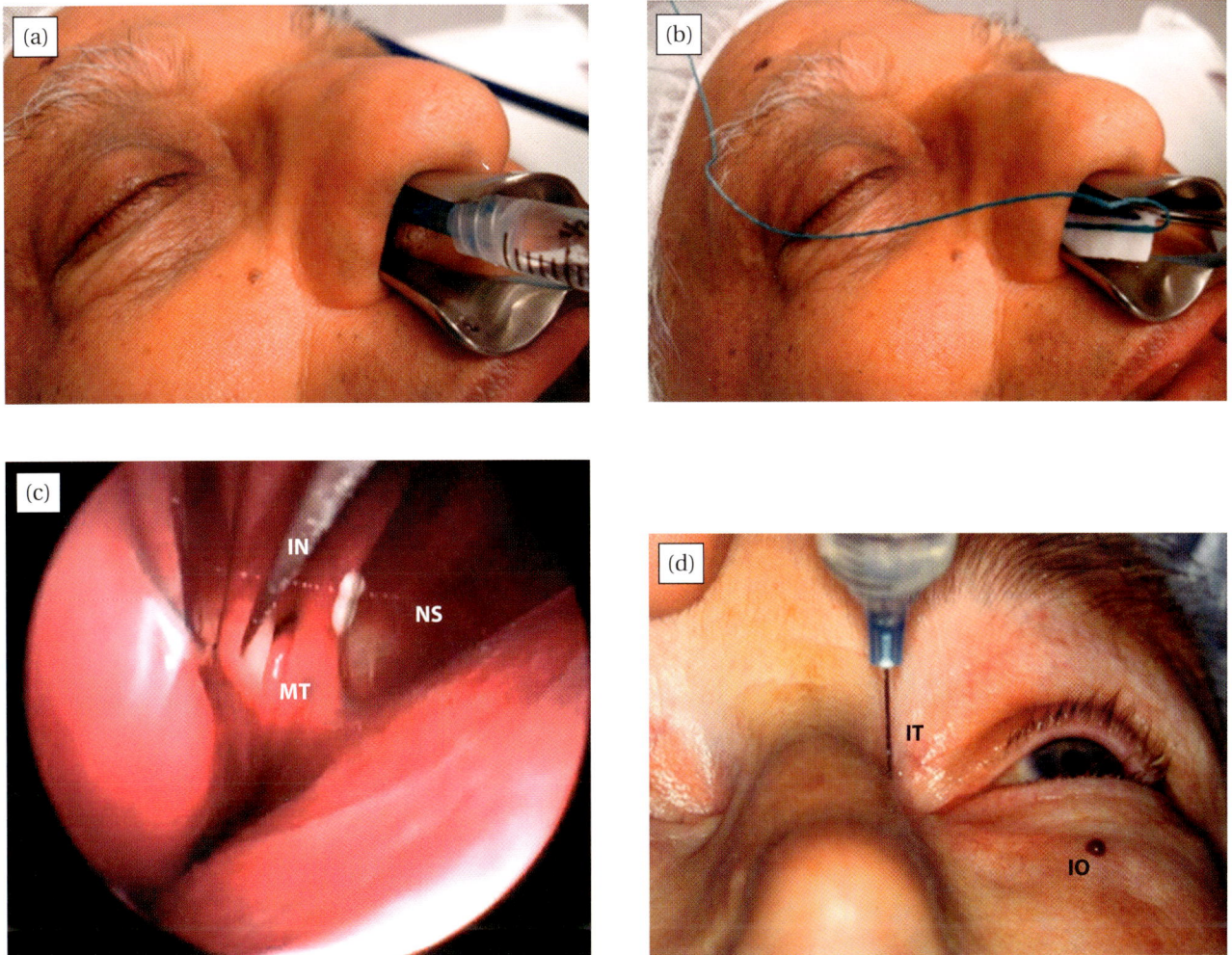

FIGURE 99.2 Hemostasis and Anesthesia. Placing the nasal speculum (NS) with the blades set vertically (rather than horizontally against the septum and lateral wall) reduces mucosal bleeding (a, b). Care should be taken to avoid dragging or pushing surgical equipment (including the suction) on areas not injected with epinephrine. The lateral wall nasal mucosa anterior to the middle turbinate (MT) and the tip of the middle turbinate (a, c) can be injected with Lidocaine with epinephrine, using a long 25 gauge needle or spinal needle (IN). The mucosa blanches with the injection. Neuropaddies, or strip gauze soaked in cocaine 4% or epinephrine (b) can be placed in the middle meatus to decongest the nasal mucosa, inwardly rotate the turbinate, and improve visualization. The anesthetist should approve the use of combined cocaine and/or epinephrine, because of the possibility of secondary tachycardia or hypertension. Local anesthesia consists of infratrochlear (d, needle site) and infraorbital blocks (d, blood spot from needle site) using lidocaine 1%–2% with 1/100,000 epinephrine and monitored sedation. Intranasal anesthesia is provided by the mucosal injection and cocaine soaks. General anesthesia is recommended for nervous patients, for cases where communication is challenging, or for surgeons learning the technique. Some surgeons prefer general anesthesia, as it is well tolerated because of the brief duration of the surgery (10–20 minutes).

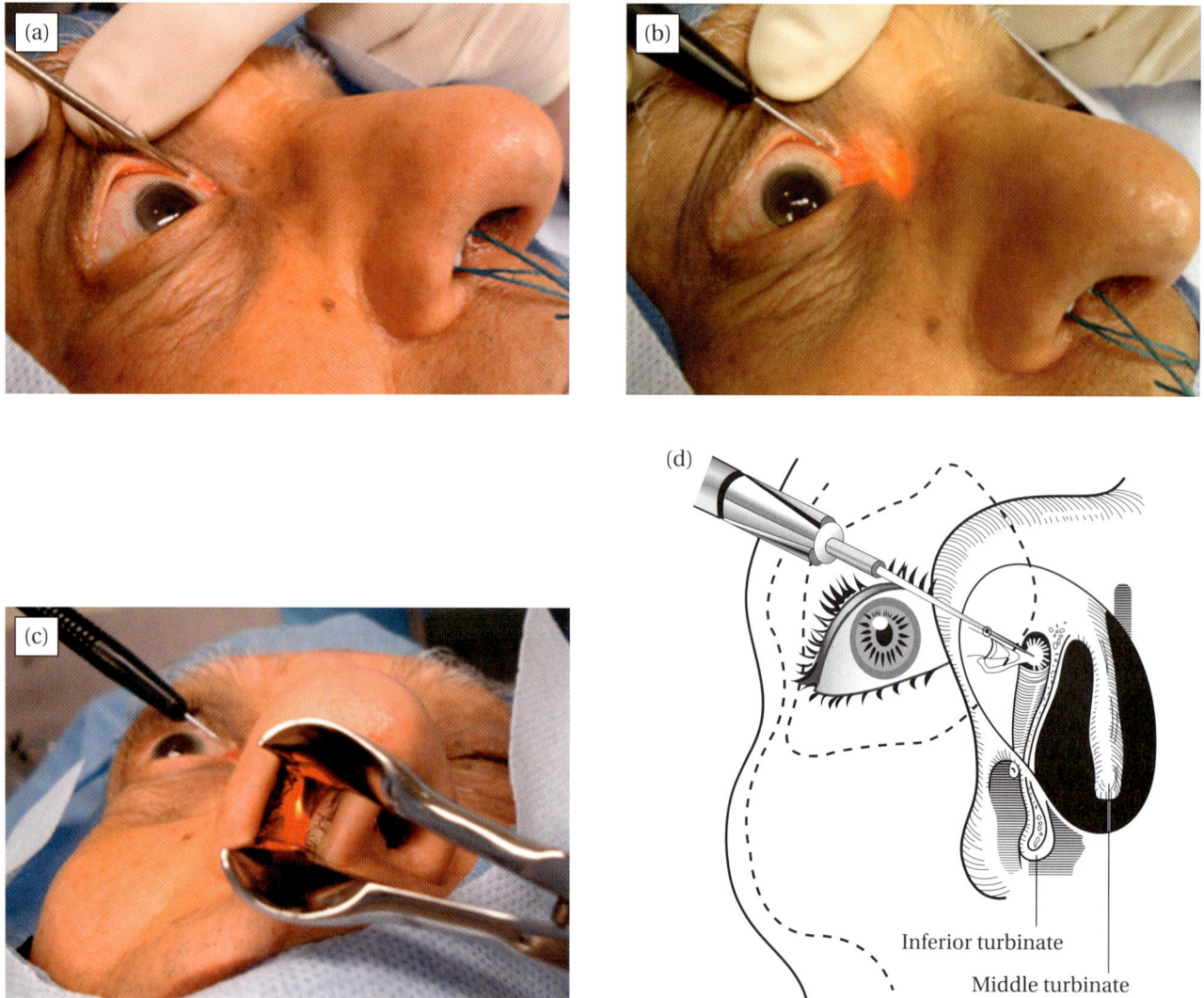

FIGURE 99.3 Placing the Light Target. After dilating the upper punctum (a), a standard disposable 20 gauge vitrectomy light pipe is threaded through the canaliculus parallel to the direction of the lid margin, until it hits the firm bone of the medial wall of the lacrimal sac (b). It is easier to enter the punctum with the light off (to prevent glare), and important to keep the lid on firm lateral traction to avoid traumatizing the delicate walls of the canaliculus during advancement. The light target is easily seen transilluminating through the thin lacrimal bone behind the thicker maxillary ridge, just lateral to the anterior tip of the middle turbinate (c, d).

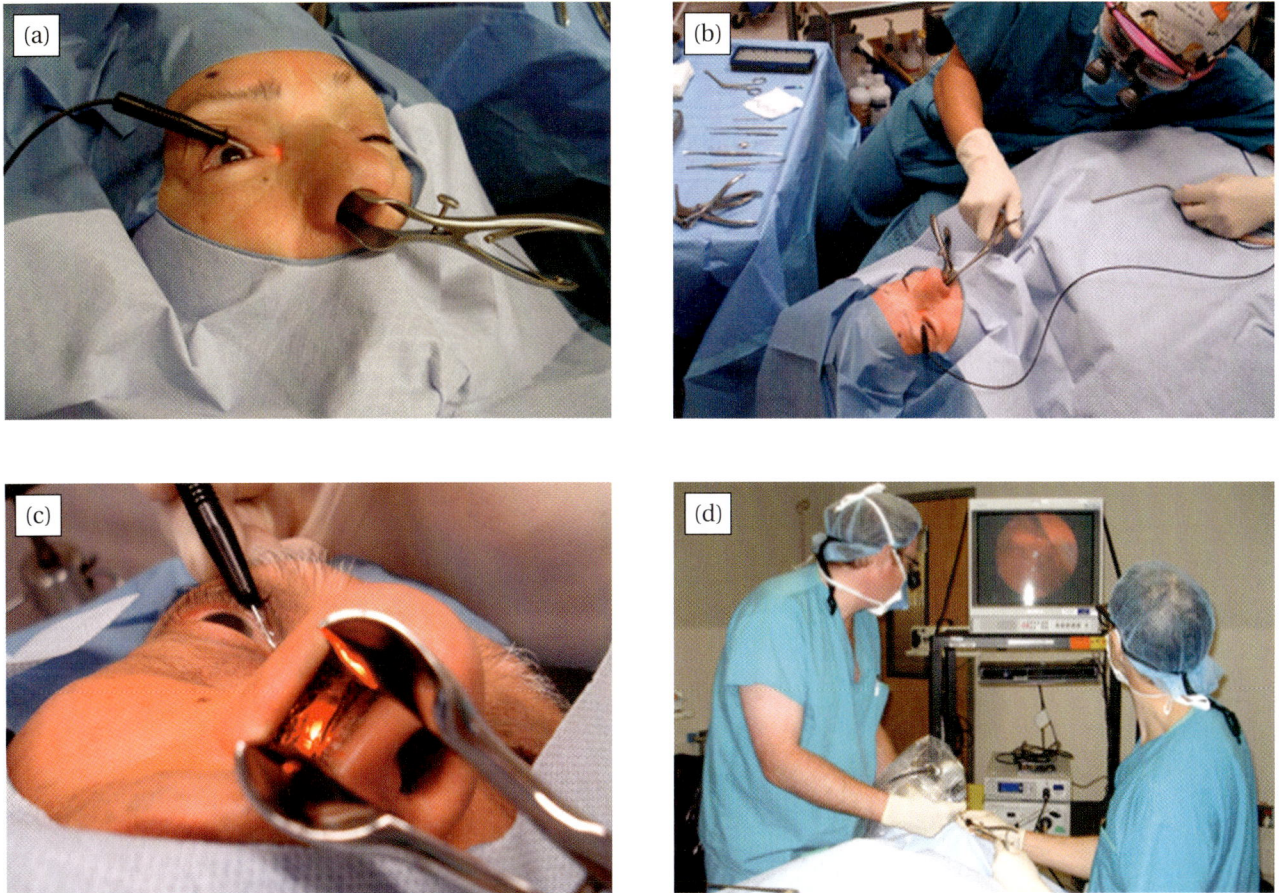

FIGURE 99.4 Viewing the Surgical Site. (a, b, c) In the non-endoscopic EN DCR, a 5 cm long blade nasal speculum with a side-locking burl can be balanced hands-free with the handles over the face. The assistant can also hold the speculum, but must be careful not to scrape the blades along the nasal mucosa and cause bleeding. The light pipe can be held against the medial bony wall of the sac by an assistant, or balanced. The surgeon wears surgical loupes and sits on the side opposite the surgical site, to facilitate a direct view along the lateral wall of the nose. No headlight is necessary, as the light target provides sufficient illumination. (d) In the endoscopic EN DCR, a right-handed surgeon sits or stands on the right side of the patient, regardless of the side being operated. The endoscope is held in the left hand and instruments are introduced below the endoscope shaft with the right hand. The operator may view the site directly with the endoscope, or indirectly through video. Anti-fog solution helps keep the endoscope clear.

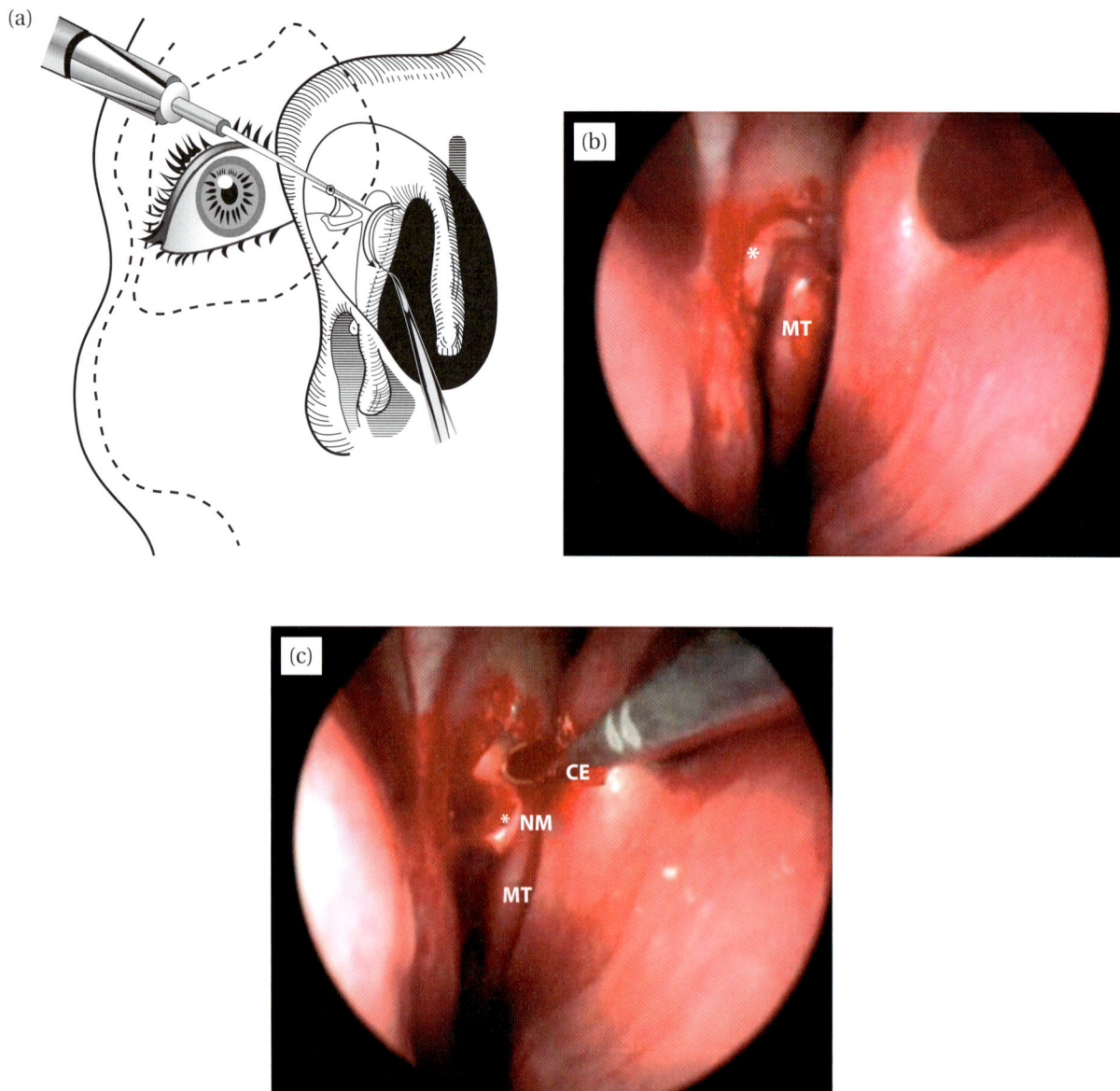

FIGURE 99.5 **Incising and Removing Nasal Mucosa.** (a, b) A myringotomy sickle knife or cataract crescent blade is used to outline a 1cm diameter ellipse of nasal mucosa (within the area injected with epinephrine) centered around the light target. The anterior incision is usually well visualized along the maxillary ridge, and should be at least 5 mm anterior to the light **(*)**. The posterior incision may be harder to visualize in cases where the maxillary ridge is prominent. Take care not to injure the mucosa along the middle turbinate (MT) during these maneuvers. Alternative instruments for cutting the nasal mucosa include lasers (holmium YAG, CO2 or KTP) and a radiofrequency unit. (c) The Cottle elevator (CE) is then used to strip the nasal mucosa (NM) off the underlying bone (maxillary ridge and thinner posterior lacrimal bone) from the incision lines toward the center. This helps prevent inadvertent tears of the nasal mucosa into an area not injected with epinephrine.

(d)

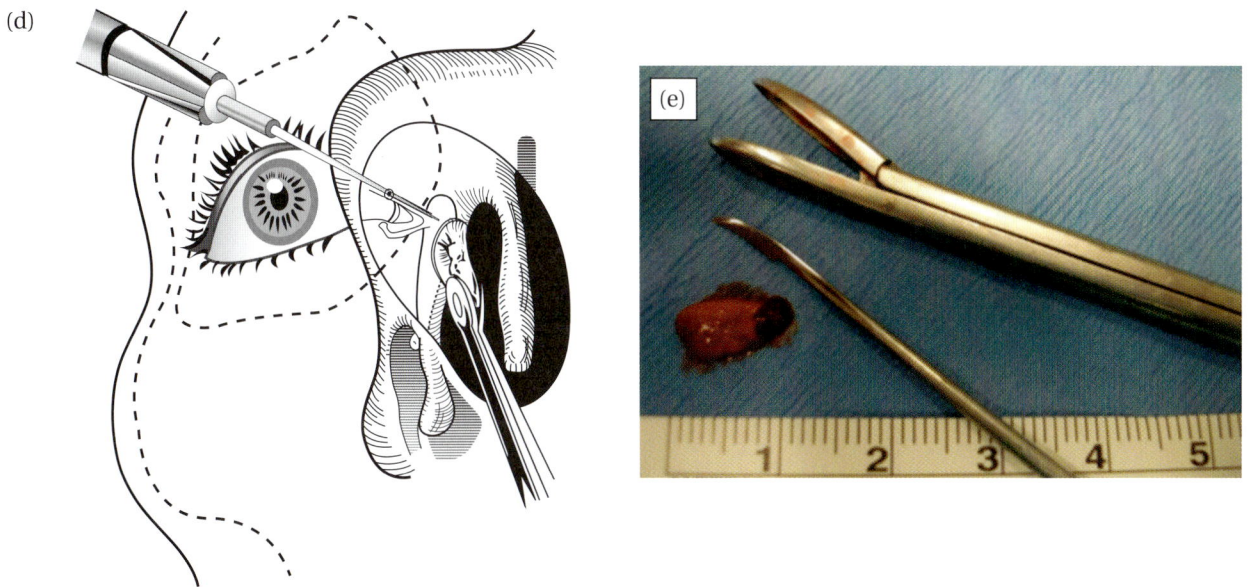

(e)

FIGURE 99.5 (*continued*) (d, e) An ethmoid forceps can then be used to peel off the 1 cm diameter nasal mucosal ellipse. The light target can be seen shining brighter through the exposed bone. The brightness of the light target reflects the thickness of the underlying bone, and highlights where the bone is thinnest for initiating its removal.

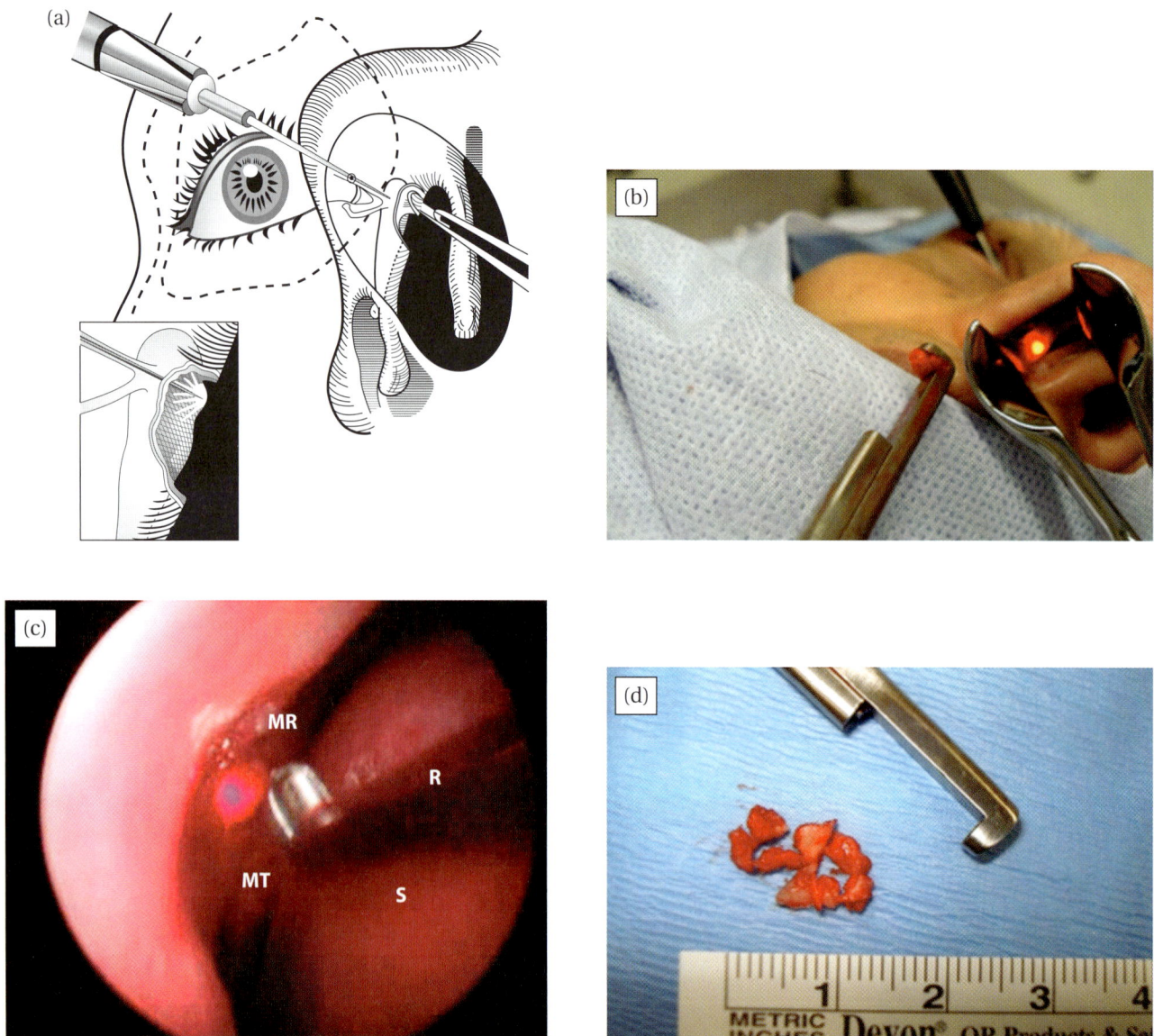

FIGURE 99.6 Creating the Bony Ostium. (a, b, c) A 3 mm Kerrison upbiting rongeur (R) with a flat distal end is slipped behind the vertical bony ridge of the internal frontal process of the maxilla. Here, it will push aside the wafer-thin lacrimal bone against the sac, and permit the rongeur to engage the posterior lip of the maxillary ridge (MR). The light target helps define where the bone is thinnest; occasionally, the rongeur may need to be slipped more inferior or posterior to penetrate the thinner bone. The bone is nibbled anteriorly through the thicker maxillary bone at one level until the lacrimal sac can be seen being tented by the light pipe, thus defining the correct plane for ongoing bone removal. Bone is then rongeured superiorly, where it becomes increasingly dense as it curves toward the root of the middle turbinate (MT). An attempt is made to rongeur sufficient bone superiorly to allow the light pipe to be seen indenting the lacrimal sac mucosa, when held horizontally within the superior canaliculus (a inset). The anterior and lateral aspect of most of the length of the sac, and superior aspect of the duct, should be freed of bone equivalent to a 1 cm ostium (d, c). The head of the middle turbinate occasionally is trimmed in cases where Jones tubes are placed (see chapter on CDCR), but this is seldom required for a primary EN DCR. A 2 mm Kerrison rongeur can be used in areas where the bone is very thick; although it removes smaller fragments than the 3 mm rongeur, it can crack through thicker bone. Mechanized drills and powered microdebriders may also be used. Various lasers have been tried to create the bony ostium, including the argon blue-green, Nd:YAG, carbon dioxide, KTP-YAG, and holmium YAG, but these create thermal char and generally cannot remove the thicker anterior and superior bone of the maxillary ridge, thus resulting in poorer outcomes.

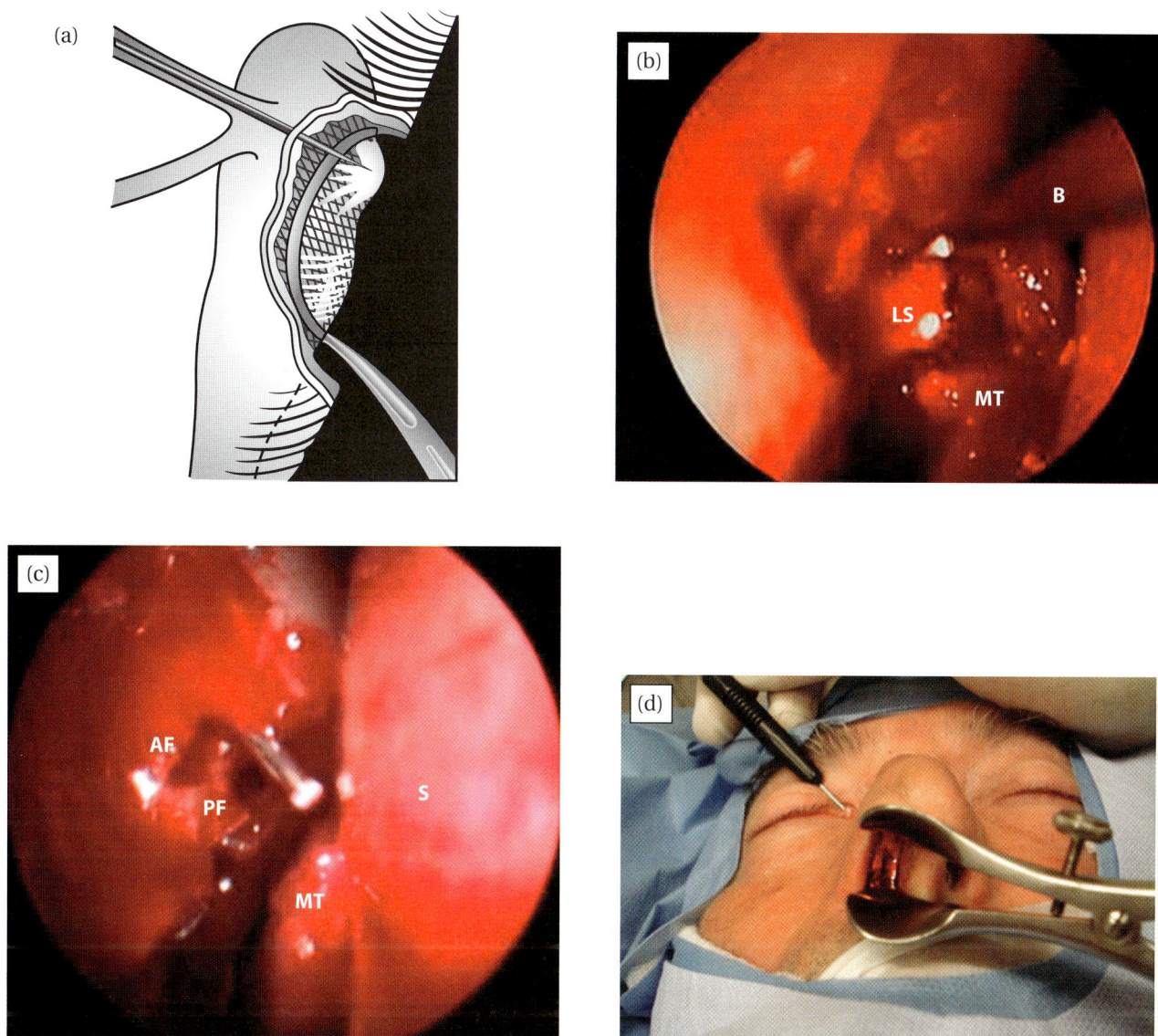

FIGURE 99.7 Fenestrating the Lacrimal Sac. (a–d) This is one of the more challenging aspects of EN DCR. The light pipe can be used to tent the exposed sac (LS) wall medially. The myringotomy or crescent blade (B) is used to puncture the sac superiorly, closest to the anterior aspect of the ostium. Once the sac has been penetrated so that the light pokes through (see Fig. 99.7c), the light pipe is withdrawn and redirected to vault the inferior sac medially, while the blade is drawn inferiorly along the lacrimal sac anterior border. Relaxing incisions can be made posteriorly, both superiorly and inferiorly, to create a posteriorly hinged flap (PF). Care is taken to limit the size of the anterior flap (AF) by cutting it close to the anterior aspect of the ostium. Avoid making a simple vertical slit in the sac, as the cut ends will readily seal. Careful tenting of the sac, and being careful to cut anteriorly, help reduce the risk of violating the lateral sac wall, herniating orbital fat or damaging orbital structures. If necessary, dacryoliths or pus can be flushed out of the sac lumen, and a biopsy of the mucosa or lumen contents should be taken from the posterior flap if disease is suspected. As throughout the surgery, avoid trauma to mucosa of the septum (S) and middle turbinate (MT) to limit the risk of adhesions forming between these structures and the lacrimal sac (LS) opening.

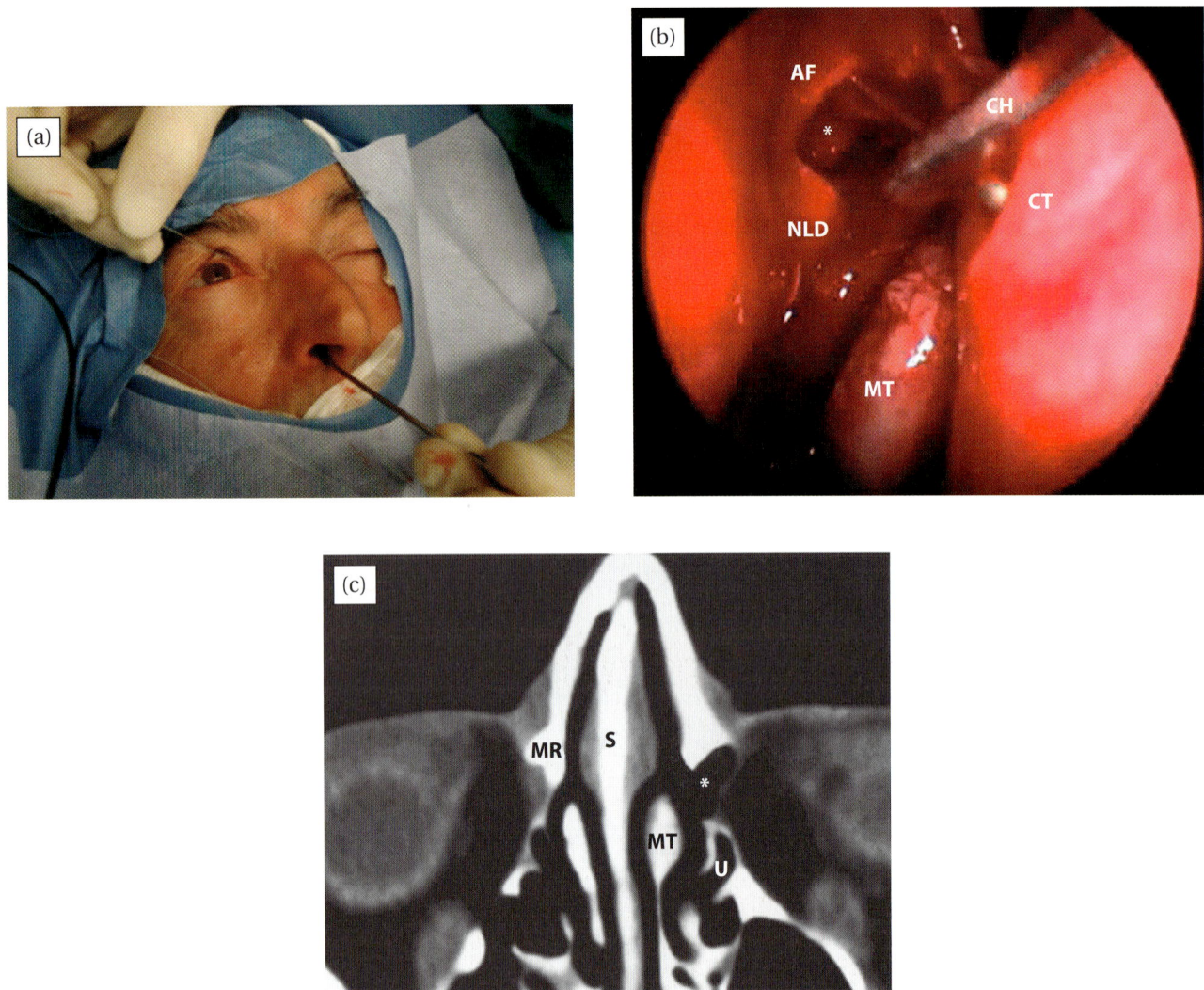

FIGURE 99.8 **Placing the Stents.** (a, b) Bicanalicular silicone stents are typically used in EN DCR because the mucosal edges of the ostium are unsutured and heal secondarily. The Crawford hook (CH) can be used to retrieve the tube (CT) through the marsupialized lacrimal sac (*) helping separate the posterior and anterior flaps (AF). The distal ends should be secured with a surgical clip or silicone bolster and tied with sufficient tension that they can't prolapse nor cause cheese-wiring of the canaliculi. (c) Axial CT Scan demonstrates a left bony ostium from a non-endoscopic EN DCR with removal of the lacrimal bone and a significant portion of the anterior maxillary ridge with marsupialization of the sac into the nose.

TABLE 99.6 *Adjunctive Measures*

- Mitomycin-C inhibits fibroblast proliferation, and some surgeons promote its use in both EN and EX DCR. While its safety has been shown, there are no convincing studies of its benefit for surgical success.
- Antibiotics: Cefazolin or trimethoprim-sulfamethoxazole for MRSA dacryocystitis can be administered, but antibiotics are not required for routine EN DCR.

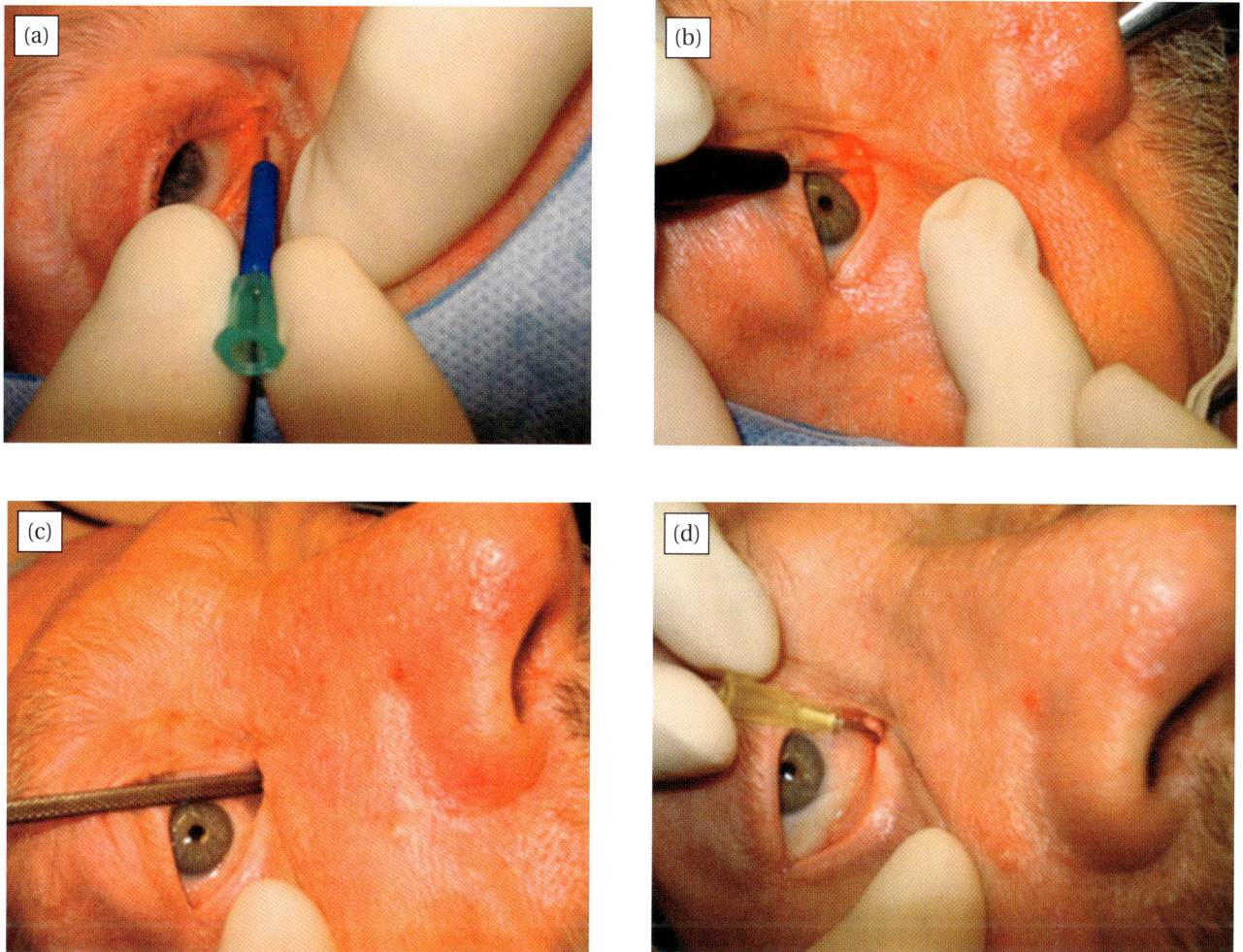

FIGURE 99.9 Canalicular Stenosis. Discrete scars involving the common canaliculus or adjoining canaliculus may be treated with a lacrimal microtrephine and stent (a). Broad symptomatic canalicular occlusions, or symptomatic epiphora from facial nerve palsy refractory to lid surgery, may require placement of a Jones tube. The light target is directed inferonasally behind the lower lid (b), and a small bony ostium is created by removing nasal mucosa and bone. A 20 gauge needle can be used as a sound to determine the correct length of pyrex tube to fit within the nasal cavity without abutting middle turbinate or septum. The soft tissues are dilated with a Bowman or gold dilator (**c**) and the tube threaded into place (d).

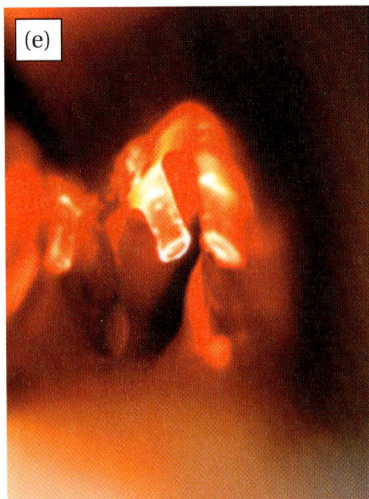

FIGURE 99.9 (*continued*) Its distal tip should be seen hanging freely in the nasal cavity (e), and water irrigated on the ocular surface should pass through it spontaneously.

TABLE 99.7 *Surgery in the Pediatric Population*

- Pediatric EN DCR is indicated for rare cases of congenital NLD obstruction that persist in spite of probing and stenting, or for cases of acquired dacryostenosis.
- Visualization remains excellent in spite of the smaller nasal cavity.

TABLE 99.8 *Postoperative Care*

- Avoid exertion and nose-blowing for one week (to avoid epistaxis and orbital emphysema).
- Patients are instructed how to manage nose bleeds and to seek help if uncontrolled bleeding occurs.
- Steroid-antibiotic drops are prescribed for two weeks, and a steroid or saline nasal spray once daily for one week to prevent dry crusts forming around ostium site.
- Oral antibiotics are prescribed for acute dacryocystitis.
- Follow-up visits are arranged for 2 weeks, 12 weeks, and six months. The ostium may be inspected and cleaned (especially in laser DCR where char may accumulate) and the passage irrigated. Longer-term follow-up may be arranged for research purposes and in cases of failure.
- The silicone stents may be removed at 6–12 weeks, or earlier if too loose or tight.

TABLE 99.9 *Complications*

- **Surgical failures** usually occur in the first three months postoperatively. Leading causes include:
  - Adhesions between the ostium site and middle turbinate or septum—avoid this by minimizing trauma to these structures and resecting the tip of the middle turbinate if it lies too close to the ostium.
  - Insufficient exposure of superior lacrimal sac from inadequate bone removal—remove sufficient bone from the superior maxillary ridge so the light pipe can be seen tenting the sac while held horizontally.
  - Scarring of the soft tissues overlying the lacrimal sac opening or common internal punctum—creation of a large posterior based lacrimal flap helps prevent the two cut ends from resealing.
- **Postoperative epistaxis** is treated with nasal compression, cold compresses on the nasal bridge, control of hypertension, and sitting upright. Nasal packs may rarely be required and are usually removed on the first postoperative day.
- **Silicone stent complications** include lateral displacement, lid cheese-wiring and pyogenic granulomas are best treated with early removal of the stent.
- **Orbital injuries:** transgression of the lateral wall of the sac may result in orbital fat herniation with possible surgical failure, medial rectus trauma, orbital hemorrhage and orbital emphysema.
- **CSF leaks** may result from disruption of the fovea ethmoidalis or cribriform plate, especially with rotational injuries to the middle turbinate.

SELECTED REFERENCES

Bartley GB. The pros and cons of laser dacryocystorhinostomy. *Am J Ophthalmol.* 1994;117:103–106.

Caldwell GW. Two new operations for obstruction of the nasal duct with preservation of the canaliculi and an incidental description of a new lacrymal probe. *New York Med J.* 1893;57:581–582.

Camara JG, Bengzon AU, Henson RD. The safety and efficacy of mitomycin C in endonasal endoscopic laser-assisted dacryocystorhinostomy. *Ophthalmic Plastic Reconstr Surg.* 2000;16:114–118.

Cunningham MJ, Woog JJ. Endonasal endoscopic dacryocystohinostomy in children. *Arch Otolaryngol Head Neck Surg.* 1998;124:328–333.

Dolman PJ. Comparison of external dacryocystorhinostomy with nonlaser endonasal dacryocysto-rhinostomy. *Ophthalmology.* 2003;110:78–84.

Dolman PJ, Alas E. *Prospective comparison of adjunctive mitomycin-C for non-endoscopic endonasal DCR.*[abstract]. Presented at the American Society of Ophthalmic Plastic and Reconstructive Surgeons, Los Angeles, 2004.

Dupuy-Dutemps MM, Bourget ET. Note preliminaire sur un proded de dacryocystorhinostomie. Ann D'Ocul (Paris) 1920;157:1445–1447.

Fayet B, Racy E, Halhal M, et al. Endonasal dacryocystorhinostomy (DCR) with protected drill. *J Fr. Ophthalmol.* 2000;23(4):321–326.

Goldberg RA. Endonasal dacryocystorhinostomy. Is it really less successful? *Arch Ophthalmol.* 2004;122:108–110.

Leone CR. Gelfoam-thrombin dacryocystorhinostomy stent. *Am J Ophthalmol.* 1982; 94:412.

Massaro BM, Gonnering RS, Harris GJ. Endonasal laser dacryocystorhinostomy: a new approach to nasolacrimal duct obstruction. *Arch Ophthalmol.* 1990;108:1172–1176.

McDonogh M, Meiring JH. Endoscopic transnasal dacryocystorhinostomy. *J Laryngol Otol.* 1989;103:585–587.

Olver J. *Colour atlas of lacrimal surgery.* Boston Butterworth-Heinemann; 2001.

Watkins LM, Janfaza P, Rubin PAD. The evolution of endonasal dacryocystorhinostomy. *Surv Ophthalmol.* 2003;48(1):73–84.

Woog JJ, Kennedy RH, Custer PL, et al. Endonasal dacryocystorhinostomy. A report by the American Academy of Ophthalmology. *Ophthalmology.* 2001;108:2369–2377.

100 Conjunctivodacryocystorhinostomy

Roger A. Dailey, MD, FACS and Douglas P. Marx, MD

TABLE 100.1 *Indications for Conjunctivodacryocystorhinostomy*

Symptomatic epiphora with one or more of the following:
* Both canaliculi either absent or obliterated
* Canaliculi are patent but "flaccid" and do not function properly
* Lacrimal pump malfunction

TABLE 100.2 *Preoperative Evaluation and Considerations*

Jones dye testing consistent with indications in Table 100.1.

Nasal exam to rule out tumors, other causes for obstruction, and nasal septal deviation (need to have room for tube to extend into nasal cavity and not be obstructed)

Systemic conditions (i.e., Wegener's granulomatosis) associated with nasolacrimal dysfunction

Medications (i.e., Taxotere or 5 FU) associated with nasolacrimal duct obstruction

Predisposing bleeding conditions should be identified and addressed

All anticoagulants should be discontinued prior to surgery if possible

Clearance by primary care physician in appropriate cases

Pertinent Background

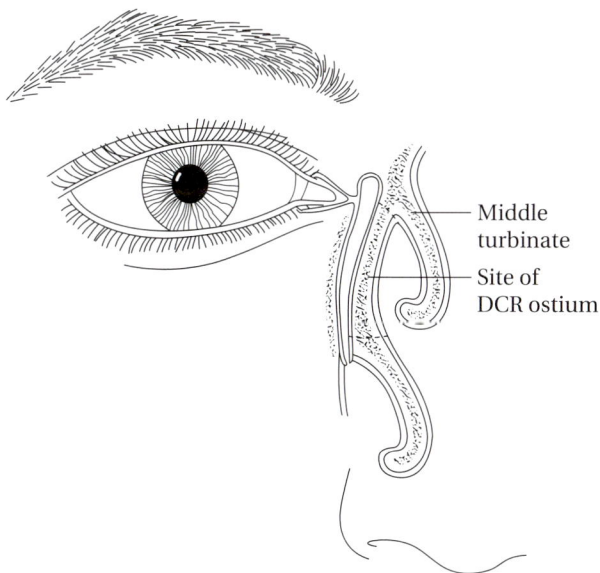

FIGURE 100.1 Diagram of nasal anatomy.

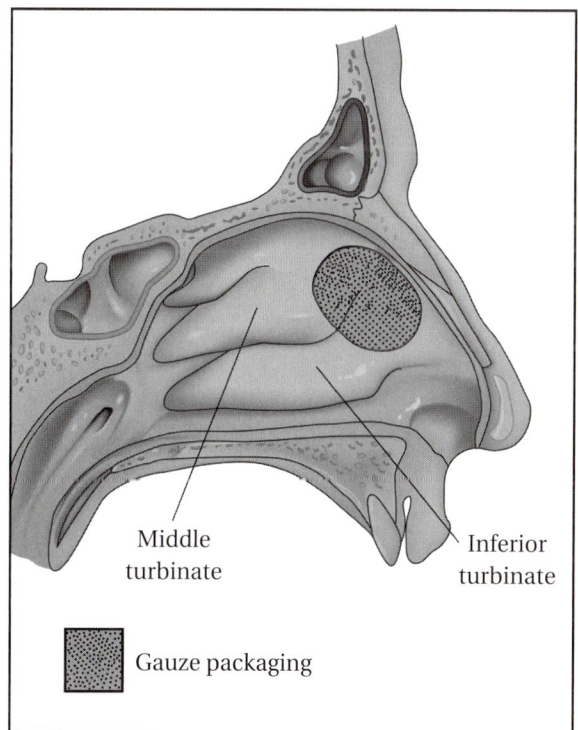

FIGURE 100.2 Diagram of nasal packing placement prior to surgery.

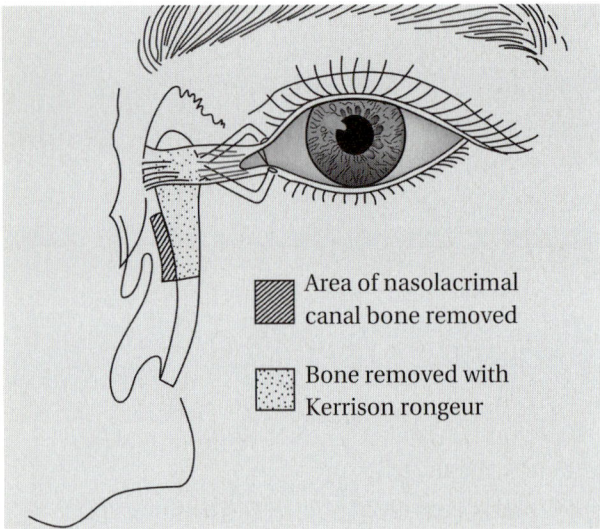

FIGURE 100.3 (a) Diagram of bone removed.
(b) Diagram of bone removed (lateral view).

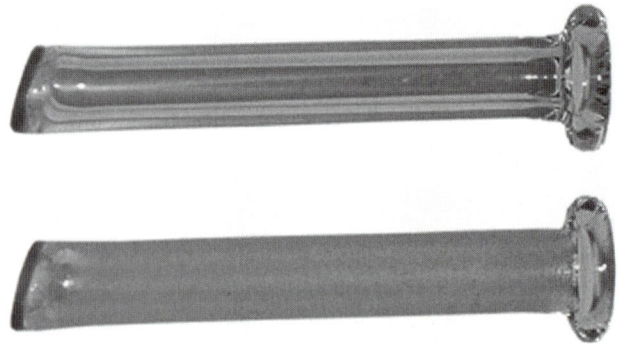

FIGURE 100.4 Standard and frosted Jones tubes.

External Conjunctivodacryocystorhinostomy

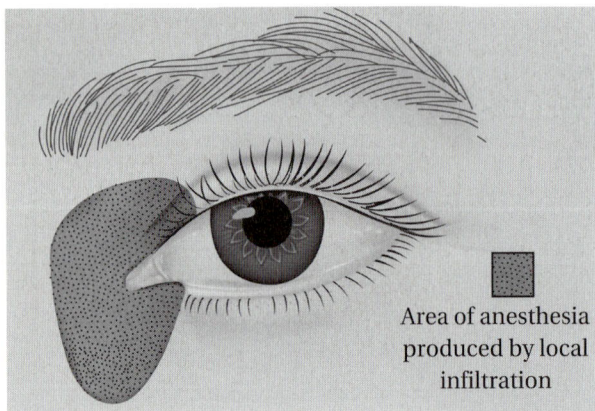

FIGURE 100.5 The nose is packed with cottonoids soaked in cocaine or oxymetazoline. Local anesthesia and epinephrine are then injected in the medial canthal region.

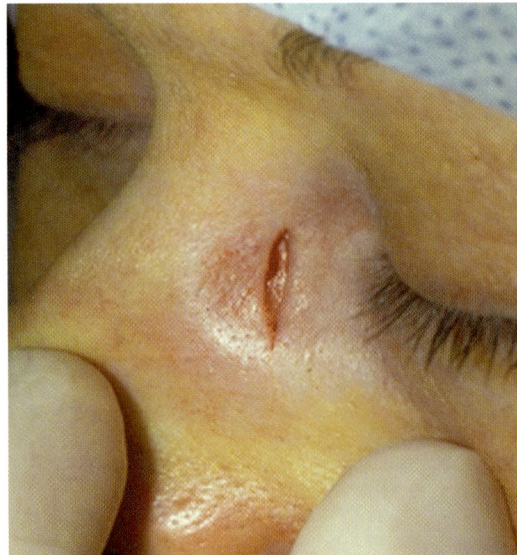

FIGURE 100.6 A skin incision is then made 11 mm medial to the medial commissure, and extended inferiorly and slightly laterally for approximately 20 mm.

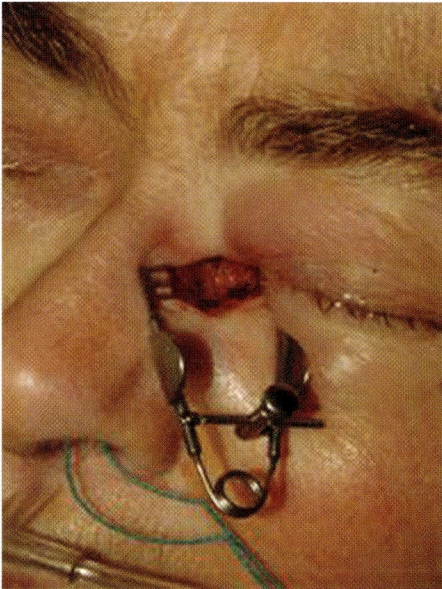

FIGURE 100.7 Sharp Stevens scissors are used to perform an incision through the remaining subcutaneous tissue. A self-retaining Agricola retractor is then inserted.

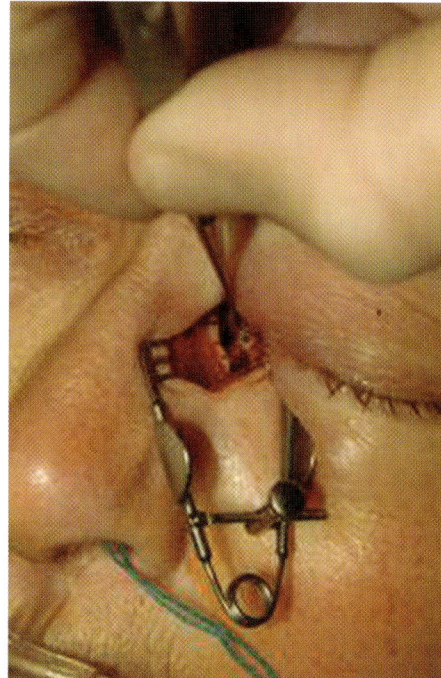

FIGURE 100.8 The periosteum medial to the anterior lacrimal crest is then incised and elevated with a Freer elevator.

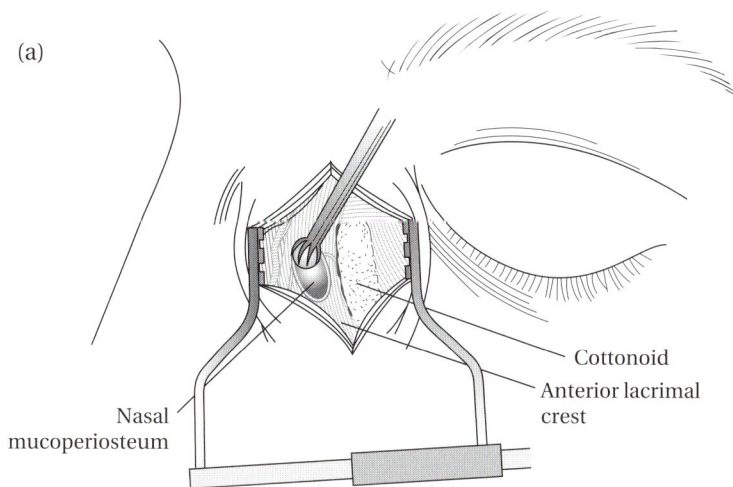

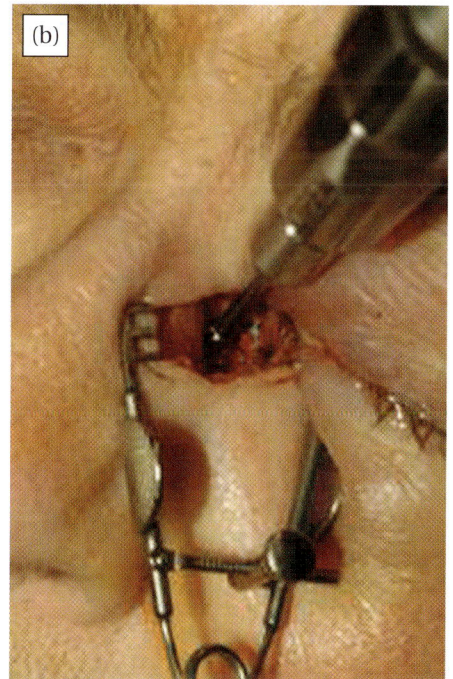

(a)

(b)

Cottonoid

Anterior lacrimal crest

Nasal mucoperiosteum

FIGURE 100.9 (a, b) An oblong area of bone anterior to the lacrimal crest is removed with a dental burr.

(a)

(b)

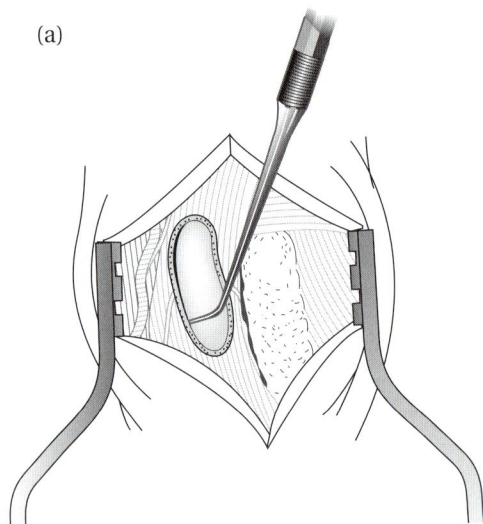

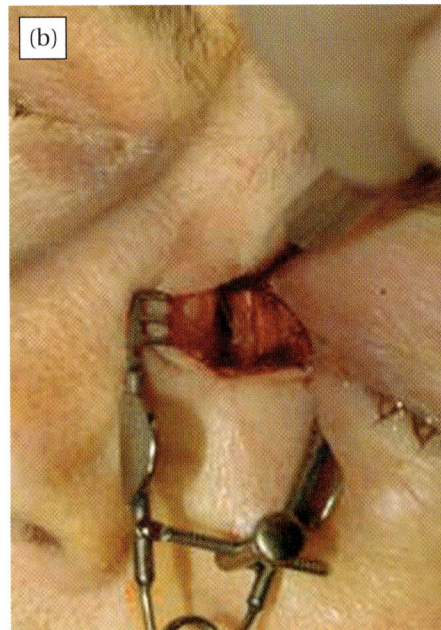

FIGURE 100.10 (a, b) The nasal mucoperiosteum is separated from the underside of the bone using a dental burnisher.

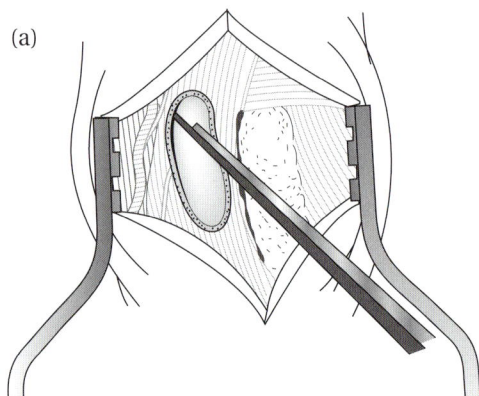

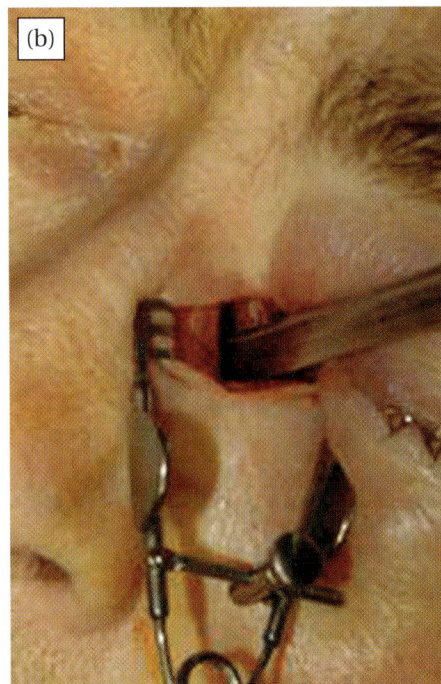

(b)

(a)

FIGURE 100.11 (a, b) A Kerrison punch and rongeurs are used to enlarge the osteotomy.

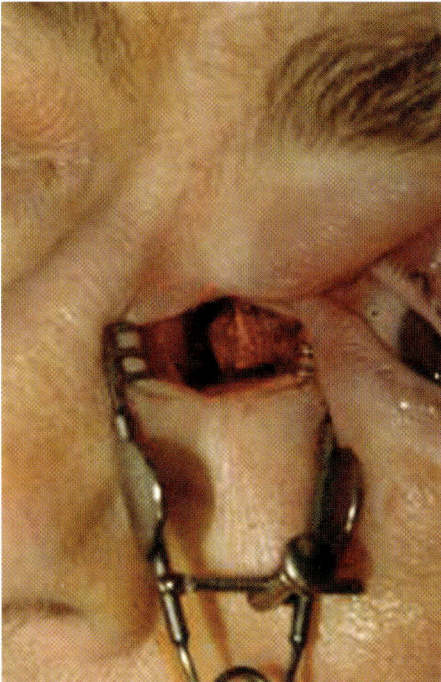

FIGURE 100.12 A zero Bowman probe is inserted into either canaliculus, to "tent" the medial wall of the lacrimal sac toward the nasal mucoperiosteum.

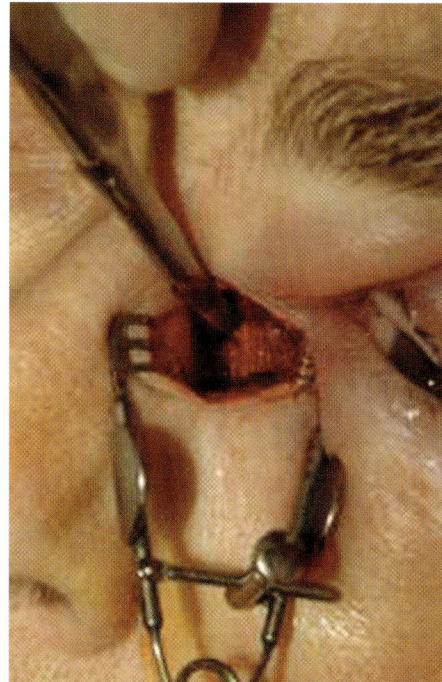

FIGURE 100.13 A No. 11 Bard-Parker blade is then used to cut through both the periosteal and the mucosal layers of the medial wall of the sac, slightly lateral to the tip of the probe.

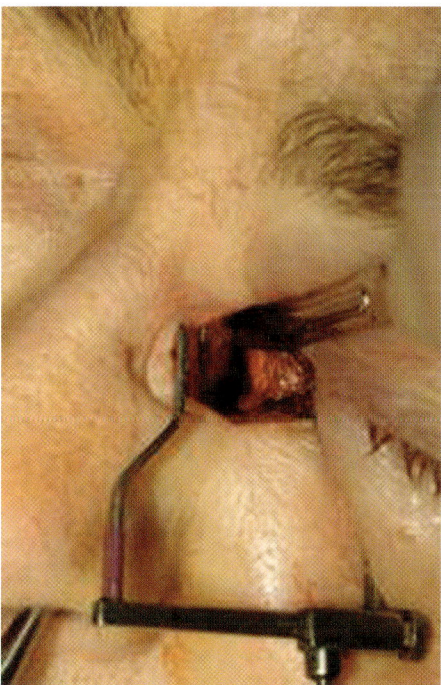

FIGURE 100.14 A similar incision is then made in the nasal mucoperiosteum.

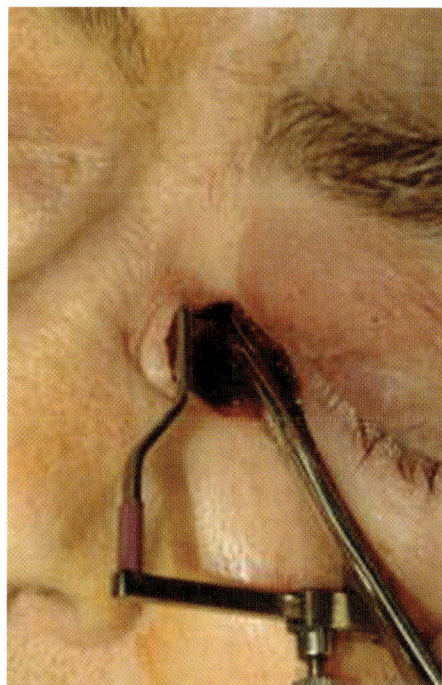

FIGURE 100.15 The posterior flaps of the tear sac and the nasal mucoperiosteum are then removed with scissors.

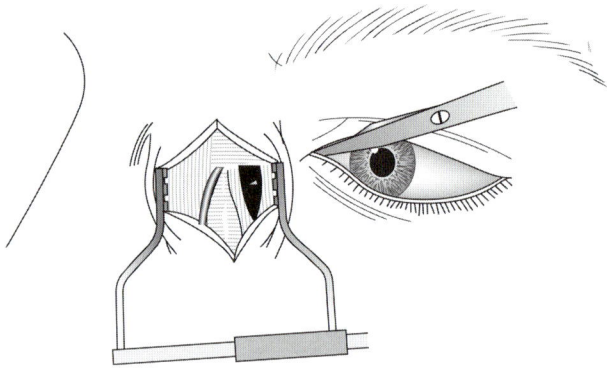

FIGURE 100.16   A sharp Stevens scissors is inserted into the region of the lacus lacrimalis just medial to the caruncle, and is advanced inferomedially until the blades are visualized extending through the opened lacrimal sac.

(a)

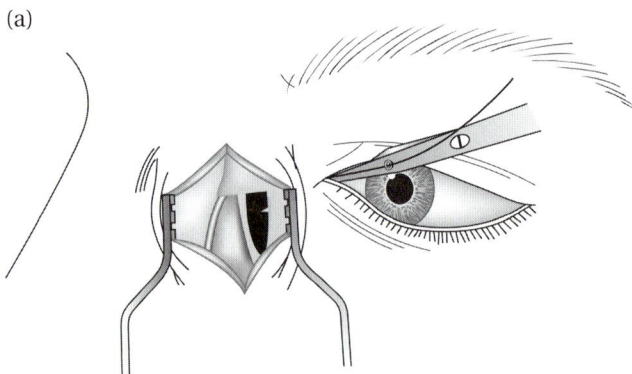

(b)

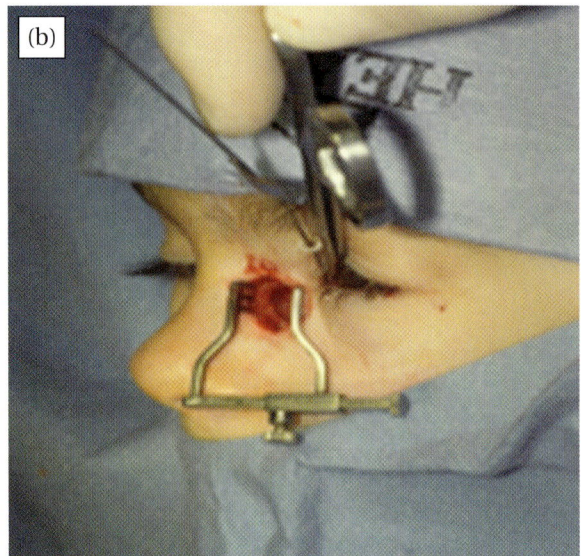

FIGURE 100.17   (a, b) The appropriately sized Pyrex tube is then placed on a zero probe. The zero probe is passed just above the scissors, between the opened blades, into the opened sac. The scissors are then removed while simultaneously pushing the Pyrex tube down the course of the probe into the nasal cavity. The collar of the tube should fit nicely in the medial canthus, and the tip of the tube should be centrally located in the nasal airway without obstruction. The caruncle is occasionally debulked. The tube is anchored in place with a 5-0 polyglactin suture wrapped around the tube and fixed to the skin in the same fashion as a surgical drain would be fixated.

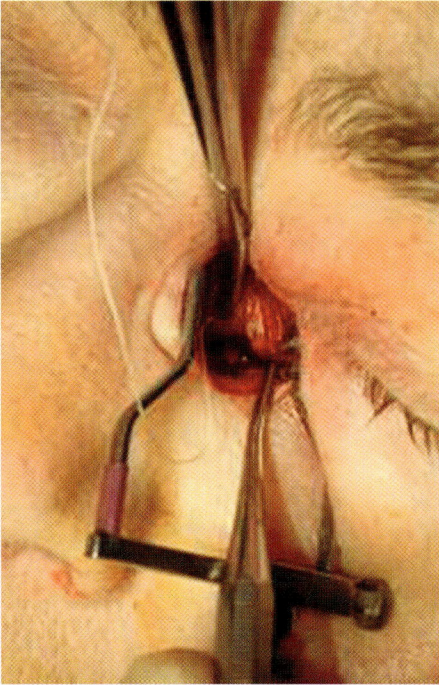

FIGURE 100.18 The anterior flaps are then closed with interrupted 5-0 polyglactin sutures.

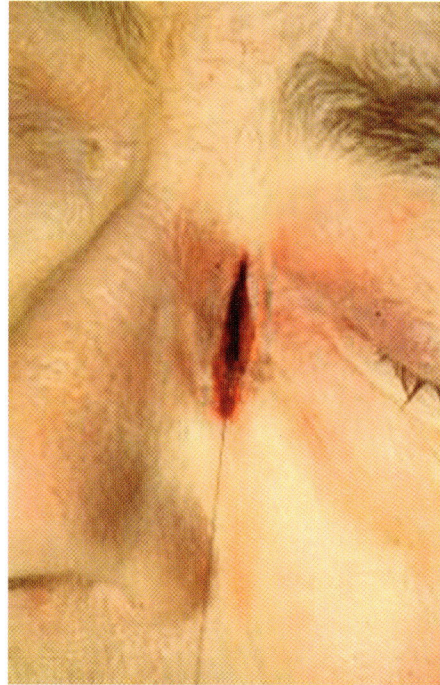

FIGURE 100.19 The orbicularis is then closed with a running 5-0 polyglactin suture.

Endoscopic Conjunctivocystorhinostomy

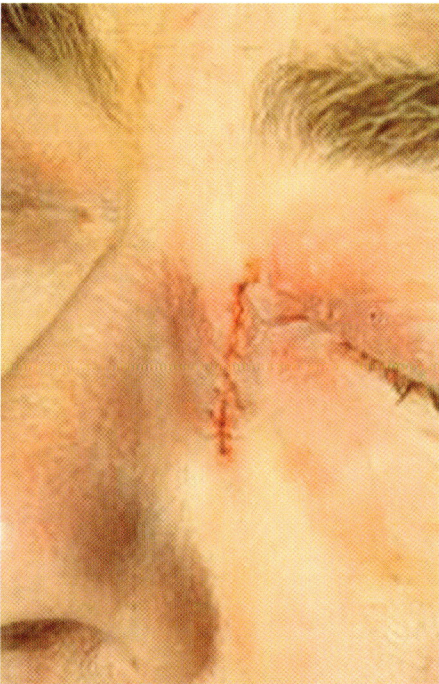

FIGURE 100.20 The overlying skin is then closed with a running horizontal mattress 5-0 plain fast-absorbing gut suture.

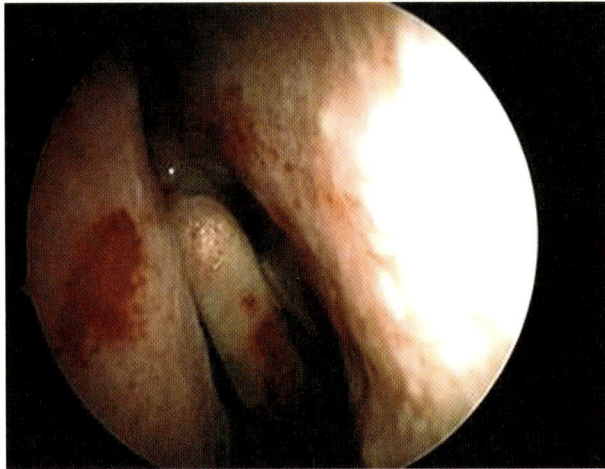

FIGURE 100.21 Following injection of the nasal mucosa and middle turbinate with local anesthesia and epinepherine, a 4mm endoscope with a zero-degree angle is introduced into the nose (left side). If necessary, a Freer elevator can be used to displace the middle turbinate gently toward the septum.

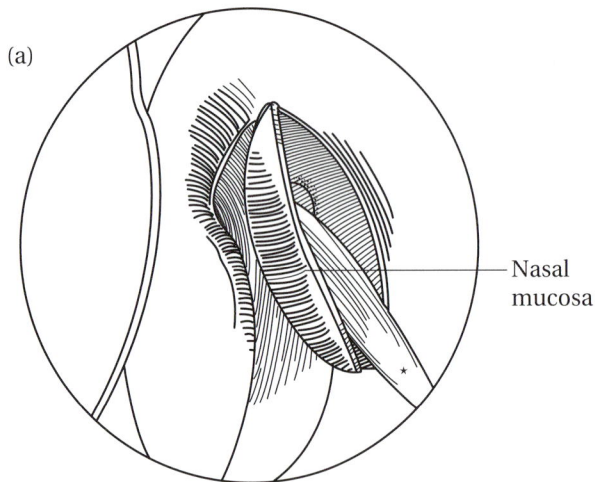

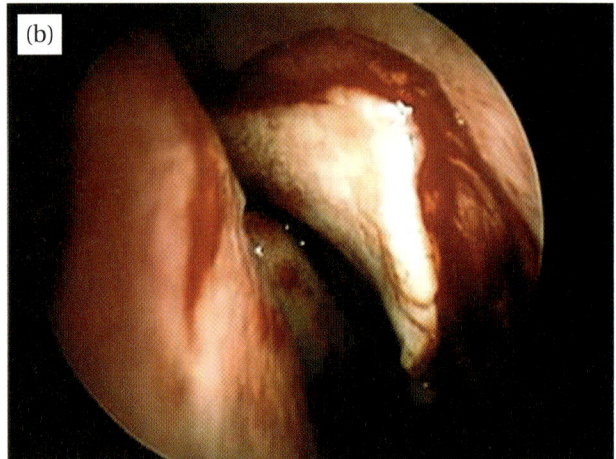

FIGURE 100.22 (a, b) A keratome is used to create an incision anterior and inferior to the middle turbinate, and the mucosa is removed using a grasping forceps.

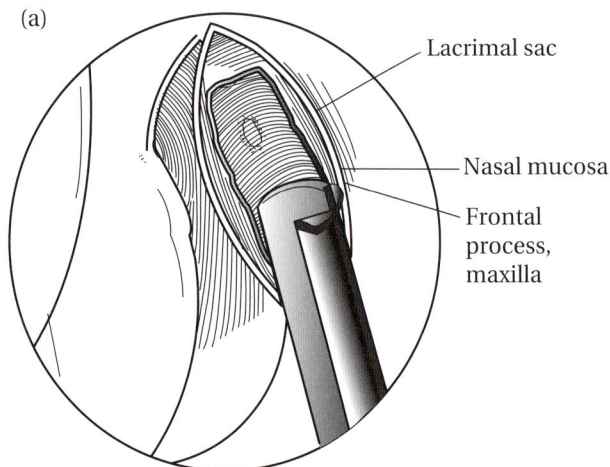

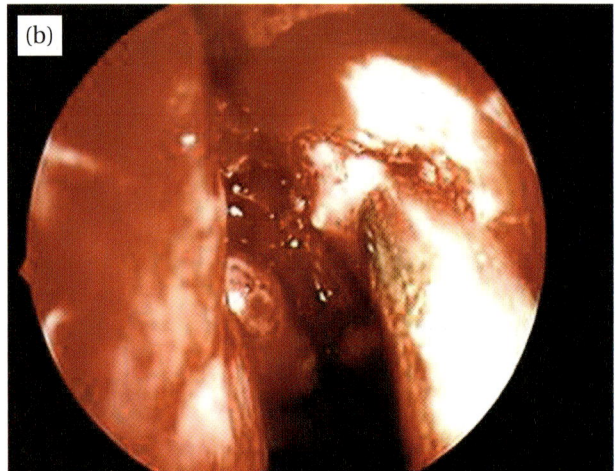

FIGURE 100.23 (a, b) A 90 degree Kerrison rongeur is then used to remove the frontal process of the maxilla until the lacrimal sac is exposed. A Xomed (curved 15 degree) (high-speed) burr can also be used to increase the osteotomy especially superiorly where the rongeur can be less effective.

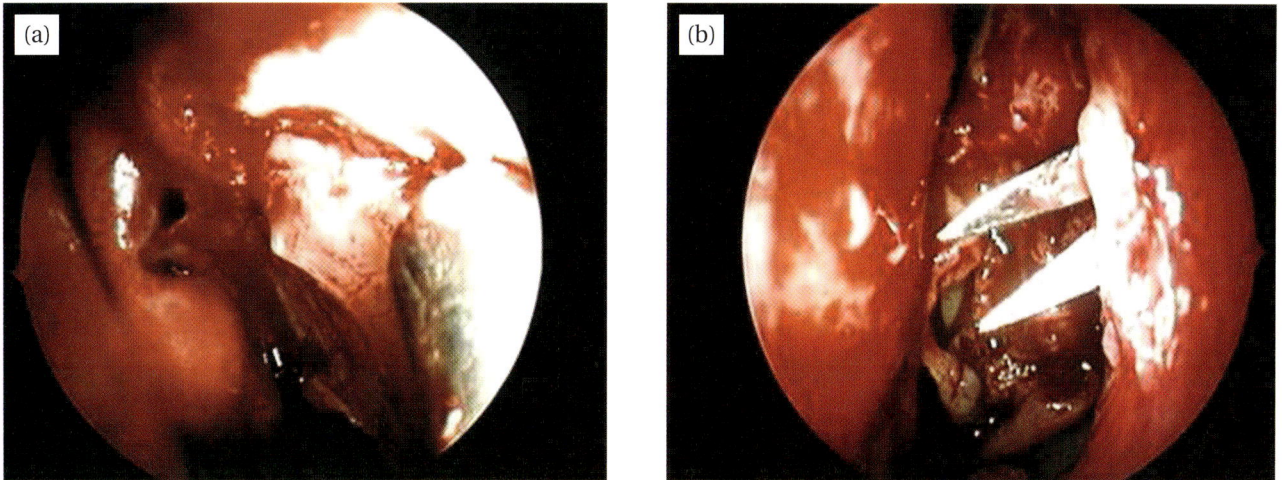

FIGURE 100.24 (a, b) A sharp Stevens scissors is inserted into the region of the lacus lacrimalis, and is advanced until the tear sac becomes tented out by the tips of the scissors. A keratome blade is then used to open the lacrimal sac, and the posterior flap is removed with "through biting" Blakely forceps.

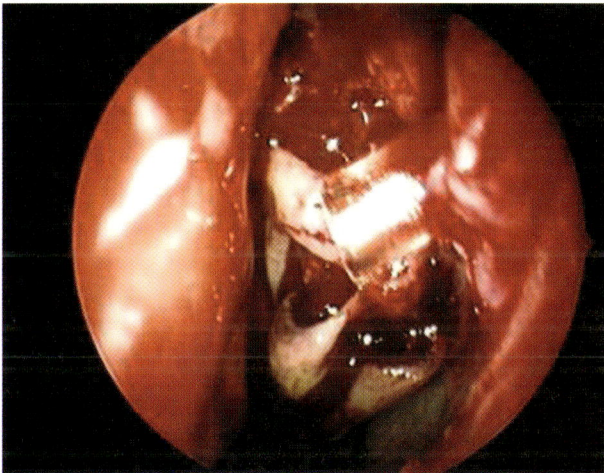

FIGURE 100.25 The appropriately sized Pyrex tube is then placed on a zero probe. The zero probe is passed just above the scissors, between the opened blades, into the opened sac. The scissors are then removed, while simultaneously pushing the Pyrex tube down the course of the probe into the nasal cavity. If the tube touches the septum, a shorter one must be used.

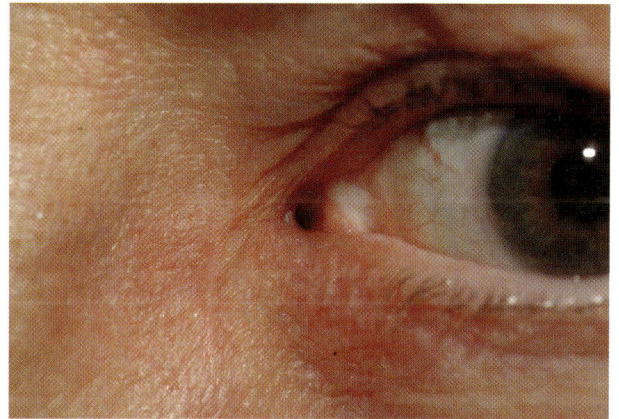

FIGURE 100.26 A 5-0 polyglactin 910 suture is then wrapped around the collar of the tube and sutured into the medial canthal region, as previously described.

TABLE 100.3 *Postoperative Management*

Preventing Extrusion of Pyrex Tube	Patient is taught to "sniff" rather than "blow" his or her nose.
	Eyelids should be tightly squeezed together when the patient needs to sneeze or blow his or her nose.
	Manual occlusion can also be performed by the patient when blowing nose.
Preventing a Clogged Pyrex Tube	A saline eye drop should be placed in the eye once a day and "snuffed" through the tube.
	If congestion is present, a vigorous treatment of the nasal condition should be performed with nasal irrigation and decongestants to prevent plugging of the tube.
Managing a Clogged Pyrex Tube	Place artificial tears or normal saline drops with a medicine dropper into the medial corner of the eyelids.
	Have the patient sniff vigorously while occluding the nose.
	Run a 00 Bowman probe through the Pyrex tube.
Cleaning Pyrex Tubes	Despite proper Jones tube hygiene, additional cleaning of the tube is occasionally required. See below.

Cleaning Pyrex Tubes

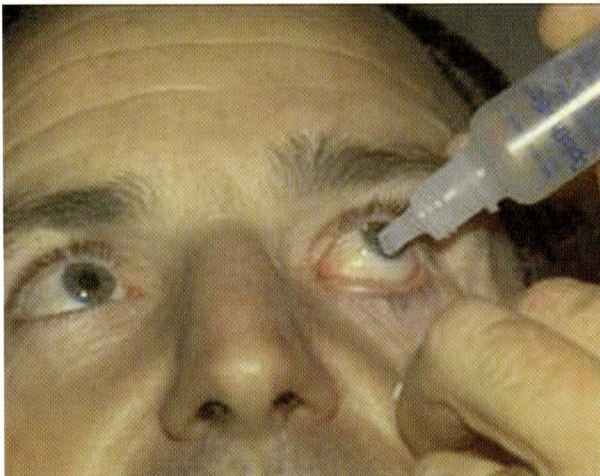

FIGURE 100.27 Topical anesthetic is placed onto the appropriate eye.

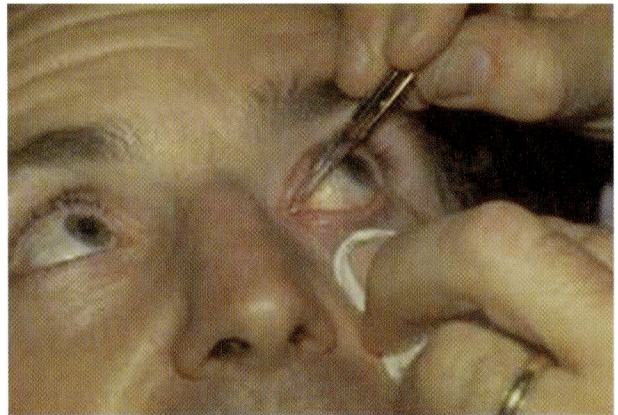

FIGURE 100.28 The tube is then grasped with forceps and carefully removed.

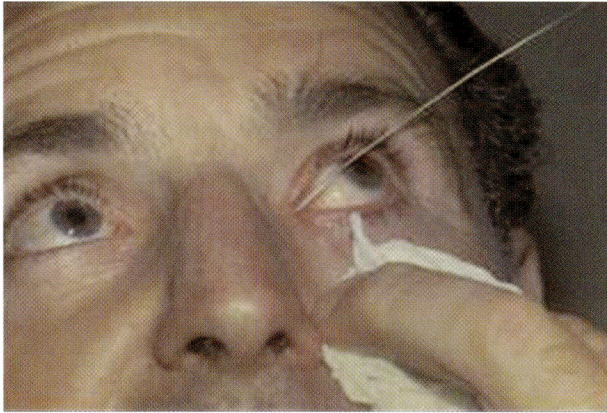

FIGURE 100.29 A small piece of cotton is tightly wrapped around a probe and soaked in a 50:50 mixture of 2% lidocaine and 0.025% oxymetazolone. The probe is then placed in the tract.

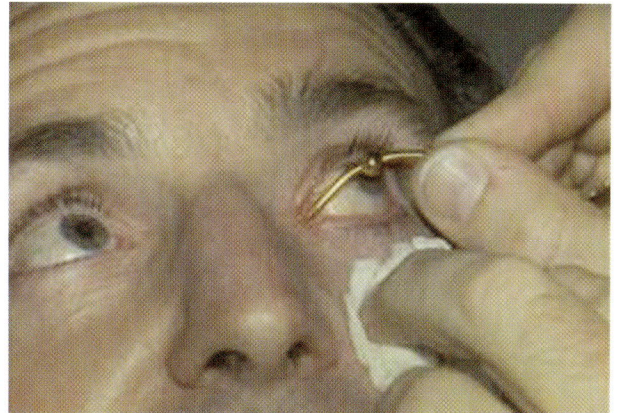

FIGURE 100.30 A Weiss (gold) dilator is then inserted.

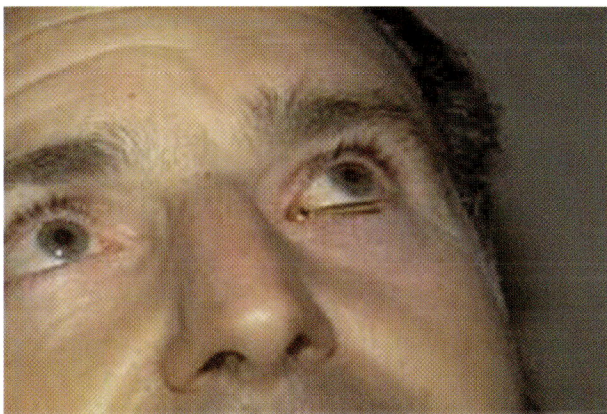

FIGURE 100.31 The Weiss dilator is left in the appropriate position while the tube is cleaned, so that the fistula doesn't occlude.

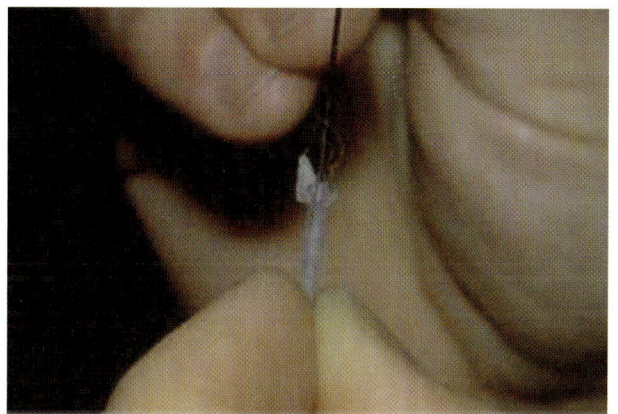

FIGURE 100.32 The Pyrex tube is cleaned with alcohol-soaked cotton in an ultrasonic cleaner.

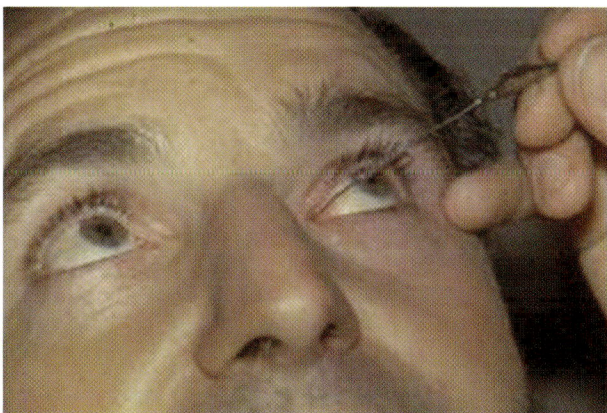

FIGURE 100.33 The cleaned and rinsed Pyrex tube is placed on a Bowman probe. The Bowman probe is then advanced into the appropriate position after the Weiss dilator has been removed.

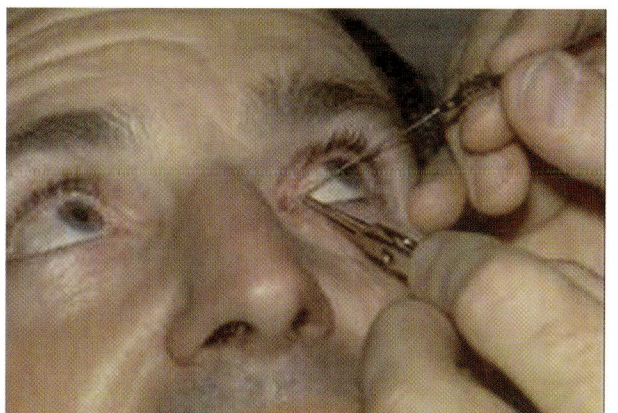

FIGURE 100.34 The Pyrex tube is reinserted with the use of forceps, while simultaneously removing the Bowman probe.

Complications and Treatments

TABLE 100.4 *Complications and Treatments*

Complications	Treatment
Pyrex tube extrusion	Replace as soon as possible
Conjunctivitis	Remove and clean tube
	Topical antibiotic/steroid drops
Granulation tissue	Remove and clean tube
Collar of tube protrudes	Replace tube with smaller sized collar
Tube repeatedly extrudes	Replace standard tube with a frosted tube

SELECTED REFERENCES

Dailey RA, Tower RN. Frosted pyrex Jones tubes. *Ophthal Plast Reconstr Surg.* 2005;21:185–187.

Jones LT. Conjunctivodacryocystorhinostomy. *Am J Ophthalmol.* 1965;59:773–783.

Steele EA, Dailey RA. Conjunctivodacryocystorhinostomy with the frosted Jones pyrex tube. *Ophthal Plast Reconstr Surg.* 2009;25:42–43.

Trotter WL, Meyer DR. Endoscopic conjunctivodacryocystorhinostomy with Jones tube placement. *Ophthalmology.* 2000;107:1206–1209

Wobig JL, Dailey RA: Surgery of the tear sac. In *Oculofacial plastic surgery.* (pp. 167–182) New York: Thieme; 2004.

Woog JJ, Sindwani R. Endoscopic dacryocystorhinostomy and conjunctivodacryocystorhinostomy. *Otolaryngol Clin North Am.* 2006;39:1001–1017.

INDEX